DIAGNOSTIC AND SURGICAL
IMAGING ANATOMY
CHEST • ABDOMEN • PELVIS

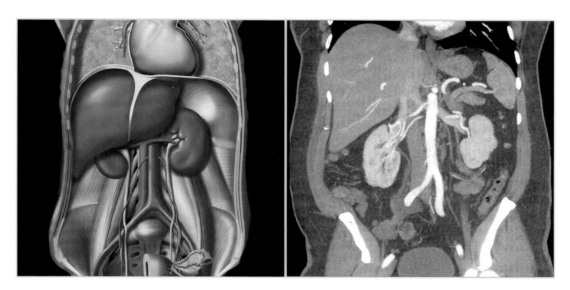

DIAGNOSTIC AND SURGICAL
IMAGING ANATOMY
CHEST • ABDOMEN • PELVIS

Michael P. Federle, MD, FACR

Professor of Radiology
Chief, Abdominal Imaging
University of Pittsburgh Medical Center
Pittsburgh, PA

Melissa L. Rosado-de-Christenson, MD

Clinical Professor of Radiology
The Ohio State University College of Medicine
Columbus, OH

Adjunct Professor of Radiology
The Uniformed Services University of the Health Sciences
Bethesda, MD

Paula J. Woodward, MD

Professor of Radiology
Adjunct Professor of Obstetrics and Gynecology
University of Utah School of Medicine
Salt Lake City, UT

Gerald F. Abbott, MD

Director of Chest Radiology
Rhode Island Hospital

Associate Professor of Diagnostic Imaging
Brown Medical School
Providence, RI

Managing Editor
Akram M. Shaaban, MBBCh

Assistant Professor of Radiology (Clinical)
University of Utah Medical Center
Salt Lake City, UT

AMIRSYS®

Names you know, content you trust

AMIRSYS®

Names you know, content you trust®

First Edition

Second Printing - December 2007

Composition by Amirsys Inc, Salt Lake City, Utah

Printed in Canada by Friesens, Altona, Manitoba, Canada

ISBN-13: 978-1-931884-33-4
ISBN-10: 1-931884-33-1
ISBN-13: 978-1-931884-34-1 (International English Edition)
ISBN-10: 1-931884-34-X (International English Edition)

Library of Congress Cataloging-in-Publication Data

Diagnostic and surgical imaging anatomy : chest, abdomen, pelvis /
  Michael P. Federle ... [et al.] ; managing editor, Akram M. Shaaban.
  — 1st ed.
    p. ; cm.
  ISBN-13: 978-1-931884-33-4
  ISBN-10: 1-931884-33-1
  ISBN-13: 978-1-931884-34-1 (international English ed.)
  ISBN-10: 1-931884-34-X (international English ed.)
  1. Diagnostic imaging—Atlases. 2. Chest—Anatomy—Atlases.
 3. Abdomen—Anatomy—Atlases. 4. Pelvis—Anatomy—Atlases.
 5. Imaging systems in medicine—Atlases. I. Federle, Michael P.
II. Title: Chest, abdomen, pelvis.
  [DNLM: 1. Thorax—anatomy & histology—Atlases. 2. Abdomen
—anatomy & histology—Atlases. 3. Magnetic Resonance Spectro-
scopy—Atlases. 4. Pelvis—anatomy & histology—Atlases. 5. Tomography, X-Ray Computed—Atlases. WE 17 D536 2006]
 RC78.7.D53D534 2006
 616.07'54—dc22

                     2006030831

To Mort Meyers, whose pioneering work opened my eyes to the
value of understanding abdominal anatomy and pathophysiology.
MPF

I dedicate this work to my family, especially my husband Dr. Paul J. Christenson, and my daughters
Jennifer and Heather who encouraged and supported me throughout this work. I learned a great deal
from my good friend and co-author Dr. Gerry Abbott, my co-author Dr. Akram Shaaban and our most
gifted illustrator, Mr. Lane Bennion.
MRdC

To all my residents (past, present and future) who have endured endless
hours of being "pimped" on anatomy. Here are all the answers!
PJW

To my great friend, mentor, and co-author, Melissa Rosado de Christenson; and,
to her husband, Dr. Paul Christenson for his patience, support and good friendship.
GFA

To my parents, I truly owe you everything
To my wife Inji, son Karim and daughter May, the jewels of my life, thanks for your
understanding and tremendous support.
AMS

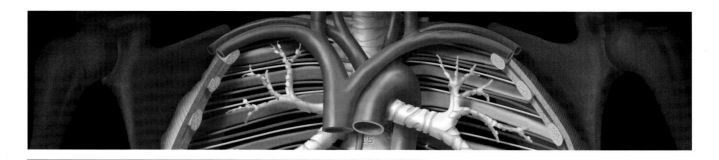

DIAGNOSTIC AND SURGICAL IMAGING ANATOMY: CHEST, ABDOMEN, PELVIS

We at Amirsys, together with our distribution colleagues at LWW, are proud to present *Diagnostic and Surgical Imaging Anatomy: Chest, Abdomen, Pelvis*, the third in our brand-new series of anatomy reference titles. All books in this best-selling series are designed specifically to serve clinicians in medical imaging and each area's related surgical subspecialties. We focus on anatomy that is generally visible on imaging studies, crossing modalities and presenting bulleted anatomy descriptions along with a glorious, rich offering of color normal anatomy graphics together with in-depth multimodality, multiplanar high-resolution imaging.

Each imaging anatomy textbook contains over 2,500 labeled color graphics and high resolution radiologic images, with heavy emphasis on 3 Tesla MR and state-of-the-art multi-detector CT. It is designed to give the busy medical professional rapid answers to imaging anatomy questions. Each normal anatomy sequence provides detailed views of anatomic structures never before seen and discussed in an anatomy reference textbook. For easy reference, each major area (chest, abdomen, pelvis) is subdivided into separate sections that cover detailed normal anatomy of all its constituents.

In summary, *Diagnostic and Surgical Imaging Anatomy: Chest, Abdomen, Pelvis* is a product designed with you, the reader, in mind. Today's typical radiologic, and surgical practice settings demand both accuracy and efficiency in image interpretation for clinical decision-making. We think you'll find this new approach to anatomy a highly efficient and wonderfully rich resource that will be the core of your reference collection in anatomy. The new *Diagnostic and Surgical Imaging Anatomy: Musculoskeletal* is also now available. Coming in 2007 are volumes on Ultrasound as well as a subspecialty- and podiatry-oriented text on Knee, Ankle, and Foot.

We hope that you will sit back, dig in, and enjoy seeing anatomy and imaging with a whole different eye.

Anne G. Osborn, MD
Executive Vice President and Editor-in-Chief, Amirsys Inc.

H. Ric Harnsberger, MD
CEO & Chairman, Amirsys Inc.

Paula J. Woodward, MD
Senior Vice President & Medical Director, Amirsys Inc.

B.J. Manaster, MD
Vice President & Associate Medical Director, Amirsys Inc.

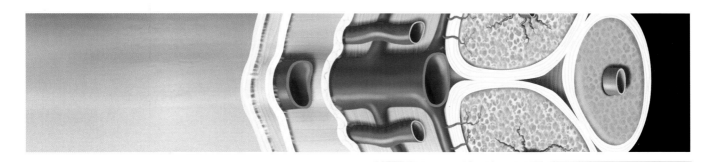

FOREWORD

As in the great age of exploration when the coastal contours of a continent were first outlined and thereafter its rivers, mountains, and valleys penetrated, so was the terra incognita of the human body explored.

A work published in 1543 influenced the annals of Western medicine forever. *De Humani Corporis Fabrica, Libri Septum* by Andreas Vesalius, usually referred to as the *Fabrica*, was one of the first anatomy texts to systematically provide descriptions derived from actual dissection of the human body. In controverting the ancient theory of Galen, the second-century Greek who had cast his shadow on medical science for over a thousand years, the *Fabrica* was an incontestable breakthrough. Vesalius is regarded as the Columbus of the human body, as a man who literally discovered a new world.

Anatomy was the stepping-stone to the understanding of not only the body's structure but also its functions and malfunctions.

It was other investigations in the sixteenth century on the vascular system and the venous valves complete with their mechanical implications that were crucial for William Harvey's demonstration of the blood circulation. Harvey's 1628 publication *De Motu Cordis* ("On the Motion of the Heart") established that the heart is a pump which causes the blood to circulate through the body, passing from the arteries to the veins. It would remain for Marcello Malpighi, founder of microscopic anatomy, decades later in 1660, to discover the capillaries. These insights marked the step from anatomy to physiology.

In 1761, the Italian physician and anatomist Giovanni Morgagni published *On the Sites and Causes of Disease*, finally establishing the direct relevance of anatomy to clinical medicine. Rudolph Virchow, the father of clinical pathology, declared in 1894 that, with Morgagni, "The new medicine begins".

Over time, surgeons became most adept in the knowledge of anatomy. By the early decades of the 20th century, the eminent surgeon Harvey Cushing could testify that "from the publication of the *Fabrica* almost to the present day the intimate pursuit of ... anatomy has constituted the high road for entry into the practice of surgery."

Today, it is the radiologist who is most facile with highly detailed anatomy and who – it must be emphasized – demonstrates this *in vivo*. This has been brought about by the revolution in diagnostic imaging. *Dis*sectional anatomy has been superseded by *cross*-sectional imaging.

This volume which deals with anatomy of the chest, abdomen and pelvis is authored by recognized experts with wide experience and keen insight including: Melissa Rosado-de-Christenson and Gerald Abbott (chest), Michael Federle (abdomen), and Paula Woodward (pelvis). It not only reveals the complex mysteries of the body's structure but further indicates why anatomical applications are still being made today. The information is presented in an engaging and reader-friendly style. Convoluted descriptions are abandoned as key anatomic principles are outlined in succinct format. Medical illustrations of exquisite museum quality are combined with state-of-art diagnostic imaging. A distinctive feature is the frequent use of pathologic examples to highlight certain anatomic structures or features that might otherwise be obscure. The exciting capabilities of ultrasonography, computed tomograpy, and magnetic resonance imaging are beyond the wildest dreams of Andreas Vesalius or Harvey Cushing. The reader cannot but be struck by the realization that the state-of-art images often rival and sometimes surpass the artist's depiction in accurate display.

Anatomy is so intimately linked to physiology and pathology that this textbook is a gem for any student or practitioner involved with the human body in modern medicine.

Morton A. Meyers, MD
Emeritus Professor of Radiology and Medicine
Distinguished University Professor
State University of New York at Stony Brook

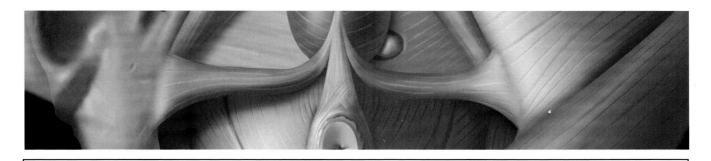

PREFACE

While in medical school, I hated "Anatomy." Working with cadavers was not only unpleasant but was relatively uninformative as well. Structures of vital importance, such as various ducts and blood vessels, were difficult to identify by dissection. The anatomic drawings in our textbooks seemed to have little or no bearing on what I was observing in the anatomy lab or operating room, and had even less apparent relevance to the practice of medicine or surgery.

When CT came along at the end of my residency, we all had to scramble to learn how to interpret these new cross-sections of the body. Existing texts were of limited help in interpretation of axial CT images, and even less help when MR arrived with its new planes of section and unfamiliar display sequences. Once we gained familiarity with these imaging tools, however, we realized that we had access to detailed anatomic information inaccessible to even the most experienced anatomist. Experience interpreting thousands of CT and MR interpretations has also made us appreciate the considerable variability from "conventional" depictions of anatomy found in standard textbooks.

We feel that the combination of vibrant medical illustrations and multiplanar, high resolution, cross sectional imaging is the ideal way to teach anatomy today. We have included depictions of common anatomic variations and pathological process to make the reader aware of the appearance and relevance of altered morphology.

We hope that the efforts of our talented medical illustrators and radiologist/authors will make the anatomy of the chest, abdomen and pelvis "come alive" for our readers.

Michael P. Federle, MD, FACR
Professor of Radiology
Chief of Abdominal Imaging
University of Pittsburgh Medical Center

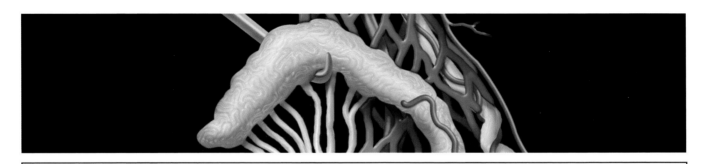

ACKNOWLEDGMENTS

Illustrations
Lane R. Bennion, MS

Contributing Illustrators
Rich Coombs, MS
James A. Cooper, MD
Walter Stuart, MFA

Image/Text Editing
Douglas Grant Jackson
Amanda Hurtado
Melanie Hall
Karen M. Pealer, BA, CCRC

Medical Text Editing
Akram M. Shaaban, MBBCh

Case Management
Roth LaFleur
Christopher Odekirk

Case Contributors
Feras Bader, MD; Salt Lake City, UT
Peter L. Choyke, MD; Bethesda, MD
Ralph Drosten, MD; Salt Lake City, UT
M. Robert Florez, BS; Colorado Springs, CO
Douglas Green, MD; Salt Lake City, UT
Jud Gurney, MD; Omaha, NE
Keyanoosh Hosseinzadeh, MD; Pittsburgh, PA
Anne Kennedy, MD; Salt Lake City, UT
Mark King, MD; Columbus, OH
Howard Mann, MD; Salt Lake City, UT
Chris McGann, MD; Salt Lake City, UT
Elizabeth Moore, MD; Davis, CA
Mohamed Salama, MD, Salt Lake City, UT
Jerry Speckman, MD; Gainesville, FL
J.Thomas Stocker, MD; Bethesda, MD
Diane C. Strollo, MD; Pittsburgh, PA
Jade J. Wong-You–Cheong, MD; Baltimore, MD

Project Leads
Melissa A. Hoopes
Kaerli Main

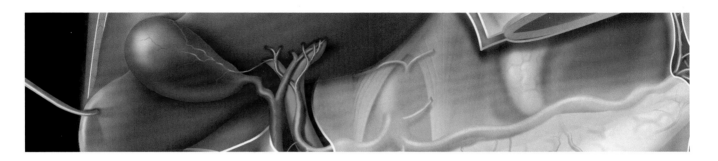

SECTIONS

PART I
Chest

PART II
Abdomen

PART III
Pelvis

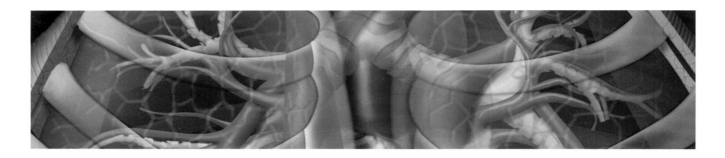

TABLE OF CONTENTS

Part III
Pelvis

DIAGNOSTIC AND SURGICAL
IMAGING ANATOMY
CHEST • ABDOMEN • PELVIS

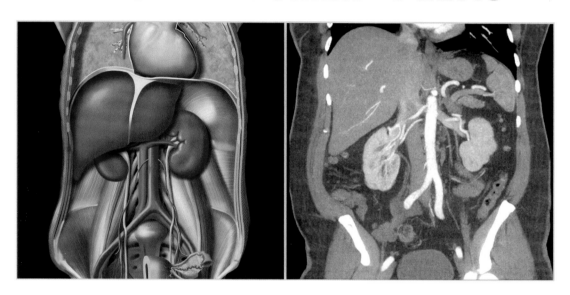

PART I
Chest

Chest Overview

Lung Development

Airway Structure

Vascular Structure

Interstitial Network

Lungs

Hila

Airways

Pulmonary Vessels

Pleura

Mediastinum

Systemic Vessels

Heart

Coronary Arteries and Cardiac Veins

Pericardium

Chest Wall

CHEST OVERVIEW

Terminology

Abbreviations
- Anteroposterior (AP)
- Posteroanterior (PA)
- Image receptor (IR)
- Source-to-image receptor distance (SID)
- Hounsfield units (HU)

General Anatomy and Function

Chest Wall
- Anatomy
  - Spine
  - Sternum
  - Ribs
  - Clavicles
  - Skeletal muscles
  - Chest wall nerves and vessels
  - Skin and subcutaneous fat
- Function
  - Provides protection for lungs, cardiovascular structures and intrathoracic organs
  - Participates in bellows-like process of respiration

Pleura
- Anatomy
  - Thin continuous membrane
  - **Parietal pleura**: Lines non pulmonary surfaces
  - **Visceral pleura**: Lines pulmonary surfaces
  - **Pleural space**: Potential space
- Function
  - Production and absorption of normal **pleural fluid**
    - **Pleural fluid** lubricates pleural surfaces
    - **Pleural fluid** facilitates lung motion during respiration
  - Clearance of abnormal **pleural fluid**

Airways
- Anatomy
  - Trachea
  - Main bronchi
  - Lobar bronchi
  - Segmental bronchi
  - Bronchioles
  - Distal airways and alveoli
- Function
  - Gas exchange during respiration
  - Protective mechanism against foreign particles
    - Ciliary escalator
    - Cough reflex
  - Air transfer to and from the alveolar-capillary interface

Heart and Great Vessels
- Anatomy
  - Venae cavae
  - Right atrium
  - Right ventricle
  - Pulmonary arteries
  - Capillary network
  - Pulmonary veins
  - Left atrium
  - Left ventricle
  - Aorta and branches
- Function
  - Pump action for systemic & pulmonary circulations
  - Transport of deoxygenated blood to capillary-alveolar interface
  - Transport of oxygenated blood to tissues

Chest Radiography

Standard Chest Radiographs
- Imaging study of choice for initial assessment of cardiopulmonary disease
- **PA** and **left lateral chest radiographs**
  - Orthogonal views (at right angles to each other)
  - Analysis of orthogonal views for anatomic localization of imaging abnormalities

Standard Radiographic Positioning
- Upright patient
- Full inspiration and breath hold near total lung capacity
- No rotation or motion
- Attempt to minimize overlying osseous structures
- Area of interest closest to IR
- Radiographic technique
  - SID of 72 inches to minimize magnification
  - Central X-ray beam centered on thorax
  - Beam collimation to include outer portion of chest wall

Radiographic Projections
- **PA chest radiograph**
  - Term **PA**: Describes posteroanterior direction of X-ray beam traversing chest toward IR
  - Anterior chest against IR
  - Head vertically positioned and chin on top of grid device
  - Dorsal wrists on hips and elbows rotated anteriorly to move scapulae laterally
  - Shoulders moved caudally and squarely against IR to bring clavicles below apices
- **Left lateral chest radiograph**
  - Term **left lateral**: Denotes that left lateral chest wall is against IR
  - X-ray beam traverses chest from right to left toward IR
  - Arms above head to move upper extremities away from lungs and mediastinum
- **AP chest radiograph**
  - Term **AP**: Describes anteroposterior direction of X-ray beam traversing chest toward IR
  - Supine and bedside (portable) radiography and imaging of sitting and semi-upright patients
    - Neonates, infants and very young children
    - Debilitated and unstable patients
    - Seriously ill and bed ridden patients
  - Distinctive features
    - Magnification of anterior structures (heart and mediastinum) farthest from IR; shorter SID
    - Clavicles course horizontally and partially obscure apices
    - Ribs assume a horizontal course

CHEST OVERVIEW

- **Lateral decubitus chest radiograph**
  - Recumbent position with right or left side down
  - Elevation of chest on radiolucent support
  - Frontal radiograph (AP or PA) with horizontal X-ray beam
  - Indications
    - Evaluation of pleural fluid in dependent pleural space (X-ray beam tangential to fluid-lung interface)
    - Evaluation of air in non-dependent pleural space (X-ray beam tangential to visceral pleura-air interface)
- **Apical lordotic** (AP or PA axial) **chest radiograph**
  - Superior angulation of X-ray beam from horizontal plane of 15-20°
  - Distinctive features
    - Anterior osseous structures (clavicles and first anterior ribs) project superiorly above lung apices
    - Ribs course horizontally
    - Magnification (foreshortening) of mediastinum
  - Indications
    - Radiographic visualization of **apex**, superior mediastinum and thoracic inlet
    - Enhanced visualization of minor fissure in suspected **right middle lobe atelectasis**
- Expiratory radiography
  - Evaluation of air trapping
  - Evaluation of pneumothorax
    - Limited value
    - No clear difference in sensitivity or specificity for diagnosis of pneumothorax

Radiographic Interpretation

- Assessment of patient's identity and proper placement of right/left markers
- Imaging of entire thorax
  - **Frontal radiographs**
    - Inclusion of all thoracic structures from larynx to costophrenic angles
    - Full inspiration with diaphragm below posterior ninth rib
  - **Lateral radiographs**
    - Inclusion of anteroposterior extent of chest wall
    - Inclusion of upper lung and posterior costodiaphragmatic sulci
- Assessment of **appropriate radiographic positioning**
  - No rotation
    - Spinous process of T3 (posterior structure) centered between medial clavicles (anterior structures) on frontal radiographs
    - Superimposition of right and left ribs posterior to vertebrae on lateral radiographs
  - Medial aspects of scapulae lateral to lungs on frontal radiographs
  - Arms above thorax without superimposition on lung and mediastinum on lateral radiographs
- **Appropriately exposed radiograph**
  - Visualization of peripheral pulmonary vasculature
  - Visualization of pulmonary vessels and thoracic vertebrae through heart on frontal radiographs
- Systematic evaluation
  - Assessment of multiple superimposed structures and tissues
  - Assessment of all visible structures including portions of neck, shoulders and upper abdomen
  - Comparison to prior studies
- Challenges
  - Evaluation of retrocardiac lung
  - Evaluation of retrodiaphragmatic lung
  - Evaluation of apical lung

Radiographic Densities

- Four basic **radiographic densities**
  - **Air**
  - **Water** (fluid, blood and soft tissue)
  - **Fat**
  - **Metal** (calcium, contrast, metallic medical devices, foreign bodies)
- **Silhouette sign**
  - An intrathoracic process (mass, consolidation, pleural fluid) that touches mediastinum or diaphragm obscures visualization of their borders on radiography
  - Critical for radiographic diagnosis of
    - **Atelectasis**
    - **Consolidation**
    - **Pulmonary edema/hemorrhage**
    - **Pleural effusion**

Computed Tomography

General Concepts

- Imaging based on X-ray absorption by tissues with differing atomic numbers
- Display of differences in X-ray absorption in cross-sectional format
- Excellent **spatial resolution**
- Enhanced visualization of structures of different tissue density based on display of a wide range of HU measurements
  - **Window width** refers to number of HU displayed; **window level** refers to median (center) HU
  - **Lung window** (width of 1500 HU; level of -600 HU)
    - Evaluation of lungs, airways and air-containing portions of gastrointestinal tract
  - **Soft tissue or mediastinal window** (width of 300-500 HU; level of 30-50 HU)
    - Evaluation of vascular structures and soft tissues of mediastinum and chest wall
  - **Bone window** (widest width; level of +30 HU)
    - Evaluation of skeletal and calcified structures and metallic objects

Conventional CT

- Evaluation, localization and characterization of abnormalities detected on radiography
- Localization of lesions in preparation for CT-guided biopsy/drainage

Contrast-Enhanced CT

- Administration of intravenous contrast
  - Evaluation of normal vessels
  - Evaluation of vascular abnormalities
  - Distinction of vascular structures from adjacent soft tissues
  - Determination of lesion/tissue enhancement

CHEST OVERVIEW

- Administration of enteric contrast
  - Evaluation of gastrointestinal tract
  - Evaluation of gastrointestinal perforations/leaks

CT Angiography
- Vascular imaging
  - Timing of contrast bolus
  - Imaging of specific vascular structures
    - **CT pulmonary angiography** for evaluation of **thromboembolic disease**
    - **CT aortography** for evaluation of **traumatic aortic injury**, **dissection** and **aneurysm**

High-Resolution CT
- Technique
  - **Thin-sections** to minimize partial volume effects
  - **High-resolution reconstruction algorithm**
- Indications
  - Evaluation of **diffuse infiltrative lung disease**
  - Evaluation of patients with **dyspnea** and normal radiographs
- Special techniques
  - **Prone imaging** for evaluation of peripheral basilar lung disease
  - **Expiratory imaging** for evaluation of distal airways disease

Special Techniques
- **Multiplanar imaging** with **coronal and sagittal reformations**
  - Evaluation of axially oriented structures and abnormalities
  - Evaluation of anatomic location of lung lesions in relation to fissures
  - Evaluation of chest wall and mediastinal involvement by adjacent pulmonary lesions
- **Surface-rendered techniques** for evaluation of airway and vascular lumens
  - **Virtual bronchoscopy**
  - **Virtual angioscopy**
- **Volume-rendered techniques** for problem solving and education

Magnetic Resonance Imaging

General Concepts
- Application of radiofrequency to excite protons within a magnetic field
- Detection of signal emitted by nuclei as they relax to their original alignment with generation of an image of their spatial distribution
- Advantages of MR
  - Excellent **contrast resolution**
  - **Multiplanar imaging**
  - Intrinsic vascular "contrast"
  - Increased soft tissue contrast

Technique
- **Spin-echo** sequences typically used in chest imaging
  - **T1 weighted images**
  - **T2 weighted images**
- **Bright blood** sequences

Indications
- Imaging of the heart and great vessels
- Distinction of vascular structures from adjacent soft tissues without the use of contrast
- Evaluation of mediastinum and hila
- Evaluation of chest wall and diaphragm

Angiography

Pulmonary Angiography
- Venous catheterization
- Cannulation of pulmonary arterial system
- Indications
  - Evaluation of congenital and acquired pulmonary vascular abnormalities
  - Evaluation of thromboembolic disease
    - Decreasing utilization

Aortography
- Arterial catheterization
- Cannulation of proximal aorta
- Indications
  - Evaluation of traumatic aortic and great vessel injury
  - Evaluation of congenital arterial vascular anomalies
  - Evaluation of caliber and integrity of aortic and great vessel lumens

Bronchial Artery & Intercostal Arteriography
- Arterial catheterization
- Selective cannulation of bronchial/intercostal arteries
- Indications
  - Diagnosis and treatment of **hemoptysis**

Other Chest Imaging Modalities

Radionuclide Imaging
- **Ventilation-perfusion imaging**
  - Evaluation of thromboembolic disease
  - Evaluation of pre- and post-operative lung function
- **Positron-emission tomography**
  - Determination of metabolic activity of lesions
  - Staging of malignant neoplasms
  - Use of integrated **PET-CT imaging**

Ultrasound
- Evaluation of **pleural effusion**
  - Free vs. loculated
  - Thoracentesis planning
  - Biopsy planning
- Evaluation of **diaphragmatic motion**

CHEST OVERVIEW

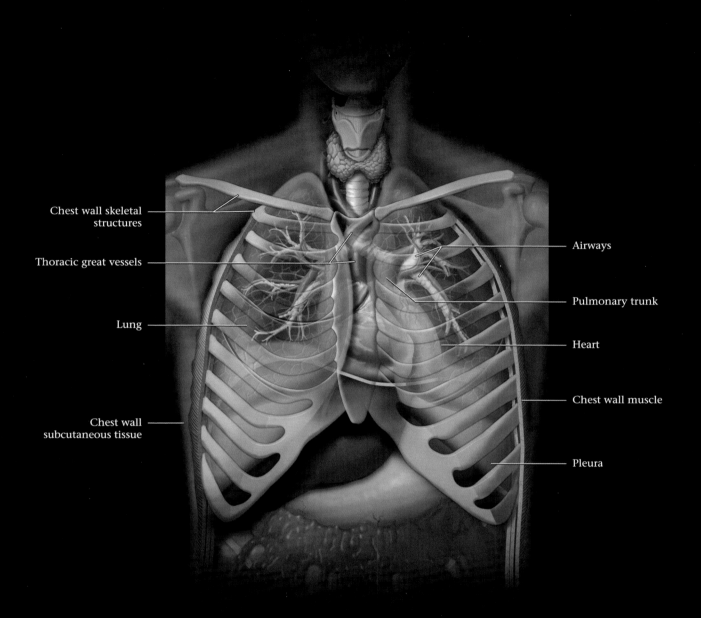

Chest wall skeletal structures

Thoracic great vessels

Lung

Chest wall subcutaneous tissue

Airways

Pulmonary trunk

Heart

Chest wall muscle

Pleura

Graphic shows the complex and diverse structures and organs in the thorax. The chest wall skeletal and soft tissue structures surround and protect the primary organs of respiration, the thoracic cardiovascular system, and the proximal gastrointestinal tract. The apposed pleural surfaces create a potential space that normally contains a small amount of fluid which lubricates the pleura and reduces friction during respiratory motion. The airways deliver oxygen to the alveolar-capillary interface and carry carbon dioxide out to the environment. The heart and vessels deliver deoxygenated blood to the capillary-alveolar interface and oxygenated blood to the peripheral organs and tissues.

CHEST OVERVIEW

PA CHEST RADIOGRAPH

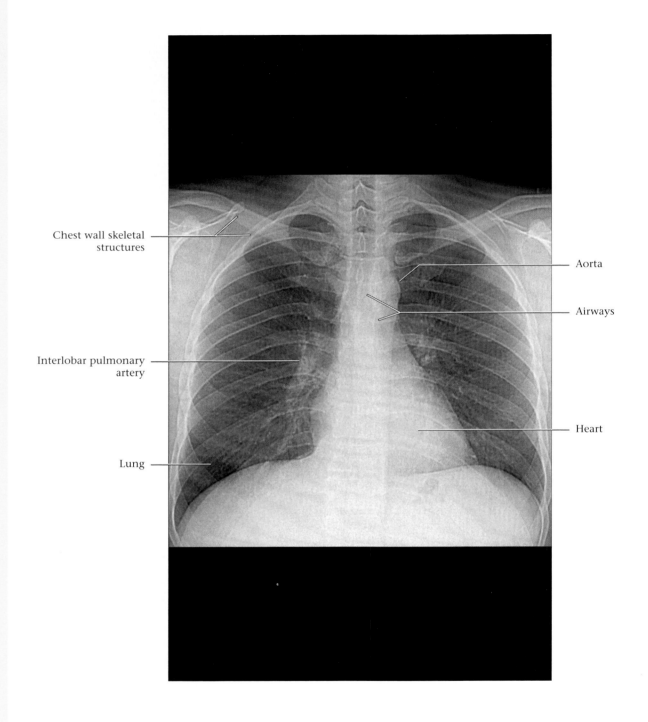

Chest wall skeletal structures

Aorta

Airways

Interlobar pulmonary artery

Heart

Lung

Normal posteroanterior chest radiograph shows the challenges inherent in the interpretation of radiographs of the thorax. Chest radiographs display a wide range of structures and tissue types with significant superimposition of structures of different radiographic density. Portions of the lung may be obscured by overlying mediastinal soft tissues and skeletal structures. Attention to radiographic image quality is of paramount importance for accurate diagnosis of subtle abnormalities.

CHEST OVERVIEW

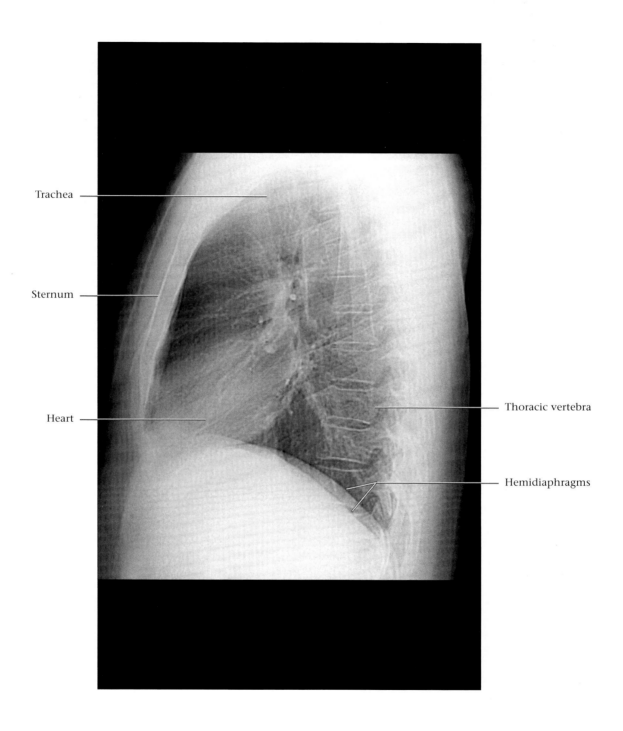

Trachea

Sternum

Heart

Thoracic vertebra

Hemidiaphragms

The left lateral chest radiograph is orthogonal (at 90°) to the PA chest radiograph. It is a complementary view that allows visualization of the retrocardiac left lower lobe and the retrodiaphragmatic lung bases. It also allows evaluation of the thoracic vertebrae. As in the PA chest radiograph, multiple structures of various densities are superimposed and must be evaluated in a systematic manner.

CHEST OVERVIEW

PA CHEST RADIOGRAPHY, POSITIONING & COLLIMATION

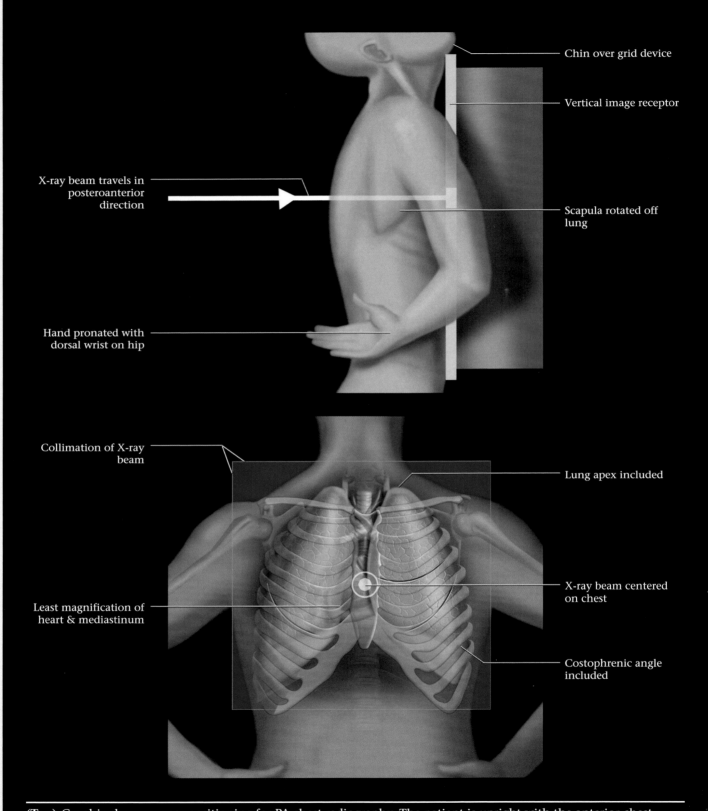

Chin over grid device

Vertical image receptor

X-ray beam travels in posteroanterior direction

Scapula rotated off lung

Hand pronated with dorsal wrist on hip

Collimation of X-ray beam

Lung apex included

X-ray beam centered on chest

Least magnification of heart & mediastinum

Costophrenic angle included

(Top) Graphic shows proper positioning for PA chest radiography. The patient is upright with the anterior chest against the vertical IR, the chin over the top of the device, the arms flexed with the backs of the hands on the hips and the shoulders internally rotated to move the scapulae off the lungs. The X-ray beam travels through the patient in a posteroanterior direction. **(Bottom)** Graphic shows proper PA chest radiographic collimation for imaging the lungs and mediastinum. The white target sign shows the centering of the X-ray beam. The blue overlay represents the collimated X-ray beam that extends from the cervical airway superiorly to below the costophrenic angles inferiorly and includes the left and right skin surfaces. The anterior structures of the chest (shown in color) are closest to the IR and experience the least magnification.

CHEST OVERVIEW

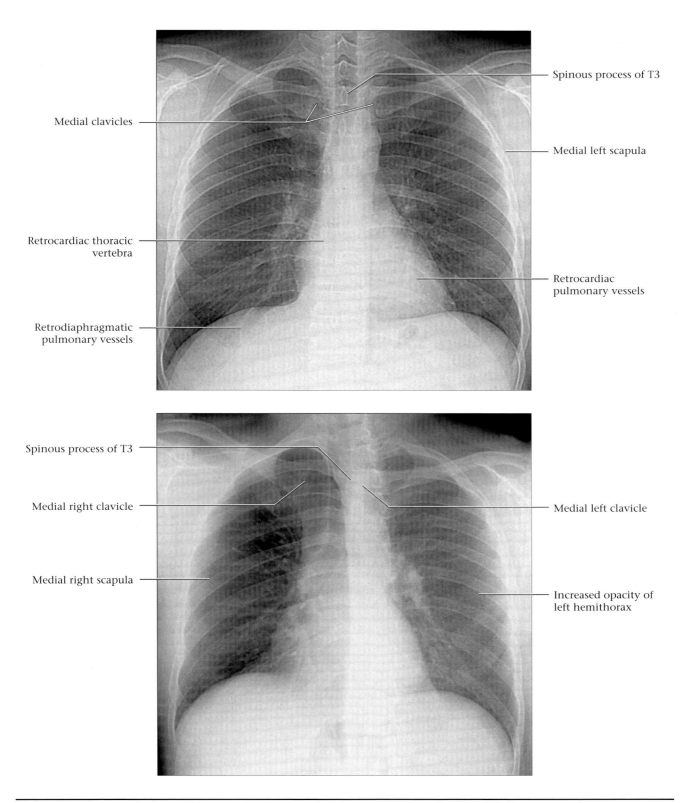

Medial clavicles

Spinous process of T3

Medial left scapula

Retrocardiac thoracic vertebra

Retrocardiac pulmonary vessels

Retrodiaphragmatic pulmonary vessels

Spinous process of T3

Medial right clavicle

Medial left clavicle

Medial right scapula

Increased opacity of left hemithorax

(Top) Well-positioned normal PA chest radiograph. The scapulae are rotated off the lungs. The spinous process of T3 is equidistant from the medial clavicles. Proper collimation spans from the cervical trachea superiorly to below the costophrenic angles inferiorly and includes the lateral aspects of the chest wall. Optimal exposure allows visualization of the peripheral pulmonary vessels, the vertebral bodies (visible through the mediastinum), and the retrocardiac and retrodiaphragmatic pulmonary vessels. **(Bottom)** Poorly positioned PA chest radiograph with marked rotation to the right. The left medial clavicle overlies the spinous process of T3 and the right medial clavicle is displaced to the right of midline. Increased density of the left hemithorax results from X-ray penetration of a greater thickness of left-sided chest wall soft tissues due to rotation.

CHEST OVERVIEW

LEFT LATERAL CHEST RADIOGRAPHY, POSITIONING & COLLIMATION

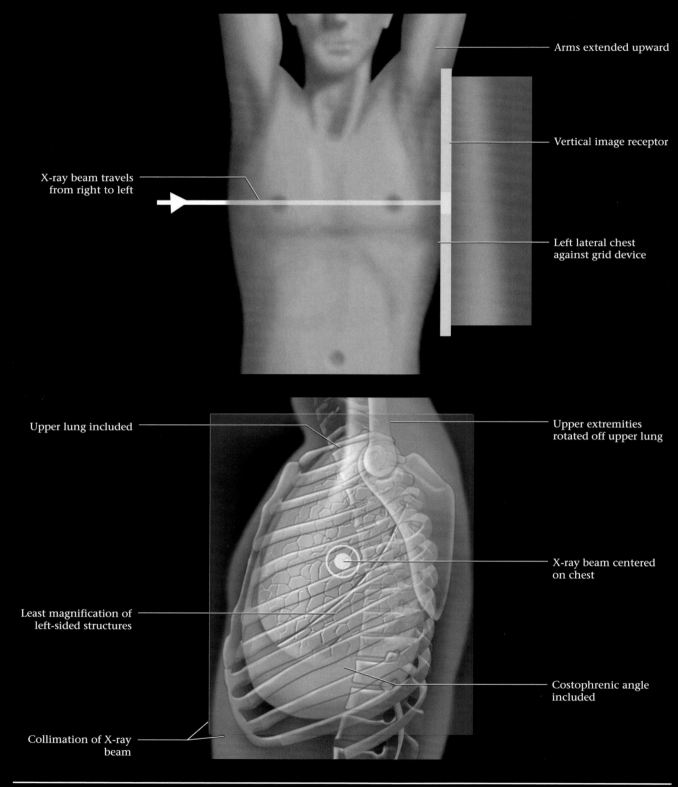

Arms extended upward

Vertical image receptor

X-ray beam travels from right to left

Left lateral chest against grid device

Upper lung included

Upper extremities rotated off upper lung

X-ray beam centered on chest

Least magnification of left-sided structures

Costophrenic angle included

Collimation of X-ray beam

(Top) Graphic shows proper positioning for left lateral chest radiography. The patient is upright with the left lateral chest against the vertical image receptor and the arms extended upward for unobstructed visualization of the upper lungs. The X-ray beam travels through the patient from right to left for a left lateral chest radiograph. **(Bottom)** Graphic shows proper left lateral chest radiographic collimation for imaging the lungs and mediastinum. The white target sign shows the centering of the X-ray beam. The blue overlay represents the collimated X-ray beam that extends from the cervical airway superiorly to below the costophrenic angles inferiorly and includes the anterior and posterior skin surfaces. The structures of the left chest (shown in color) are closest to the image receptor and experience the least magnification.

CHEST OVERVIEW

LEFT LATERAL CHEST RADIOGRAPHY

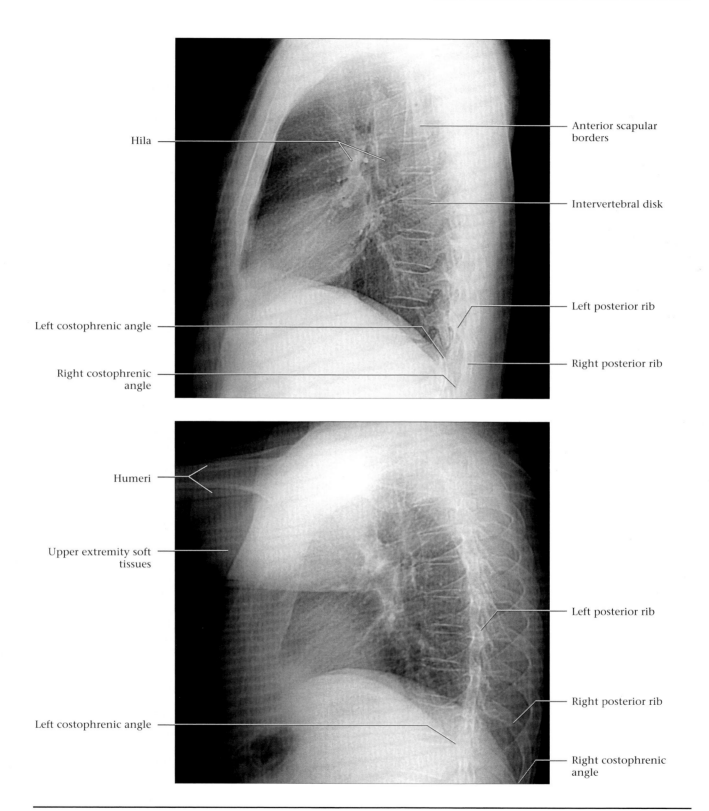

Hila

Anterior scapular borders

Intervertebral disk

Left costophrenic angle

Right costophrenic angle

Left posterior rib

Right posterior rib

Humeri

Upper extremity soft tissues

Left costophrenic angle

Left posterior rib

Right posterior rib

Right costophrenic angle

(Top) Well-positioned normal left lateral chest radiograph. The upper extremities are not visible. The hila are centrally located. The thoracic intervertebral disks are visible. The posterior ribs are superimposed and project behind the vertebrae. There is minimal magnification of the left posterior ribs, which appear sharper and smaller than the right posterior ribs. Proper collimation allows inclusion of the lung apices, the posterior costophrenic angles and the anterior and posterior skin surfaces. **(Bottom)** Poorly positioned left lateral chest radiograph. The skeletal and soft tissue structures of the upper extremities obscure the anterior lungs and mediastinum. Rotation prevents superimposition of the posterior ribs. The right posterior ribs appear larger and project behind the left posterior ribs. The right costophrenic angle projects posterior to the left.

CHEST OVERVIEW

AP CHEST RADIOGRAPHY, POSITIONING & COLLIMATION

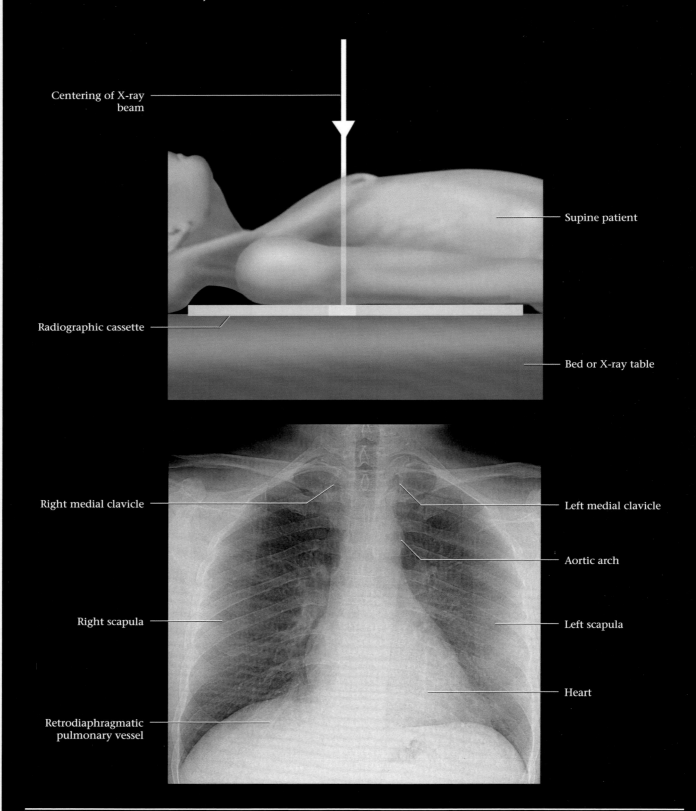

Centering of X-ray beam

Supine patient

Radiographic cassette

Bed or X-ray table

Right medial clavicle

Left medial clavicle

Aortic arch

Right scapula

Left scapula

Heart

Retrodiaphragmatic pulmonary vessel

(Top) Graphic shows proper positioning for supine AP chest radiography. The patient's back is against the radiographic cassette, the upper extremities are by the patient's sides. Internal rotation of the shoulders will minimize the degree of superimposition of the scapulae on the lateral upper lungs. The X-ray beam travels through the patient in an anteroposterior direction. The heart and anterior chest structures are farthest from the cassette and experience some magnification. **(Bottom)** Normal AP chest radiograph. The heart and great vessels appear mildly magnified. The clavicles show a horizontal course and their medial portions obscure the lung apices. The medial scapulae project over the lateral aspects of the lungs. Note that exposure factors and collimation are optimal with visualization of retrocardiac vertebrae and vessels and retrodiaphragmatic vessels.

CHEST OVERVIEW

PORTABLE AP CHEST RADIOGRAPHY, TRAUMA & INTENSIVE CARE

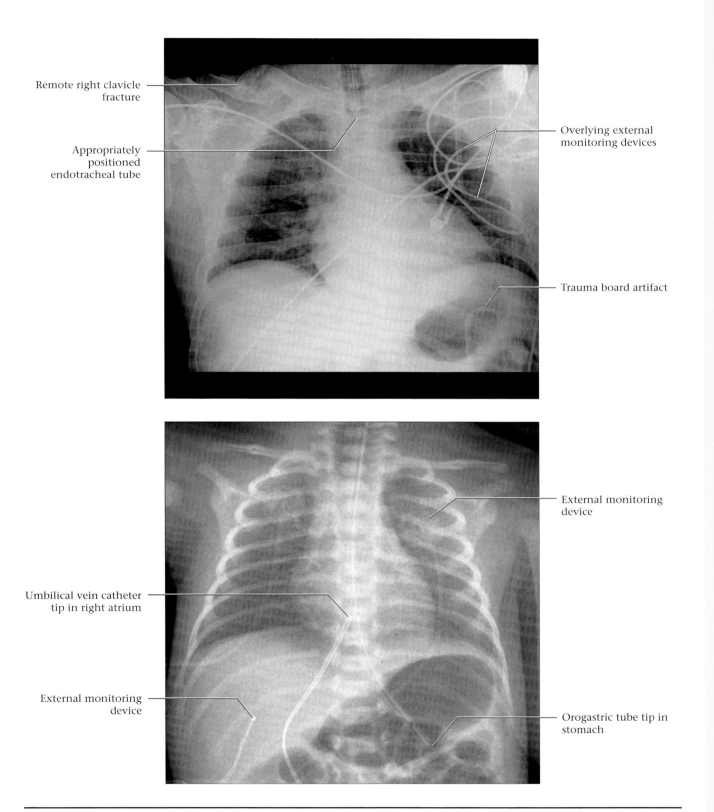

Remote right clavicle fracture

Appropriately positioned endotracheal tube

Overlying external monitoring devices

Trauma board artifact

Umbilical vein catheter tip in right atrium

External monitoring device

External monitoring device

Orogastric tube tip in stomach

(Top) Supine bedside (portable) AP chest radiograph. Portable radiographs are used for imaging debilitated, seriously ill and traumatized patients. AP chest radiographs in the setting of trauma are often compromised by technical factors related to overlying radio-opaque monitoring and stabilizing devices. However, they provide a quick assessment of the integrity of the thoracic structures and the position of life support devices. **(Bottom)** Bedside AP chest radiography is optimal for imaging neonates and infants, particularly those who are seriously ill due to congenital lesions and/or prematurity. One day old infant born at 31 weeks gestation is undergoing treatment for prematurity and mild respiratory distress syndrome. Portable radiography allows assessment of life support devices (endotracheal tube, umbilical artery/vein catheters) and pulmonary parenchyma.

CHEST OVERVIEW

PA & AP CHEST RADIOGRAPHS

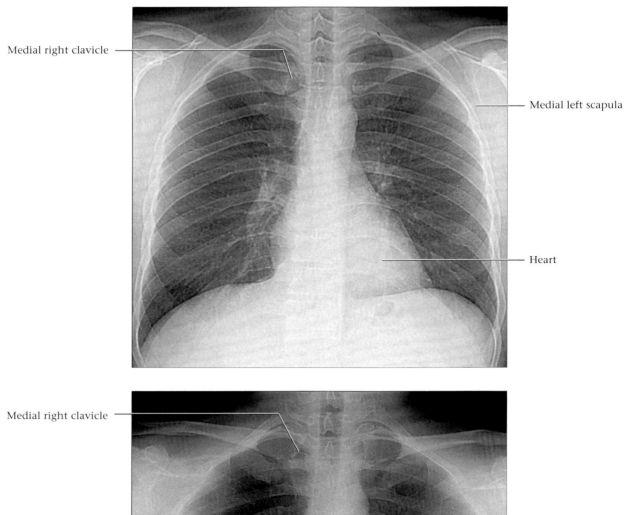

Medial right clavicle

Medial left scapula

Heart

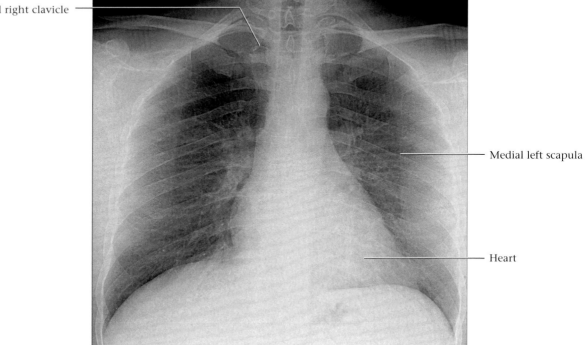

Medial right clavicle

Medial left scapula

Heart

(Top) First of four normal radiographs of the same patient. On the PA chest radiograph, the heart and mediastinum are closest to the image receptor and undergo the least magnification. The medial clavicles curve inferiorly and do not obscure the lung apices. The scapulae are rotated laterally and do not obscure the lateral aspects of the lungs. **(Bottom)** On the AP chest radiograph, the heart and mediastinum appear slightly larger as they are farthest from the image receptor and undergo some magnification. The clavicles exhibit a horizontal course and their medial aspects obscure the lung apices. The medial portions of the scapulae overlie the lateral aspects of the lungs.

CHEST OVERVIEW

INSPIRATORY AND EXPIRATORY CHEST RADIOGRAPHS

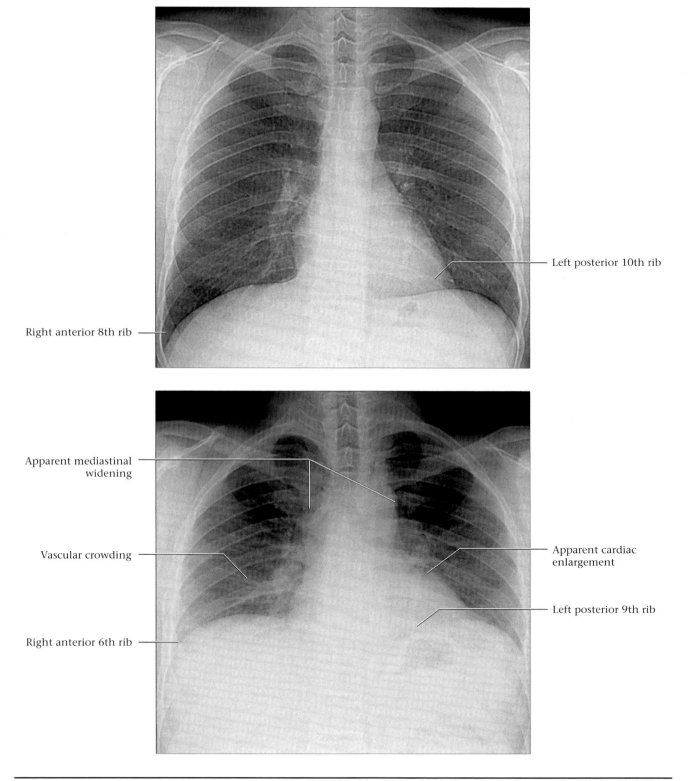

Left posterior 10th rib

Right anterior 8th rib

Apparent mediastinal widening

Vascular crowding

Right anterior 6th rib

Apparent cardiac enlargement

Left posterior 9th rib

(Top) Normal PA chest radiograph obtained at full inspiration shows optimal visualization of the lung bases and the retrocardiac and retrodiaphragmatic lung. A portion of the 8th anterior right rib is visible through the lung and projects above the hemidiaphragm. A portion of the 10th posterior left rib is visible through the lung and projects above the hemidiaphragm. **(Bottom)** Normal PA chest radiograph obtained at end expiration shows low lung volumes. The lung bases are partially obscured with increased basilar density and vascular crowding with resultant poor visualization of the retrodiaphragmatic lung. A portion of the right 6th anterior rib is visible through the lung and projects above the hemidiaphragm. A portion of the left 9th posterior rib is visible through the lung and projects above the hemidiaphragm.

CHEST OVERVIEW

LATERAL DECUBITUS CHEST RADIOGRAPHY, POSITIONING & COLLIMATION

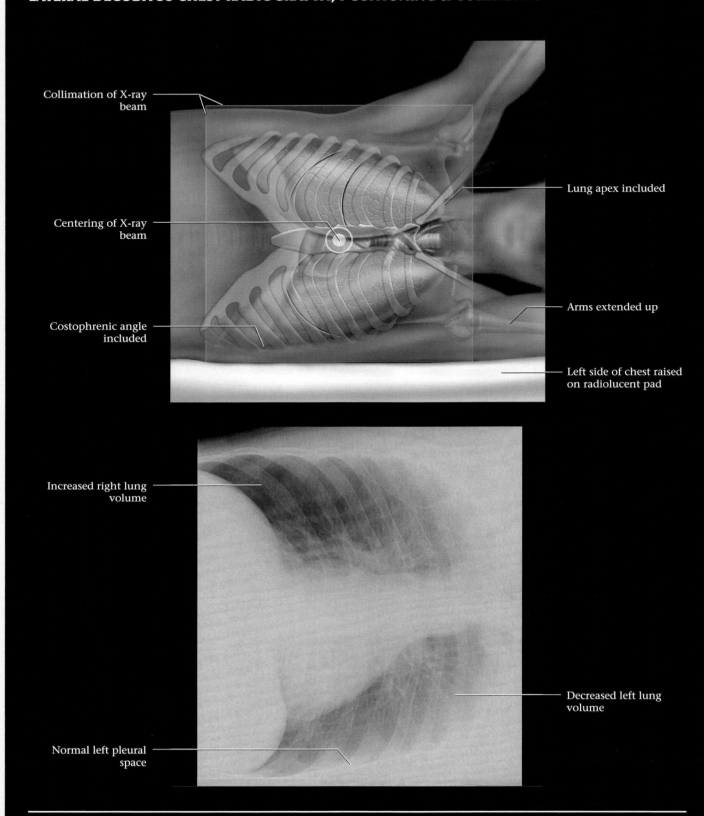

Collimation of X-ray beam

Centering of X-ray beam

Costophrenic angle included

Lung apex included

Arms extended up

Left side of chest raised on radiolucent pad

Increased right lung volume

Decreased left lung volume

Normal left pleural space

(Top) Graphic shows proper lateral decubitus PA radiographic collimation for imaging the lungs and mediastinum. The white target sign shows the centering of the X-ray beam. The blue overlay represents the collimated X-ray beam that extends from the cervical airway superiorly to below the costophrenic angles inferiorly and includes the left and right skin surfaces. The thorax is elevated on a radiolucent pad to ensure inclusion of the dependent pleural surface and chest wall. The anterior structures of the chest (shown in color) are closest to the image receptor and experience the least magnification. **(Bottom)** Normal left lateral decubitus radiograph shows a larger lung volume in the non-dependent right lung and volume loss manifesting as increased density in the dependent left lung. There is no pleural thickening or fluid.

CHEST OVERVIEW

APICAL LORDOTIC CHEST RADIOGRAPHY, POSITIONING

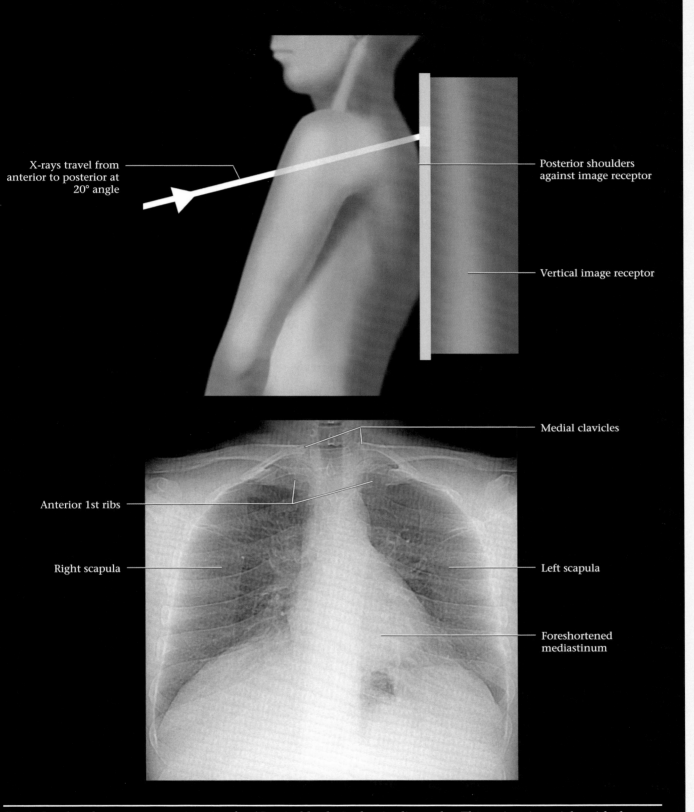

X-rays travel from anterior to posterior at 20° angle

Posterior shoulders against image receptor

Vertical image receptor

Medial clavicles

Anterior 1st ribs

Right scapula

Left scapula

Foreshortened mediastinum

(Top) Graphic shows proper positioning for AP apical lordotic chest radiography. The patient is upright with the posterior shoulders against the vertical image receptor, the arms are internally rotated to move scapulae away from the lungs. The X-ray beam travels through the patient from anterior to posterior and is centered at the manubrium sternum and oriented superiorly at a 20° angle from the horizontal plane. (Bottom) Normal apical lordotic chest radiograph projects the medial aspects of the clavicles off the lung apices. Note that the apex is partly obscured by the anterior aspects of the first ribs and their costochondral junctions in this case. The mediastinum is foreshortened and mildly magnified. The scapulae overlie a significant portion of the lateral lungs.

CHEST OVERVIEW

RADIOGRAPHIC DENSITIES

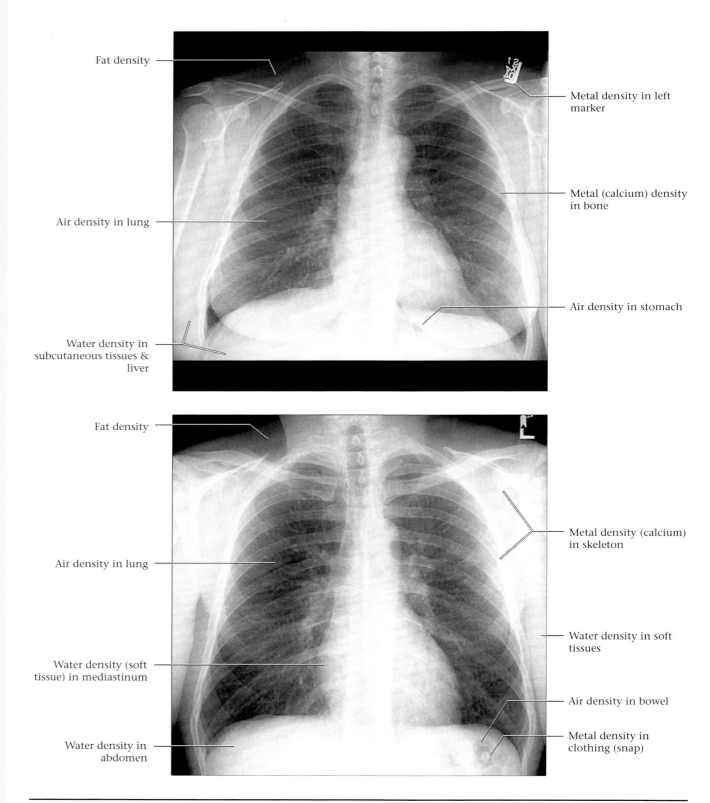

Fat density

Metal density in left marker

Metal (calcium) density in bone

Air density in lung

Air density in stomach

Water density in subcutaneous tissues & liver

Fat density

Metal density (calcium) in skeleton

Air density in lung

Water density in soft tissues

Water density (soft tissue) in mediastinum

Air density in bowel

Metal density in clothing (snap)

Water density in abdomen

(Top) Normal PA chest radiograph shows the four radiographic densities. Air is present in the lungs bilaterally and within the stomach. Water (or soft tissue) density is seen in the mediastinum, abdomen and subcutaneous tissues. Fat density is visible between the normal soft tissues of the upper thorax. Metal density is noted in the skeletal structures (calcium) and the metallic left marker. **(Bottom)** Normal PA chest radiograph shows the four radiographic densities. Air density is present in the lungs cnd within bowel. Water (soft tissue) density is seen in the mediastinum, abdomen and subcutaneous soft tissues. Fat is more difficult to demonstrate in this thin patient but is present between the normal soft tissues of the upper chest. Metal is represented by the skeletal structures (calcium), the metallic left marker and a snap on the patient's gown.

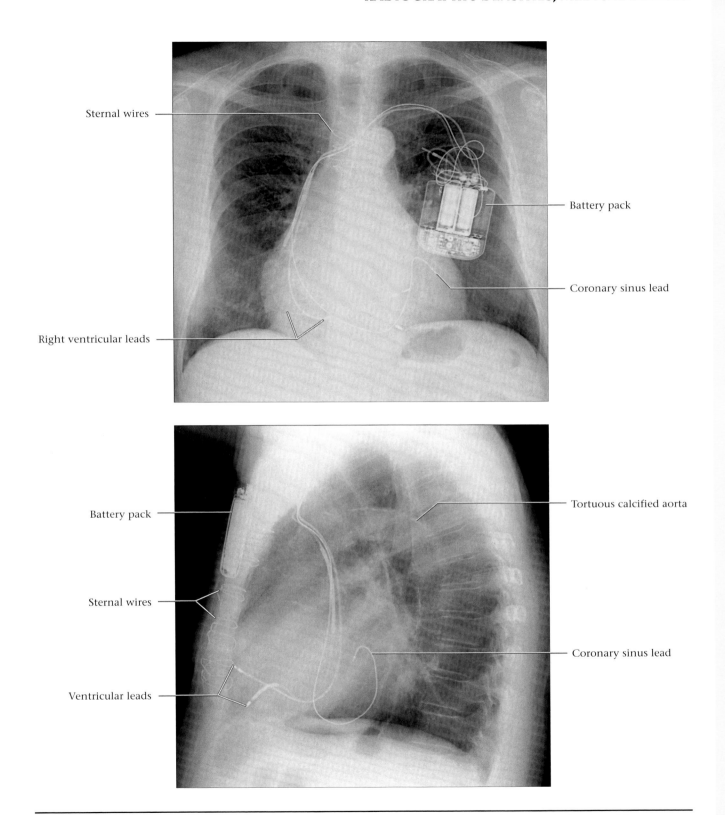

Sternal wires

Battery pack

Coronary sinus lead

Right ventricular leads

Battery pack

Tortuous calcified aorta

Sternal wires

Coronary sinus lead

Ventricular leads

(Top) First of two chest radiographs of a patient with a biventricular pacemaker and automatic implantable cardioverter defibrillator with a battery pack. Orthogonal radiographs allow accurate assessment of the integrity and position of medical devices. PA chest radiograph shows two pacer leads in the right ventricle and one in the coronary sinus. The metallic battery pack obscures visualization of the left mid lung. There is cardiomegaly and tortuosity and calcification of the thoracic aorta. The lungs are clear. Sternal wires are present. **(Bottom)** Left lateral chest radiograph shows two right ventricular leads and a third lead in the coronary sinus. The left lung behind the battery pack is now visible although superimposed on the contralateral right lung. Cardiomegaly, aortic tortuosity and calcification and sternal wires are again noted.

CHEST OVERVIEW

SILHOUETTE SIGN

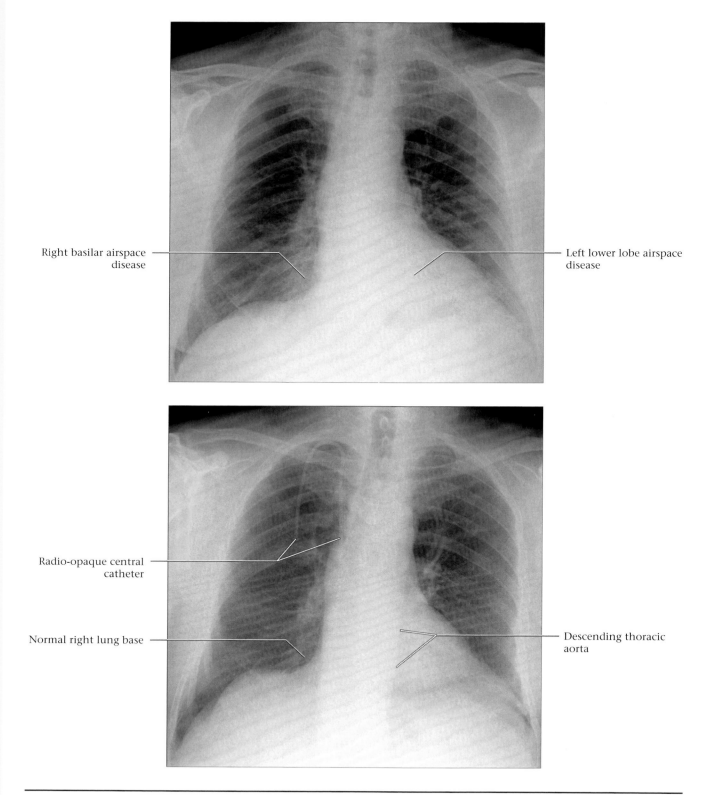

Right basilar airspace disease

Left lower lobe airspace disease

Radio-opaque central catheter

Normal right lung base

Descending thoracic aorta

(Top) First of two chest radiographs of a patient with multifocal pneumonia who presented with fever. AP chest radiograph shows right basilar airspace disease manifesting as increased basilar opacity and obscuration of the right cardiac border. Left lower lobe airspace disease manifests with obscuration of the retrocardiac descending aorta. Multifocal pneumonia was suspected clinically and was confirmed on chest CT. **(Bottom)** PA chest radiograph obtained two years earlier shows a normal appearance of the right lung base, visualization of the right cardiac border and a normal left lower lobe with visualization of the retrocardiac descending aorta. A right internal jugular catheter is also present. This case illustrates the value of the silhouette sign and the value of comparison with prior studies in the diagnosis of subtle radiographic abnormalities.

CHEST OVERVIEW

ANATOMIC LOCALIZATION WITH ORTHOGONAL RADIOGRAPHS

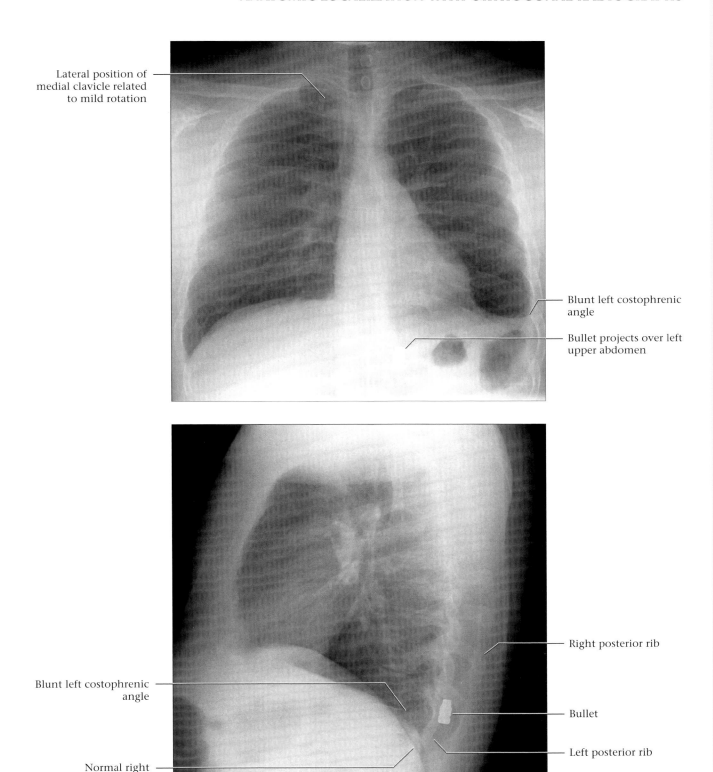

Lateral position of medial clavicle related to mild rotation

Blunt left costophrenic angle

Bullet projects over left upper abdomen

Blunt left costophrenic angle

Right posterior rib

Bullet

Left posterior rib

Normal right hemidiaphragm

(Top) First of two radiographs of the same patient. PA chest radiograph shows a bullet over the soft tissues of the upper abdomen to the left of the midline. There is blunting of the left costophrenic angle related to remote trauma. (Bottom) The orthogonal left lateral chest radiograph allows anatomic localization of the bullet in the soft tissues of the posterior left chest wall. The patient is rotated. Note that the bullet projects posterior to the sharper, smaller and anteriorly located left posterior ribs. The right posterior ribs appear less sharp and larger as they are farther from the IR. The right and left hemidiaphragms can be confidently identified based on their relationship to the corresponding ipsilateral ribs. PA and lateral radiographs allow anatomic localization of imaging abnormalities.

CHEST OVERVIEW

DECUBITUS RADIOGRAPHY FOR EVALUATION OF COMPLEX PLEURAL DISEASE

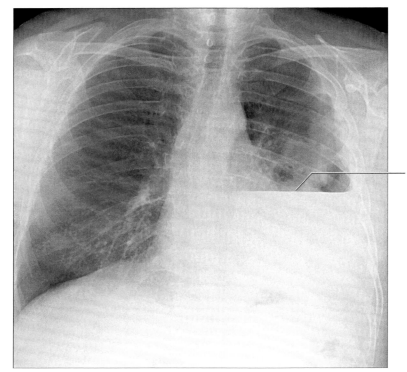

Air-fluid level in left hemithorax

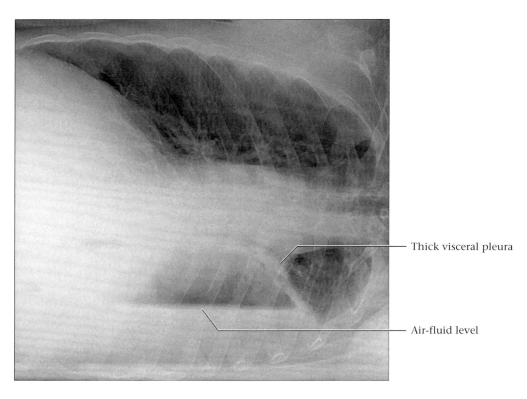

Thick visceral pleura

Air-fluid level

(Top) First of two chest radiographs of a patient with a left empyema. PA chest radiograph shows a large air-fluid level in the left inferior hemithorax. **(Bottom)** Left lateral decubitus chest radiograph shows a discrepant length of the air-fluid level (it appears longer than on the PA radiograph) indicating that the collection has an elongate shape. Note the thick medial wall of the air and fluid collection. The findings are characteristic of a loculated pleural collection. The presence of air indicates a communication with the tracheobronchial tree (bronchopleural fistula) and the findings are diagnostic of a complicated empyema. In this case, the lateral decubitus radiograph allows pleural localization of the abnormality and distinction from parenchymal disease.

CHEST OVERVIEW

LORDOTIC CHEST RADIOGRAPHY FOR EVALUATION OF APICAL LESION

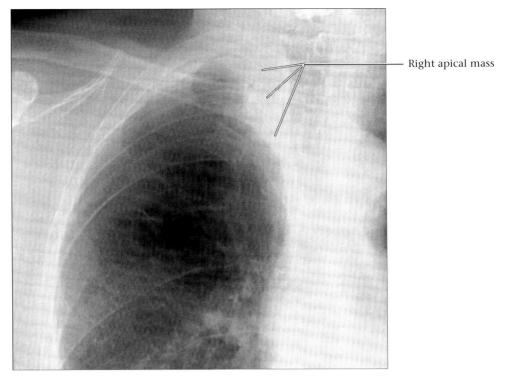

Right apical mass

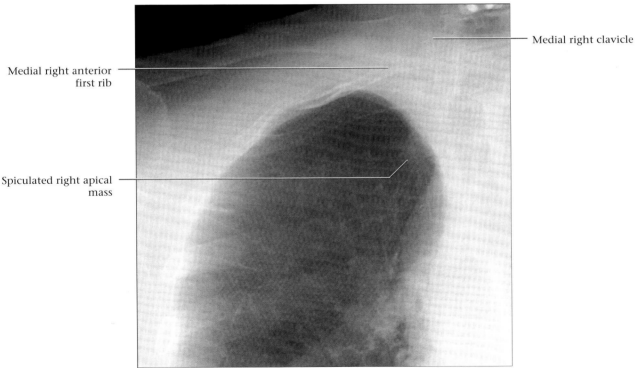

Medial right clavicle

Medial right anterior first rib

Spiculated right apical mass

(Top) First of two radiographs of a patient with a right apical mass. PA chest radiograph coned-down to the right apex demonstrates an abnormal irregular apical mass and thickening of the medial aspect of the right apical pleura. (Bottom) AP apical lordotic radiograph coned to the right upper lobe allows visualization of the medial aspect of the right apical lung by projecting the right medial clavicle and right first anterior rib above the lung apex. The spiculated lateral border of this right apical non-small cell lung cancer is now visible.

SILHOUETTE SIGN, LEFT LOWER LOBE AIRSPACE DISEASE

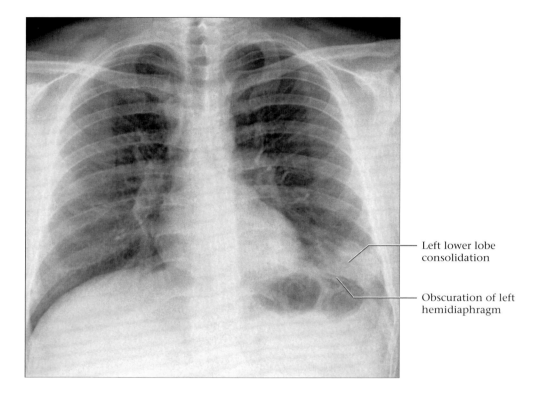

Left lower lobe consolidation

Obscuration of left hemidiaphragm

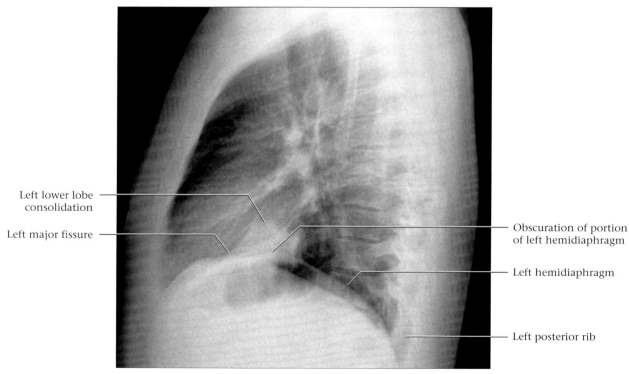

Left lower lobe consolidation

Left major fissure

Obscuration of portion of left hemidiaphragm

Left hemidiaphragm

Left posterior rib

(Top) First of two chest radiographs of a patient with left lower lobe consolidation. PA chest radiograph shows a left basilar air space opacity that obscures the left hemidiaphragm. While the left hemidiaphragm is not visible, its location is inferred by the presence of adjacent abdominal air-filled loops of bowel. The alveolar air in the left lower lobe has been replaced by an inflammatory process producing the silhouette sign. **(Bottom)** Lateral chest radiograph shows that the consolidation abuts the oblique fissure anteriorly and is located in the anteromedial basal segment of the left lower lobe. The left lateral chest radiograph allows identification of the left (least magnified) ribs that are closest to the IR and the ipsilateral left hemidiaphragm.

CHEST OVERVIEW

SILHOUETTE SIGN, RIGHT MIDDLE LOBE AIRSPACE DISEASE

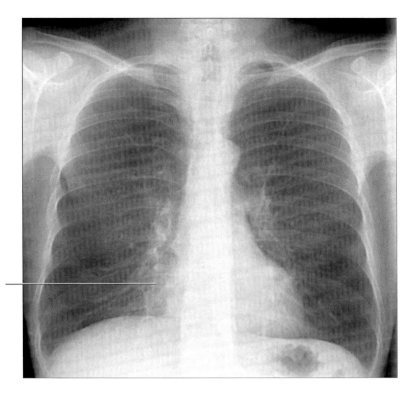

Right middle lobe
opacity obscures right
cardiac border

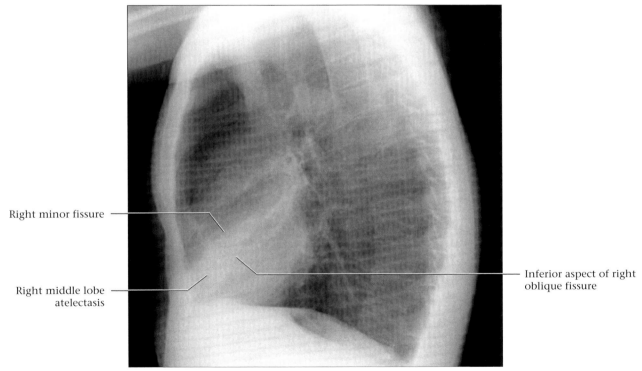

Right minor fissure

Right middle lobe
atelectasis

Inferior aspect of right
oblique fissure

(Top) First of two chest radiographs of a patient with right middle lobe atelectasis. PA chest radiograph shows air space opacity in the medial aspect of the right lower lung zone which obscures the right cardiac border. The location of the process can be inferred by the inability to visualize the right cardiac border while the right hemidiaphragm is visualized. Atelectasis has resulted in evacuation of the alveolar air from the right middle lobe producing the silhouette sign. **(Bottom)** Lateral chest radiograph shows a triangular opacity that projects over the heart and represents the atelectatic right middle lobe. Postero-inferior displacement of the minor fissure and antero-superior displacement of the inferior aspect of the right major fissure are typical of right middle lobe volume loss and distinguish atelectasis from consolidation.

CHEST OVERVIEW

CROSS-SECTIONAL ANATOMY

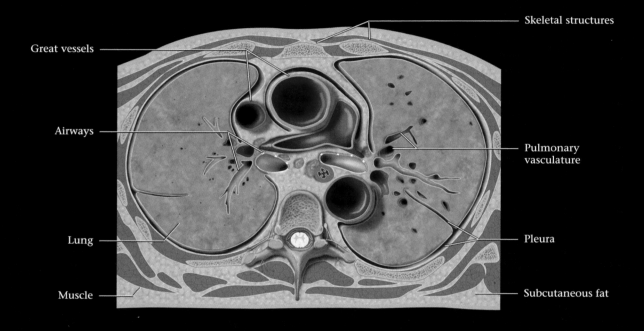

Great vessels

Skeletal structures

Airways

Pulmonary vasculature

Lung

Pleura

Muscle

Subcutaneous fat

Graphic shows the cross-sectional appearance of the mid thorax and illustrates visualization of numerous organs and tissues in cross-section. Cross-sectional imaging allows assessment of the various and diverse organs, structures and tissues of the chest. The soft tissues of the chest wall consist of skin, subcutaneous fat and chest wall muscles. Together with the skeletal structures, the soft tissues of the chest wall surround and protect the thoracic cavity and its internal organs and tissues. The apposed pleural surfaces form the pleural space. The pulmonary arteries and veins course through the lungs. The mediastinal fat, mediastinal vascular structures, esophagus, central tracheobronchial tree and lymph nodes are also depicted.

CHEST OVERVIEW

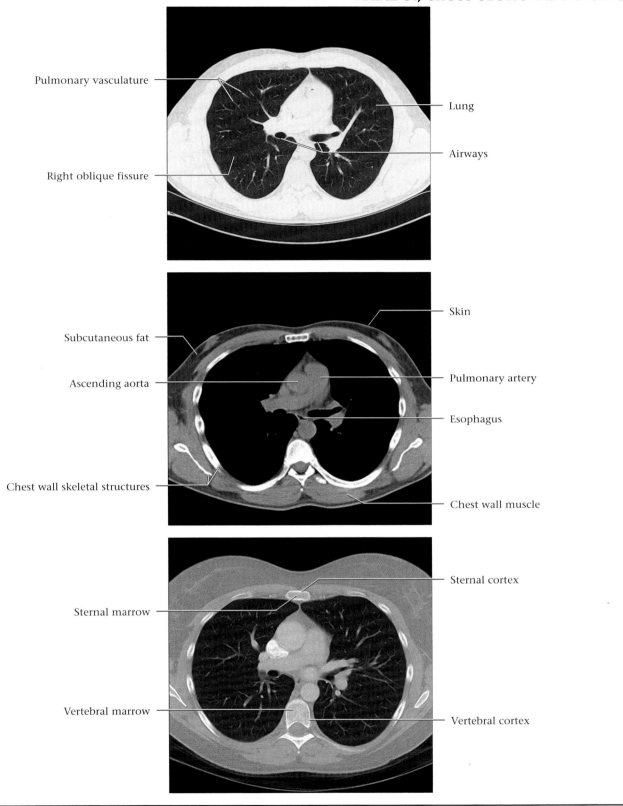

(Top) Normal contrast-enhanced chest CT (lung window) allows evaluation of the lungs, pulmonary vasculature, central tracheobronchial tree and pleural surfaces. The mediastinum and chest wall are poorly evaluated in this window setting. (Middle) Normal unenhanced chest CT (mediastinal window) allows evaluation of the soft tissue structures of the mediastinum and the soft tissues and skeletal structures of the chest wall. The pulmonary parenchyma, pleura and central tracheobronchial tree are not well evaluated. (Bottom) Normal contrast-enhanced chest CT (bone window) allows optimal assessment of the skeletal structures with visualization of their cortices and marrow spaces. Note improved skeletal visualization when compared to the mediastinal window image (previous image). This window setting is also useful for evaluation of calcifications and metallic medical devices.

CHEST OVERVIEW

UNENHANCED & CONTRAST-ENHANCED CT

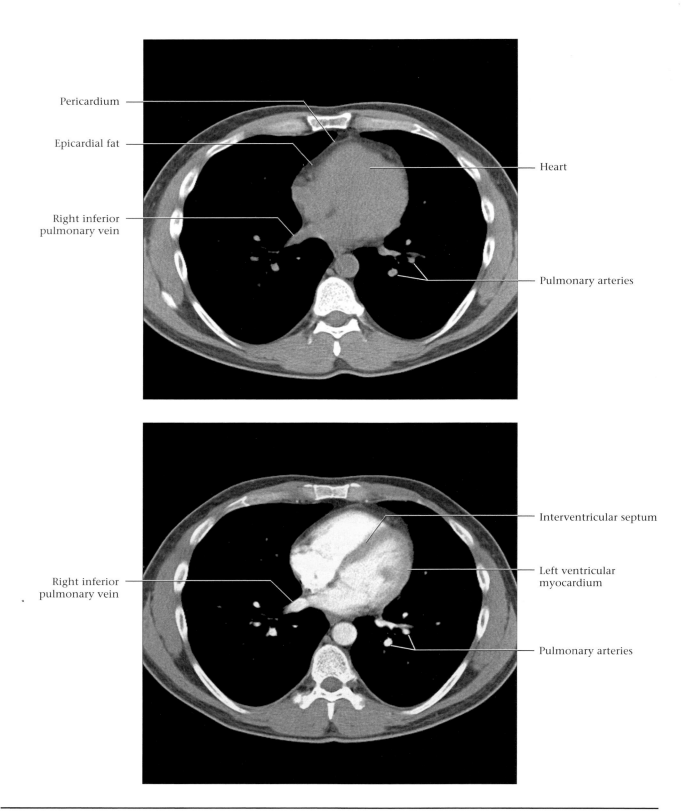

Pericardium

Epicardial fat

Heart

Right inferior
pulmonary vein

Pulmonary arteries

Interventricular septum

Left ventricular
myocardium

Right inferior
pulmonary vein

Pulmonary arteries

(Top) First of two normal chest CT images through the heart. Unenhanced chest CT (mediastinal window) shows the heart surrounded by epicardial fat and contained within the pericardium. The inferior pulmonary veins are visible bilaterally. Note that individual cardiac chambers cannot be resolved. **(Bottom)** Contrast-enhanced chest CT (mediastinal window) shows excellent visualization of the inferior pulmonary veins, pulmonary arteries and cardiac chambers. The interventricular septum and the left ventricular myocardium are well demonstrated.

CHEST OVERVIEW

SECTION THICKNESS & HIGH-RESOLUTION CT

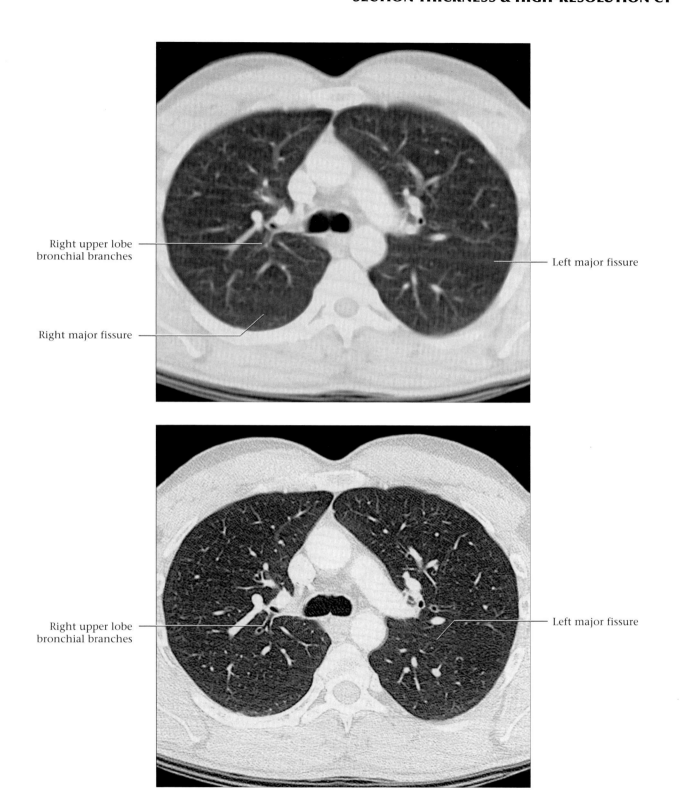

Right upper lobe bronchial branches

Left major fissure

Right major fissure

Right upper lobe bronchial branches

Left major fissure

(Top) First of two images of a normal contrast-enhanced chest CT. Conventional chest CT (lung window) with 5 mm slice thickness shows adequate visualization of the lung parenchyma, pulmonary vasculature and tracheobronchial tree. The major fissures are visible as avascular bands coursing obliquely through the lungs. (Bottom) HRCT with 1.2 mm slice thickness at the same level as the previous image shows improved visualization of pulmonary detail. The left major fissure is now seen as a distinct line. There is improved visualization of the bronchial walls and sharper outlines of the pulmonary vessels.

CHEST OVERVIEW

SUPINE & PRONE HRCT

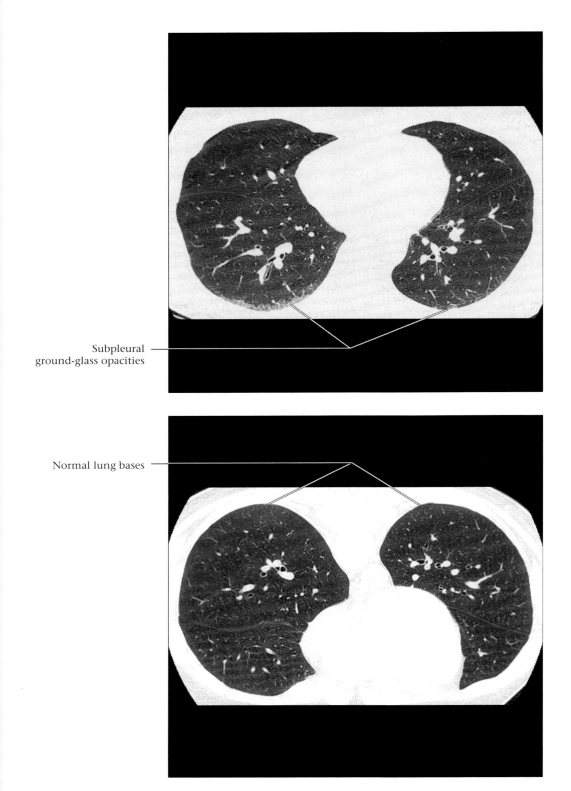

Subpleural ground-glass opacities

Normal lung bases

(Top) First of two images of a normal HRCT in a patient with mild dyspnea. Supine HRCT shows posterior subpleural ground-glass opacity that is more prominent on the right. There is no architectural distortion or other abnormality. **(Bottom)** Prone HRCT image shows complete clearance of basilar subpleural ground-glass opacities and confirms that they related to dependent or supine atelectasis.

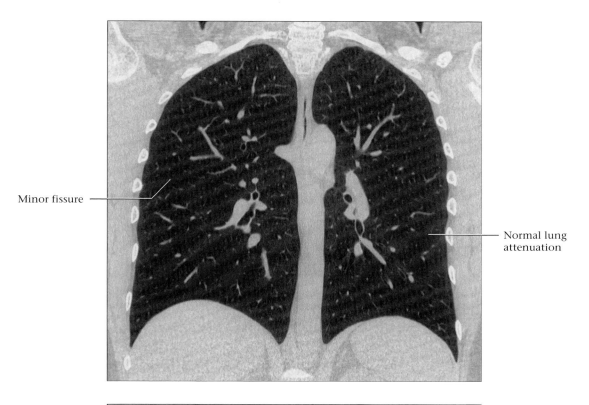

Minor fissure

Normal lung attenuation

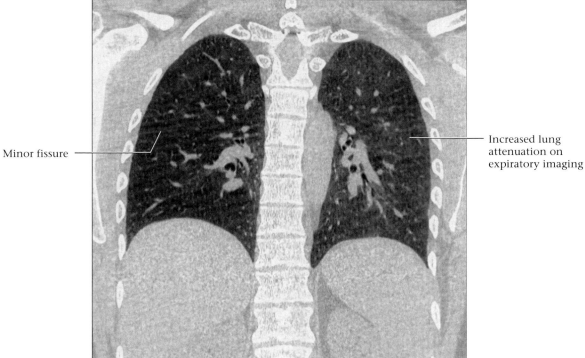

Minor fissure

Increased lung attenuation on expiratory imaging

(Top) First of two images from a normal HRCT. Inspiratory high-resolution CT (coronal reconstruction) shows normal homogeneous pulmonary attenuation. Note excellent visualization of vascular structures, central bronchi and pleural surfaces. **(Bottom)** Expiratory HRCT (coronal reconstruction) at the same level as the previous image shows elevation of the hemidiaphragms, decrease in lung volume and increased heterogeneous attenuation of the lung parenchyma. Although lung attenuation is heterogeneous, there is no evidence of air trapping. In this case, the right lung appears slightly more lucent than the left on expiratory imaging.

CHEST OVERVIEW

CT ANGIOGRAPHY, CORONAL & SAGITTAL RECONSTRUCTIONS

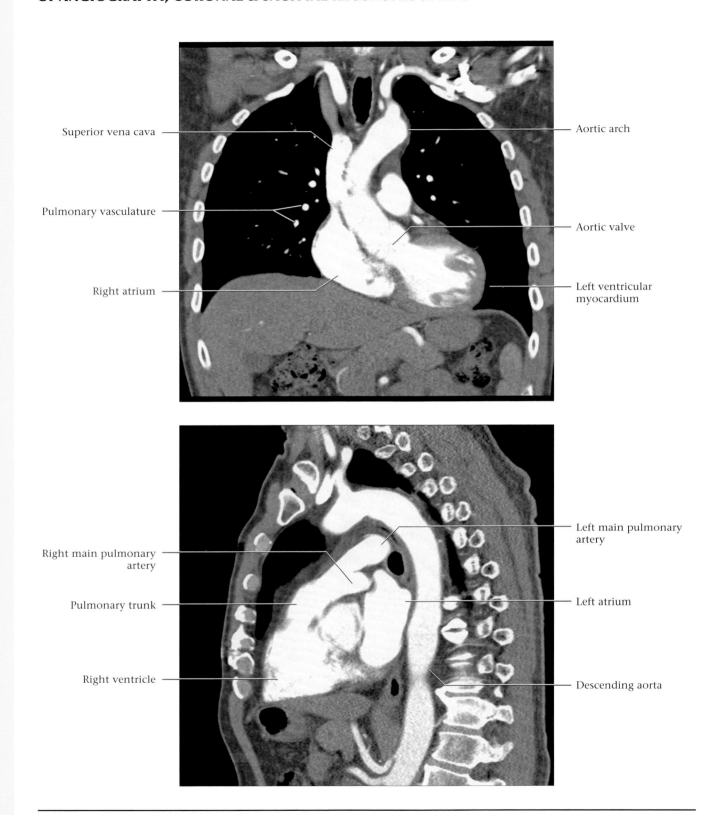

Superior vena cava

Pulmonary vasculature

Right atrium

Aortic arch

Aortic valve

Left ventricular myocardium

Right main pulmonary artery

Pulmonary trunk

Right ventricle

Left main pulmonary artery

Left atrium

Descending aorta

(Top) First of two images from a normal CT angiogram of the chest. Coronal CT angiogram (mediastinal window) allows visualization and evaluation of the cardiac chambers and the vascular lumens of the thoracic great vessels. CT angiography also allows assessment of the peripheral pulmonary vasculature for exclusion of pulmonary thromboembolic disease. **(Bottom)** Sagittal CT angiogram (mediastinal window) allows visualization of the descending thoracic aorta and its branches. Note visualization of the right ventricle, the right ventricular outflow tract, and the right and left main pulmonary arteries. Multiplanar reconstructions of CT angiograms allow exquisite visualization of the vascular lumens and cardiac chambers for evaluation of luminal enlargement, endoluminal thrombus or tumor, vascular disruption and congenital anomalies.

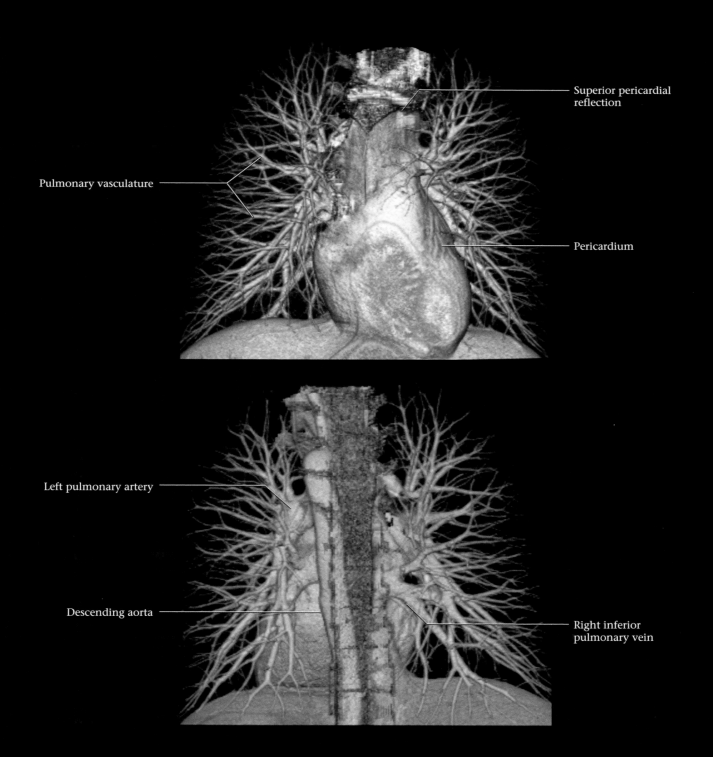

Superior pericardial reflection

Pulmonary vasculature

Pericardium

Left pulmonary artery

Descending aorta

Right inferior pulmonary vein

(Top) First of two volume rendered CT images of the chest. The coronal volume rendered CT image of the anterior chest shows the pulmonary vasculature and the superior extent of the pericardium. **(Bottom)** Posterior coronal volume rendered CT image display allows distinction of pulmonary veins from pulmonary arteries and shows portions of the descending thoracic aorta.

CHEST OVERVIEW

AXIAL MR, CROSS-SECTIONAL IMAGING

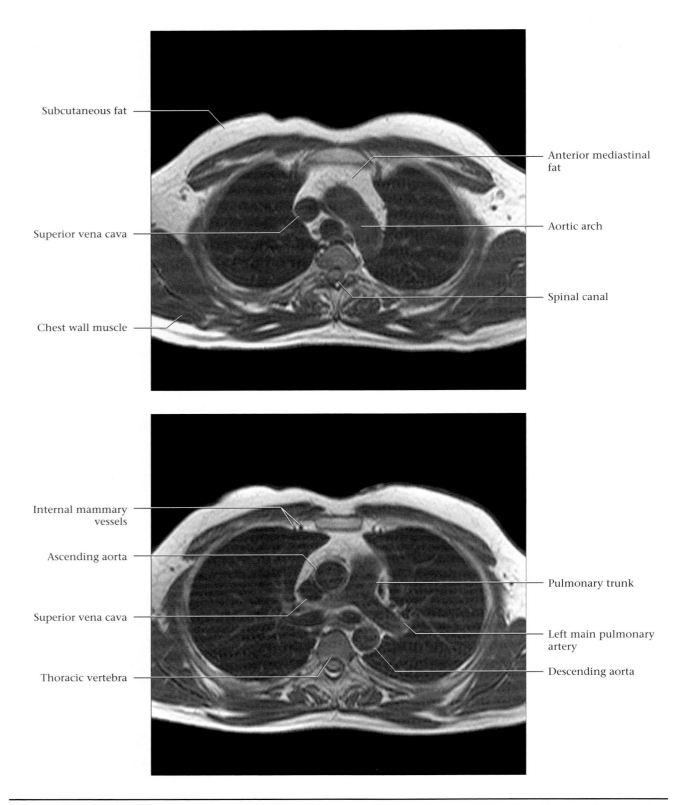

(Top) Axial cardiac gated MR through the aortic arch shows excellent contrast resolution that allows evaluation of mediastinal and chest wall structures. Note the distinction of the mediastinal and subcutaneous fat from adjacent soft tissue structures. Visualization of the lungs is less optimal and is mildly compromised by motion. **(Bottom)** Axial cardiac gated MR through the pulmonary trunk shows the value of MR in the evaluation of thoracic vascular structures without the use of iodinated contrast. The internal mammary vessels are also demonstrated.

CHEST OVERVIEW

CORONAL & SAGITTAL MR, CROSS-SECTIONAL IMAGING

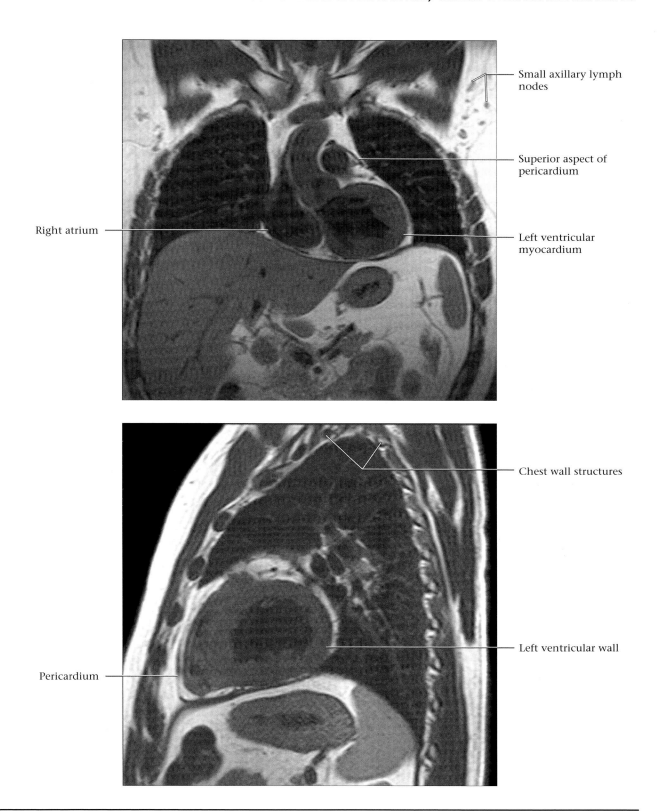

Small axillary lymph nodes

Superior aspect of pericardium

Right atrium

Left ventricular myocardium

Chest wall structures

Left ventricular wall

Pericardium

(Top) Coronal cardiac gated chest MR shows outstanding imaging of the mediastinum and diaphragm. Note the excellent visualization of the cardiac chambers and ventricular myocardium. The pericardium is particularly well visualized in this case. **(Bottom)** Sagittal cardiac gated chest MR shows exquisite visualization of soft tissue structures in the chest wall. MR is used as a problem solving modality for assessment of mediastinal and chest wall tumor invasion and is particularly useful for staging apical tumors.

CHEST OVERVIEW

CT EVALUATION OF APICAL LESIONS

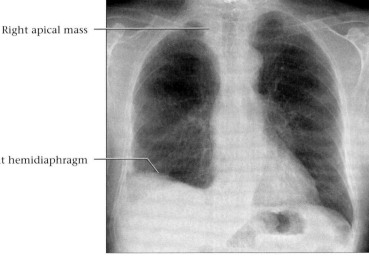

Right apical mass

Elevated right hemidiaphragm

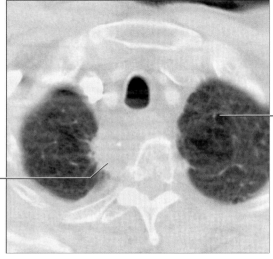

Centrilobular emphysema

Right apical mass

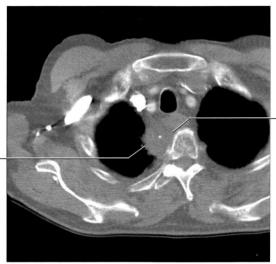

Absent tissue plane between mass & mediastinum

Right apical soft tissue mass

(Top) First of three images of a patient with a right apical non-small cell lung cancer. PA chest radiograph shows the right apical mass and elevation of the ipsilateral right hemidiaphragm. While this lesion can be better visualized with apical lordotic radiography, CT is the method of choice for the evaluation of thoracic malignancies. (Middle) Chest CT (lung window) shows the right apical tumor and its spiculated lateral border. Note bilateral upper lobe centrilobular emphysema. (Bottom) Chest CT (mediastinal window) demonstrates the soft tissue mass with punctate internal calcification. There is no tissue plane between the mass and the adjacent mediastinum, a finding that suggests direct mediastinal involvement by the lesion. CT allows lesion localization and characterization and is used for pre-operative staging of patients with lung cancer.

CHEST OVERVIEW

CT EVALUATION OF SUBTLE RADIOGRAPHIC ABNORMALITIES

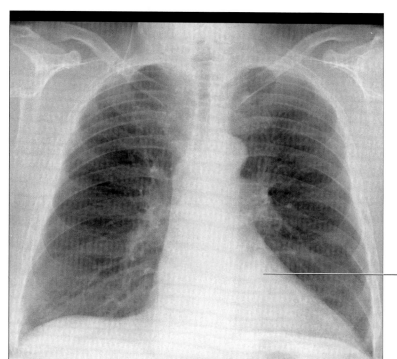

Subtle retrocardiac lesion

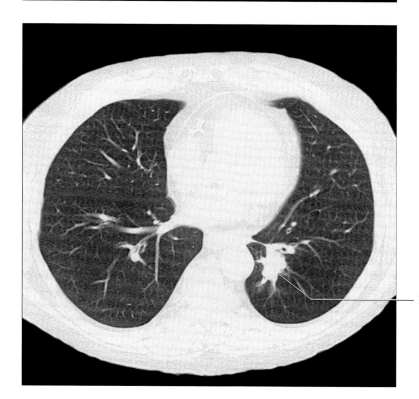

Left lower lobe mass

(Top) First of two images of an asymptomatic man with an incidentally discovered radiographic abnormality. PA chest radiograph shows a subtle left lower lobe retrocardiac opacity. (Bottom) Chest CT (lung window) shows a left lower lobe nodule which represented a primary lung adenocarcinoma. CT allows accurate assessment of subtle radiographic abnormalities, and may facilitate early diagnosis of primary malignancy as in this case.

LUNG DEVELOPMENT

General Concepts

Overview of Lung Development
- **Larynx** and **trachea**
  - Origin of primitive larynx from **laryngotracheal groove**
  - Formation of **tracheal bud** and primitive trachea
  - Separation of primitive trachea from foregut and developing esophagus
- **Bronchi**
  - Tracheal bud branches into two primitive **bronchial buds**
  - **Bronchial buds** are precursors of bilateral **main bronchi**
- **Lungs**
  - Sequential branching of primitive **bronchi**
  - Formation of distinct pulmonary **lobes**
  - Formation of distinct pulmonary **segments**
- **Distal airways** and **lung parenchyma**
  - Interaction of **endodermal** and **mesodermal** elements allow normal lung development
  - Continued **branching** of primitive airways
  - Progressive **vascularization** of surrounding mesenchyme
  - Development of **alveolar-capillary interface**
  - Postnatal airway development and maturation

Concurrent Developmental Processes
- Pleural and diaphragmatic development
  - Developing lungs protrude into coelomic cavity
  - Separation of pleural and pericardial cavities
  - Diaphragmatic development
  - Pleural investment of lungs within bilateral hemithoraces
- Vascular development
  - Pulmonary arterial development along developing airways
  - Vasculogenesis within primitive mesenchyme to form **capillary network**
  - Pulmonary vein and lymphatic development along segmental boundaries

Developmental Stages
- **Embryonic stage**
- **Pseudoglandular stage**
- **Canalicular stage**
- **Saccular stage**
- **Alveolar stage**

Embryonic Stage (26 Days-6 Weeks)

Laryngotracheal Groove
- Develops **26-28 days** after fertilization
- Arises caudal to primitive pharynx and fourth pair of pharyngeal pouches
- Longitudinal growth
- **Endodermal** derived structures
  - Tracheobronchial and pulmonary epithelium
  - Tracheobronchial glands
- **Mesodermal** derived structures
  - Tracheobronchial cartilage
  - Tracheobronchial connective tissue
  - Tracheobronchial smooth muscle

Respiratory Diverticulum or Lung Bud
- Develops **four weeks** after fertilization
- Pouch-like outgrowth from caudal aspect of **laryngotracheal groove**
- Caudal growth
- Invested in mesodermal derived splanchnic mesenchyme

Tracheal Bud
- Globular enlargement of distal lung bud
- Caudal growth from primordial pharynx
- Proximal communication with foregut through primordial laryngeal inlet

Tracheoesophageal Septum
- Longitudinal **tracheoesophageal folds** form on either side of developing tracheal bud
- Medial growth of bilateral tracheoesophageal folds
- Formation of **tracheoesophageal septum** from midline fusion of **tracheoesophageal folds**
- Separation of primitive trachea from developing esophagus

Primary Bronchial Buds and Branches
- Branching of primitive tracheal bud into right and left branches (**fifth week** after fertilization)
  - **Right bronchial bud:** Larger and vertically oriented
  - **Left bronchial bud:** Smaller and horizontally oriented
- Branching of primary bronchial buds into two **primitive lobar bronchi**
  - **Right superior lobar bronchus:** Right upper lobe bronchus
  - **Right inferior lobar bronchus:** Primitive bronchus intermedius
    - Right middle lobe bronchus
    - Right lower lobe bronchus
  - **Left superior lobar bronchus:** Left upper lobe bronchus
  - **Left inferior lobar bronchus:** Left lower lobe bronchus
- Branching of primitive lobar bronchi into primitive segmental bronchi

Pseudoglandular Stage (6-16 Weeks)

Microscopic Morphology
- Gland-like appearance of lung
- Formation of tracheobronchial cartilages, mucus glands and cilia by **thirteen weeks** after fertilization
- Primitive airways lined by **endodermal derived columnar epithelium**
- Primitive airways surrounded by **mesodermal derived mesenchymal tissue**
- Absent alveolar-capillary interface

Important Events
- Formation of all major airway elements
  - Bronchial development complete to level of terminal bronchioles

LUNG DEVELOPMENT

- All bronchopulmonary segments formed by **seven weeks** after fertilization

Physiologic Implications
- Respiration not possible
- No possibility of extrauterine survival

Canalicular Stage (16-28 Weeks)

Microscopic Morphology
- Continued enlargement of primitive airway lumens
- Continued thinning of airway epithelium
- Epithelial differentiation into **type 1 and type 2 cells**
- Airways separated by reduced but significant mesenchymal tissue

Important Events
- Continued vascularization of lung
- Continued development of primitive airways
  - **Terminal bronchioles** give rise to two or more **respiratory bronchioles**
  - **Respiratory bronchioles** give rise to 3-6 **alveolar ducts**
  - Development of a small number of **terminal saccules**
- Lamellar inclusions within **type 2 pneumocytes** in terminal saccules with potential for surfactant production

Physiologic Implications
- Limited surfactant production
- Respiration is possible in late canalicular stage
- Possibility of neonatal survival with intensive care and appropriate life support

Saccular Stage (28-36 Weeks)

Microscopic Morphology
- Continued airway differentiation
- Continued thinning of airway epithelium
- Some capillaries abut and bulge into developing alveoli
- Terminal sacs begin to approach the morphology of adult alveoli

Important Events
- Development of increasing numbers of **terminal saccules**
- Establishment of **primitive alveolar-capillary interface**
- Increased potential for **surfactant production**

Physiologic Implications
- Respiration with adequate gas exchange is possible
- Survival of premature neonates with appropriate life support

Alveolar Stage (36 Weeks-8 Years)

Microscopic Morphology
- Continued thinning of epithelial lining of terminal sacs

- Formation of **primordial alveoli**
- Adjacent capillaries bulge into terminal saccules

Important Events
- Continued development of distal airways with primordial alveoli forming along respiratory bronchioles and terminal saccules
- Development of **thin alveolar-capillary membrane**

Physiologic Implications
- Presence of nearly mature alveolar-capillary interface
- Adequate surfactant production
- Respiration possible without external support

Important Factors for Normal Prenatal Lung Development

Volume Requirements
- Adequate **intrathoracic volume** required for normal pulmonary development
- Factors predisposing to **pulmonary hypoplasia**
  - **Intrathoracic masses** and lesions producing mass effect
    - **Pleural effusion**
    - **Space occupying thoracic congenital anomalies**
  - **Thoracic wall** abnormalities
  - **Extrathoracic masses** and lesions producing mass effect
    - **Abdominal masses**
    - **Ascites**
  - **Intrauterine volume reduction**
    - **Oligohydramnios**

Circulatory Requirements
- Circulation affects pulmonary development
- Abnormal circulation may result in pulmonary hypoplasia

Neonatal Lung

Clearance of Retained Fluid
- External clearance
  - Mouth
  - Nasal cavity
- Internal clearance
  - Lymphatics
  - Capillaries

First Breath
- Diaphragmatic contraction
- Role of **surfactant**
  - Alveolar expansion results in **surfactant discharge** by **type 2 pneumocytes**
  - Decreased surface tension of remaining intra-alveolar fluid
  - Increased surfactant activity with decreased surface area
  - **Prevention of alveolar collapse** during expiration
- Pulmonary vascular changes
  - Fluid-filled lungs result in high resistance of pulmonary circulation

LUNG DEVELOPMENT

- Small portion of cardiac output goes to lungs prior to birth
  - Pulmonary expansion with first breath
    - Vascular vasodilatation
    - Increased pulmonary blood flow

Postnatal Lung Development
- **Twenty four million terminal sacs and alveoli present at birth** compared to **three hundred million in adult lungs**
- Five-fold increase of alveolar numbers within first year of life
- Formation of 95% of adult alveoli by 8 years of age

Disorders of Lung Immaturity

Transient Tachypnea of Newborn
- Also known as **retained fetal lung fluid**
- Neonatal respiratory distress in **term** or **pre-term infants**
- Imaging
  - Normal volume
  - Small pleural effusions
  - Increased interstitial opacities
  - Resolution within one or two days

Respiratory Distress Syndrome
- Impaired capacity of **type 2 pneumocytes** to replenish **surfactant** prior to 36 weeks of gestation
- Symptoms occur shortly after birth in premature infants
- Imaging
  - Low lung volumes
  - Opaque lung parenchyma with air bronchograms
  - Volume loss related to surfactant insufficiency
- Treatment
  - Prenatal steroids to accelerate lung maturation
  - Mechanical ventilatory support
  - Surfactant administration
  - Nitric oxide gas

Disorders Related to Tracheobronchial Morphology

Central Tracheobronchial Tree
- Horizontal course of left main bronchus
- Vertical course of right main bronchus
- Propensity for **aspiration** into right side
  - Oral secretions
  - Ingested material
  - **Foreign bodies**

Developmental Disorders

Abnormal Tracheo-Esophageal Development
- **Tracheal aplasia/agenesis**
  - **Abnormal course** and **anomalous ventral location** of **tracheoesophageal folds** in early embryonic development

- Interruption of proximal tracheal lumen
  - Foregut derived bronchi may communicate with each other or arise directly from esophagus
- **Esophageal atresia** and **tracheoesophageal fistula**
  - **Abnormal course** and **anomalous dorsal location** of **tracheoesophageal folds** in early embryonic development
    - Interruption of primitive proximal esophagus
  - Tracheoesophageal fistula with communication between distal trachea and distal esophageal segment
- **Tracheoesophageal fistula**
  - **Failure of complete midline fusion** of tracheoesophageal folds
  - Abnormal communication between proximal trachea and esophagus

Abnormalities of Foregut Budding
- **Extralobar sequestration**
  - **Supernumerary foregut bud** induces primitive mesenchyme to form lung parenchyma
    - Supernumerary lung tissue (sequestration) develops in thorax, diaphragm or abdomen
    - No communication with normal tracheobronchial tree
  - Neonatal respiratory distress from mass effect and/or pulmonary hypoplasia
  - Imaging
    - Homogeneous soft tissue mass typically located in left hemithorax
    - Systemic arterial supply
- **Bronchogenic cyst**
  - **Supernumerary or anomalous foregut bud** that does not induce development of lung parenchyma
    - **Middle mediastinal mass** in **subcarinal** location
    - **Unilocular thin-walled cyst**
  - Symptomatic or asymptomatic older children and young adults
  - Imaging
    - Subcarinal middle mediastinal spherical mass
    - Thin-walled cystic lesion with fluid characteristics
    - May exhibit soft tissue characteristics because of character of fluid content

Abnormalities of Distal Airway Development
- **Bronchial atresia**
  - **Focal in-utero vascular compromise** of portion of distal bronchial wall
    - Focal bronchial atresia
    - Near normal distal airway development
  - Asymptomatic adults
  - Imaging
    - Round, tubular or branching opacity representing mucocele distal to atretic airway
    - Surrounding hyperlucent lung

LUNG DEVELOPMENT

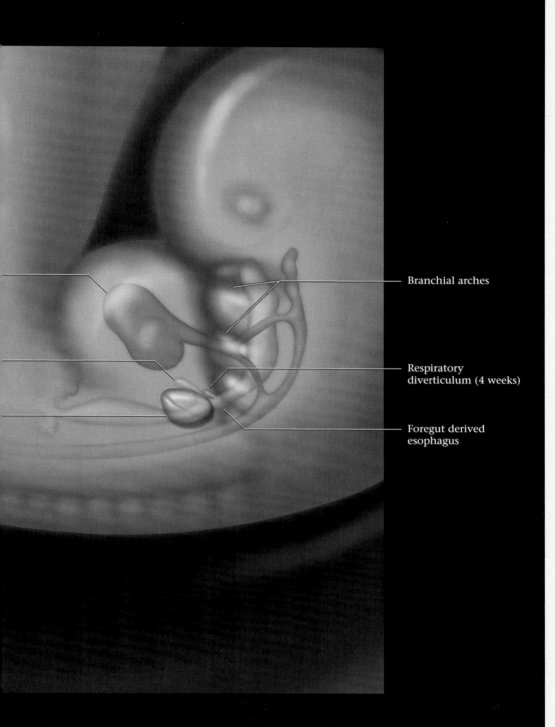

Branchial arches

Respiratory diverticulum (4 weeks)

Foregut derived esophagus

opment of the primitive lung. The respiratory diverticulum arises from the laryngotracheal
al esophagus caudal to the 4th pharyngeal pouches. The sequential evolution of the
to the tracheal bud and the primitive lung is shown. Note the close relationship of the
hial tree and lungs to the primitive esophagus.

LUNG DEVELOPMENT

EMBRYONIC STAGE

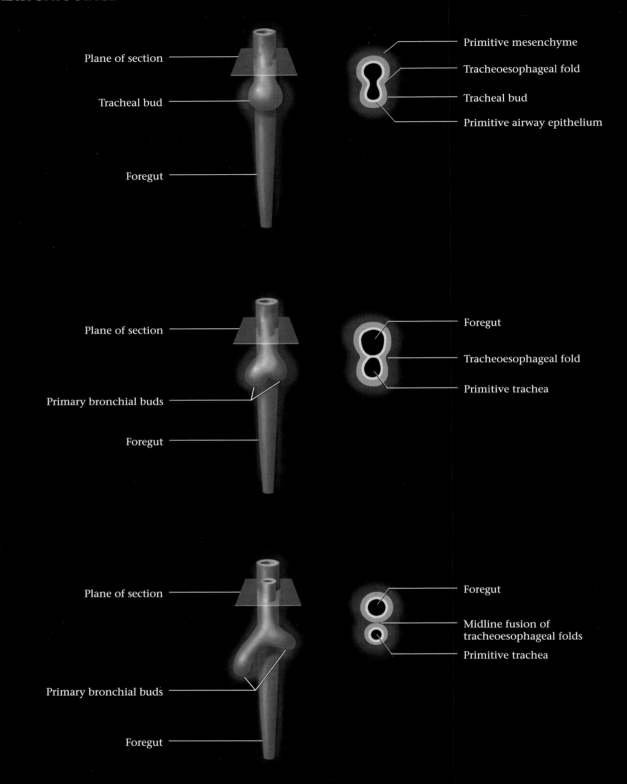

Plane of section

Tracheal bud

Foregut

Primitive mesenchyme

Tracheoesophageal fold

Tracheal bud

Primitive airway epithelium

Plane of section

Primary bronchial buds

Foregut

Foregut

Tracheoesophageal fold

Primitive trachea

Plane of section

Primary bronchial buds

Foregut

Foregut

Midline fusion of tracheoesophageal folds

Primitive trachea

(Top) Graphic shows the tracheal bud, a ventral outpouching of the foregut surrounded by mesodermal derived mesenchyme and lined by endodermal derived epithelium. The axial plane of section (right) shows communication between the tracheal bud and the foregut. The formation of bilateral longitudinal tracheoesophageal folds is shown. (Middle) Graphic shows early branching of the tracheal bud into primary bronchial buds which will form the right and left main bronchi. The longitudinal tracheoesophageal folds (right) continue to migrate medially to fuse in the midline. (Bottom) Graphic shows further vertical development of the primary bronchial buds. Note that the right bronchial bud is vertically oriented and the left follows a more horizontal course. The tracheoesophageal folds fuse in the midline to separate the trachea from the esophagus.

LUNG DEVELOPMENT

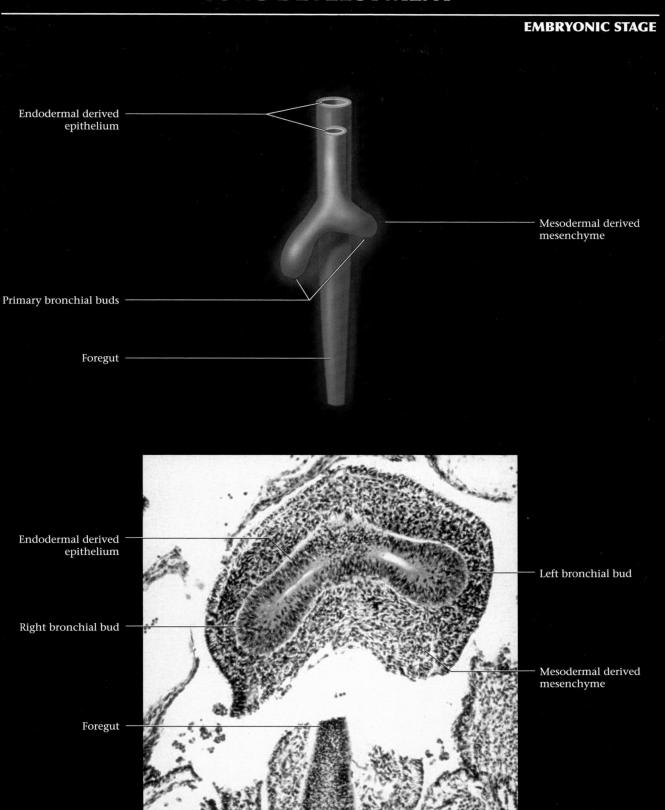

Endodermal derived epithelium

Mesodermal derived mesenchyme

Primary bronchial buds

Foregut

Endodermal derived epithelium

Left bronchial bud

Right bronchial bud

Mesodermal derived mesenchyme

Foregut

(Top) Graphic shows the development and morphology of the bronchial buds as they invaginate into the primitive mesenchyme. The bronchial buds are the precursors of the main bronchi and determine their anatomic orientation in adulthood. **(Bottom)** Photomicrograph (Hematoxylin and Eosin stain) of a coronal section through the primitive thorax of a 4 mm embryo shows the bronchial buds invaginating into the surrounding mesenchyme. The foregut is located dorsal to the plane of section. Note that the right bronchial bud is larger and courses in a more vertical direction than the left bronchial bud. These structures are the precursors of the central tracheobronchial tree. (Courtesy J. Thomas Stocker, MD, Uniformed Services University of the Health Sciences, Bethesda, MD).

LUNG DEVELOPMENT

EMBRYONIC & PSEUDOGLANDULAR STAGES

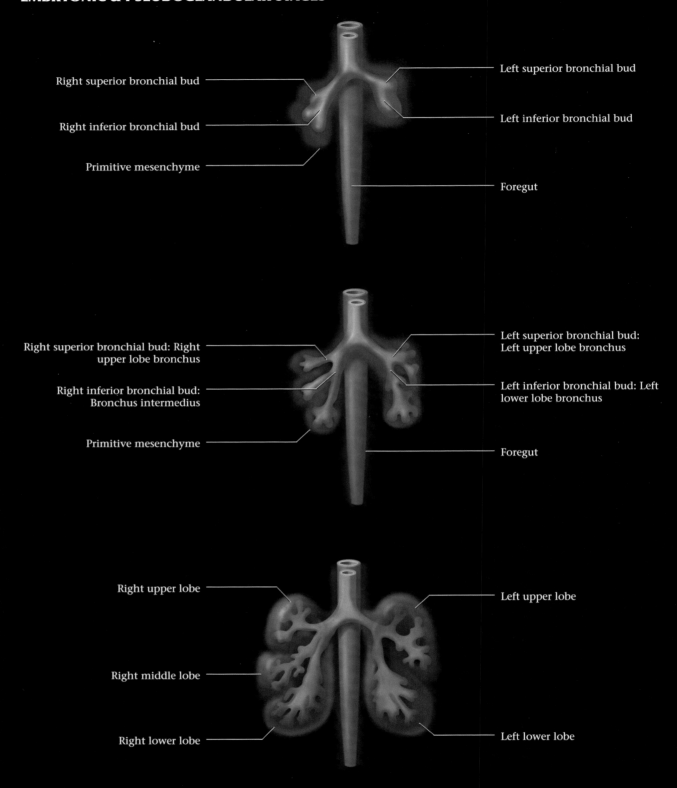

Right superior bronchial bud

Right inferior bronchial bud

Primitive mesenchyme

Left superior bronchial bud

Left inferior bronchial bud

Foregut

Right superior bronchial bud: Right upper lobe bronchus

Right inferior bronchial bud: Bronchus intermedius

Primitive mesenchyme

Left superior bronchial bud: Left upper lobe bronchus

Left inferior bronchial bud: Left lower lobe bronchus

Foregut

Right upper lobe

Right middle lobe

Right lower lobe

Left upper lobe

Left lower lobe

(Top) Graphic shows the developing tracheobronchial tree at 28 days of gestation. The right and left bronchial buds begin to divide into right and left superior and inferior bronchial buds. The developing tracheobronchial tree is surrounded by primitive mesenchyme. **(Middle)** Graphic shows developing tracheobronchial tree at 42 days of gestation with continued elongation and branching of the bronchial buds to form rudimentary lobar bronchi. Further growth and branching of the distal primitive airway forms rudimentary segmental bronchi. The rudimentary bronchus intermedius gives rise to primitive right middle and right lower lobe bronchi. **(Bottom)** Graphic shows tracheobronchial development at 56 days of gestation with continued branching of the primitive airways. The primitive mesenchyme surrounds the developing airways forming rudimentary lung lobes.

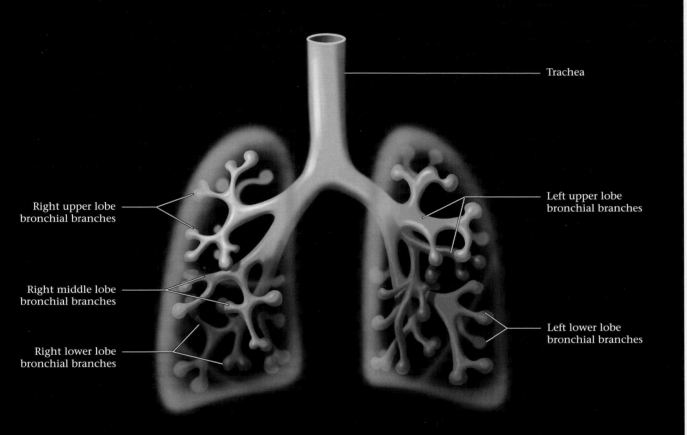

Trachea

Right upper lobe
bronchial branches

Right middle lobe
bronchial branches

Right lower lobe
bronchial branches

Left upper lobe
bronchial branches

Left lower lobe
bronchial branches

Graphic shows tracheobronchial development at approximately 10 weeks of gestation. Note airway differentiation into rudimentary lobar bronchial branches (shown in different colors) and segmental bronchial branches. Note that the green and red bronchial branches represent different portions of the primitive left upper lobe. Recognizable lung lobes are present. By the end of the pseudoglandular stage of lung development all major elements of the airways are formed. The interaction between the primitive tracheobronchial tree and the surrounding primitive mesenchyme induces the development of lung parenchyma.

LUNG DEVELOPMENT

PSEUDOGLANDULAR & CANALICULAR STAGES

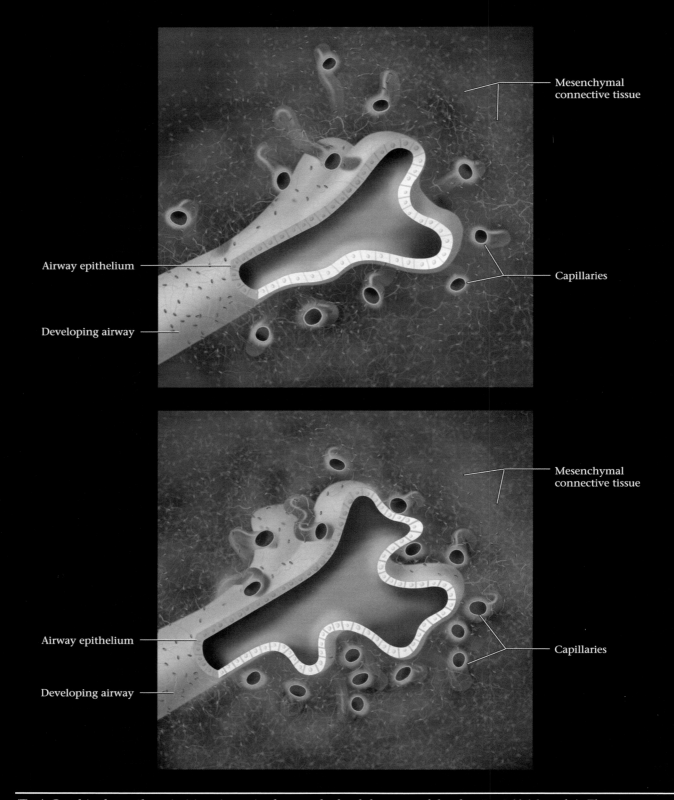

Mesenchymal
connective tissue

Airway epithelium

Developing airway

Capillaries

Mesenchymal
connective tissue

Airway epithelium

Developing airway

Capillaries

(Top) Graphic shows the primitive airway in the pseudoglandular stage of development (6-16 weeks). The airways are blind ending tubules. There is no alveolar-capillary interface as connective tissue separates the thick-walled primitive airway from the pulmonary capillaries. Respiration is not possible. **(Bottom)** Graphic shows the primitive airway in the canalicular stage of development (16-28 weeks). The airway lumen has enlarged and the airway epithelium has thinned. There is an increased number of vessels within the primitive mesenchyme and some of the vessels abut the airway wall. Respiration is possible at the end of this stage of lung development, but these infants require intensive care and support for survival.

LUNG DEVELOPMENT

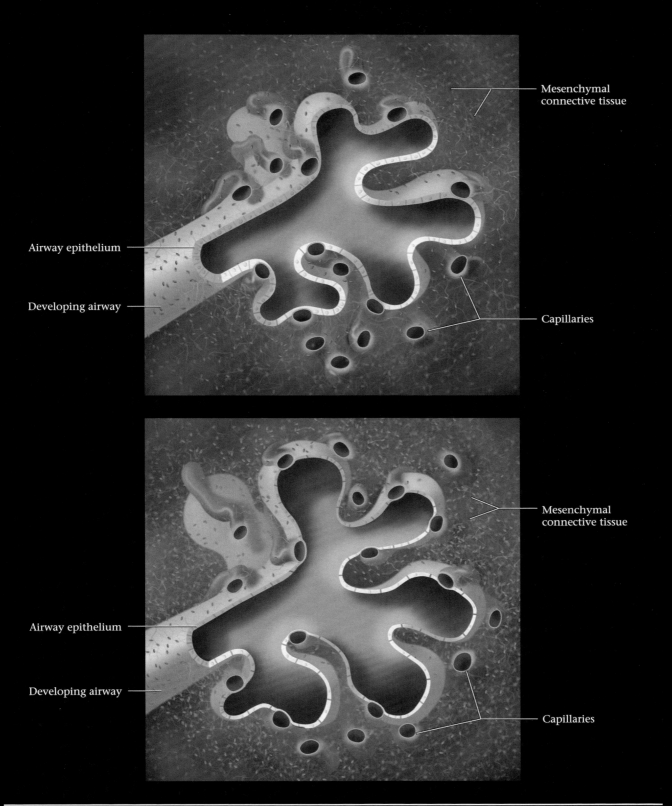

Mesenchymal connective tissue

Airway epithelium

Developing airway

Capillaries

Mesenchymal connective tissue

Airway epithelium

Developing airway

Capillaries

(Top) Graphic shows the developing airway in the saccular stage of lung development (28-36 weeks). The airway lumen continues to enlarge. The lining epithelium continues to thin. More numerous capillaries abut the wall of the primitive airway and some bulge into the airway lumen. The alveolar-capillary interface continues to mature. Respiration is possible and many infants born at this stage of pulmonary development survive with proper medical management and support. **(Bottom)** Graphic shows the developing airway in the alveolar stage of pulmonary development (36 weeks-8 years). The airway lumen continues to enlarge and there is less surrounding connective tissue. The airway epithelium is thin and many capillaries bulge into the airway lumen establishing mature alveolar-capillary interfaces. Airway development continues after birth and into childhood.

PSEUDOGLANDULAR AND CANALICULAR STAGES

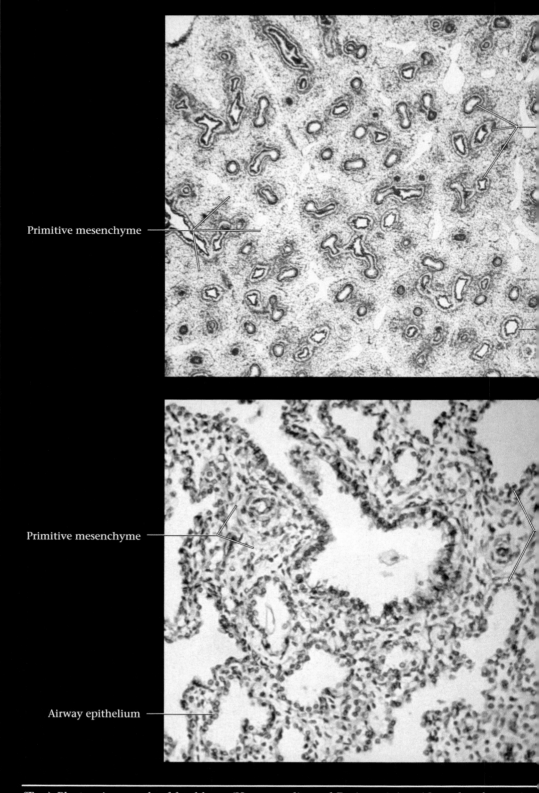

Primitive mesenchyme

Primitive mesenchyme

Airway epithelium

(Top) Photomicrograph of fetal lung (Hematoxylin and Eosin stain) at 10 weeks of gestation stage of lung development shows the gland-like microscopic morphology of the lung. The p lined by columnar epithelium and separated by a significant quantity of primitive mesench Stocker, MD, Uniformed Services University of the Health Sciences, Bethesda, MD). **(Bottom** fetal lung (Hematoxylin and Eosin stain) at 24 weeks of gestation in the canalicular stage of the enlarging airway lumens. Some of the airway epithelium has thinned and there is less in mesenchyme. (Courtesy I. Thomas Stocker, MD, Uniformed Services University of the Healt

Alveoli

Alveolar-capillary interface

Capillary network

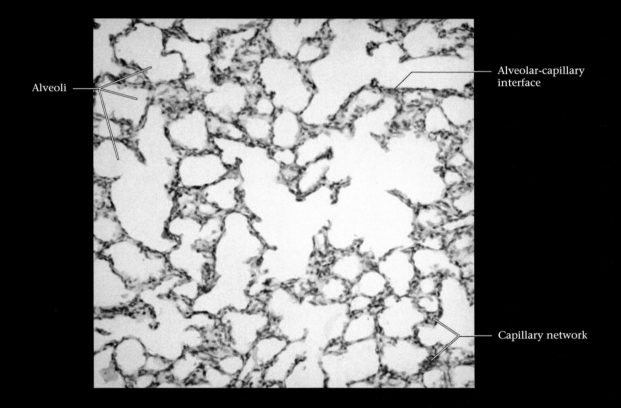

Photomicrograph (Hematoxylin and Eosin stain) of normal lung at 38 weeks of gestation in the alveolar stage of lung development demonstrates formation of adult-like alveoli and alveolar-capillary interfaces that allow the process of respiration. (Courtesy J. Thomas Stocker, MD, Uniformed Services University of the Health Sciences, Bethesda, MD).

LUNG DEVELOPMENT

NORMAL NEONATAL LUNG

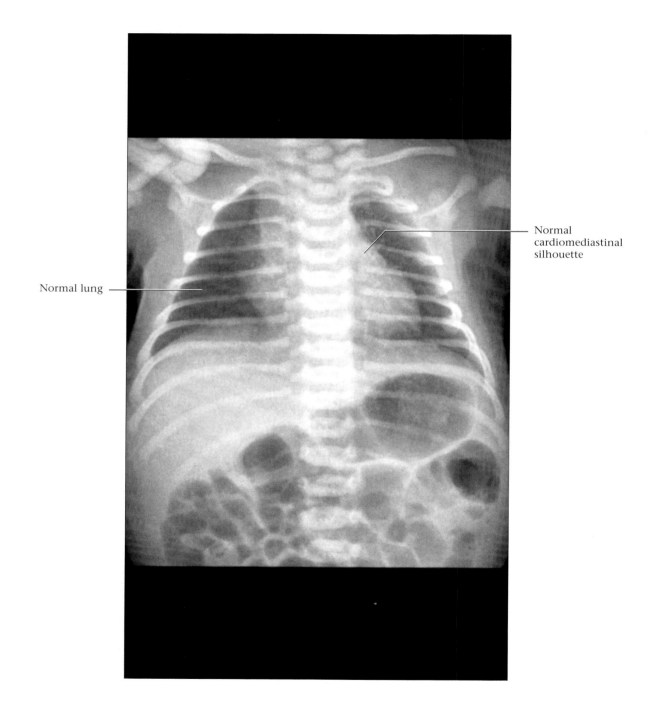

Normal lung

Normal
cardiomediastinal
silhouette

Asymptomatic term infant imaged shortly after birth for evaluation of a holosystolic murmur. AP chest radiograph shows normal lung volumes and a normal cardiomediastinal silhouette. The patient was diagnosed with mild aortic stenosis.

LUNG DEVELOPMENT

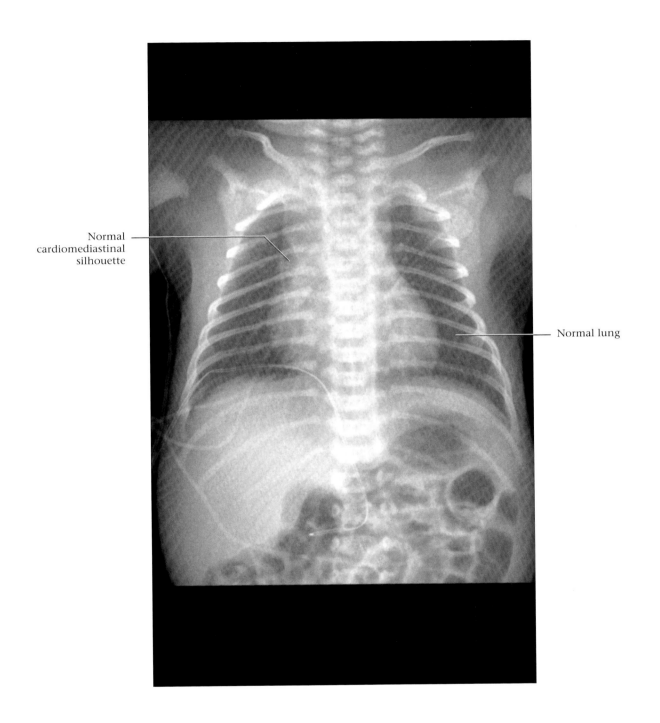

Normal
cardiomediastinal
silhouette

Normal lung

Mildly symptomatic premature infant born at 33 weeks of gestation. AP chest radiograph shows normal lung volumes and a normal cardiomediastinal silhouette. The patient responded to conservative management and required no further imaging.

LUNG DEVELOPMENT

IMMATURE LUNG, TRANSIENT TACHYPNEA OF NEWBORN

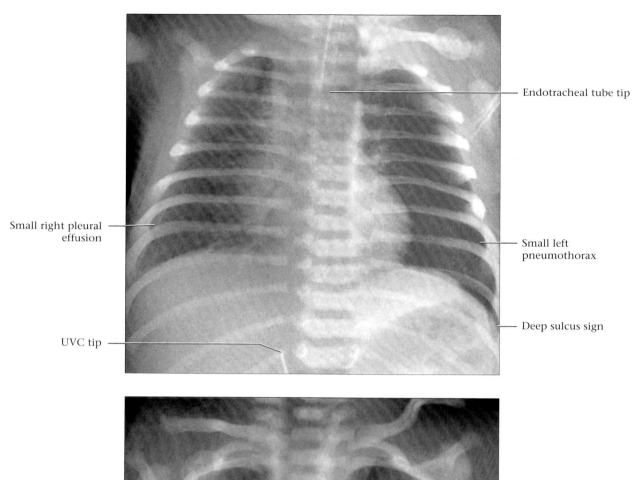

Endotracheal tube tip

Small right pleural effusion

Small left pneumothorax

Deep sulcus sign

UVC tip

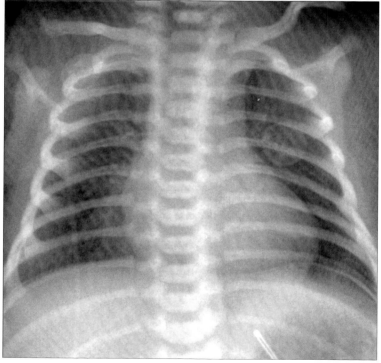

(Top) First of two radiographs of a term infant with retained fetal fluid who presented with tachypnea and respiratory distress at birth. AP chest radiograph shows coarse linear opacities in the perihilar regions and a small right pleural effusion. A small left pneumothorax manifests with a subtle pleural line and a deep sulcus sign. The endotracheal tube is appropriately positioned. The tip of the umbilical vein catheter (UVC) is visualized. (Bottom) AP chest radiograph obtained 48 hours later shows that the patient has been extubated. The lungs are clear and have normal volume. The pleural effusion and pneumothorax have resolved. The findings are consistent with retained fetal fluid or transient tachypnea of the newborn. While the etiology of this condition is not completely understood, lung immaturity is thought to play a role in its pathogenesis.

LUNG DEVELOPMENT

IMMATURE LUNG, RESPIRATORY DISTRESS SYNDROME

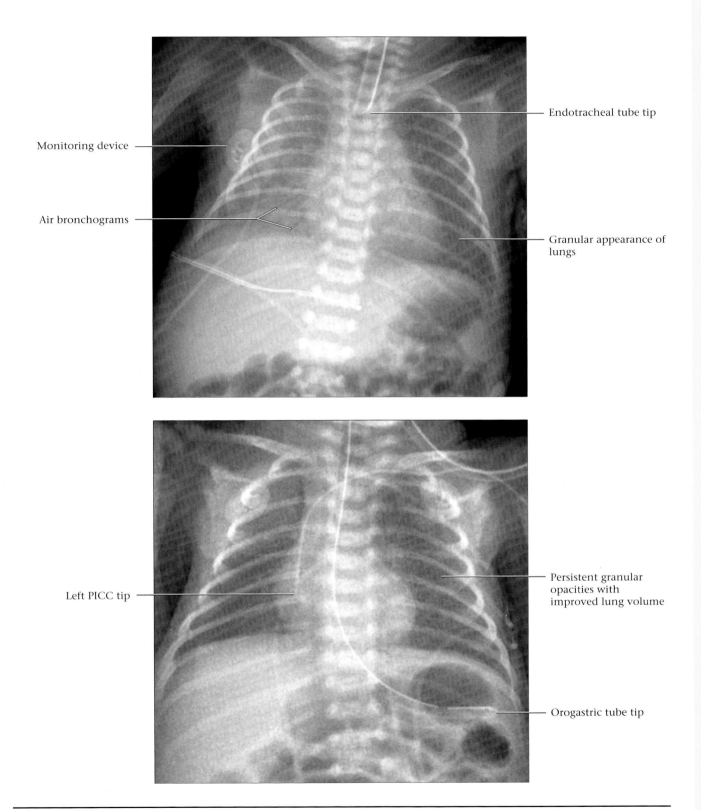

Monitoring device

Air bronchograms

Endotracheal tube tip

Granular appearance of lungs

Left PICC tip

Persistent granular opacities with improved lung volume

Orogastric tube tip

(Top) First of two portable chest radiographs of a pre-term infant born at 26 weeks of gestation who developed respiratory distress syndrome. AP chest radiograph shows a granular appearance of the lungs and air bronchograms. The pulmonary opacities result from a combination of atelectasis and retained fluid. There is no pleural effusion. The endotracheal tube is appropriately positioned. **(Bottom)** AP chest radiograph at ten days of age shows that the patient has been extubated. The lung volumes have improved with residual granular appearance. An orogastric tube and a peripherally inserted central catheter (PICC) are noted. Approximately 60-80% of pre-term infants born before 28 weeks of gestation develop respiratory distress syndrome.

LUNG DEVELOPMENT

MORPHOLOGY & ORIENTATION OF MAIN BRONCHI

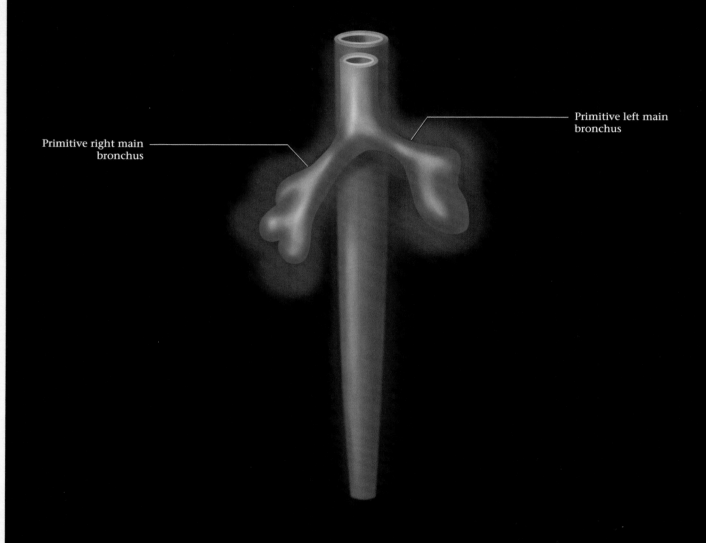

Primitive right main bronchus

Primitive left main bronchus

Graphic shows the morphology and orientation of the central airways at 28 days of gestation. Note that the primordial right main bronchus is more vertically oriented and larger than the left. As a result, the right lung is more susceptible to aspiration of foreign bodies and secretions.

LUNG DEVELOPMENT

BRONCHIAL ORIENTATION, ASPIRATED MOLAR IN THE BRONCHUS INTERMEDIUS

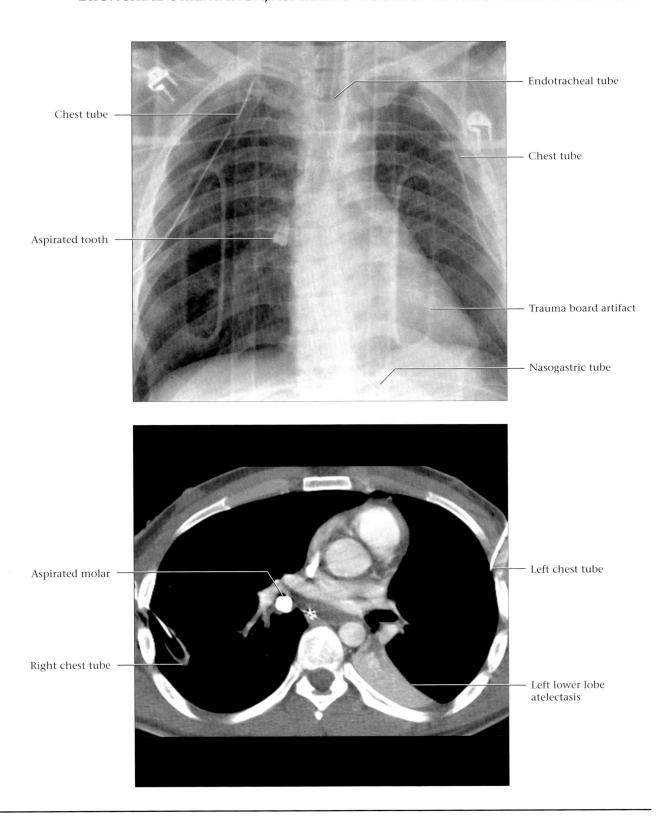

(Top) First of two images of a patient who was involved in a motor vehicle collision and aspirated a dislodged molar. AP portable chest radiograph demonstrates a molar within the bronchus intermedius. Note bilateral chest tubes, appropriately positioned life support devices and trauma board artifacts. The vertical orientation of the right main bronchus makes it susceptible to aspiration of foreign bodies and secretions. (Bottom) Contrast-enhanced chest CT (mediastinal window) demonstrates a dense round calcification in the lumen of the bronchus intermedius representing the aspirated molar. Bilateral chest tubes and a nasogastric tube are also present. Note atelectasis of the left lower lobe. (Courtesy Diane C. Strollo, MD, University of Pittsburgh, Pittsburgh, PA).

LUNG DEVELOPMENT

EMBRYONIC STAGE, EXTRALOBAR SEQUESTRATION

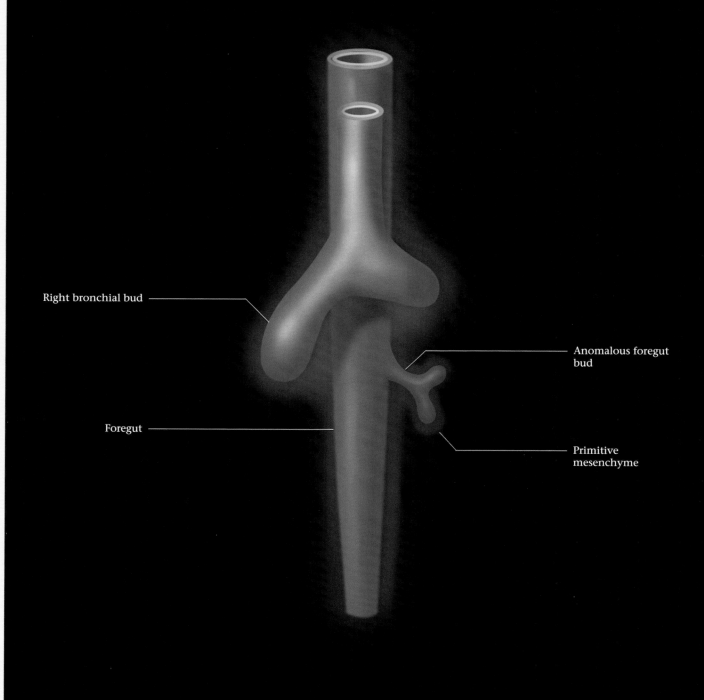

Right bronchial bud

Anomalous foregut bud

Foregut

Primitive mesenchyme

Graphic shows the proposed pathogenesis of extralobar sequestration. An anomalous supernumerary bud from the primitive foregut comes in contact with the surrounding primitive mesenchyme and induces the development of lung parenchyma. In most cases of extralobar sequestration the original connection with the foregut involutes resulting in "sequestered" but otherwise normal lung tissue that has a systemic blood supply.

LUNG DEVELOPMENT

EMBRYONIC STAGE, EXTRALOBAR SEQUESTRATION

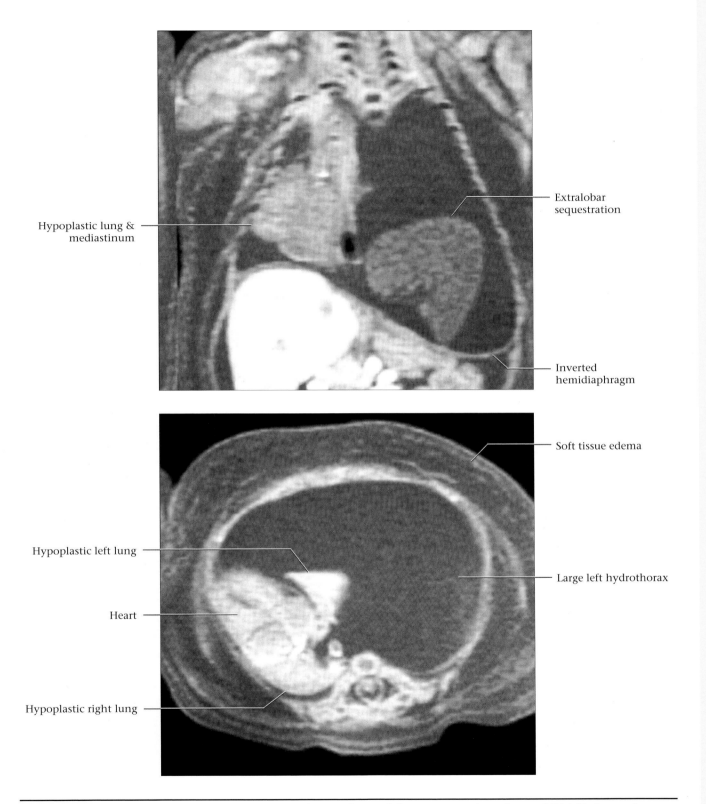

Hypoplastic lung & mediastinum

Extralobar sequestration

Inverted hemidiaphragm

Soft tissue edema

Hypoplastic left lung

Large left hydrothorax

Heart

Hypoplastic right lung

(Top) First of two post mortem MR images of an infant with extralobar sequestration. Coronal T1 MR shows the sequestered lung in the left hemithorax. A large left pleural effusion and a smaller right pleural effusion are also noted. There is severe pulmonary hypoplasia with most of the lung and the mediastinum located within the right hemithorax. Note inversion of the left hemidiaphragm by the large hydrothorax. Abdominal ascites and edema of the soft tissues of the chest wall are consistent with fetal hydrops. **(Bottom)** Axial T1 MR shows the large left hydrothorax and severe pulmonary hypoplasia. Severe soft tissue edema is again noted. Normal lung development requires adequate intrathoracic volume. In this case, mass effect from the large extralobar sequestration and hydrothorax interfered with normal lung development and resulted in pulmonary hypoplasia.

LUNG DEVELOPMENT

EMBRYONIC STAGE, BRONCHOGENIC CYST

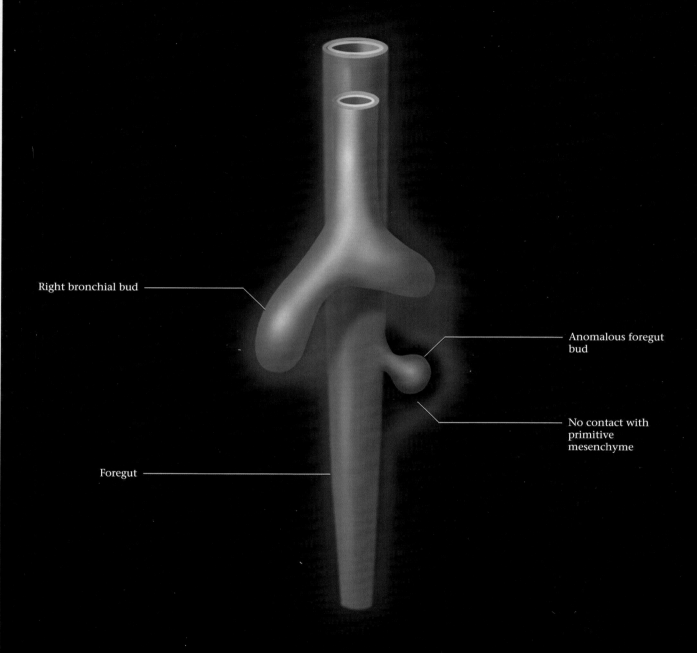

Right bronchial bud

Anomalous foregut bud

No contact with primitive mesenchyme

Foregut

Graphic shows the proposed pathogenesis of bronchogenic cyst. An anomalous supernumerary bud from the primitive foregut does not come in contact with the surrounding primitive mesenchyme and fails to induce the formation of lung parenchyma. The original communication with the foregut typically involutes resulting in a blind ending pouch or cyst. Because the anomalous bud develops in the same way as the primitive central airways, its wall contains bronchial components, hence the term "bronchogenic".

LUNG DEVELOPMENT

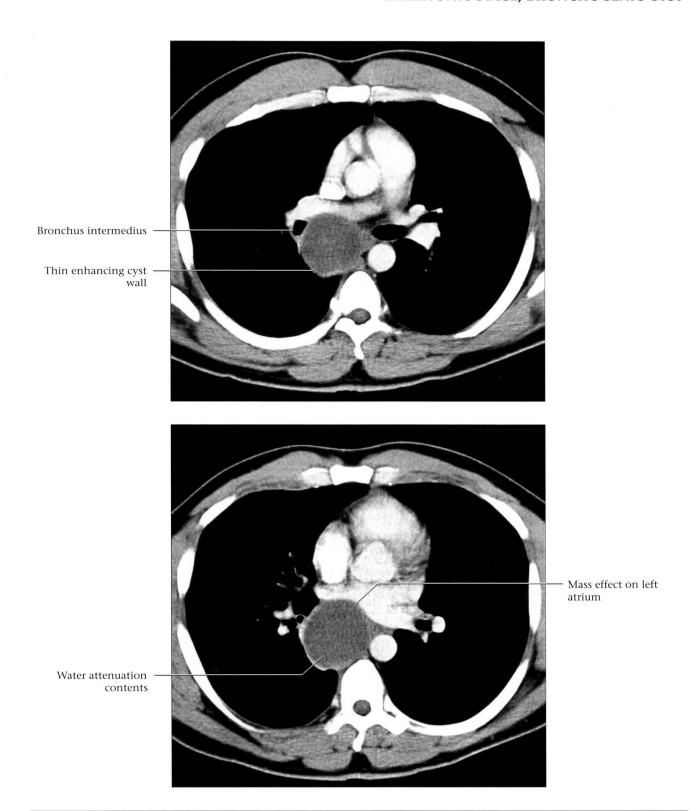

Bronchus intermedius

Thin enhancing cyst wall

Mass effect on left atrium

Water attenuation contents

(Top) First of two axial CT images of a young man with a middle mediastinal (subcarinal) bronchogenic cyst. Contrast-enhanced chest CT (mediastinal window) at the level of the carina demonstrates a thin-walled spherical cyst with water attenuation contents in the subcarinal region. The cyst produces mass effect on the right pulmonary artery and the bronchus intermedius. **(Bottom)** Contrast-enhanced chest CT (mediastinal window) at the level of the left atrium shows the spherical subcarinal cystic lesion with nonenhancing water attenuation contents and a thin enhancing wall. The lesion produces mass effect on the left atrium. The morphology and location of the lesion are characteristic of bronchogenic cyst.

LUNG DEVELOPMENT

PSEUDOGLANDULAR STAGE, BRONCHIAL ATRESIA

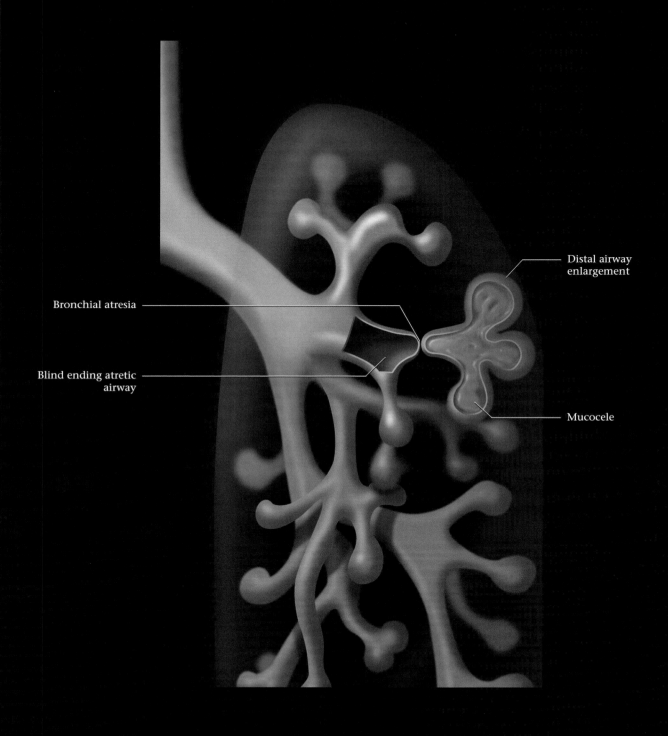

Bronchial atresia

Blind ending atretic airway

Distal airway enlargement

Mucocele

Graphic shows the proposed pathogenesis of bronchial atresia. This anomaly probably develops during the pseudoglandular stage of lung development when all the elements of the tracheobronchial tree are present and is thought to result from compromise of the blood supply to a small length of the airway wall. The atretic bronchus ends blindly at the point of atresia. The distal airway is not immediately affected but its secretions cannot be cleared. With time a mucus plug or mucocele develops and enlarges the airway lumen. After birth, air trapping occurs distally around the mucocele resulting in hyperlucent lung parenchyma.

LUNG DEVELOPMENT

PSEUDOGLANDULAR STAGE, BRONCHIAL ATRESIA

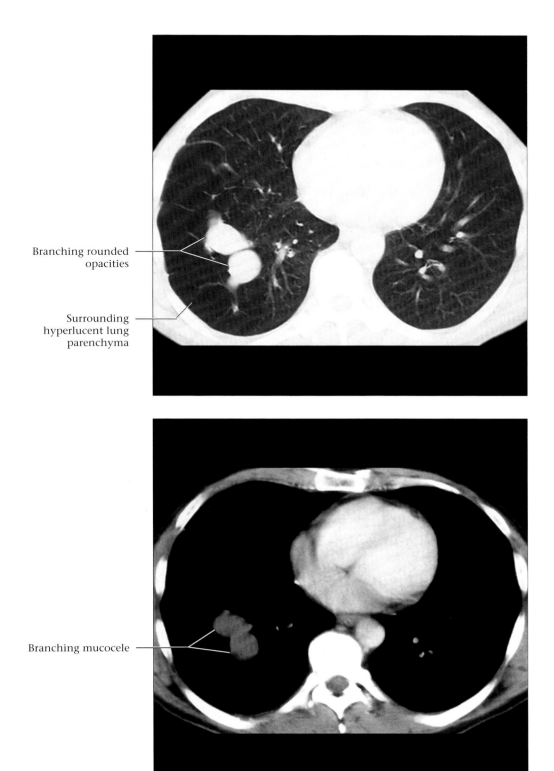

Branching rounded opacities

Surrounding hyperlucent lung parenchyma

Branching mucocele

(Top) First of two axial CT images of an asymptomatic young man with bronchial atresia. Contrast-enhanced chest CT (lung window) demonstrates branching rounded opacities located centrally in the right lower lobe and surrounded by hyperlucent lung parenchyma. Air distal to the bronchial atresia and around the mucocele is thought to reach the distal lung via collateral air drift. **(Bottom)** This image shows that the branching opacities exhibit intrinsic low attenuation and do not enhance with contrast. The branching opacities represent the mucocele that develops distal to the point of atresia. The findings are diagnostic of bronchial atresia.

AIRWAY STRUCTURE

General Anatomy and Function

Airways
- Tubular, pipe-like structures
- Conduct air through their lumens
- Anatomic components (proximal to distal)
  - Trachea
  - Bronchi
  - Bronchioles
  - Terminal bronchioles
  - Respiratory bronchioles
  - Alveolar ducts
  - Alveolar sacs
  - Alveoli

Airway Branches
- Airway generations
  - 23 generations of dichotomous branching beyond tracheal carina
  - 2-12 generations (typically 6-8) between terminal bronchioles and alveolar sacs
  - 4-29 (typically 10) alveoli per alveolar sac
- Airway types
  - **Bronchi**
    - Larger than 1 mm in diameter
    - Taper and branch
    - Give rise to non-cartilaginous bronchioles
  - **Bronchioles**
    - 1 mm or less in diameter
    - Most distal bronchiole lined by respiratory epithelium is terminal bronchiole
  - **Terminal bronchioles**
    - Most distal conducting airway
    - Give rise to approximately three generations of respiratory bronchioles
  - **Respiratory bronchioles**
    - Increasing numbers of alveoli extend from their walls
    - Give rise to three generations of alveolar ducts
  - **Alveolar ducts**
    - Series of alveoli adjacent to one another
    - Terminate in alveolar sacs
  - **Alveolar sacs**
    - Groups or clusters of most distal alveoli
  - **Alveoli**

Airway Function
- Air conduction through airway lumens
- Exchange of gas between inspired air and blood
  - Delivery of oxygen to alveoli
  - Delivery of carbon dioxide to atmosphere

Functional and Structural Airway Zones
- **Conducting zone**
  - Function
    - Air conduction only
  - Components
    - **Trachea**
    - **Bronchi**
    - **Bronchioles**
  - Branching pattern
    - **Dichotomous**: Parent airway divides into two
    - **Asymmetric**: Variable diameter
  - Structure
    - No alveoli in airway walls
    - No gas exchanging epithelium
- **Transitional zone**
  - Function
    - Air conduction
    - Respiration
  - Components
    - **Respiratory bronchioles**
    - **Alveolar ducts**
  - Branching pattern
    - **Dichotomous**
    - **Symmetric**
    - Frequently **trichotomous** or **quadrivial**
  - Structure
    - Airway walls contain alveoli
    - Enable gas exchange
- **Respiratory zone**
  - Function
    - Respiration only
    - Gas exchange
  - Components
    - **Alveoli**
    - **Alveolar sacs**
  - Branching pattern
    - Dichotomous
  - Structure
    - Thin walls
    - Contact with capillary membrane

Airway Structure

Trachea
- Connects larynx to main bronchi
- Microscopic anatomy
  - Epithelium
    - **Pseudostratified ciliated columnar epithelium**
    - **Goblet cells**
  - Submucosal structures
    - Submucosal seromucinous glands
  - Mural horseshoe-shaped incomplete **cartilage** rings (16-20)
  - Posterior membranous portion with transverse **smooth muscle bundles**
- Functional anatomy
  - **Cilia** propel mucus to laryngeal inlet
  - Submucosal **seromucinous glands** secrete water, electrolytes and mucin into airway lumen

Bronchi
- Connect trachea to muscular bronchioles
- Microscopic anatomy
  - Epithelium
    - **Pseudostratified ciliated columnar epithelium**
    - **Goblet cells**
  - Submucosal structures
    - **Seromucinous glands**
    - **Smooth muscle bundles**
  - Crescent-shaped masses of **cartilage**

Muscular Bronchioles
- Less than 1 mm in diameter
- Microscopic anatomy

AIRWAY STRUCTURE

- Epithelium
  - Pseudostratified ciliated columnar epithelium transitions to **ciliated cuboidal epithelium**
- Submucosal structures
  - Spirally arranged smooth muscle
  - Connective tissue
- Absence of cartilage

Terminal Bronchioles
- Last conducting bronchioles
- Thin walls, decreased diameter
- Microscopic anatomy
  - Lined with **ciliated columnar to cuboidal epithelium**
  - No goblet cells
  - Smooth muscle and connective tissue in walls

Respiratory Bronchioles
- Between terminal bronchioles and alveolar ducts
- Microscopic anatomy
  - Lined with ciliated simple cuboidal epithelium (non-ciliated in distal portions)
  - Smooth muscle and connective tissue in walls
  - Walls interrupted by delicate air pockets (alveoli)

Alveolar Ducts
- Between respiratory bronchioles and proximal alveoli/alveolar sacs
- Straight tubular spaces bounded entirely by alveoli
- Microscopic anatomy
  - Bands of smooth muscle in walls distinguish them from alveoli

Alveoli and Alveolar Sacs
- Small, cup-shaped structures
  - Outpouchings of respiratory bronchioles, alveolar ducts, alveolar sacs
  - Demarcated by thin walls (septa)
- Adult lungs contain approximately **300 million alveoli**
- Microscopic anatomy of alveolar septa
  - Continuous flattened squamous epithelium
    - **Type 1 epithelial cells** (squamous pneumocytes) cover 93% of alveolar surface
    - **Type 2 cells** (rounded nuclei) produce **surfactant**
  - Alveolar macrophages
    - Intra-alveolar migratory cells
    - Participate in lung defense mechanisms
  - Overlying capillaries
  - Intervening interstitial tissue

Fundamental Units of Lung Structure

Primary Pulmonary Lobule
- All alveolar ducts, alveolar sacs, and alveoli distal to the last respiratory bronchiole
  - Includes blood vessels, nerves and connective tissue
  - **20-25 million primary pulmonary lobules** in human lungs
- No clinical or imaging significance

Acinus
- Portion of lung distal to terminal bronchiole including

- Respiratory bronchioles
- Alveolar ducts
- Alveolar sacs
- Alveoli
- Accompanying vessels and connective tissue
- Pulmonary functional unit of gas exchange
- Acinar diameter of 6-10 mm
- 25,000 acini in a lung volume of 5.25 L

Secondary Pulmonary Lobule
- Smallest discrete unit of lung surrounded by connective tissue and interlobular septa
- Structure
  - Supplied by lobular bronchiole: A pre-terminal bronchiole that gives rise to
    - Smaller pre-terminal bronchioles
    - Terminal bronchioles
    - Respiratory bronchioles
  - Supplied by lobular artery and branches
  - Marginated by interlobular septa containing pulmonary veins and lymphatics
- Morphology
  - Irregularly polyhedral shape
  - 1.0-2.5 cm in diameter

Collateral Channels

Alveolar Pores (Pores of Kohn)
- Round or oval fenestrations
- Measure approximately 2-10 microns
- Allow communication between adjacent alveoli

Canals of Lambert
- Direct communication between alveoli and respiratory, terminal and pre-terminal bronchioles
- Function
  - May provide only intra-acinar accessory communication
  - May provide inter-acinar communication facilitating collateral ventilation

Imaging-Anatomic Correlations

Trachea
- Posterior wall configuration on CT indicates phase of respiration
  - Bows outward during suspended inspiration
  - Flattens and bows inward during expiration

Bronchi/Bronchioles
- Bronchi < 2 mm in diameter not normally visible on HRCT
- Bronchioles rarely visible within 1 cm of pleural surface on HRCT

Secondary Pulmonary Lobule
- Not generally visible in normal individuals
- Most developed and most apparent in lung periphery
- Interlobular septa at lower limits of thin-section CT resolution
  - Subpleural septa are approximately 0.1 mm thick

AIRWAY STRUCTURE

- ○ Most often seen in apices, anteriorly and near mediastinal pleura
- ○ Location may be inferred by identification of septal veins
- Lobular bronchioles at lower limits of thin-section CT resolution
  - ○ Not normally visible
  - ○ Lobular bronchiole measures approximately 1 mm in diameter
  - ○ Visibility correlates with wall thickness (0.15 mm)
  - ○ Location may be inferred by identification of centrilobular artery

Acinus
- Normal acini are not visible on imaging
- Experimental filling of a single acinus results in a rosette appearance and progresses to a spherical opacity
  - ○ Acinar/airspace nodule

Anatomic Distribution of Selected Diseases

Centrilobular Nodules: Infectious Bronchiolitis
- CT features
  - ○ Small nodules
    - ▪ Variable attenuation
    - ▪ Size range from a few mm to 1 cm
  - ○ Centrilobular location
    - ▪ Situated 5-10 mm from pleural surface
- Pathologic correlation
  - ○ **Inflammatory** (cellular) **bronchiolitis**
    - ▪ Inflammation/infiltration of centrilobular bronchioles
    - ▪ Involvement of surrounding interstitium and alveoli
  - ○ Etiologies: **Bacterial, mycobacterial, fungal** and **viral infections**

Tree-in-Bud Opacities: Small Airways Infection
- CT features
  - ○ Peripheral linear branching
  - ○ Associated centrilobular nodules
    - ▪ Variable attenuation
    - ▪ Clustering of nodules
    - ▪ Situated several mm from pleural surface
  - ○ Findings resemble the appearance of a **tree-in-bud**
- Pathologic correlation
  - ○ Small airways infection
  - ○ Dilated centrilobular bronchioles
    - ▪ Filling of bronchiolar lumens with inflammatory fluid/cells
  - ○ Peribronchiolar inflammation
  - ○ Etiologies: **Mycobacterial infection, bronchopneumonia, infectious bronchiolitis**

Centrilobular Low Attenuation: Centrilobular Emphysema
- CT features

- ○ Foci (3-10 mm) of centrilobular low attenuation
- ○ Low attenuation surrounding centrilobular artery
- ○ Imperceptible walls
- Pathologic correlation
  - ○ **Centrilobular (proximal acinar, centriacinar) emphysema**
    - ▪ Involves proximal acinus
    - ▪ Distention and destruction of respiratory bronchioles
    - ▪ Enlarged airspace in central acinus with relatively normal distal acinus
  - ○ Most severe involvement of upper lobes and superior segments of lower lobes

Lobular Low Attenuation: Panlobular Emphysema
- CT features
  - ○ Diffuse extensive areas of low attenuation
  - ○ Reduced size of pulmonary vessels
- Pathologic correlation
  - ○ **Panlobular (panacinar) emphysema**
    - ▪ Affects entire acinus and all acini in secondary pulmonary lobule
    - ▪ Diffuse or lower lobe predominance
    - ▪ Association with α-1-antitrypsin deficiency

Lobular Low Attenuation: Paraseptal Emphysema
- CT features
  - ○ Juxtapleural cystic areas near interlobular septa, large vessels and bronchi
  - ○ Frequent association with centrilobular emphysema
- Pathologic correlation
  - ○ Affects periphery of pulmonary acinus and subpleural secondary pulmonary lobules
  - ○ Enlarged alveolar ducts
  - ○ Predominant upper lobe involvement
  - ○ Association with **bullous disease**

Lobular Low Attenuation: Constrictive Bronchiolitis
- CT features
  - ○ Mosaic attenuation; mosaic perfusion
  - ○ Patchy distribution
  - ○ **Air-trapping** on expiratory CT
- Pathologic correlation
  - ○ Concentric narrowing of membranous bronchioles by fibrosis with resultant air flow obstruction
    - ▪ **Air-trapping**
    - ▪ **Mosaic attenuation/perfusion**

Acinar Nodules: Infection
- CT features
  - ○ 6-10 mm fluffy nodular opacities
- Pathologic correlation
  - ○ Inflammation of terminal and respiratory bronchioles
  - ○ Sparing of distal air spaces
  - ○ Airway dissemination of infection
    - ▪ **Tuberculosis**
    - ▪ Early **varicella pneumonia**

AIRWAY STRUCTURE

OVERVIEW OF AIRWAY STRUCTURE

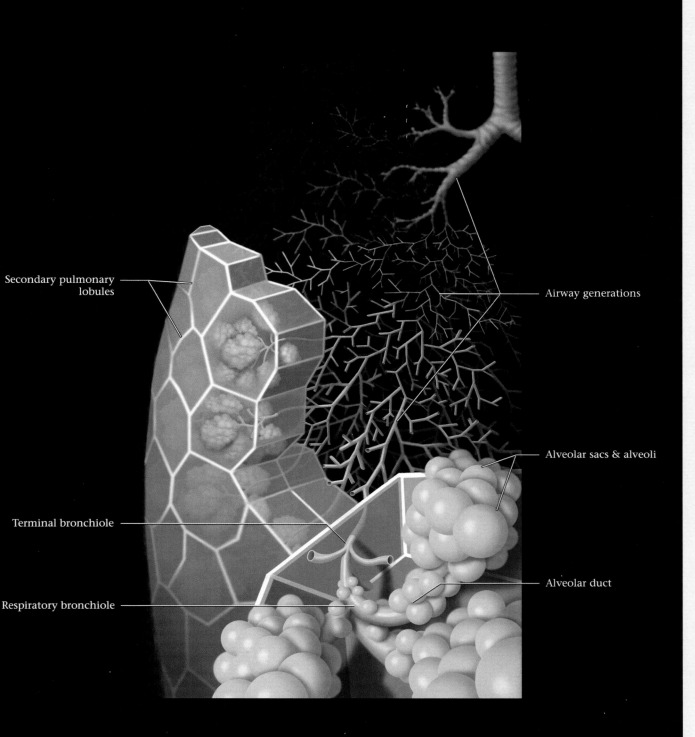

Secondary pulmonary lobules

Airway generations

Alveolar sacs & alveoli

Terminal bronchiole

Alveolar duct

Respiratory bronchiole

Graphic representation of 24 airway generations branching dichotomously from the trachea to the most distal airways that comprise the secondary pulmonary lobule (SPL). The SPL is the smallest unit of lung surrounded by connective tissue septa and has a polyhedral shape. Each SPL contains the distal branches of a lobular bronchiole and its accompanying pulmonary (lobular) artery. The acinus is comprised of the airways distal to a terminal bronchiole with each SPL containing twelve or fewer acini. The terminal bronchiole gives rise to two or three respiratory bronchioles which in turn give rise to three alveolar ducts each terminating in alveolar sacs and alveoli. The respiratory bronchiole is characterized by its alveolated wall. The alveolar duct wall is covered with alveoli. The alveolar sacs terminate in clustered alveoli.

AIRWAY STRUCTURE

BRONCHI, BRONCHIOLES & ACINI

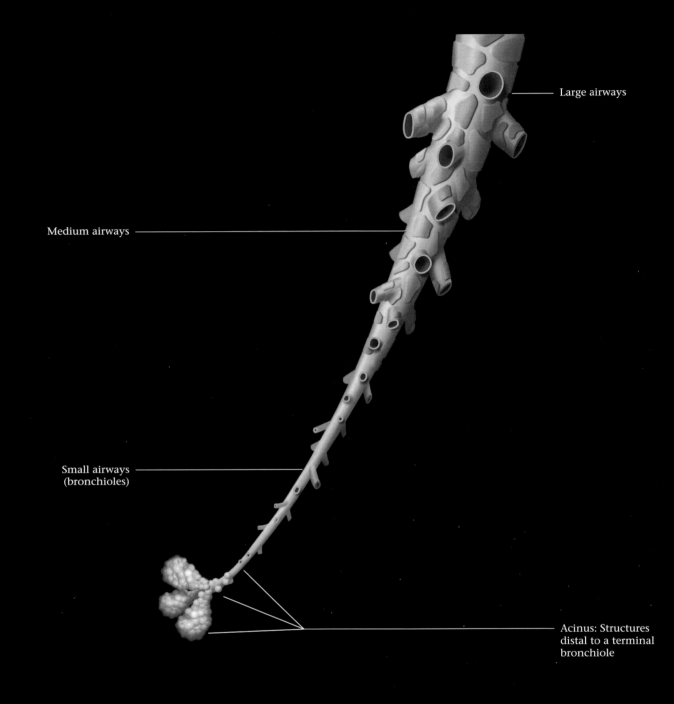

Large airways

Medium airways

Small airways
(bronchioles)

Acinus: Structures
distal to a terminal
bronchiole

Graphic telescoping depiction of an airway illustrating the decreasing size of the different airway types and the structural changes of the airway wall with a decreasing number and size of cartilage plates. Cartilage plates are present in large and medium-size airways but gradually become smaller and less numerous in the medium bronchi. The walls of small airways (bronchioles) do not contain cartilage. Distal clusters of alveoli and alveolar sacs form acini, the pulmonary functional unit of gas exchange. The acinus is defined as the airways, vessels and supporting structures distal to a terminal bronchiole.

AIRWAY STRUCTURE

MICROSCOPIC STRUCTURE OF THE TRACHEA, BRONCHI & BRONCHIOLES

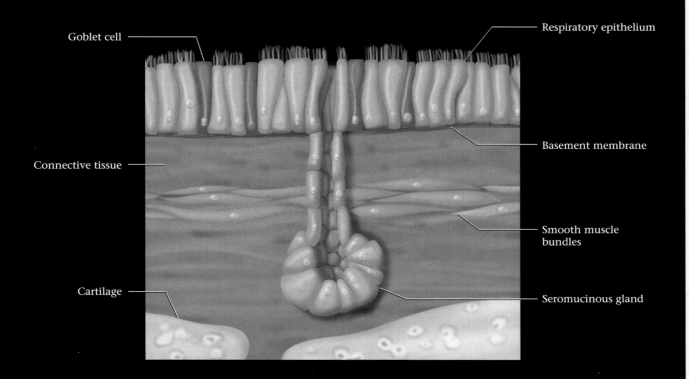

Goblet cell

Respiratory epithelium

Connective tissue

Basement membrane

Smooth muscle bundles

Cartilage

Seromucinous gland

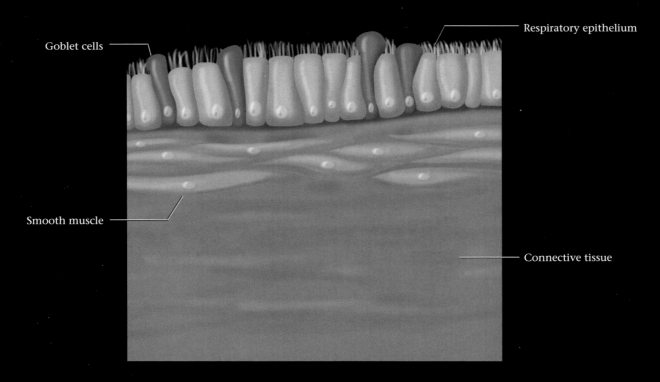

Respiratory epithelium

Goblet cells

Smooth muscle

Connective tissue

(Top) Graphic shows the microscopic structure of the large cartilaginous airways. These airways are lined by pseudostratified ciliated columnar (respiratory) epithelium that rests on a basement membrane. The cilia participate in the mucociliary escalator that pushes overlying mucin in a cephalad direction and provides clearance of secretions and particulate matter. Submucosal loose connective tissue beneath the basement membrane contains smooth muscle bundles and seromucinous glands. Cartilage plates are found beneath the submucosal layer. (Bottom) Graphic shows the microscopic structure of the bronchioles which are lined by respiratory epithelium. Goblet cells contribute to airway mucus production and are interspersed between columnar ciliated cells. Smooth muscle bundles are spirally arranged in the submucosa. There are no cartilage plates or bronchial glands.

AIRWAY STRUCTURE

CT IMAGING ANATOMY OF THE LARGE AIRWAYS

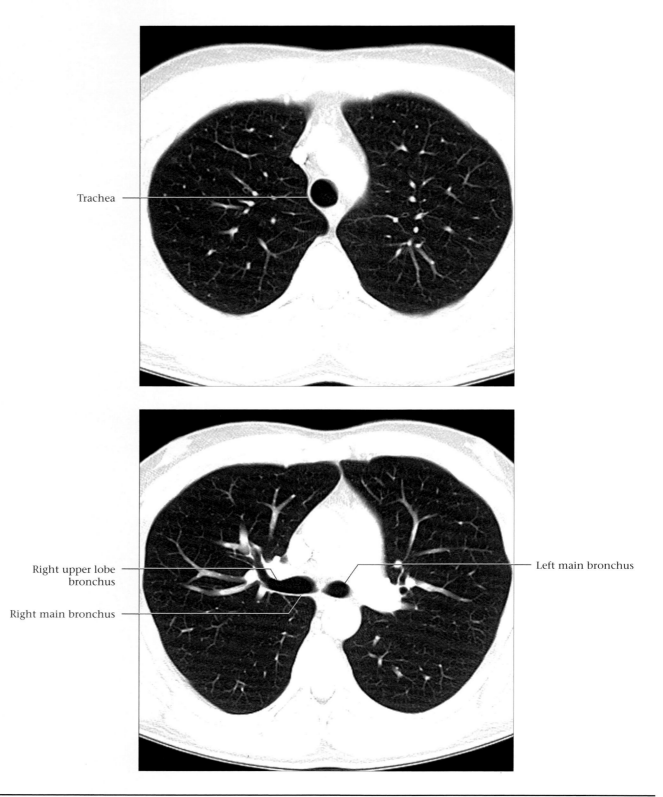

Trachea

Right upper lobe bronchus

Right main bronchus

Left main bronchus

(Top) First of four normal CT images of the large airways. The trachea is the largest conducting airway. Its thin wall is supported by anterolateral "C"-shaped cartilages with a posterior membranous portion. The cartilaginous rings contribute to the round morphology exhibited by the trachea during inspiration. **(Bottom)** Right and left main bronchi arise from the trachea at the tracheal carina. The main bronchi give rise to lobar bronchi.

AIRWAY STRUCTURE

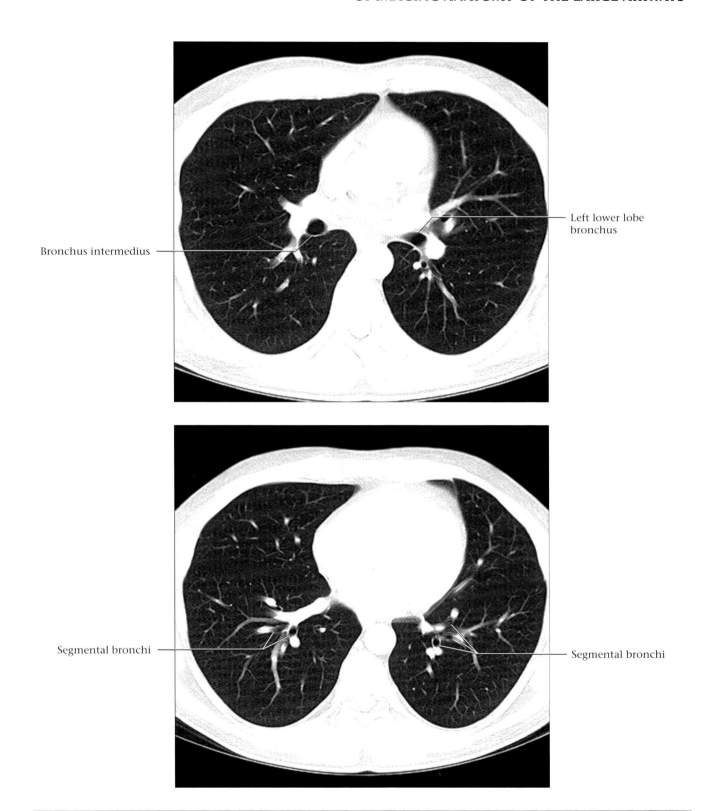

(Top) The right main bronchus gives rise to the right upper lobe bronchus and the bronchus intermedius. The left main bronchus gives rise to left upper and left lower lobe bronchi. **(Bottom)** Each lobar bronchus gives rise to segmental bronchi which in turn continue to branch into bronchioles. The smallest normally visible airways are bronchioles. The small airways distal to the muscular bronchioles are not visible with current imaging modalities.

AIRWAY STRUCTURE

RADIOGRAPHY, LARGE AIRWAY CARTILAGE CALCIFICATION

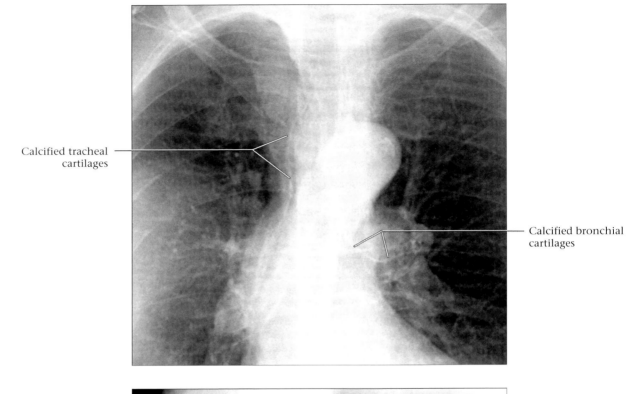

Calcified tracheal cartilages

Calcified bronchial cartilages

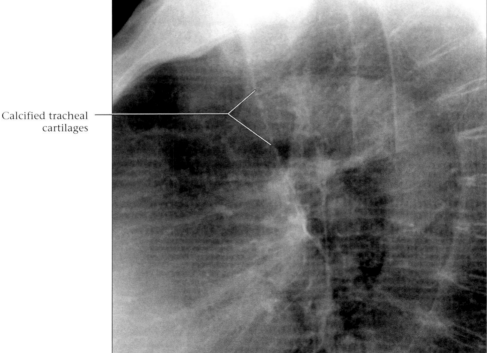

Calcified tracheal cartilages

(Top) First of four images of an elderly patient with normal tracheal calcification. Coned down PA chest radiograph shows calcified tracheal and bronchial cartilages manifesting as thin white lines along the airway walls. **(Bottom)** Coned down lateral chest radiograph shows calcification of the tracheal wall manifesting as a thin white line that is best seen along the anterior tracheal wall. The corrugated appearance of the calcification likely relates to the discontinuous nature of the individual "C"-shaped tracheal cartilages along the length of the airway.

AIRWAY STRUCTURE

CT, LARGE AIRWAY CARTILAGE CALCIFICATION

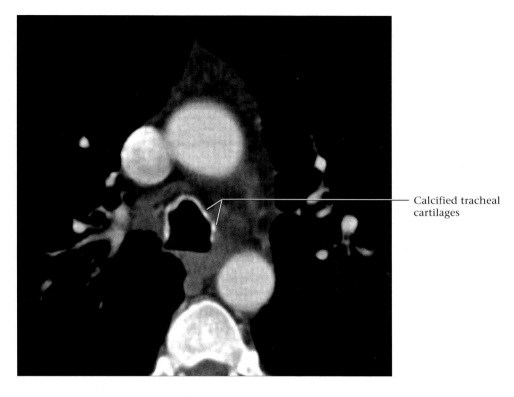

Calcified tracheal cartilages

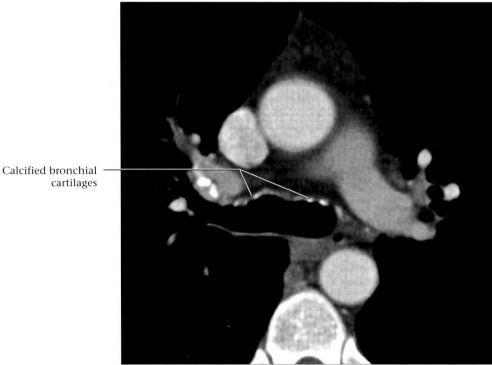

Calcified bronchial cartilages

(Top) Contrast-enhanced chest CT (mediastinal window) coned-down to the mediastinum shows calcification of individual tracheal cartilages. **(Bottom)** Contrast-enhanced chest CT (mediastinal window) coned-down to the mediastinum shows calcification of individual bronchial cartilages. An axial image just below the tracheal carina shows calcified cartilages in the main bronchi. Calcification of tracheal and bronchial cartilages may occur normally in elderly individuals, enhance visualization of the airway strall on radiography, and allow identification of individual calcified cartilages on CT.

AIRWAY STRUCTURE

SMALL AIRWAY STRUCTURE & THE SECONDARY PULMONARY LOBULE

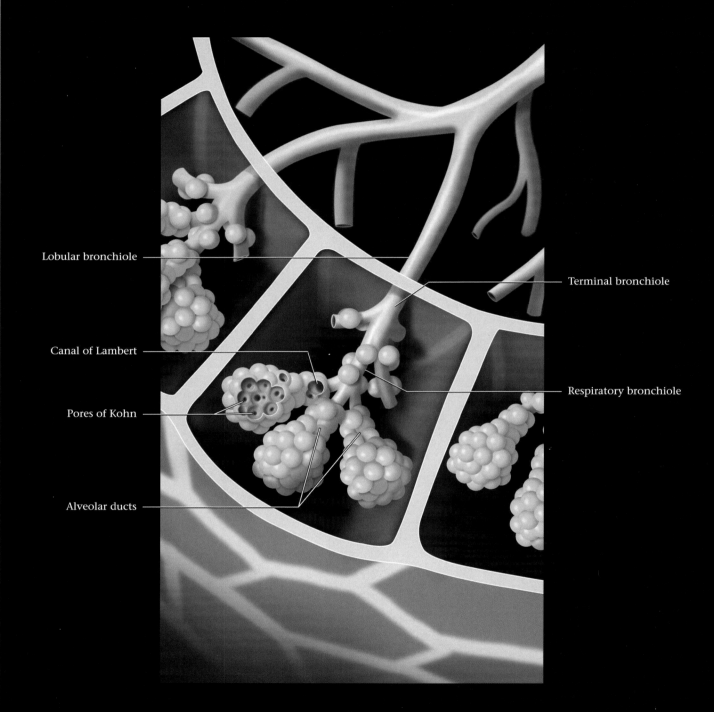

Lobular bronchiole

Terminal bronchiole

Canal of Lambert

Respiratory bronchiole

Pores of Kohn

Alveolar ducts

Graphic shows the structure of a portion of a pulmonary acinus within the secondary pulmonary lobule. The acinus is comprised of the structures distal to a terminal bronchiole. The terminal bronchiole is the last conducting airway and gives rise to two or more respiratory bronchioles, which are transitional airways characterized by their alveolated walls. Each respiratory bronchiole gives rise to three alveolar ducts which are airways lined by alveoli. Alveolar ducts terminate in alveolar sacs and alveoli. Pores of Kohn provide communication between adjacent alveoli. Canals of Lambert provide communication between various airways within an acinus as well as between adjacent acini and facilitate collateral ventilation.

AIRWAY STRUCTURE

MICROSCOPIC STRUCTURE OF THE SMALL AIRWAYS

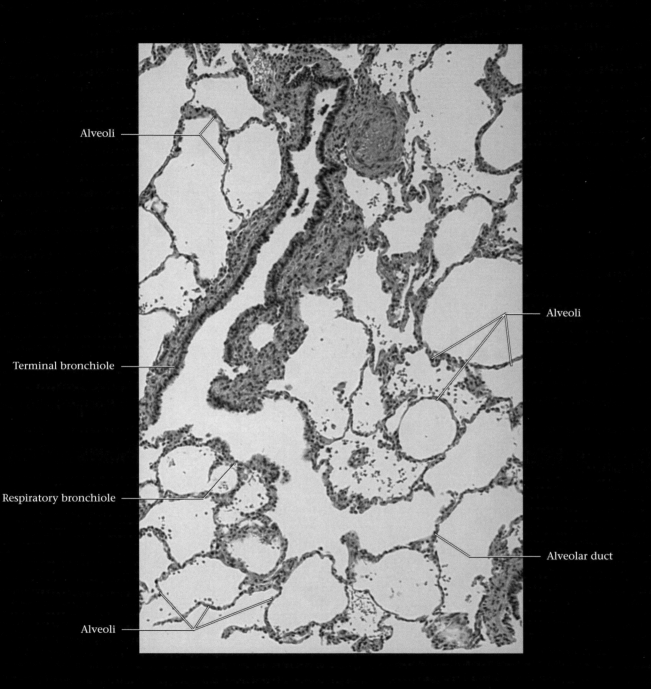

Alveoli

Terminal bronchiole

Respiratory bronchiole

Alveoli

Alveoli

Alveolar duct

High-power photomicrograph (Hematoxylin and Eosin stain) shows the microscopic structure of the small airways. The terminal bronchiole is the last purely conducting airway and gives rise to respiratory bronchioles which are characterized by their partially alveolated walls. The alveolar duct is a tubular space lined by alveoli.

AIRWAY STRUCTURE

MICROSCOPIC STRUCTURE OF THE ALVEOLI

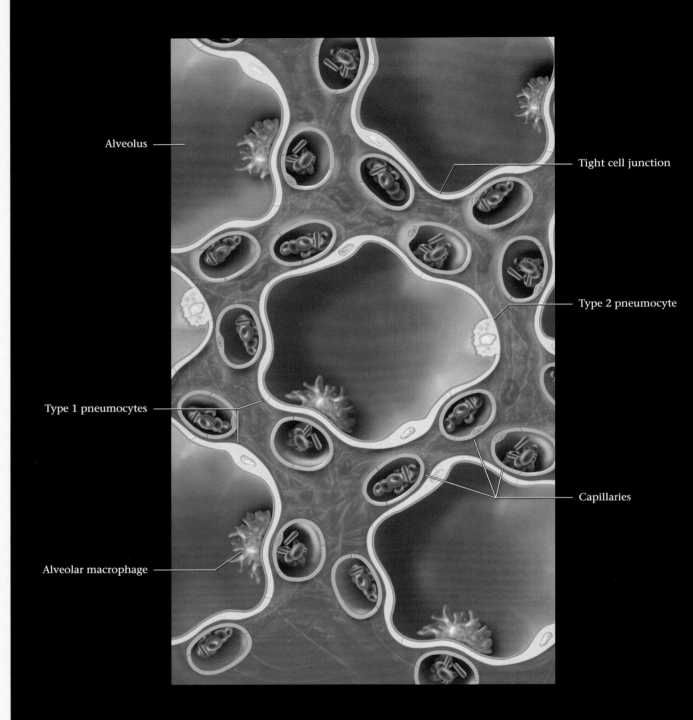

Alveolus

Tight cell junction

Type 2 pneumocyte

Type 1 pneumocytes

Capillaries

Alveolar macrophage

Graphic shows the microscopic structure of the alveoli. The alveolar-capillary interface is the principal site of respiration where the alveoli come in contact with the rich capillary network of the lung. Inspired oxygen is delivered to the capillaries and carbon dioxide is delivered to the airway. The type 1 pneumocyte is a flat cell with tight cell junctions that lines the alveolar surface. The tight cell junctions prevent permeability of fluid into the alveolar space. The type 2 pneumocyte is a larger polygonal cell that produces surfactant and processes circulating vasoactive substances. The alveolar macrophage is a migratory cell that forms part of the defense mechanisms of the lung.

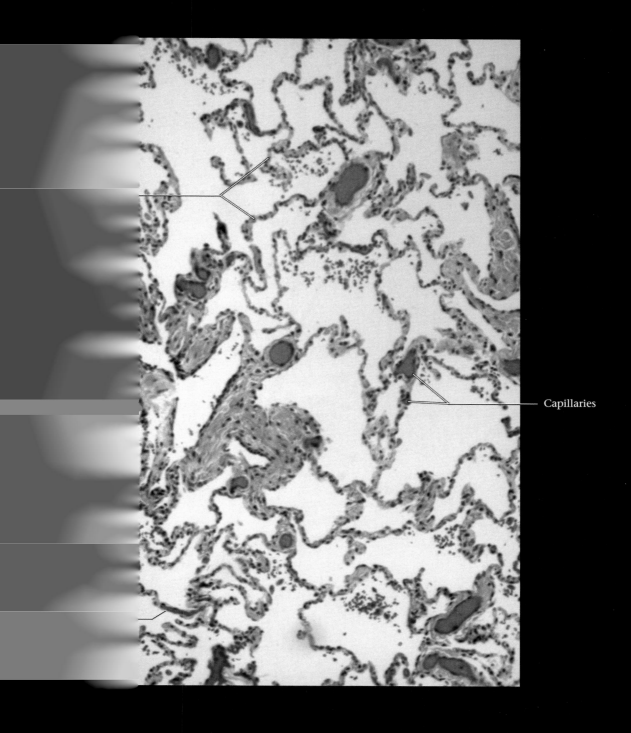

Capillaries

graph (Hematoxylin and Eosin stain) shows the microscopic structure of the alveoli. The flat
ar pneumocytes facilitates gas exchange with adjacent capillaries at the alveolar capillary
red million alveoli in human lungs provide an enormous surface area (70 meters squared)

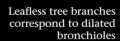

TREE-IN-BUD

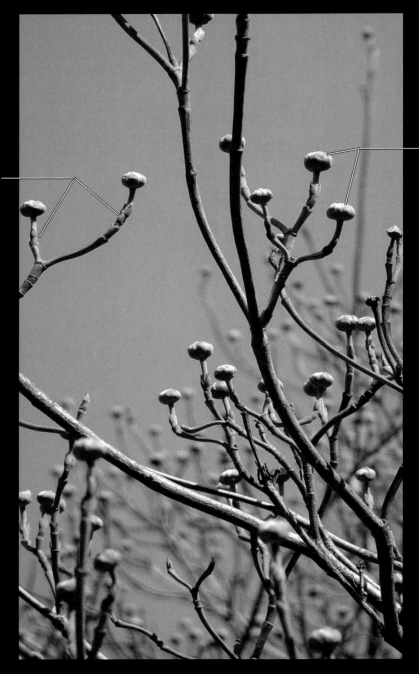

Leafless tree branches correspond to dilated bronchioles

Buds correspond to peribronchiolar inflammatory tissue

Photograph of a leafless tree-in-bud illustrates the origin of the term "tree-in-bud" opacities used to describe the CT findings of cellular bronchiolitis. The small tree branches correspond to dilated centrilobular bronchioles filled with inflammatory cells and/or fluid on HRCT; the round buds correspond to peribronchiolar inflammatory tissue. Photograph by Gerald F. Abbott, MD

AIRWAY STRUCTURE

TREE-IN-BUD OPACITIES, INFECTIOUS BRONCHIOLITIS

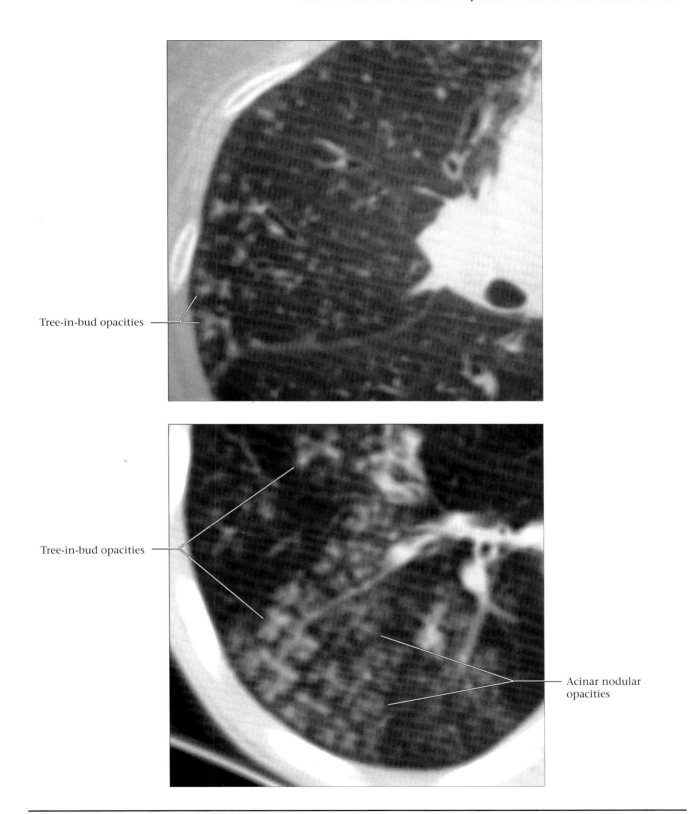

Tree-in-bud opacities

Tree-in-bud opacities

Acinar nodular opacities

(Top) Coned down HRCT of an immune compromised patient with tuberculosis shows multifocal tree-in-bud opacities (short linear opacities with terminal nodular opacities). This finding is a direct sign of bronchiolitis that results from thickening and filling of the lumens of terminal bronchioles with associated cellular infiltration and inflammation of the surrounding distal airways. **(Bottom)** Coned down thin-section chest CT of a patient with bronchopneumonia shows exuberant tree-in-bud opacities that form early acinar nodules in the right lower lobe.

AIRWAY STRUCTURE

CENTRILOBULAR & PANLOBULAR LOW ATTENUATION, EMPHYSEMA

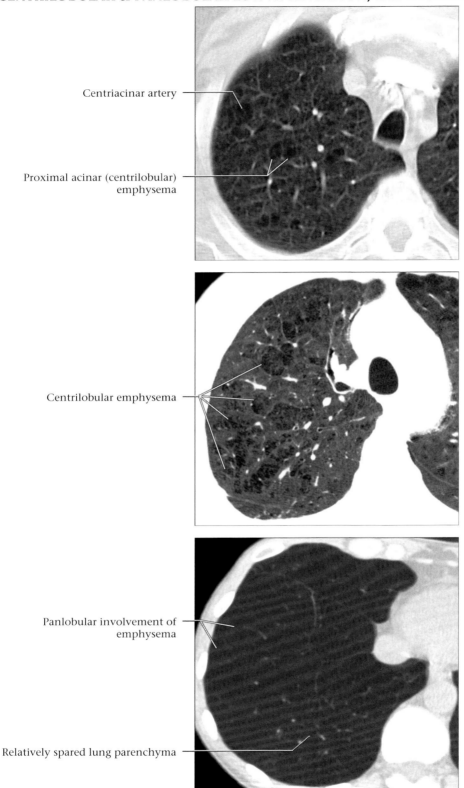

Centriacinar artery

Proximal acinar (centrilobular) emphysema

Centrilobular emphysema

Panlobular involvement of emphysema

Relatively spared lung parenchyma

(Top) HRCT of the right lung apex shows round foci of low attenuation with imperceptible walls representing centrilobular (proximal acinar) emphysema. The hyperlucent foci are confined to the center of the secondary pulmonary lobule. The centrilobular artery may manifest as a dot in the center of the emphysematous space. **(Middle)** HRCT of the right upper lobe shows more advanced centrilobular emphysema with larger areas of centrilobular lucency. **(Bottom)** HRCT of the right lung base of a 45 year old man with panacinar emphysema secondary to alpha-1-antitrypsin deficiency shows hyperlucent lung parenchyma with a paucity of normal vessels. The entire acinus is affected by the lung destruction. Lung parenchyma of higher attenuation indicates areas of relative sparing. Contributed by Mark A. King, MD, The Ohio State university, Columbus, OH.

AIRWAY STRUCTURE

PANLOBULAR LOW ATTENUATION, PARASEPTAL EMPHYSEMA & BULLOUS DISEASE

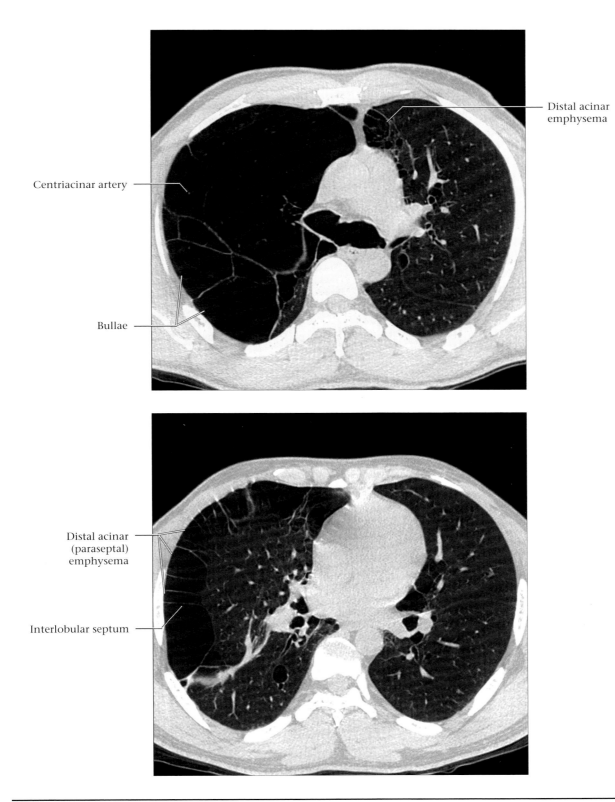

Distal acinar emphysema

Centriacinar artery

Bullae

Distal acinar (paraseptal) emphysema

Interlobular septum

(Top) First of two HRCT images of 45 year old man with dyspnea shows extensive paraseptal (distal acinar) emphysema and bullous disease. Section through the carina shows extensive right upper lobe bullae. There is also mild paraseptal emphysema in the medial left upper lobe and along the left major fissure. In spite of extensive lung destruction, centrilobular arteries are still visible as dot-like opacities in the central portion of secondary pulmonary lobules. **(Bottom)** HRCT image through the lung bases shows the characteristic appearance of paraseptal emphysema manifesting as a peripheral arcade of cystic structures with well-defined walls in the subpleural aspect of the right upper lobe. The destroyed secondary pulmonary lobules are marginated by interlobular septa. Paraseptal emphysema may be associated with bullous disease.

AIRWAY STRUCTURE

LOBULAR LOW ATTENUATION, CONSTRICTIVE BRONCHIOLITIS

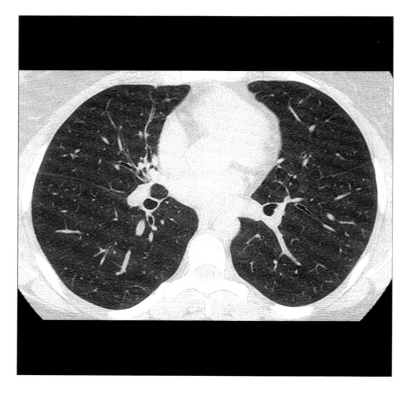

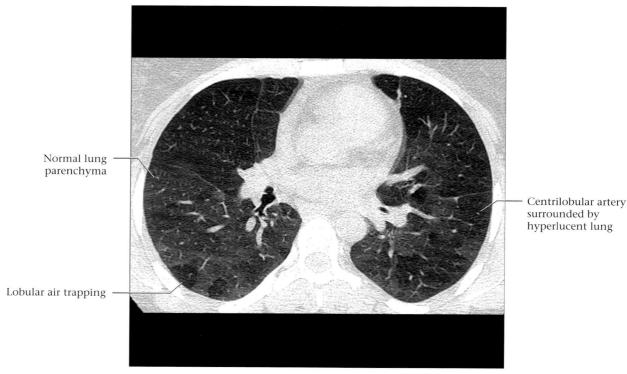

Normal lung parenchyma

Centrilobular artery surrounded by hyperlucent lung

Lobular air trapping

(Top) First of four CT images of a patient with constrictive bronchiolitis secondary to smoke inhalation injury. Inspiratory axial HRCT shows very subtle heterogeneity of lung attenuation. **(Bottom)** Expiratory axial HRCT shows mosaic attenuation secondary to air trapping. The normal lung parenchyma exhibits increased attenuation on expiratory imaging. Abnormal lung parenchyma manifests with multifocal bilateral areas of lobular air trapping. Some of these exhibit polyhedral shapes and represent air strapping in adjacent secondary pulmonary lobules. The central lobular artery is visible in association with some of the affected secondary pulmonary lobules.

AIRWAY STRUCTURE

LOBULAR LOW ATTENUATION, CONSTRICTIVE BRONCHIOLITIS

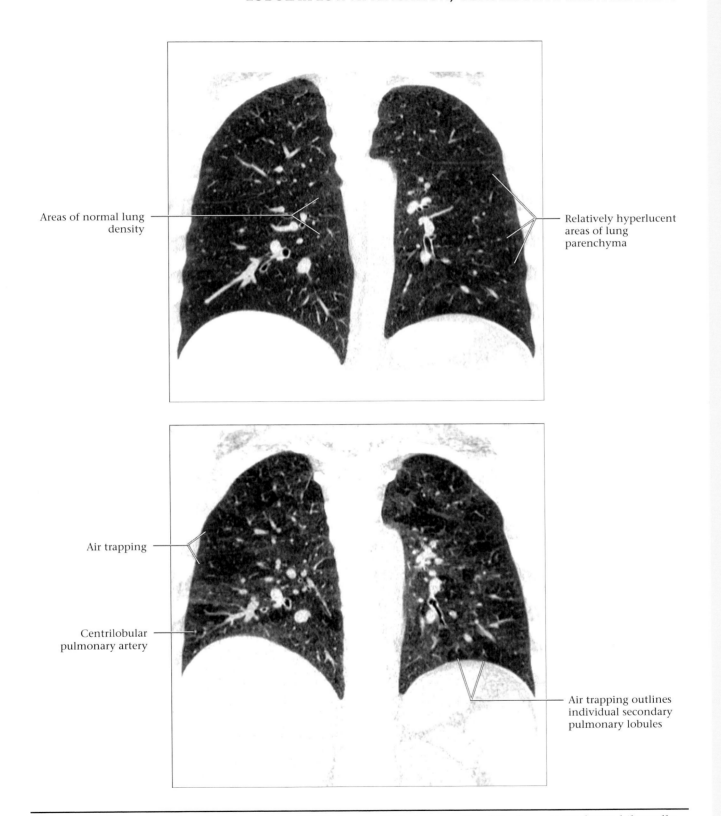

Areas of normal lung density

Relatively hyperlucent areas of lung parenchyma

Air trapping

Centrilobular pulmonary artery

Air trapping outlines individual secondary pulmonary lobules

(Top) Coronal reconstruction of an inspiratory HRCT shows mild heterogeneity of the lung parenchyma bilaterally. Areas of hyperlucency are interspersed with areas of normal lung density resulting in mosaic attenuation of the lung parenchyma. **(Bottom)** Coronal reconstruction of an expiratory HRCT accentuates the pulmonary heterogeneity by demonstrating multifocal areas of lobular air trapping. These manifest as polyhedral foci of hyperlucent lung parenchyma. Several affected individual secondary pulmonary lobules exhibit hyperlucency on expiratory imaging. Central "dots" within the secondary pulmonary lobules represent centrilobular pulmonary arteries. The findings are characteristic of constrictive bronchiolitis.

AIRWAY STRUCTURE

ACINAR NODULES, BRONCHOPNEUMONIA

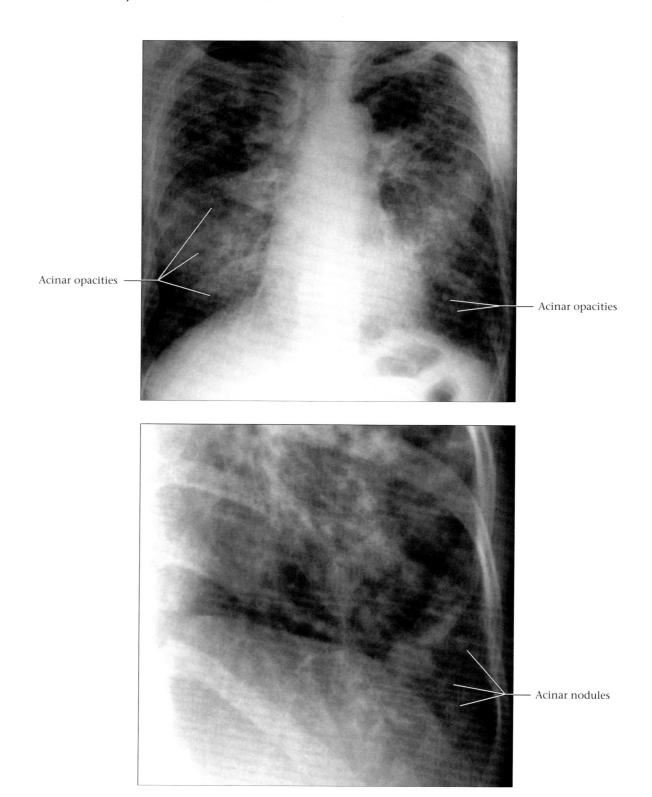

Acinar opacities

Acinar opacities

Acinar nodules

(Top) First of two radiographs of a patient with active tuberculosis shows the imaging appearance of the abnormal acinus. PA chest radiograph shows bilateral areas of consolidation predominantly involving the upper lobes and superior segments of the lower lobes. Multiple indistinctly margined acinar nodular opacities result from bronchogenic spread of the infection. (Bottom) PA chest radiograph coned-down to the left lower lobe shows multiple indistinctly margined round opacities representing intra-acinar inflammatory exudate. Acinar nodules are a radiographic manifestation of bronchogenic spread of infection, characteristic of tuberculosis.

AIRWAY STRUCTURE

ACINAR NODULES, BARIUM ASPIRATION

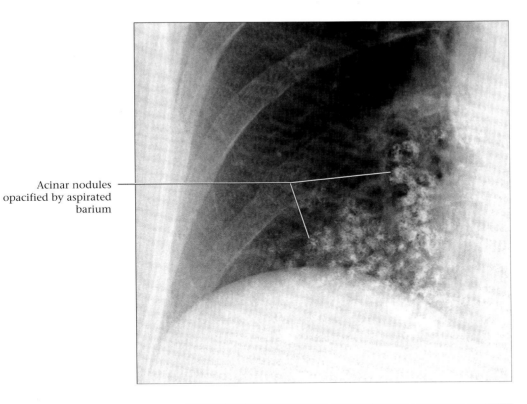

Acinar nodules opacified by aspirated barium

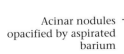
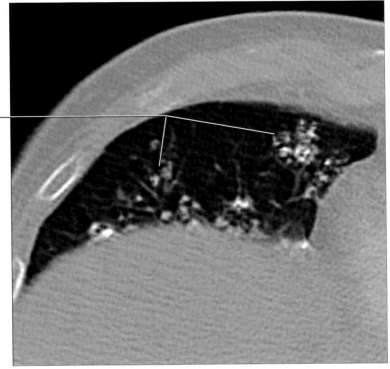

Acinar nodules opacified by aspirated barium

(Top) First of two images of a patient who aspirated barium contrast agent shows multiple high attenuation acinar nodular opacities in the right middle lobe. PA chest radiograph coned-down to the right lower lung shows acinar rosettes of metallic density representing barium within the pulmonary acini. Each acinar nodule measures 6-10 mm in diameter. **(Bottom)** Unenhanced chest CT (bone window) coned-down to the right middle lobe shows barium-opacified acinar nodules, some forming clusters within secondary pulmonary lobules. The normal pulmonary acinus is not visible on imaging studies and is only identified when filled with fluid, cells or barium.

VASCULAR STRUCTURE

Overview of Pulmonary Vascular Structure

Arteries
- **Dual arterial supply** with pulmonary and systemic components
- **Pulmonary arterial system**
  - Pulmonary circulation
  - Conduit from right ventricle to capillary-alveolar interface
- **Bronchial arterial system**
  - Systemic circulation
  - Conduit from aorta to airway walls, vessel walls and visceral pleura

Veins
- **Dual venous drainage** with pulmonary and systemic components
- **Pulmonary venous system**
  - Pulmonary circulation
  - Conduit from alveolar-capillary interface to left atrium
  - Venous drainage of the lung
- **True bronchial venous system**
  - Conduit from perihilar bronchi and vessels to the azygos venous system
  - Venous drainage of the walls of central vessels and tracheobronchial tree

Other Systemic Vessels
- Sources of collateral blood supply to the lung from the systemic circulation
- **Pulmonary ligament arteries**
  - Aortic branches located in the pulmonary ligament
  - Supply esophageal plexus
  - Supply medial visceral pleura
  - May supply adjacent lung parenchyma
    - **Potential source of blood supply to intralobar sequestrations**
- Subclavian and axillary arteries
- Intercostal arteries
- Inferior phrenic arteries

Lymphatics
- Vascular channels
- Collection of lymphatic fluid
- Conduit of lymphatic fluid towards hila

Relationship of Vascular Structures
- Anatomy
  - **Bronchoarterial bundle** is a single connective tissue sheath that contains
    - Pulmonary arteries
    - Bronchi
    - Bronchial arteries
  - **Lymphatics** located along
    - Bronchi to level of respiratory bronchioles
    - Pulmonary arteries
    - Pulmonary veins
    - Interlobular and connective tissue septa
    - Visceral pleural connective tissue
- **Vascular anastomoses**
  - **Pulmonary to bronchial arteries**

- Communication between pulmonary and systemic circulations
  - Located in the walls of larger airways
  - Functionally closed in normal individuals
  - May become patent in disease states
- **Bronchial arteries to pulmonary veins**
  - Communication between systemic and pulmonary circulations
  - Communication between capillary bed of bronchial wall and pulmonary veins
- **Pulmonary veins to lymphatics**
  - Communication with arterial channels
  - Communication with venous channels

General Anatomy and Function

Anatomy
- **Pulmonary circulation**
  - Pulmonary arteries
  - Capillary network
  - Pulmonary veins
- **Systemic circulation**
  - Bronchial arteries
  - Non-bronchial systemic arteries
  - True bronchial veins
- **Pulmonary lymphatics**
  - Complex network of vascular channels
    - **Reservoir lymphatics:** Broad, ribbon-like
    - **Conduit lymphatics:** Tubular
    - **Saculotubular lymphatics:** Plexiform complex around vessels and bronchi
  - **Bronchus-associated lymphoid tissue (BALT)**
  - **Intrapulmonary lymph nodes**
  - **Intrapulmonary peribronchial lymph nodes**

Function
- **Pulmonary circulation**
  - **Pulmonary arteries**
    - Collection of deoxygenated blood from the right cardiac chambers
    - Conduit of deoxygenated blood to pulmonary capillary-alveolar interface
  - **Pulmonary alveolar-capillary network**
    - Gas exchange
  - **Pulmonary veins**
    - Collection of oxygenated blood from the alveolar-capillary network and conduit of oxygenated blood to left atrium and systemic circulation
    - Collection of blood from capillary beds of bronchial/bronchiolar walls, vessel walls and visceral pleura and conduit to left atrium
- **Systemic circulation**
  - **Bronchial arteries**
    - Conduit of oxygenated blood from the aorta to the airway walls, vessel walls and visceral pleura
  - **True bronchial veins**
    - Conduit of de-oxygenated blood from central vessel/bronchial walls to azygos system
- **Lymphatics**
  - Drainage of lymphatic fluid towards the hila

VASCULAR STRUCTURE

○ Occasional lymphatic drainage to abdominal lymph nodes

Pulmonary Arteries

General Concepts
- **Pulmonary trunk** arises from the right ventricle
- Dichotomous branching into right and left main pulmonary arteries
- Pulmonary artery branches
  ○ **Lobar**
  ○ **Segmental**
  ○ **Subsegmental**

Physiology
- **Low pressure pulmonary circulation**
- Minimal flow through lung apices
  ○ Rapid increase in cardiac output accommodated through recruitment of closed capillaries in underperfused upper lung zones
- Muscular arteries constrict in response to hypoxia
  ○ **Ventilation-perfusion matching** to prevent hypoxemia

Microscopic Anatomy
- **Proximal large arteries**
  ○ Elastic arteries
- **Distal small arteries**
  ○ Transition to **muscular arteries** at level of bronchioles
  ○ **External elastic lamina**
  ○ **Muscular media**
  ○ **Internal elastic lamina**
- **Smallest arteries**: Loss of smooth muscle in vessel wall
  ○ Muscle in media thins as artery size decreases
  ○ **Single elastic lamina** distally
  ○ Difficult distinction between arteries and arterioles due to varying amounts of muscle in vessel walls
    - Term "arteriole" not applicable to the pulmonary circulation

Imaging Anatomy
- Pulmonary arteries course alongside the bronchi
  ○ Medial to bronchi in the upper lobes
  ○ Lateral to bronchi in the middle lobe, lingula and lower lobes
- Accessory branches directly penetrate the lung
- **Lobular arteries** of the secondary pulmonary lobule
  ○ Typically dominant lobular branch in center of lobule (centrilobular)
  ○ Manifest as central dot-like opacities within 1 cm of pleural surfaces

Capillary Network

Anatomy
- Origin from distal most pulmonary arteries
- Surround alveoli of respiratory bronchioles, alveolar ducts, alveolar sacs and alveoli
- Respiratory surface with enormous surface area
  ○ Approximately **300 million alveoli**
  ○ Approximately **1000 capillaries per alveolus**

○ **Surface area of 70 m²**

Microscopic Anatomy
- Lined by flat endothelial cells on a basement membrane
- Loose endothelial cell junctions
  ○ Permit passage of low molecular weight proteins

Imaging Anatomy
- Below the resolution of clinical CT scanners

Pulmonary Veins

General Concepts
- Right and left pulmonary veins
- Sources of venous drainage
  ○ Efferent alveolar capillaries
  ○ Bronchial/vascular wall capillary networks
  ○ Visceral pleura

Microscopic Anatomy
- Small pulmonary veins indistinguishable from small arteries
- Mural smooth muscle cells and elastic lamina

Imaging Anatomy
- **Pulmonary veins** travel in the **periphery of lung units**
  ○ **Acinus**
  ○ **Lobule**
  ○ **Segment**
- Pulmonary vein branches
  ○ **Septal veins** in periphery of secondary pulmonary lobule
    - Visible along interlobular septa; help define the boundaries of secondary pulmonary lobules
    - 0.5 mm in diameter
    - Arcuate or branching structures identified 1.0-1.5 cm from pleural surface
  ○ Veins in periphery of subsegments and segments
  ○ Veins in periphery of lobes
  ○ **Superior pulmonary veins**
    - Drainage of upper lobes and right middle lobe
  ○ **Inferior pulmonary veins**
    - Drainage of lower lobes
  ○ Variable anatomy of central pulmonary veins at anastomosis with left atrium

Bronchial Arteries

General Concepts
- Variable origin from systemic circulation
  ○ Single **right bronchial artery** from third intercostal artery
  ○ Two **left bronchial arteries** from descending aorta
- Vascular supply to
  ○ Subepithelial capillary plexus along airway length from trachea to terminal bronchioles
  ○ Peribronchial, perivascular connective tissue
  ○ Vessel walls: Great vessels, pulmonary arteries and veins

VASCULAR STRUCTURE

○ Paratracheal, carinal, hilar and intrapulmonary lymphoid tissue
○ Visceral pleura
○ Esophagus
• Numerous anastomoses to other systemic mediastinal vessels
• Travel in close relationship to (within) walls of bronchi and bronchioles

Microscopic Anatomy
• **Muscular media**
  ○ **High pressure systemic circulation**
• Prominent **internal elastic lamina**
• No external elastic lamina

Imaging Anatomy
• Typically inapparent
• Visualization of central bronchial arteries in several disease states with collateral circulation to the lung

Bronchial Veins

General Concepts
• True bronchial veins only in the perihilar regions
• Drainage to azygos and hemiazygos systems

Imaging Anatomy
• Generally not visible on imaging studies

Pulmonary Lymphatics

General Concepts
• Diffuse and complex pulmonary lymphatic network
• Lymphatic channels along
  ○ Bronchi
    ▪ To level of respiratory bronchioles
  ○ Vessels
    ▪ Pulmonary arteries
    ▪ Pulmonary veins
  ○ Connective tissue septa
    ▪ Interlobular septa
  ○ Intralobular interstitium
  ○ Visceral pleura

Microscopic Anatomy
• Thin endothelium
• Endoluminal valves direct flow towards hila
• Not normally visible on histologic specimens
  ○ May become prominent in certain disease states

Imaging Anatomy
• Generally not visible on imaging studies

Vascular Structure of Secondary Pulmonary Lobule

Lobular Pulmonary Artery
• Each lobular pulmonary artery supplies a single lobule
• Courses alongside the distal airway
• Ramifies as the alveolar capillary network
• Imaging

○ Lobular artery: Central dot-like structure approximately 1 mm in diameter
○ Intralobular acinar arteries: Vessels as small as 0.2 mm in diameter resolved on thin-section CT

Bronchial Artery
• Courses within airway wall
• Ramifies as airway wall (subepithelial) capillary network

Pulmonary Vein
• **Intralobular pulmonary veins** drain into **septal pulmonary veins**
  ○ Septal veins are visible on CT and measure approximately 0.5 mm in diameter
  ○ Located approximately 5-10 mm from arteries
• Each lobular (septal) pulmonary vein drains two or more adjacent lobules
• Tributaries from
  ○ Alveolar capillary network
  ○ Bronchial artery-derived airway wall (subendothelial) capillary network
  ○ Visceral pleural capillaries

Lymphatics
• Peribronchovascular lymphatics
  ○ Alongside lobular pulmonary arteries and airways
• Perilobular lymphatics
  ○ Along interlobular septa and pulmonary veins
• Visceral pleural lymphatics
• Intercommunication via anastomotic channels
  ○ Peribronchovascular to perilobular
  ○ Peribronchovascular to pleural

Anatomic Correlates of Selected Diseases

Random Pulmonary Nodules
• Diseases
  ○ **Hematogenous metastases**
  ○ **Miliary infection**
• CT features
  ○ Nodules randomly distributed in relation to the structures of the secondary pulmonary lobule
  ○ Some nodules may exhibit a relationship to small pulmonary arteries
    ▪ Helpful finding to suggest hematogenous mechanism of dissemination

Perilymphatic Pulmonary Nodules
• Diseases
  ○ **Sarcoidosis**
  ○ **Lymphangitic carcinomatosis**
• CT features
  ○ Nodules located along the lymphatic channels of the secondary pulmonary lobule
    ▪ **Peribronchovascular**
    ▪ **Interlobular septal**
    ▪ **Subpleural**
    ▪ **Centrilobular**

VASCULAR STRUCTURE

PULMONARY VASCULAR STRUCTURE, PULMONARY ARTERIES

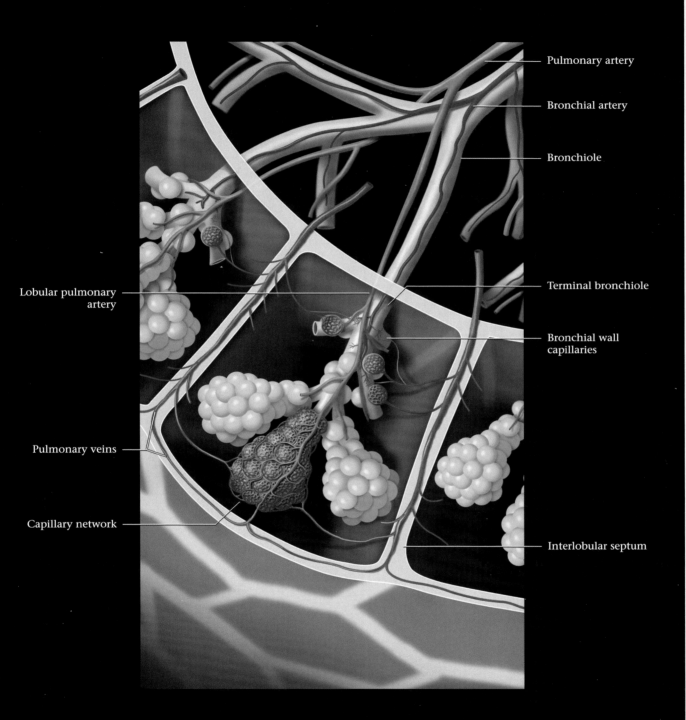

Pulmonary artery

Bronchial artery

Bronchiole

Terminal bronchiole

Bronchial wall capillaries

Lobular pulmonary artery

Pulmonary veins

Capillary network

Interlobular septum

Graphic shows the complexity of the vascular components of the secondary pulmonary lobule which reproduces (in miniature) the structural morphology of the lung with respect to the organization of vascular structures, airways and lymphatics. The pulmonary arteries travel alongside the airways, supply the capillary network that surrounds the alveoli and bring deoxygenated blood to the capillary-alveolar interface. The bronchial arteries travel within the airway wall and supply the capillary networks within the walls of the airways.

VASCULAR STRUCTURE

CT, PULMONARY VASCULATURE

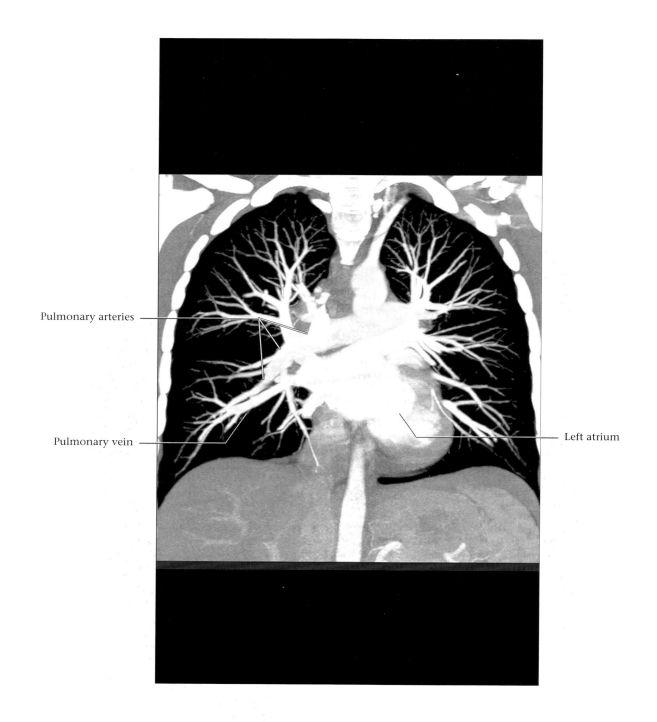

First of two contrast-enhanced maximum intensity projection CT images of the lungs shows the complex nature of the pulmonary vasculature. Coronal image shows visualization of numerous overlapping blood vessels. Peripheral pulmonary arteries are identified by visualization of their origin from the main pulmonary arteries. Peripheral pulmonary veins are identified by visualization of their drainage into the central pulmonary veins and the left atrium.

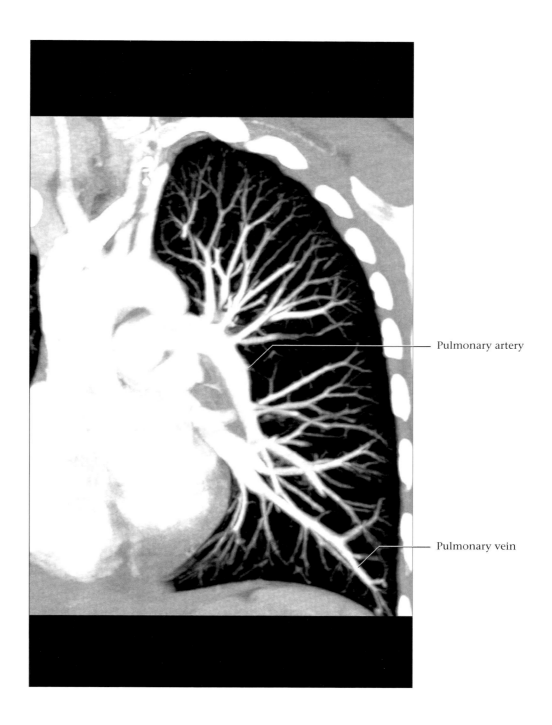

Pulmonary artery

Pulmonary vein

Contrast-enhanced oblique coronal maximum intensity projection CT image of the left pulmonary vascular tree. Pulmonary arteries are distinguished from pulmonary veins based on visualization of their central vascular connections. Note the near vertical course of the large pulmonary arteries of the left lower lobe and the more horizontal course of the major left lower lobe pulmonary veins.

VASCULAR STRUCTURE

CT ANGIOGRAPHY, PULMONARY ARTERIES

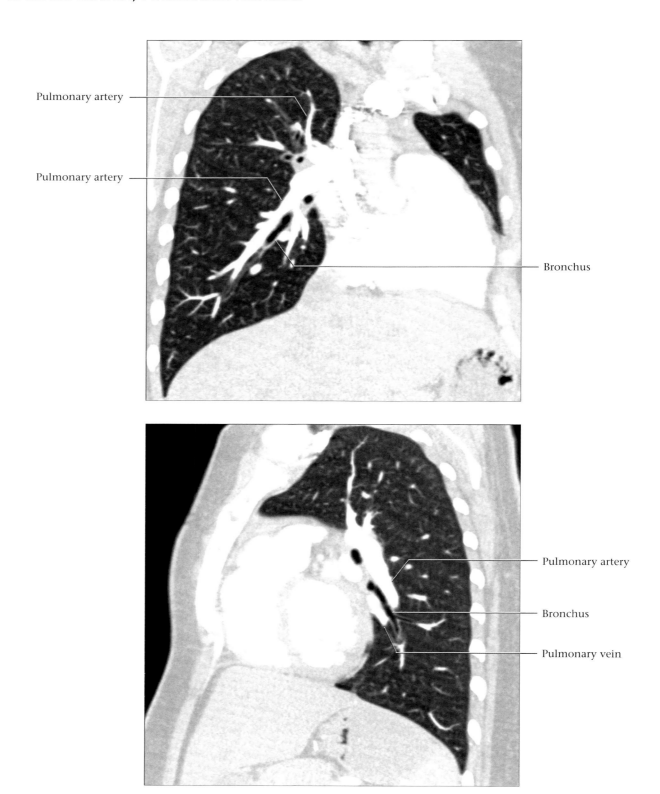

Pulmonary artery

Pulmonary artery

Bronchus

Pulmonary artery

Bronchus

Pulmonary vein

(Top) First of two oblique coronal reconstructions from a normal CT pulmonary angiogram (lung window) of a 21 year old woman with chest pain shows the relationship of the pulmonary arteries to the adjacent bronchi. CT of the right pulmonary arterial tree shows that the arteries course medial to the bronchi in the right upper lobe and lateral to the bronchi in the lower lobes. **(Bottom)** CT pulmonary angiogram of the left pulmonary arterial tree shows the left interlobar pulmonary artery located posterolateral to a left lower lobe bronchus. The adjacent pulmonary vein is located anteromedial to the bronchus. The pulmonary arteries carry deoxygenated blood from the right ventricle to the capillary-alveolar interface.

VASCULAR STRUCTURE

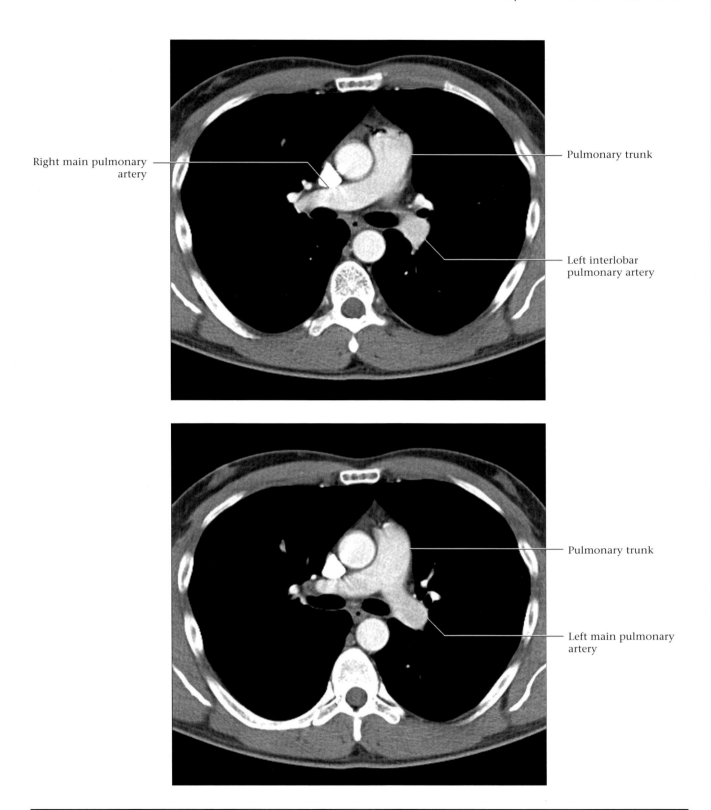

Right main pulmonary artery

Pulmonary trunk

Left interlobar pulmonary artery

Pulmonary trunk

Left main pulmonary artery

(Top) First of two images from a normal contrast-enhanced chest CT (mediastinal window) shows adequate enhancement of the vascular structures of the mediastinum. The pulmonary trunk gives rise to the right and left main pulmonary arteries. The right main pulmonary artery is visualized in its entirety as it courses anterior to the bronchus intermedius and posterior to the ascending aorta and superior vena cava. Note a small amount of air in the non-dependent portion of the pulmonary trunk that resulted from the intravenous contrast injection. **(Bottom)** CT section obtained below the tracheal carina demonstrates the bifurcation of the pulmonary trunk into right and left main pulmonary arteries. Note the horizontal course of the left main pulmonary artery into the left lung.

VASCULAR STRUCTURE

MICROSCOPIC FEATURES, PULMONARY & BRONCHIAL ARTERIES

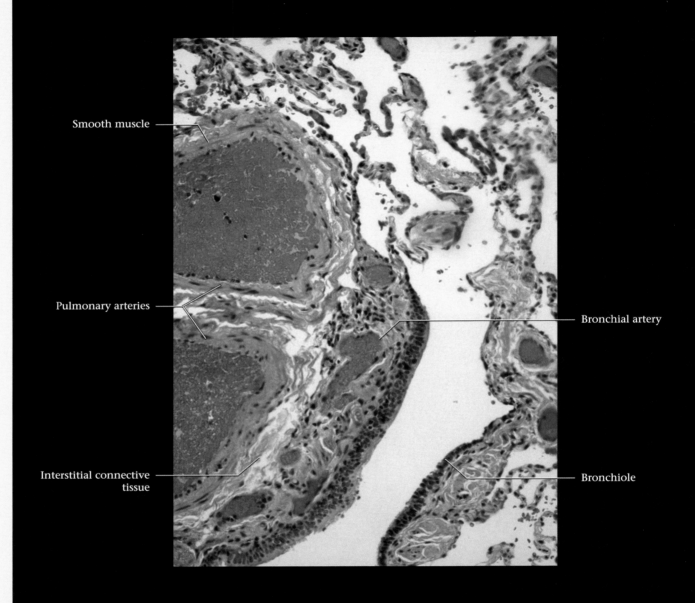

Smooth muscle

Pulmonary arteries

Interstitial connective tissue

Bronchial artery

Bronchiole

High-power photomicrograph (Hematoxylin and Eosin stain) of normal lung demonstrates a bronchiole lined by pseudostratified cuboidal epithelium. Note the adjacent pulmonary artery branches which travel alongside the bronchus in the bronchovascular sheath and the intervening loose interstitial connective tissue. The muscular pulmonary arteries exhibit circularly oriented smooth muscle located between internal and external elastic laminae. Bronchial arteries are intimately related to their corresponding airway walls and are described as traveling within them.

VASCULAR STRUCTURE

RELATIONSHIP OF PULMONARY ARTERIES TO AIRWAYS

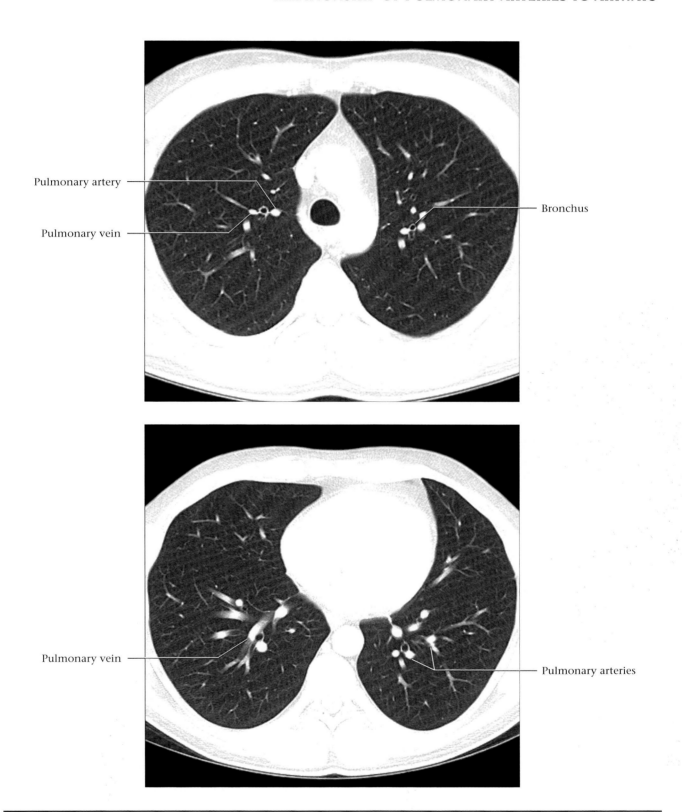

(Top) First of two images from a normal contrast-enhanced chest CT (lung window) shows the relationship of the pulmonary arteries and veins to the adjacent airways. CT section at the level of the aortic arch shows the vascular structures of the upper lobes. The pulmonary arteries are located medial to the adjacent bronchi. The pulmonary veins are located lateral to the bronchi. (Bottom) CT image at the level of the heart shows that the lower lobe pulmonary arteries are located lateral to adjacent bronchi. The strulmonary veins course along connective tissue septa that surround the pulmonary segments. In clinical practice, scrolling through sequential stacks of images permits tracing the peripheral vessels to their central portions to distinguish arteries from veins.

VASCULAR STRUCTURE

THE CAPILLARY-ALVEOLAR INTERFACE

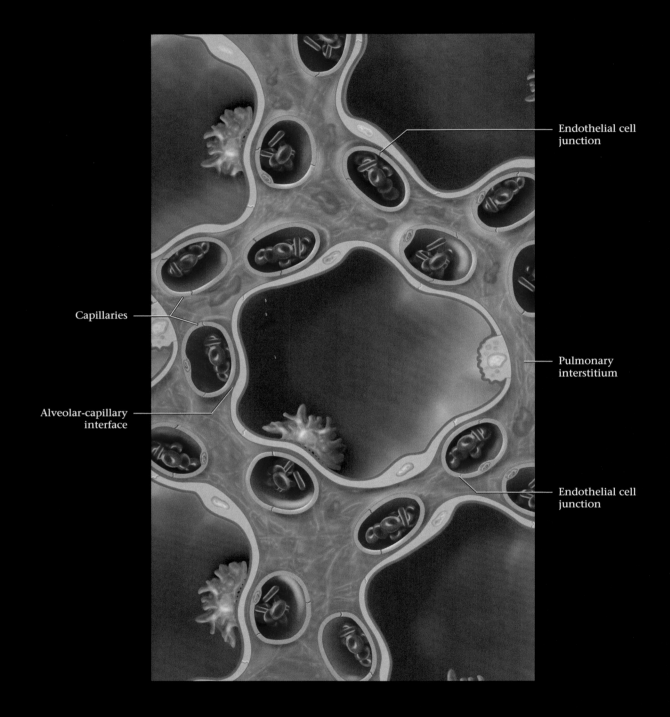

Endothelial cell junction

Capillaries

Pulmonary interstitium

Alveolar-capillary interface

Endothelial cell junction

Graphic shows the relationship of the capillary network to the alveoli. The capillary-alveolar interface is the site of gas exchange. The large number of capillaries provides an enormous surface area for respiration. The thin vascular endothelium and the thin alveolar wall cells facilitate the process of gas exchange. Loose endothelial cell junctions permit passage of intravascular low molecular weight substances.

VASCULAR STRUCTURE

MICROSCOPIC FEATURES OF CAPILLARY-ALVEOLAR INTERFACE

Capillary network

Alveolar wall

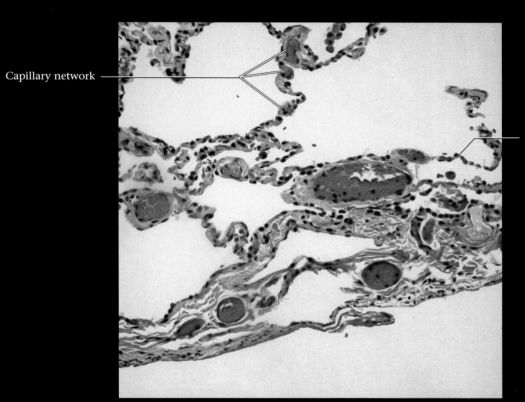

High-power photomicrograph (Hematoxylin and Eosin stain) of normal lung shows the thin alveolar walls and the numerous capillaries associated with each alveolus. The capillaries and other vascular structures are easily identified as they contain red blood cells in their lumens. The many capillaries associated with each alveolus provide an enormous surface area for respiration.

CT ANGIOGRAPHY, PULMONARY VEINS

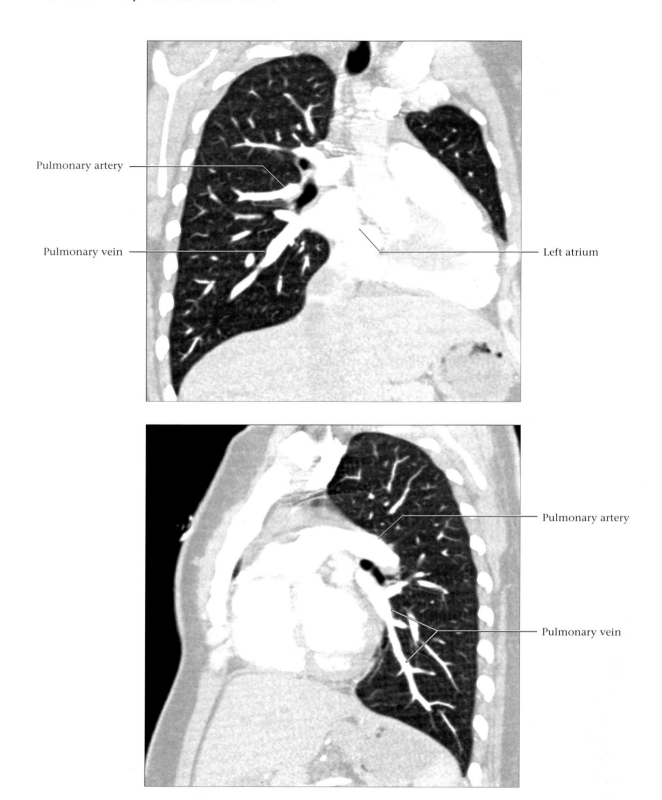

Pulmonary artery

Pulmonary vein

Left atrium

Pulmonary artery

Pulmonary vein

(Top) First of two oblique coronal reconstructions from a normal CT pulmonary angiogram (lung window) of a 21 year old woman with chest pain shows the right central pulmonary veins as they enter the left atrium. The pulmonary veins carry oxygenated blood from the lungs to the left cardiac chambers for delivery to the tissues. **(Bottom)** Oblique coronal CT of the left lung demonstrates the left central pulmonary veins located medial to an adjacent bronchus. The left pulmonary artery is easily identified by noting its connection to the pulmonary trunk as it arises from the right ventricle. The left pulmonary artery courses over the left main bronchus to supply the left lung.

VASCULAR STRUCTURE

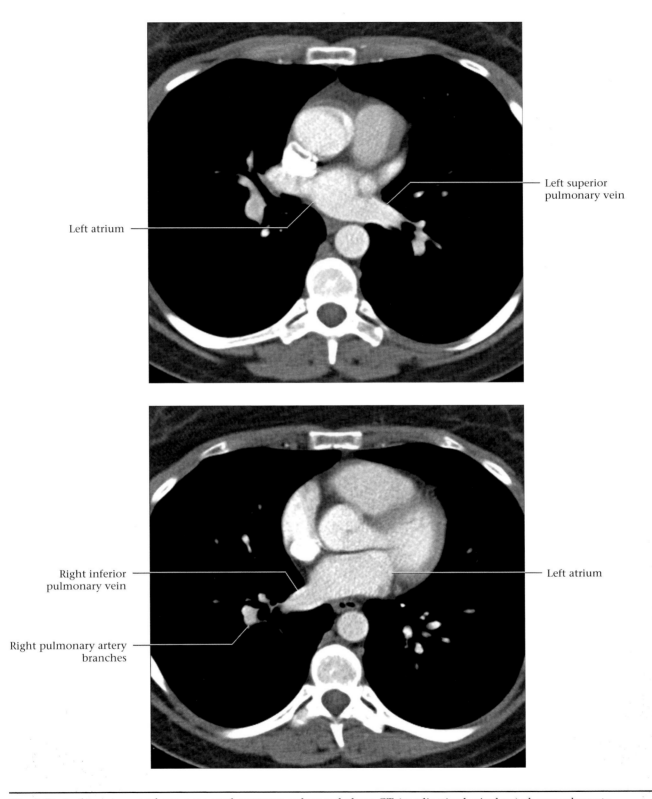

Left superior pulmonary vein

Left atrium

Right inferior pulmonary vein

Left atrium

Right pulmonary artery branches

(Top) First of two images from a normal contrast-enhanced chest CT (mediastinal window) shows adequate enhancement of the central vascular structures. CT section at the level of the left atrium shows the left superior pulmonary vein. There are characteristically two left and two right pulmonary veins although the number and morphology of the central pulmonary veins are variable. **(Bottom)** CT section at the level of the inferior aspect of the left atrium shows the right inferior pulmonary vein. Note the branches of the right pulmonary artery located lateral to the right lower lobe bronchi.

VASCULAR STRUCTURE

VEINS OF SECONDARY PULMONARY LOBULE

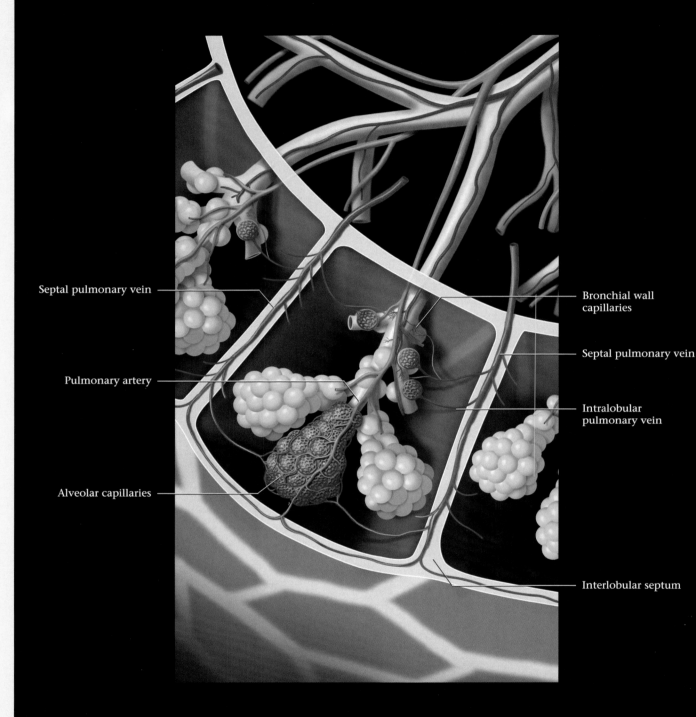

Septal pulmonary vein

Pulmonary artery

Alveolar capillaries

Bronchial wall capillaries

Septal pulmonary vein

Intralobular pulmonary vein

Interlobular septum

Graphic shows the vascular anatomy of the secondary pulmonary lobule (SPL). The veins are found in the interlobular septa that define the boundaries of the SPL. Intralobular pulmonary veins arise from the capillary network that surrounds the alveoli and drain into septal veins. The septal pulmonary veins drain more than one SPL. The pulmonary veins also drain the subendothelial capillary network of the airway walls and the visceral pleura.

VASCULAR STRUCTURE

CT, NORMAL SECONDARY PULMONARY LOBULE

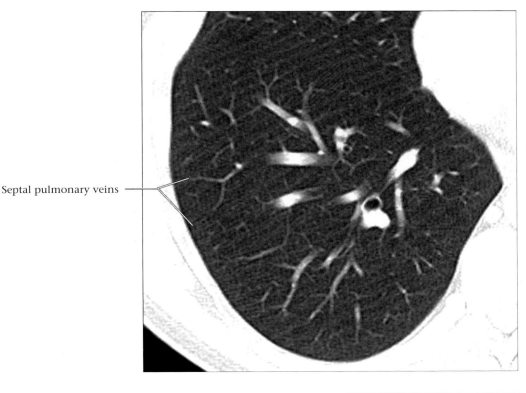

Septal pulmonary veins

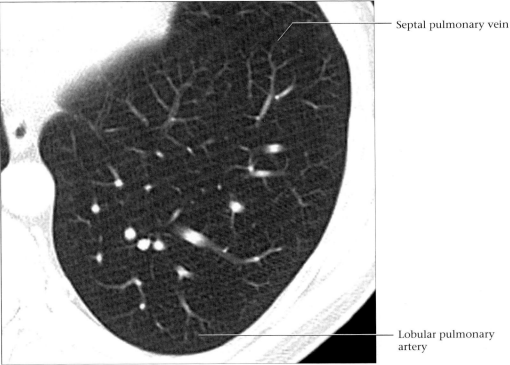

Septal pulmonary vein

Lobular pulmonary artery

(Top) First of two axial images of a normal contrast-enhanced chest CT (lung window) shows the vessels of the normal secondary pulmonary lobule. Coned down CT of the right lower lobe shows the peripheral pulmonary vein branches that demarcate the boundaries of the secondary pulmonary lobules. Note that the interlobular septa are not always visible in normal individuals but their location can be inferred through identification of the septal veins.
(Bottom) Coned down CT of the left lower lobe shows pulmonary veins outlining secondary pulmonary lobules. The vessels in the center of the space bound by the septal veins represent the central lobular arteries of the secondary pulmonary lobules. Note that vascular structures are not visible in the subpleural lung parenchyma.

VASCULAR STRUCTURE

THE PULMONARY LYMPHATICS

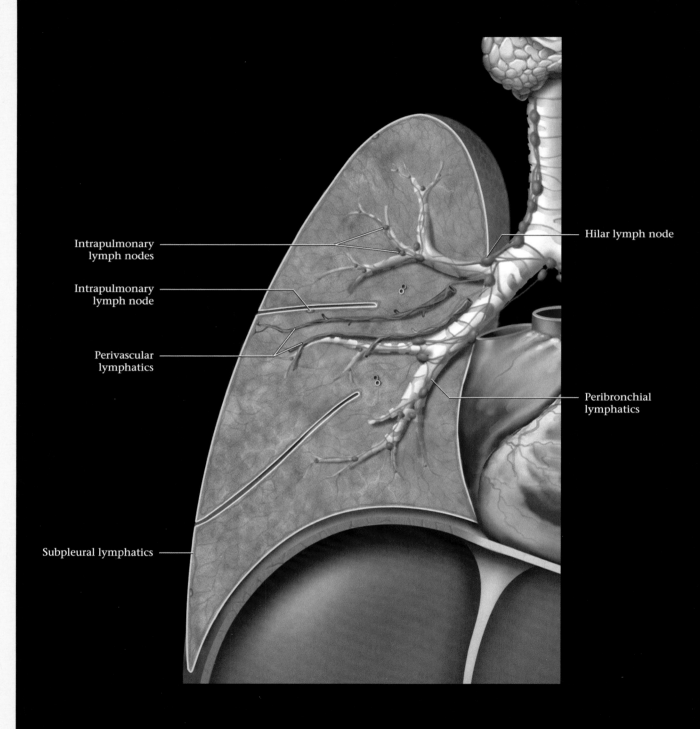

Intrapulmonary
lymph nodes

Intrapulmonary
lymph node

Perivascular
lymphatics

Subpleural lymphatics

Hilar lymph node

Peribronchial
lymphatics

Graphic shows the complex lymphatic network of the lungs. The pulmonary lymphatics are found along bronchi, vessels, and in the subpleural connective tissue. Collecting lymphatics also course within the pulmonary connective tissue septa. The lymphatic network becomes organized as small intrapulmonary lymph nodes that typically occur at the bifurcations of large airways.

VASCULAR STRUCTURE

LYMPHATICS OF SECONDARY PULMONARY LOBULE

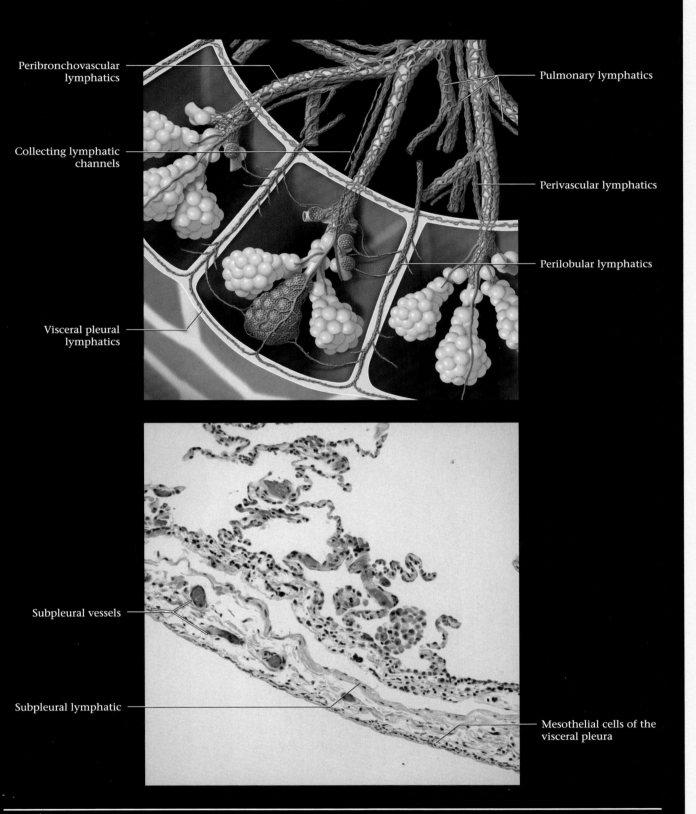

Peribronchovascular lymphatics

Pulmonary lymphatics

Collecting lymphatic channels

Perivascular lymphatics

Perilobular lymphatics

Visceral pleural lymphatics

Subpleural vessels

Subpleural lymphatic

Mesothelial cells of the visceral pleura

(Top) Graphic shows the complex lymphatic channels within the secondary pulmonary lobule (SPL). Peribronchovascular lymphatics course along the airway walls to the level of the respiratory bronchioles. Perilobular lymphatics course in the interlobular septa and surround the pulmonary veins. Visceral pleural lymphatics are also illustrated. Pulmonary lymphatics are numerous and complex interconnecting vascular structures. Understanding the structure and anatomic location of the lymphatics of the SPL is important in identifying a perilymphatic distribution of disease on thin-section CT. **(Bottom)** High-power photomicrograph (Hematoxylin and Eosin stain) shows a visceral pleural lymphatic channel surrounded by loose connective tissue and visceral pleural vessels, likely pulmonary veins.

VASCULAR STRUCTURE

RANDOM NODULES & NODULES RELATED TO SMALL VESSELS, PULMONARY METASTASES

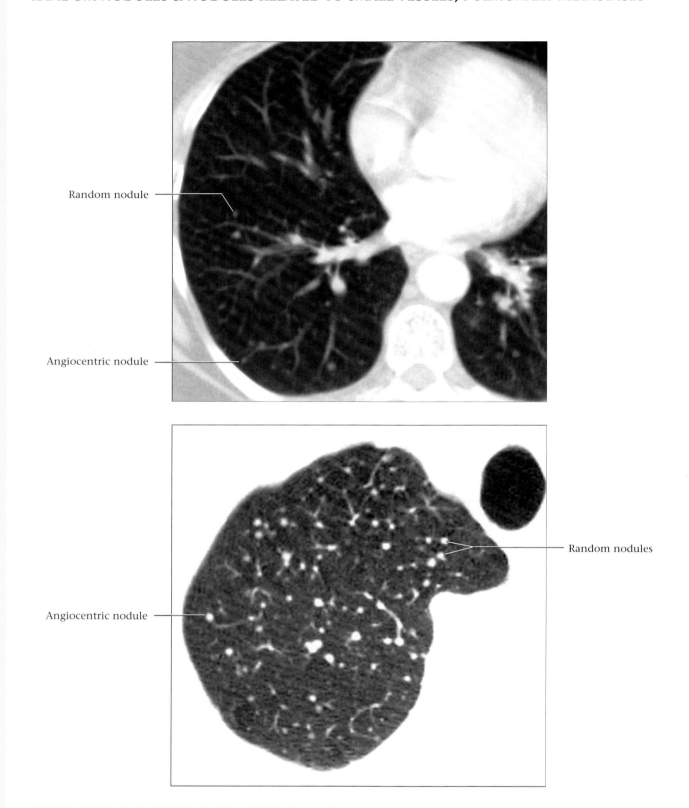

Random nodule

Angiocentric nodule

Random nodules

Angiocentric nodule

(Top) Contrast-enhanced chest CT (lung window) of a patient with metastatic thyroid carcinoma demonstrates the random distribution of hematogenous metastatic nodules. Some of the nodules exhibit a relationship to small pulmonary vessels occurring at the distal ends of small pulmonary artery branches. This finding is characteristic of hematogenous dissemination of disease and can be seen in secondary neoplasia, hematogenous infection, vasculitis and embolic disease. **(Bottom)** HRCT of a patient with metastatic colon cancer demonstrates tiny spherical well-defined metastatic pulmonary nodules that exhibit a random distribution. Some of the nodules occur at the distal ends of pulmonary arteries denoting their hematogenous route of dissemination.

VASCULAR STRUCTURE

RANDOM NODULES, MILIARY TUBERCULOSIS

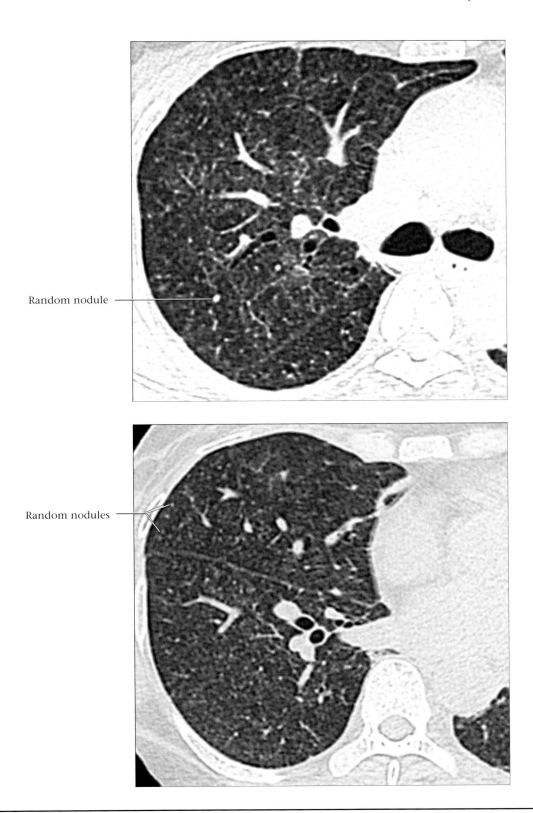

Random nodule

Random nodules

(Top) First of two sections from a high-resolution CT (lung window) of a patient with miliary tuberculosis. HRCT through the right upper lobe shows multifocal tiny pulmonary nodules throughout the lung that exhibit a random distribution. In this case some of the nodules are located in the subpleural lung parenchyma and along interlobular septa. (Bottom) HRCT through the right lower and right middle lobes shows profuse micronodules that exhibit a random distribution although some of the nodules are located in the subpleural lung parenchyma along the interlobar fissure. Although the mode of disease dissemination in this case is hematogenous it is difficult to associate the nodules to small pulmonary vessels.

VASCULAR STRUCTURE

PERILYMPHATIC NODULES, SARCOIDOSIS

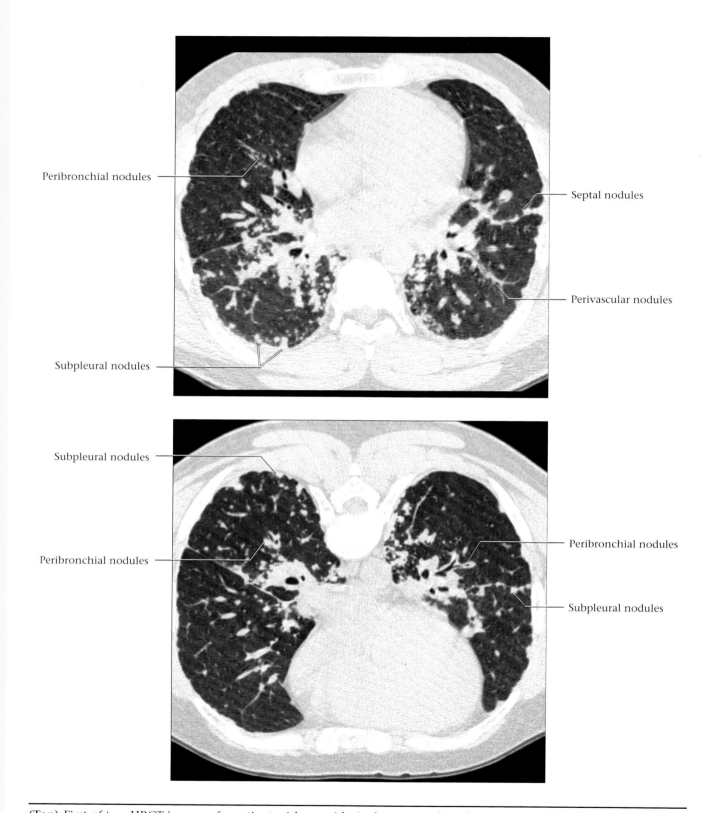

Peribronchial nodules

Septal nodules

Perivascular nodules

Subpleural nodules

Subpleural nodules

Peribronchial nodules

Peribronchial nodules

Subpleural nodules

(Top) First of two HRCT images of a patient with sarcoidosis shows a perilymphatic distribution of pulmonary nodules representing granulomas. Supine HRCT shows nodules arranged in the anatomic distribution of the pulmonary lymphatics and located along vascular structures, along airways and along the pleural surfaces and the interlobular septa. **(Bottom)** Prone HRCT shows persistence of posterior subpleural micronodules. The beaded appearance of the left interlobar fissure results from micronodules situated along subpleural lymphatics. Note the irregular thickening of the bronchial walls consistent with peribronchial nodules. This case is representative of the characteristic perilymphatic distribution of the granulomas seen in patients with sarcoidosis. Silicosis and coal worker's pneumoconiosis can produce similar findings.

VASCULAR STRUCTURE

PERILYMPHATIC NODULES, LYMPHANGITIC CARCINOMATOSIS

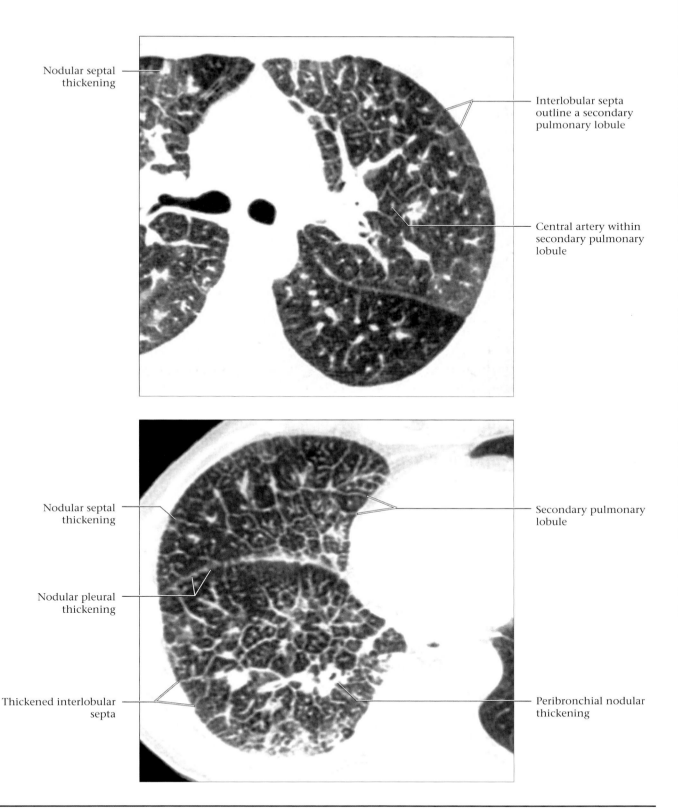

Nodular septal thickening

Interlobular septa outline a secondary pulmonary lobule

Central artery within secondary pulmonary lobule

Nodular septal thickening

Secondary pulmonary lobule

Nodular pleural thickening

Thickened interlobular septa

Peribronchial nodular thickening

(Top) HRCT (lung window) of a patient with lymphangitic carcinomatosis shows smooth and nodular thickening of the interlobular septa, which demarcate the boundaries of the secondary pulmonary lobules. The central dot-like structures within the secondary pulmonary lobules represent the lobular arteries. (Bottom) HRCT (lung window) through the right lower and middle lobes of a patient with lymphangitic carcinomatosis shows a beaded appearance of the right interlobar fissure, smooth and nodular thickening of the interlobular septa and peribronchial thickening. Lymphangitic carcinomatosis is characterized by tumor in pulmonary lymphatics and desmoplasia in the surrounding interstitium, and exhibits a perilymphatic distribution on CT. Lymphoma, leukemia and other lymphoproliferative disorders can also produce these findings.

INTERSTITIAL NETWORK

Terminology

Abbreviations
- High-resolution CT (HRCT)

Overview of Pulmonary Interstitium

Embryology
- Embryologic remnant of splanchnopleuric mesenchymal bed
  - Site of airway and vessel ingrowth during lung morphogenesis

Anatomy
- Continuum of loose connective tissue
  - Extends from pulmonary hila to visceral pleura
    - Anchored at hila
    - Under tension by negative visceral pleural (intrapleural) pressure

Microscopic Features
- Fine reticulin fibers
- Fine elastin fibers
- Coarser collagen fibers
- Most prominent around large bronchovascular structures

Components of Pulmonary Interstitium
- Matrix components
  - Fibrous network of collagen and elastin fibers
    - Collagen fibers: Inextensible
    - Elastin fibers: Extensible
- Cellular components
  - Fibroblasts
  - Mast cells
  - Tissue macrophages
  - Lymphocytes
- Continuous epithelial and endothelial basement membranes
  - Form barriers defining outer borders of interstitium

Function of Pulmonary Interstitium
- Provides lung with structural integrity
- Permits lung deformation during respiration

Interstitial Fiber Network

Three Subdivisions Forming a Continuum
- **Axial (bronchoarterial)**
- **Parenchymal (intralobular)**
- **Peripheral (subpleural)**

Axial (Bronchoarterial)
- Surrounds bronchoarterial bundles
- Extends from hila to respiratory bronchioles in lung periphery

Parenchymal (Intralobular)
- Fine network of very thin connective tissue fibers within alveolar walls
- Situated between alveolar and capillary basement membranes
- Supports structures of secondary pulmonary lobule

Peripheral (Subpleural)
- Situated between pleura and lung parenchyma
- Continuous with interlobular septa and perivenous interstitial space
- Extends from lung periphery to hila

Imaging Normal Pulmonary Interstitium

Radiographs
- Typically invisible
- Thin or imperceptible fissural lines demarcate subpleural interstitium
- Visualization of interstitium on radiography should suggest interstitial lung disease

HRCT
- Typically invisible
- Occasional visualization of interlobular septa
  - Typically located along peripheral pulmonary veins
- Imperceptible axial interstitial network
  - Along bronchovascular bundles

Imaging of Interstitial Lung Disease

Chest Radiography
- Limited by spatial resolution and overlapping parenchymal structures
- Useful for depicting distribution and temporal progression of interstitial abnormalities

HRCT
- General concepts
  - Individual HRCT scans sample lung at spaced levels
  - Multidetector HRCT allows volumetric HRCT of entire lungs during single breath-hold
- Technical factors
  - Thin collimation
    - 1-1.5 mm
  - High-resolution algorithm for image reconstruction
  - Full inspiration
  - Optional prone imaging
  - Optional expiratory imaging
- Utility of HRCT
  - Greater sensitivity and specificity than chest radiography
  - Demonstrates gross lung anatomy
  - Characterizes abnormal findings better than chest radiography

Chest Radiography of Abnormal Pulmonary Interstitium

Linear (Septal) Opacities
- Thickening of **interlobular septa**
- Classified by location, extent and orientation as **Kerley lines**
- **Kerley A lines**
  - Straight linear opacities in upper lung

INTERSTITIAL NETWORK

- 2-6 cm in length
- 1-3 mm in width
- Point toward hilum centrally; directed towards lung periphery
- Extend towards but not to pleural surface
- **Kerley B lines**
  - Straight linear opacities predominantly in lower lung
    - 1.5-2 cm in length
    - 1-2 mm in width
  - Perpendicular to and in contact with the pleura
- **Kerley C lines**
  - Branching linear opacities seen at lung bases
  - Fine and net-like
  - Represent Kerley B lines seen en face

Peribronchial Cuffing

- Thickening of axial (bronchoarterial) interstitium
- Seen as apparent bronchial wall thickening when visualized end-on
- Most apparent in perihilar regions

Perihilar Haze

- Interstitial edema surrounding bronchoarterial bundles
- Results in blurring of vascular borders
- Best appreciated in comparison to prior radiographs

Reticular and Nodular Opacities

- **Reticular opacities**
  - Multiple intersecting irregular lines
    - Fine: < 3 mm thick
    - Medium: 3-10 mm thick
    - Coarse: > 10 mm thick
- **Nodular opacities**
  - Interstitial nodules
  - Characteristically small
    - 1-2 mm
  - Typically well-defined borders
- **Reticulonodular opacities**
  - Perceived combination of lines and dots; often artifactual
  - Superimposition of lines/reticulation may mimic nodules
  - Superimposition of nodules may mimic reticulation

HRCT of Abnormal Pulmonary Interstitium

Reticular Opacities

- Multiple intersecting irregular lines with a net-like appearance
- **Interlobular septal thickening**
  - Smooth
    - Pulmonary edema
    - Lymphangitic carcinomatosis (often nodular)
  - Nodular
    - Lymphangitic carcinomatosis
    - Sarcoidosis
  - Irregular
    - Fibrosis
    - Associated with architectural distortion and traction bronchiectasis

- **Intralobular interstitial thickening**
  - Fine, reticular mesh-like opacities
  - Often represents early fibrosis
- **Honeycomb lung** (end-stage lung disease)
  - Indicates extensive lung fibrosis
  - Thick-walled, air-filled cysts
    - 3 mm to 3 cm
  - Cysts share walls, occur in several layers in subpleural lung
  - Associated with traction bronchiectasis/bronchiolectasis resulting from lung fibrosis
    - Fibrous tissue produces outward traction on bronchial walls; resultant irregular bronchial dilatation
    - Traction bronchiolectasis involves small airways in peripheral lung
    - Associated with reticular opacities, parenchymal distortion, honeycombing

Nodules

- Interstitial nodules are characteristically small (1-2 mm) and well-defined
- Anatomic distribution may suggest diagnosis

Anatomic Correlates of Specific Interstitial Lung Diseases

Interstitial Pulmonary Edema

- **Radiography**
  - Axial interstitium
    - Prominence of bronchovascular bundles
    - Blurring of bronchial and vascular margins
    - Peribronchial cuffing when visualized end-on
  - Peripheral interstitium
    - Prominence and thickening of interlobar fissures
    - Prominent minor fissure on frontal chest radiograph
    - All fissures prominent on lateral chest radiographs
    - Kerley lines (A and/or B)
- **CT**
  - Axial interstitium
    - Thickening of bronchovascular bundles
  - Peripheral interstitium
    - Smooth thickening of interlobular septa

Lymphangitic Carcinomatosis

- **Radiography**
  - Axial interstitium
    - Smooth and nodular thickening of bronchovascular bundles
    - Kerley A lines
  - Peripheral interstitium
    - Smooth and nodular thickening of interlobar fissures
    - Kerley B lines
- **CT**
  - Axial interstitium
    - Smooth and nodular thickening of bronchovascular bundles
    - Centrilobular peribronchovascular thickening
    - Centrilobular nodules

INTERSTITIAL NETWORK

- ○ Peripheral interstitium
  - Smooth and nodular thickening of interlobular septa
  - Smooth and nodular thickening of interlobar fissures

Sarcoidosis
- **Radiography**
  - ○ Axial interstitium
    - Thickening of bronchovascular bundles
    - Reticular and nodular opacities may emanate from lung hila
    - Predominant involvement of mid and upper lung zones
  - ○ Peripheral interstitium
    - Thickening, nodularity of interlobular septa and interlobar fissures
- **CT**
  - ○ Axial interstitium
    - Small nodules along bronchovascular bundles
    - Thickening of bronchovascular bundles
  - ○ Peripheral interstitium
    - Small nodules along interlobular septa
    - Small nodules along interlobar fissures
    - Small subpleural nodules

Interstitial Fibrosis
- **Radiography**
  - ○ Peripheral interstitium
    - Reticular opacities
    - Predominantly involve peripheral and basilar lungs
  - ○ Parenchymal interstitium
    - Fine basilar reticular opacities
    - Volume loss with progressive lung fibrosis
- **CT**
  - ○ Peripheral interstitium
    - Irregular thickening of interlobular septa
    - Irregular thickening of interlobar fissures
    - Irregular interface with mediastinal pleural surface
  - ○ Parenchymal interstitium
    - Intralobular reticular opacities
    - Associated traction bronchiectasis

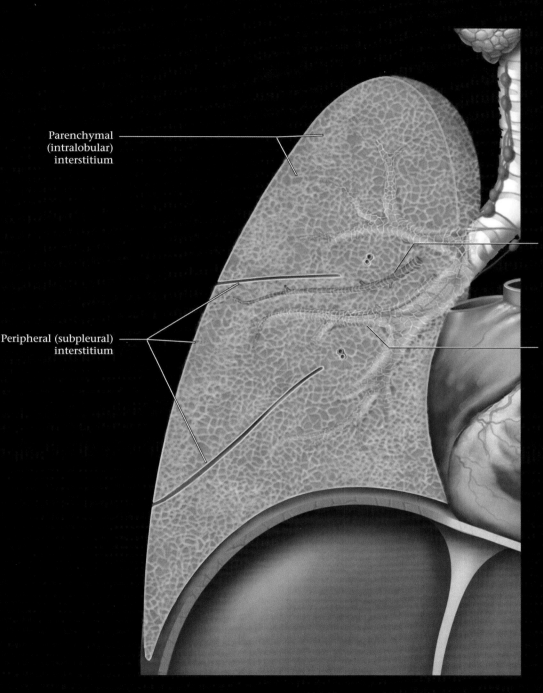

Parenchymal (intralobular) interstitium

Interstitial sheath around pulmonary vein

Peripheral (subpleural) interstitium

Axial interstitium along bronchovascular bundle

Graphic shows axial (bronchoarterial) interstitium extending along the bronchovascular structures from the hilum to the lung periphery. The peripheral (subpleural/interlobular septal) interstitium extends along the subpleural region, including the interlobar fissures, and contiguously along interlobular septa, extending back to the lung hila with the pulmonary veins and lymphatics. The fine interstitial network of the parenchymal (intralobular) interstitium is seen throughout the lung.

INTERSTITIAL NETWORK

AXIAL, PARENCHYMAL & PERIPHERAL INTERSTITIUM

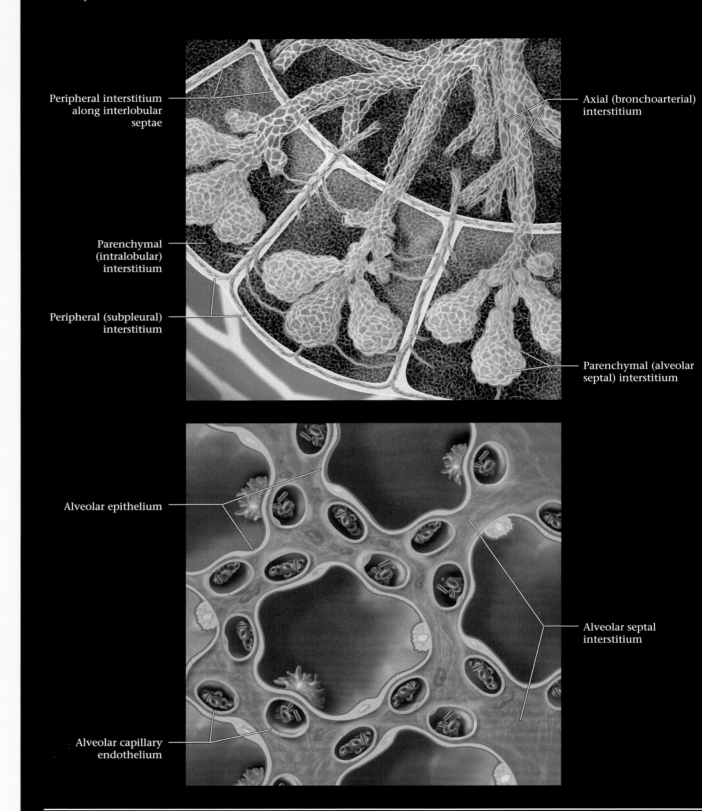

Peripheral interstitium along interlobular septae

Axial (bronchoarterial) interstitium

Parenchymal (intralobular) interstitium

Peripheral (subpleural) interstitium

Parenchymal (alveolar septal) interstitium

Alveolar epithelium

Alveolar septal interstitium

Alveolar capillary endothelium

(Top) Graphic shows the parenchymal and peripheral interstitium of the secondary pulmonary lobule. The peripheral interstitium extends along the subpleural regions and along the interlobular septa with the pulmonary veins and lymphatics towards the pulmonary hilum. The most distal portions of the axial interstitial sheath are shown along the bronchovascular structures as they enter secondary pulmonary lobules. The parenchymal interstitium forms a meshwork around clusters of alveoli and alveolar sacs. A continuous interstitial fiber network within the secondary pulmonary lobule extends to the interlobular septa. **(Bottom)** The parenchymal interstitium is interposed between the capillary endothelium and the alveolar epithelium and is seen within adjacent alveolar septa.

MICROSCOPIC FEATURES OF NORMAL PULMONARY INTERSTITIUM

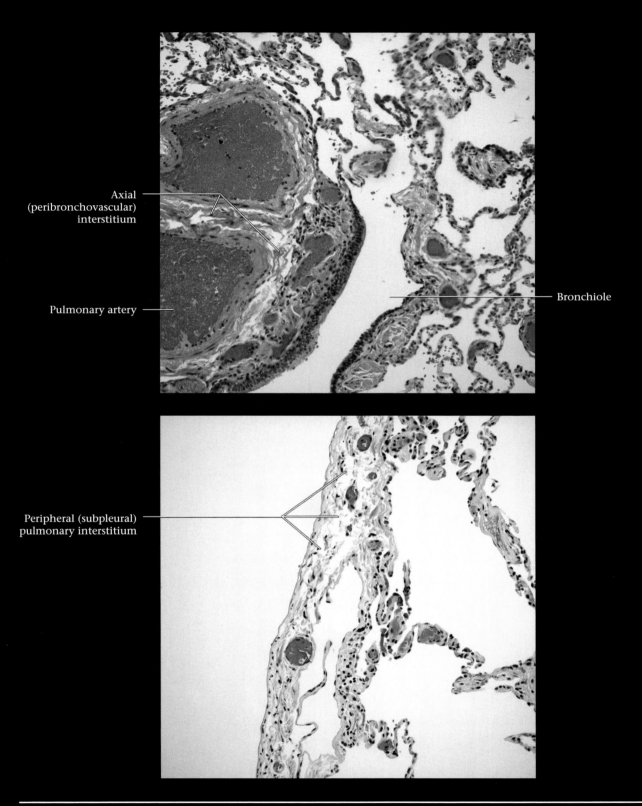

Axial (peribronchovascular) interstitium

Pulmonary artery

Bronchiole

Peripheral (subpleural) pulmonary interstitium

(Top) High-power photomicrograph (Hematoxylin and Eosin stain) shows the fine connective tissue elements that compose the axial (peribronchovascular) interstitium surrounding the pulmonary vessels and the airways. **(Bottom)** High-power photomicrograph (Hematoxylin and Eosin stain) shows the peripheral (subpleural) pulmonary interstitium. Fine collagen and elastin fibers occupy the subpleural region and surround subpleural vessels and lymphatics.

INTERSTITIAL NETWORK

RADIOGRAPHY OF NORMAL PULMONARY INTERSTITIUM

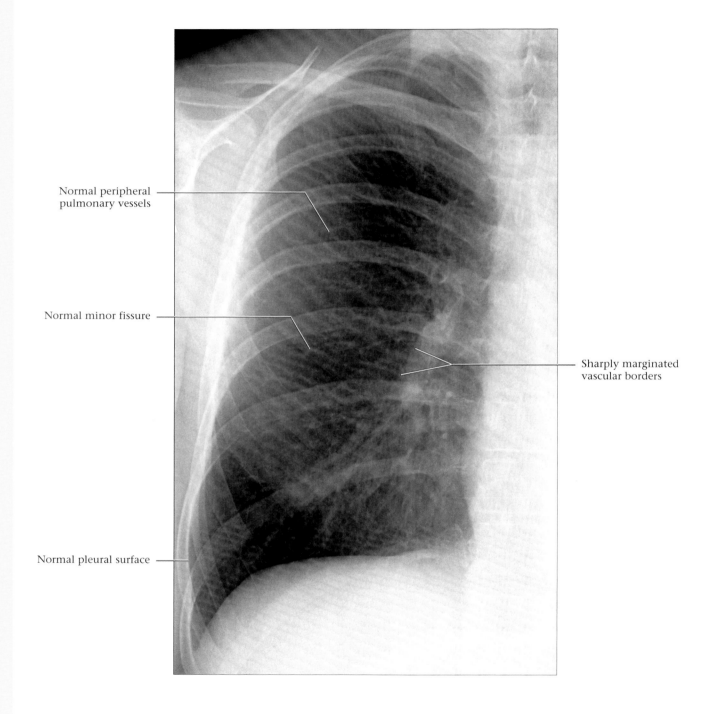

Normal peripheral pulmonary vessels

Normal minor fissure

Sharply marginated vascular borders

Normal pleural surface

First of two normal chest radiographs of the same patient. PA chest radiograph coned down to the right lung shows normal pulmonary markings. The pulmonary vascular structures taper normally towards the lung periphery. The borders of the vascular structures are sharp. The pleural surfaces are imperceptible and the minor fissure is poorly visualized.

INTERSTITIAL NETWORK

RADIOGRAPHY OF NORMAL PULMONARY INTERSTITIUM

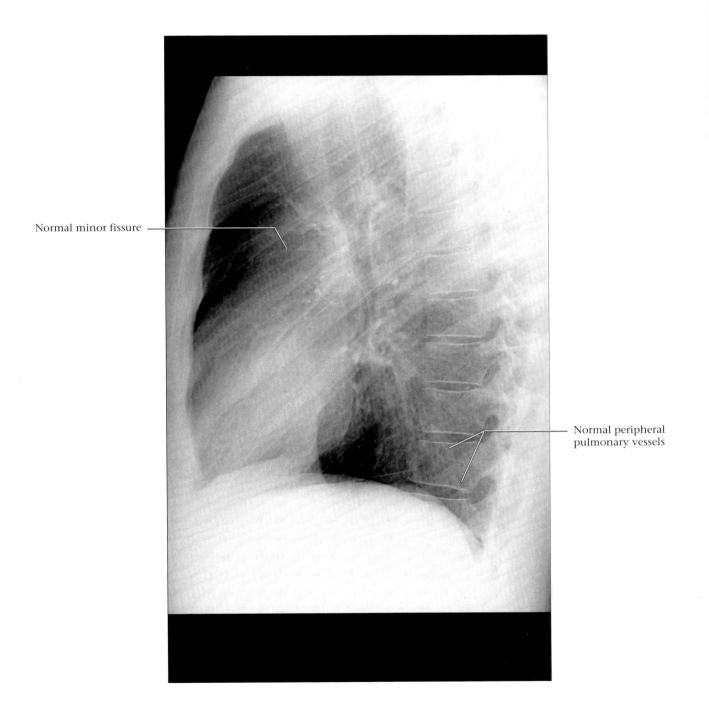

Normal minor fissure

Normal peripheral pulmonary vessels

Left lateral chest radiograph shows normal vasculature in the lung periphery. The normal minor fissure is visible as a thin white line. Ill-definition of pulmonary vessels, thickening of the fissures and pleural surfaces, thickening of bronchovascular bundles and visualization of interstitial opacities should suggest interstitial lung disease.

INTERSTITIAL NETWORK

ANATOMIC-HRCT CORRELATION

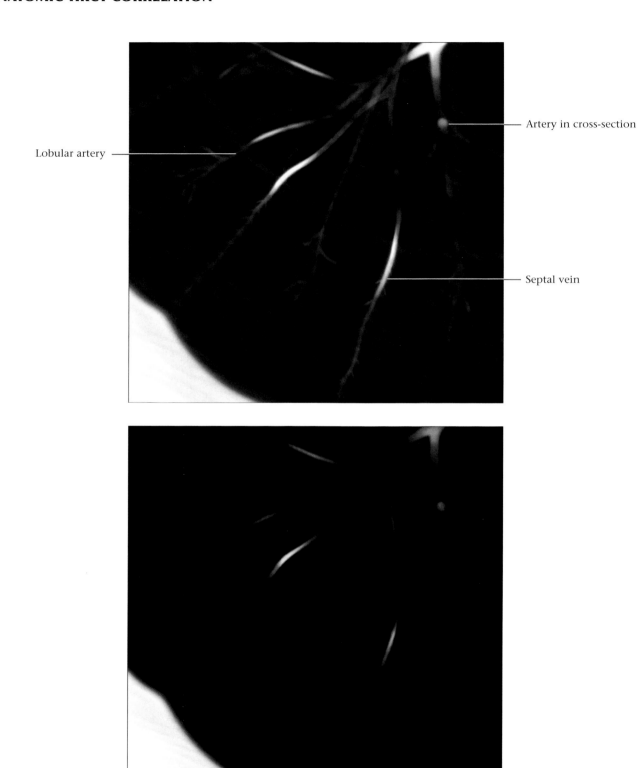

Lobular artery

Artery in cross-section

Septal vein

(Top) Graphic shows the anatomy of the peripheral lung at the level of the secondary pulmonary lobule. Acinar structures within the secondary pulmonary lobule are supplied by branching pulmonary arteries and drained by pulmonary veins and lymphatics. The central vascular structures of the pulmonary lobule and the peripheral vascular structures within the interlobular septa are highlighted. These are the structures that can be resolved with HRCT. **(Bottom)** Graphic shows the portions of the underlying anatomy that are typically visible on normal HRCT. Short segments of tapering arteries and veins may be visualized. Small portions of interlobular septa are occasionally visualized in normal individuals.

INTERSTITIAL NETWORK

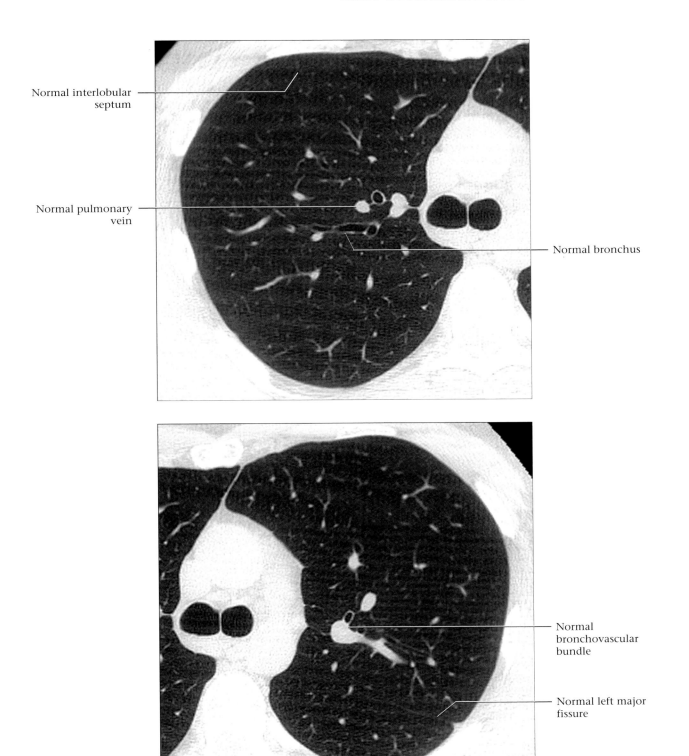

Normal interlobular septum

Normal pulmonary vein

Normal bronchus

Normal bronchovascular bundle

Normal left major fissure

(Top) First of two normal axial HRCT images of the same patient show the CT appearance of the interstitium which is not visible in normal subjects. HRCT through the right upper lobe shows normal vascular and bronchial structures. Peripheral subpleural linear structures perpendicular to the pleural surface likely represent interlobular septa containing normal septal veins and their surrounding interstitium. **(Bottom)** HRCT through the left upper lobe shows normal vessels, bronchi and pleural markings. The left major fissure is partially visualized and manifests as a thin delicate line that separates the left upper lobe from the left lower lobe. The normal subpleural interstitium is not visible.

INTERSTITIAL NETWORK

RADIOGRAPHY OF INTERSTITIAL PULMONARY EDEMA

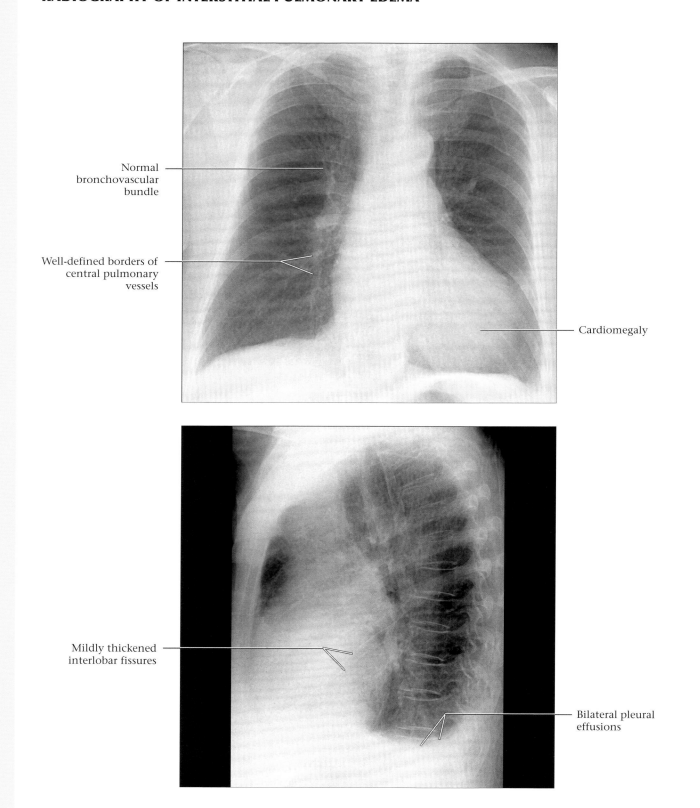

Normal bronchovascular bundle

Well-defined borders of central pulmonary vessels

Cardiomegaly

Mildly thickened interlobar fissures

Bilateral pleural effusions

(Top) First of four chest radiographs of a patient with chronic heart failure shows the radiographic appearance of the abnormal pulmonary interstitium. PA chest radiograph shows cardiomegaly, an atherosclerotic partially calcified aorta and a relatively normal pulmonary interstitium. The vascular structures of the lung are normal in caliber and distribution and their borders are well-defined. A bronchovascular bundle in the right upper lobe exhibits no bronchial wall thickening. **(Bottom)** Lateral chest radiograph shows mild thickening of the interlobar fissures and bilateral pleural effusions that manifest as blunting of the posterior costodiaphragmatic recesses.

INTERSTITIAL NETWORK

RADIOGRAPHY OF INTERSTITIAL PULMONARY EDEMA

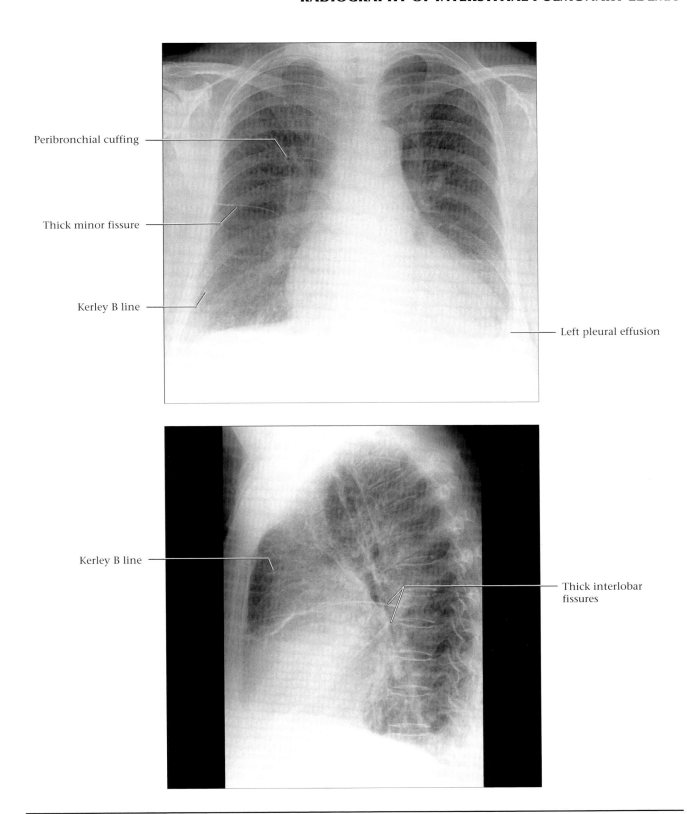

Peribronchial cuffing

Thick minor fissure

Kerley B line

Left pleural effusion

Kerley B line

Thick interlobar fissures

(Top) PA chest radiograph obtained after exacerbation of interstitial pulmonary edema shows engorgement of pulmonary vascular structures with blurring of vessel margins in the perihilar regions. Note thickening of the minor fissure and "peribronchial cuffing" around the bronchovascular bundle seen end-on in the right suprahilar region. Kerley B lines (septal lines) are demonstrated in the lower lungs, extending inward from and perpendicular to the pleural surface. Bilateral pleural effusions are larger. **(Bottom)** Lateral chest radiograph shows engorgement of pulmonary vessels with blurring of their margins and generalized prominence and smooth thickening of interlobar fissures. Note Kerley B lines (septal lines) in the retrosternal region.

INTERSTITIAL NETWORK

CT OF ABNORMAL INTERSTITIUM, INTERSTITIAL EDEMA

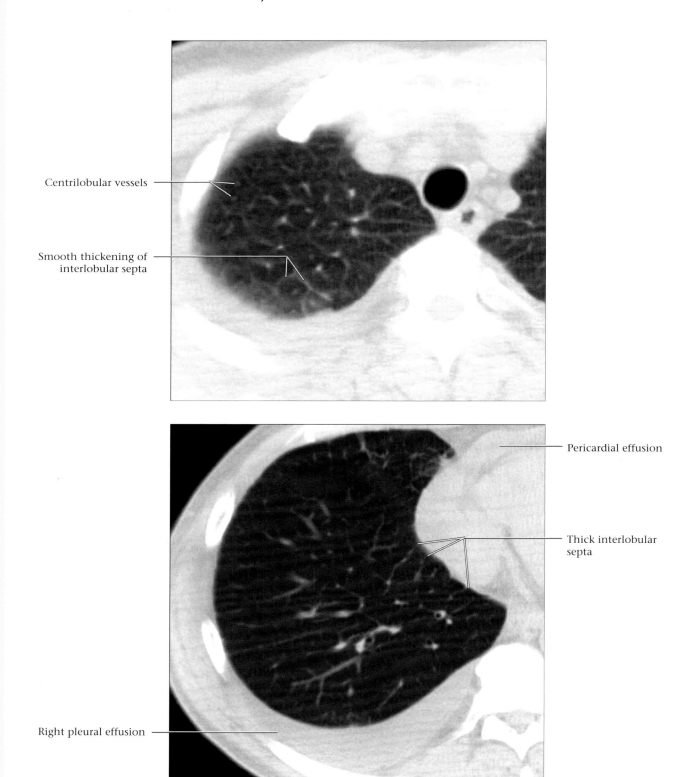

Centrilobular vessels

Smooth thickening of interlobular septa

Pericardial effusion

Thick interlobular septa

Right pleural effusion

(Top) First of four images of an unenhanced chest CT (lung window) of a 49 year old man with interstitial edema and a right pleural effusion shows characteristic CT findings of thickening of the peripheral (interlobular septal) interstitium. CT through the right lung apex shows smooth thickening of the interlobular septa outlining the boundaries of several secondary pulmonary lobules. **(Bottom)** CT image through the right lower and middle lobes shows a right pleural effusion and a pericardial effusion. Smooth septal thickening partially outlines the boundaries of several secondary pulmonary lobules.

INTERSTITIAL NETWORK

CT OF ABNORMAL INTERSTITIUM, INTERSTITIAL EDEMA

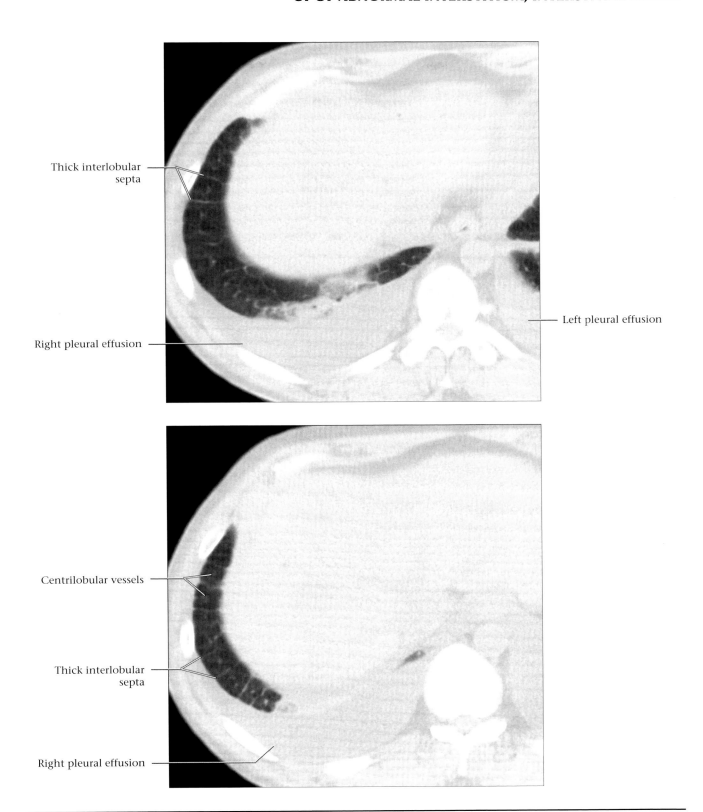

Thick interlobular septa

Right pleural effusion

Left pleural effusion

Centrilobular vessels

Thick interlobular septa

Right pleural effusion

(Top) Image through the right lung base shows bilateral pleural effusions and relaxation atelectasis of the right lower lobe. There is smooth thickening of interlobular septa. **(Bottom)** Image through the right lung base shows prominent smooth thickening of interlobular septa outlining the peripheral boundaries of an arcade of subpleural secondary pulmonary lobules in the inferior aspect of the right lower lobe. Each secondary pulmonary lobule contains a central dot-like opacity that represents the lobular pulmonary artery.

INTERSTITIAL NETWORK

RADIOGRAPHY OF ABNORMAL INTERSTITIUM, SARCOIDOSIS

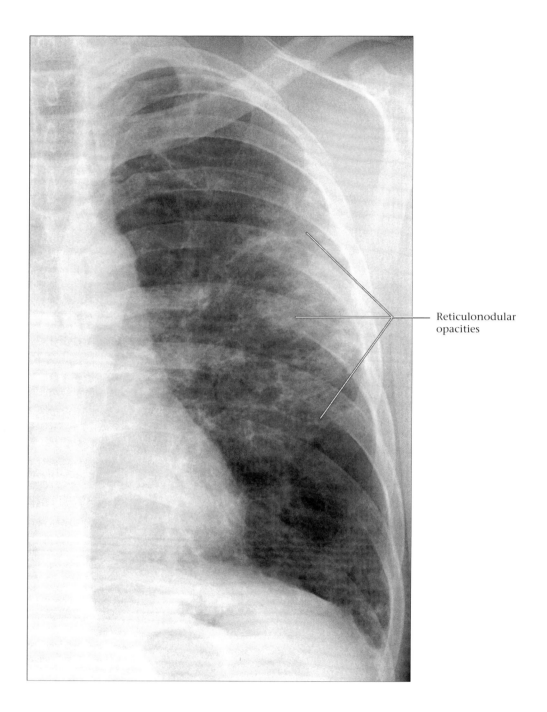

Reticulonodular
opacities

PA chest radiograph of a young man with sarcoidosis coned down to the left lung shows reticulonodular opacities predominantly involving the mid- and upper lung zones and the central portions of the lung.

INTERSTITIAL NETWORK

CT OF ABNORMAL INTERSTITIUM, INTERSTITIAL EDEMA

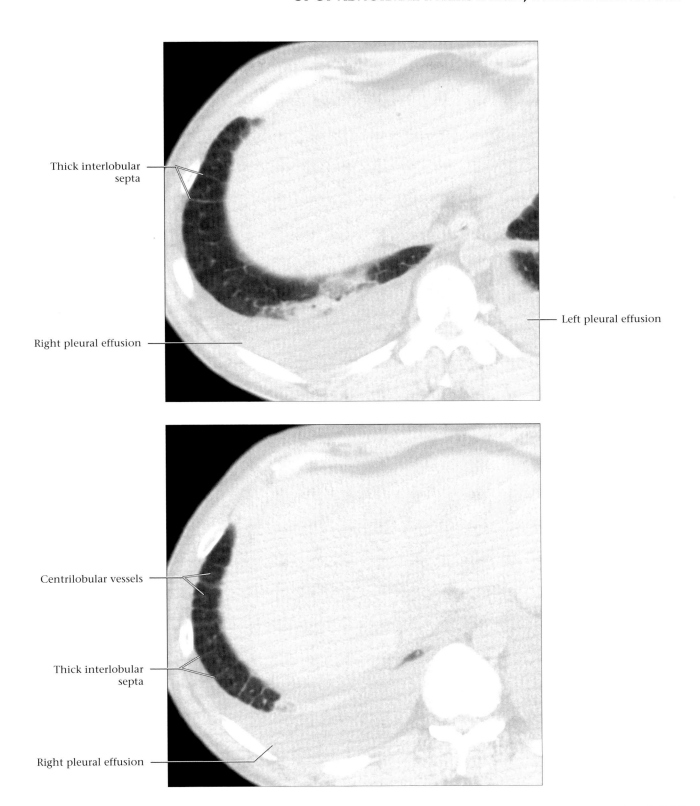

Thick interlobular septa

Right pleural effusion

Left pleural effusion

Centrilobular vessels

Thick interlobular septa

Right pleural effusion

(Top) Image through the right lung base shows bilateral pleural effusions and relaxation atelectasis of the right lower lobe. There is smooth thickening of interlobular septa. **(Bottom)** Image through the right lung base shows prominent smooth thickening of interlobular septa outlining the peripheral boundaries of an arcade of subpleural secondary pulmonary lobules in the inferior aspect of the right lower lobe. Each secondary pulmonary lobule contains a central dot-like opacity that represents the lobular pulmonary artery.

INTERSTITIAL NETWORK

RADIOGRAPHY OF ABNORMAL INTERSTITIUM, LYMPHANGITIC CARCINOMATOSIS

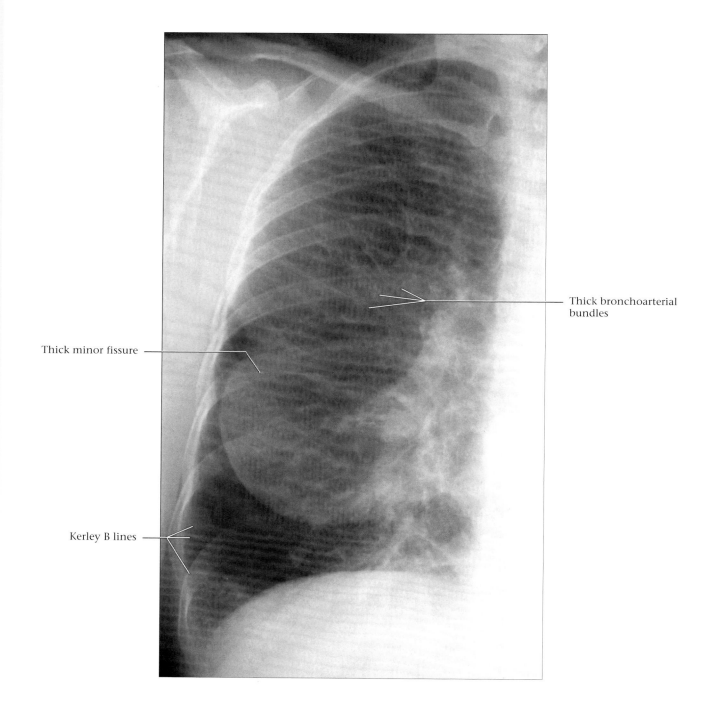

Thick bronchoarterial bundles

Thick minor fissure

Kerley B lines

First of three images of a 46 year old woman with lymphangitic carcinomatosis manifesting with thickening of the interlobular septa. PA chest radiograph coned down to the right lung shows thickening of the bronchoarterial bundles and numerous Kerley B lines that course perpendicularly towards the right visceral pleura. Thickening of the minor fissure reflects involvement of the subpleural interstitium.

INTERSTITIAL NETWORK

HRCT OF ABNORMAL INTERSTITIUM, LYMPHANGITIC CARCINOMATOSIS

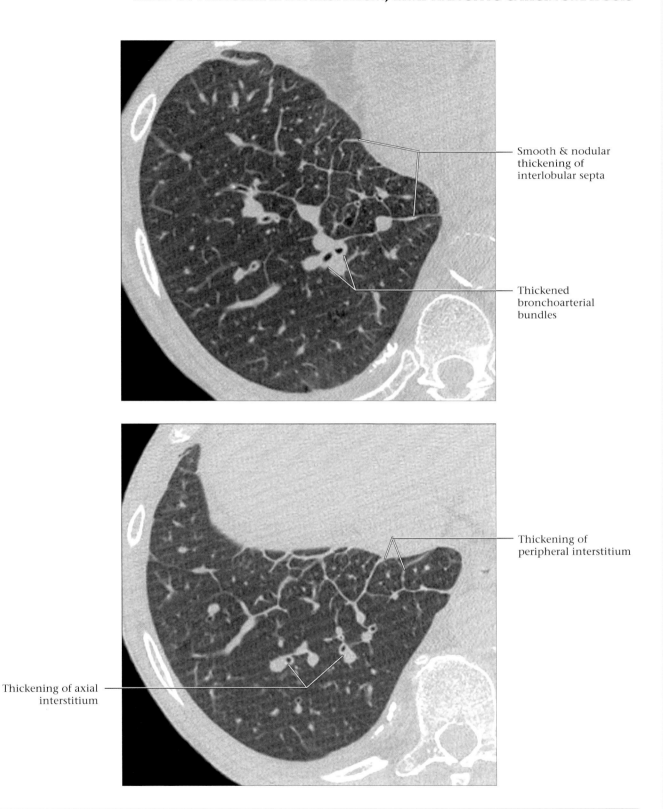

Smooth & nodular thickening of interlobular septa

Thickened bronchoarterial bundles

Thickening of peripheral interstitium

Thickening of axial interstitium

(Top) Axial HRCT of the right lung base shows smooth and nodular thickening of the interlobular septa outlining secondary pulmonary lobules. There is also tumor involvement of the axial interstitium that manifests with thickening of the bronchial walls and bronchoarterial bundles. **(Bottom)** Axial HRCT of the right lung base shows thickening of the axial and peripheral interstitial tissues. The axial interstitium is located along bronchoarterial bundles. The peripheral interstitium is located in the subpleural region and in the interlobular septa.

INTERSTITIAL NETWORK

RADIOGRAPHY OF ABNORMAL INTERSTITIUM, SARCOIDOSIS

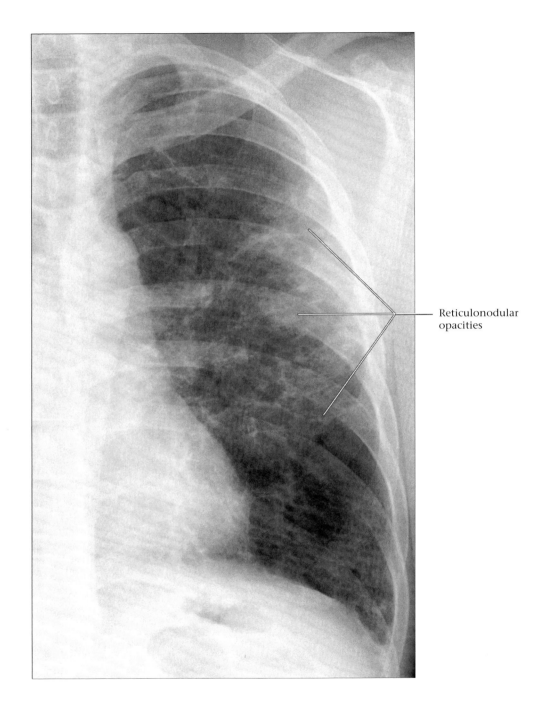

Reticulonodular
opacities

PA chest radiograph of a young man with sarcoidosis coned down to the left lung shows reticulonodular opacities predominantly involving the mid- and upper lung zones and the central portions of the lung.

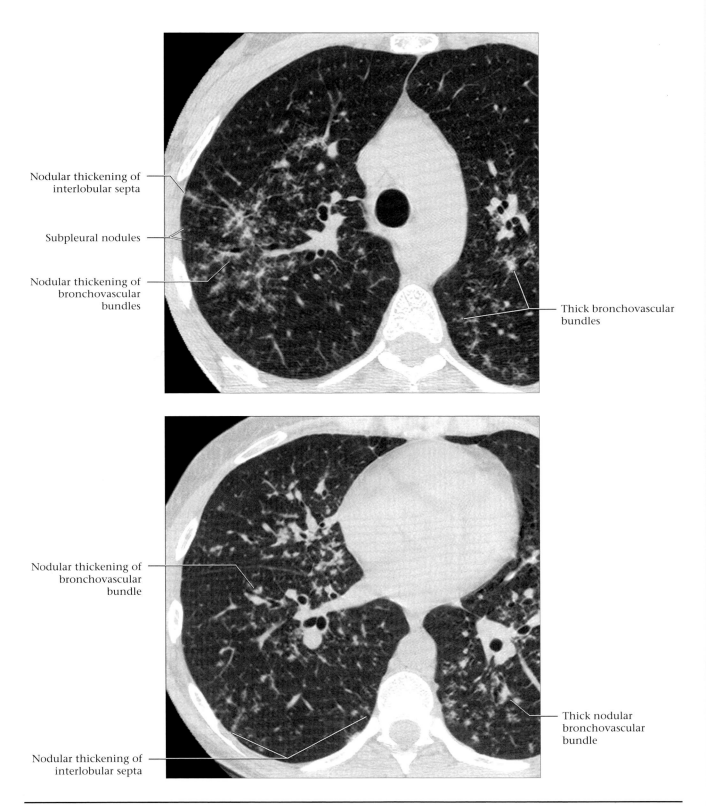

Nodular thickening of interlobular septa

Subpleural nodules

Nodular thickening of bronchovascular bundles

Thick bronchovascular bundles

Nodular thickening of bronchovascular bundle

Thick nodular bronchovascular bundle

Nodular thickening of interlobular septa

(Top) First of two axial HRCT scans of a patient with sarcoidosis shows nodular thickening of bronchovascular/bronchoarterial bundles (axial interstitium) and interlobular septa (peripheral interstitium) with several subpleural nodules (peripheral interstitium). **(Bottom)** Image through the lower lungs shows nodular thickening of bronchovascular bundles and interlobular septa.

INTERSTITIAL NETWORK

RADIOGRAPHY OF ABNORMAL INTERSTITIUM, IDIOPATHIC PULMONARY FIBROSIS

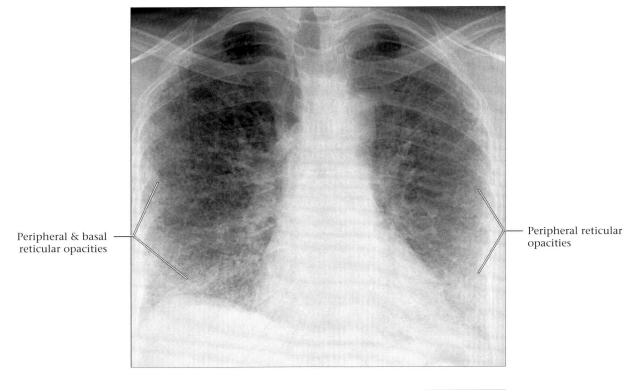

Peripheral & basal reticular opacities

Peripheral reticular opacities

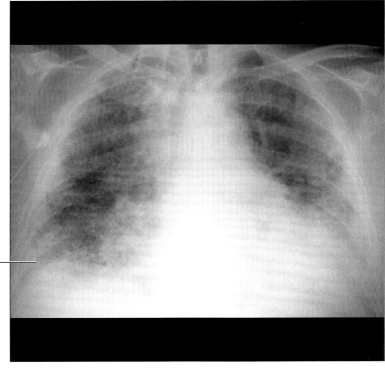

Coarse peripheral reticular opacities

(Top) PA chest radiograph of a patient with idiopathic pulmonary fibrosis (IPF) shows reticular opacities that predominantly involve the peripheral and basal aspects of both lungs. (Bottom) PA chest radiograph of a patient with advanced idiopathic pulmonary fibrosis shows moderate to coarse reticular opacities that predominantly involve the peripheral and basal aspects of both lungs.

INTERSTITIAL NETWORK

HRCT OF ABNORMAL INTERSTITIUM, IDIOPATHIC PULMONARY FIBROSIS

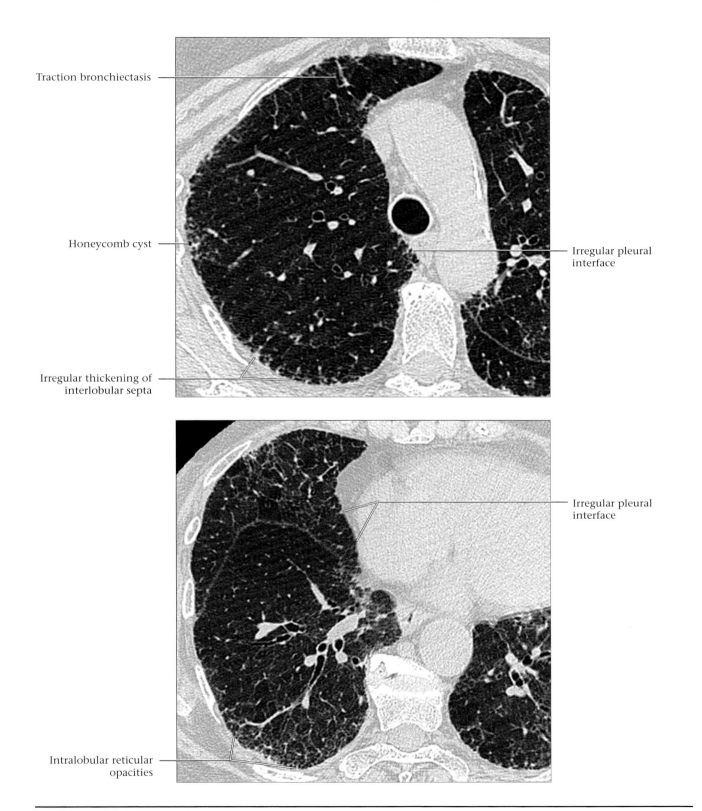

Traction bronchiectasis

Honeycomb cyst

Irregular pleural interface

Irregular thickening of interlobular septa

Irregular pleural interface

Intralobular reticular opacities

(Top) First of two axial HRCT images of a patient with early idiopathic pulmonary fibrosis shows diffuse involvement of the peripheral and parenchymal interstitium. HRCT through the right upper lobe shows irregular thickening of interlobular septa that results in irregular pleural interfaces. The diagnosis of underlying fibrosis is supported by the presence of traction bronchiectasis and subtle subpleural honeycombing manifesting with tiny subpleural cystic changes. (Bottom) HRCT through the lower lungs shows irregular thickening of interlobular septa, intralobular reticular opacities and irregular pleural interfaces. Interstitial fibrosis results in visualization of an abnormal pulmonary interstitium.

LUNGS

Terminology

Abbreviations
- Right upper lobe (**RUL**)
- Middle lobe (**ML**)
- Right lower lobe (**RLL**)
- Left upper lobe (**LUL**)
- Left lower lobe (**LLL**)

Definitions
- **Middle lobe:** Frequently used to refer to right middle lobe as there is normally no left middle lobe
- **Lingula:** Tongue like morphology of inferior aspect of left upper lobe, equivalent to contralateral middle lobe

Anatomy

General Anatomy
- Two lungs, each on either side of the mediastinum
- Each lung lined by visceral pleura
- Each lung freely mobile within pleural space with medial attachments at hilum and pulmonary ligament
- **Right lung**
  - Largest
    - Three lobes
    - Some spatial medial encroachment by adjacent right mediastinal structures
  - Lobes
    - **Right upper lobe**
    - **Middle lobe**
    - **Right lower lobe**
- **Left lung**
  - Smallest
    - Two lobes
    - Larger spatial medial encroachment by left mediastinal structures

Surface Anatomy
- Shape
  - Each lung resembles a half a cone morphologically
- Anatomic landmarks of the lung
  - One apex
  - One base
  - Two surfaces
  - Three borders
- **Apex**
  - Most superior extent of the lung
    - Level with posteromedial first rib
    - Apex 3-4 cm above first costal cartilage
    - Apex 2.5 cm above medial clavicle
- **Base**
  - Concave semilunar morphology adapted to the shape of adjacent diaphragm
    - Deeper concavity in right lung base
  - Slight vertical orientation posteriorly
    - Posterolateral inferior extension into costodiaphragmatic recesses
- Surfaces
  - **Costal surface**
    - Convex morphology
    - Indented by the ribs
  - **Mediastinal** or **medial surface**

- Mediastinal (anterior) and vertebral (posterior) components
- Surrounds the hilum
- Anterior concavity to accommodate mediastinal structures
- Right cardiac indentation, predominantly from right atrium
- Left cardiac indentation, predominantly from left ventricle
- Right lung indented by superior and inferior venae cavae, azygos vein, esophagus, right brachiocephalic vein
- Left lung indented by aortic arch, descending aorta, esophagus, left brachiocephalic vein, left subclavian artery
- Borders
  - **Inferior border**
    - Separates base from costal surface
  - **Posterior border**
    - Separates costal surface from mediastinal surface
  - **Anterior border**
    - Separates costal surface from mediastinal surface
    - Right anterior border is vertically oriented
    - Left anterior border exhibits an inferior concavity or **left cardiac notch**

Lobes

Boundaries
- Lobar boundaries defined by adjacent pleural fissures
- **Right major fissure**
  - Separates upper and middle lobes from lower lobe
- **Minor fissure**
  - Separates anterior upper lobe from middle lobe
- **Left major fissure**
  - Separates upper lobe from lower lobe
- **Accessory azygos fissure**
  - Gives rise to anomalous lobe within right upper lobe

Internal Structure
- Lobar anatomy related to lobar bronchial branches and corresponding pulmonary arteries that supply the lobes

Right Lung
- **Right upper lobe** (right superior lobe)
- **Middle lobe**
- **Right lower lobe** (right inferior lobe)

Left Lung
- **Left upper lobe** (left superior lobe)
- **Left lower lobe** (left inferior lobe)

Azygos Lobe
- Normal variant seen in approximately 0.5% of chest radiographs
- Reported 2:1 male to female ratio
- Embryology
  - Anomalous development of azygos vein forms accessory **azygos fissure**
- Imaging
  - Visualization of azygos fissure

LUNGS

- Thin curvilinear opacity oriented obliquely in medial right upper lobe
  - Terminates in "teardrop" opacity representing the azygos vein
  - Variable size and morphology of azygos lobe and azygos vein
  - Typically supplied by apical bronchus or its branches

Segments

Internal Structure
- Segmental anatomy related to segmental bronchial branches and corresponding pulmonary arteries that supply the segments

Right Upper Lobe
- **Apical segment**
- **Posterior segment**
  - Abuts superior major and posterolateral minor fissures
  - Abuts posterolateral costal and posterosuperior mediastinal surfaces
- **Anterior segment**
  - Abuts anterior minor fissure
  - Abuts anterolateral costal and mid anterior mediastinal surfaces

Middle Lobe
- **Lateral segment**
  - Abuts inferolateral major and lateral minor fissures
  - Abuts inferior anterolateral costal surface
- **Medial segment**
  - Abuts inferomedial major and anteromedial minor fissures
  - Abuts mid anterior costal and inferior anterior mediastinal (right heart border) surfaces

Right Lower Lobe
- **Superior segment**
  - Abuts superior major fissure
  - Abuts mid posterolateral costal and mid posterior mediastinal surfaces
- **Medial basal segment**
  - Abuts inferomedial major fissure
  - Abuts mid inferior mediastinal surface
- **Anterior basal segment**
  - Abuts inferolateral major fissure
  - Abuts inferior lateral costal surface
- **Lateral basal segment**
  - Abuts posterolateral major fissure
  - Abuts inferior posterolateral costal surface
- **Posterior basal segment**
  - Abuts inferior posteromedial costal and inferior posterior mediastinal surfaces

Left Upper Lobe
- **Apicoposterior segment**
  - Abuts superior major fissure
- **Anterior segment**
  - Abuts anteromedial costal and mid anterior mediastinal surfaces
- **Superior lingular segment**

- Abuts mid lateral major fissure
- Abuts inferior anterolateral costal and mid anterior mediastinal (superior left heart border) surfaces
- **Inferior lingular segment**
  - Abuts inferior major fissure
  - Abuts inferior anteromedial costal and inferior anterior mediastinal (inferior left heart border) surfaces

Left Lower Lobe
- **Superior segment**
  - Abuts superior major fissure
  - Abuts mid posteromedial costal and mid posterior mediastinal surfaces
- **Anteromedial basal segment**
  - Abuts inferior major fissure
  - Abuts inferior mid lateral costal and mid inferior mediastinal surfaces
- **Lateral basal segment**
  - Abuts inferior posterolateral costal surface
- **Posterior basal segment**
  - Abuts inferior posteromedial costal and inferior posterior mediastinal (descending aorta) surfaces

Anatomy Based Imaging Abnormalities

General Principles
- Utilization of lobar/segmental anatomy for **localization of disease**
  - Use of **orthogonal radiographs** to localize lesions within a lobe or segment
- Determination of **volume loss** based on **fissural displacement**
- CT localization of lesions within a lobe or segment
  - Multiplanar reconstructions for accurate localization with respect to fissures
  - **Preoperative assessment** and **staging** of patients with **lung cancer**
    - Lesion localization and exclusion of involvement of adjacent lobes
- Determination of segmental vs. non-segmental abnormalities on ventilation/perfusion nuclear scintigraphy

Sign of the Silhouette
- Obscuration of **right superior mediastinum**
  - **Right upper lobe** airspace disease
- Obscuration of **right cardiac border**
  - **Middle lobe** airspace disease
  - **Middle lobe medial segment** airspace disease
- Obscuration of **left cardiac border**
  - **Lingular** airspace disease
    - Superior and/or inferior lingular segments
- Obscuration of **left superior mediastinum**
  - **Left upper lobe** airspace disease
- Obscuration of **hemidiaphragm**
  - **Lower lobe** airspace disease
- Obscuration of **descending aorta**
  - **Left lower lobe** airspace disease
    - Superior and/or posterior basal segments

LUNGS

OVERVIEW OF THE LUNGS

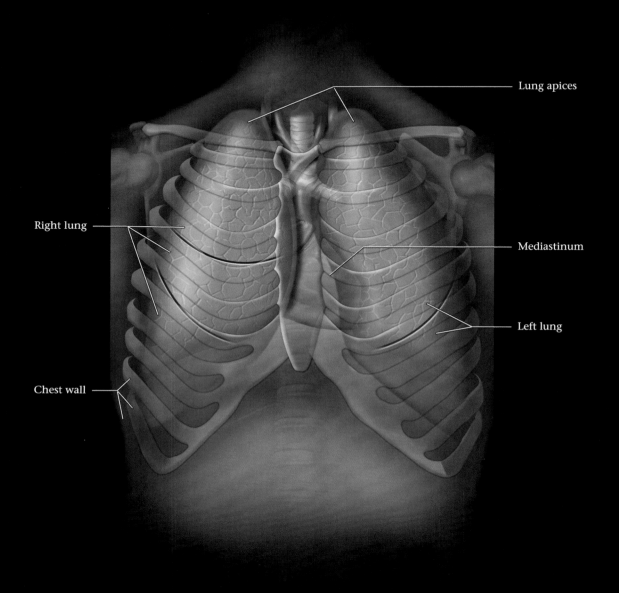

Lung apices

Right lung

Mediastinum

Left lung

Chest wall

Graphic depicts the anatomy of the anterior lungs. The lungs are surrounded by the pleura and the skeletal and soft tissue structures of the chest wall. The two lungs are located on either side of the mediastinum. Each lung is freely mobile within its surrounding pleural space and is attached to the mediastinum at the hilum and pulmonary ligament. The lung apices project above the medial clavicles and anterior first ribs and course towards the roots of the neck. The right lung has three lobes and is larger than the left lung. The left lung has two lobes.

LUNGS

SURFACE ANATOMY, ANTERIOR AND POSTERIOR LUNGS

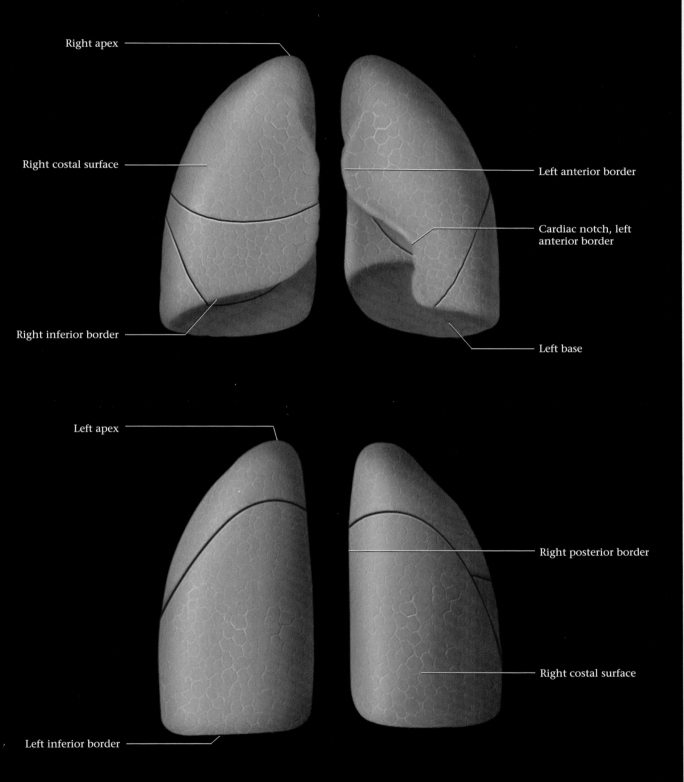

Right apex

Right costal surface

Right inferior border

Left anterior border

Cardiac notch, left anterior border

Left base

Left apex

Right posterior border

Right costal surface

Left inferior border

(Top) Graphic depicts the surface anatomy of the anterior lungs. The shape of each lung resembles that of a half cone. The lung surface anatomy is characterized by an apex, a base, two surfaces and three borders. The apices represent the highest extent of the lungs. The anterior borders separate the anterior costal surfaces from the mediastinal (medial) surfaces. Note the arcuate morphology of the inferior aspect of the left anterior border, the cardiac notch. The costal surfaces are adjacent to the chest wall. The inferior borders separate the costal surfaces from the bases. **(Bottom)** Graphic depicts the posterior lung surfaces. The inferior lung borders separate the costal surfaces from the lung bases. The posterior borders separate the costal surfaces from the mediastinal (medial) surfaces.

LUNGS

SURFACE ANATOMY, LATERAL LUNGS

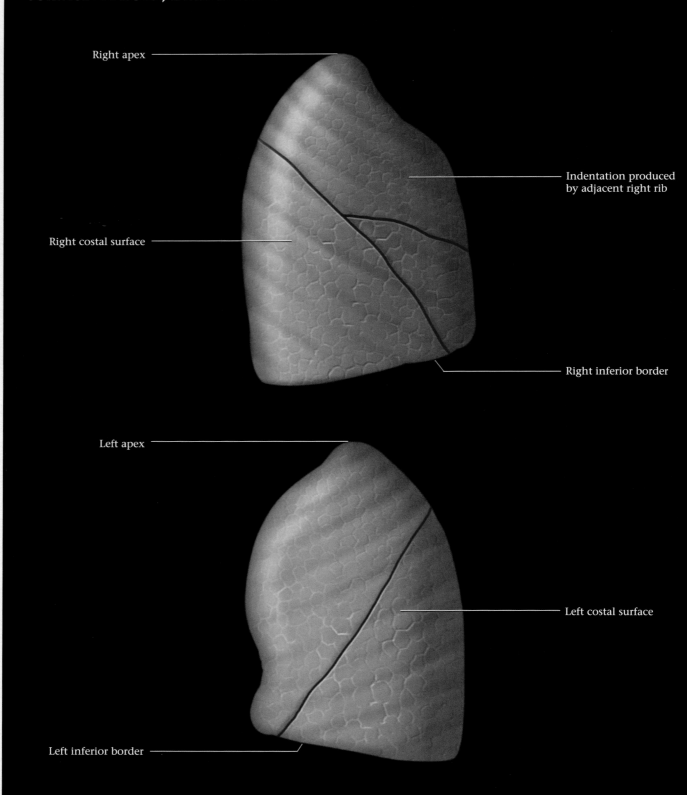

Right apex

Indentation produced by adjacent right rib

Right costal surface

Right inferior border

Left apex

Left costal surface

Left inferior border

(Top) Graphic depicts the lateral surface anatomy of the right lung. The lateral lung surface forms part of the costal surface named for the adjacent ribs (and intercostal spaces) which produce obliquely oriented indentations on the lung parenchyma. The inferior border separates the lateral costal surface from the base. **(Bottom)** Graphic depicts the lateral surface anatomy of the left lung. The lateral surface forms part of the costal surface. The inferior border separates the costal surface from the base.

LUNGS

SURFACE ANATOMY, MEDIAL LUNGS

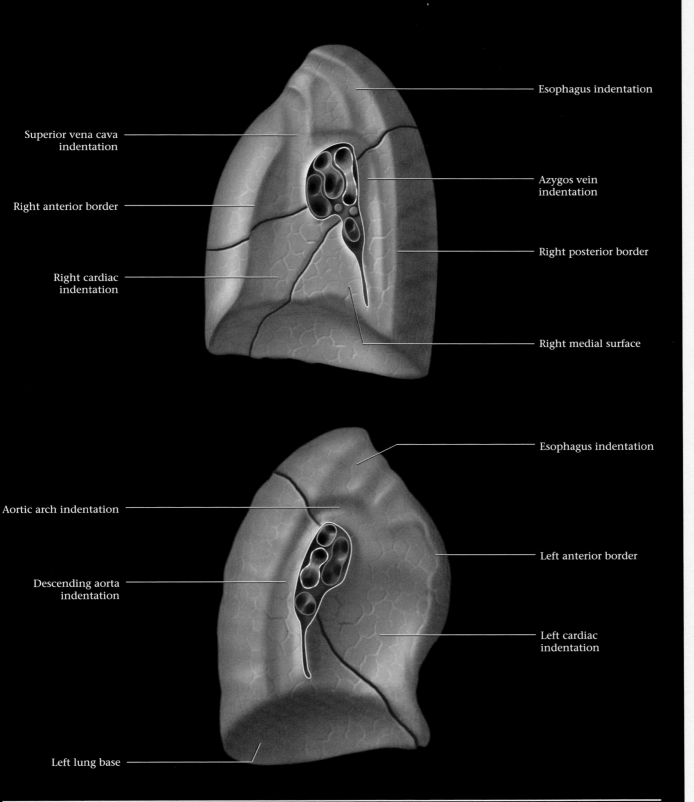

Esophagus indentation

Superior vena cava indentation

Azygos vein indentation

Right anterior border

Right posterior border

Right cardiac indentation

Right medial surface

Esophagus indentation

Aortic arch indentation

Left anterior border

Descending aorta indentation

Left cardiac indentation

Left lung base

(Top) Graphic depicts the surface anatomy of the medial right lung. The mediastinal surface is concave and exhibits indentations produced by adjacent mediastinal structures, including vessels and organs. The right cardiac indentation is produced predominantly by the right atrium. The anterior border separates the mediastinal surface from the costal surface. The right hilum is located centrally on the mediastinal surface. **(Bottom)** Graphic depicts the surface anatomy of the medial left lung. The mediastinal surface exhibits indentations produced by adjacent mediastinal structures. The left cardiac indentation is predominantly produced by the left ventricle. The descending aorta indents the left lower lobe and correlates with visualization of the retrocardiac descending aorta on frontal chest radiographs.

LUGS

RADIOGRAPHY, SURFACE ANATOMY OF THE LUNGS

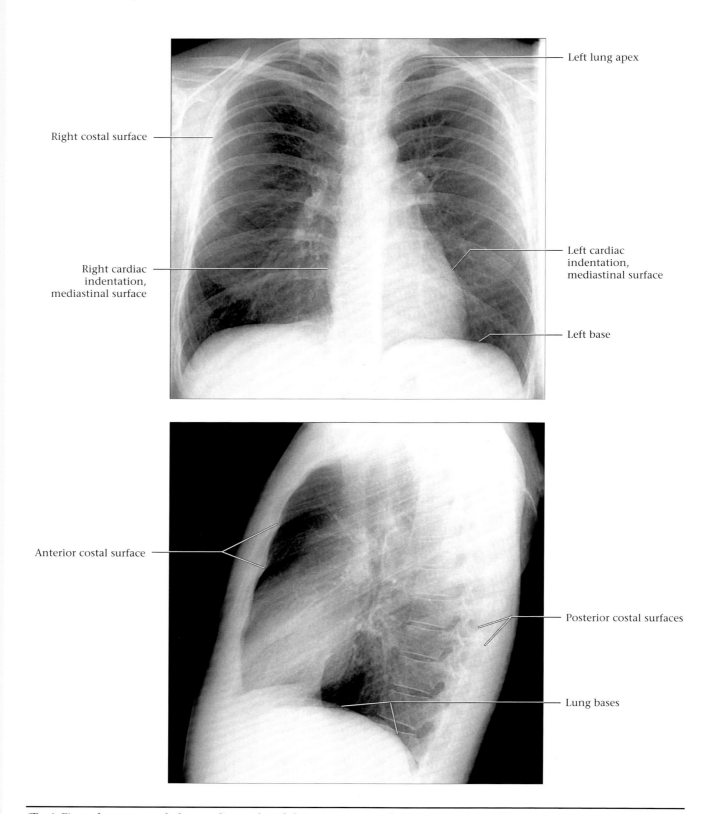

(Top) First of two normal chest radiographs of the same patient demonstrates the radiographic surface anatomy of the lungs. PA chest radiograph shows the costal and mediastinal lung surfaces, the lung bases and the apices. Note the left cardiac indentation on the mediastinal surface produced predominantly by the left ventricle. The right cardiac indentation on the right medial surface is produced predominantly by the right atrium. (Bottom) Left lateral chest radiograph demonstrates the anterior and posterior aspects of the costal surfaces and the morphology of the lung bases. Note the indentations made on the costal surface by the adjacent anterior ribs. The bases exhibit a convex morphology with a more horizontal orientation anteriorly and a near vertical orientation posteriorly.

LUNGS

CT, SURFACE ANATOMY OF THE LUNGS

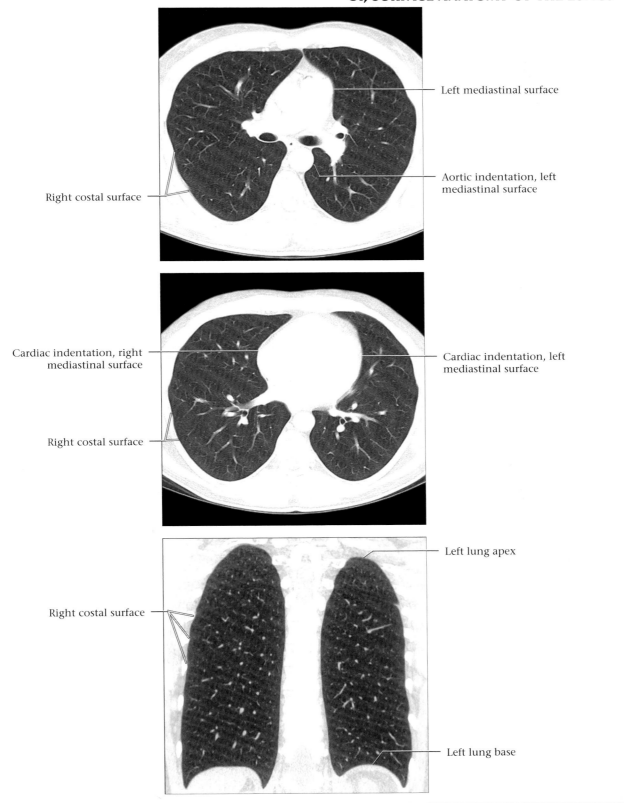

Left mediastinal surface

Aortic indentation, left mediastinal surface

Right costal surface

Cardiac indentation, right mediastinal surface

Cardiac indentation, left mediastinal surface

Right costal surface

Left lung apex

Right costal surface

Left lung base

(Top) First of three normal chest CT images (lung window) depicting the CT surface anatomy of the lungs. Axial CT below the carina demonstrates the undulating morphology of the costal lung surfaces related to indentations produced by adjacent ribs. The left mediastinal surface is indented by the descending thoracic aorta. (Middle) Axial CT at the level of the heart demonstrates the surface anatomy of the inferior lungs. The costal surfaces exhibit an undulating morphology produced by adjacent ribs. Note the larger left cardiac indentation on the mediastinal surface produced by the left ventricle and the smaller contralateral indentation produced by the right atrium. (Bottom) HRCT with coronal reconstruction demonstrates the morphology of the apices and the bases. Note the undulating morphology of the costal surfaces and the superiorly convex morphology of the bases.

LUNGS

LOBES

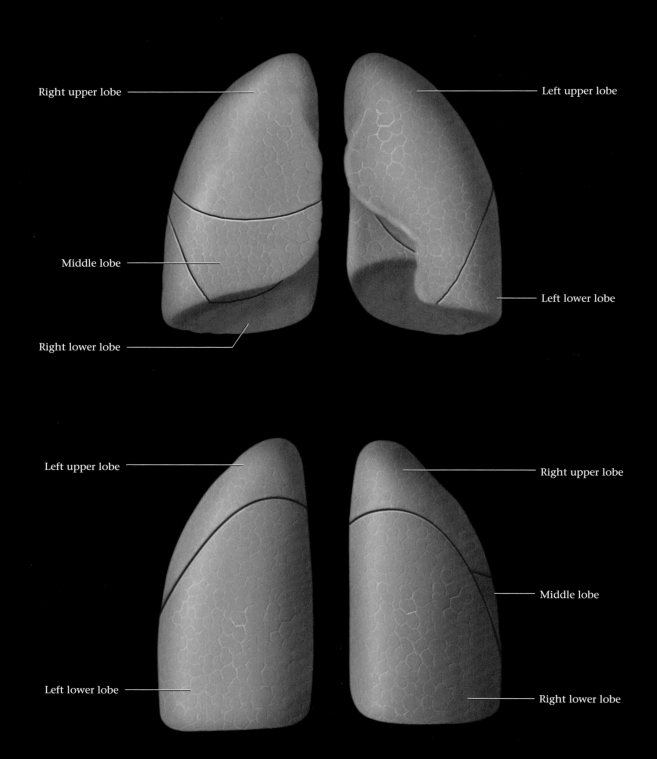

Right upper lobe

Left upper lobe

Middle lobe

Left lower lobe

Right lower lobe

Left upper lobe

Right upper lobe

Middle lobe

Left lower lobe

Right lower lobe

(Top) Graphic depicts the anatomy of the anterior lung lobes. The right lung has three lobes and is larger than the left. Visceral pleura lines each of the lobes which are compartmentalized by the interlobar fissures. **(Bottom)** Graphic depicts the anatomy of the posterior lung lobes. The lobar boundaries are demarcated by the interlobar fissures. Note the superior extent of the posterior lower lobes.

LUNGS

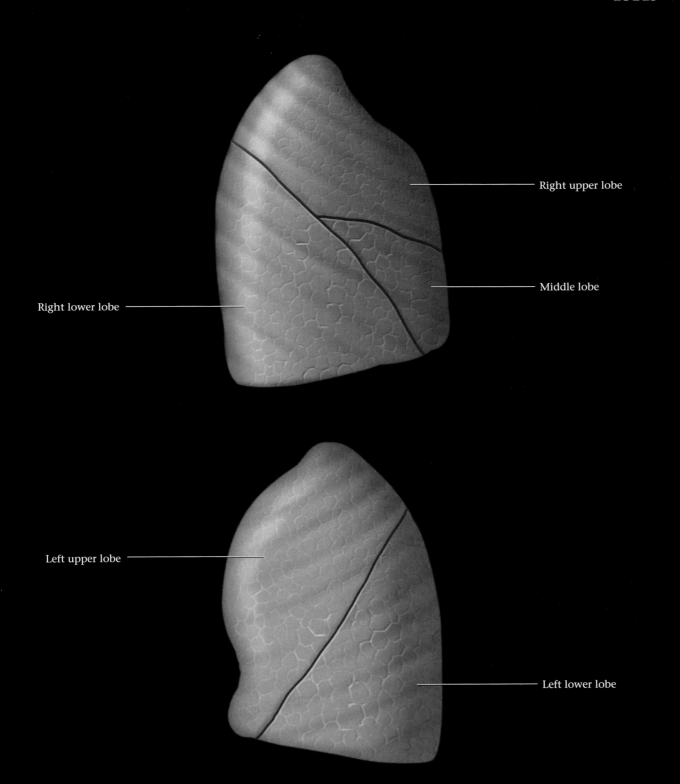

Right upper lobe

Middle lobe

Right lower lobe

Left upper lobe

Left lower lobe

(Top) Graphic shows the lateral right lung surface and the location of the three right lung lobes demarcated by the interlobar (major and minor) fissures. The right upper and middle lobes occupy the anterior right lung. The right lower lobe occupies the posterior inferior right lung. Note the superior extent of the posterior right lower lobe. **(Bottom)** Graphic shows the lateral left lung surface and the location of the two left lung lobes separated by the left major fissure. The left upper lobe occupies the anterior superior left lung. The left lower lobe occupies the posterior inferior left lung. Note the superior extent of the posterior left lower lobe.

LUNGS

RADIOGRAPHY, LOBES

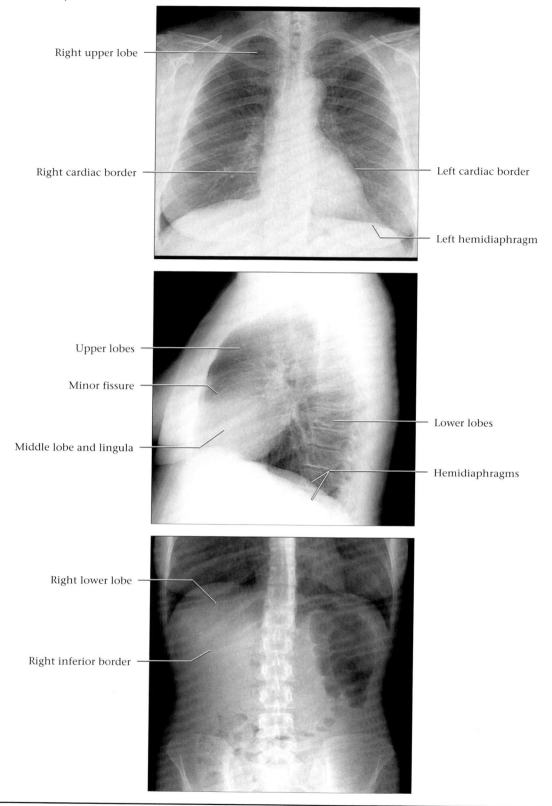

Right upper lobe

Right cardiac border

Left cardiac border

Left hemidiaphragm

Upper lobes

Minor fissure

Lower lobes

Middle lobe and lingula

Hemidiaphragms

Right lower lobe

Right inferior border

(Top) First of two normal chest radiographs of the same patient illustrating the location of the lung lobes. PA chest radiograph shows the right and left cardiac borders that abut the middle and left upper lobes respectively. The lower lobes abut the hemidiaphragms. The relationship of the right upper and middle lobes can be evaluated on radiography when the minor fissure is visible. (Middle) Left lateral radiograph shows the lower lobes in the posterior inferior thorax above the posterior hemidiaphragms. The middle lobe and lingula project over the heart. The right upper lobe is superior to the minor fissure. The right and left upper lobes and the middle lobe are located anterior to the major fissures. (Bottom) Normal upright abdominal radiograph shows the inferior extent of the posterior lower lobes with pulmonary vessels visible through the right hemidiaphragm.

LUNGS

CORONAL & OBLIQUE SAGITTAL CT, LOBES

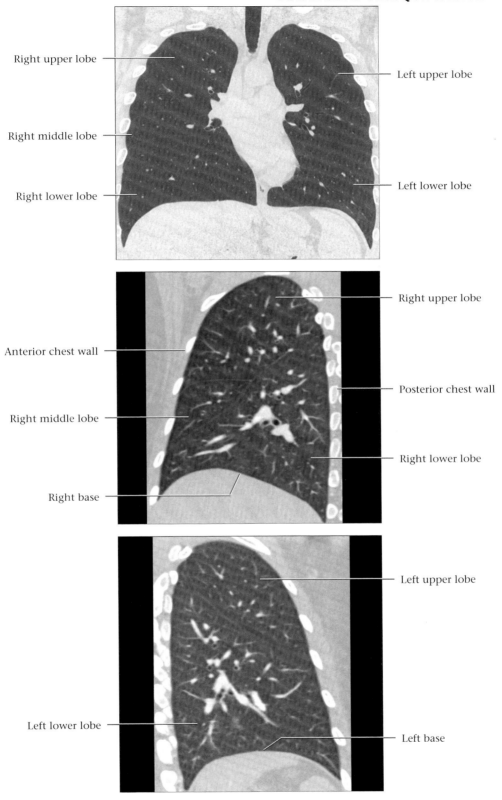

(Top) Normal coronal HRCT (lung window) demonstrates the five lung lobes and their relationships to adjacent structures. Visualization of the interlobar fissures allows identification of the boundaries of each lobe. **(Middle)** First of two normal oblique coronal chest CT images (lung window) demonstrating the relationship of the lung lobes. Image of the right lung shows that the right upper lobe forms the right apex and occupies the anterosuperior and posterosuperior right lung. The middle lobe occupies the mid anterior right lung. The right lower lobe occupies the posterior right lung and exhibits superior concavity at the base. **(Bottom)** Image of the left lung shows the anterosuperior location of the left upper lobe and the superior extent of the left lower lobe. The left lower lobe forms the concave left lung base.

LUNGS

AXIAL CT, LOBES

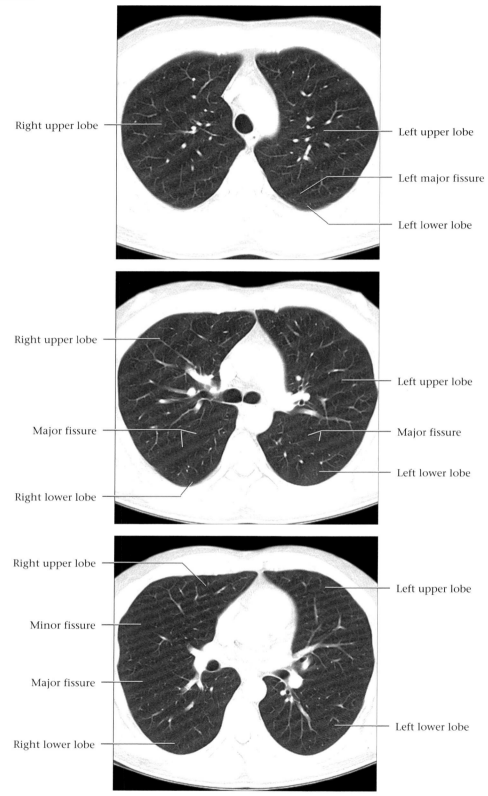

Right upper lobe — Left upper lobe — Left major fissure — Left lower lobe

Right upper lobe — Left upper lobe — Major fissure — Major fissure — Left lower lobe — Right lower lobe

Right upper lobe — Left upper lobe — Minor fissure — Major fissure — Left lower lobe — Right lower lobe

(**Top**) First of six normal thin section chest CT images (lung window) of the same patient demonstrates the axial anatomy of the lung lobes. Image through the aortic arch shows that the upper lobes occupy the superior aspects of the lungs. Visualization of the fissures allows identification of the different lobes. A very small portion of the superior left lower lobe is anteriorly bound by the major fissure. (**Middle**) Axial image through the carina demonstrates the anterior location of the upper lobes and the posterior location of the lower lobes. The major fissures manifest as avascular bands between the lobes. (**Bottom**) Axial image through the bronchus intermedius shows portions of the three right lung lobes. The minor fissure is seen as an avascular band. The lower lobes are located posteriorly, the upper lobes and middle lobe are located anteriorly.

LUNGS

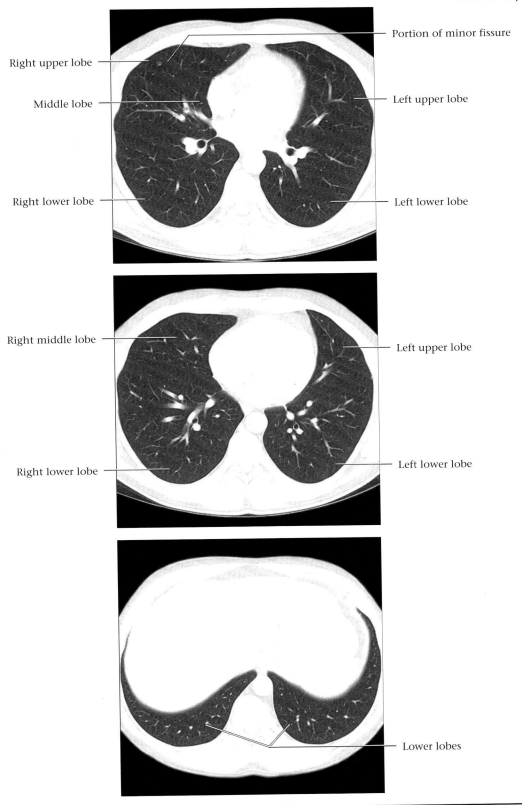

Right upper lobe

Middle lobe

Right lower lobe

Portion of minor fissure

Left upper lobe

Left lower lobe

Right middle lobe

Right lower lobe

Left upper lobe

Left lower lobe

Lower lobes

(Top) Axial image through the lower lobe bronchi demonstrates that the middle lobe abuts the right cardiac border. The minor fissure is barely visible as is a tiny portion of the right upper lobe. **(Middle)** Axial image through the heart demonstrates its relationship to the middle and left upper lobes. The inferior left upper lobe abuts the left ventricle. The right middle lobe abuts the right atrium. While the middle lobe and the left upper lobe have a significant inferior extent, the lower lobes occupy the greatest lung volume at this level. **(Bottom)** Axial image through the posterior lung bases demonstrates the retrodiaphragmatic and posteroinferior extent of the lower lobes and highlight the concave morphology of the lung bases.

LUNGS

SEGMENTS OF THE RIGHT LUNG

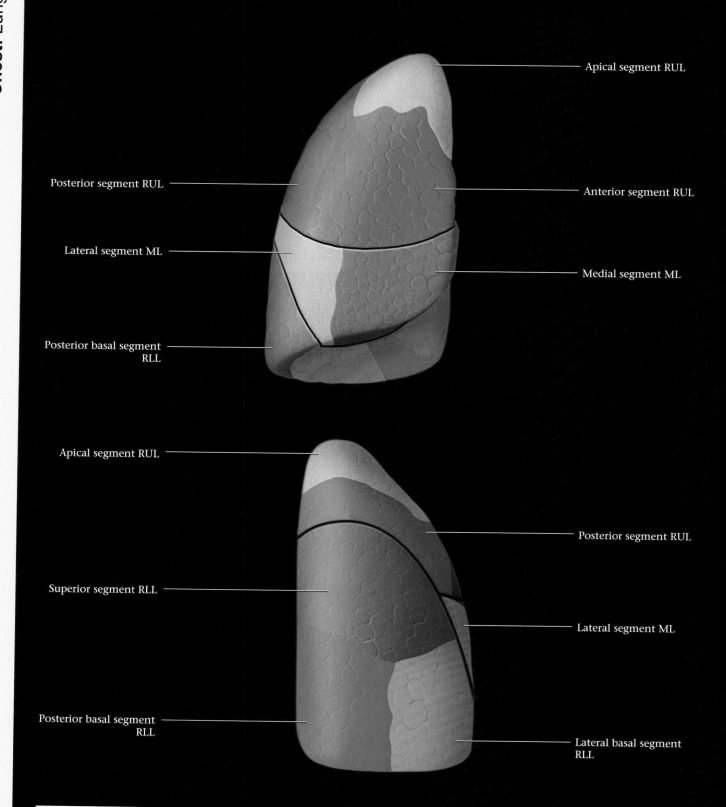

Apical segment RUL

Posterior segment RUL

Anterior segment RUL

Lateral segment ML

Medial segment ML

Posterior basal segment RLL

Apical segment RUL

Posterior segment RUL

Superior segment RLL

Lateral segment ML

Posterior basal segment RLL

Lateral basal segment RLL

(Top) First of four graphics depicting the segmental anatomy of the right lung. The anterior view shows the three right upper lobe segments named after their respective segmental bronchi. As the nomenclature would suggest, the apical, anterior and posterior segments occupy the corresponding regions of the right upper lobe. The anterior segment of the right upper lobe abuts the minor fissure. The middle lobe has medial and lateral segments. The medial segment abuts the right atrium. **(Bottom)** The posterior view shows the posterior segment of the right upper lobe abutting the posterosuperior major fissure. The superior segment occupies the apex of the right lower lobe. The basal segments are located inferior to the superior segment. The lateral basal segment of the right lower lobe is located lateral to the posterior basal segment.

LUNGS

SEGMENTS OF THE RIGHT LUNG

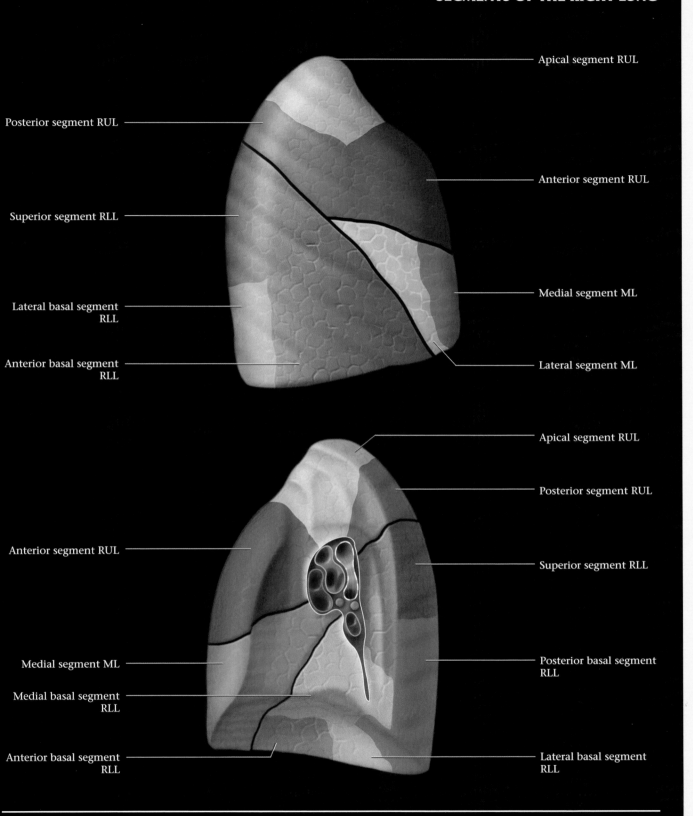

Apical segment RUL

Posterior segment RUL

Anterior segment RUL

Superior segment RLL

Medial segment ML

Lateral basal segment RLL

Anterior basal segment RLL

Lateral segment ML

Apical segment RUL

Posterior segment RUL

Anterior segment RUL

Superior segment RLL

Medial segment ML

Posterior basal segment RLL

Medial basal segment RLL

Anterior basal segment RLL

Lateral basal segment RLL

(Top) Lateral view of the right lung shows the location of the right upper lobe segments (posterior, apical and anterior) corresponding to their anatomic positions within the lobe. The anterior segment of the right upper lobe abuts the anterior minor fissure. The medial segment of the middle lobe is located anterior to the lateral segment. Note the relationship of the anterior basal and lateral basal segments below the superior segment of the lower lobe. **(Bottom)** Medial view shows the anatomic location of the right upper lobe segments. The anterior segment abuts the minor fissure. The posterior segment abuts the superior major fissure. The medial segment of the middle lobe abuts the right atrium. Note the relationship between the medial and posterior basal segments of the right lower lobe situated below the superior segment, which abuts the superior major fissure.

SEGMENTS OF THE LEFT LUNG

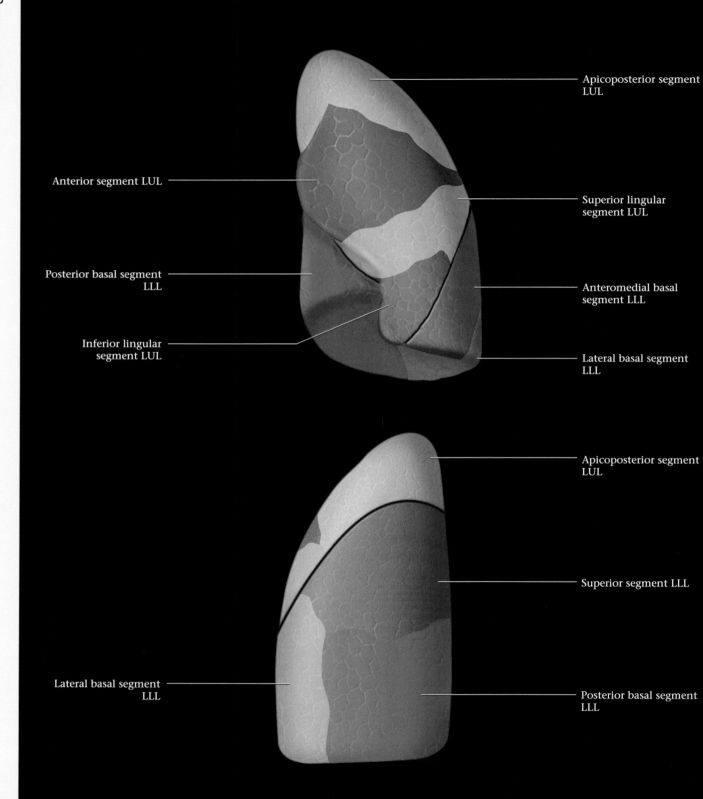

Apicoposterior segment LUL

Anterior segment LUL

Superior lingular segment LUL

Posterior basal segment LLL

Anteromedial basal segment LLL

Inferior lingular segment LUL

Lateral basal segment LLL

Apicoposterior segment LUL

Superior segment LLL

Lateral basal segment LLL

Posterior basal segment LLL

(Top) First of four graphics depicting the segmental anatomy of the left lung. The anterior view shows the four segments of the left upper lobe. The apicoposterior segment forms the apex and is located above the anterior segment which in turn is located above the lingula. The superior and inferior lingular segments abut the superior and inferior aspects of the left cardiac border respectively. Note the anterior and medial location of the anteromedial basal segment of the left lower lobe and the posteromedial location of the posterior basal segment. **(Bottom)** The posterior view shows the apicoposterior segment of the left upper lobe above the posterior major fissure. The superior segment of the left lower lobe also abuts the posterior major fissure. The posterior basal segment of the left lower lobe is located medial to the lateral basal segment.

LUNGS

SEGMENTS OF THE LEFT LUNG

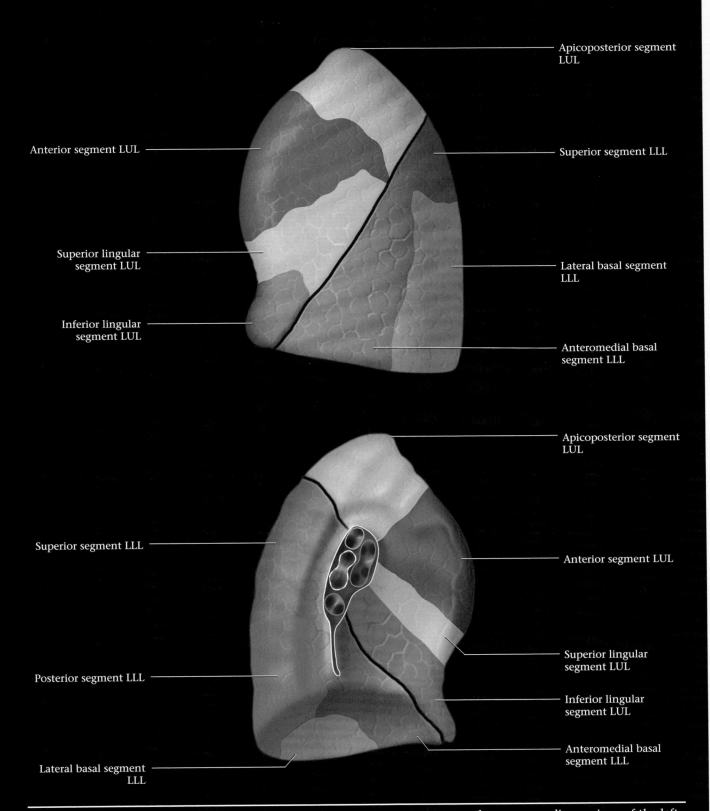

Apicoposterior segment LUL

Anterior segment LUL

Superior segment LLL

Superior lingular segment LUL

Lateral basal segment LLL

Inferior lingular segment LUL

Anteromedial basal segment LLL

Apicoposterior segment LUL

Superior segment LLL

Anterior segment LUL

Posterior segment LLL

Superior lingular segment LUL

Inferior lingular segment LUL

Lateral basal segment LLL

Anteromedial basal segment LLL

(Top) Lateral view shows that the apicoposterior and anterior segments occupy the corresponding regions of the left upper lobe. The superior lingular segment abuts the mid portion of the left major fissure and a small portion of the inferior lingular segment abuts the inferior left major fissure. Note the anterior location of the anteromedial basal segment of the left lower lobe with respect to the lateral basal segment. The apex of the lower lobe is formed by the superior segment. **(Bottom)** Medial view shows the relative locations of the segments of the upper lobe (apicoposterior, anterior, superior lingular and inferior lingular). The superior segment of the lower lobe abuts the superior major fissure and is situated above the basal segments. Note the relationship between the posterior and anteromedial basal segments of the lower lobe.

LUNGS

CT, LUNG SEGMENTS

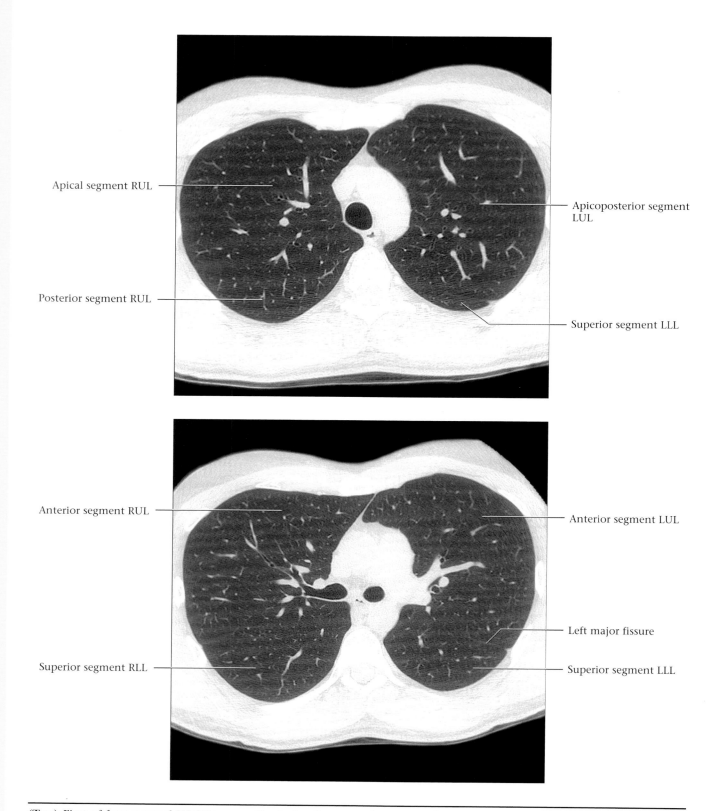

Apical segment RUL

Posterior segment RUL

Apicoposterior segment LUL

Superior segment LLL

Anterior segment RUL

Superior segment RLL

Anterior segment LUL

Left major fissure

Superior segment LLL

(Top) First of four normal HRCT images illustrates the general anatomic locations of the different lung segments. CT segmental anatomy is determined using the fissural and bronchial anatomy to determine the location of a specific lung segment. Axial image through the aortic arch shows the location of the apical and posterior right upper lobe segments. These are combined into a single apicoposterior segment in the left upper lobe based on the underlying bronchial anatomy. Visualization of the left major fissure allows identification of a small portion of the superior segment of the left lower lobe. (Bottom) Axial image below the carina demonstrates the location of the anterior segments of the right and left upper lobes. The superior segments of the lower lobes are located posterior to the superior aspects of the bilateral major fissures.

LUNGS

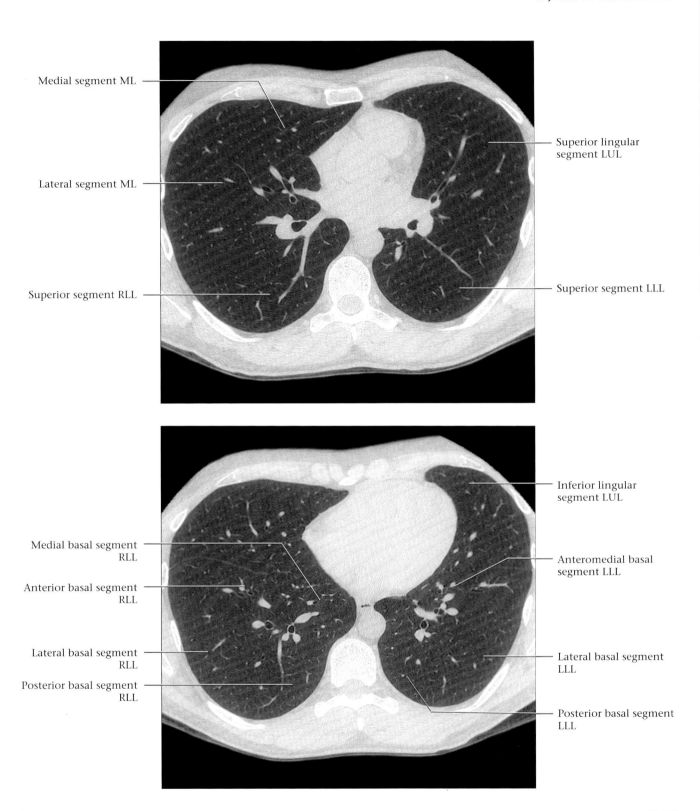

Medial segment ML

Lateral segment ML

Superior segment RLL

Superior lingular segment LUL

Superior segment LLL

Inferior lingular segment LUL

Medial basal segment RLL

Anterior basal segment RLL

Lateral basal segment RLL

Posterior basal segment RLL

Anteromedial basal segment LLL

Lateral basal segment LLL

Posterior basal segment LLL

(Top) Axial image through the segmental middle lobe and lingular bronchi demonstrates the relative locations of the medial and lateral segments of the middle lobe. The superior lingular segment of the left upper lobe is also shown. The superior segments of the right and left lower lobes are located posterior to the superior aspects of the bilateral major fissures. **(Bottom)** Axial image through the basal lower lobe segments demonstrates the relative locations of the medial, anterior, lateral and posterior basal segments of the right lower lobe. The inferior lingular segment of the left upper lobe is located anterior to the inferior aspect of the left major fissure. The left lower lobe has three basal segments designated anteromedial, lateral and posterior. Note their relative locations inferred from the location of their respective segmental bronchi.

LUNGS

PERFUSION SCINTIGRAPHY, LUNGS

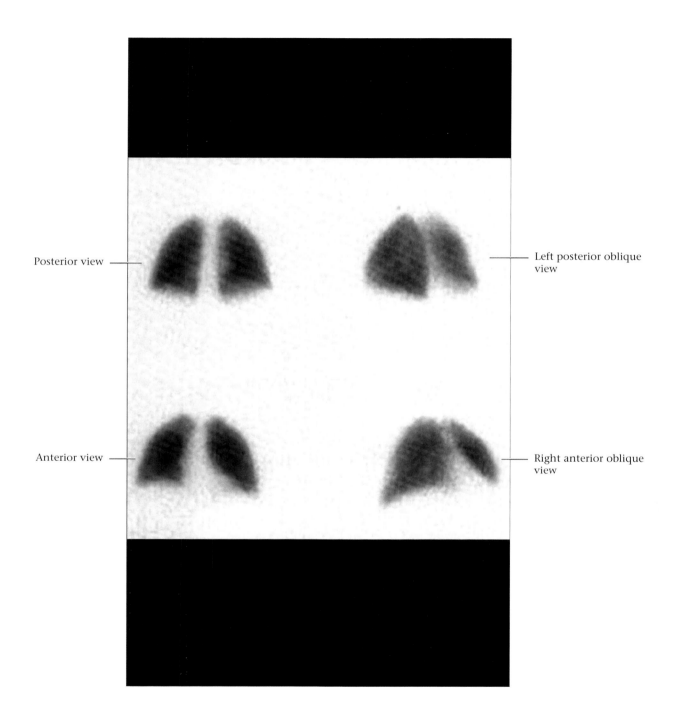

Posterior view

Left posterior oblique view

Anterior view

Right anterior oblique view

First of two images from a normal perfusion lung scan shows homogeneous distribution of activity throughout the pulmonary lobes and segments indicating normal lung perfusion. Understanding the segmental anatomy of the lungs in various projections is crucial for accurate interpretation of pulmonary nuclear scintigraphy. Note the inferior extent of the lungs on the posterior view. The cardiac notch of the left upper lobe is nicely depicted on the anterior view. The right anterior oblique view shows the concave morphology of the right base.

LUNGS

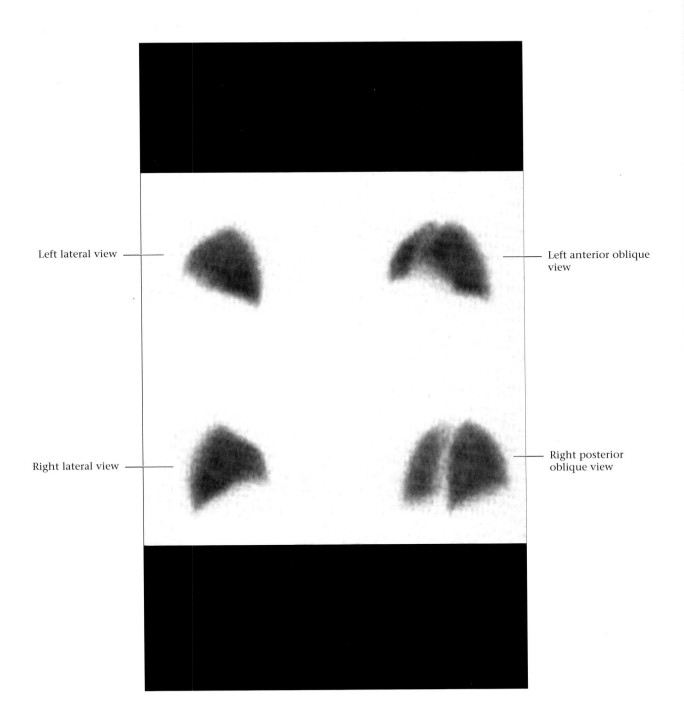

Left lateral view

Left anterior oblique view

Right lateral view

Right posterior oblique view

Additional views demonstrate homogeneous distribution of activity throughout the lungs indicating normal pulmonary perfusion and no evidence of thromboembolic disease. The left lateral view shows relative absence of activity in the anterior inferior left lung corresponding to the cardiac notch of the left anterior lung border. The right lateral view shows the concave morphology of the right base. The right posterior oblique view shows the inferior extent of the posterior right lower lobe.

LUNGS

RADIOGRAPHY, AZYGOS LOBE

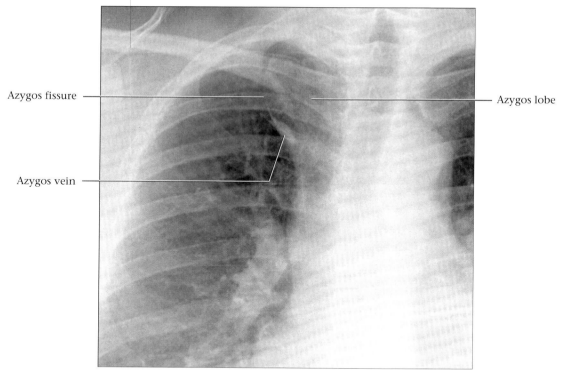

Azygos fissure

Azygos lobe

Azygos vein

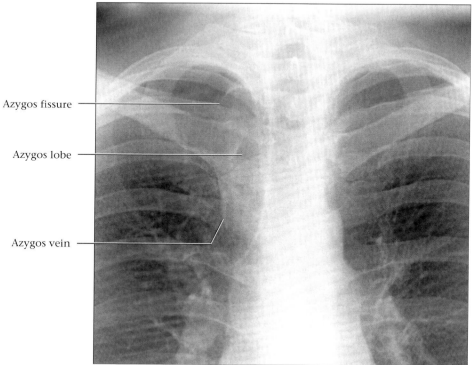

Azygos fissure

Azygos lobe

Azygos vein

(Top) PA chest radiograph coned-down to the right upper lung demonstrates an azygos lobe. The thin accessory azygos fissure terminates inferiorly as a teardrop opacity that represents the anomalous azygos vein. The azygos fissure divides the superior aspect of the upper lobe and demarcates the lateral boundary of the anomalous azygos lobe. **(Bottom)** First of four images of an asymptomatic young man with an incidentally discovered azygos lobe. PA chest radiograph coned-down to the upper lobes demonstrates the characteristic morphology of the accessory azygos fissure. The azygos lobe in this example is slightly smaller and the anomalous azygos vein is less apparent. There is great variability in the size and configuration of the azygos lobe, the course of the azygos fissure and the course, size and morphology of the anomalous azygos vein.

LUNGS

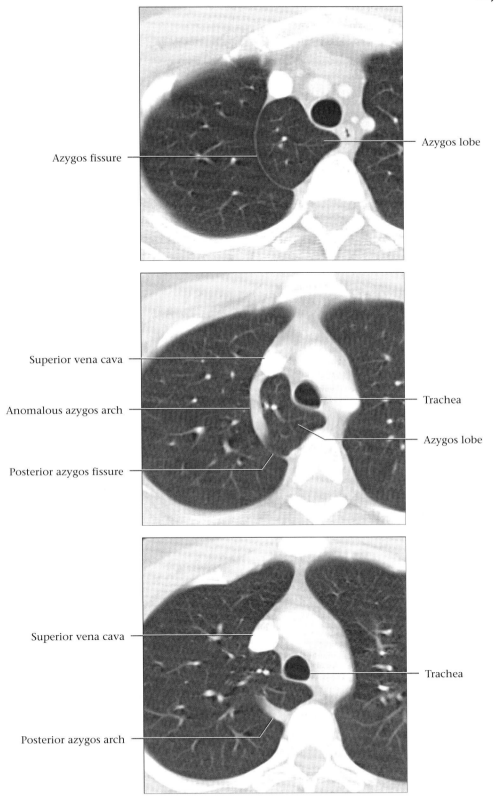

Azygos fissure — Azygos lobe

Superior vena cava — Trachea

Anomalous azygos arch — Azygos lobe

Posterior azygos fissure

Superior vena cava — Trachea

Posterior azygos arch

(Top) Contrast-enhanced chest CT (lung window) demonstrates the cross-sectional morphology of the azygos lobe. Axial image through the superior aspect of the azygos lobe demonstrates the thin accessory azygos fissure that demarcates the lateral boundary of the azygos lobe which extends behind the trachea. (Middle) Axial image through the aortic arch demonstrates the anomalous azygos arch that courses within the accessory azygos fissure and anastomoses anteriorly with the superior vena cava. (Bottom) Axial image through the inferior aortic arch demonstrates the posterior aspect of the anomalous azygos arch. Note that the azygos fissure is no longer seen in its entirety. The medial aspect of the azygos lobe is still evident.

LUNGS

RADIOGRAPHY, LOBAR PNEUMONIA

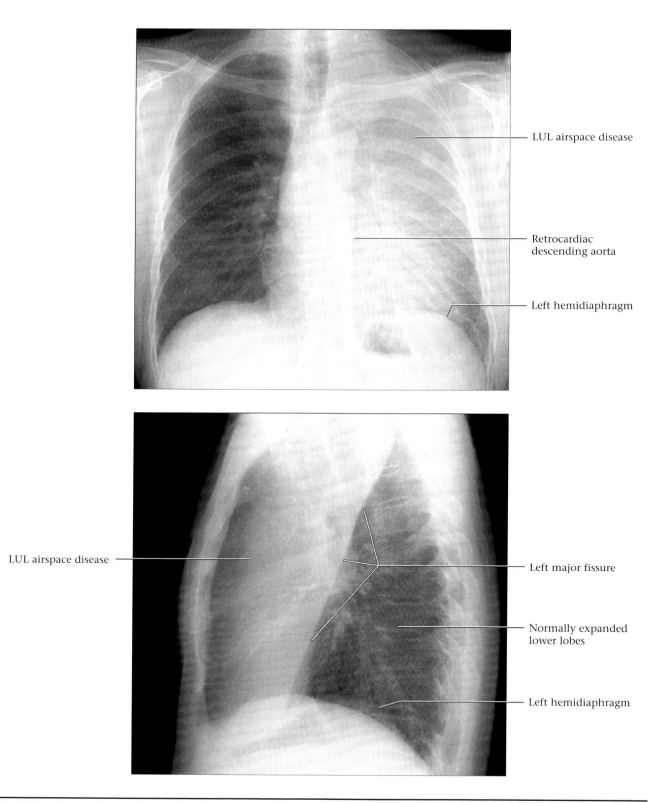

LUL airspace disease

Retrocardiac descending aorta

Left hemidiaphragm

LUL airspace disease

Left major fissure

Normally expanded lower lobes

Left hemidiaphragm

(Top) First of two chest radiographs of a 42 year old man with left upper lobe pneumonia demonstrates complete opacification of the left upper lobe. PA chest radiograph demonstrates obscuration of the left anterior mediastinal structures. The left hemidiaphragm and retrocardiac descending aorta are visible indicating that the left lower lobe is not involved. The radiographic findings are consistent with left upper lobe airspace disease. **(Bottom)** Left lateral chest radiograph confirms that the consolidation is located in the left upper lobe and involves it in its entirety. The airspace disease is located anterior to the major fissure. The left lower lobe is normally expanded and of normal opacity. The left hemidiaphragm is not obscured indicating that the left lower lobe is not involved.

LUNGS

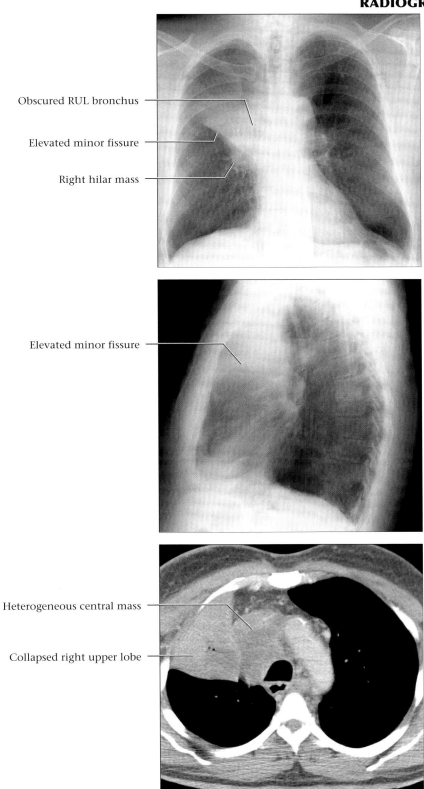

Obscured RUL bronchus

Elevated minor fissure

Right hilar mass

Elevated minor fissure

Heterogeneous central mass

Collapsed right upper lobe

(Top) First of three images of a 72 year old man who presented with hemoptysis. PA chest radiograph demonstrates right upper lobe volume loss manifesting with elevation of the minor fissure and a central convexity produced by a right hilar mass. The central mass prevents complete right upper lobe atelectasis and produces the S-sign of Golden. The right upper lobe bronchus is obscured. (Middle) Left lateral chest radiograph demonstrates a triangular anterior opacity representing the atelectatic right upper lobe. A portion of the elevated minor fissure is also visible. (Bottom) Contrast-enhanced chest CT (mediastinal window) shows the atelectatic right upper lobe manifesting as a triangular anterolateral soft tissue structure. The right upper lobe bronchus (not shown) was obstructed by a heterogeneous central mass that represented a primary lung cancer.

LUGS

RADIOGRAPHY, LOBAR ATELECTASIS

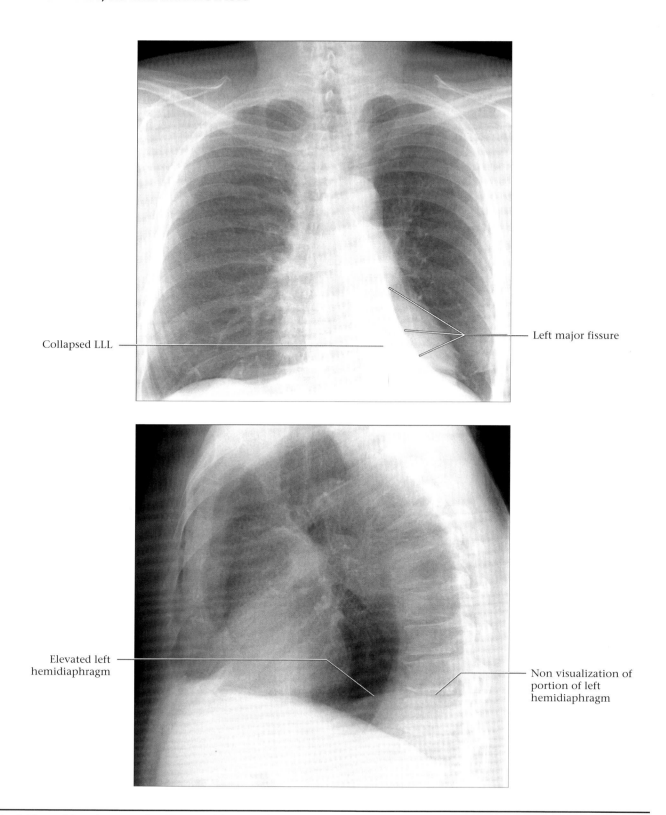

Collapsed LLL

Left major fissure

Elevated left hemidiaphragm

Non visualization of portion of left hemidiaphragm

(Top) First of four images of a 67 year old man who presented with hemoptysis. PA chest radiograph demonstrates shift of the midline structures to the left in association with relative hyperlucency of the aerated left lung. An elongate triangular retrocardiac opacity obscures the distal descending aorta and the medial left hemidiaphragm localizing the process to the left lower lobe. The triangular morphology of the abnormality and the associated findings are consistent with left lower lobe atelectasis. **(Bottom)** Left lateral chest radiograph demonstrates elevation of the left hemidiaphragm consistent with left lung volume loss. The posterior aspect of the left hemidiaphragm is obscured by the adjacent atelectatic left lower lobe.

LUNGS

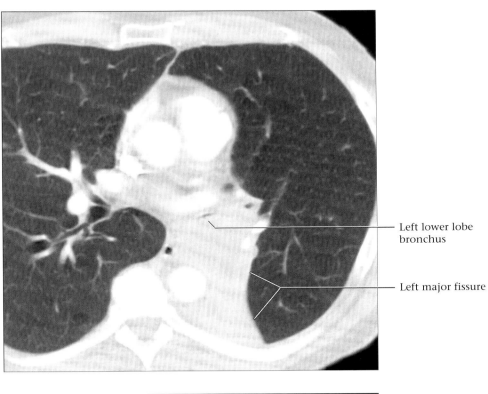

Left lower lobe bronchus

Left major fissure

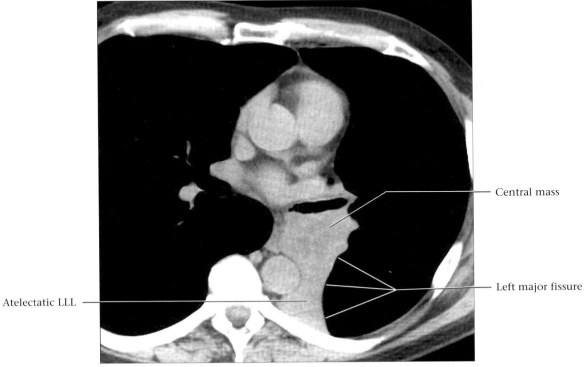

Central mass

Left major fissure

Atelectatic LLL

(Top) Contrast-enhanced chest CT (lung window) confirms the presence of left lower lobe atelectasis. There is mass effect on and narrowing of the lumen of the left lower lobe bronchus consistent with an obstructive process. The atelectatic left lower lobe abuts the descending aorta and obscures its lateral border on the frontal chest radiograph. The medially displaced left major fissure outlines the border of the atelectatic left lower lobe. Note the relative hyperlucency of the left upper lobe as compared to the right lung. **(Bottom)** Unenhanced chest CT (mediastinal window) demonstrates the soft tissue attenuation of the atelectatic left lower lobe, which abuts the descending aorta. A heterogeneous central mass representing a bronchogenic carcinoma obstructs the left lower lobe bronchus.

LUNGS

RADIOGRAPHY, SEGMENTAL AIRSPACE DISEASE

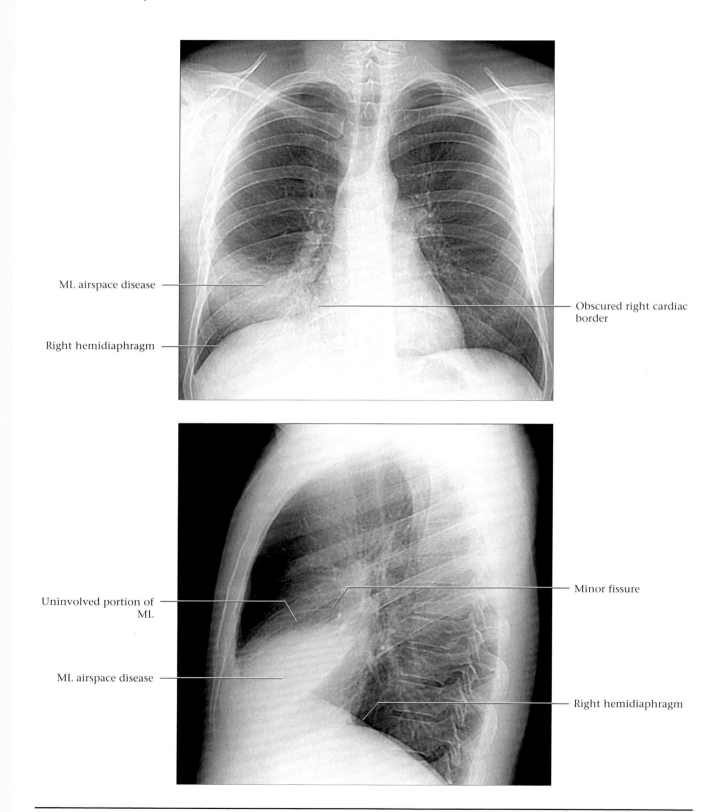

ML airspace disease

Right hemidiaphragm

Obscured right cardiac border

Uninvolved portion of ML

ML airspace disease

Minor fissure

Right hemidiaphragm

(Top) First of four images of a 35 year old man with right middle lobe pneumonia. PA chest radiograph demonstrates airspace disease in the right lower lung zone. The airspace abnormality obscures the right cardiac border indicating its right middle lobe anatomic location. **(Bottom)** Left lateral chest radiograph shows that the process overlies the heart and confirms its middle lobe location. The consolidation abuts the major fissure posteriorly. A portion of the middle lobe below the minor fissure is still aerated indicating that the entire middle lobe is not affected. The lungs posterior to the major fissures are well aerated and the hemidiaphragms are visible indicating that the right lower lobe is not affected.

LUNGS

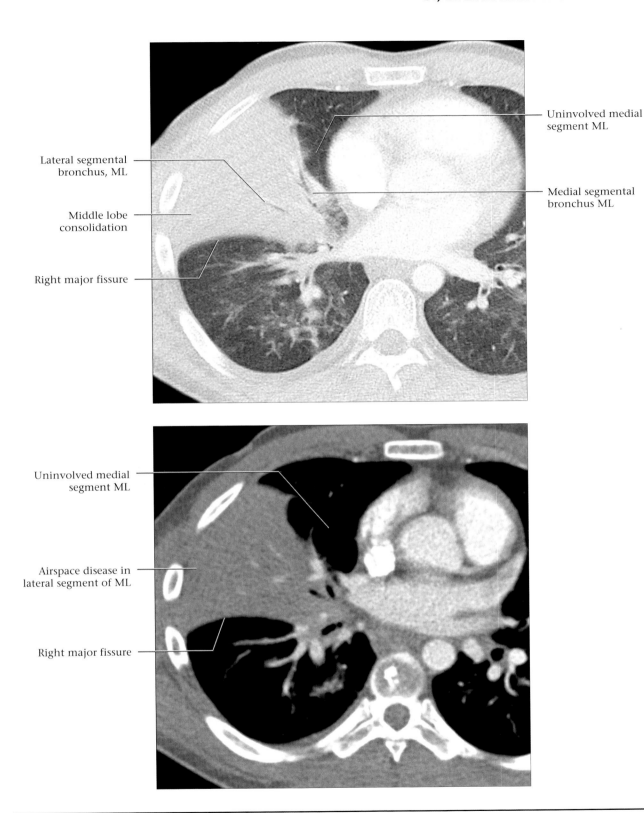

Uninvolved medial segment ML

Lateral segmental bronchus, ML

Medial segmental bronchus ML

Middle lobe consolidation

Right major fissure

Uninvolved medial segment ML

Airspace disease in lateral segment of ML

Right major fissure

(Top) Contrast-enhanced chest CT (lung window) demonstrates the middle lobe consolidation. Portions of the medial and lateral segmental middle lobe bronchi are visible. A portion of the medial segment of the middle lobe is aerated and uninvolved. The posterior boundary of the right middle lobe process is demarcated by the major fissure. **(Bottom)** Contrast-enhanced chest CT (mediastinal window) demonstrates the middle lobe consolidation which affects the lateral segment of the middle lobe in its entirety. The airspace process abuts the right major fissure posteriorly. A portion of the medial segment of the middle lobe remains uninvolved.

LUNGS

RADIOGRAPHY, SEGMENTAL AIRSPACE DISEASE

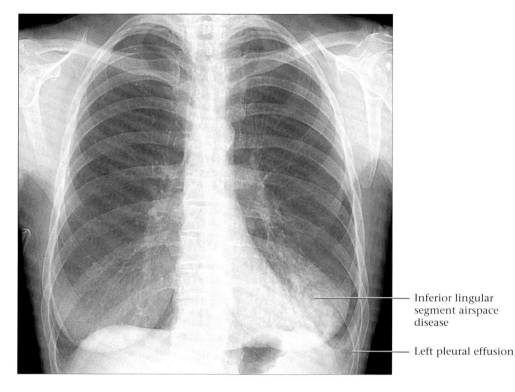

Inferior lingular segment airspace disease

Left pleural effusion

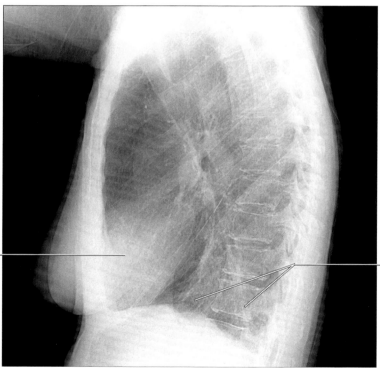

Subtle lingular airspace disease

Anteromedial & posterior basal segmental opacities

(**Top**) First of two chest radiographs of a 44 year old woman with multifocal pneumonia. PA chest radiograph demonstrates airspace disease in the left lower lung zone. The process obscures the inferior left cardiac border consistent with involvement of the inferior lingular segment of the left upper lobe. There is a small pleural effusion. (**Bottom**) Left lateral chest radiograph demonstrates subtle opacity projecting over the heart and confirms left upper lobe involvement by pneumonia. The increased opacity in the left lower lobe corresponded to subtle involvement of the anteromedial basal and posterior basal segments of the left lower lobe.

LUNGS

RADIOGRAPHY, SEGMENTAL AIRSPACE DISEASE

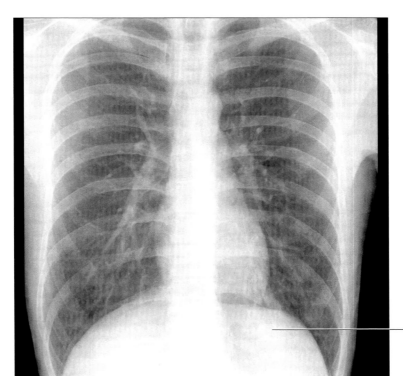

— LLL airspace disease

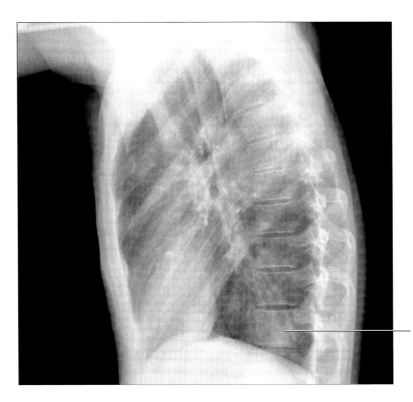

— Airspace disease in
posterior basal segment
LLL

(Top) First of two radiographs of a 28 year old man with early left lower lobe pneumonia. PA chest radiograph demonstrates subtle focal airspace disease located predominantly in the mid portion of the retrodiaphragmatic left lower lobe. **(Bottom)** Left lateral chest radiograph demonstrates abnormal opacity located posteriorly and projecting over a distal thoracic vertebral body. The thoracic vertebrae should appear increasingly lucent when examined in the cephalocaudad direction on lateral radiographs. Increased density over a distal thoracic vertebra is indicative of lower lobe airspace disease. Knowledge of the segmental anatomy of the lung and evaluation of orthogonal radiographs allows localization of the process to the posterior basal segment of the left lower lobe.

LUNGS

SCINTIGRAPHY, LOBAR & SEGMENTAL ABNORMALITIES

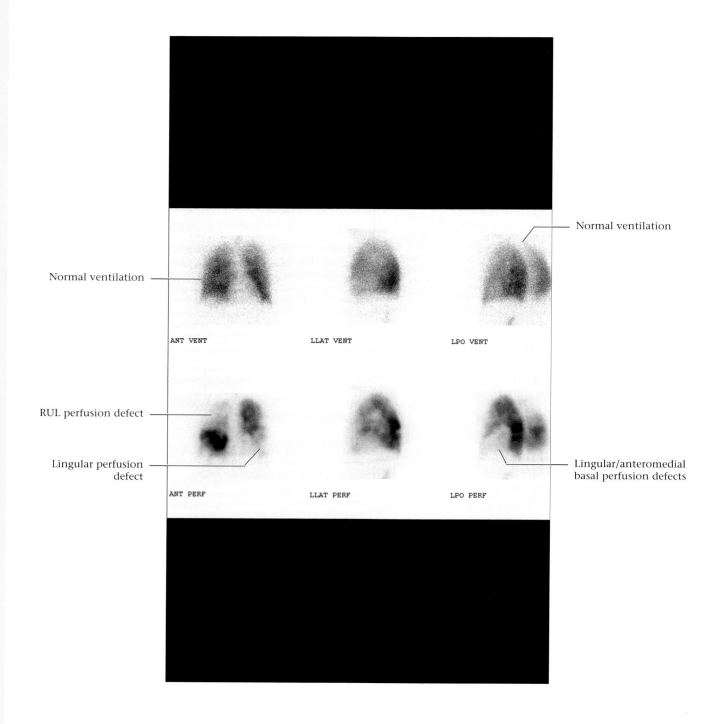

First of two images from a ventilation perfusion lung scintigraphy study of a 56 year old man with advanced prostate cancer and new onset of dyspnea demonstrate abnormal distribution of activity. Anterior, left lateral and left posterior oblique ventilation images (top row) demonstrate relatively normal distribution of activity throughout the lungs. Anterior, left lateral and left posterior oblique perfusion images (bottom row) demonstrate multifocal lobar and segmental areas of decreased activity denoting abnormal lung perfusion.

LUNGS

NUCLEAR SCINTIGRAPHY, LOBAR & SEGMENTAL ABNORMALITIES

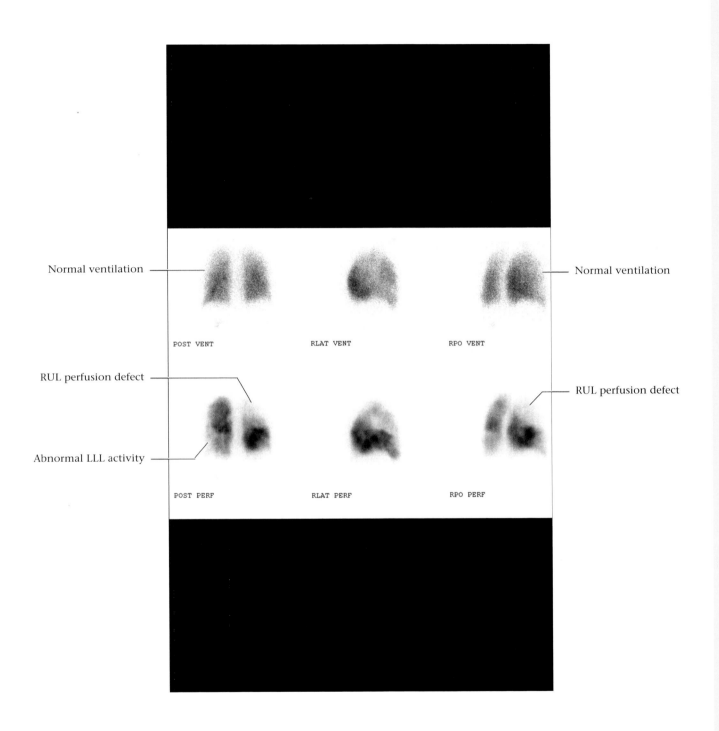

Normal ventilation

POST VENT   RLAT VENT   RPO VENT

Normal ventilation

RUL perfusion defect

RUL perfusion defect

Abnormal LLL activity

POST PERF   RLAT PERF   RPO PERF

Additional ventilation perfusion images demonstrate normal pulmonary ventilation on the posterior, right lateral and right posterior oblique views (top row). Posterior, right lateral and right posterior oblique perfusion images (bottom row) demonstrate a dominant perfusion defect affecting the right upper lobe and abnormal perfusion affecting the left lower lobe. The findings are consistent with high probability for pulmonary thromboembolic disease.

HILA

Terminology

Abbreviations
- American Thoracic Society (ATS)

Definitions
- **Hilum:** Small point of attachment of a seed to its base or support (plural; **hila**)
- **Lung hilum**
  - Point of connection between lung and mediastinum
  - Central area between the mediastinum medially and the lung laterally through which bronchi, vessels and other structures course into the lung

General Anatomy and Function

Anatomy
- **Hilum** located on central mediastinal lung surface
- Hilar structures
  - **Pulmonary arteries**
  - **Pulmonary veins**
  - **Main bronchi**
  - **Bronchial arteries/veins**
  - **Nerves**
  - **Lymph nodes**
  - **Lymphatics**
- Hilar boundaries
  - Mediastinal pleural reflections
    - Inferior extension as **pulmonary ligament**

Function
- May play a role in stabilizing the lung
- **Pulmonary ligament**
  - May play a role in stabilizing the lower lobe
  - May accommodate cephalocaudad motion of hilar structures during respiration

Hilar Anatomy

Right Hilum
- Structures
  - **Right main bronchus**
  - **Right pulmonary artery branches**
  - **Right pulmonary veins**
  - **Bronchopulmonary lymph nodes**
- Relationships
  - **Right main bronchus** located posteriorly and superiorly
    - **Eparterial bronchus**, first main branch arises superiorly and above right pulmonary artery
  - **Right pulmonary artery branches**, anterior to **right main bronchus**
  - **Right superior pulmonary vein**, anterior to **right pulmonary artery branches**
  - **Right inferior pulmonary vein**, in inferior hilum

Left Hilum
- Structures
  - **Left main bronchus**
  - **Left pulmonary artery**
  - **Left pulmonary veins**
  - **Bronchopulmonary lymph nodes**
- Relationships
  - **Left main bronchus**, located posteriorly in mid hilum
  - **Left pulmonary artery**, superior to **left main bronchus**
    - **Hyparterial bronchus**, main bronchus below **left pulmonary artery**
  - **Left superior pulmonary vein**, anterior to **left main bronchus** and **left pulmonary artery**
  - **Left inferior pulmonary vein**, in inferior hilum

Radiography of the Hila

Frontal (PA/AP) Radiography
- Superior right hilum
  - **Right ascending pulmonary artery** (**truncus anterior**) located medially
  - **Right superior pulmonary vein** located laterally
  - Centrally located **apical** and **anterior segmental bronchi**
- Hilar angle
  - Angle formed by **right superior pulmonary vein** obliquely crossing **right descending** (interlobar) **pulmonary artery**
- Inferior right hilum
  - **Right interlobar** (descending) **pulmonary artery** located lateral to **bronchus intermedius**
  - **Right inferior pulmonary vein**, minimal contribution to hilar opacity
- Superior left hilum
  - **Apical pulmonary artery** located medially
  - **Superior pulmonary vein** located laterally
  - **Anterior** and **apicoposterior segmental bronchi** located centrally
- Inferior left hilum
  - **Left interlobar pulmonary artery** lateral to **left lower lobe bronchus**
  - Minimal contribution from **left inferior pulmonary vein**
- Hilar opacity
  - Greatest contribution from **pulmonary arteries** and **superior pulmonary veins**
  - Minimal contribution from bronchial walls, lymph nodes, surrounding tissues
- Hilar height
  - Left hilum higher than right in **97%** of cases
  - Equal hilar height in **3%** of cases
  - Right hilum never higher than left in normal subjects

Lateral Radiography
- Airways
  - **Right upper lobe bronchus**
    - Superior round lucency
    - Visible in **50%** of cases
    - Circumferential visualization of bronchial walls suggests abnormal adjacent soft tissue
  - **Left upper lobe bronchus**
    - Inferior round lucency
    - Visible in **75%** of cases
    - Typically circumferential wall visualization, completely surrounded by vessels

HILA

- Intermediate stem line
  - Vertical thin linear opacity formed by posterior walls of **right main bronchus** and **bronchus intermedius**
  - Normal thickness ≤ 3 mm
  - Visible in **95%** of cases
  - Outlined by endoluminal air and retrobronchial lung in **azygoesophageal recess**
  - Courses through posterior/middle third of **left upper lobe bronchus**
  - Anterior wall of left lower lobe bronchus
    - Merges superiorly with **left upper lobe bronchus**
    - Visible in **45%** of cases
  - Left retrobronchial line
    - Formed by posterior walls of **left main bronchus** and **left lower lobe bronchus**
    - Normal thickness ≤ 3 mm
    - Terminates at origin of **left lower lobe superior segmental bronchus**
    - Shorter and posterior to **intermediate stem line**
- Vessels
  - **Right hilar vascular opacity**
    - Anterior to the hilar airways
    - Posteriorly located **right ascending** and **interlobar arteries**
    - Anteriorly located **right superior pulmonary vein**
    - Surrounding areolar tissue and lymph nodes
    - Right pulmonary artery is intramediastinal and does not form part of hilar vascular opacity
  - Left hilar vascular opacity
    - **Left pulmonary artery**, forms arcuate opacity superior and posterior to **left upper lobe bronchus**
    - Superior aspect of **left pulmonary artery** visible in **95%** of cases
  - Inferior hilar window
    - Avascular zone in anterior inferior hilum inferior to lower lobe bronchi

- Proximal bronchus intermedius/left upper lobe bronchus
  - Bronchus intermedius covered anterolaterally by horizontal and vertical portions of interlobar artery
  - Right superior pulmonary vein abuts junction of horizontal and descending interlobar artery
    - Characteristic "**elephant head-and-trunk**" morphology
  - Left distal main and upper lobe bronchi
  - Left interlobar artery posterior to bronchi
- Intermediate/lingular bronchi
  - Bronchus intermedius
  - Right interlobar artery lateral to bronchus intermedius
  - Proximal lingular upper lobe and left superior segmental lower lobe bronchi
  - Left interlobar artery lateral to bronchial bifurcation
- Middle lobe bronchus
  - Origin of middle lobe bronchus and superior segmental bronchus (the latter may arise slightly superior to this level)
  - Middle lobe artery lateral to bronchus
  - Right interlobar artery lateral to bifurcation of bronchus intermedius into middle and lower lobe bronchi
  - Anteromedial right superior pulmonary vein
  - Left interlobar pulmonary artery lateral to left lower lobe truncus basalis
- Basilar lower lobe bronchi/inferior pulmonary veins
  - Right medial basal segmental bronchus anterior to inferior pulmonary vein
  - Right anterior, lateral and posterior segmental bronchi lateral and posterior to inferior pulmonary vein
  - Left anteromedial segmental bronchus anterior to inferior pulmonary vein
  - Left lateral and posterior segmental bronchi posterior to inferior pulmonary vein

CT of the Hila

Six Characteristic Axial Levels

- **Supracarinal trachea**
  - Right apical artery medial to apical segmental bronchus
  - Right apical vein lateral to apical segmental bronchus
  - Left apicoposterior segmental bronchus and artery
  - Left apical and anterior veins anteromedial to bronchus and artery
- **Carina/right upper lobe bronchus**
  - Right upper lobe, anterior and posterior segmental bronchi
  - Right ascending artery anterior to main bronchus
  - Right anterior segmental artery medial to anterior segmental bronchus
  - Lateral location of right superior pulmonary vein
  - Left apicoposterior bronchus and artery, lateral to left pulmonary artery
  - Left superior pulmonary vein located anteromedial to bronchus and artery

Hilar Lymph Nodes

Normal Lymph Nodes

- Radiography
  - Typically not apparent
  - May be visible when calcified
- CT
  - Small soft tissue nodules, may exhibit fat attenuation centers
    - Optimal visualization on contrast-enhanced studies
    - Most prominent lymph nodes at bifurcations of right pulmonary artery, middle lobe bronchus, left upper lobe and lingular bronchi
  - Identification of subtle calcification not visible on radiography
  - Short axis measurement ≤ **1 cm**
- MR
  - Distinction of lymph nodes from adjacent vessels
  - Not sensitive to calcification

HILA

ATS Lymph Node Stations

- Lymph node classification/mapping
- Staging of lung cancer
- Terminology
  - Number relates to lymph node location (station)
  - Letter denotes location of lymph node with respect to the midline
    - R = right
    - L = left
- Hilar lymph nodes
  - Considered **intrapulmonary** for staging purposes
  - Ipsilateral hilar lymph node involvement in lung cancer; **N1** disease
  - Numeral **10** denotes hilar location
    - 10R = right hilar lymph nodes
    - 10L = left hilar lymph nodes

Hilar Signs

Hilum Overlay Sign

- Visualization of hilar structures through medial opacities that overlie the hilum on frontal radiographs
- Indicates that abnormality is not in hilum/pulmonary artery
  - Abnormality anterior or posterior to the hilum

Hilar Convergence Sign

- Convergence of pulmonary artery branches towards hilar opacity on frontal radiographs
  - Radiographic evidence of pulmonary artery enlargement

Imaging of Anatomy Based Hilar Abnormalities

Alteration of Hilar Height

- Typically seen with loss of lung volume
  - Inferior hilar displacement with lower lobe volume loss
  - Superior hilar displacement with upper lobe volume loss

Increased Hilar Density

- Calcification
  - **Granulomatous disease**
    - Frequent finding on radiography
    - Focal or multifocal discrete lymph node calcification: Punctate, irregular, diffuse
    - Association with calcified pulmonary granulomas
  - **Pneumoconiosis (silicosis, coal-workers pneumoconiosis)**
    - May exhibit peripheral (**egg-shell**) lymph node calcification
    - Association with upper/posterior lung zone predominant multifocal pulmonary silicotic nodules that may exhibit calcification
  - **Metastases**
    - Lymph node metastases from bone forming or dystrophic neoplasms
    - May be associated with calcified pulmonary metastases

- Hilar neoplasm, bronchogenic carcinoma
  - May manifest with asymmetric/subtle hilar density on radiography
    - CT evaluation for exclusion of central/hilar mass
  - Central/hilar mass with or without bronchial obstruction
    - Characteristic of **squamous cell carcinoma**
  - Hilar/mediastinal lymphadenopathy with poor visualization of primary neoplasm
    - Characteristic of **small cell carcinoma**
  - CT imaging for pre-operative staging
    - Assessment of primary neoplasm (T)
    - Assessment of lymph node involvement (N)
- Hilar neoplasm, metastatic disease
  - Primary lung cancer
  - Extrathoracic malignancy
  - Lymphoma

Bilateral Hilar Enlargement, Lymph Nodes

- **Non-neoplastic lymphadenopathy**
  - **Sarcoidosis**
    - **Bilateral symmetric hilar lymphadenopathy**
    - Associated **mediastinal lymphadenopathy (paratracheal, aortopulmonary window)**
    - Associated pulmonary nodules with **perilymphatic distribution**
- **Neoplastic lymphadenopathy**
  - **Metastases**
  - **Lymphoma**

Bilateral Hilar Enlargement, Pulmonary Arteries

- **Pulmonary arterial hypertension**
  - **Pulmonary trunk width > 3.0 cm on CT**
  - Pulmonary trunk diameter greater than diameter of adjacent ascending aorta

Unilateral Hilar Enlargement, Lymph Nodes

- Neoplastic Lymphadenopathy
  - Bronchogenic carcinoma
  - Metastases
  - Lymphoma

Unilateral Hilar Enlargement, Pulmonary Artery

- **Pulmonic stenosis**
  - Asymptomatic adults
  - Post-stenotic dilatation of left pulmonary artery related to direction of high velocity jet of blood through stenotic valve

Thick Intermediate Stem Line

- **Thickness > 3 mm** on lateral radiography
- Etiologies
  - Interstitial edema
  - Hilar/perihilar mass

HILA

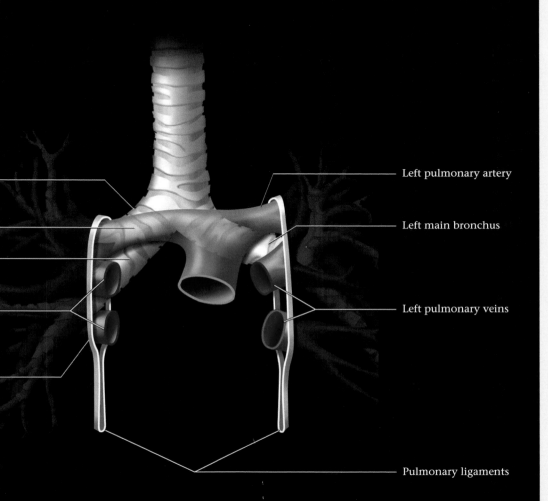

Left pulmonary artery

Left main bronchus

Left pulmonary veins

Pulmonary ligaments

al anatomy of the pulmonary hila. The hila constitute the "roots" of the lungs and are
stinal pleural reflections which extend inferiorly as the pulmonary ligaments. The hila are
rways, vessels and connective tissues travel between the mediastinum and the adjacent
ows the central bronchi, pulmonary arteries and pulmonary veins, which are the principal

RIGHT HILUM

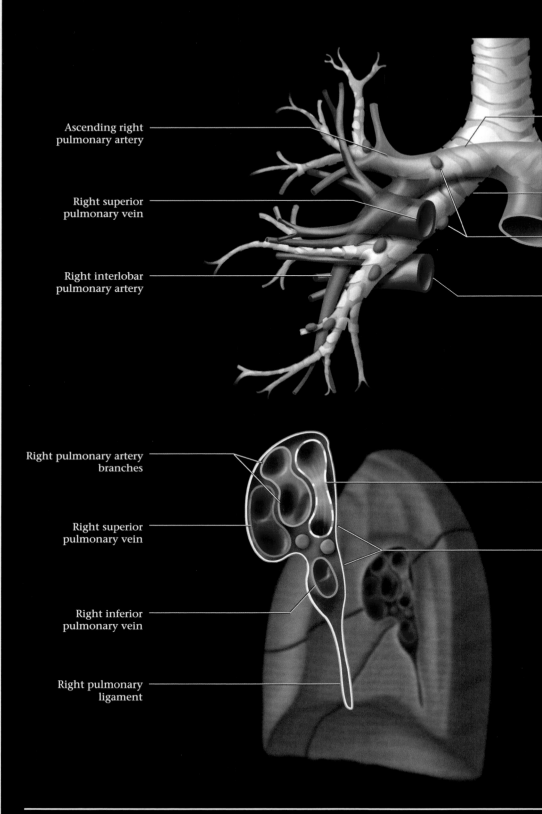

Ascending right pulmonary artery

Right superior pulmonary vein

Right interlobar pulmonary artery

Right pulmonary artery branches

Right superior pulmonary vein

Right inferior pulmonary vein

Right pulmonary ligament

(Top) First of two graphics showing the right hilar anatomy. Anterior view shows the pulmo[...] along their respective bronchi. The right bronchial morphology is eparterial, with the upper [...] pulmonary artery. The right pulmonary artery has ascending and descending branches. The [...] a horizontal course relative to that of the arteries. Hilar lymph nodes in the 10R ATS station [...] considered intrapulmonary for the purposes of lung cancer staging. (Bottom) Medial view sh[...] of the hilum on the mediastinal lung surface and the location of the hilar structures. The up[...] superior pulmonary vein, right pulmonary artery and right bronchi (from anterior to posteri[...] pulmonary vein is located inferiorly. Normal hilar lymph nodes are depicted in green.

LEFT HILUM

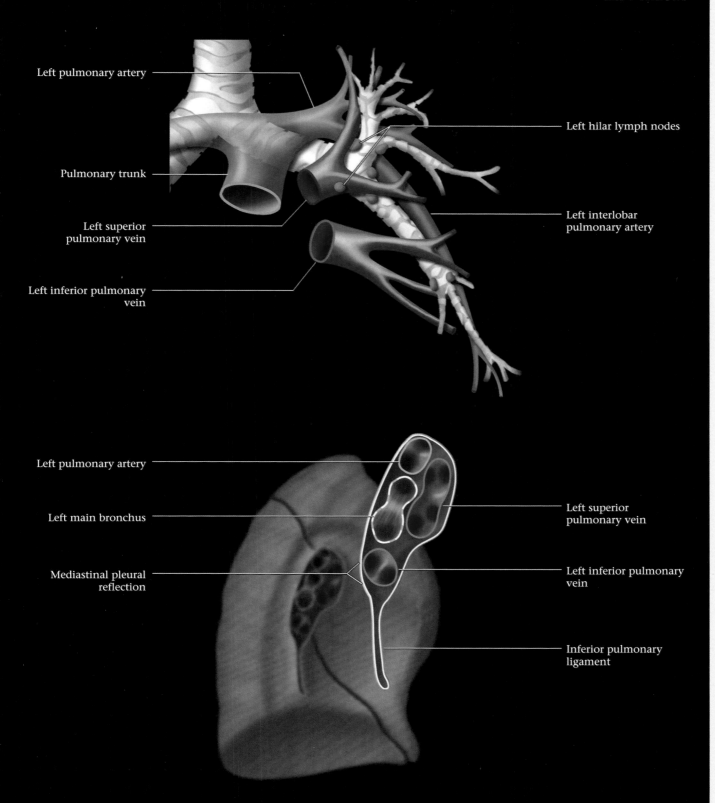

Left pulmonary artery

Pulmonary trunk

Left superior
pulmonary vein

Left inferior pulmonary
vein

Left hilar lymph nodes

Left interlobar
pulmonary artery

Left pulmonary artery

Left main bronchus

Mediastinal pleural
reflection

Left superior
pulmonary vein

Left inferior pulmonary
vein

Inferior pulmonary
ligament

(Top) First of two graphics illustrating the anatomy of the normal left hilum. Anterior view shows that the left pulmonary artery courses above the left main bronchus (hyparterial bronchus). The left interlobar pulmonary artery courses along the posterolateral aspect of the left lower lobe bronchus. Note the anterior location of the pulmonary veins. Hilar lymph nodes in the 10L ATS lymph node station are shown in green. **(Bottom)** Medial view shows the location of the left hilum on the mid portion of the mediastinal lung surface. The left bronchus is situated posteriorly within the mid hilum. The pulmonary artery is located above the hyparterial left bronchus. The superior and inferior pulmonary veins are located anterior and inferior to the left bronchus respectively.

HILA

RADIOGRAPHY, NORMAL HILA

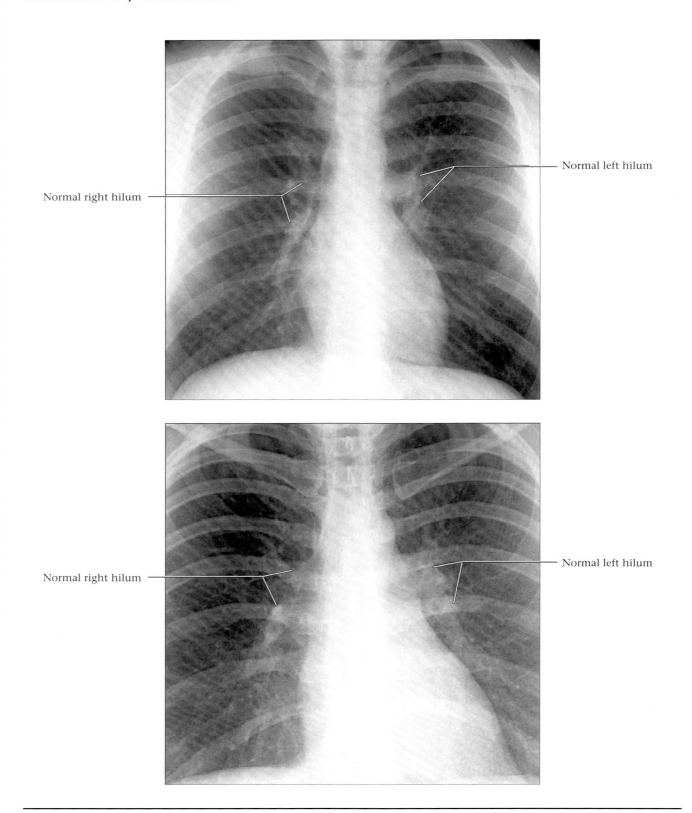

Normal right hilum

Normal left hilum

Normal right hilum

Normal left hilum

(Top) First of four normal chest radiographs of different patients demonstrating variations in the radiographic appearance of the pulmonary hila. PA chest radiograph shows that most of the hilar density visible on radiography is attributable to the pulmonary arteries and superior pulmonary veins. There is normally a mild asymmetry in hilar height with the right hilum located slightly lower than the left. This hilar configuration is seen in approximately 97% of normal subjects. **(Bottom)** Normal PA chest radiograph coned to the hila demonstrates roughly equal hilar heights. This hilar configuration is seen in approximately 3% of normal subjects.

RADIOGRAPHY, NORMAL HILA

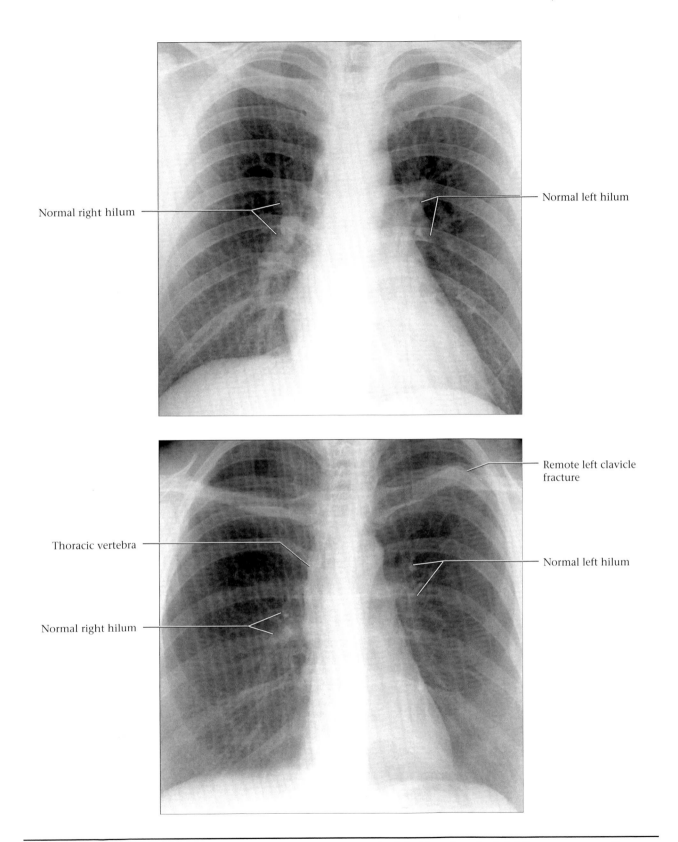

Normal right hilum

Normal left hilum

Remote left clavicle fracture

Thoracic vertebra

Normal left hilum

Normal right hilum

(Top) PA chest radiograph shows mild rotation of the patient to the left. Note that the left hilum may normally project slightly behind the left cardiac border. The hilar heights are normal with the right hilum being slightly lower than the left. **(Bottom)** PA chest radiograph of an asymptomatic adult with thoracic scoliosis and a remote healed left clavicular fracture. The chest wall deformity results in apparent displacement of the superior mediastinum to the left of the midline, hilar asymmetry and poor visualization of the right hilum. However, normal hilar height is preserved with the right hilum being slightly lower than the left.

HILA

RADIOGRAPHY, NORMAL RIGHT HILUM

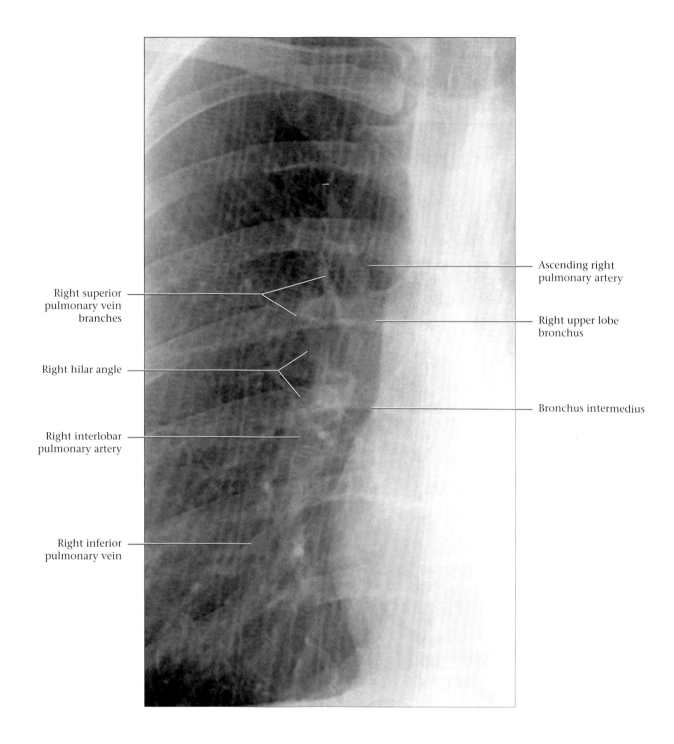

Right superior pulmonary vein branches

Right hilar angle

Right interlobar pulmonary artery

Right inferior pulmonary vein

Ascending right pulmonary artery

Right upper lobe bronchus

Bronchus intermedius

First of two coned-down images from a normal PA chest radiograph. Coned-down view of the right hilum shows that the superior hilum is characterized by the ascending right pulmonary artery located medial to the right upper lobe apical segmental bronchus. The right superior pulmonary vein is oriented obliquely and located lateral to the bronchus. The right main bronchus bifurcates into the right upper lobe bronchus and the bronchus intermedius. The right interlobar pulmonary artery is seen in the inferior right hilum and courses along the lateral aspect of the bronchus intermedius. A branch of the right inferior pulmonary vein exhibits a horizontal course relative to that of the right lower lobe pulmonary arteries.

HILA

RADIOGRAPHY, NORMAL LEFT HILUM

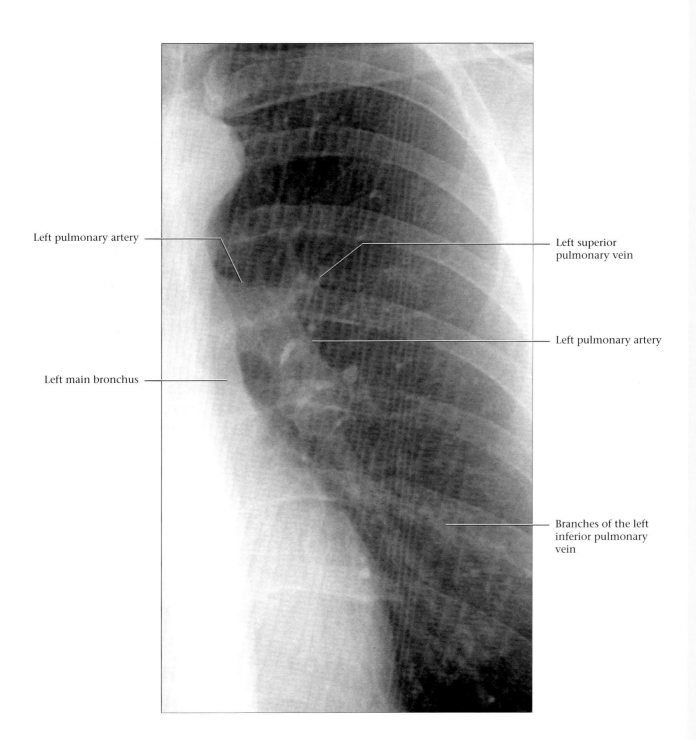

Left pulmonary artery

Left main bronchus

Left superior pulmonary vein

Left pulmonary artery

Branches of the left inferior pulmonary vein

Coned-down view of the left hilum shows the left pulmonary artery coursing above the left main bronchus. The left main bronchus is also called the hyparterial bronchus based on its relationship to the left pulmonary artery. The left superior pulmonary vein courses obliquely towards the left atrium. The left interlobar pulmonary artery courses along the posterolateral aspect of the left lower lobe bronchus. Branches of the left inferior pulmonary vein follow a relatively horizontal course when compared to that of the lower lobe pulmonary arteries.

HILA

GRAPHIC & RADIOGRAPHY, NORMAL HILA

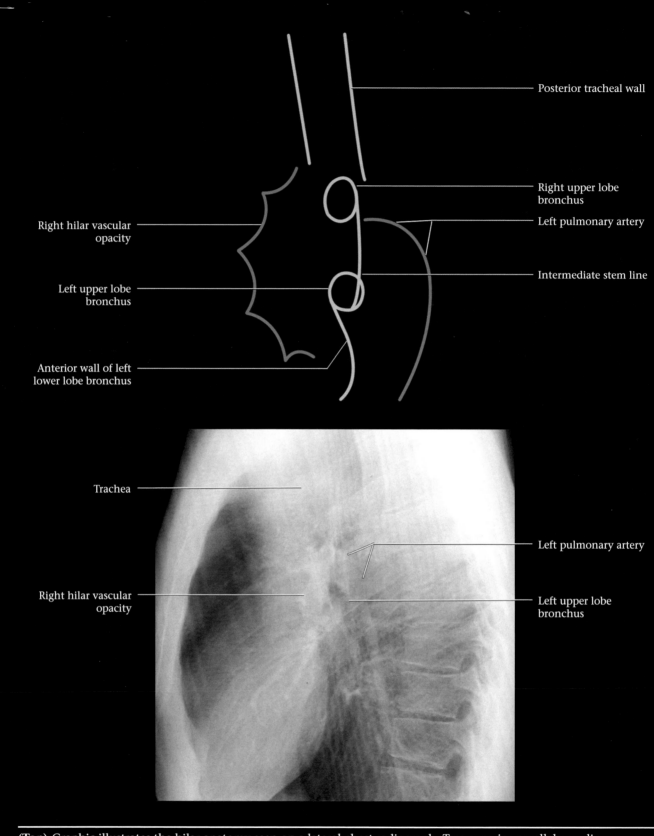

Posterior tracheal wall

Right upper lobe bronchus

Left pulmonary artery

Intermediate stem line

Right hilar vascular opacity

Left upper lobe bronchus

Anterior wall of left lower lobe bronchus

Trachea

Left pulmonary artery

Right hilar vascular opacity

Left upper lobe bronchus

(Top) Graphic illustrates the hilar anatomy seen on a lateral chest radiograph. Two superior parallel gray lines represent the trachea. Two gray circles (one superior, one inferior) represent the orifices of the right and left upper lobe bronchi respectively. A gray line drawn from the posterior superior circle intersects the posterior aspect of the inferior circle and represents the intermediate stem line. The arcuate gray line below the inferior circle represents the anterior wall of the left lower lobe bronchus. The anterior and posterior blue lines depict the right hilar vascular opacity and left pulmonary artery respectively. **(Bottom)** First of four normal lateral chest radiographs of different patients shows the anterior right hilar vascular opacity and the posterior left pulmonary artery. The left upper lobe bronchus is seen end-on in the central hilum.

HILA

RADIOGRAPHY, NORMAL HILA

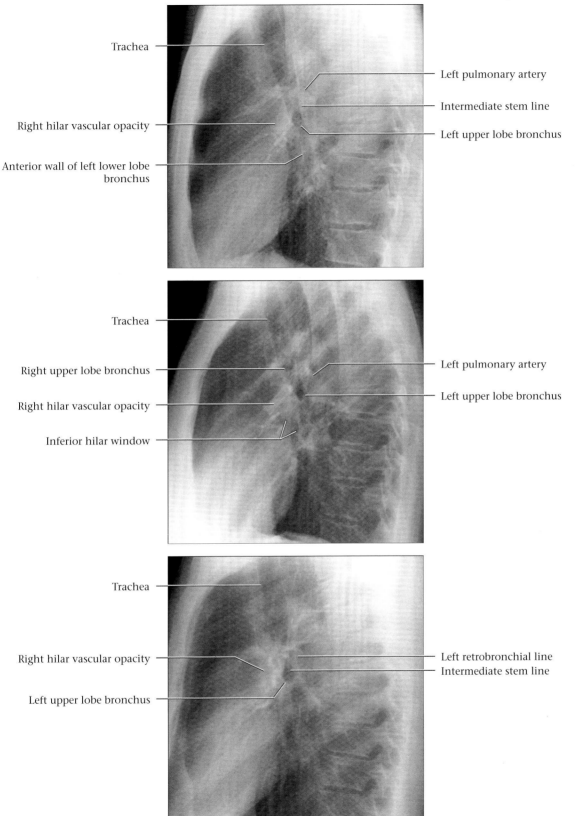

Trachea

Right hilar vascular opacity

Anterior wall of left lower lobe bronchus

Left pulmonary artery

Intermediate stem line

Left upper lobe bronchus

Trachea

Right upper lobe bronchus

Right hilar vascular opacity

Inferior hilar window

Left pulmonary artery

Left upper lobe bronchus

Trachea

Right hilar vascular opacity

Left upper lobe bronchus

Left retrobronchial line
Intermediate stem line

(Top) Left lateral chest radiograph shows the anterior right hilar vascular opacity and the posterior left pulmonary artery. The left upper lobe bronchus is seen end-on and is visible in 75% of normal subjects. The anterior wall of the left lower lobe bronchus is visible; the right upper lobe bronchus is not. **(Middle)** Left lateral chest radiograph shows partial visualization of the right upper lobe bronchus, seen in 50% of normal individuals. Typically the entire bronchial circumference is not visible. Note the avascular inferior hilar window. **(Bottom)** Left lateral chest radiograph shows the intermediate stem line (posterior walls of right main and intermediate bronchi), which normally measures 1.5 to 3 mm and is visible in 95% of normal subjects. The left retrobronchial line (posterior walls of left main and proximal lower lobe bronchi) is also visible.

HILA

AXIAL CT, NORMAL HILA

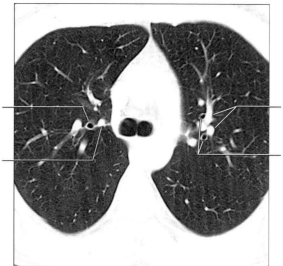

Right apical segmental bronchus

Right apical segmental artery

Left superior pulmonary veins

Branches of apicoposterior segmental bronchus

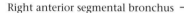

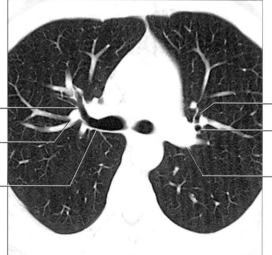

Right anterior segmental bronchus

Right posterior segmental vein

Right upper lobe bronchus

Anterior segmental bronchus

Apicoposterior segmental bronchus

Left pulmonary artery

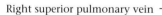

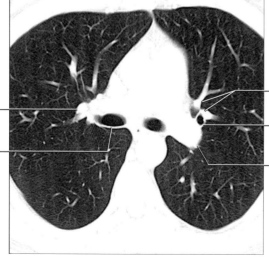

Right superior pulmonary vein

Bronchus intermedius

Left superior pulmonary vein branches

Left apicoposterior segmental bronchus

Left pulmonary artery

(Top) First of eighteen normal axial CT images (lung and mediastinal window) demonstrates the axial anatomy of the superior hila. The upper lobe bronchi and vessels form the suprahilar regions. The right apical segmental artery is medial to the apical segmental bronchus and the vein is lateral to the bronchus. Branches of the apicoposterior segmental bronchus and their corresponding veins and arteries are noted on the left. **(Middle)** Axial image shows the right upper lobe and right anterior segmental bronchi and their relationship to adjacent vessels. The left apicoposterior nord anterior segmental bronchi are anterior to the left pulmonary artery. **(Bottom)** Axial image through the bronchus intermedius shows the anterior location of the right superior pulmonary vein. The left superior pulmonary vein branches are anteromedial to the apicoposterior segmental bronchus.

AXIAL CT, NORMAL HILA

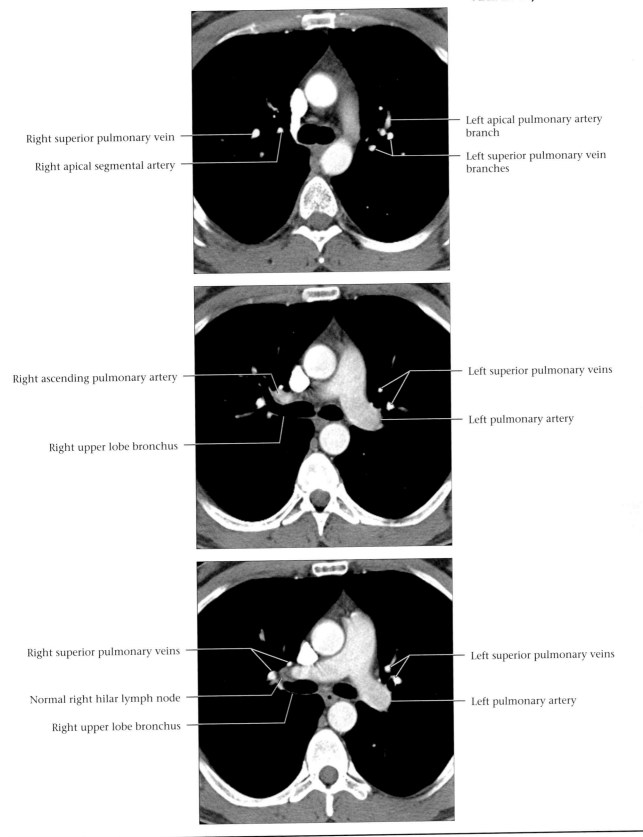

Right superior pulmonary vein

Right apical segmental artery

Left apical pulmonary artery branch

Left superior pulmonary vein branches

Right ascending pulmonary artery

Right upper lobe bronchus

Left superior pulmonary veins

Left pulmonary artery

Right superior pulmonary veins

Normal right hilar lymph node

Right upper lobe bronchus

Left superior pulmonary veins

Left pulmonary artery

(Top) Axial image demonstrates the vascular anatomy of the suprahilar regions. The upper lobe pulmonary vein branches course medially to join the left superior pulmonary vein. The upper lobe pulmonary arteries are typically medial to the bronchi (except in the lingula). **(Middle)** Axial image through the right upper lobe bronchus shows the ascending right pulmonary artery located anteriorly. The left superior pulmonary veins are located anterior to the left pulmonary artery. **(Bottom)** Axial image through the proximal aspect of the right upper lobe bronchus shows normal right hilar nodal tissue (ATS lymph node station 10R). Hilar lymph nodes are considered intrapulmonary (N1) for staging ipsilateral lung cancers. The anterior location of the pulmonary veins is again noted.

HILA

AXIAL CT, NORMAL HILA

Right superior pulmonary veins

Right interlobar pulmonary artery

Bronchus intermedius

Left superior pulmonary vein

Apicoposterior segmental bronchus

Left interlobar pulmonary artery

Right superior pulmonary veins

Right interlobar pulmonary artery

Bronchus intermedius

Left upper lobe bronchus

Left interlobar pulmonary artery

Right interlobar pulmonary artery

Bronchus intermedius

Left superior pulmonary vein

Superior lingular bronchus

Left interlobar pulmonary artery

(Top) Axial image through the bronchus intermedius demonstrates its thin posterior wall that forms part of the intermediate stem line on lateral radiography. The left pulmonary artery courses over the left main bronchus and is posterior to the apicoposterior segmental bronchus. (Middle) Axial image through the left upper lobe and intermediate bronchi shows the posterolateral location of the left interlobar pulmonary artery with respect to the left upper lobe bronchus. The proximal right interlobar pulmonary artery and right superior pulmonary veins are anterior to the bronchus intermedius. (Bottom) Axial image through the superior lingular bronchus shows the posterolateral left interlobar pulmonary artery. The right superior pulmonary veins and interlobar artery exhibit the characteristic "elephant head-and-trunk" configuration anterior to the bronchus intermedius.

HILA

AXIAL CT, NORMAL HILA

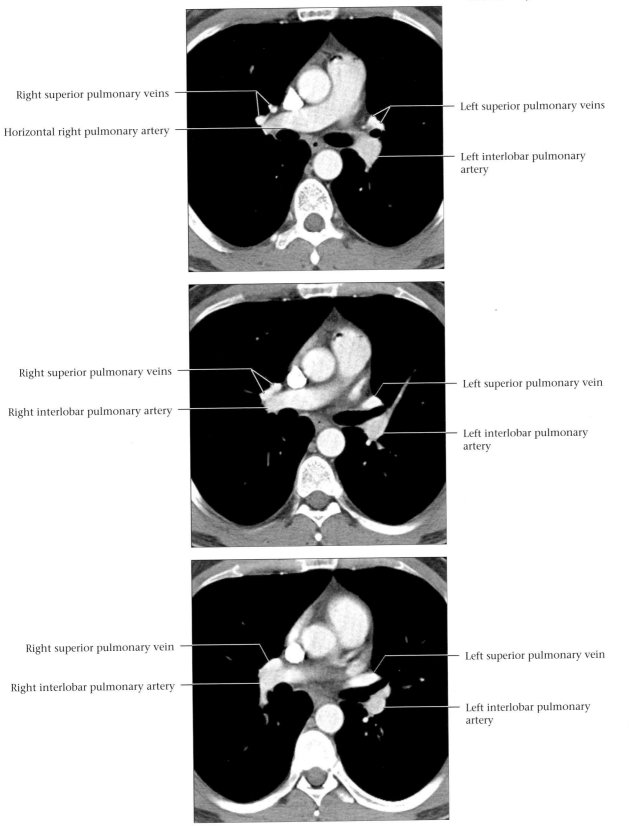

Right superior pulmonary veins

Horizontal right pulmonary artery

Left superior pulmonary veins

Left interlobar pulmonary artery

Right superior pulmonary veins

Right interlobar pulmonary artery

Left superior pulmonary vein

Left interlobar pulmonary artery

Right superior pulmonary vein

Right interlobar pulmonary artery

Left superior pulmonary vein

Left interlobar pulmonary artery

(Top) Axial image through the pulmonary trunk shows the bilateral superior pulmonary veins located anterior to the horizontal portion of the right pulmonary artery and anteromedial to the left apicoposterior segmental bronchus. The left interlobar pulmonary artery courses posterior to the bronchi. **(Middle)** Axial image through the left upper lobe bronchus shows the bilateral superior pulmonary veins located anteriorly. Note the horizontal portion of the right pulmonary artery and the vertical course of the left interlobar artery behind the left upper lobe bronchus. **(Bottom)** Axial image through the bronchus intermedius shows that the right superior pulmonary vein is closely related to the anterior aspect of the right interlobar artery as the latter curves posteriorly. These structures form the "elephant head-and-trunk" morphology of the right hilum at this level.

HILA

AXIAL CT, NORMAL HILA

Middle lobe bronchus

Right interlobar pulmonary artery

Superior segmental right lower lobe bronchus

Left interlobar pulmonary artery

Superior segmental left lower lobe bronchus

Right truncus basalis

Basal segmental right lower lobe pulmonary arteries

Left truncus basalis

Basal segmental left lower lobe pulmonary arteries

Left inferior pulmonary vein

Right inferior pulmonary vein

Right lower lobe basal segmental bronchi

Left inferior pulmonary vein

Left lower lobe basal segmental bronchi

(Top) Axial image through the middle lobe bronchus demonstrates the lateral location of the right interlobar pulmonary artery with respect to the bronchial bifurcation at this level. Note the origins and posterior course of the bilateral superior segmental lower lobe bronchi. (Middle) Axial image through the infrahilar region demonstrates the bilateral basal trunks of the lower lobe bronchi and the posterolateral location of the corresponding lower lobe basal segmental pulmonary arteries. The left inferior pulmonary vein is medial to the left basal trunk. (Bottom) Axial image through the infrahilar region demonstrates the near horizontal course of the bilateral inferior pulmonary veins. The basal segmental bronchi are located anterior and posterior to the pulmonary veins and are accompanied by their corresponding pulmonary arteries.

HILA

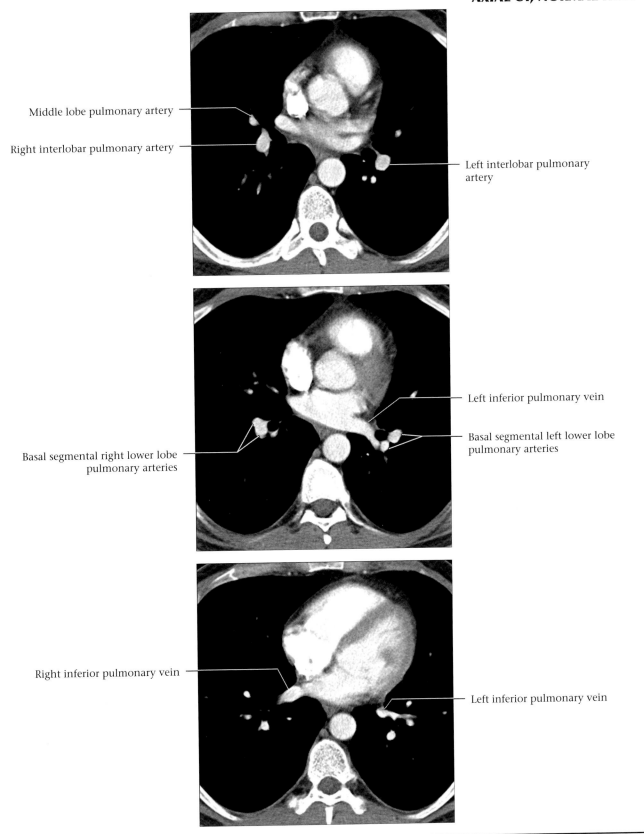

(Top) Axial image at the level of the middle lobe bronchus shows the middle lobe pulmonary artery located lateral to the bronchus. The vertical course and lateral location of the bilateral interlobar pulmonary arteries are also shown. **(Middle)** Axial image through the left inferior pulmonary vein demonstrates the characteristic lateral location of the pulmonary arteries with respect to their corresponding bronchi in the lower and middle lobes. Note the horizontal course of the left inferior pulmonary vein. **(Bottom)** Axial image through the bilateral inferior pulmonary veins demonstrates their horizontal course relative to the more vertical course of the lower lobe arteries. Note that the left inferior pulmonary vein is located posterior to the anteromedial basal segmental pulmonary artery but anterior to the lateral and posterior basal segmental pulmonary arteries.

HILA

CORONAL CT, NORMAL HILA

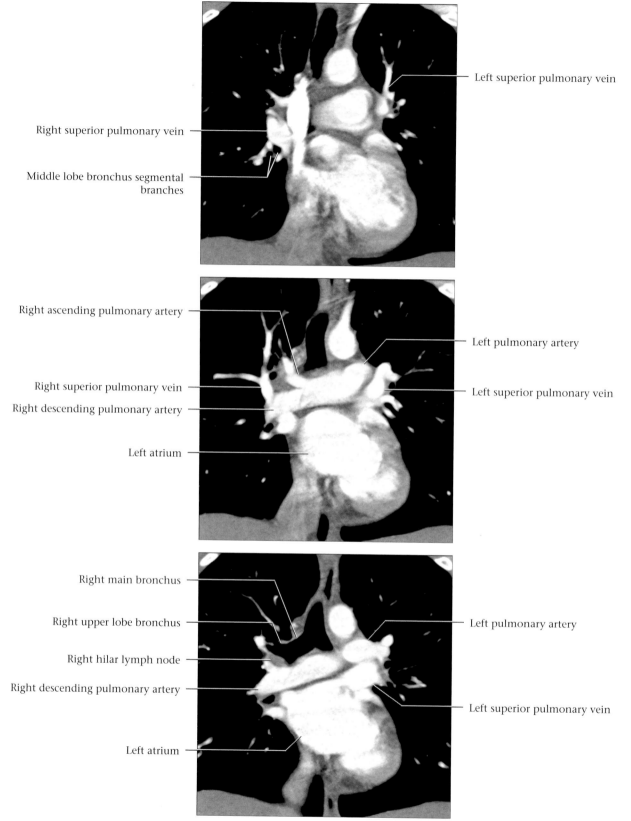

(Top) First of twelve normal coronal reconstruction images from a contrast-enhanced chest CT (mediastinal and lung window). Image through the anterior hila demonstrates the anterior location of the bilateral superior pulmonary veins and the medial and lateral segmental middle lobe bronchi seen in cross-section. (Middle) Coronal image through the horizontal portion of the right pulmonary artery shows its ascending and descending branches. The left superior pulmonary vein is seen in its vertical course into the left atrium. (Bottom) Coronal image through the carina shows the superior location of the left pulmonary artery with respect to the right. The right (eparterial) main bronchus is above the ipsilateral pulmonary artery. Note the normal hilar lymph node at the bifurcation of the right main bronchus into right upper lobe and intermediate bronchi.

HILA

CORONAL CT, NORMAL HILA

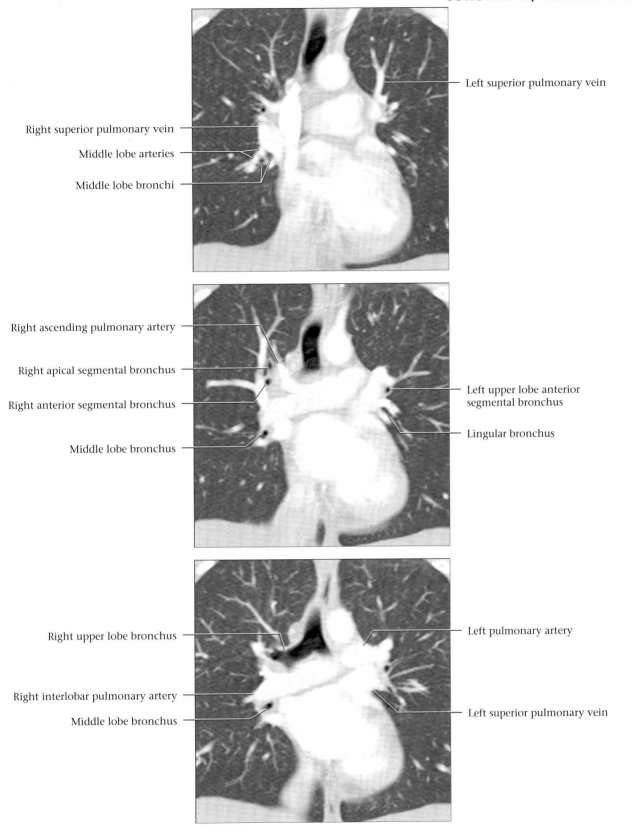

Left superior pulmonary vein

Right superior pulmonary vein

Middle lobe arteries

Middle lobe bronchi

Right ascending pulmonary artery

Right apical segmental bronchus

Left upper lobe anterior segmental bronchus

Right anterior segmental bronchus

Lingular bronchus

Middle lobe bronchus

Right upper lobe bronchus

Left pulmonary artery

Right interlobar pulmonary artery

Middle lobe bronchus

Left superior pulmonary vein

(Top) Coronal image through the anterior hila shows the segmental branches (medial and lateral) of the middle lobe bronchus and the anterior location of the bilateral superior pulmonary veins. **(Middle)** Coronal image through the horizontal right pulmonary artery demonstrates the relationship of the right upper lobe arteries and veins to the airways. The right ascending pulmonary artery is medial to the apical and anterior segmental bronchi and the right superior pulmonary vein is located laterally. The middle lobe bronchus and the right and left upper lobe anterior segmental bronchi are seen in cross-section. **(Bottom)** Coronal image through the right upper lobe bronchus demonstrates that the right (eparterial) bronchus is situated above the ipsilateral pulmonary artery. Note the superior location of the left pulmonary artery with respect to the right.

HILA

CORONAL CT, NORMAL HILA

(Top) Coronal image through the bronchus intermedius demonstrates the bilateral pulmonary veins entering the left atrium. The coronal anatomy of the left suprahilar region is demonstrated. The right interlobar pulmonary artery courses lateral to the bronchus intermedius. A normal right hilar lymph node is also seen. **(Middle)** Coronal image through the mid hila shows the lateral location of the right interlobar pulmonary artery with respect to the bronchus intermedius. Note the horizontal course of the right inferior pulmonary veins. The left pulmonary artery courses above the left (hyparterial) bronchus. **(Bottom)** Coronal image through the posterior hila shows the vertical orientation of the left interlobar pulmonary artery, seen lateral to the left lower lobe bronchus, and the horizontal course of the left inferior pulmonary vein into the left atrium.

HILA

CORONAL CT, NORMAL HILA

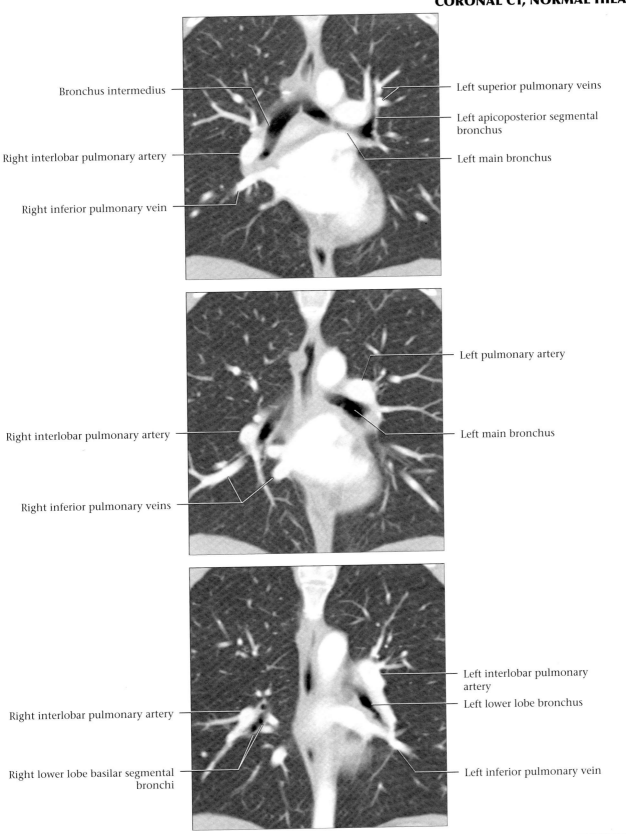

Bronchus intermedius

Right interlobar pulmonary artery

Right inferior pulmonary vein

Left superior pulmonary veins

Left apicoposterior segmental bronchus

Left main bronchus

Right interlobar pulmonary artery

Right inferior pulmonary veins

Left pulmonary artery

Left main bronchus

Right interlobar pulmonary artery

Right lower lobe basilar segmental bronchi

Left interlobar pulmonary artery

Left lower lobe bronchus

Left inferior pulmonary vein

(Top) Coronal image through the posterior aspect of the carina shows the left pulmonary artery coursing superior to the left main (hyparterial) bronchus. Note the bronchial anatomy of the left superior hilum and the relationship of the airways to adjacent vessels. The right interlobar artery courses along the lateral aspect of the bronchus intermedius. (Middle) Coronal image through the posterior hila demonstrates the relationship of the left pulmonary artery to the left main bronchus and the relationship of the right interlobar artery to the bronchus intermedius. Two right inferior pulmonary veins enter the left atrium. (Bottom) Coronal image through the posterior hila demonstrates the left interlobar pulmonary artery coursing vertically along the left lower lobe bronchus and the relatively horizontal course of the left inferior pulmonary vein.

HILA

GRAPHIC, SAGITTAL CT & MR, NORMAL RIGHT HILUM

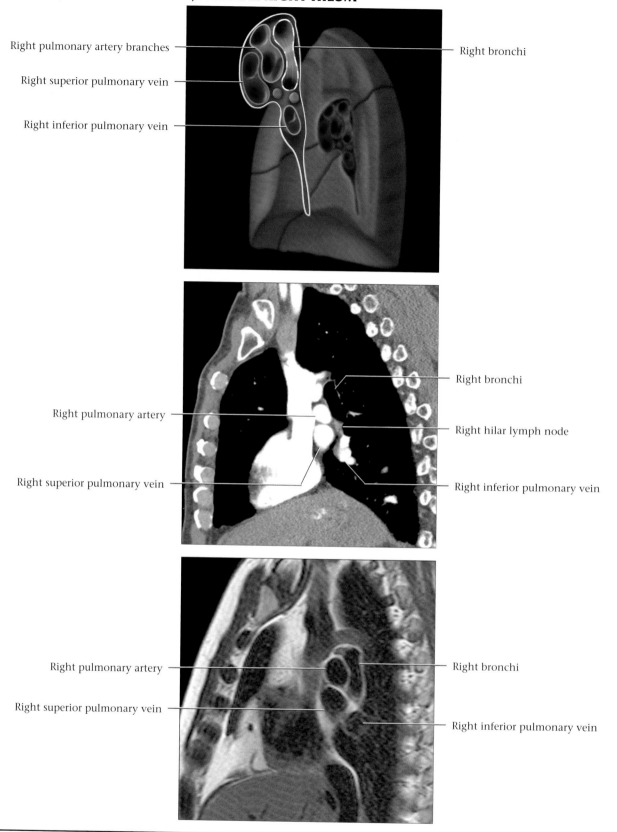

Right pulmonary artery branches

Right superior pulmonary vein

Right inferior pulmonary vein

Right bronchi

Right pulmonary artery

Right superior pulmonary vein

Right bronchi

Right hilar lymph node

Right inferior pulmonary vein

Right pulmonary artery

Right superior pulmonary vein

Right bronchi

Right inferior pulmonary vein

(Top) Graphic demonstrates the relationships of the hilar airways and vessels. The right bronchi are the most posterior structures in the upper hilum and the superior pulmonary vein the most anterior. The pulmonary artery is located centrally between the superior pulmonary vein and the bronchi, and the inferior pulmonary vein is located inferiorly. (Middle) Normal contrast-enhanced chest CT (mediastinal window) with sagittal reconstruction through the right hilum demonstrates the relationship of the airways and vascular structures depicted on the graphic. Hilar nodal tissue is often identified on thin section chest CT of normal subjects. (Bottom) Sagittal T1-weighted MR image through the right hilum shows the anterior and inferior locations of the pulmonary veins and the posterior location of the airway. The right pulmonary artery is located in the central hilum.

HILA

GRAPHIC, SAGITTAL CT & MR, NORMAL LEFT HILUM

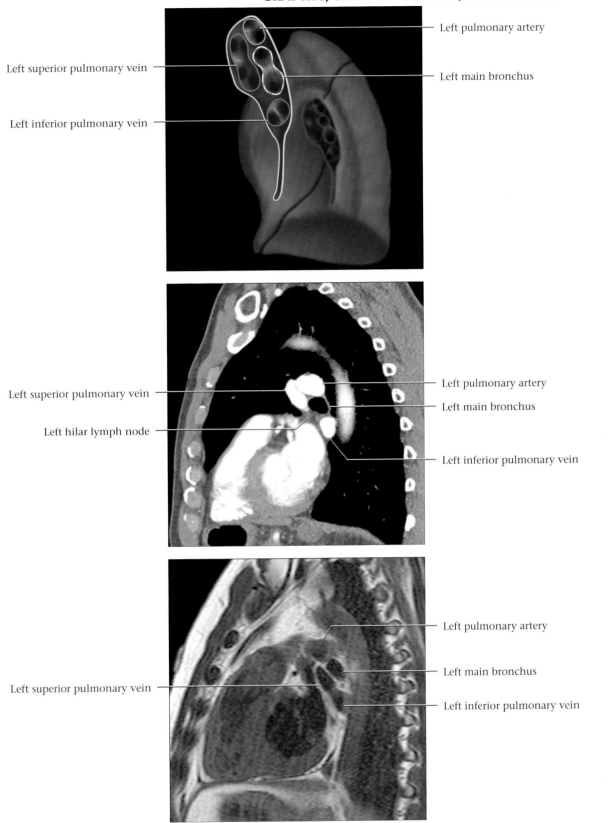

(Top) Graphic that corresponds to the sagittal CT and MR images shows the normal relationships of the left hilar vessels to the main bronchus. The pulmonary veins are located anteriorly and inferiorly and the left main bronchus is located posteriorly. The left pulmonary artery is located superiorly and courses over the left (hyparterial) bronchus. (Middle) Contrast-enhanced chest CT with sagittal reconstruction (mediastinal window) demonstrates the appearance of the normal left hilum. The left pulmonary artery courses above the left (hyparterial) bronchus. The pulmonary veins are located anteriorly and inferiorly within the hilum. The left main bronchus is located posteriorly within the mid portion of the hilum. Note left hilar lymph nodes. (Bottom) Sagittal T1-weighted MR image through the left hilum shows the anatomic relationships shown on the graphic and the CT.

HILA

AXIAL MR, NORMAL HILA

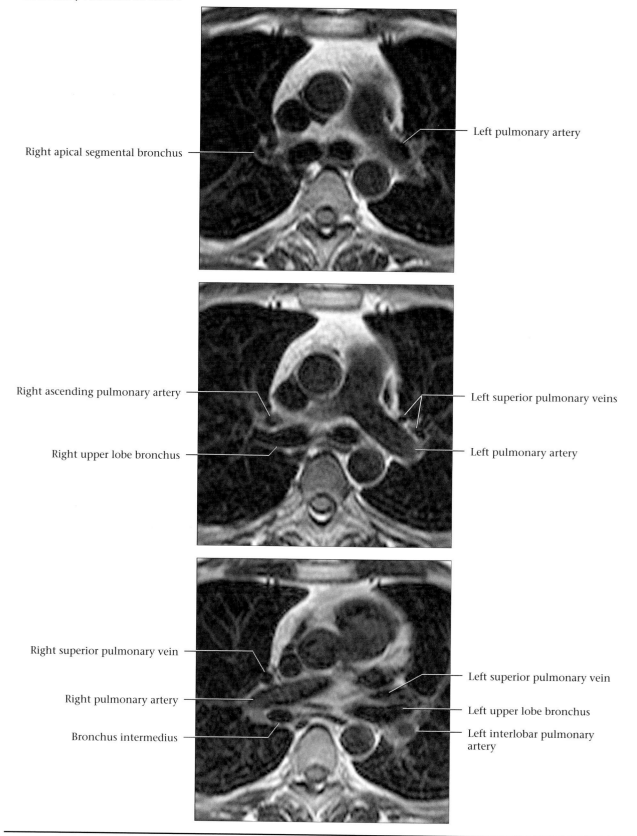

Right apical segmental bronchus

Left pulmonary artery

Right ascending pulmonary artery

Left superior pulmonary veins

Right upper lobe bronchus

Left pulmonary artery

Right superior pulmonary vein

Left superior pulmonary vein

Right pulmonary artery

Left upper lobe bronchus

Bronchus intermedius

Left interlobar pulmonary artery

(Top) First of three normal axial T1-weighted MR images demonstrates the left pulmonary artery as it courses over the (hyparterial) left bronchus. The right apical segmental bronchus is identified with its corresponding pulmonary artery. **(Middle)** Axial image below the carina demonstrates the horizontal portion of the left pulmonary artery and the anteriorly located left superior pulmonary veins. The right upper lobe bronchus and anteriorly located right ascending pulmonary artery are seen in the right hilum. **(Bottom)** Axial image at the level of the bronchus intermedius shows the horizontal portion of the right pulmonary artery coursing anterior to the bronchus intermedius and the left interlobar pulmonary artery located posterolateral to the left upper lobe bronchus. Note the anterior location of the bilateral superior pulmonary veins.

HILA

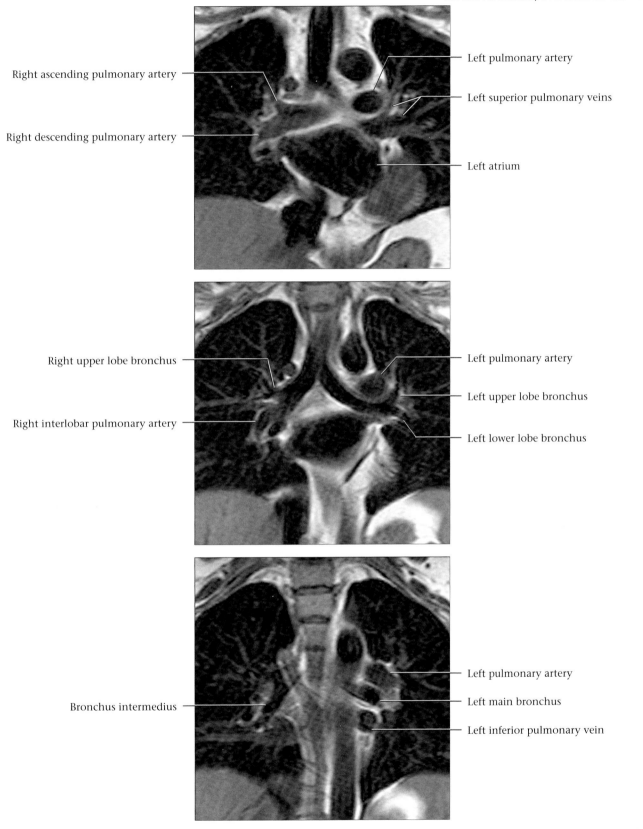

Right ascending pulmonary artery

Right descending pulmonary artery

Left pulmonary artery

Left superior pulmonary veins

Left atrium

Right upper lobe bronchus

Right interlobar pulmonary artery

Left pulmonary artery

Left upper lobe bronchus

Left lower lobe bronchus

Bronchus intermedius

Left pulmonary artery

Left main bronchus

Left inferior pulmonary vein

(Top) First of three coronal T1-weighted MR images through the mid hila shows the horizontal portion of the right pulmonary artery and its ascending and descending branches. The left superior pulmonary veins are seen coursing into the left atrium under the left pulmonary artery. (Middle) Coronal image through the carina demonstrates the relationship of the bilateral pulmonary arteries to their ipsilateral bronchi. The left pulmonary artery courses above the left main or hyparterial bronchus. The right pulmonary artery is located under the right or eparterial bronchus. (Bottom) Coronal image through the bronchus intermedius and the posterior left main bronchus demonstrates the posterior aspect of the left pulmonary artery as it begins to course inferiorly to become the interlobar pulmonary artery. Note the horizontal orientation of the left inferior pulmonary vein.

HILA

THE HILUM OVERLAY SIGN

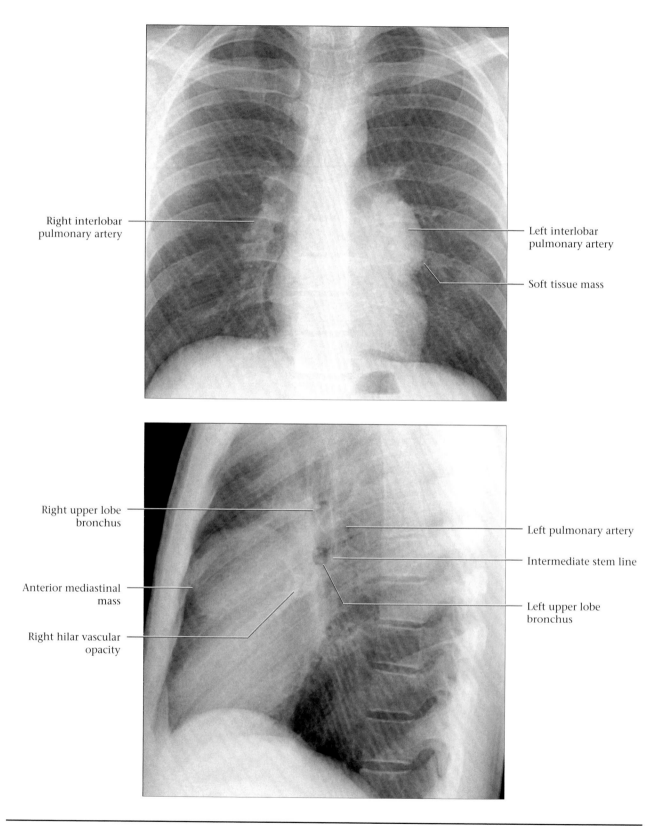

Right interlobar pulmonary artery

Left interlobar pulmonary artery

Soft tissue mass

Right upper lobe bronchus

Left pulmonary artery

Intermediate stem line

Anterior mediastinal mass

Right hilar vascular opacity

Left upper lobe bronchus

(Top) First of two radiographs of a 23 year old man with mediastinal T-cell lymphoma demonstrates the hilum overlay sign. PA chest radiograph shows an ovoid mass that projects over the left hilum and mid portion of the left mediastinal contour. The left interlobar pulmonary artery is visible through the soft tissue mass indicating that the mass is separate from the artery and the hilum. **(Bottom)** Left lateral chest radiograph demonstrates the anterior mediastinal location of the soft tissue mass. The left pulmonary artery and hilar structures appear normal. The right hilar vascular opacity is noted anterior to the hilar airways. Other normal hilar landmarks such as the bilateral upper lobe bronchi, the intermediate stem line and the left retrobronchial line are visible.

HILA

THE HILUM CONVERGENCE SIGN

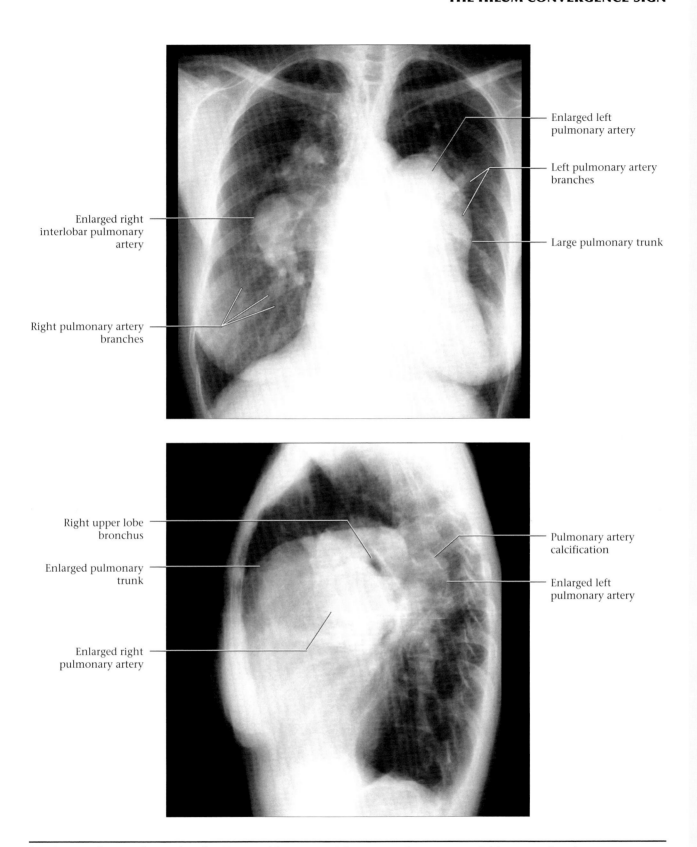

Enlarged left pulmonary artery

Left pulmonary artery branches

Large pulmonary trunk

Enlarged right interlobar pulmonary artery

Right pulmonary artery branches

Right upper lobe bronchus

Enlarged pulmonary trunk

Enlarged right pulmonary artery

Pulmonary artery calcification

Enlarged left pulmonary artery

(Top) First of two radiographs of a 45 year old woman with severe pulmonary arterial hypertension due to uncorrected atrial septal defect shows the hilar convergence sign. PA chest radiograph shows cardiomegaly and an enlarged pulmonary trunk. Enlarged pulmonary arteries converge towards bilateral hilar masses indicating their vascular etiology. Reproduced with permission from Parker MS, Rosado-de-Christenson ML, Abbott GF. Teaching Atlas of Chest Imaging. New York: Thieme, 2005. (Bottom) Left lateral chest radiograph shows massive pulmonary trunk and pulmonary artery enlargement with posterior displacement of the hilar airways. The orifice of the right upper lobe bronchus is well visualized due to the surrounding enlarged vessels. Mural pulmonary artery calcification indicates severe long standing pulmonary arterial hypertension.

HILA

ABNORMAL HILAR POSITION, VOLUME LOSS

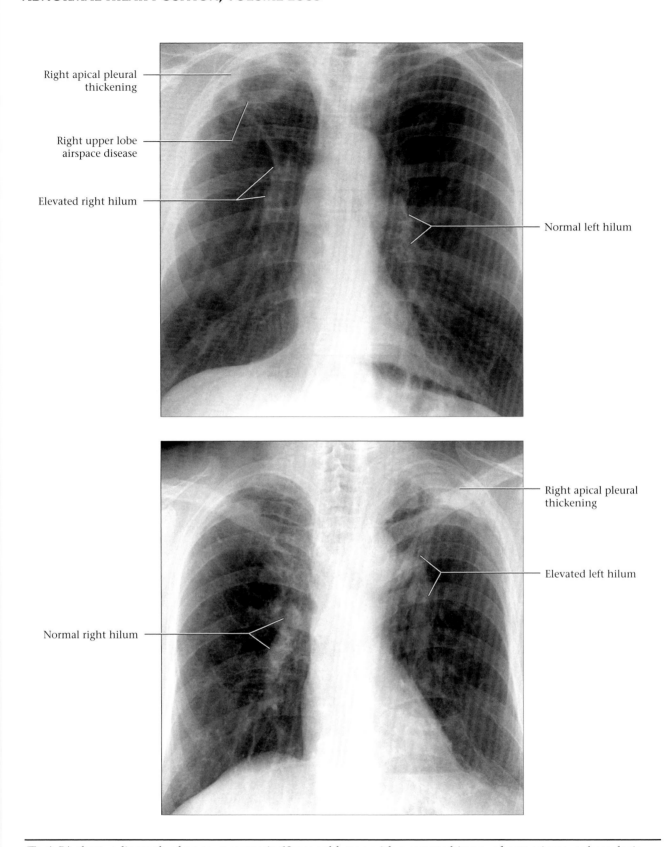

Right apical pleural thickening

Right upper lobe airspace disease

Elevated right hilum

Normal left hilum

Right apical pleural thickening

Elevated left hilum

Normal right hilum

(Top) PA chest radiograph of an asymptomatic 60 year old man with a remote history of postprimary tuberculosis demonstrates elevation of the right hilum secondary to right apical fibrosis manifesting with right upper lobe airspace disease and adjacent pleural thickening. The normal right hilum is typically slightly lower than the left. **(Bottom)** PA chest radiograph of a 57 year old man with asymmetric left apical pleural thickening and left upper lobe fibrosis secondary to prior post primary tuberculosis demonstrates elevation and distortion of the left hilum. Although the left hilum is typically higher than the right, the asymmetry of hilar height is not normally this pronounced. The right hilum is of normal size and position.

HILA

BILATERAL HILAR CALCIFICATION, PNEUMOCONIOSIS

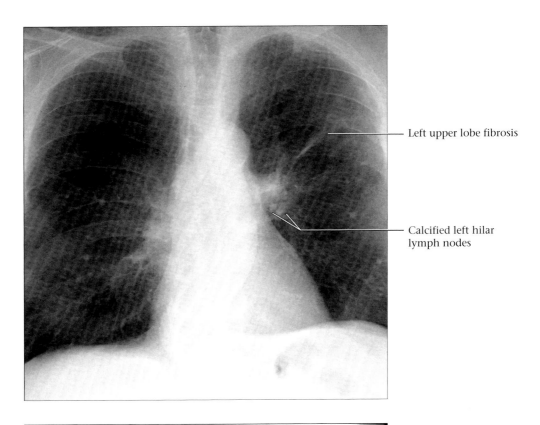

Left upper lobe fibrosis

Calcified left hilar lymph nodes

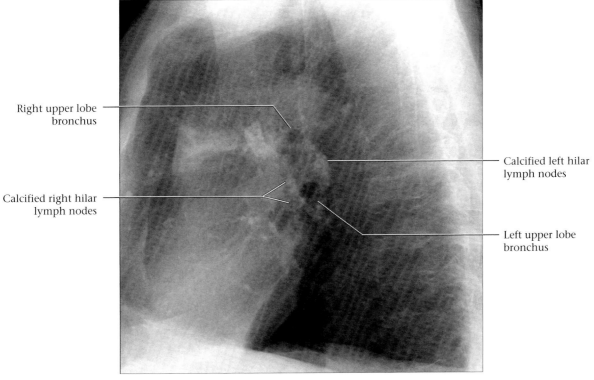

Right upper lobe bronchus

Calcified right hilar lymph nodes

Calcified left hilar lymph nodes

Left upper lobe bronchus

(Top) First of two images of an asymptomatic 64 year old man with silicosis. PA chest radiograph demonstrates mild elevation of the left hilum with associated left suprahilar pulmonary linear opacity secondary to focal fibrosis. There are multifocal foci of hilar lymph node calcification secondary to silicosis. Note multifocal small bilateral calcified lung nodules related to pulmonary involvement by silicosis. (Bottom) Left lateral chest radiograph demonstrates bilateral hilar lymph node calcification. Note exquisite visualization of the entire circumference of the right upper lobe bronchial orifice which suggests an increase in adjacent soft tissue likely related to adjacent lymph node enlargement. Mediastinal lymph node calcification is also noted.

HILA

HILAR CALCIFICATION, REMOTE GRANULOMATOUS INFECTION

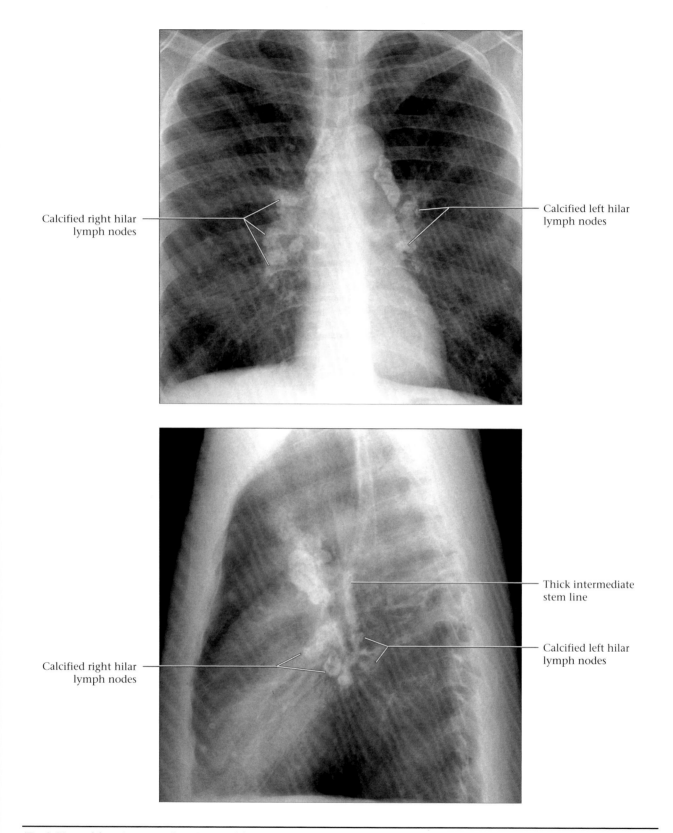

Calcified right hilar lymph nodes

Calcified left hilar lymph nodes

Thick intermediate stem line

Calcified left hilar lymph nodes

Calcified right hilar lymph nodes

(Top) First of four images of a 46 year old man with known remote granulomatous infection and past episodes of broncholithiasis. PA chest radiograph demonstrates bilateral abnormal hilar density with exuberant bilateral multifocal calcifications of ovoid and spherical morphology consistent with calcification in bilateral hilar and mediastinal lymph nodes. There are bilateral small nodular calcified granulomas in the lungs. **(Bottom)** Left lateral chest radiograph demonstrates bilateral hilar and mediastinal lymph node calcifications as well as calcified pulmonary granulomas. There is thickening of the intermediate stem line. Calcified mediastinal granulomas are noted projecting anterior to the central airways. Note that there are calcified lymph nodes in the inferior hilar window.

HILAR CALCIFICATION, REMOTE GRANULOMATOUS INFECTION

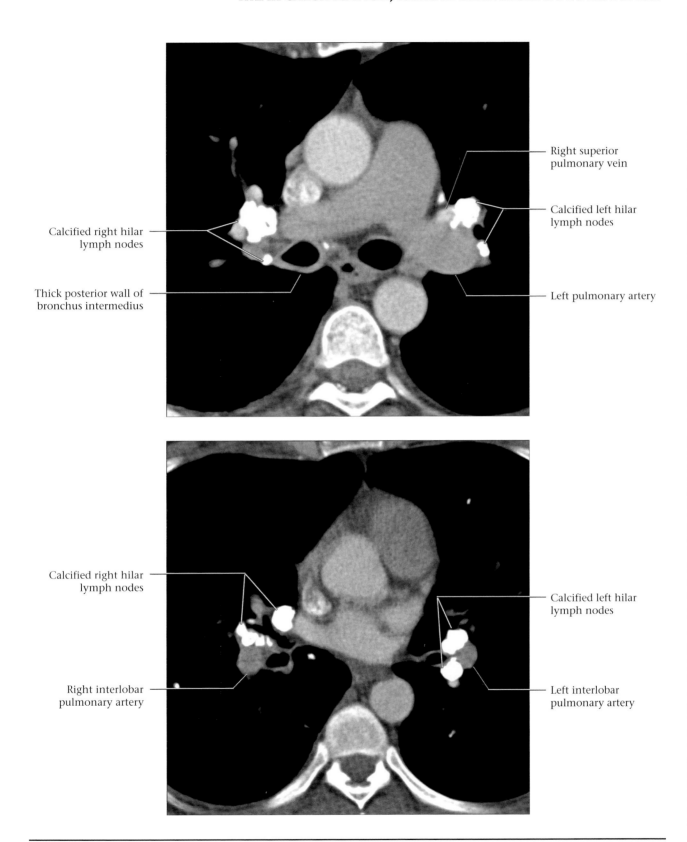

Right superior pulmonary vein

Calcified left hilar lymph nodes

Calcified right hilar lymph nodes

Thick posterior wall of bronchus intermedius

Left pulmonary artery

Calcified right hilar lymph nodes

Calcified left hilar lymph nodes

Right interlobar pulmonary artery

Left interlobar pulmonary artery

(Top) Contrast-enhanced chest CT (mediastinal window) at the level of the pulmonary trunk demonstrates bilateral lobular densely calcified hilar nodules representing calcified lymph nodes secondary to remote granulomatous infection. The posterior wall of the bronchus intermedius is thick and correlates with the finding seen on the lateral chest radiograph. **(Bottom)** Contrast-enhanced chest CT (mediastinal window) at the level of the left atrium shows bilateral densely calcified hilar/infrahilar lymph nodes. Calcification in intrathoracic lymph nodes typically relates to benign processes, usually remote granulomatous infection.

HILA

THICK INTERMEDIATE STEM LINE, BRONCHOGENIC CARCINOMA

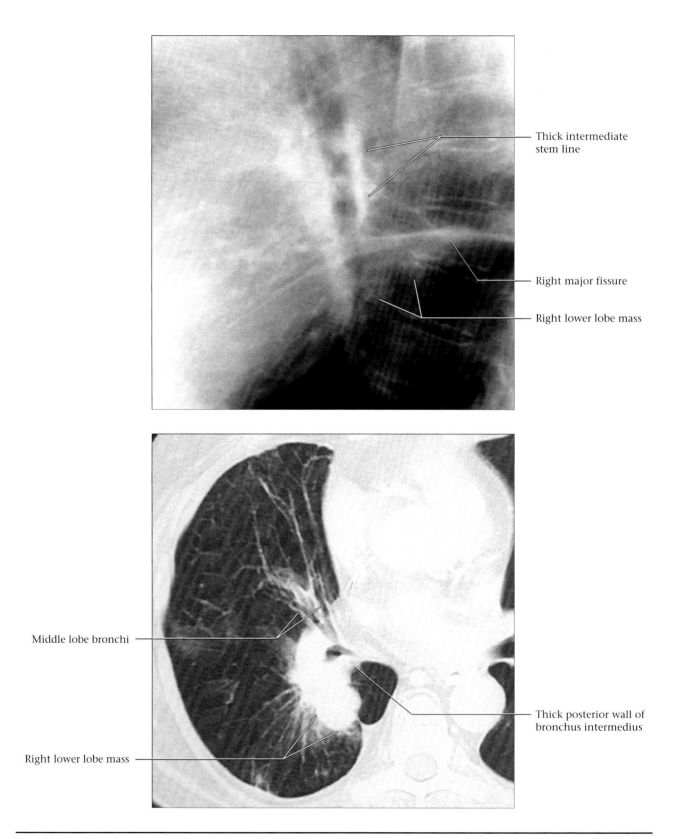

Thick intermediate stem line

Right major fissure

Right lower lobe mass

Middle lobe bronchi

Thick posterior wall of bronchus intermedius

Right lower lobe mass

(Top) First of two images of a 41 year old man with a central right lower lobe squamous cell carcinoma. Left lateral chest radiograph coned-down to the hila demonstrates lobular thickening of the intermediate stem line. Note inferior displacement and thickening of the major fissure secondary to right lower lobe volume loss and the lobular right lower lobe mass. **(Bottom)** Contrast-enhanced chest CT (lung window) demonstrates a large lobular right lower lobe mass with spiculated borders and a pleural tag. The bronchus intermedius is deformed by peribronchial and endoluminal involvement by the neoplasm and adjacent affected intrapulmonary lymph nodes. Note associated middle and right lower lobe volume loss secondary to bronchial obstruction.

HILA

UNILATERAL HILAR ENLARGEMENT, BRONCHOGENIC CARCINOMA

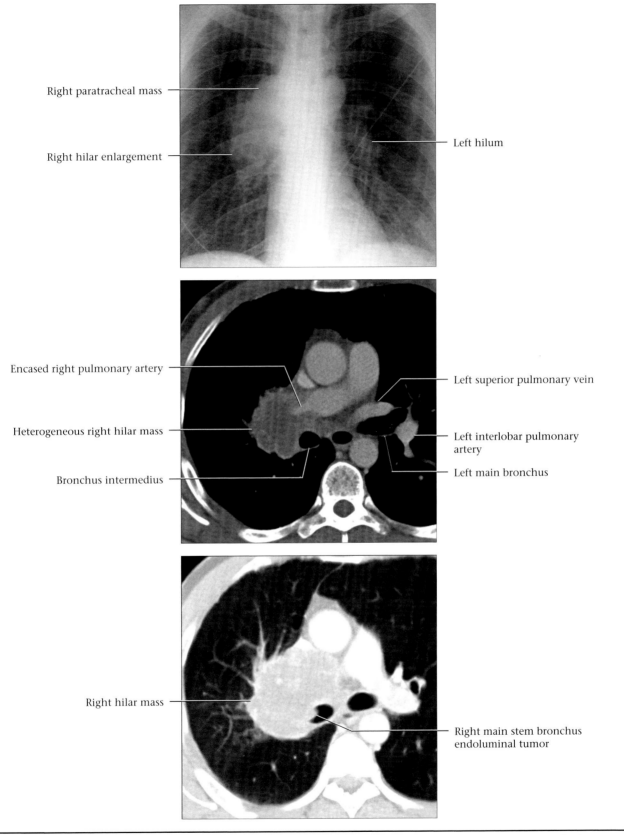

Right paratracheal mass

Right hilar enlargement

Left hilum

Encased right pulmonary artery

Left superior pulmonary vein

Heterogeneous right hilar mass

Left interlobar pulmonary artery

Bronchus intermedius

Left main bronchus

Right hilar mass

Right main stem bronchus endoluminal tumor

(Top) First of three images of a 50 year old man who presented with advanced lung cancer metastatic to the brain. AP chest radiograph coned to the hila demonstrates unilateral right hilar enlargement and a right paratracheal mass. The right upper lobe bronchial lumen is obscured. (Middle) Contrast-enhanced chest CT (mediastinal window) demonstrates a heterogeneously enhancing right hilar mass that encases, narrows and obstructs the right pulmonary artery and abuts the anterolateral wall of the bronchus intermedius. The left hilum appears normal. (Bottom) Contrast-enhanced chest CT (lung window) shows a large right hilar mass that invades the adjacent mediastinum, obstructs the right upper lobe bronchus and is associated with endoluminal tumor in the right main bronchus. Endoscopic biopsy revealed non-small cell lung cancer.

HILA

BILATERAL HILAR ENLARGEMENT, LYMPHADENOPATHY

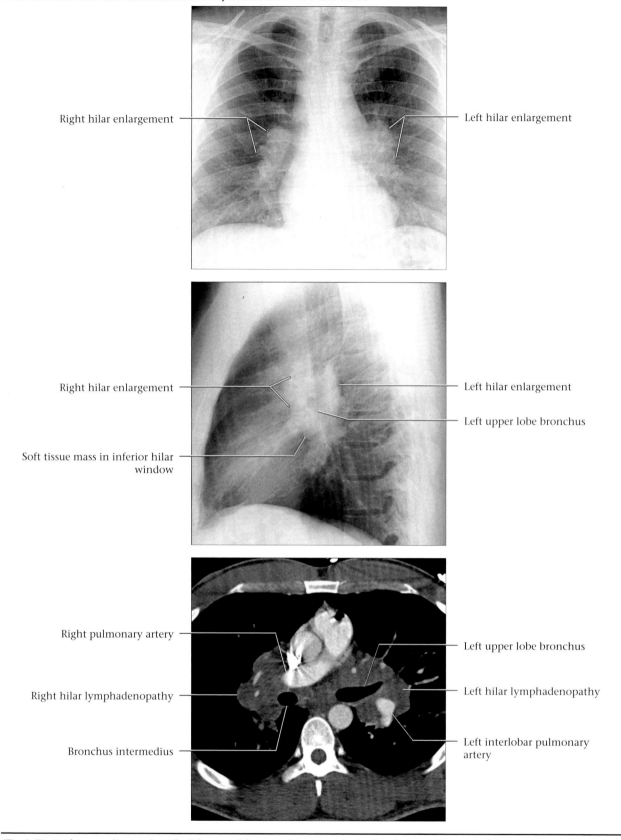

Right hilar enlargement — Left hilar enlargement

Right hilar enlargement — Left hilar enlargement

Left upper lobe bronchus

Soft tissue mass in inferior hilar window

Right pulmonary artery — Left upper lobe bronchus

Right hilar lymphadenopathy — Left hilar lymphadenopathy

Bronchus intermedius — Left interlobar pulmonary artery

(Top) First of two radiographs of a 38 year old man with sarcoidosis. PA chest radiograph demonstrates bilateral hilar enlargement secondary to lymphadenopathy. The superior mediastinum is wide consistent with associated right paratracheal and aortopulmonary window lymphadenopathy. (Middle) Left lateral chest radiograph demonstrates bilateral lobular hilar enlargement secondary to lymphadenopathy. Note the abnormal lobular soft tissue in the inferior hilar window related to lymphadenopathy. (Bottom) Contrast-enhanced chest CT (mediastinal window) of a 32 year old man with sarcoidosis demonstrates marked bilateral hilar and subcarinal lymphadenopathy. The enlarged lymph nodes encase the vascular structures and airways.

BILATERAL HILAR ENLARGEMENT, PULMONARY HYPERTENSION

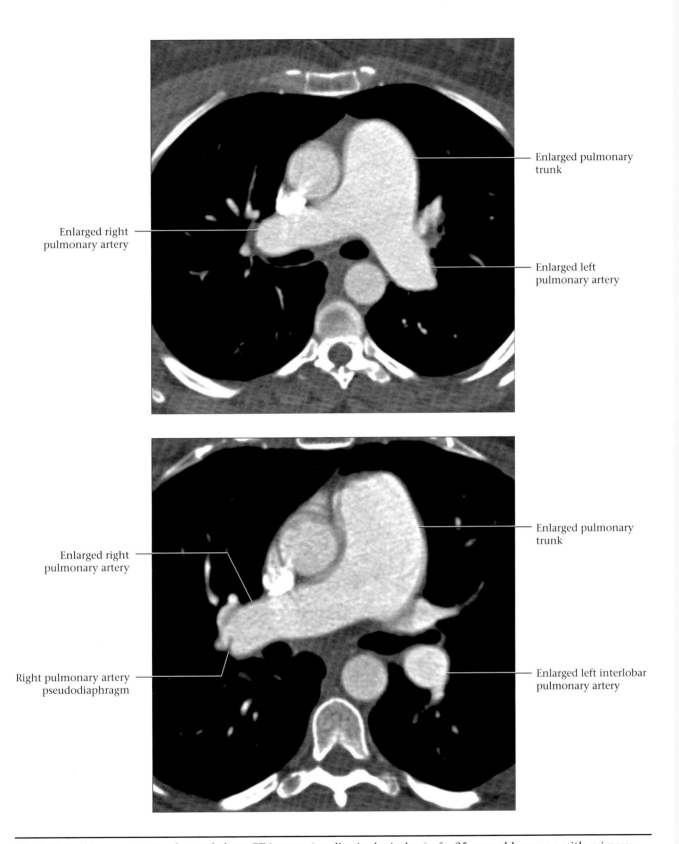

Enlarged pulmonary trunk

Enlarged right pulmonary artery

Enlarged left pulmonary artery

Enlarged pulmonary trunk

Enlarged right pulmonary artery

Enlarged left interlobar pulmonary artery

Right pulmonary artery pseudodiaphragm

(Top) First of two contrast-enhanced chest CT images (mediastinal window) of a 35 year old woman with primary pulmonary arterial hypertension. Axial image below the carina demonstrates enlargement of the pulmonary trunk and the bilateral pulmonary arteries. Pulmonary hypertension should be suspected when the diameter of the pulmonary trunk is larger than that of the adjacent ascending aorta as in this case. **(Bottom)** Axial image obtained 10 mm caudally demonstrates an enlarged pulmonary trunk and enlargement of the bilateral pulmonary arteries. Note the linear endoluminal filling defect in the right pulmonary artery which represents a "pseudodiaphragm" secondary to marked vascular dilatation. This finding may be misinterpreted as imaging evidence of chronic pulmonary thromboembolism.

HILA

UNILATERAL HILAR ENLARGEMENT, PULMONIC STENOSIS

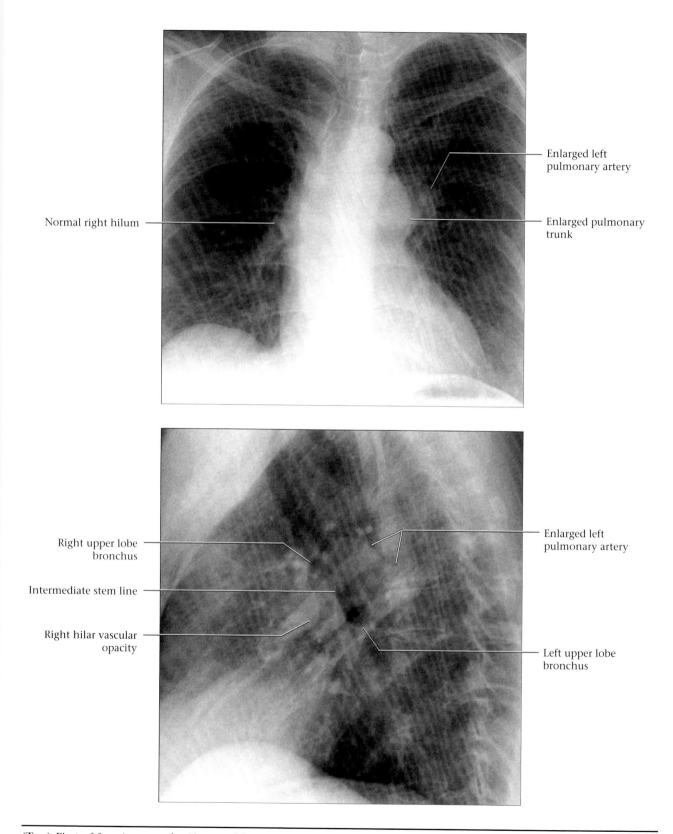

Normal right hilum

Enlarged left pulmonary artery

Enlarged pulmonary trunk

Right upper lobe bronchus

Intermediate stem line

Right hilar vascular opacity

Enlarged left pulmonary artery

Left upper lobe bronchus

(Top) First of four images of a 49 year old woman with pulmonic stenosis and a heart murmur. PA chest radiograph demonstrates asymmetric left hilar enlargement affecting the pulmonary trunk and the left pulmonary artery. The right hilum exhibits normal height, size and opacity. (Bottom) Left lateral chest radiograph coned-down to the hila demonstrates unilateral enlargement and lobular morphology of the left pulmonary artery. Poor positioning and rotation result in an unusual anterior location of the normal intermediate stem line. Note visualization of the bronchus intermedius and its bifurcation into middle and right lower lobe bronchi. The left upper lobe bronchus is visualized as is the normal right hilar vascular opacity.

HILA

UNILATERAL HILAR ENLARGEMENT, PULMONIC STENOSIS

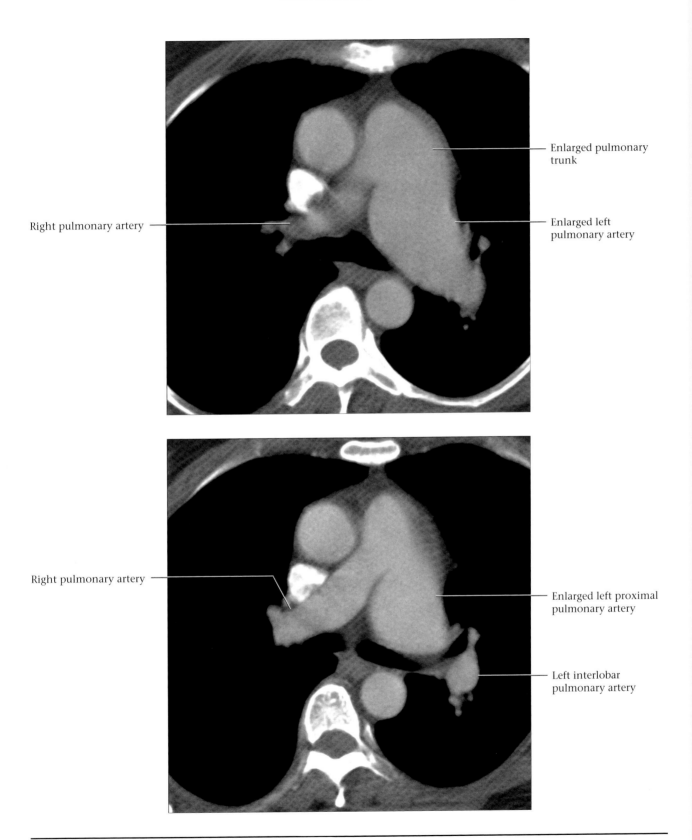

Right pulmonary artery

Enlarged pulmonary trunk

Enlarged left pulmonary artery

Right pulmonary artery

Enlarged left proximal pulmonary artery

Left interlobar pulmonary artery

(Top) Contrast-enhanced chest CT (mediastinal window) through the carina demonstrates enlargement of the pulmonary trunk and asymmetric enlargement of the left pulmonary artery. The right pulmonary artery is of normal size. **(Bottom)** Contrast-enhanced chest CT (mediastinal window) obtained just below the carina demonstrates enlargement of the left pulmonary artery. The right pulmonary artery and left interlobar pulmonary artery are grossly normal. Patients with pulmonic stenosis are often asymptomatic and exhibit asymmetric enlargement of the pulmonary trunk and the left pulmonary artery due to post stenotic dilatation related to the direction of the high velocity jet of blood that courses through the stenotic valve.

AIRWAYS

Terminology

Definitions
- Spurs
  - Precise anatomic landmarks of airway origins
  - Thin septum/triangular density along bronchial edge at points of bifurcation

Nomenclature

System of Jackson and Huber (1943)
- Describes segmental lung anatomy

System of Boyden (1961)
- Designates segmental bronchi (B)
- Followed by a number (e.g., B1, B2, etc.)
- Numbered sequentially, progressing distally from trachea

Overview of Airway Anatomy

Trachea
- See below

Bronchi
- Right main bronchus
- Left main bronchus

Lobar and Segmental Bronchi
- Right upper lobe bronchus
  - Apical segmental bronchus (B1)
  - Posterior segmental bronchus (B2)
  - Anterior segmental bronchus (B3)
- Middle lobe bronchus
  - Lateral segmental bronchus (B4)
  - Medial segmental bronchus (B5)
- Right lower lobe bronchus
  - Superior segmental bronchus (B6)
  - Basilar segmental bronchi
    - Medial segmental bronchus (B7)
    - Anterior segmental bronchus (B8)
    - Lateral segmental bronchus (B9)
    - Posterior segmental bronchus (B10)
- Left upper lobe bronchus
  - Apical-posterior segmental bronchus (B1+2)
  - Anterior segmental bronchus (B3)
  - Lingular bronchus
    - Superior segmental bronchus (B4)
    - Inferior segmental bronchus (B5)
- Left lower lobe bronchus
  - Superior segmental bronchus (B6)
  - Basilar segmental bronchi
    - Anteromedial segmental bronchus (B7+8)
    - Lateral segmental bronchus (B9)
    - Posterior segmental bronchus (B10)

Trachea

General Anatomy
- Midline structure, 10-12 cm in length; intrathoracic portion 6-9 cm in length
- Extends caudally from inferior aspect of cricoid cartilage (level of C6 vertebral body)
- Bifurcates at carina (level of T5 vertebral body) into right and left main bronchi
- Diameters
  - Coronal **13-25 mm** (men); **10-21 mm** (women)
  - Sagittal **13-27 mm** (men); **10-23 mm** (women)

Relationships
- Thyroid gland lies on anterior and both lateral aspects of upper trachea, above thoracic inlet
- Esophagus lies posterior to trachea, interposed between trachea and vertebral column
- Aorta lies along anterior and left lateral aspect of trachea
- Brachiocephalic artery lies along anterior and right lateral aspect of trachea
- Aerated lung (right upper lobe) lies adjacent to right lateral tracheal wall

Right Bronchial Anatomy

Right Main Bronchus
- Origin anterior to esophagus; courses inferolaterally posterior to right pulmonary artery
- **Eparterial** (i.e., "situated above an artery"); refers to its relationship to adjacent **right pulmonary artery**
- Relatively short; more vertical than left main bronchus; more prone to foreign body aspiration
- Divides into **right upper lobe bronchus** and **bronchus intermedius**

Right Upper Lobe Bronchus
- Origin from lateral aspect of right main bronchus at or just below carina; more cephalad than left upper lobe bronchus
- Courses horizontally and laterally (1-2 cm) before branching
- Posterior wall an important anatomic landmark; in direct contact with aerated lung (< 3 mm thick)
  - Thickened by tumor, lymphadenopathy; prominent posteromedial azygos vein may mimic thickening

Right Upper Lobe Bronchial Segments
- Apical segmental bronchus
  - First branch of right upper lobe bronchus identified when scanning in a cephalocaudal direction
  - Seen as circular lucency in cross section; superimposed on distal portion of right upper lobe bronchus
- **Posterior** and **anterior** segmental bronchi
  - Typically horizontal, parallel to axial plane
  - Posterior segmental bronchus courses cephalad and posteriorly; anterior segmental bronchus courses anteriorly

Bronchus Intermedius
- Origin at level of right upper lobe bronchus
- Courses obliquely (3-4 cm); directly posterior to right pulmonary artery
- Posterior wall in contact with aerated lung; should be thin, uniform in thickness (< 3 mm)

AIRWAYS

○ Thickening suggests tumor infiltration, lymphadenopathy, edema
- Branches into **middle lobe** and **right lower lobe bronchi**
- Obstruction may produce combined volume loss/pneumonitis in middle and right lower lobes

Middle Lobe Bronchus
- Origin from anterolateral wall of **bronchus intermedius**; same level as origin of lower lobe bronchus; origins separated by a spur
- Courses anterolaterally, caudally, and obliquely
- Branches into **lateral** and **medial segmental bronchi**; equal in size in 50% of individuals; medial segment larger than lateral in most other individuals
- Lateral segmental bronchus more horizontal; visualized over a great length

Right Lower Lobe Bronchus
- **Superior segmental bronchus** originates posteriorly from short proximal portion of right lower lobe bronchus
- Right lower lobe bronchus continues 5-10 mm as **truncus basalis**; divides into four basilar segmental bronchi
  ○ **Medial, anterior, lateral** and **posterior basilar segmental bronchi** arise on CT in counterclockwise order
  ○ Supply medial, anterior, lateral and posterior basilar lung segments, respectively
  ○ Identified by relative position to each other; course toward respective lung segments

Left Bronchial Anatomy

Left Main Bronchus
- Origin anterior to esophagus; courses inferolaterally
- **Hyparterial** (i.e., "situated below an artery"); refers to its relationship to adjacent **left pulmonary artery**
- Longer, more horizontal than right main bronchus; less prone to aspiration
- Divides into **left upper** and **left lower lobe bronchi**

Left Upper Lobe Bronchus
- Origin from left main bronchus; bifurcates or trifurcates
- Most commonly branches into superior and lingular divisions

Left Upper Lobe Bronchial Segments
- Superior portion divides into **apicoposterior** and **anterior segmental bronchi**
- Inferior (lingular) portion courses obliquely, inferiorly and anterolaterally; analogous to middle lobe bronchus
  ○ Bifurcates into **superior** and **inferior segmental bronchi**

Left Lower Lobe Bronchus
- Same general branching pattern as right lower lobe bronchus

Left Lower Lobe Bronchial Segments
- **Superior segmental bronchus** courses posteriorly, at or near level of lingular bronchus
- Left lower lobe bronchus continues as **truncus basalis**; divides into three basilar segmental bronchi
- **Anteromedial, lateral** and **posterior segmental bronchi**; arise on CT in clockwise order
- Course toward and supply respective lung segments

Variants of Bronchial Anatomy

Anomalous Bronchi
- Arise at lower level than normal in bronchial tree

Supernumerary Bronchi
- Supply same segment of lung as respective normal segmental bronchus

Axillary Bronchus
- Supernumerary airway supplying lateral aspect of right upper lobe

Accessory Tracheal Bronchus
- Syn.: Pig bronchus
- Rare; 1-2% prevalence in adults
- Upper lobe bronchus or segmental bronchus; arises from right lateral tracheal wall
- May be occluded by endotracheal intubation; possible resultant infection

Accessory Cardiac Bronchus
- Rare supernumerary bronchus; 0.5% prevalence in adults
- Arises from medial aspect of right main bronchus or bronchus intermedius
- Courses caudally toward mediastinum and heart (hence "cardiac" designation); typically blind-ending

Situs Abnormalities
- Bilateral right-sided airway anatomy; associated with asplenia, congenital heart disease; rare in adults
- Bilateral left-sided airway anatomy; isolated finding or associated with hypogenetic lung syndrome, less commonly with polysplenia

Imaging of the Airways

Radiography
- Tracheal air column visible on PA and lateral chest radiography; smooth, parallel intraluminal borders
- **Right paratracheal stripe**
  ○ Thin line (1-4 mm) represents right lateral tracheal wall on PA chest radiography
  ○ Extends from clavicle to arch of azygos vein in tracheobronchial angle
  ○ Visible in 2/3 of normal individuals; should be of uniform thickness
  ○ Thickening suggests paratracheal lymphadenopathy
- Bronchoarterial pairs may be visualized in perihilar region; seen in cross-section on PA chest radiograph
- Normal bronchi not visualized in mid-to-peripheral lungs on radiography

AIRWAYS

CT

- Imaging optimized by thin-section and/or helical CT, HRCT
- Bronchi paired with respective pulmonary arteries as bronchoarterial bundle
- Throughout their length, bronchi and accompanying pulmonary arteries approximately equal in diameter
- **Bronchoarterial (B/A) ratio** calculated by dividing internal (luminal) diameter of bronchus (B) by outer diameter of adjacent pulmonary artery (A)
  - B/A ratio in normal individuals ranges from **0.65-0.7**
- Expiratory CT/HRCT may reveal air-trapping; evidence of small airway disease
- Virtual bronchoscopy simulates visualization through a bronchoscope
  - 3D internal surface rendering of spiral CT data

Anatomy Based Imaging Abnormalities

Tracheal Narrowing

- Tracheal stenosis (narrowing of normal diameter by > 10%); trauma is most common benign etiology
  - May result from endotracheal intubation or tracheostomy; may cause dyspnea on exertion, stridor, and wheezing
  - Thyroid enlargement related to goiter or neoplasm may cause tracheal narrowing and/or displacement
  - Extrinsic compression by vascular anomalies (double aortic arch, aberrant right subclavian artery, pulmonary artery sling)
- Focal narrowing
  - Postintubation stenosis, postinfectious stenosis, neoplasia, systemic diseases (Crohn disease, sarcoidosis, Behcet syndrome)
- Diffuse narrowing
  - Wegener granulomatosis, relapsing polychondritis, tracheobronchopathia osteochondroplastica, amyloidosis, papillomatosis, rhinoscleroma

Tracheomalacia

- Abnormal degree of compliance of tracheal wall and supporting cartilage; flaccidity usually apparent during forced expiration

Saber Sheath Trachea

- Deformity limited to intrathoracic portion of trachea; coronal diameter of two-thirds or less than sagittal diameter at same level
- Common finding in men > 50 years of age; associated with chronic obstructive pulmonary disease (COPD); usually of no clinical significance

Foreign Body Inhalation

- Foreign bodies typically lodge in right or left main bronchi; less commonly in trachea or lobar bronchi
- Predilection for inhalation into right main bronchus due to its more vertical course

Bronchiectasis

- Chronic, irreversible dilatation of bronchi, usually associated with inflammation (transient airway dilatation described in pneumonia and atelectasis)
- Diameter of normal bronchi approximately equal to diameter of accompanying (homologous) pulmonary artery; **bronchoarterial (BA) ratio > 1**
- **Reid classification** based on gross, bronchographic, and CT/HRCT appearances
  - **Cylindrical** (mild) characterized by relatively straight, parallel walls (may resemble tram tracks on radiography/CT); may form **signet ring sign** on CT when imaged in cross-section
  - **Varicose** (moderate) appears irregular; foci of luminal constriction alternating with areas of dilatation; resultant beaded bronchial morphology
  - **Cystic/saccular** (severe) appears balloon-like; > 1 cm in diameter; reduced number of bronchial divisions
- CT/HRCT demonstrates dilatation of bronchi, with or without bronchial wall thickening
- Mucoid impaction of bronchiectatic airways may result in nodular and/or tubular opacities on radiography and CT; branching tubular opacities may occur
- **Traction bronchiectasis** refers to airway dilatation resultant from retractile interstitial fibrosis

Mounier-Kuhn (Tracheobronchomegaly)

- Rare; unknown etiology; dilatation of trachea and main bronchi; corrugated appearance may result from mucosal prolapse between adjacent cartilaginous rings

Endoluminal Tumor

- Primary (benign or malignant) and secondary (metastatic) tumors may narrow, deform and/or occlude bronchi; with or without distal effects (atelectasis, pneumonitis, mucoid impaction, lung abscess)
- Atelectasis/pneumonitis affecting pulmonary lobes or segments should prompt CT assessment of associated bronchi for tumor detection
- Combined changes (atelectasis/pneumonitis) affecting middle lobe and right lower lobe suggests involvement of bronchus intermedius

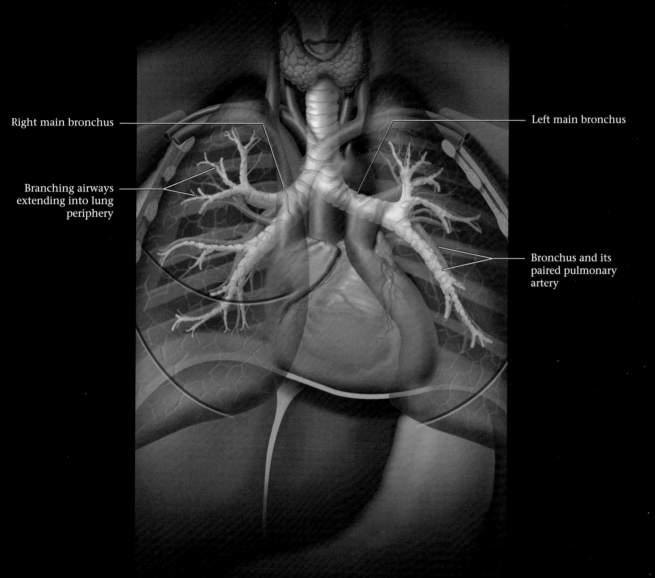

Right main bronchus

Left main bronchus

Branching airways
extending into lung
periphery

Bronchus and its
paired pulmonary
artery

Overview of the airways shows the tracheobronchial tree extending bilaterally from the tracheal bifurcation at the carina. Lobar and segmental bronchi emanate from the right and left main bronchi as they branch, taper and extend into the lung periphery. Each airway beyond the lung hila is accompanied by its paired, homologous pulmonary artery.

AIRWAYS

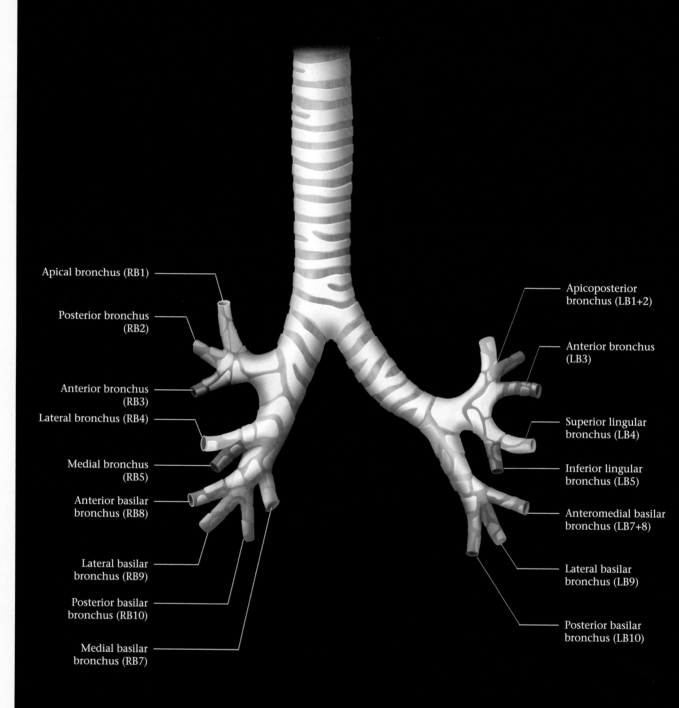

Apical bronchus (RB1)

Posterior bronchus (RB2)

Anterior bronchus (RB3)

Lateral bronchus (RB4)

Medial bronchus (RB5)

Anterior basilar bronchus (RB8)

Lateral basilar bronchus (RB9)

Posterior basilar bronchus (RB10)

Medial basilar bronchus (RB7)

Apicoposterior bronchus (LB1+2)

Anterior bronchus (LB3)

Superior lingular bronchus (LB4)

Inferior lingular bronchus (LB5)

Anteromedial basilar bronchus (LB7+8)

Lateral basilar bronchus (LB9)

Posterior basilar bronchus (LB10)

Graphic of anterior view of tracheobronchial tree depicts color-coded segmental bronchial origins that correspond to color-coded lung segments (see "Lungs" section).

AIRWAYS

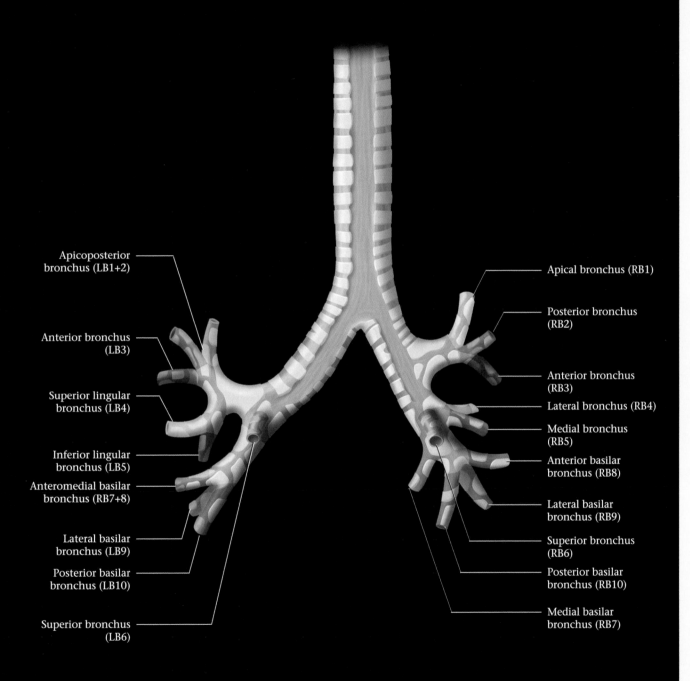

Apicoposterior
bronchus (LB1+2)

Anterior bronchus
(LB3)

Superior lingular
bronchus (LB4)

Inferior lingular
bronchus (LB5)

Anteromedial basilar
bronchus (RB7+8)

Lateral basilar
bronchus (LB9)

Posterior basilar
bronchus (LB10)

Superior bronchus
(LB6)

Apical bronchus (RB1)

Posterior bronchus
(RB2)

Anterior bronchus
(RB3)

Lateral bronchus (RB4)

Medial bronchus
(RB5)

Anterior basilar
bronchus (RB8)

Lateral basilar
bronchus (RB9)

Superior bronchus
(RB6)

Posterior basilar
bronchus (RB10)

Medial basilar
bronchus (RB7)

Graphic of posterior view of tracheobronchial tree depicts color-coded segmental bronchial origins that correspond to color-coded lung segments (see "Lungs" section).

AIRWAYS

RADIOGRAPHY, CENTRAL AIRWAYS

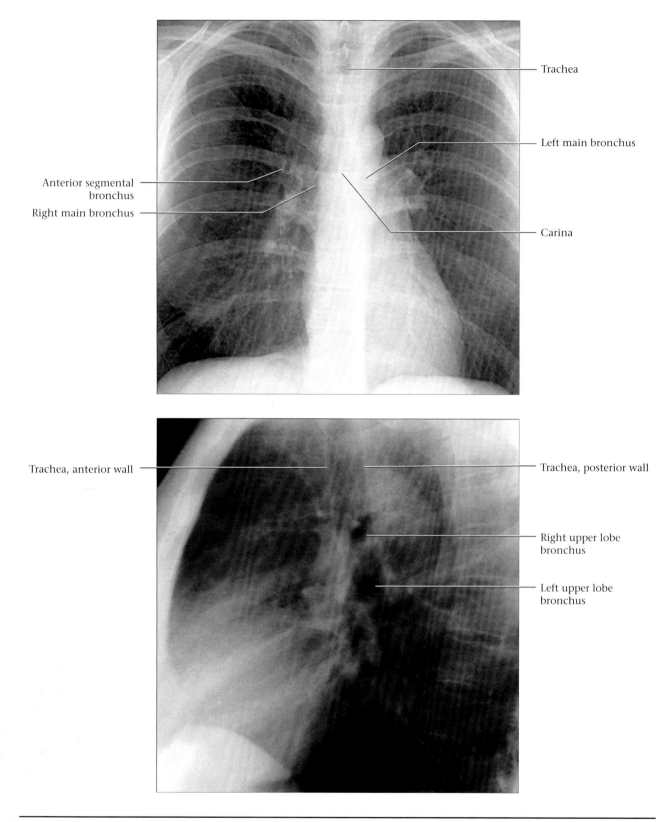

(**Top**) PA chest radiograph demonstrates the midline tracheal air column. The trachea bifurcates at the carina, supplying the right main and left main bronchi. The anterior segmental bronchus of the right upper lobe is frequently visible on PA chest radiographs. (**Bottom**) Left lateral chest radiograph demonstrates the tracheal air column and the characteristic oval lucencies of the right upper lobe bronchus and left upper lobe bronchus.

AIRWAYS

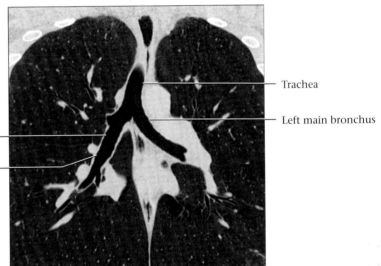

Apical segmental bronchi — Apicoposterior segmental bronchi

Trachea

Right upper lobe bronchus — Anterior segmental bronchi

Posterior segmental bronchus, right upper lobe

Right main bronchus — Carina

Trachea

Left main bronchus

Bronchus intermedius

Right lower lobe bronchus

(Top) First of two axial HRCT scans of the central airways demonstrates the trachea as a midline structure with sharply defined luminal margins. The posterior, membranous tracheal wall bows outward on scans obtained during full, suspended inspiration. The most cephalad segmental airways imaged in axial sections through the upper lungs are the apical segmental bronchi on the right and the apicoposterior segmental bronchi on the left. **(Middle)** HRCT at the level of the carina demonstrates the midline carina, the right main bronchus, and the origin of the right upper lobe bronchus. Note the thin posterior wall of the right main bronchus, a characteristic appearance in normal individuals. **(Bottom)** Volumetric HRCT, coronal reformation, demonstrates the relatively vertical course of the right main bronchus in comparison to the more oblique course of the left main bronchus.

AIRWAYS

SEGMENTAL ANATOMY, RIGHT LUNG

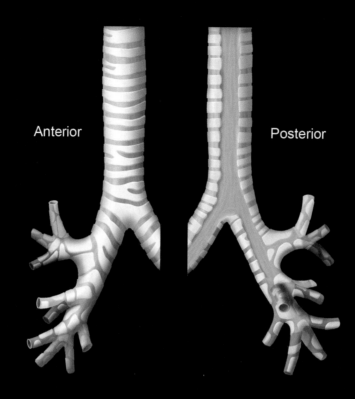

Anterior   Posterior

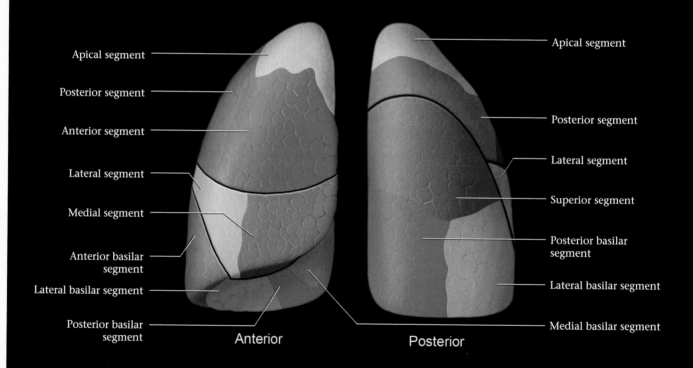

Apical segment

Posterior segment

Anterior segment

Lateral segment

Medial segment

Anterior basilar segment

Lateral basilar segment

Posterior basilar segment

Anterior

Apical segment

Posterior segment

Lateral segment

Superior segment

Posterior basilar segment

Lateral basilar segment

Medial basilar segment

Posterior

(Top) Graphic of anterior and posterior views of the trachea and right portion of the tracheobronchial tree depicts color-coded segmental bronchial origins that correspond to color-coded lung segments. **(Bottom)** Graphic of anterior and posterior views of the right lung. Lung segments of each lobe are color-coded to correspond to the segmental bronchial origins depicted in the top graphic.

AIRWAYS

CT, RIGHT LUNG SEGMENTAL BRONCHI

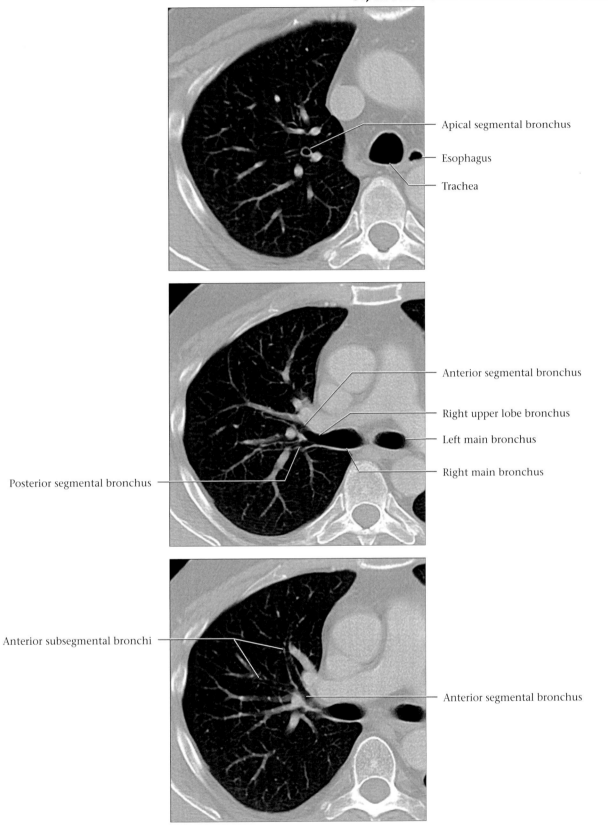

Apical segmental bronchus

Esophagus

Trachea

Anterior segmental bronchus

Right upper lobe bronchus

Left main bronchus

Right main bronchus

Posterior segmental bronchus

Anterior subsegmental bronchi

Anterior segmental bronchus

(Top) First of nine axial HRCT scans demonstrating segmental bronchi of the right lung. The apical segmental bronchus is characteristically seen in cross-section as a circular lucency. **(Middle)** Axial HRCT scan at the level of the carina demonstrates the characteristic horizontal orientation of the anterior and posterior segmental bronchi. **(Bottom)** Axial HRCT scan at the level of the right pulmonary artery demonstrates branching of the anterior segmental bronchus into subsegmental airways that are well visualized by virtue of their horizontal orientation, parallel to the HRCT scan plane.

CT, RIGHT LUNG SEGMENTAL BRONCHI

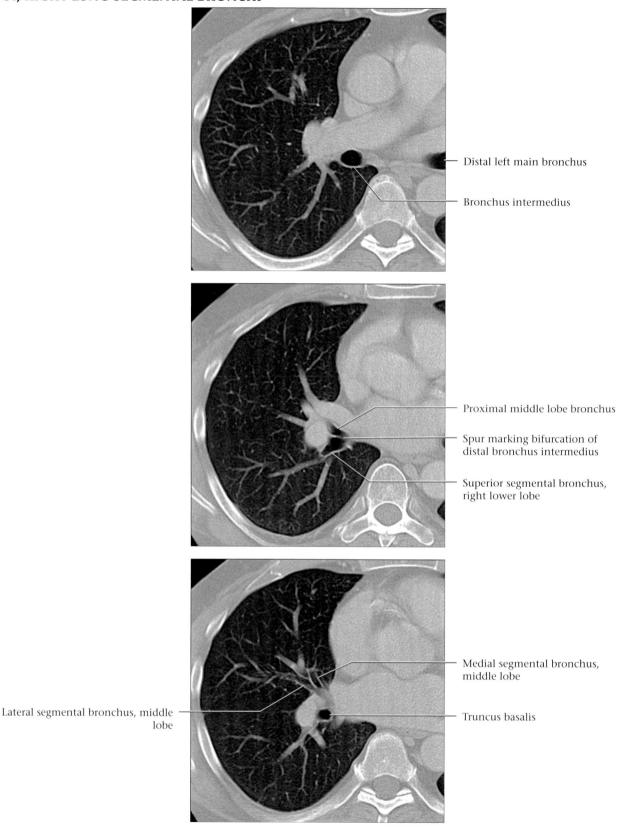

(Top) The bronchus intermedius lies immediately posterior to the right pulmonary artery. Its posterior wall is characteristically thin and uniform, measuring < 3 mm in thickness. **(Middle)** At the distal end of the bronchus intermedius, axial HRCT section demonstrates the distinctive thin septum (spur) demarcating the point of bifurcation of the bronchus intermedius at the origins of the middle lobe bronchus and the superior segmental bronchus of the right lower lobe. **(Bottom)** A more caudal axial HRCT section demonstrates the horizontal portions of the medial segmental and lateral segmental bronchi of the middle lobe and the truncus basalis supplying the right lower lobe distal to the origin of the superior segmental bronchus.

AIRWAYS

CT, RIGHT LUNG SEGMENTAL BRONCHI

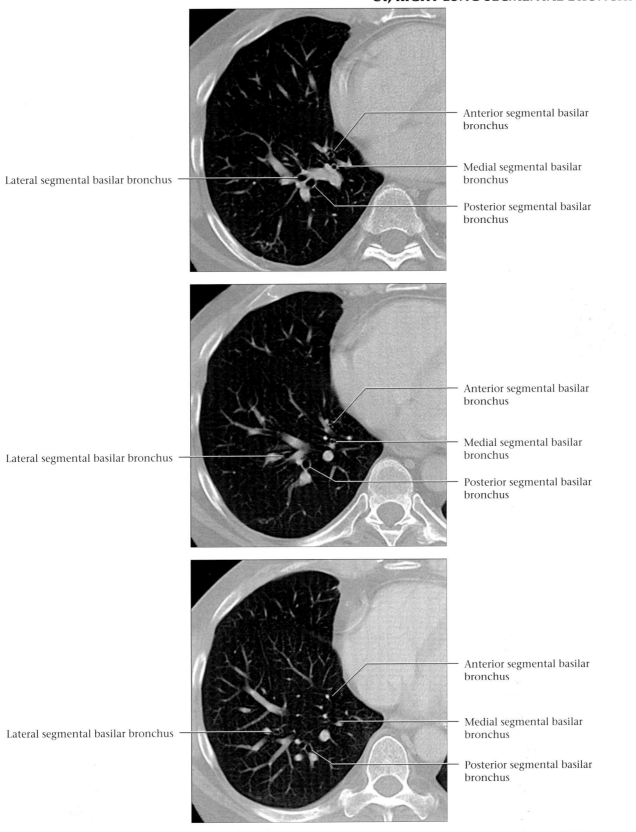

Anterior segmental basilar bronchus

Medial segmental basilar bronchus

Posterior segmental basilar bronchus

Lateral segmental basilar bronchus

Anterior segmental basilar bronchus

Medial segmental basilar bronchus

Posterior segmental basilar bronchus

Lateral segmental basilar bronchus

Anterior segmental basilar bronchus

Medial segmental basilar bronchus

Posterior segmental basilar bronchus

Lateral segmental basilar bronchus

(Top) The four basilar segmental bronchi of the right lower lobe originate distal to the truncus basalis. **(Middle)** The medial, anterior, lateral, and posterior basilar segmental bronchi arise in counterclockwise order and course toward their respective lung segment. Each bronchus is accompanied by its paired, homologous, segmental pulmonary artery. **(Bottom)** The four basilar segmental bronchi begin to diverge and course peripherally within their respective basilar lung segments.

AIRWAYS

SEGMENTAL ANATOMY, LEFT LUNG

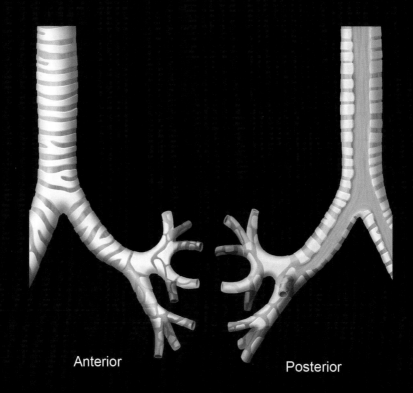

Anterior

Posterior

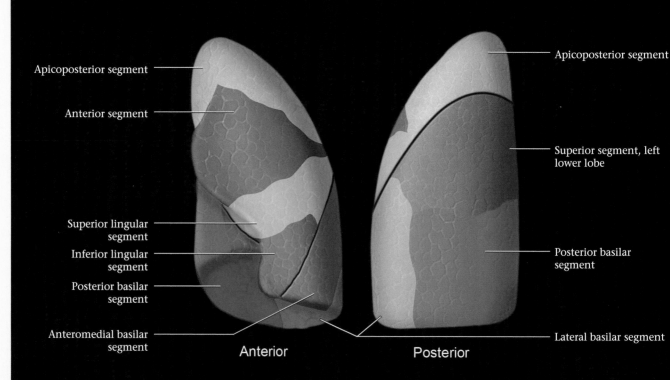

Apicoposterior segment

Anterior segment

Superior lingular segment

Inferior lingular segment

Posterior basilar segment

Anteromedial basilar segment

Anterior

Apicoposterior segment

Superior segment, left lower lobe

Posterior basilar segment

Lateral basilar segment

Posterior

(Top) Graphic depicts anterior and posterior views of the trachea and left portion of the tracheobronchial tree. Segmental airway origins are color-coded to correspond to lung segments. (Bottom) Graphic of anterior and posterior views of the left lung. Lung segments of each lobe are color-coded to correspond to the segmental bronchial origins depicted in the top graphic.

AIRWAYS

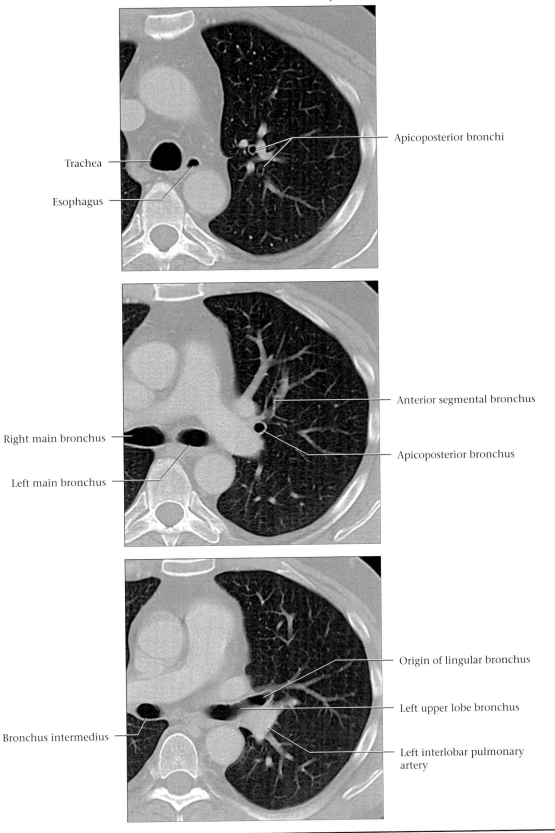

Trachea

Esophagus

Apicoposterior bronchi

Right main bronchus

Left main bronchus

Anterior segmental bronchus

Apicoposterior bronchus

Bronchus intermedius

Origin of lingular bronchus

Left upper lobe bronchus

Left interlobar pulmonary artery

(Top) First of nine axial HRCT scans demonstrating segmental bronchi of the left lung. The vertically oriented apical and posterior branches of the apicoposterior bronchus are seen in cross-section, each adjacent to its accompanying homologous pulmonary artery. **(Middle)** The apicoposterior bronchus is seen in cross-section, in contradistinction to the horizontal orientation and longitudinal display of the anterior segmental bronchus. The anterior segmental bronchus is usually easily identified on axial CT sections because of its characteristic horizontal course in the same plane as the CT scan. **(Bottom)** HRCT scan demonstrates the left upper lobe bronchus. A circular lucency overlying its distal aspect indicates the origin of the lingular bronchus. The lower portion of the left upper lobe bronchus is marginated laterally by the left interlobar pulmonary artery.

AIRWAYS

CT, LEFT LUNG SEGMENTAL BRONCHI

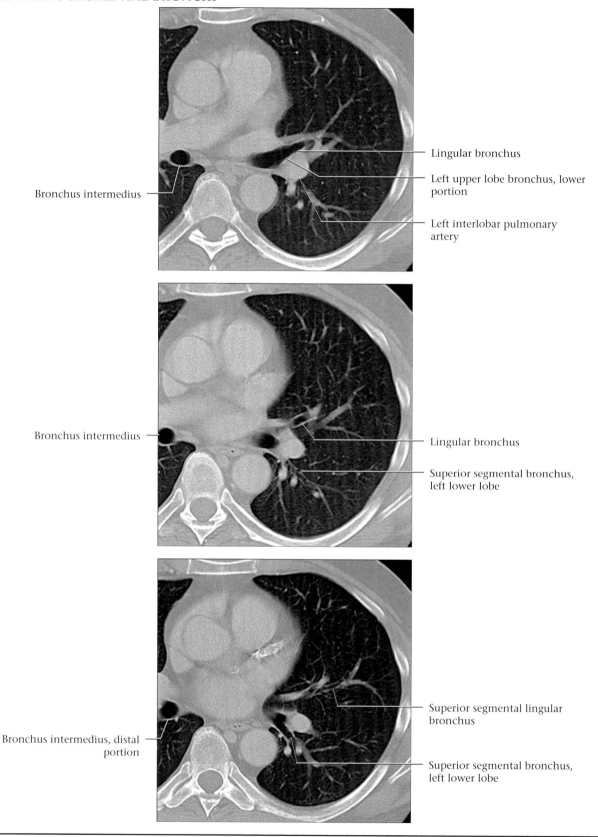

Bronchus intermedius —

Lingular bronchus

Left upper lobe bronchus, lower portion

Left interlobar pulmonary artery

Bronchus intermedius —

Lingular bronchus

Superior segmental bronchus, left lower lobe

Bronchus intermedius, distal portion

Superior segmental lingular bronchus

Superior segmental bronchus, left lower lobe

(Top) The lower portion of the left upper lobe bronchus is marginated laterally by the left interlobar pulmonary artery. The proximal portion of the lingular bronchus courses anterolaterally. **(Middle)** The lingular bronchus courses obliquely, inferiorly, and anterolaterally and is analogous to the middle lobe bronchus of the right lung. The origin of the superior segmental bronchus of the left lower lobe is normally at or near the same level of origin as the lingular bronchus. **(Bottom)** More caudally, the superior segmental lingular bronchus courses horizontally within the left upper lobe, characteristically at or near the same level as the superior segmental bronchus of the left lower lobe.

AIRWAYS

CT, LEFT LUNG SEGMENTAL BRONCHI

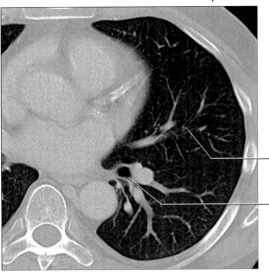

Superior segmental lingular bronchus

Truncus basalis, left lower lobe

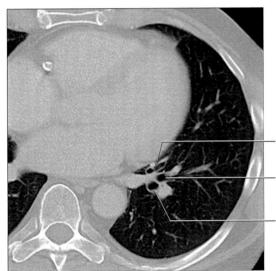

Anteromedial segmental basilar bronchus

Lateral segmental basilar bronchus

Posterior segmental basilar bronchus

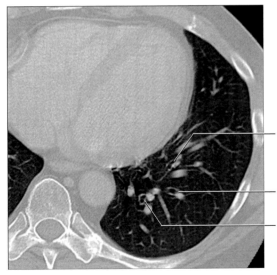

Anteromedial segmental basilar bronchus

Lateral segmental basilar bronchus

Posterior segmental basilar bronchus

(Top) The left lower lobe bronchus continues as the truncus basalis for a short distance before dividing into three basilar segmental bronchi. (Middle) Distal to the truncus basalis, the anteromedial, lateral, and posterior basilar segmental bronchi arise in clockwise order. (Bottom) The anteromedial, lateral, and posterior basilar segmental bronchi diverge and course toward their respective lung segments. Each bronchus is accompanied by its paired, homologous segmental pulmonary artery.

AIRWAYS

CORONAL CT, AIRWAY ANATOMY

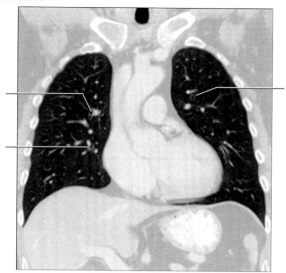

Anterior segmental bronchus, right upper lobe

Medial segmental bronchus, middle lobe

Anterior segmental bronchus, left upper lobe

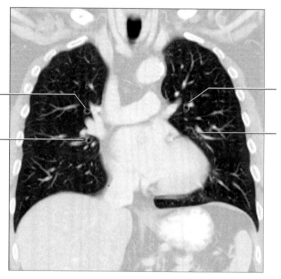

Anterior segmental bronchus, right upper lobe

Medial segmental bronchus, middle lobe

Anterior segmental bronchus, left upper lobe

Superior segmental lingular bronchus

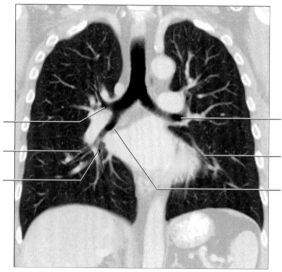

Right upper lobe bronchus

Lateral segmental bronchus, middle lobe

Medial segmental bronchus, middle lobe

Left upper lobe bronchus

Inferior lingular segmental bronchus

Bronchus intermedius

(Top) First of six coronal CT images of normal bronchi. In this most anterior section, right and left anterior segmental bronchi and the medial segmental bronchus of the middle lobe are demonstrated in cross-section. Each bronchus is adjacent to its paired, homologous pulmonary artery and both are approximately equal in diameter. (Middle) More posteriorly, in the plane of the right pulmonary artery, the superior segmental lingular bronchus is demonstrated. The lingular bronchi are analogous to the contralateral middle lobe bronchi. (Bottom) In the plane of the tracheal carina, the origins of the right upper and left upper lobe bronchi are demonstrated. The origins of the medial and lateral segmental bronchi of the middle lobe are seen arising beyond the distal end of the bronchus intermedius.

AIRWAYS

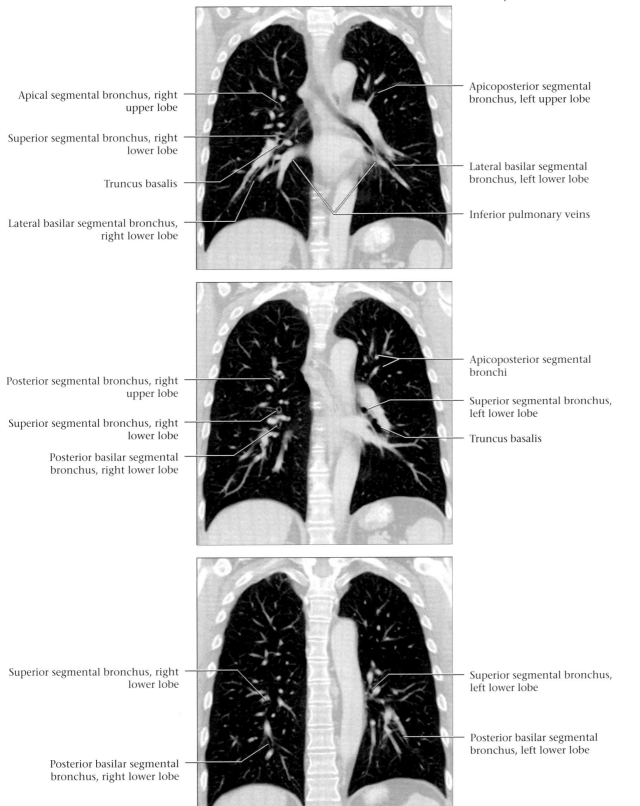

Apical segmental bronchus, right upper lobe

Superior segmental bronchus, right lower lobe

Truncus basalis

Lateral basilar segmental bronchus, right lower lobe

Apicoposterior segmental bronchus, left upper lobe

Lateral basilar segmental bronchus, left lower lobe

Inferior pulmonary veins

Posterior segmental bronchus, right upper lobe

Superior segmental bronchus, right lower lobe

Posterior basilar segmental bronchus, right lower lobe

Apicoposterior segmental bronchi

Superior segmental bronchus, left lower lobe

Truncus basalis

Superior segmental bronchus, right lower lobe

Posterior basilar segmental bronchus, right lower lobe

Superior segmental bronchus, left lower lobe

Posterior basilar segmental bronchus, left lower lobe

(Top) In the plane of the inferior pulmonary veins, the right truncus basalis and right and left basilar segmental bronchi are demonstrated. (Middle) In the prevertebral plane, right posterior and left apicoposterior bronchi are demonstrated in the upper lobes and superior segmental bronchi are shown in both lower lobes. (Bottom) The most posterior section demonstrates superior segmental bronchi and posterior basilar segmental bronchi of both lower lobes.

AIRWAYS

VIRTUAL BRONCHOSCOPY

Bronchus intermedius

Carina

Right upper lobe bronchus

Right main bronchus

Left main bronchus

Superior segmental bronchus, right lower lobe

Truncus basalis and basilar segmental bronchi

Bronchus intermedius

Medial segmental bronchus, middle lobe

Soft tissue ridge manifests as spur on CT

Lateral segmental bronchus, middle lobe

Middle lobe bronchus

Left lower lobe bronchus

Left upper lobe bronchus

(Top) First of three virtual bronchoscopic images of normal airways. Each image is aligned with the anterior aspect of the patient at the bottom of the image. The midline carina marks the bifurcation of the distal trachea to form the right and left main bronchi. **(Middle)** In the distal aspect of the bronchus intermedius, a ridge of soft tissue demarcates the origins of the lower lobe bronchus (above) and the middle lobe bronchus (below) and manifests on CT as a thin septum (spur). **(Bottom)** The left main bronchus bifurcates to form the left upper lobe bronchus and left lower lobe bronchus.

AIRWAYS

BRONCHOARTERIAL RATIO

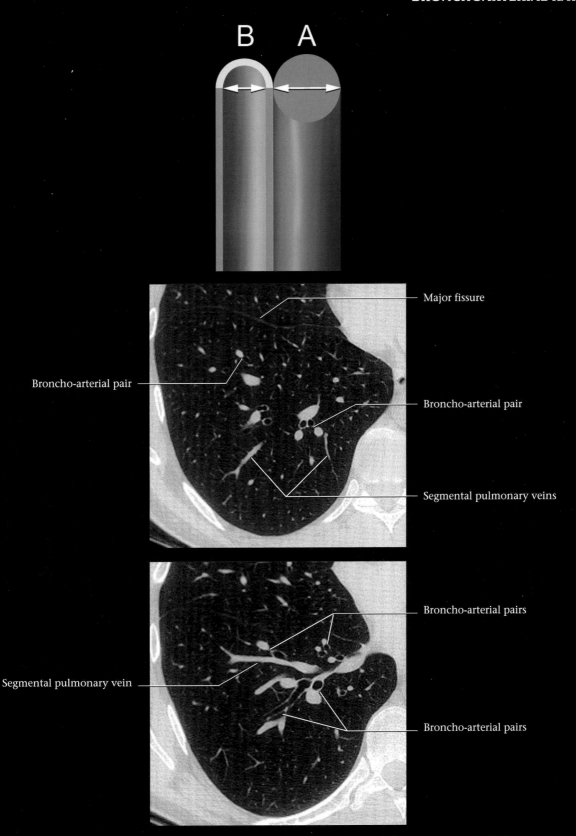

Major fissure

Broncho-arterial pair

Broncho-arterial pair

Segmental pulmonary veins

Broncho-arterial pairs

Segmental pulmonary vein

Broncho-arterial pairs

(Top) Graphic demonstrates the broncho-arterial ratio (B/A), determined by dividing the inner luminal diameter of an airway by the outer diameter of its accompanying (homologous) pulmonary artery. The B/A ratio in normal individuals ranges from 0.65-0.7. (Middle) CT of right lower lobe demonstrates broncho-arterial pairs, each comprised of a bronchus and its adjacent (homologous) pulmonary artery seen in cross-section. (Bottom) CT of the right lower lobe demonstrates broncho-arterial pairs seen longitudinally.

AIRWAYS

RADIOGRAPHY, BRONCHIECTASIS

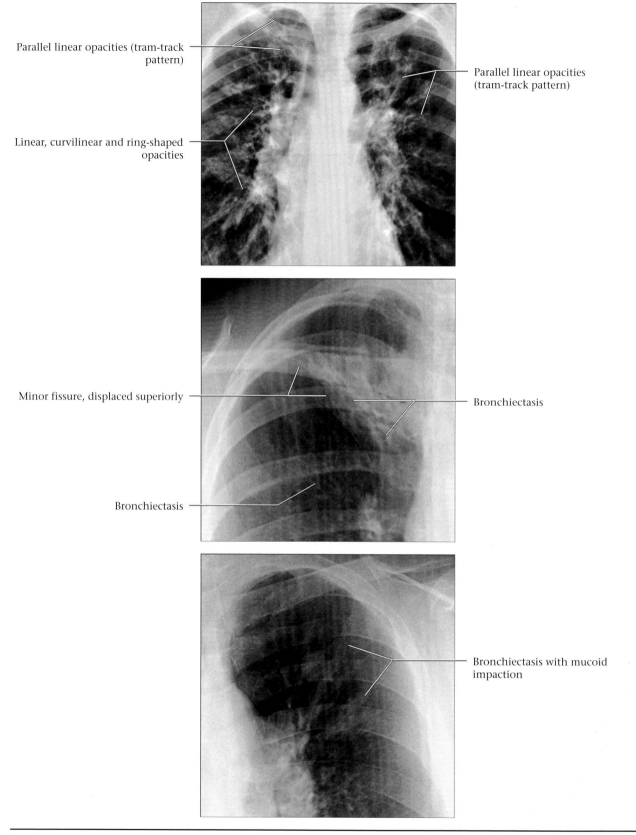

Parallel linear opacities (tram-track pattern)

Parallel linear opacities (tram-track pattern)

Linear, curvilinear and ring-shaped opacities

Minor fissure, displaced superiorly

Bronchiectasis

Bronchiectasis

Bronchiectasis with mucoid impaction

(Top) PA chest radiograph of a patient with cystic fibrosis demonstrates extensive changes of bronchiectasis manifesting as parallel linear opacities emanating from both hila and curvilinear and ring shaped opacities. (Middle) Coned down PA chest radiograph demonstrates bronchiectasis and loss of volume in the right upper lobe. Subtle bronchiectasis in the superior segment of the right lower lobe manifests as parallel linear opacities emanating from the hilum (tram-track pattern). (Bottom) Coned down PA chest radiograph demonstrates mucoid impaction within bronchiectatic airways in the left upper lobe, manifesting as tubular opacities emanating from the hilum.

CT, BRONCHIECTASIS

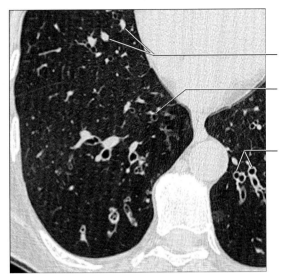

Mucoid impaction forming nodular opacities

Signet ring pattern of bronchiectasis

Bronchiectasis with airway wall thickening

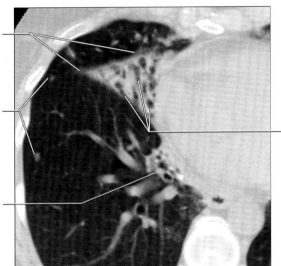

Atelectatic middle lobe

Small parenchymal nodules

Bronchiectasis and retractile scarring, right lower lobe

Bronchiectasis

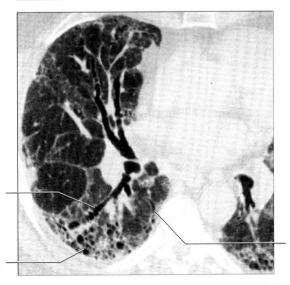

Traction bronchiectasis

End-stage (honeycomb) lung

Traction bronchiectasis

(Top) Chest CT (lung window) of a patient with a history of recurrent pneumonia demonstrates scattered areas of bronchiectasis in the lung bases, manifested by dilated airways and airway wall thickening. Small nodular opacities represent mucoid impaction of bronchiectatic airways. **(Middle)** Chest CT (lung window) of the right lower lung demonstrates bronchiectasis within an atelectatic middle lobe and focal bronchiectasis in the anteromedial aspect of the right lower lobe. Small nodular opacities are noted in the lung periphery. This combination of features is suggestive of atypical mycobacterial infection. Bronchoscopic cultures yielded Mycobacterium avium intracellulare (MAI). **(Bottom)** HRCT (lung window) of the right lower lobe demonstrates traction bronchiectasis within areas of interstitial fibrosis and honeycomb (end-stage) lung.

AIRWAYS

TRACHEAL NARROWING

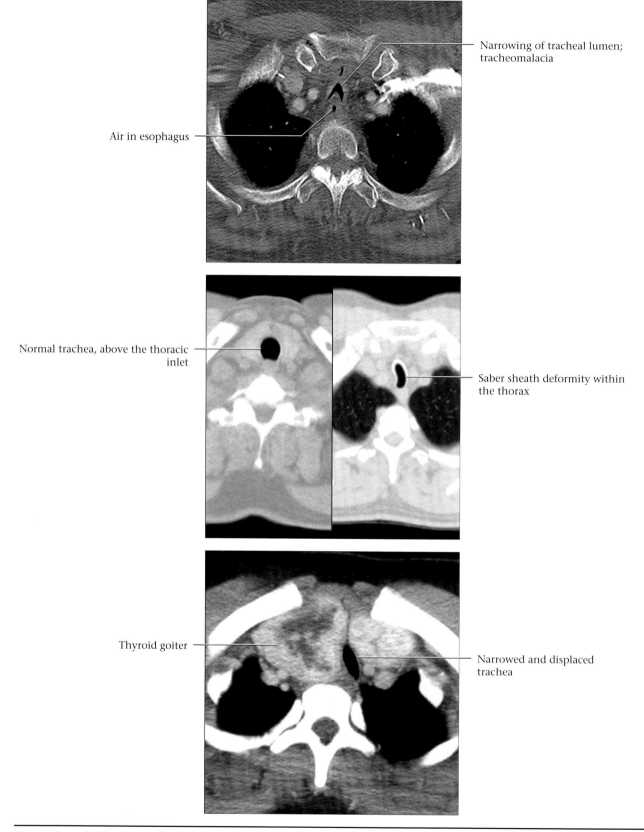

Narrowing of tracheal lumen; tracheomalacia

Air in esophagus

Normal trachea, above the thoracic inlet

Saber sheath deformity within the thorax

Thyroid goiter

Narrowed and displaced trachea

(Top) Chest CT (bone window) demonstrates tracheomalacia at the level of a previous percutaneous tracheostomy complicated by fracture of tracheal cartilaginous rings. **(Middle)** Chest CT (lung window) demonstrates saber sheath tracheal deformity of the intrathoracic portion of the trachea (right). The extrathoracic trachea (left) is normal in size and configuration. **(Bottom)** Contrast-enhanced chest CT (mediastinal window) shows a moderately large thyroid goiter that narrows the trachea at the thoracic inlet and displaces it to the left of midline.

AIRWAYS

BRONCHIAL ANOMALIES, TRACHEAL BRONCHUS

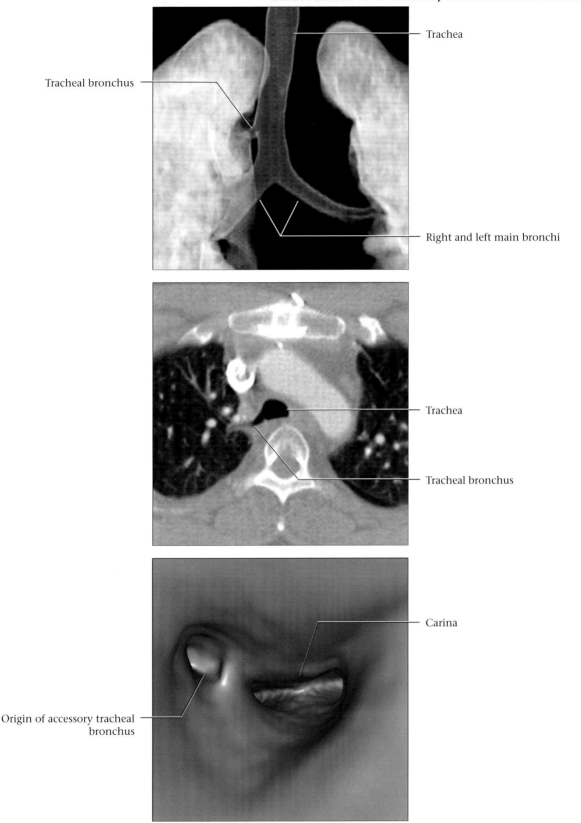

Trachea

Tracheal bronchus

Right and left main bronchi

Trachea

Tracheal bronchus

Carina

Origin of accessory tracheal bronchus

(Top) First of three images of a patient with an incidentally discovered tracheal bronchus. 3D rendered CT image of the central airways and adjacent upper lungs demonstrates the accessory tracheal bronchus arising from the right lateral aspect of the trachea. (Middle) Contrast-enhanced chest CT (lung window) demonstrates an accessory tracheal bronchus arising from the right lateral wall of the trachea and supplying adjacent lung parenchyma in the right upper lobe. (Bottom) Virtual bronchoscopic image demonstrates the origin of the accessory tracheal bronchus arising from the right lateral tracheal wall. The anterior tracheal wall is at the bottom of the virtual bronchoscopic image.

AIRWAYS

ENDOBRONCHIAL TUMORS

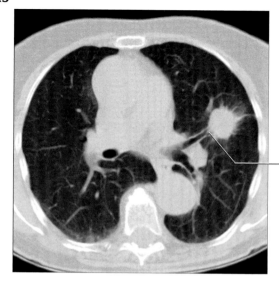

Adenocarcinoma obstructing
superior lingular bronchus

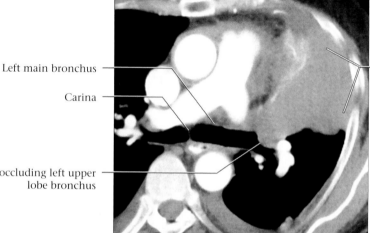

Left main bronchus

Carina

Lung cancer occluding left upper
lobe bronchus

Atelectatic left upper lobe

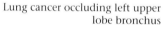

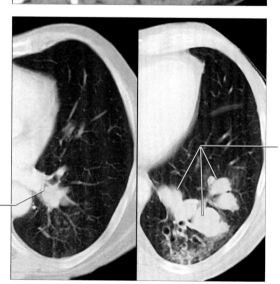

Mucoid impaction within
obstructed, dilated bronchi

Lung cancer obstructing left lower
lobe bronchus

(Top) First of three cases. Chest CT (lung window) demonstrates endobronchial obstruction of the superior lingular bronchus by a primary adenocarcinoma of the lung. Presumed collateral ventilation of parenchyma distal to the point of obstruction prevents development of atelectasis or other distal effects of endobronchial obstruction. **(Middle)** Contrast-enhanced chest CT (mediastinal window) demonstrates total occlusion of the left upper lobe bronchus by a primary lung cancer (squamous cell carcinoma) with resultant atelectasis of the left upper lobe. Lack of air bronchograms within an atelectatic lobe suggests the presence of proximal airway obstruction. **(Bottom)** Composite of two CT images of the left lower lobe (lung window) demonstrates endobronchial tumor obstructing the left lower bronchus and associated distal mucoid impaction within distended bronchi.

AIRWAYS

WEGENER GRANULOMATOSIS

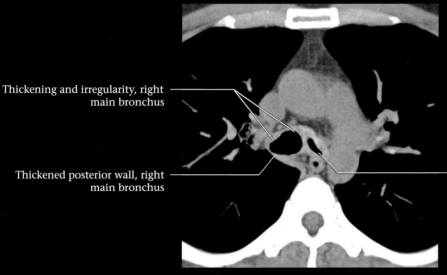

Thickening and irregularity, right main bronchus

Thickened posterior wall, right main bronchus

Narrowing and irregularity of left main bronchus

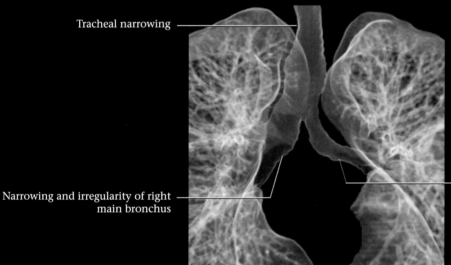

Tracheal narrowing

Narrowing and irregularity of right main bronchus

Narrowing and irregularity of left main bronchus

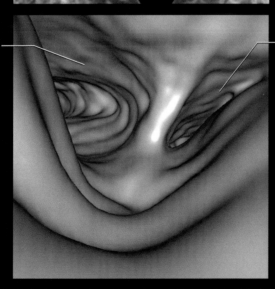

Narrowing and irregularity of right main bronchus

Narrowing and irregularity of left main bronchus

(Top) First of three images of a patient with Wegener granulomatosis involving the central airways. Chest CT (mediastinal window) at the level of the carina demonstrates thickening of airway walls with involvement of right and left main bronchi and the carina. **(Middle)** 3D CT rendering of the central airways demonstrates narrowing and irregularity of the distal trachea and the right and left main bronchi. **(Bottom)** Virtual bronchoscopic image of the carina and right and left main bronchi demonstrates narrowing and irregularity of the central airways.

PULMONARY VESSELS

Pulmonary Arteries

Function
- Conduit of de-oxygenated blood to capillary-alveolar interface

Pulmonary Trunk
- Arises from **right ventricular outflow tract**; anterior and to the left of **ascending aorta**
- Posterosuperior course toward the left and posterior to **ascending aorta**
- Contained in **pericardium**
  - Common serous pericardial sheath contains proximal **pulmonary trunk** and **ascending aorta**

Right Pulmonary Artery and Branches
- **Right pulmonary artery**
  - Longer and larger than **left pulmonary artery**
  - Horizontal intramediastinal course
  - Relationships
    - Posterior to **ascending aorta, superior vena cava,** and **right superior pulmonary vein**
  - Branches
    - **Ascending trunk** or **truncus anterior**, supplies right upper lobe
    - **Descending trunk** or **interlobar pulmonary artery**, supplies middle and right lower lobes
    - Peripheral branches located medial to bronchi in upper lobes and lateral to bronchi in middle and lower lobes

Left Pulmonary Artery and Branches
- **Left pulmonary artery**
  - Shorter and smaller than **right pulmonary artery**
  - Slightly posterior to **right pulmonary artery**
  - Courses superior to left main bronchus
  - Branches
    - Short **ascending branch**, supplies left upper lobe
    - **Descending** or **interlobar pulmonary artery**, supplies left lower lobe and lingula
    - Peripheral pulmonary arteries located medial to bronchi in anterior and apicoposterior segments of left upper lobe and lateral to bronchi in lingula and lower lobe

Pulmonary Veins

Function
- Conduit of oxygenated blood from capillary-alveolar interface to left heart chambers

Embryologic Anatomy
- Left atrium partially derived from **primitive common pulmonary vein**
- Atrial expansion with incorporation of primitive common pulmonary vein into atrial chamber
- Two pairs of **superior** and **inferior pulmonary veins** with frequent variations in number
  - 70% of population has four pulmonary veins
  - Underincorporation of pulmonary veins into atrium
    - More common on the left
    - Common trunk for **superior** and **inferior pulmonary veins** in 12-25% of subjects
  - Overincorporation of pulmonary veins into atrium resulting in supernumerary/accessory veins
    - More common on the right
  - Frequent variations in central anastomosis of **middle lobe pulmonary vein**
    - **Middle lobe pulmonary vein** draining into **right superior pulmonary vein** in 53-69% of normal subjects
    - **Middle lobe pulmonary vein** draining directly into left atrium in 17-23% of normal subjects
    - **Middle lobe pulmonary vein** draining into **inferior pulmonary vein** in 3-8% of normal subjects
  - Above data per Ghaye B et al: Percutaneous ablation for atrial fibrillation: the role of cross-sectional imaging. RadioGraphics. 23:S19-S33, 2003
- Clinical significance
  - Identification of normal anatomic variants
  - Pre-ablation imaging of patients with atrial fibrillation due to ectopic arrhythmogenic foci

General Anatomy
- Pulmonary veins course along peripheral aspects of subsegments, segments and lobes
- **Superior pulmonary veins** exhibit an oblique course into left atrium
- **Inferior pulmonary veins** exhibit an oblique course into left atrium
- **Right pulmonary veins**
  - **Superior pulmonary vein**
    - Drains upper and middle lobes
  - **Inferior pulmonary vein**
    - Drains lower lobe
- **Left pulmonary veins**
  - **Superior pulmonary vein**
    - Drains upper and lower divisions of upper lobe
  - **Inferior pulmonary vein**
    - Drains lower lobe

Nomenclature of Pulmonary Arteries and Veins

General Concepts
- **Boyden** nomenclature of tracheobronchial tree (see "Airways" section)
- **Jackson and Huber** systematization of segmental lung anatomy (See "Lungs" section)
- Right (R); left (L)
- Arteries (A); veins (V)
- Numerical descriptor, analogous to bronchial nomenclature (see "Airways" section)
- Typical branching pattern
  - 10 segmental pulmonary arteries, second order branches
  - 20 subsegmental pulmonary arteries, third order branches
  - Subsegmental pulmonary arteries, fourth order branches; dichotomous division of segmental arteries
  - Subsequent dichotomous divisions into fifth and sixth order branches

PULMONARY VESSELS

- Nomenclature that follows is based on: Remy-Jardin M: CT Angiography of the Chest. Philadelphia, Lippincott Williams & Wilkins, 2001

Right Upper Lobe Pulmonary Arteries
- **Ascending trunk (truncus anterior)**
  - **Apical segmental artery; RA1**
    - Posteriorly located apical and anterior subsegmental branches
  - **Anterior segmental artery; RA2**
    - Laterally located posterior and anterior subsegmental branches
- **Posterior segmental artery; RA3**
  - Originates from interlobar pulmonary artery
  - Laterally located apical and posterior subsegmental branches

Middle Lobe Pulmonary Arteries
- Origin from **right interlobar pulmonary artery**
  - May arise as a single vessel
  - May arise as two distinct vessels
  - Origin slightly superior to origin of **right lower lobe superior segmental artery**
- **Lateral segmental artery; RA4**
  - Posterior and anterior subsegmental branches
- **Medial segmental artery; RA5**
  - Superior and inferior subsegmental branches

Right Lower Lobe Pulmonary Arteries
- **Lower lobe pulmonary artery**
  - Continuation of interlobar pulmonary artery distal to origin of middle lobe arteries
  - **Superior segmental artery; RA6**
    - Posterior origin
    - Combined medial/superior and lateral subsegmental branches
  - **Common basal artery**
    - Gives rise to basal segmental arteries
  - **Medial basal segmental artery; RA7**
    - Anterolateral and anteromedial subsegmental branches
  - **Anterior basal segmental artery; RA8**
    - Lateral and basal subsegmental branches
  - **Lateral basal segmental artery; RA9**
    - Lateral and basal subsegmental branches
  - **Posterior basal segmental artery; RA10**
    - Laterobasal and mediobasal subsegmental branches

Left Upper Lobe Pulmonary Arteries
- Greater number of separate subsegmental branches
- **Upper division**
  - Independent origin of apical and posterior segmental arteries, unlike bronchial divisions
  - **Apical segmental artery; LA1**
  - **Anterior segmental artery; LA2**
    - Lateral and anterior subsegmental arteries
  - **Posterior segmental artery; LA3**
- **Lower division**
  - Single lingular artery gives rise to two segmental arteries
  - **Superior lingular segmental artery; LA4**
    - Posterior and anterior subsegmental branches
  - **Inferior lingular segmental artery; LA5**

- Superior and inferior subsegmental branches

Left Lower Lobe Pulmonary Arteries
- **Superior segmental artery; LA6**
  - Posterior origin, superior to that of lingular artery
  - Superomedial and lateral subsegmental branches
- **Anteromedial basal segmental artery; LA7+8**
  - Anterior, medial, lateral and basal subsegmental branches
- **Lateral basal segmental artery; LA9**
  - Lateral and basal subsegmental branches
- **Posterior basal segmental artery; LA10**
  - Lateral and basal subsegmental branches

Right Upper Lobe Pulmonary Veins
- **Apical segmental vein; RV1**
  - Apical and anterior subsegmental tributaries
- **Anterior segmental vein; RV2**
  - Inferior and superior tributaries
- **Posterior segmental vein; RV3**
- RV1, RV2 and RV3 join to form a large vein anterior to interlobar pulmonary artery

Middle Lobe Pulmonary Veins
- **Lateral segmental vein; RV4**
- **Medial segmental vein; RV5**
- Form common trunk that courses below middle lobe bronchus and joins **superior pulmonary vein**

Right Lower Lobe Pulmonary Veins
- **Superior segmental vein; RV6**
  - Drains into inferior pulmonary vein
- **Medial basal segmental vein; RV7**
- **Anterior basal segmental vein; RV8**
- **Lateral basal segmental vein; RV9**
- **Posterior basal segmental vein; RV10**
- Common basal vein draining basal segments

Left Upper Lobe Pulmonary Veins
- **Upper Division**
  - Apicoposterior segmental vein: LV1+3
  - Anterior segmental vein: LV2
- **Lower Division**
  - Superior lingular segmental vein; LV4
  - Inferior lingular segmental vein; LV5

Left Lower Lobe Pulmonary Veins
- **Superior segmental vein; LV6**
- **Anteromedial basal segmental vein; LV7+8**
- **Lateral basal segmental vein; LV9**
- **Posterior basal segmental vein; LV10**

Imaging of Pulmonary Arteries

Radiography
- **Pulmonary trunk**
  - Prominent in normal children, adolescents, young adults
- **Right interlobar pulmonary artery**
  - Lateral to bronchus intermedius on frontal radiographs
  - Normal transverse measurements
    - **15 mm in women; 16 mm in men**

PULMONARY VESSELS

Angiography

- Assessment of endoluminal integrity and luminal size
- Visualization of branching patterns and distal arterial tree (including capillary bed)
- Visualization of abnormal vascular connections

CT

- **Pulmonary trunk**
  - Normal transverse diameter of **up to 28.6 mm** (24.2 mm ± 2.2)
  - Measured in **scan plane of bifurcation** on **axial images, perpendicular to vascular long axis**
- **Interlobar pulmonary artery**
  - Normal transverse diameter of **up to 16.8 mm** (13 ± 1.9 mm)

Pulmonary Lymphatics

Anatomy

- Pulmonary lymphatic channels
- **Pulmonary lymph nodes**
  - **Peripheral intrapulmonary**
  - **Subsegmental; station 14**
  - **Segmental; station 13**
  - **Lobar; station 12**
  - **Interlobar; station 11**
- **Bronchopulmonary (hilar) lymph nodes**
  - **Hilar; station 10**

Imaging

- Normal pulmonary lymphatic channels not visible on imaging studies
- Normal intrapulmonary lymph nodes visible on CT
  - Elongate subpleural small pulmonary nodules; intrapulmonary lymph nodes
  - Normal sized lymph nodes at bronchial bifurcations

Anatomic-Imaging Correlations

Pulmonary Venous Hypertension

- **Vascular equalization** (mean pulmonary venous pressure; 13-15 mm Hg)
  - Earliest radiographic manifestation; equal size of upper and lower lobe vessels
- **Vascular redistribution** (mean pulmonary venous pressure; 15-18 mm Hg)
  - Upper lobe vessels more dilated than lower lobe vessels

Pulmonary Arterial Hypertension

- **Mean pulmonary artery pressure > 25 mm Hg at rest; > 30 mm Hg during exercise**
- Imaging
  - **Enlarged pulmonary trunk, diameter > 2.8 cm**

Arteriovenous Malformations

- **Congenital pulmonary arteriovenous malformation**
  - Direct communication between pulmonary artery(ies) and vein(s) without intervening capillary bed
  - Hereditary hemorrhagic telangiectasia (Rendu-Osler-Weber syndrome)
  - Imaging
    - **Nodular opacity with feeding and draining vessels**
    - Single or multiple
    - Arteriography for exclusion of multifocal disease and embolotherapy
- **Hepatopulmonary syndrome**
  - Acquired pulmonary arteriovenous malformations in patients with end-stage liver disease
  - Characterized by hepatic dysfunction, hypoxemia and pulmonary vascular dilatation
  - Imaging
    - Dilated peripheral lower lobe pulmonary vessels extending to the pleura
    - Direct visualization of abnormal arteriovenous connections

Anomalous Pulmonary Venous Drainage

- **Partial anomalous pulmonary venous drainage, left upper lobe**
  - Imaging
    - Left upper lobe venous drainage to **anomalous vertical vein** coursing along left superior mediastinum and draining into **left brachiocephalic vein**
    - Absence of normal left superior pulmonary vein at hilum
- **Scimitar syndrome (congenital venolobar syndrome)**
  - Partial anomalous right lung pulmonary venous drainage into inferior vena cava, hepatic or portal veins
  - Associated with **right pulmonary hypoplasia**, bronchopulmonary malformations, systemic arterial supply to right lung
  - Imaging
    - Visualization of abnormal vein with **scimitar shape**
    - Identification of site of venous drainage
    - Evaluation of associated anomalies

Pulmonary Vein Varix

- Congenital or acquired **enlargement of central pulmonary vein or veins**
- Associated with chronic elevation of left atrial pressures
- Imaging
  - Nodular opacity on radiography corresponds to enlarged pulmonary vein on CT

Pulmonary Thromboembolic Disease

- Common disease with significant morbidity/mortality
- Symptomatic patients; post-operative/bed-ridden, patients with malignant neoplasms
- Imaging of acute thromboembolic disease
  - Acute dilatation of pulmonary trunk as sign of pulmonary arterial hypertension
  - Visualization of partial/complete filling defects within contrast opacified pulmonary arteries
- Imaging of chronic thromboembolic disease
  - Findings of pulmonary arterial hypertension
  - Partial/complete filling defects in vascular lumen with **eccentric location** and **irregular borders**
  - **Recanalization/calcification** of emboli

PULMONARY VESSELS

OVERVIEW OF THE PULMONARY VESSELS

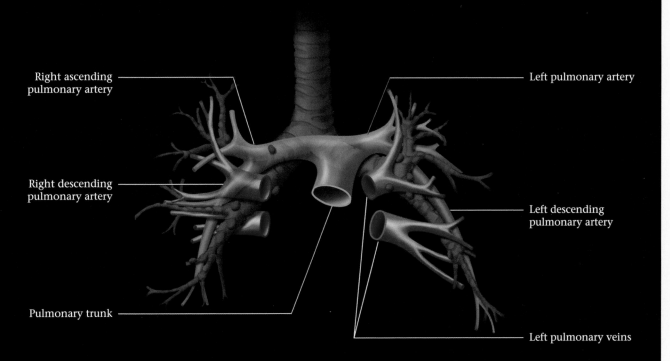

Right ascending pulmonary artery

Right descending pulmonary artery

Pulmonary trunk

Left pulmonary artery

Left descending pulmonary artery

Left pulmonary veins

Graphic depicts the anatomy and relationships of the pulmonary vessels. The pulmonary arteries (in blue) accompany the bronchi and carry deoxygenated blood to the capillary-alveolar interface. The pulmonary veins travel along the periphery of the pulmonary units (secondary pulmonary lobules, pulmonary segments and pulmonary lobes) and carry oxygenated blood from the alveolar capillaries to the left-sided circulation. Pulmonary lymphatics (not shown) course along the vascular structures and the tracheobronchial tree and are focally organized into lymph nodes in the lungs, along the airways and in the hila. The bronchopulmonary and hilar lymph nodes are considered intrapulmonary lymph nodes for the purpose of lung cancer staging.

PULMONARY VESSELS

RADIOGRAPHY, NORMAL PULMONARY VESSELS

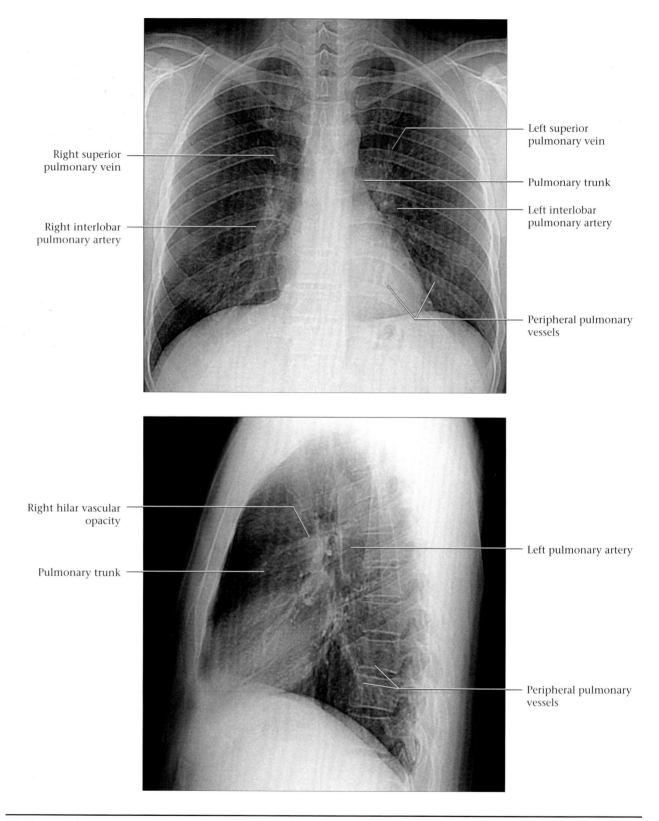

Right superior pulmonary vein

Right interlobar pulmonary artery

Left superior pulmonary vein

Pulmonary trunk

Left interlobar pulmonary artery

Peripheral pulmonary vessels

Right hilar vascular opacity

Pulmonary trunk

Left pulmonary artery

Peripheral pulmonary vessels

(Top) First of two normal chest radiographs illustrating the radiographic appearance of the normal pulmonary vessels. PA chest radiograph demonstrates that the pulmonary arteries provide the greatest contribution to the hilar opacities. The bilateral interlobar (descending) pulmonary arteries are typically well visualized. Normal peripheral pulmonary vessels are also seen. The pulmonary arteries undergo dichotomous branching and are least perceptible in the subpleural lung periphery. The superior pulmonary veins are seen in the suprahilar central lungs. The pulmonary lymphatics are not visible on normal radiographs. (Bottom) Left lateral chest radiograph shows the normal pulmonary vessels. The pulmonary trunk is barely apparent. The right hilar vascular opacity is produced by pulmonary veins and arteries. The left pulmonary artery is visible in most normal subjects.

PULMONARY VESSELS

RADIOGRAPHY, NORMAL PULMONARY VESSELS

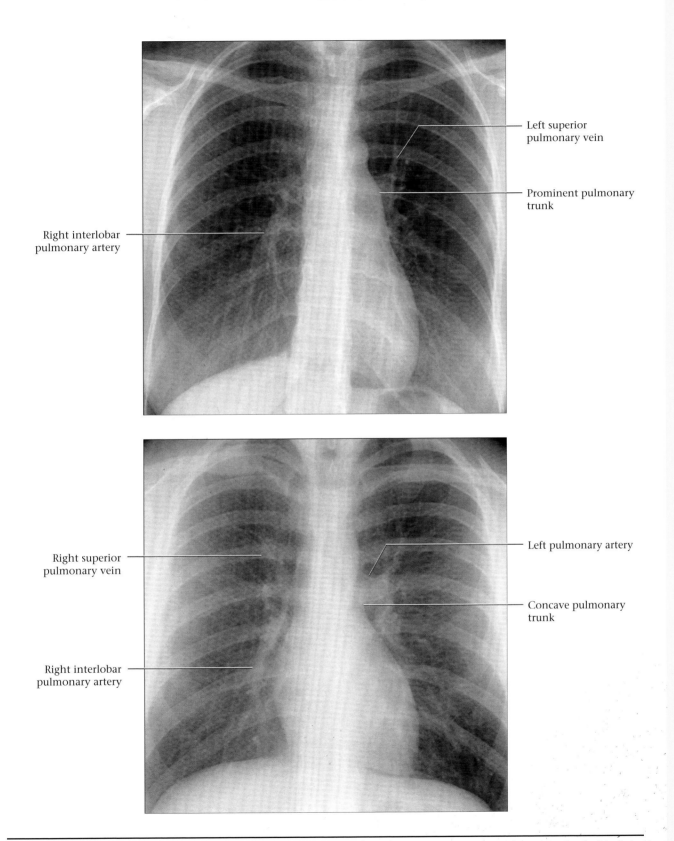

(Top) First of two normal chest radiographs demonstrating the variable appearance of the pulmonary trunk. PA chest radiograph of a 23 year old woman shows a prominent pulmonary trunk. The pulmonary trunk may be prominent in chest radiographs of children, adolescents and young adults. **(Bottom)** PA chest radiograph of a 15 year old boy demonstrates the normal medially concave pulmonary trunk configuration typically seen in adult patients.

PULMONARY VESSELS

ANATOMY OF THE PULMONARY ARTERIES AND VEINS

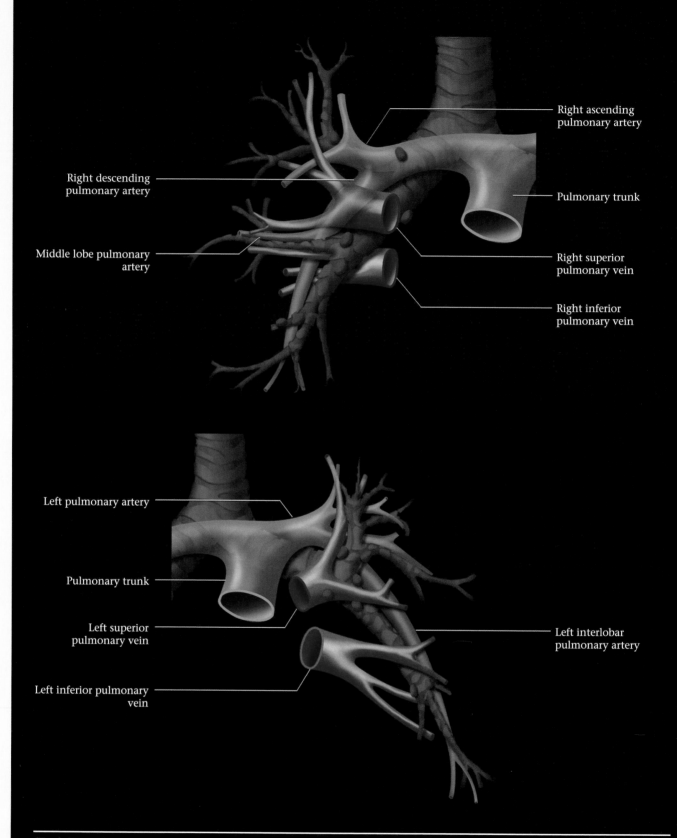

Right ascending pulmonary artery

Right descending pulmonary artery

Pulmonary trunk

Middle lobe pulmonary artery

Right superior pulmonary vein

Right inferior pulmonary vein

Left pulmonary artery

Pulmonary trunk

Left superior pulmonary vein

Left interlobar pulmonary artery

Left inferior pulmonary vein

(Top) First of two graphics depicting the anatomy of the pulmonary vessels. Anterior view of the right pulmonary vasculature shows the right pulmonary artery arising from the pulmonary trunk and bifurcating into ascending and descending branches. Pulmonary arteries generally course medial to vessel bronchi in the right upper lobe and lateral to the bronchi in the middle and lower lobes. The right superior pulmonary vein courses anterior to the bronchi and pulmonary artery. The right inferior pulmonary vein courses posterior to the bronchi in the inferior portion of the hilum. (Bottom) Anterior view of the left pulmonary vessels shows the left pulmonary arteries coursing along the bronchi. The left pulmonary artery courses over the ipsilateral main bronchus. The pulmonary veins course anterior to the bronchi. Note bronchopulmonary and hilar lymph nodes (in green).

PULMONARY VESSELS

ANGIOGRAPHY, NORMAL PULMONARY ARTERIES

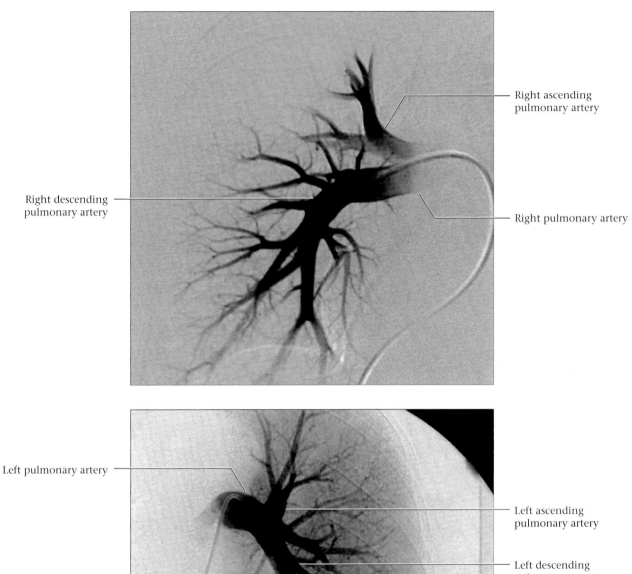

Right ascending pulmonary artery

Right descending pulmonary artery

Right pulmonary artery

Left pulmonary artery

Left ascending pulmonary artery

Left descending pulmonary artery

(Top) First of two images from a normal pulmonary arteriogram. Right pulmonary arteriogram shows an endovascular catheter that courses from the inferior vena cava through the right atrium, right ventricle, pulmonary trunk and right pulmonary artery to terminate in the proximal right vescending (interlobar) pulmonary artery. Note the superior course of the right ascending pulmonary artery, the arcuate course of the interlobar pulmonary artery and the horizontal course of the proximal right pulmonary artery. (Bottom) Left pulmonary arteriogram shows the endovascular catheter coursing from the right atrium through the right ventricle and pulmonary trunk to terminate in the interlobar left pulmonary artery. The left pulmonary artery is shorter and smaller than the right and courses over the left main bronchus.

PULMONARY VESSELS

AXIAL CT, NORMAL CENTRAL PULMONARY ARTERIES & VEINS

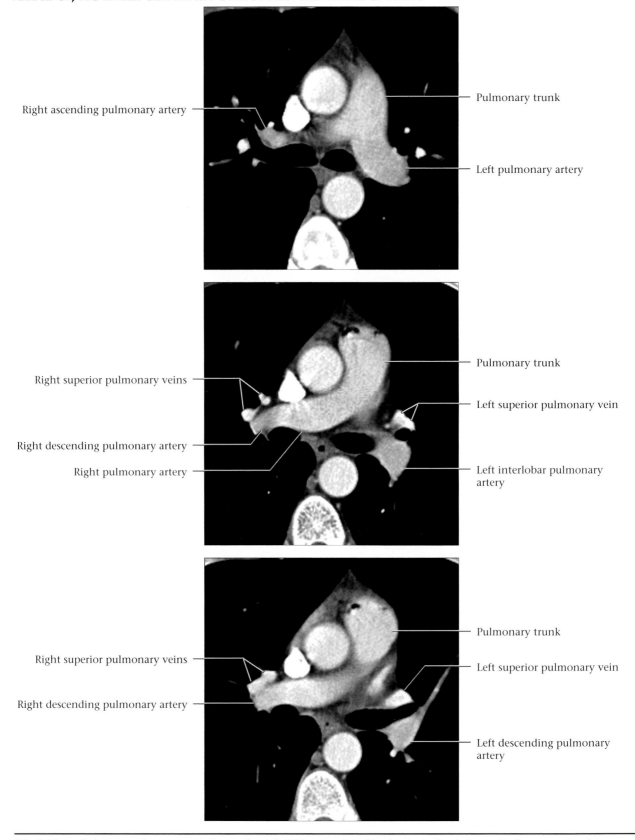

Right ascending pulmonary artery

Pulmonary trunk

Left pulmonary artery

Right superior pulmonary veins

Pulmonary trunk

Left superior pulmonary vein

Right descending pulmonary artery

Right pulmonary artery

Left interlobar pulmonary artery

Right superior pulmonary veins

Pulmonary trunk

Left superior pulmonary vein

Right descending pulmonary artery

Left descending pulmonary artery

(Top) First of six normal contrast-enhanced axial CT images (mediastinal window) through the central pulmonary vessels. Image through the left pulmonary artery shows that it is located superior to the right pulmonary artery and courses posteriorly over the left main bronchus. Note the right ascending (truncus anterior) pulmonary artery. **(Middle)** Image through the pulmonary trunk shows its posterior course and relationship to the ascending aorta. The left pulmonary artery courses over the left main (hyparterial) bronchus continuing as the interlobar artery. Note the horizontal course of the proximal right pulmonary artery behind the ascending aorta and superior vena cava. **(Bottom)** Image through the proximal pulmonary trunk shows that it is the most anteriorly located vascular structure at this level. Note the anterior location of the bilateral superior pulmonary veins at the hila.

PULMONARY VESSELS

AXIAL CT, NORMAL CENTRAL PULMONARY ARTERIES & VEINS

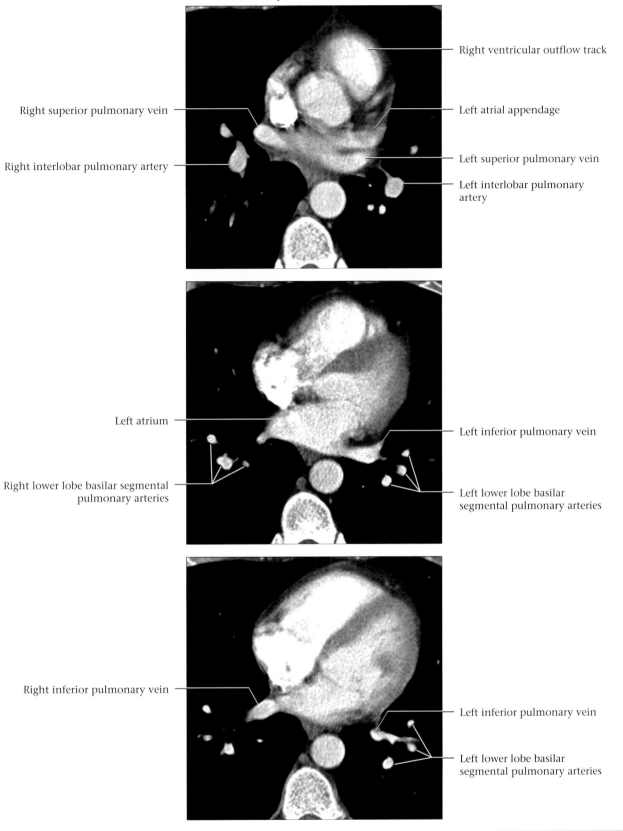

Right ventricular outflow track

Right superior pulmonary vein

Left atrial appendage

Right interlobar pulmonary artery

Left superior pulmonary vein

Left interlobar pulmonary artery

Left atrium

Left inferior pulmonary vein

Right lower lobe basilar segmental pulmonary arteries

Left lower lobe basilar segmental pulmonary arteries

Right inferior pulmonary vein

Left inferior pulmonary vein

Left lower lobe basilar segmental pulmonary arteries

(Top) Image through the superior aspect of the left atrium demonstrates the constant relationship between the left superior pulmonary vein and the left atrial appendage. The right superior pulmonary vein is located anterior to the bronchus intermedius. The bilateral interlobar pulmonary arteries are located posterolateral to the bronchi. (Middle) Image through the mid portion of the left atrium shows the left inferior pulmonary vein and the bilateral basilar segmental pulmonary arteries which follow a relatively vertical course with respect to the pulmonary veins. (Bottom) Image through the inferior left atrium demonstrates the normal right inferior pulmonary vein and the more distal basilar segmental lower lobe pulmonary arteries. This patient has four separate central pulmonary veins.

PULMONARY VESSELS

ANGIOGRAPHY, NORMAL PULMONARY VEINS

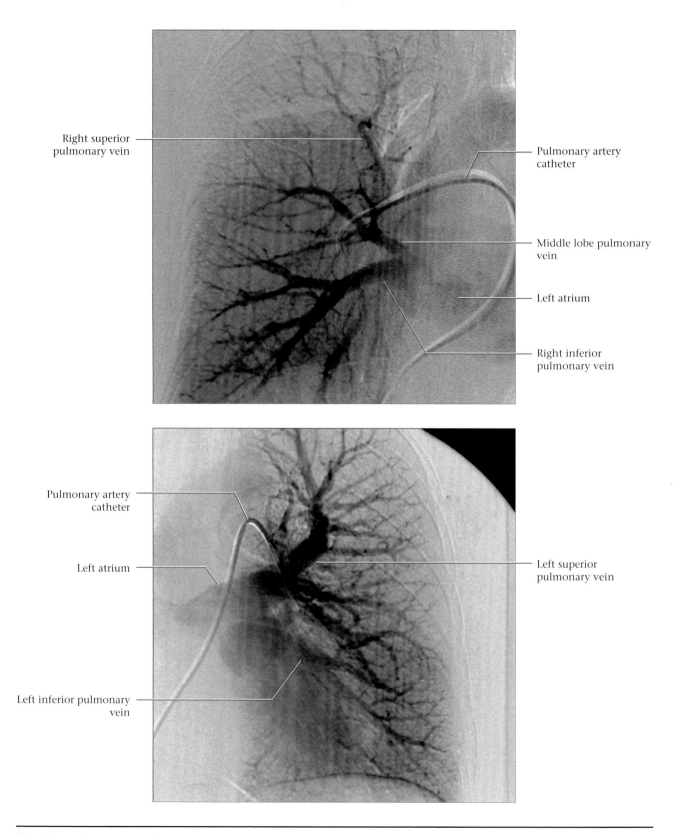

(Top) First of two images from a normal pulmonary arteriogram showing the normal anatomy of the pulmonary veins. Venous phase of a right pulmonary arteriogram shows the catheter tip within the right interlobar pulmonary artery. The delayed image shows the morphology of the pulmonary veins as they enter the left atrium. In this case, the middle lobe pulmonary vein drains into the right inferior pulmonary vein. The right superior pulmonary vein is not well opacified. (Bottom) Venous phase of normal left pulmonary arteriogram demonstrates the pulmonary veins draining into the left atrium. The arterial catheter travels through the right atrium, right ventricle, pulmonary trunk and left pulmonary artery to terminate in the interlobar artery. The normal left superior pulmonary vein is well opacified. The left inferior pulmonary vein is less clearly visualized.

PULMONARY VESSELS

CORONAL CT, NORMAL VARIANTS OF PULMONARY VENOUS ANATOMY

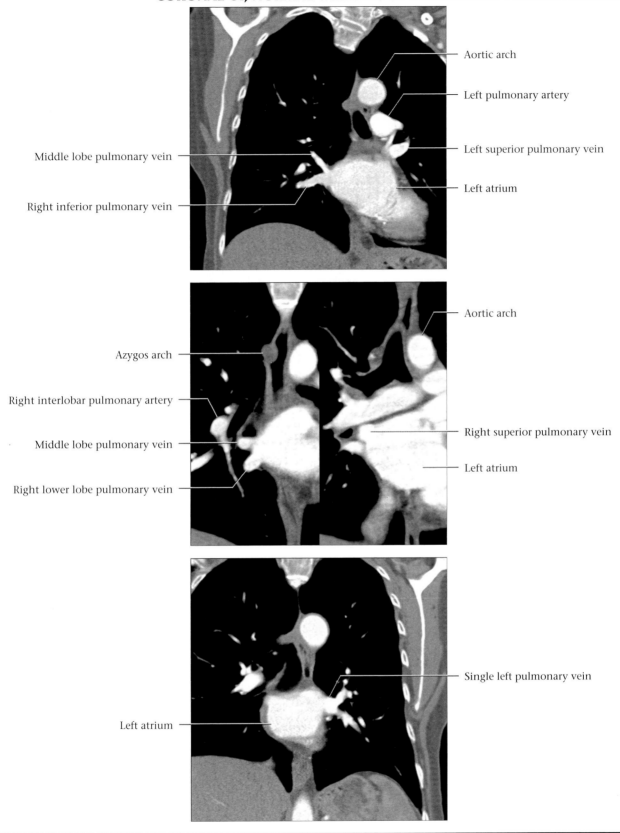

(Top) First of three contrast-enhanced chest CT images (mediastinal window) of different patients illustrating variations in the normal anatomy of the central pulmonary veins. Oblique coronal reconstruction demonstrates the middle lobe pulmonary vein draining into the right inferior pulmonary vein. (Middle) Composite image of two oblique coronal sections through the right side of the left atrium demonstrates a supernumerary right pulmonary vein. The middle lobe pulmonary vein drains directly into the left atrium between the ostia of the superior and inferior pulmonary veins. Supernumerary pulmonary veins are more common on the right and result from overincorporation during embryogenesis. (Bottom) Coronal image through the posterior left atrium shows that the superior and inferior left pulmonary veins have a single trunk, the result of underincorporation.

PULMONARY VESSELS

CORONAL CT, CENTRAL PULMONARY ARTERIES & VEINS

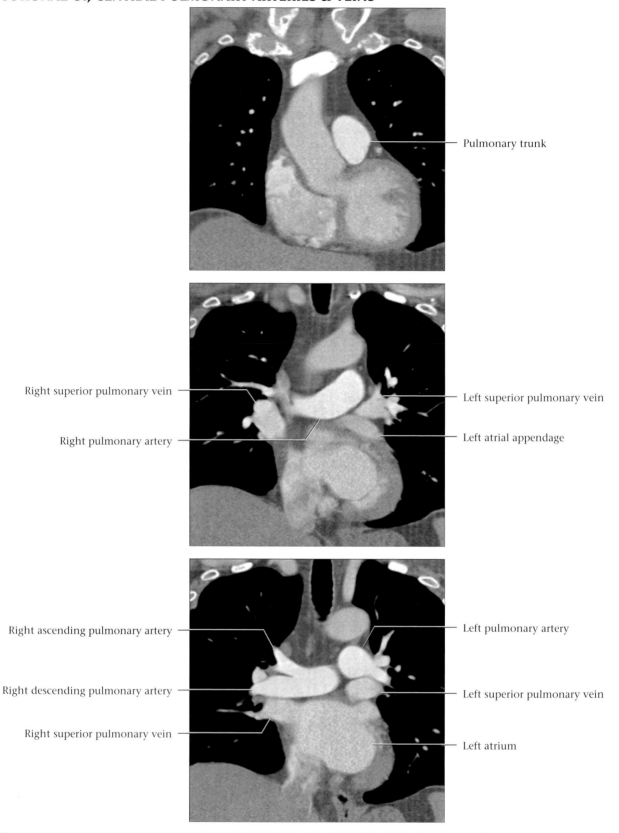

Pulmonary trunk

Right superior pulmonary vein — — Left superior pulmonary vein

Right pulmonary artery — — Left atrial appendage

Right ascending pulmonary artery — — Left pulmonary artery

Right descending pulmonary artery — — Left superior pulmonary vein

Right superior pulmonary vein — — Left atrium

(Top) First of six normal contrast-enhanced chest CT images (mediastinal window) shows the normal anatomy of the pulmonary vessels. The pulmonary trunk courses posteriorly and to the left of the ascending aorta and is seen in cross-section. (Middle) Image through the right pulmonary artery shows its horizontal intramediastinal course. Note the constant relationship of the left superior pulmonary vein and the left atrial appendage. The bilateral superior pulmonary veins course obliquely into the left atrium and are anteriorly located structures. (Bottom) Image through the left atrium shows the bifurcation of the right pulmonary artery into ascending and descending branches and shows the proximal left pulmonary artery.

PULMONARY VESSELS

CORONAL CT, CENTRAL PULMONARY ARTERIES & VEINS

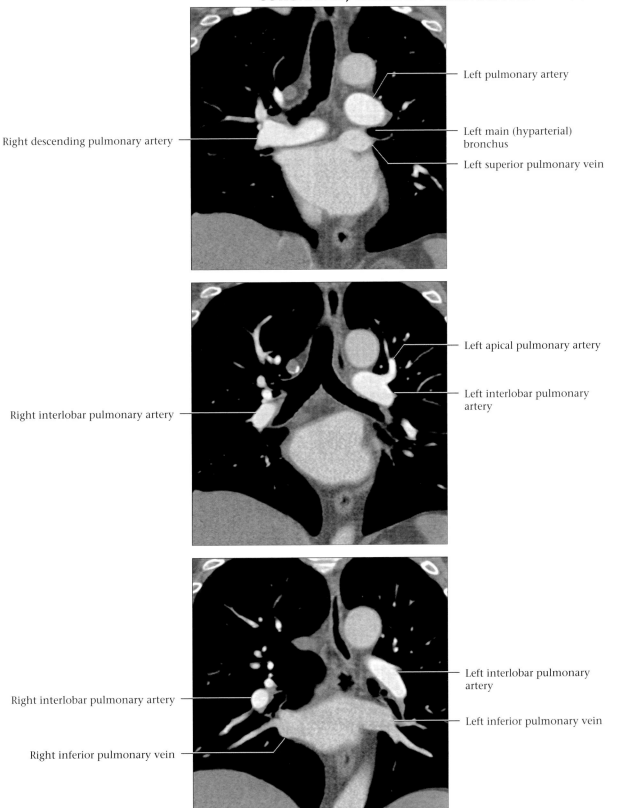

Right descending pulmonary artery

Left pulmonary artery

Left main (hyparterial) bronchus

Left superior pulmonary vein

Right interlobar pulmonary artery

Left apical pulmonary artery

Left interlobar pulmonary artery

Right interlobar pulmonary artery

Left interlobar pulmonary artery

Right inferior pulmonary vein

Left inferior pulmonary vein

(Top) Image through the mid portion of the left atrium shows that the left pulmonary artery is higher than the right and courses over the ipsilateral left main (hyparterial) bronchus. The lateral aspect of the horizontal portion of the right pulmonary artery is also shown. (Middle) Image through the carina shows the bilateral interlobar pulmonary arteries. Note the left apical pulmonary artery arising as a branch of the distal left pulmonary artery. (Bottom) Coronal image through the posterior aspect of the left atrium shows the bilateral inferior pulmonary veins entering the posterior left atrium. The bilateral interlobar pulmonary arteries and their relative vertical course with respect to the pulmonary veins are also shown.

PULMONARY VESSELS

SAGITTAL MR, NORMAL CENTRAL PULMONARY ARTERIES & VEINS

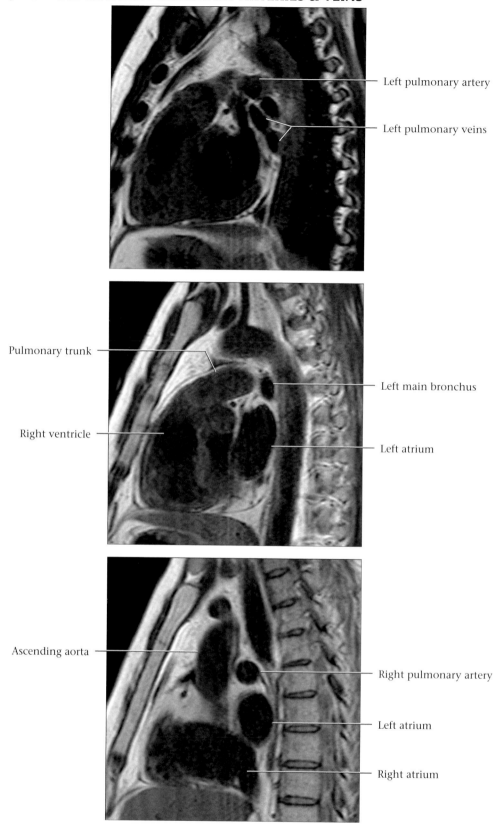

Left pulmonary artery

Left pulmonary veins

Pulmonary trunk

Left main bronchus

Right ventricle

Left atrium

Ascending aorta

Right pulmonary artery

Left atrium

Right atrium

(Top) First of three normal sagittal T1 MR images through the central pulmonary vessels showing the normal vascular relationships in this imaging plane. Image obtained to the left of midline shows the left superior and inferior pulmonary veins located anterior to the left main bronchus. Note that the left pulmonary artery courses over the left main (hyparterial) bronchus. (Middle) Image through the aortic arch demonstrates that the pulmonary trunk arises from the right ventricular outflow track and courses posteriorly and to the left prior to bifurcating into right and left pulmonary arteries. (Bottom) Image obtained to the right of midline shows a portion of the ascending aorta and the horizontal course of the right pulmonary artery. The pulmonary trunk is located anterior and to the left of the ascending aorta.

PULMONARY VESSELS

AXIAL CT, NORMAL RIGHT SEGMENTAL PULMONARY ARTERIES

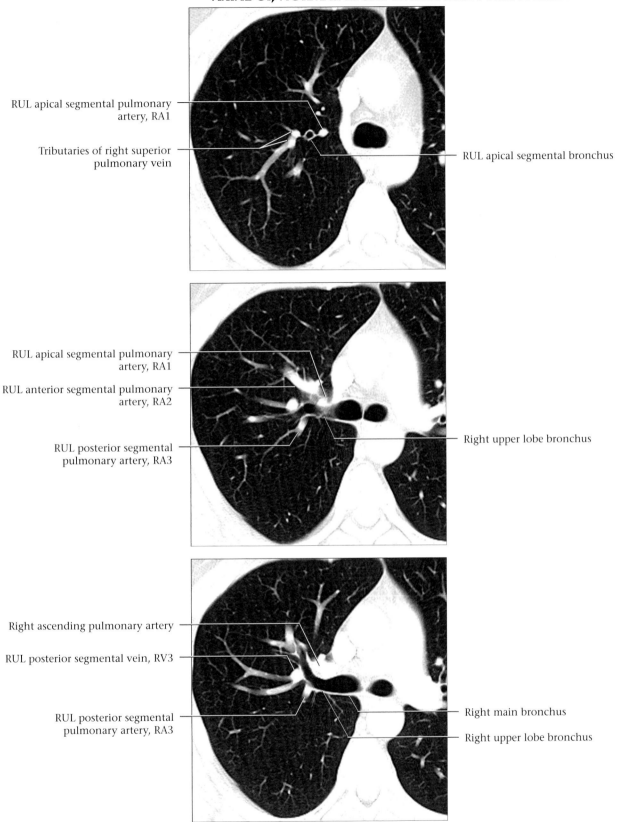

RUL apical segmental pulmonary artery, RA1

Tributaries of right superior pulmonary vein

RUL apical segmental bronchus

RUL apical segmental pulmonary artery, RA1

RUL anterior segmental pulmonary artery, RA2

RUL posterior segmental pulmonary artery, RA3

Right upper lobe bronchus

Right ascending pulmonary artery

RUL posterior segmental vein, RV3

RUL posterior segmental pulmonary artery, RA3

Right main bronchus

Right upper lobe bronchus

(Top) First of nine axial contrast-enhanced chest CT images (lung window) through the right lung showing the normal anatomy of the segmental pulmonary arteries. Image obtained above the carina shows the right apical segmental pulmonary artery (RA1) located medial to the right upper lobe (RUL) apical segmental bronchus. Tributaries of the right superior pulmonary vein are located lateral to the bronchus. **(Middle)** Image through the right upper lobe bronchus shows the apical segmental (RA1) and anterior segmental (RA2) pulmonary arteries. Tributaries of the right superior pulmonary vein are seen lateral to the bronchi. **(Bottom)** Image through the right upper lobe anterior segmental bronchus shows the right ascending pulmonary artery. The right posterior segmental pulmonary artery (RA3) typically arises from the right interlobar pulmonary artery.

PULMONARY VESSELS

AXIAL CT, NORMAL RIGHT SEGMENTAL PULMONARY ARTERIES

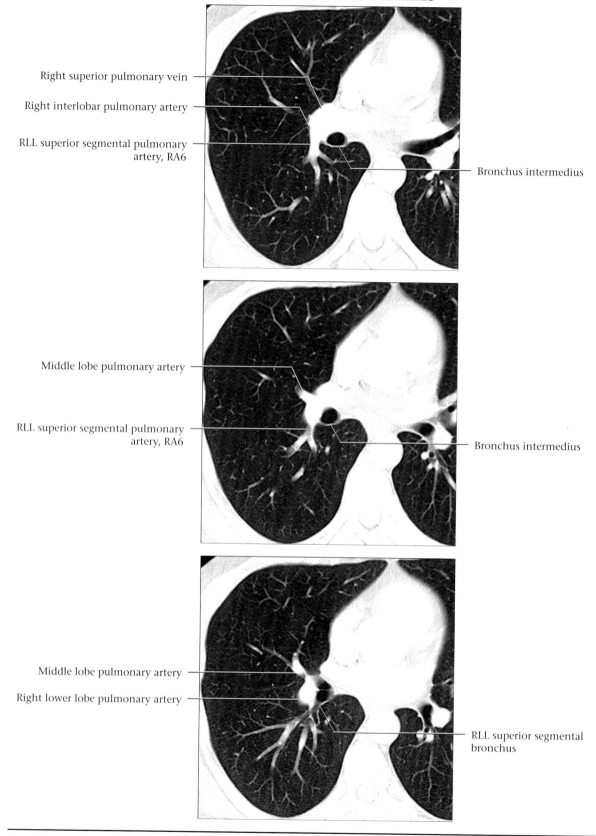

Right superior pulmonary vein

Right interlobar pulmonary artery

RLL superior segmental pulmonary artery, RA6

Bronchus intermedius

Middle lobe pulmonary artery

RLL superior segmental pulmonary artery, RA6

Bronchus intermedius

Middle lobe pulmonary artery

Right lower lobe pulmonary artery

RLL superior segmental bronchus

(Top) Image through the bronchus intermedius shows the origin of the right lower lobe (RLL) superior segmental pulmonary artery (RA6) arising from the right interlobar pulmonary artery. Although it is difficult to resolve, the right superior pulmonary vein is located immediately anterior to the right pulmonary artery at this level. (Middle) Image through the proximal middle lobe pulmonary artery shows the inferior aspect of the right lower lobe superior segmental pulmonary artery (RA6). This vessel typically arises just superior to its corresponding segmental bronchus. The middle lobe (ML) pulmonary artery arises as a single trunk from the right interlobar pulmonary artery. (Bottom) Image through the origin of the right lower lobe superior segmental bronchus shows the middle lobe pulmonary artery prior to its bifurcation and the right lower lobe pulmonary artery.

PULMONARY VESSELS

AXIAL CT, NORMAL RIGHT SEGMENTAL PULMONARY ARTERIES

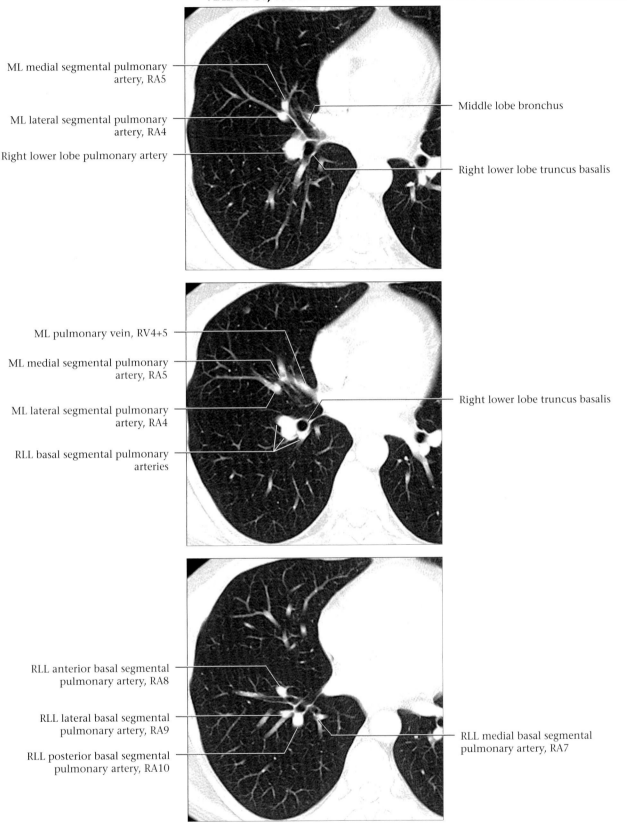

ML medial segmental pulmonary artery, RA5

ML lateral segmental pulmonary artery, RA4

Right lower lobe pulmonary artery

Middle lobe bronchus

Right lower lobe truncus basalis

ML pulmonary vein, RV4+5

ML medial segmental pulmonary artery, RA5

ML lateral segmental pulmonary artery, RA4

RLL basal segmental pulmonary arteries

Right lower lobe truncus basalis

RLL anterior basal segmental pulmonary artery, RA8

RLL lateral basal segmental pulmonary artery, RA9

RLL posterior basal segmental pulmonary artery, RA10

RLL medial basal segmental pulmonary artery, RA7

(Top) Image through the origin of the middle lobe bronchus shows the bifurcation of the middle lobe pulmonary artery into lateral (RA4) and medial (RA5) segmental pulmonary arteries. The right lower lobe pulmonary artery is the caudal continuation of the interlobar pulmonary artery after the take off of the middle lobe pulmonary artery. (Middle) Image through the truncus basalis shows the middle lobe segmental pulmonary arteries and the right lower lobe basal segmental artery branches. The middle lobe pulmonary vein (RV4+5) courses inferomedially to drain into the right superior pulmonary vein. (Bottom) Image through the basal segmental bronchi shows the right lower lobe basal segmental pulmonary arteries located lateral to the corresponding bronchi. These are the medial (RA7), anterior (RA8), lateral (RA9) and posterior (RA10) basal segmental pulmonary arteries.

PULMONARY VESSELS

AXIAL CT, NORMAL LEFT SEGMENTAL PULMONARY ARTERIES

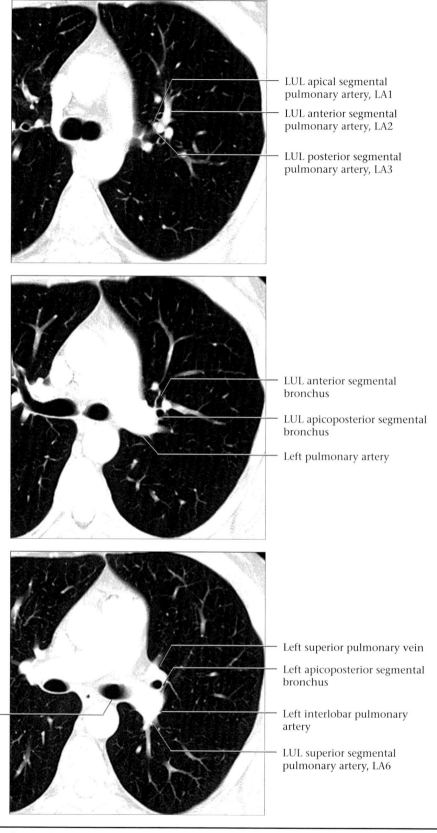

LUL apical segmental pulmonary artery, LA1

LUL anterior segmental pulmonary artery, LA2

LUL posterior segmental pulmonary artery, LA3

LUL anterior segmental bronchus

LUL apicoposterior segmental bronchus

Left pulmonary artery

Left superior pulmonary vein

Left apicoposterior segmental bronchus

Left main bronchus

Left interlobar pulmonary artery

LUL superior segmental pulmonary artery, LA6

(Top) First of nine axial contrast-enhanced chest CT images (lung window) showing the normal anatomy of the left segmental pulmonary arteries. Image through the carina shows the bifurcation of LA1+3 into medially located apical (LA1) and laterally located posterior segmental pulmonary arteries. The left upper lobe (LUL) anterior segmental pulmonary artery (LA2) is also demonstrated. **(Middle)** Image through the left upper lobe anterior segmental bronchus shows the left pulmonary artery coursing over the left main (hyparterial) bronchus. **(Bottom)** Image through the left main bronchus shows the origin of the left lower lobe superior segmental pulmonary artery (LA6) from the interlobar artery. The anteriorly located left superior pulmonary vein is also demonstrated.

PULMONARY VESSELS

AXIAL CT, NORMAL LEFT SEGMENTAL PULMONARY ARTERIES

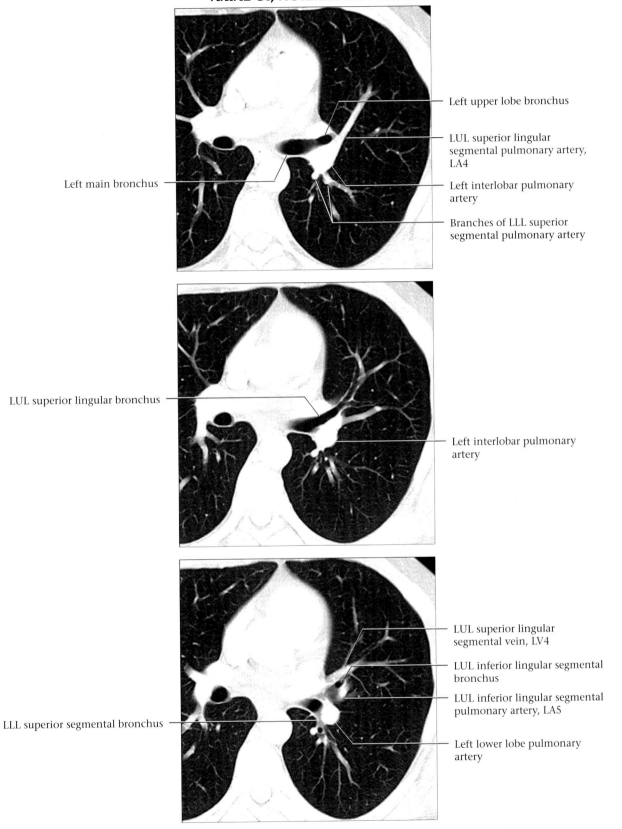

Left upper lobe bronchus

LUL superior lingular segmental pulmonary artery, LA4

Left main bronchus

Left interlobar pulmonary artery

Branches of LLL superior segmental pulmonary artery

LUL superior lingular bronchus

Left interlobar pulmonary artery

LUL superior lingular segmental vein, LV4

LUL inferior lingular segmental bronchus

LUL inferior lingular segmental pulmonary artery, LA5

LLL superior segmental bronchus

Left lower lobe pulmonary artery

(Top) Image through the left upper lobe bronchus shows the origin of the superior lingular segmental pulmonary artery (LA4) from the interlobar pulmonary artery. This artery is typically seen superior to its accompanying segmental bronchus. Branches of the left lower lobe superior segmental pulmonary artery are also demonstrated. **(Middle)** Image through the left upper lobe superior lingular segmental bronchus demonstrates the posterolateral location of the left interlobar pulmonary artery. **(Bottom)** Image through the superior aspect of the left lower lobe superior segmental bronchus shows the proximal left upper lobe inferior lingular segmental pulmonary artery (LA5) coursing lateral to its corresponding bronchus. The left upper lobe superior lingular vein courses medial to the bronchus.

PULMONARY VESSELS

AXIAL CT, NORMAL LEFT SEGMENTAL PULMONARY ARTERIES

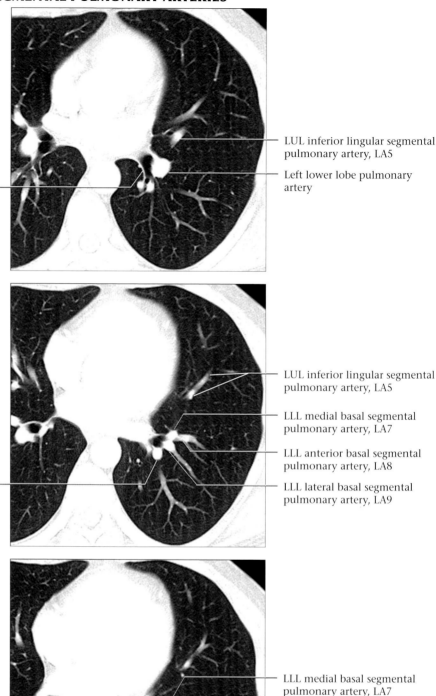

LLL superior segmental bronchus

LUL inferior lingular segmental pulmonary artery, LA5

Left lower lobe pulmonary artery

LUL inferior lingular segmental pulmonary artery, LA5

LLL medial basal segmental pulmonary artery, LA7

LLL anterior basal segmental pulmonary artery, LA8

LLL posterior basal segmental pulmonary artery, LA10

LLL lateral basal segmental pulmonary artery, LA9

LLL medial basal segmental pulmonary artery, LA7

LLL anterior basal segmental pulmonary artery, LA8

LLL posterior basal segmental pulmonary artery, LA10

LLL lateral basal segmental pulmonary artery, LA9

(Top) Image through the left lower lobe (LLL) superior segmental bronchus shows the course of the left upper lobe inferior lingular segmental pulmonary artery (LA5) lateral to the corresponding segmental bronchus. **(Middle)** Image through the proximal left lower lobe basal segmental bronchi shows the anteriorly located left lower lobe medial (LA7) and lateral (LA8) basal segmental pulmonary arteries. These vessels typically arise from a common trunk (LA7+8). The left lower lobe lateral (LA9) and posterior (LA10) segmental pulmonary arteries are also shown. **(Bottom)** Image through the left lower lobe basilar segmental bronchi shows the basilar segmental pulmonary arteries. These are (clockwise from anterior to posterior) the left lower lobe medial (LA7), anterior (LA8), lateral (LA9) and posterior (LA10) basal segmental pulmonary arteries.

GRAPHIC & CT, NORMAL INTRAPULMONARY LYMPH NODES

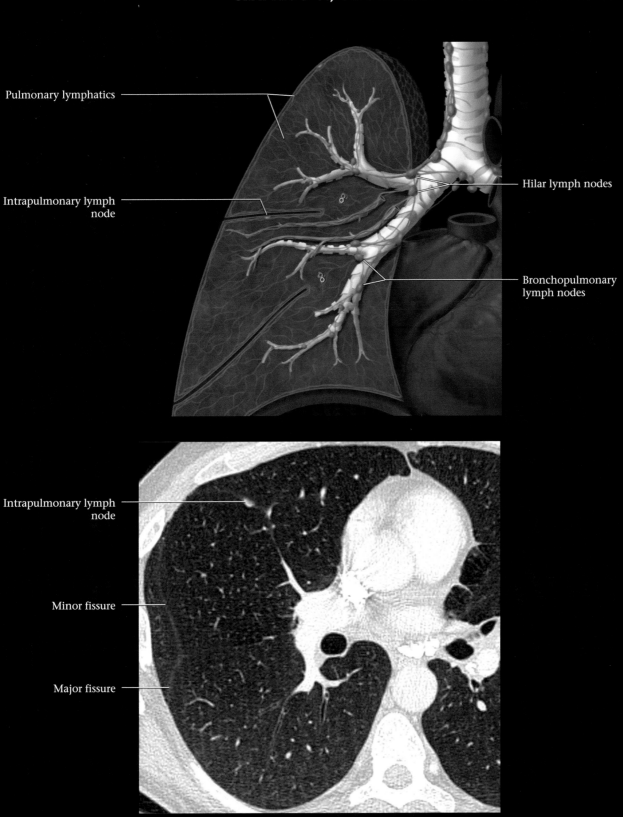

Pulmonary lymphatics

Intrapulmonary lymph node

Hilar lymph nodes

Bronchopulmonary lymph nodes

Intrapulmonary lymph node

Minor fissure

Major fissure

(Top) Graphic depicts the normal anatomy of the pulmonary lymphatic vessels. These small structures are not visible on normal imaging studies. They course centripetally towards the hilum and form aggregates of lymphoid tissue or lymph nodes. These typically occur at bronchial bifurcations. The bronchopulmonary lymph nodes and hilar lymph nodes are considered intrapulmonary for the purpose of lung cancer staging. **(Bottom)** Normal high-resolution chest CT shows a peripheral subpleural ovoid soft tissue nodule along the minor fissure. With increasing utilization of thin section multidetector chest CT, small pulmonary nodules are often identified. Many nodules under 4 mm in size relate to benign conditions such as remote granulomatous infection. Ovoid elongate small subpleural nodules likely represent intrapulmonary lymph nodes.

PULMONARY VESSELS

CT, PULMONARY LYMPH NODES

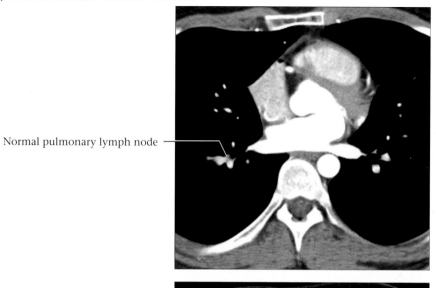

Normal pulmonary lymph node —

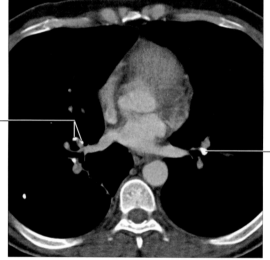

Granulomatous pulmonary lymph nodes —

— Normal sized calcified pulmonary lymph node

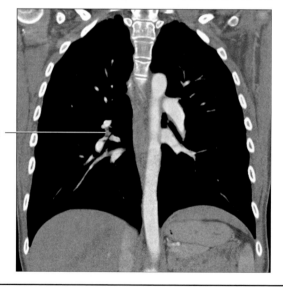

Normal pulmonary lymph node —

(Top) Normal axial contrast-enhanced chest CT (mediastinal window) demonstrates non-enhancing soft tissue adjacent to the basilar segmental right lower lobe pulmonary arteries near the bronchovascular sheath representing a normal pulmonary lymph node. **(Middle)** Axial contrast-enhanced chest CT of a patient with remote granulomatous infection demonstrates granulomatous calcification in normal-sized pulmonary lymph nodes. These lymph nodes are easily identified by virtue of their complete calcification. Note their intimate relationship to the structures in the bronchovascular sheath. **(Bottom)** Normal coronal contrast-enhanced chest CT (mediastinal window) demonstrates non-enhancing soft tissue representing a normal pulmonary lymph node located at a bronchial bifurcation.

PULMONARY VESSELS

VASCULAR REDISTRIBUTION; PULMONARY VENOUS HYPERTENSION

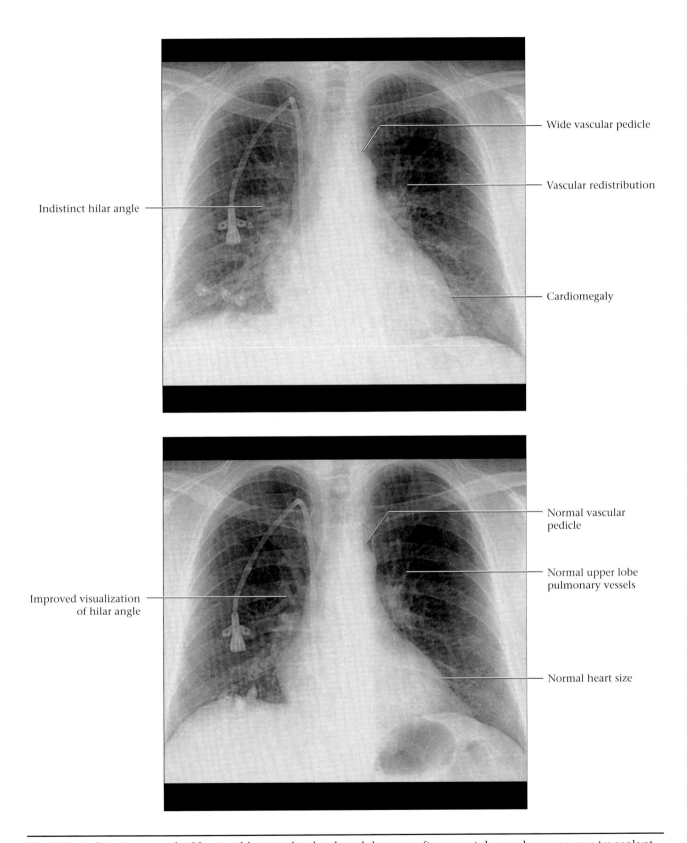

Indistinct hilar angle

Wide vascular pedicle

Vascular redistribution

Cardiomegaly

Improved visualization of hilar angle

Normal vascular pedicle

Normal upper lobe pulmonary vessels

Normal heart size

(Top) First of two images of a 52 year old man who developed dyspnea after an autologous bone marrow transplant. PA chest radiograph demonstrates redistribution of pulmonary vascular flow to the upper lung zones and indistinctness of the hilar angle. There is cardiomegaly and a wide vascular pedicle. The findings indicate the presence of pulmonary venous hypertension. (Bottom) Follow-up PA chest radiograph demonstrates resolution of vascular redistribution, visualization of distinct vascular margins, visualization of the hilar angle, a normal vascular pedicle and resolution of previously demonstrated cardiomegaly. Note the right internal jugular catheter tip in the right atrium.

PULMONARY VESSELS

ABNORMAL VASCULAR CONNECTIONS, ARTERIOVENOUS MALFORMATION

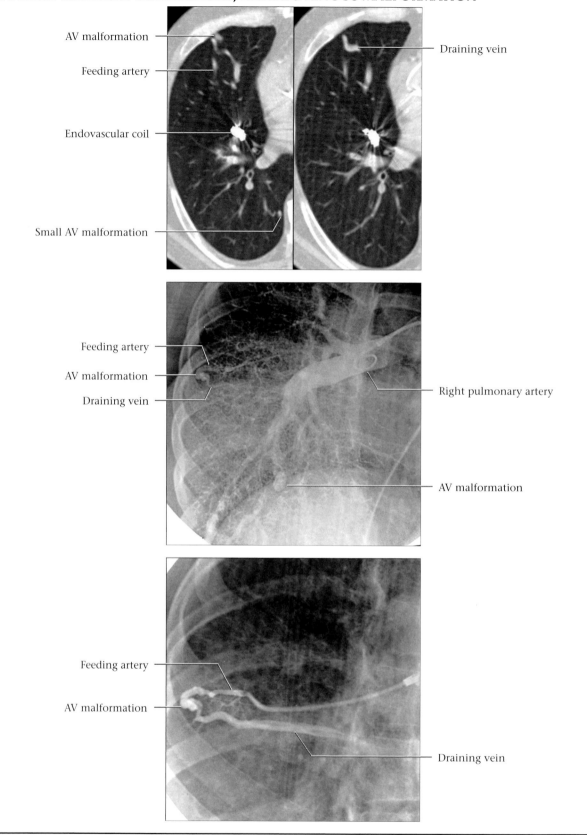

(Top) Composite axial nonenhanced chest CT (lung window) of a 58 year old man with hereditary hemorrhagic telangiectasia and multifocal pulmonary arteriovenous (AV) malformations shows metallic material within the lumen of a previously embolized lesion and at least two additional AV malformations. **(Middle)** First of two images of a 37 year old woman with hereditary hemorrhagic telangiectasia. Right pulmonary arteriogram shows at least two pulmonary AV malformations. Angiography is performed for identification of multifocal lesions and for evaluation prior to embolotherapy. **(Bottom)** Selective injection from a pulmonary arteriogram into the feeding artery of an AV malformation shows the smaller feeding artery and the larger draining vein. AV malformations provide direct communication between the pulmonary arterial and venous systems without an intervening capillary bed.

PULMONARY VESSELS

ABNORMAL VASCULAR CONNECTIONS, HEPATOPULMONARY SYNDROME

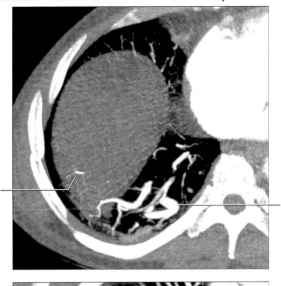

Pleural based AV malformation ———

——— Dilated right lower lobe vessels

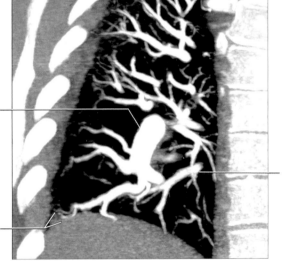

Dilated interlobar pulmonary artery ———

——— Pulmonary vein

AV malformations ———

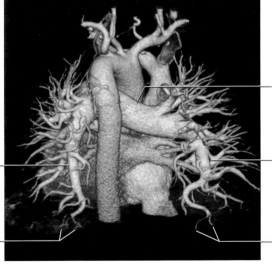

——— Right pulmonary artery

Left interlobar pulmonary artery ———

——— Right interlobar pulmonary artery

Subpleural AV malformations ———

——— Dilated peripheral pulmonary arteries

(Top) First of three contrast-enhanced chest CT images of a 48 year old man with end-stage liver disease and hepatopulmonary syndrome. Axial image through the right lung base shows markedly dilated right lower lobe pulmonary arteries and veins and pleural based acquired AV communications. Note visualization of subpleural enlarged vascular structures. **(Middle)** Coronal image demonstrates marked enlargement of the right pulmonary arteries and veins. Peripheral AV malformations or communications are visualized in the right lung base. **(Bottom)** Coronal posterior volume rendered CT image through the thorax shows the large size of the pulmonary arteries, particularly the bilateral lower lobe pulmonary arteries. The interlobar pulmonary arteries are also enlarged. Subpleural AV communications and dilated peripheral pulmonary vessels are also noted.

PULMONARY VESSELS

ABNORMAL VASCULAR CONNECTIONS, PARTIAL ANOMALOUS PULMONARY VENOUS RETURN

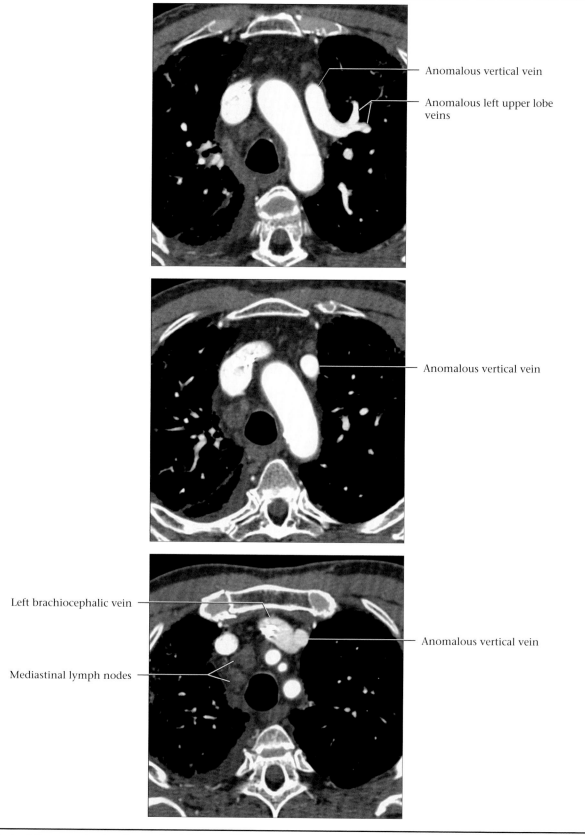

(Top) First of three contrast-enhanced axial chest CT images (mediastinal window) of a 63 year old man with partial anomalous pulmonary venous return of the left upper lobe. Anomalous left upper lobe pulmonary veins drain into an anomalous vein in the left superior mediastinum. **(Middle)** Image through the superior aspect of the aortic arch demonstrates the anomalous vertical vein coursing along the left lateral aspect of the aortic arch. **(Bottom)** Axial image at the level of the left brachiocephalic vein demonstrates its anastomosis with the anomalous vertical vein. Mediastinal lymphadenopathy is also noted in the right paratracheal region. Patients with this anomaly exhibit absence of the normal superior pulmonary vein in the left hilum (not shown).

PULMONARY VESSELS

ABNORMAL VASCULAR CONNECTIONS, SCIMITAR SYNDROME

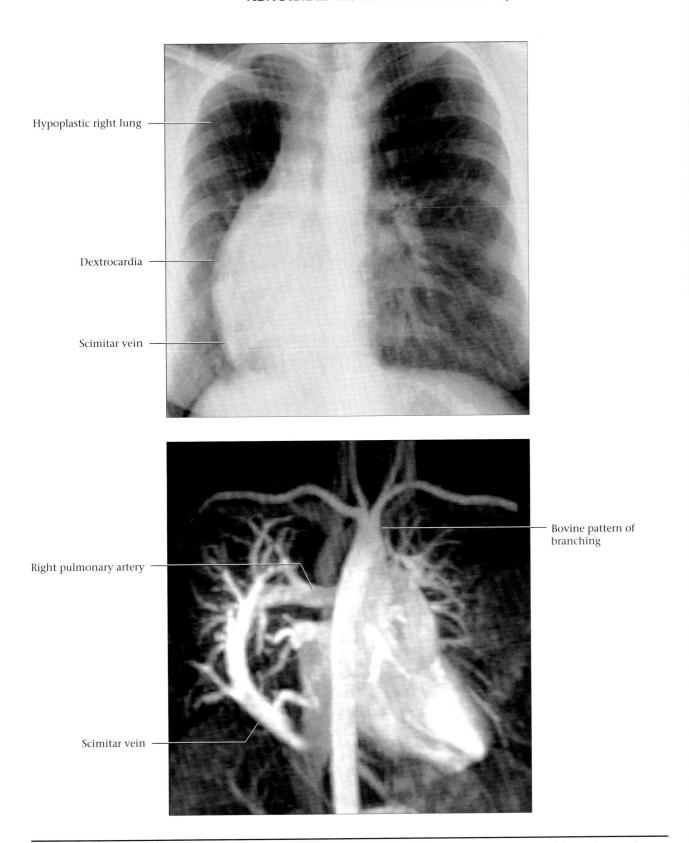

Hypoplastic right lung

Dextrocardia

Scimitar vein

Bovine pattern of branching

Right pulmonary artery

Scimitar vein

(Top) PA chest radiograph of a woman with congenital venolobar (scimitar) syndrome shows mild rotation to the right. There is dextrocardia related to right pulmonary hypoplasia. An arcuate right-sided vascular structure represents the anomalous scimitar vein that drains into the inferior vena cava. **(Bottom)** Magnetic resonance angiography of another patient with congenital venolobar syndrome demonstrates a right aortic arch with bovine pattern of great vessel branching. An anomalous arcuate (scimitar) vein drains portions of the right lung and anastomoses with the inferior vena cava. Patients with scimitar syndrome may be asymptomatic or may have symptoms related to congenital heart disease. The syndrome may be associated with right pulmonary hypoplasia, systemic blood supply to the right lung and anomalies of the tracheobronchial tree.

PULMONARY VESSELS

PULMONARY VEIN ENLARGEMENT, PULMONARY VARIX

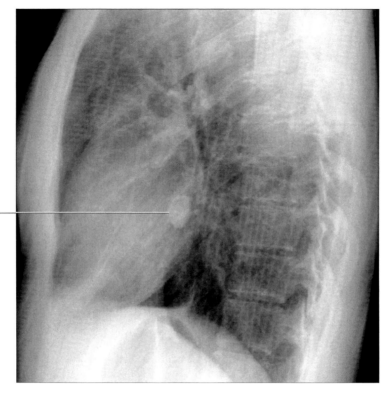

Ovoid pulmonary nodule

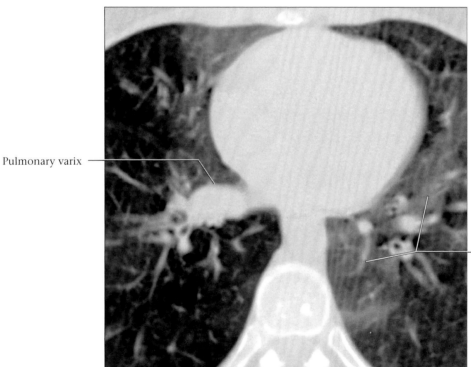

Pulmonary varix

Paramediastinal ground glass opacity

(Top) First of two images of a patient with a right pulmonary varix. Lateral chest radiograph shows an ovoid soft tissue nodule that projects over the left atrium and the anatomic location of the pulmonary veins. The lesion was poorly visualized on PA chest radiograph (not shown). **(Bottom)** Unenhanced chest CT (lung window) shows that the pulmonary nodule seen on radiography represented an enlarged right inferior pulmonary vein. There is also heterogeneous attenuation of the surrounding lung parenchyma with high attenuation in the paramediastinal aspects of the lung. Pulmonary varices can be congenital or acquired lesions. Acquired varices are often related to elevated left atrial pressures and are typically found incidentally on radiography. Images courtesy of Jerry Speckman, MD, University of Florida, Gainesville, Florida.

PULMONARY VESSELS

PULMONARY ARTERY ENLARGEMENT, PULMONARY ARTERIAL HYPERTENSION

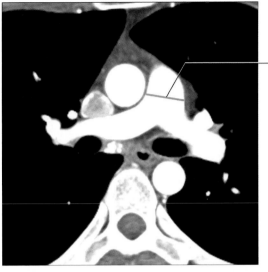

Measurement of the pulmonary trunk

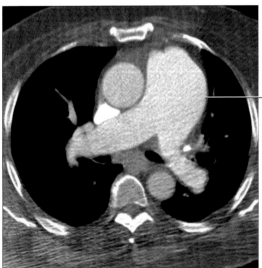

Enlarged pulmonary trunk

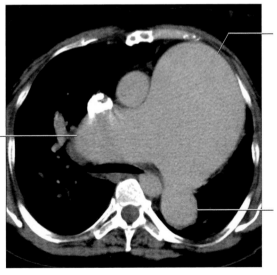

Massively enlarged pulmonary trunk

Enlarged right pulmonary artery

Enlarged left pulmonary artery

(Top) Normal contrast-enhanced axial gated chest CT image (mediastinal window) shows the method of measurement of the pulmonary trunk (blue line) on CT, performed perpendicular to the vascular long axis at the bifurcation. The normal size of the pulmonary trunk is up to 28.6 mm. (Middle) First of two axial contrast-enhanced chest CT images (mediastinal window) through the pulmonary trunks of two different patients. CT of a 74 year old woman with pulmonary arterial hypertension and multiple prior episodes of pulmonary thromboembolic disease demonstrates enlargement of the pulmonary artery trunk measuring 5.7 cm. (Bottom) CT of a 51 year old woman with severe pulmonary hypertension shows massive enlargement of the pulmonary arteries. The pulmonary trunk measures 7.4 cm and the pulmonary artery pressure was 56 mm Hg.

PULMONARY VESSELS

ARTERIAL FILLING DEFECTS; ACUTE PULMONARY THROMBOEMBOLIC DISEASE

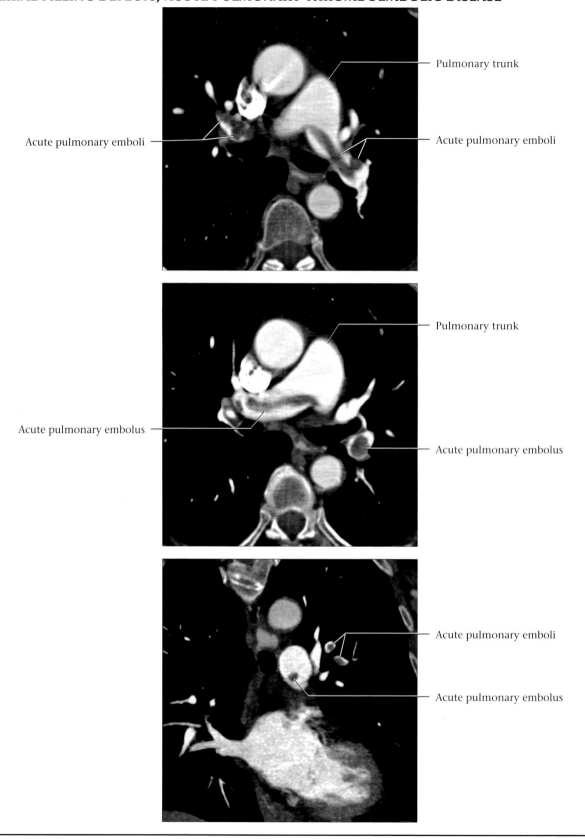

(Top) First of three images from a CT pulmonary angiogram (mediastinal window) of a 67 year old woman with acute pulmonary thromboembolic disease. Axial image shows pulmonary emboli within the left and the proximal left interlobar pulmonary arteries. A large pulmonary embolus is also noted within an enlarged right ascending pulmonary artery. **(Middle)** Axial image through the pulmonary trunk shows low attenuation filling defects surrounded by endovascular contrast within the right pulmonary artery and the left interlobar pulmonary artery. **(Bottom)** Oblique coronal image through the left pulmonary artery shows endoluminal centrally located emboli in the left pulmonary artery and in branches of the left upper lobe anterior segmental artery.

PULMONARY VESSELS

ARTERIAL FILLING DEFECTS; CHRONIC PULMONARY THROMBOEMBOLIC DISEASE

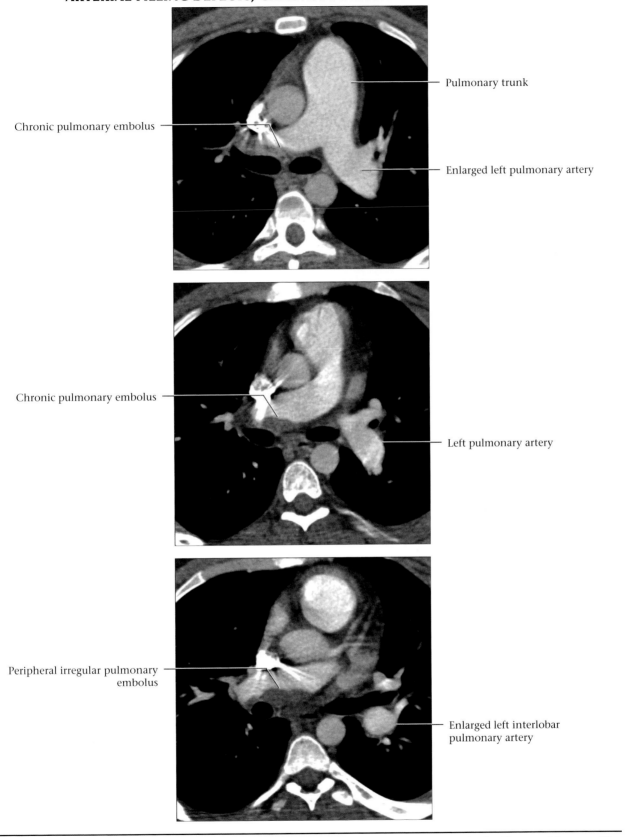

(Top) First of three axial images from a contrast-enhanced chest CT (mediastinal window) of a 20 year old man with pulmonary arterial hypertension (pulmonary artery pressure of 51 mm Hg). Image through the pulmonary trunk shows diffuse pulmonary artery enlargement. The pulmonary trunk measured 3.5 cm. Note chronic pulmonary embolus in the right pulmonary artery. (Middle) Image obtained below the carina shows eccentric soft tissue in the right pulmonary artery and enlargement of the left interlobar pulmonary artery. (Bottom) Axial image through the root of the aorta shows the posterior eccentric soft tissue filling defect in the right pulmonary artery that extends into the proximal right interlobar artery. The irregular contour of the soft tissue filling defect is consistent with known chronic pulmonary embolus. The left interlobar pulmonary artery is enlarged.

PULMONARY VESSELS

PULMONARY EMBOLISM, FOREIGN MATERIALS

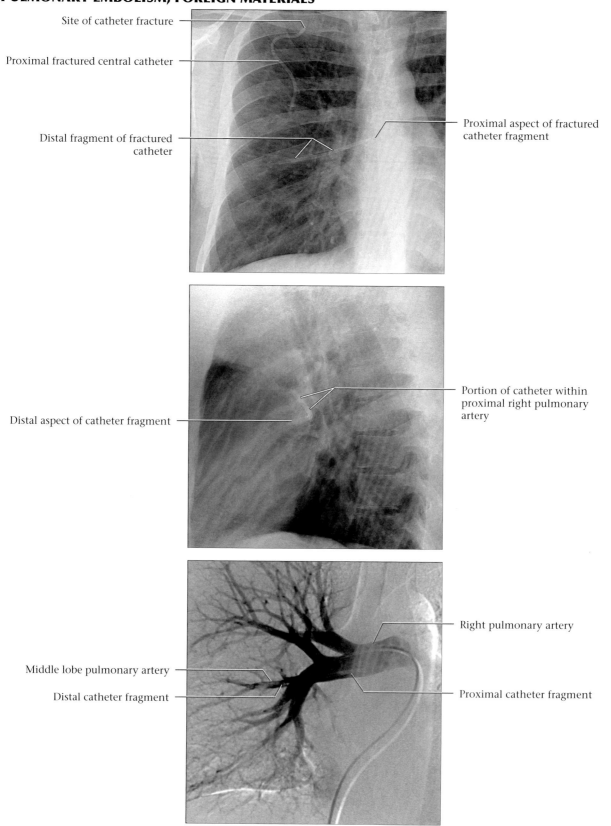

Site of catheter fracture

Proximal fractured central catheter

Distal fragment of fractured catheter

Proximal aspect of fractured catheter fragment

Distal aspect of catheter fragment

Portion of catheter within proximal right pulmonary artery

Right pulmonary artery

Middle lobe pulmonary artery

Distal catheter fragment

Proximal catheter fragment

(Top) First of three images of a 44 year old man with a fractured right subclavian central catheter which embolized to the middle lobe pulmonary artery. PA chest radiograph coned-down to the right lung shows the site of catheter fracture and the embolized catheter fragment within the middle lobe pulmonary artery. The proximal aspect of the fractured fragment is in the intramediastinal (horizontal) right pulmonary artery. (Middle) Coned-down lateral chest radiograph demonstrates the fractured catheter fragment projecting over the right hilar vascular opacity and within the proximal right pulmonary artery. (Bottom) Right pulmonary arteriogram performed prior to catheter retrieval shows the location of the catheter fragment with its proximal portion in the right pulmonary artery and its distal portion in the middle lobe pulmonary artery.

PULMONARY VESSELS

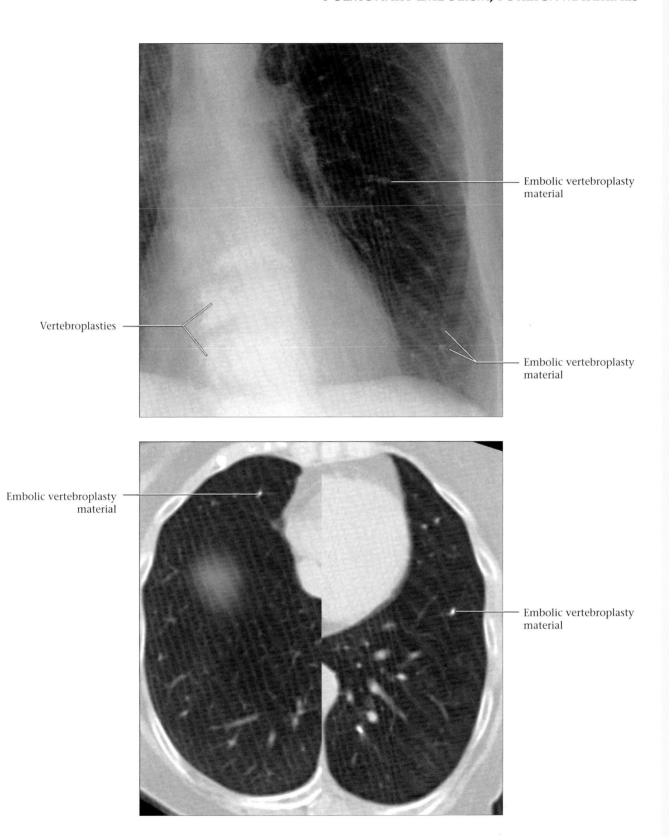

Embolic vertebroplasty material

Vertebroplasties

Embolic vertebroplasty material

Embolic vertebroplasty material

Embolic vertebroplasty material

(Top) First of two images of a 77 year old woman with metastatic breast cancer and prior multifocal thoracic vertebroplasty. PA chest radiograph coned-down to the left lung demonstrates multiple linear branching high density lesions in the bilateral lungs that follow the course of the peripheral pulmonary arteries. (Bottom) Composite of contrast-enhanced abdominal CT images through the lung bases (lung window) demonstrates endovascular vertebroplasty material manifesting as foci of high attenuation that fill the lumens of distal pulmonary arteries. Embolization of vertebroplasty material during the procedure resulted in high density foreign material lodged in the lumens of various peripheral pulmonary arteries.

PLEURA

General Anatomy and Function

General anatomy
- Parietal pleura
- Visceral pleura
- Fissures
  - Interlobar fissures
    - Right major fissure
    - Minor fissure
    - Left major fissure
  - Accessory fissures
    - Azygos fissure
    - Left minor fissure
    - Superior accessory fissure
    - Inferior accessory fissure

Pleural Structure
- Continuous surface epithelium and underlying connective tissue
- **Visceral pleura** adheres to pulmonary surfaces
- **Parietal pleura** a continuation of visceral pleura; lines corresponding half·of thoracic wall, covers ipsilateral diaphragm and ipsilateral mediastinal surface
- Visceral and parietal pleurae form right and left **pleural cavities; potential spaces** containing a small amount of serous pleural fluid
- Combined thickness of visceral and parietal pleurae and fluid-containing pleural space is **< 0.5 mm**

Function
- **Visceral pleura** directly apposes and slides freely over **parietal pleura** during respiration
- During inspiration, muscles of respiration and diaphragm increase intrathoracic volume; create negative pressure within pleural space and lung
  - Resultant lung expansion causes reduction in intra-alveolar pressure; prompts conduction of air through upper respiratory tract and airways into alveoli

Pleural Space
- Potential space; normally contains 2-10 mL of fluid
- Fluid **production capacity, 100 mL/hr;** fluid **absorption capacity, 300 mL/hr**
- Fluid flux normally **from parietal pleura capillaries** to **pleural space;** absorbed by microscopic stomata in **parietal pleura**

Parietal Pleura

Nomenclature
- Covers nonparenchymal surfaces; forms lining of thoracic cavities
- **Costal** portion extends along ribs and intercostal spaces; **diaphragmatic** portion covers the diaphragm; **mediastinal** portion covers the mediastinum

Blood Supply and Drainage
- **Supply** from adjacent chest wall (intercostal, internal mammary, diaphragmatic arteries)
- **Drainage** to bronchial veins (diaphragmatic pleural drainage to inferior vena cava and brachiocephalic trunk)

Innervation
- **Intercostal nerves** (costal and peripheral diaphragmatic pleura) and **phrenic nerves** (mediastinal and central diaphragmatic pleura)
- Irritation of costal or peripheral diaphragmatic pleura **refers pain along intercostal nerves to thoracic or abdominal wall**
- Irritation of mediastinal or central diaphragmatic pleura **refers pain to lower neck and shoulder**

Histology
- Single layer of parietal **mesothelial cells** over **loose, fat-containing areolar connective tissue;** bounded externally by endothoracic fascia

Visceral Pleura

Layers
- **Mesothelial layer, thin connective tissue layer, chief layer of connective tissue, vascular layer, limiting lung membrane** (connected to chief layer by collagen and elastic fibers)
  - Histology reveals single layer of flat mesothelial cells separated by basal lamina from underlying lamina propria of loose connective tissue

Blood Supply and Drainage
- Supply by **systemic bronchial vessels**, drainage by **pulmonary and bronchial veins**
- Lymphatic drainage to deep pulmonary plexus within interlobar and peribronchial spaces toward hilum

Innervation
- Visceral afferent nerves traveling along bronchial vessels; lacks pain fibers

Pleural Reflections

Pulmonary Ligament
- Formed by mediastinal pleura extending inferiorly, as a double layer, below the hilum (see "Hila" section)

Costodiaphragmatic Recesses
- Pleura extends caudally beyond inferior lung border
- Costal and diaphragmatic pleura separated by narrow slit, the costodiaphragmatic recess
- Extends approximately 5 cm below inferior border of the lung during quiet inspiration; caudal extent at 12th rib posteromedially

Interlobar Fissures

General Concepts
- **Complete fissures** extend from the lung surface to the hilum
- **Incomplete fissures** fail to extend to the hilum; allow **parenchymal communication** and collateral air drift between adjacent lobes
  - Frequency **12.5-73% (major fissures); 60-90% (minor fissure); more frequent on right than left**

PLEURA

Major (Oblique) Fissures

- Originate posteriorly, near level of T5 vertebral body; left major fissure originates near T4 in 75% of individuals
- Terminate along anterior diaphragmatic pleural surface, 3-4 cm posterior to anterior chest wall
- **Right major fissure** separates **right upper lobe** and **middle lobe** from **right lower lobe**
- **Left major fissure** separates **left upper lobe** from **left lower lobe**
- Change in contour from **upper portion (concave anterior aspect)** to **lower portion (convex anterior aspect)**; termed propeller-like morphology

Minor (Horizontal) Fissure

- Separates superior aspect of **middle lobe** from **right upper lobe; incomplete in > 80% of individuals**

Accessory Fissures

General Concepts

- Clefts of varying depth in outer surface of lung; occur in **22-32% of individuals**

Azygos Fissure

- **Right-sided**; results from failure of normal migration of azygos vein to tracheobronchial angle
- Invaginated visceral and parietal pleura form fissure (**four layers of pleura**) in medial aspect of right lung apex (see "Lungs" section)

Left Minor Fissure

- Separates **lingula** from remainder of **left upper lobe**; frequency of **8-18%** but rarely detected on PA chest radiography (frequency of 1.6%)

Superior Accessory Fissure

- Separates **superior segment of lower lobe** from **basal segments**; horizontal or oblique in orientation

Inferior Accessory Fissure

- Incompletely separates **medial basal segment** from **rest of basal segments of lower lobe; right more common than left**
- Frequency of **5-10% on chest radiographs, 16-21% of chest CT studies, and 30-50% of anatomic specimens**

Imaging

Radiography

- **Major fissures**
  - Not normally seen on PA chest radiographs
  - Portions of major fissures typically visible on lateral chest radiographs; identified by continuity with respective hemidiaphragm
- **Minor fissure**
  - Visible in **50-80% of PA chest radiographs** as a horizontal linear opacity at or near anterior 4th rib; variable contour
  - Contacts lateral chest wall near axillary portion of right 6th rib; ends medially at interlobar pulmonary artery; never crosses hilar vessels
  - Curves gently downward in anterior and lateral portions
- **Azygos fissure**
  - Thin, curvilinear opacity coursing from right lung apex toward hilum; characteristic **tear-drop configuration of inferior end (azygos vein)**
- **Left minor fissure**
  - Thin linear opacity, **more cephalad and oblique than minor fissure**
- **Superior accessory fissure**
  - Projected below and medial to minor fissure on PA chest radiograph
- **Inferior accessory fissure**
  - Thin linear opacity extending obliquely from medial hemidiaphragm toward hilum on PA chest radiograph; occasionally seen on lateral chest radiograph

CT

- Normal pleura not imaged by CT/HRCT
- **Intercostal stripe**
  - Thin, linear opacity (1-2 mm thick) in normal individuals; overlies intercostal spaces; connects inner aspects of ribs
  - Produced by two layers of pleura, extrapleural fat, endothoracic fascia, and innermost intercostal muscle (see "**Chest Wall**" section)
  - Disappears on inner aspect of ribs (innermost intercostal muscle absent); may be mimicked by intercostal veins in paravertebral region
- **Major fissures**
  - Thin linear opacities; curvilinear in upper and lower thorax (concave and convex anterior aspects, respectively); may appear as thin bands of ground-glass opacity when oblique to axial plane
- **Minor fissure**
  - Variable appearance; thin, curvilinear opacity; ground-glass opacity; area devoid of vessels (roughly triangular)

Ultrasound

- Differentiation of solid pleural masses from fluid; assessment of echogenicity and morphology (may change shape with respiration) of fluid collections, visualization of echogenic line of visceral pleura
- Anechoic effusions usually transudative (see below); echoic effusions with septations typically exudative (see below)

Imaging Anatomic Correlations

Pleural Effusion

- Categorized as **transudates** or **exudates**; based on composition of fluid obtained by thoracentesis; determined by **Light's criteria**
  - **Transudates** not associated with pleural disease; **systemic abnormalities** (cardiac failure, pericardial disease, cirrhosis, pregnancy, hypoalbuminemia, overhydration, renal failure)

PLEURA

- **Exudates** indicate presence of **pleural disease** (pneumonia, empyema, tuberculosis, neoplasm, pulmonary embolism, collagen vascular disease)
- **Radiography**
  - Blunt costophrenic angle (focal opacification, meniscus-shaped upper border)
    - PA detection of at least **200 mL in lateral costophrenic angle**; lateral detection of at least **75 mL in posterior costophrenic angle**
    - Lateral decubitus radiograph detection of > 10 mL
  - Small to moderate effusions manifest as opacities with meniscus-shaped upper borders; lateral aspect more cephalad than medial portion; **obscure diaphragm if > 500 mL**; large effusions may opacify hemithorax, displace mediastinum, invert diaphragm
  - **Supine radiography:** Increased density of affected hemithorax, veil-like opacity, apical cap, thickening of paravertebral stripe
  - **Subpulmonic effusion:** Accumulation of fluid in subpulmonic pleural space
    - Lateral displacement of dome or peak of pseudodiaphragm on PA radiograph
    - Flattening, elevation of undersurface of posterior lung on lateral radiograph; flattening of inferior lung contour anterior to major fissure; sharp fissural downward angulation (resembles profile of **Rock of Gibraltar**)
    - Left subpulmonic effusion > 2 cm distance between lung base and superior border of gastric air bubble
  - **Pseudotumor**
    - **Interlobar pleural fluid**; most associated with **cardiac decompensation**; typical after treatment of heart failure; spontaneous resolution
    - Focal elliptical/lenticular opacity within interlobar fissure; **minor fissure most commonly affected**
    - Peripheral margins of opacity typically taper as they merge with affected fissure
  - **Loculation** associated with exudative pleural effusion; limited by pleural adhesions
    - Fixed, non-mobile mass-like opacity; typically elliptical or lenticular
    - Typically sharply defined on chest radiographs when surface is tangential (parallel) to X-ray beam; ill-defined when imaged en face
  - **Empyema**
    - **Infected pleural effusion**; association with pneumonia; loculation (see above)
    - Air-fluid levels within loculated effusion suggest **empyema** with **bronchopleural fistula**
- **CT**
  - Not useful for distinguishing transudate from exudate; most effusions near water attenuation on CT (20-30 HU) regardless of cause; range from 0 HU to 100 HU
  - Small effusions initially in posterior costodiaphragmatic recess; maintain concave/meniscoid anterior margin
  - Large effusions track anteriorly and cephalad; may extend into fissures

- **Empyema**: Elliptical or lenticular fluid collection; often bounded by smooth, uniform thick visceral and parietal pleurae ("**split pleura**" sign)
  - Thick pleura may enhance with contrast; air-fluid levels within pleural effusion suggest **bronchopleural fistula**
  - Nondependent location, sharp demarcation from adjacent lung, compression/displacement of adjacent lung and vessels
- **Ultrasound**
  - **Anechoic effusions** may be **transudative** or **exudative**
  - **Septations** suggestive exudative effusion

Pneumothorax
- Air or gas within pleural space; spontaneous (associated with blebs, bullae); primary (no underlying lung disease) or secondary (underlying lung disease)
- Radiographic features vary with degree of volume loss, presence of tension (pleural pressure exceeds alveolar pressure), and patient position
- Thin linear opacity represents outer margin of visceral pleura; separated from parietal pleura and chest wall by lucent space devoid of pulmonary vessels; findings at lung apex in upright patient
- Lucency extending into costodiaphragmatic sulcus in supine patients (**deep sulcus sign**)

Pleural Thickening
- Focal thickening
  - **Pleural plaques** occur **15-20 years after asbestos exposure**; focal collections of acellular collagen on parietal pleura (costal, diaphragmatic and mediastinal pleura)
    - Imaging, discontinuous areas of pleural thickening, predominantly along 6th-8th ribs, on parietal pleura at domes of diaphragms, along mediastinal pleura; spare apices and costophrenic sulci; non-calcified or calcified
  - **Localized fibrous tumor**, solitary lenticular, round, or lobulated neoplasm; benign (80%) or malignant
  - **Bronchogenic carcinoma** may focally invade pleura or produce diffuse pleural thickening
- Diffuse thickening may be benign (fibrothorax) or malignant (metastases, mesothelioma, lymphoma, invasive thymoma)

Pleural Calcification
- Focal (pleural plaques) or diffuse (fibrothorax, healed hemothorax)

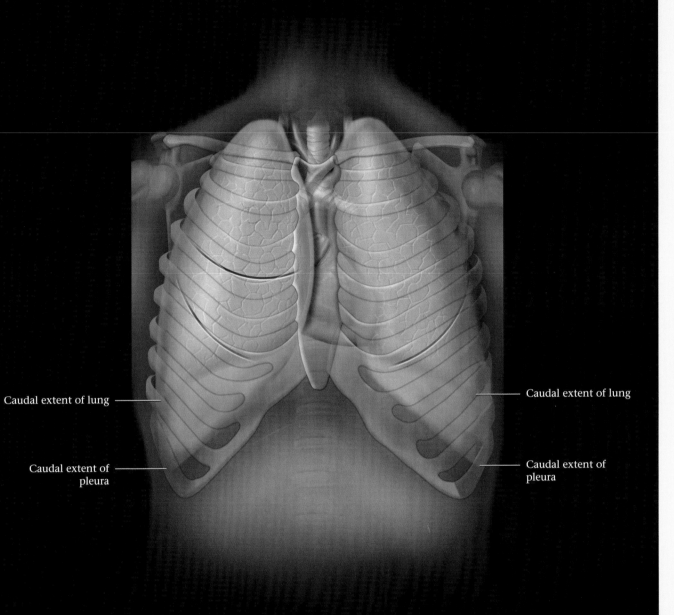

Caudal extent of lung

Caudal extent of lung

Caudal extent of pleura

Caudal extent of pleura

Graphic shows the anatomy of the pleura. The visceral pleura covers the pulmonary surfaces. The parietal pleura covers the non-pulmonary surfaces within the thoracic cavity and extends more caudally than the lungs. The inferior reflection of parietal pleura extends within the costophrenic sulci to the level of the upper kidneys.

PLEURA

CORONAL SECTION, ANATOMY OF PLEURAL REFLECTIONS

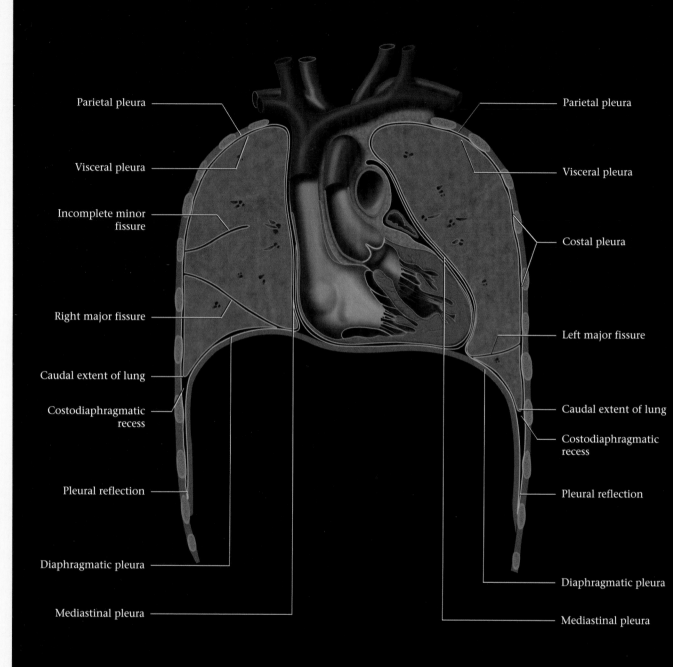

Parietal pleura

Visceral pleura

Incomplete minor fissure

Right major fissure

Caudal extent of lung

Costodiaphragmatic recess

Pleural reflection

Diaphragmatic pleura

Mediastinal pleura

Parietal pleura

Visceral pleura

Costal pleura

Left major fissure

Caudal extent of lung

Costodiaphragmatic recess

Pleural reflection

Diaphragmatic pleura

Mediastinal pleura

Graphic shows the extensive distribution of the pleura as visualized in the coronal plane. Visceral pleura covers the surfaces of both lungs and forms interlobar fissures that may be complete or incomplete in their extension to the hila. Parietal pleura lines both thoracic cavities and may be designated by its location as costal, diaphragmatic or mediastinal pleurae. Inferiorly, the parietal pleura extends deeply into the costodiaphragmatic recesses where costal and diaphragmatic pleura are in apposition.

PLEURA

SAGITTAL SECTION, ANATOMY OF PLEURAL REFLECTIONS

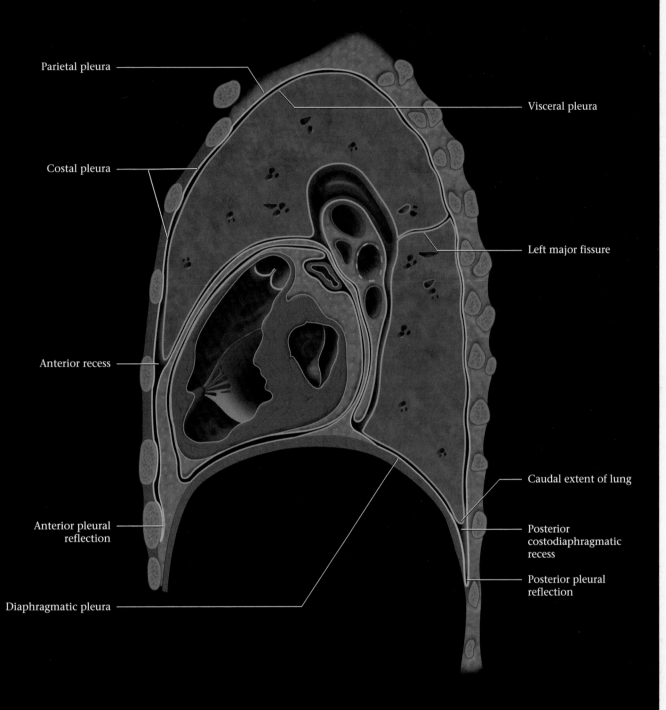

Parietal pleura

Visceral pleura

Costal pleura

Left major fissure

Anterior recess

Anterior pleural
reflection

Caudal extent of lung

Posterior
costodiaphragmatic
recess

Posterior pleural
reflection

Diaphragmatic pleura

Graphic shows the extent of parietal and visceral pleura as visualized in the sagittal plane in the left mid-clavicular zone. The posterior pleural reflection in the costodiaphragmatic recess extends caudally to the level of the 12th rib.

PLEURA

ANATOMY OF PLEURAL FISSURES

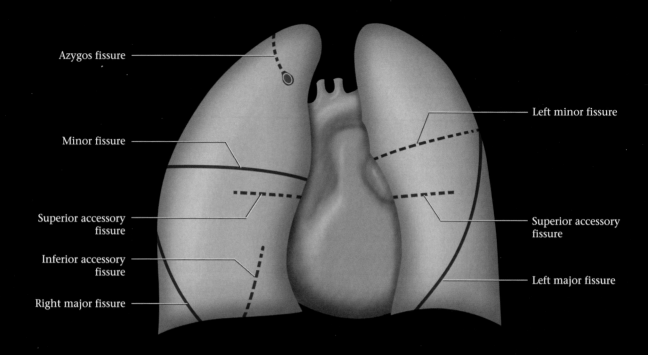

Azygos fissure

Minor fissure

Superior accessory fissure

Inferior accessory fissure

Right major fissure

Left minor fissure

Superior accessory fissure

Left major fissure

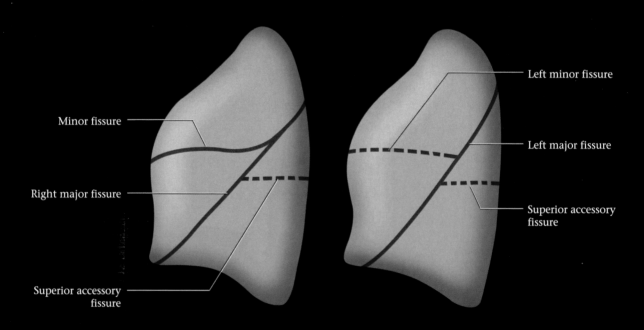

Minor fissure

Right major fissure

Superior accessory fissure

Left minor fissure

Left major fissure

Superior accessory fissure

(Top) Graphic shows standard interlobar fissures as solid lines and the most common accessory fissures as dashed lines. (Bottom) The minor fissure is typically slightly convex superiorly and its anterior aspect courses inferiorly.

PLEURA

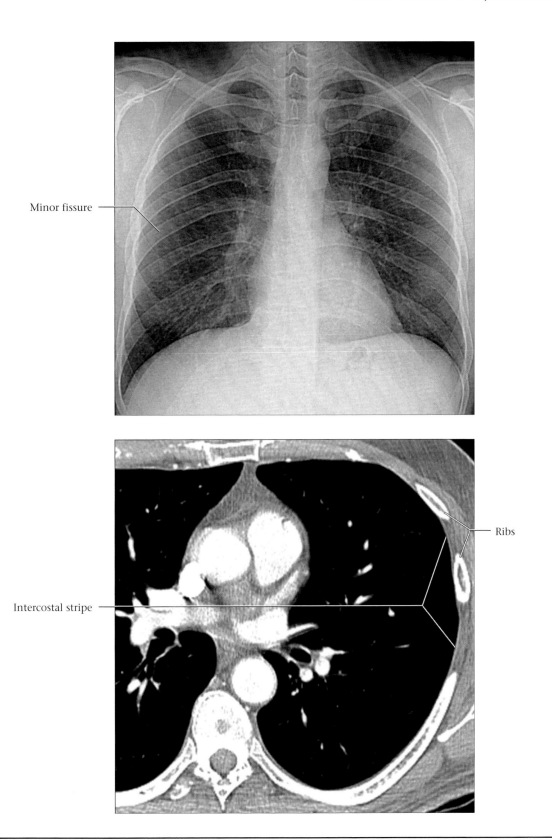

Minor fissure

Ribs

Intercostal stripe

(Top) Normal PA chest radiograph shows a subtle thin, curvilinear opacity overlying the posterolateral aspect of the right 7th rib representing the normal minor fissure. The major fissures are not visualized. **(Bottom)** Contrast-enhanced chest CT (mediastinal window) shows the intercostal stripe manifesting as a thin, linear opacity (1-2 mm) along the inner margin of the intercostal spaces. The stripe appears to connect the inner aspects of the ribs and is produced by two layers of pleura, extrapleural fat, endothoracic fascia, and innermost intercostal muscle. The stripe is not shown on the inner aspect of the ribs because the innermost intercostal muscle is absent at that location. The stripe becomes more apparent in the paravertebral region, particularly in obese individuals.

PLEURA

RADIOGRAPHY, STANDARD FISSURES

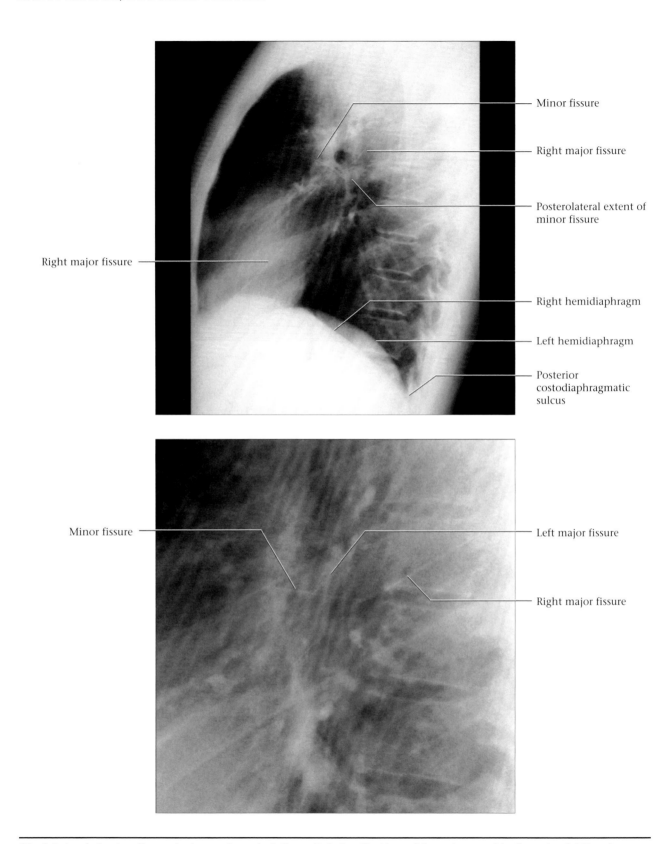

(Top) Lateral chest radiograph shows characteristic partial visualization of the minor and both major (oblique) fissures on this projection. The posterior aspect of the minor fissure curves inferiorly and intersects the right major fissure. **(Bottom)** Lateral chest radiograph coned-down to the hila shows the minor fissure extending posteriorly to its intersection with the right major fissure. The left major fissure (shown anterior to that intersection) usually courses more steeply than the right major fissure and originates posteriorly at the level of the 4th thoracic vertebral body. The right major fissure typically originates at the level of the 5th thoracic vertebral body.

CT, STANDARD FISSURES

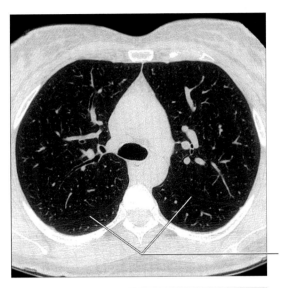

Upper major fissures, concave anteriorly

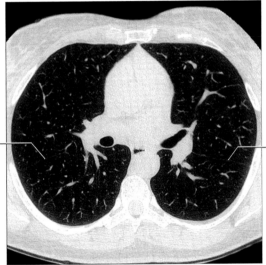

Mid portion of right major fissure

Mid portion of left major fissure

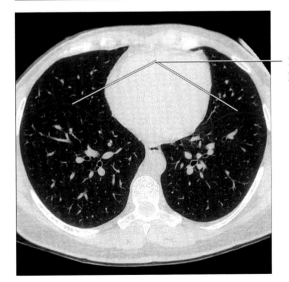

Lower major fissures, concave posteriorly

(Top) First of three axial chest CT images (lung window) demonstrates the right and left major fissures in the upper thorax manifesting as thin curvilinear structures with concave anterior aspects. **(Middle)** In their mid-portions, near the hilar levels, both major fissures are nearly straight in configuration. **(Bottom)** In the lower thorax, the contour of the major fissures has changed and the anterior aspects of both major fissures are convex. This shift in configuration along the vertical axis of the major fissure has been described as a "propeller-like" morphology. Alterations of this normal shift in configuration may occur with atelectasis.

PLEURA

RADIOGRAPHY, MINOR FISSURE

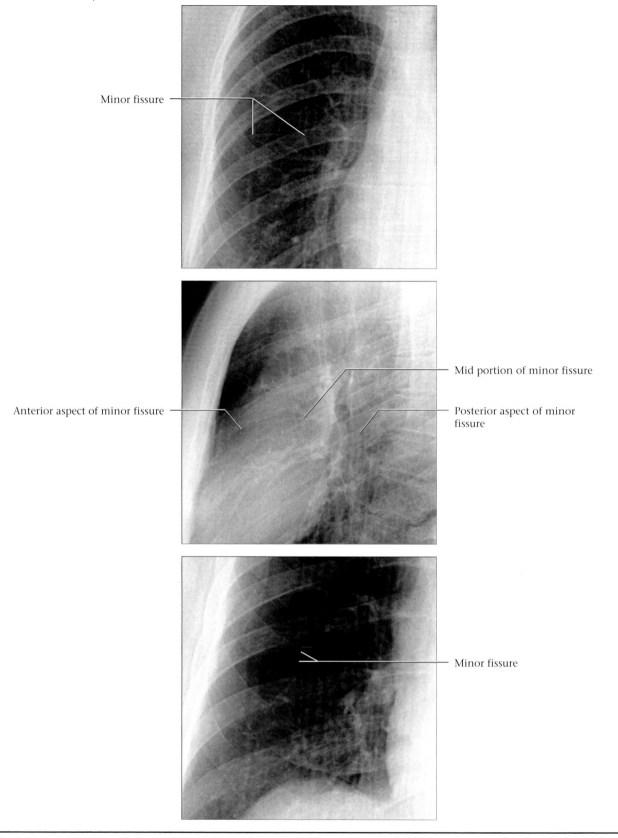

Minor fissure

Anterior aspect of minor fissure

Mid portion of minor fissure

Posterior aspect of minor fissure

Minor fissure

(Top) First of three coned-down chest radiographs showing the anatomy of the minor fissure. On the PA chest radiograph the fissure manifests as a thin linear opacity extending across the mid-right hemithorax, originating near the axillary portion of right 6th rib and ending medially at the interlobar artery. Note that the linear opacity never crosses hilar vessels. (Middle) On the lateral view, the anterior and posterior portions of the minor fissure curve gently downward in characteristic fashion. (Bottom) PA chest radiograph shows the fissure manifesting as two adjacent and roughly parallel linear opacities. Because of its curving configuration, the minor fissure often manifests as a double-line on frontal radiographs, produced by the X-ray beam encountering tangential components of the fissure at two locations along its course.

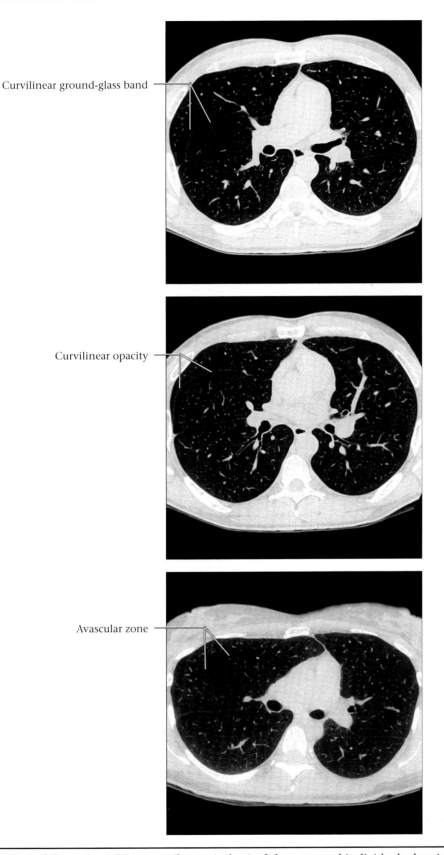

Curvilinear ground-glass band

Curvilinear opacity

Avascular zone

(Top) First of three chest CT images (lung window) of three normal individuals showing the variable appearance of the minor fissure on axial CT sections. In this example, the fissure manifests as a curvilinear band of ground-glass opacity. **(Middle)** The minor fissure may also manifest as a discrete curvilinear opacity. Note the incomplete minor fissure that allows parenchymal communication and collateral air drift between the right upper and middle lobes. **(Bottom)** In many individuals, the minor fissure may manifest as a zone of relative avascularity that is often roughly triangular in morphology.

PLEURA

CORONAL CT, STANDARD FISSURES

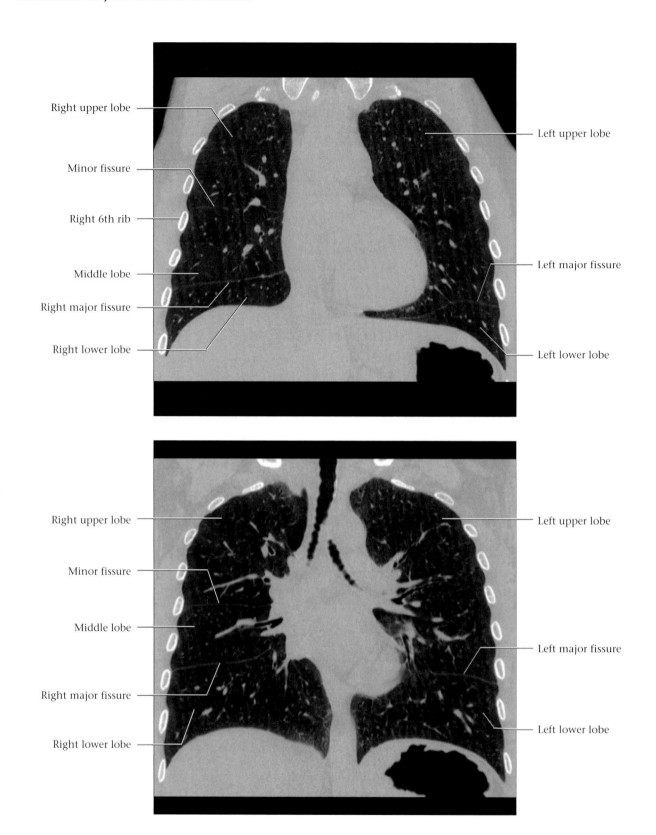

Right upper lobe

Minor fissure

Right 6th rib

Middle lobe

Right major fissure

Right lower lobe

Left upper lobe

Left major fissure

Left lower lobe

Right upper lobe

Minor fissure

Middle lobe

Right major fissure

Right lower lobe

Left upper lobe

Left major fissure

Left lower lobe

(Top) First of four coronal chest CT images (lung window) showing the normal coronal fissural anatomy. In this most anterior section, the minor fissure is seen originating near the axillary portion of right 6th rib. The major fissures are slightly oblique in orientation. (Bottom) At the hilar level, the minor fissure terminates medially at the right interlobar artery and separates the right upper lobe from the middle lobe. The right major fissure separates the right lower from the right upper and middle lobes; the left major fissure separates the left upper and left lower lobes.

PLEURA

CORONAL CT, STANDARD FISSURES

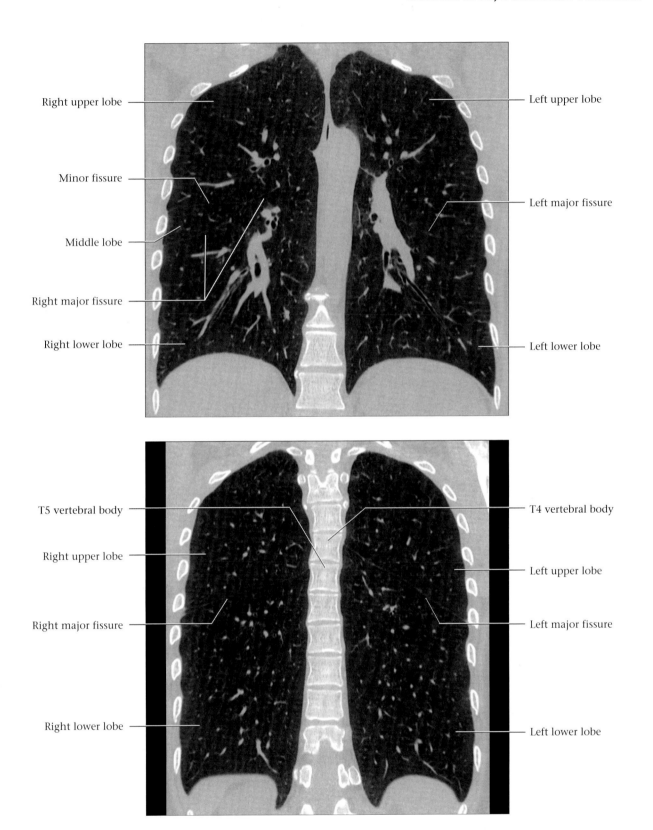

Right upper lobe

Minor fissure

Middle lobe

Right major fissure

Right lower lobe

Left upper lobe

Left major fissure

Left lower lobe

T5 vertebral body

Right upper lobe

Right major fissure

Right lower lobe

T4 vertebral body

Left upper lobe

Left major fissure

Left lower lobe

(Top) In the coronal plane of the aorta, the medial aspect of the minor fissure intersects the major fissure posterolateral to the right hilum. **(Bottom)** The right major fissure originates posteriorly at the level of the T5 vertebral body; the left major fissure originates at the level of the T4 vertebral body. The middle lobe is no longer visualized in this posterior coronal plane.

PLEURA

ANATOMY, CT & RADIOGRAPHY, INCOMPLETE FISSURES

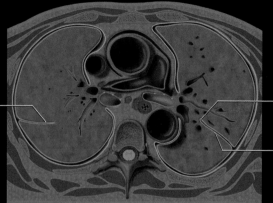

Incomplete right major fissure

Visceral pleural reflection forms incomplete fissure

Incomplete left major fissure

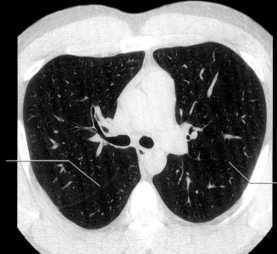

Incomplete right major fissure

Complete left major fissure

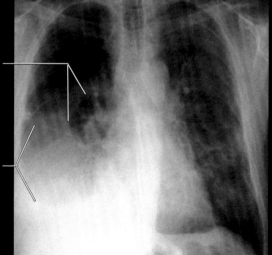

Incomplete fissure manifests as sharp interface

Moderate-sized pleural effusion

(Top) Graphic shows bilateral incomplete major fissures that extend inward from the lung surface but fail to reach the hila. Visceral pleura reflects upon itself at the medial termination of each incomplete fissure. **(Middle)** Axial HRCT (lung window) shows an incomplete right major fissure and a complete left major fissure. The incomplete fissures allow parenchymal communication between the right upper and right lower lobes. **(Bottom)** PA chest radiograph shows an incomplete right major fissure. A moderate sized pleural effusion extends into the right major fissure and produces a sharp interface where the visceral pleura reflects upon itself to form the medial termination of the incomplete fissure.

PLEURA

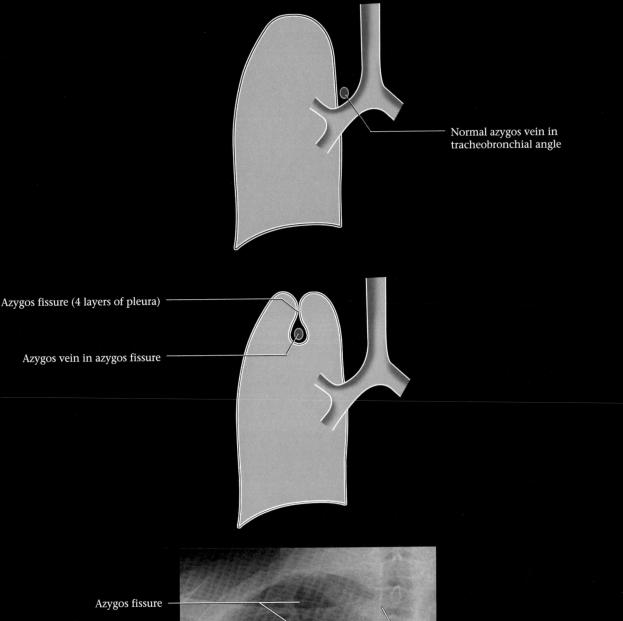

Normal azygos vein in tracheobronchial angle

Azygos fissure (4 layers of pleura)

Azygos vein in azygos fissure

Azygos fissure

Right paratracheal stripe

Azygos vein terminates azygos fissure (tear-drop)

(Top) First of two graphics shows the result of normal migration of the primitive posterior cardinal vein to the tracheobronchial angle to form the azygos vein. **(Middle)** Early migration of azygos vein coursing inferiorly from the lung apex results in formation of an azygos fissure, composed of four layers of pleura. **(Bottom)** PA chest radiograph coned-down to the right upper lung shows an azygos fissure manifesting as a curvilinear opacity extending inferomedially from the right lung apex. The teardrop-shaped opacity at the inferior aspect of the fissure represents the azygos vein. Lung parenchyma medial to the fissure ("azygos lobe") shares communication and collateral drift with adjacent parenchyma in the right upper lobe.

PLEURA

RADIOGRAPHY & CT, INFERIOR ACCESSORY FISSURES

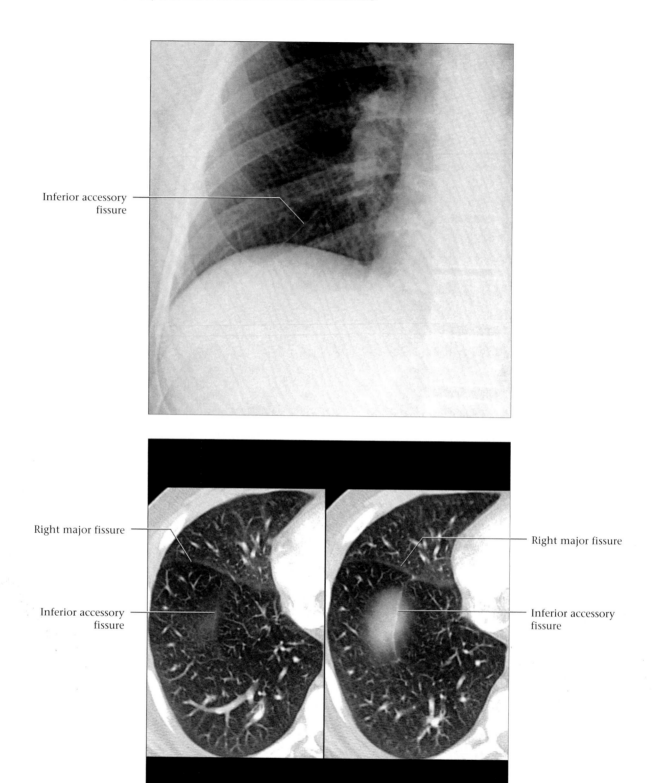

Inferior accessory fissure

Right major fissure

Inferior accessory fissure

Right major fissure

Inferior accessory fissure

(Top) PA chest radiograph coned-down to the right lower hemithorax shows an inferior accessory fissure manifesting as a thin linear opacity extending obliquely from the medial aspect of the hemidiaphragm toward the hilum.
(Bottom) Composite of two adjacent chest CT images (lung window) of the right lung base demonstrates an inferior accessory fissure manifesting as a gently curving linear opacity separating the medial basal segment from the remainder of the basal segments of the right lower lobe.

PLEURA

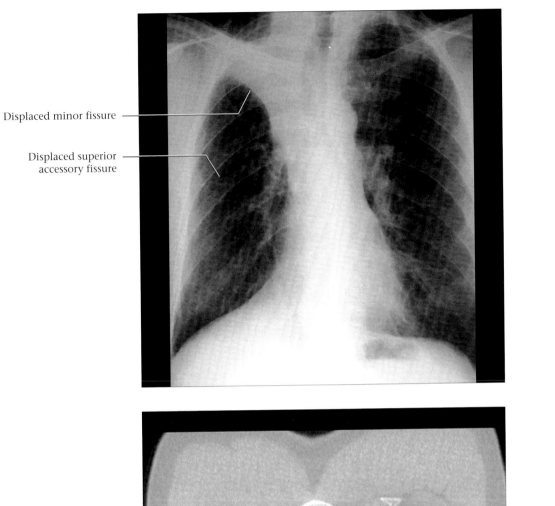

Displaced minor fissure —

Displaced superior accessory fissure —

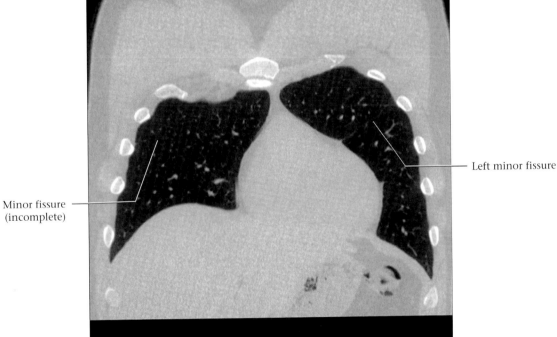

Minor fissure (incomplete) —

— Left minor fissure

(Top) PA chest radiograph shows right upper lobe atelectasis resulting from a central obstructing squamous cell carcinoma. The minor fissure manifests as a sharp interface between the airless right upper lobe superiorly and the aerated lung inferiorly. The superior accessory fissure is displaced superolaterally and mimics the normal appearance of a non-displaced minor fissure. The right hemidiaphragm is elevated, an indirect sign of right upper lobe atelectasis. (Bottom) Coronal HRCT (lung window) shows an incomplete minor fissure on the right and a left minor fissure. The left minor fissure separates the lingula from the remainder of the left upper lobe.

PLEURA

RADIOGRAPHY & CT, PNEUMOTHORAX

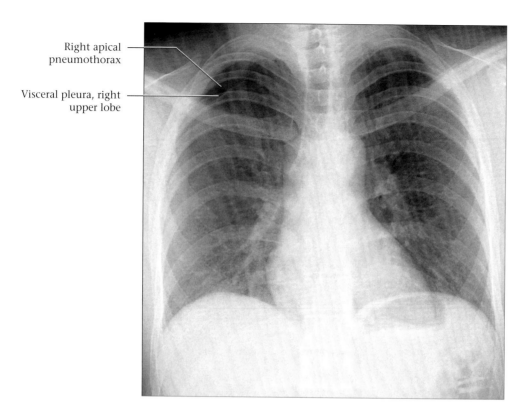

Right apical pneumothorax

Visceral pleura, right upper lobe

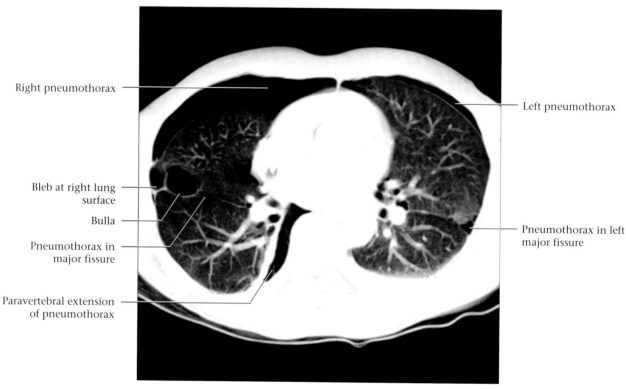

Right pneumothorax

Left pneumothorax

Bleb at right lung surface

Bulla

Pneumothorax in major fissure

Pneumothorax in left major fissure

Paravertebral extension of pneumothorax

(Top) PA chest radiograph shows air in the right apical pleural space (pneumothorax) manifesting as abnormal lucency peripheral to the visceral pleural surface of the right upper lobe. **(Bottom)** Chest CT (lung window) shows bilateral pneumothoraces following trauma, manifesting as abnormal air attenuation within the bilateral pleural spaces. The right pneumothorax extends into the right major fissure and along the paravertebral pleural space. A superficial bleb and adjacent bulla are also demonstrated. The left pneumothorax extends into the lateral aspect of the left major fissure and along the anterior pleural space.

PLEURA

AZYGOS FISSURE, PNEUMOTHORAX & PLEURAL EFFUSION

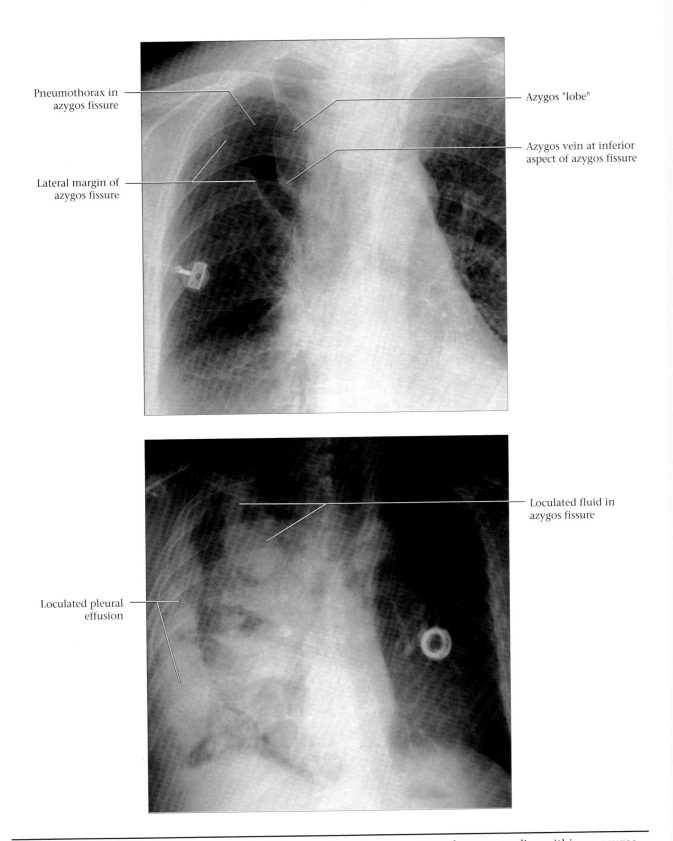

Pneumothorax in azygos fissure

Lateral margin of azygos fissure

Azygos "lobe"

Azygos vein at inferior aspect of azygos fissure

Loculated fluid in azygos fissure

Loculated pleural effusion

(Top) PA chest radiograph coned-down to the right upper lung shows a pneumothorax extending within an azygos fissure and separating the medial and lateral portions of the fissure. (Bottom) PA chest radiograph of a patient with malignant pleural effusion shows a loculated pleural effusion along the lateral right hemithorax and within an azygos fissure. The expanded fissure roughly maintains its characteristic configuration with a tear-drop morphology of its inferior termination.

PLEURA

RADIOGRAPHY, PLEURAL EFFUSION

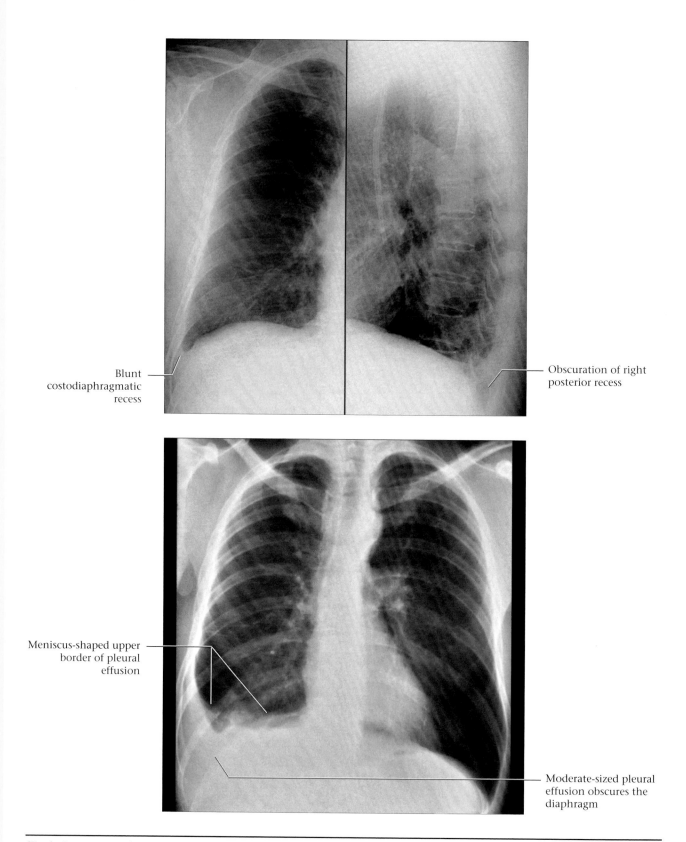

Blunt costodiaphragmatic recess

Obscuration of right posterior recess

Meniscus-shaped upper border of pleural effusion

Moderate-sized pleural effusion obscures the diaphragm

(Top) Composite of PA and lateral radiographs shows a small right pleural effusion manifesting on the PA radiograph as blunting of the right costodiaphragmatic recess. On the lateral radiograph the effusion manifests as hazy opacity obscuring the right posterior costodiaphragmatic recess. **(Bottom)** PA chest radiograph of a 57-year old man with right lower lobe pneumonia shows a small-to-moderate pleural effusion manifesting as a dense opacity with a meniscus-shaped upper border that obscures the right diaphragm (> 500 mL). The lateral aspect of the opacity is more cephalad than its medial portion.

PLEURA

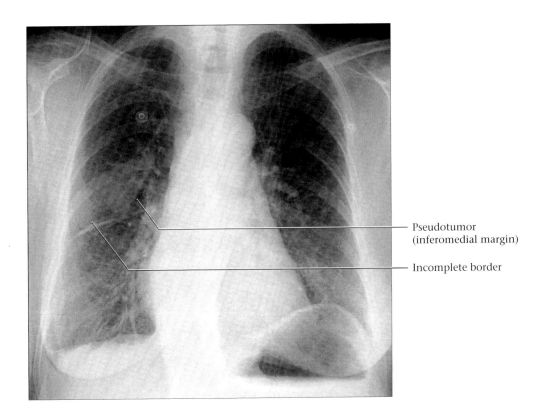

Pseudotumor
(inferomedial margin)

Incomplete border

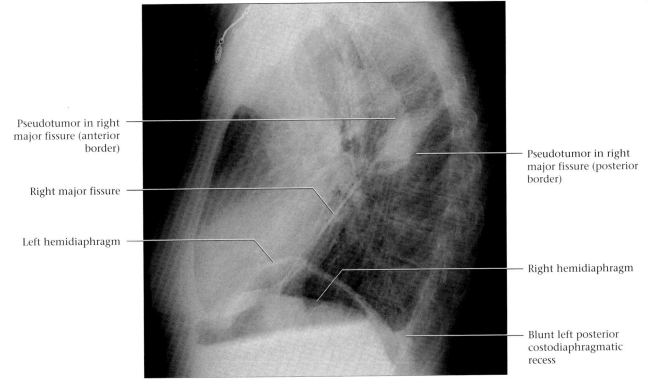

Pseudotumor in right
major fissure (anterior
border)

Right major fissure

Left hemidiaphragm

Pseudotumor in right
major fissure (posterior
border)

Right hemidiaphragm

Blunt left posterior
costodiaphragmatic
recess

(Top) First of two chest radiographs of a patient recently treated for heart failure. PA chest radiograph shows a focal opacity in the right mid-hemithorax that has both well-defined and ill-defined (incomplete) borders, suggesting an extraparenchymal lesion. **(Bottom)** Lateral radiograph shows the lenticular shape of the same opacity. The anterior and posterior borders of the opacity taper and form obtuse margins as they merge with the involved right major fissure. Following further diuresis and treatment of the patient's underlying cardiac failure, the opacity ("pseudotumor") resolved completely.

PLEURA

RADIOGRAPHY & CT, PLEURAL EFFUSION

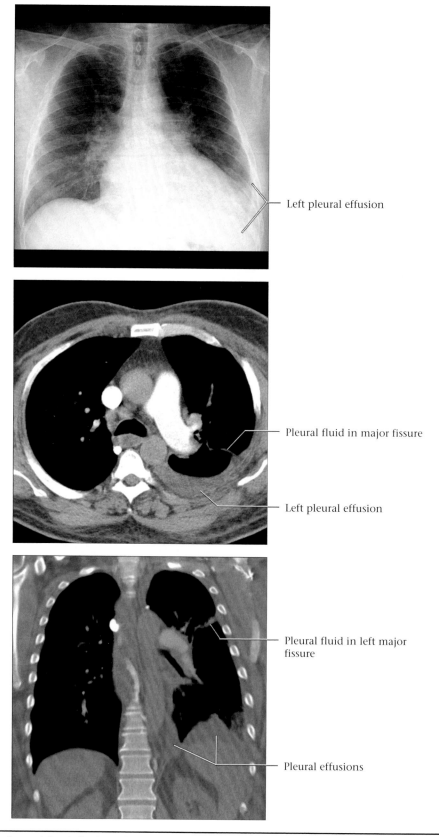

Left pleural effusion

Pleural fluid in major fissure

Left pleural effusion

Pleural fluid in left major fissure

Pleural effusions

(Top) First of three images of a patient with a left pleural effusion. PA chest radiograph shows a small-to-moderate left pleural effusion manifesting as a hazy opacity that obscures the ipsilateral diaphragm. (Middle) Axial contrast-enhanced chest CT (mediastinal window) shows that the effusion layers posteriorly in the dependent aspect of the left pleural space. The fluid collection has a concave/meniscoid anterior margin and extends into the adjacent major fissure. (Bottom) Coronal contrast-enhanced chest CT (mediastinal window) shows the left pleural effusion extending across the left hemidiaphragm and along the paravertebral pleural space. The effusion also extends into the major fissure superiorly.

PLEURA

RADIOGRAPHY & CT, LOCULATED PLEURAL EFFUSION

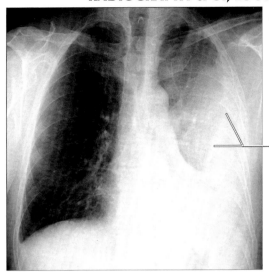

Well-defined margins of loculated pleural effusion

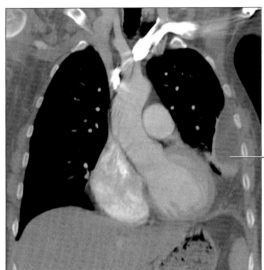

Loculated pleural effusion

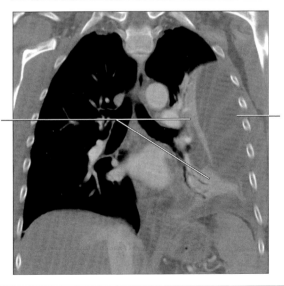

Relaxation atelectasis of left upper and left lower lobes

Loculated pleural effusion

(Top) First of three images of a patient with a loculated pleural effusion. PA chest radiograph shows a dense lenticular opacity extending along the lateral aspect of the left hemithorax. The opacity appeared fixed and nonmobile on lateral decubitus radiographs (not shown). (Middle) Coronal contrast-enhanced chest CT (mediastinal window; first of two images) shows the characteristic lenticular morphology of a loculated pleural effusion. (Bottom) Coronal contrast-enhanced chest CT (mediastinal window; last of two images) shows extension of the loculated fluid along the hemidiaphragm and relaxation atelectasis of the left upper and left lower lobes.

PLEURA

RADIOGRAPHY, CT & ULTRASOUND, EMPYEMA & BRONCHOPLEURAL FISTULA

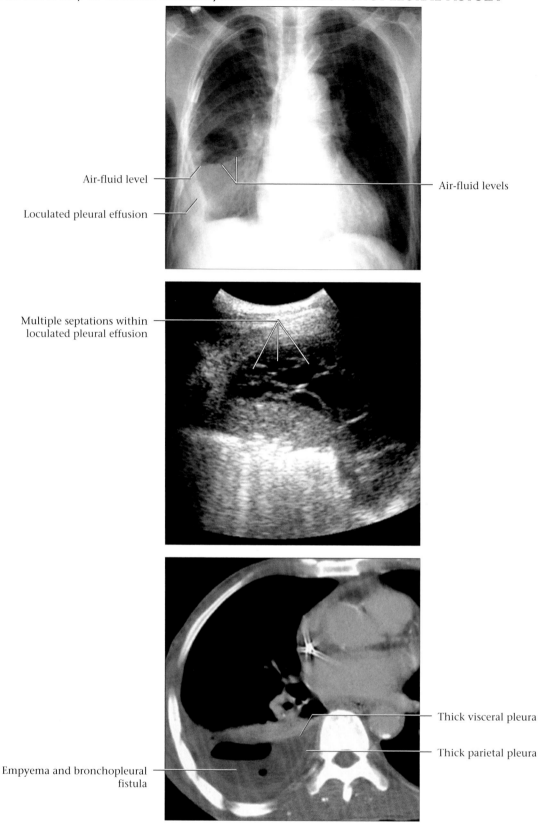

(Top) First of three images of a patient with right empyema and bronchopleural fistula. PA chest radiograph shows a loculated right pleural effusion with associated air-fluid levels indicating bronchopleural fistula. **(Middle)** Ultrasound reveals multiple septations within the loculated fluid collection suggesting an exudative pleural effusion. **(Bottom)** Unenhanced chest CT (mediastinal window) shows a loculated fluid collection in the posterior aspect of the right hemithorax. Small pockets of air within the fluid collection are consistent with a bronchopleural fistula and multiple internal septations. Thoracentesis confirmed empyema. Smoothly thickened parietal and visceral pleurae diverge to surround the empyema and form the "split pleura" sign.

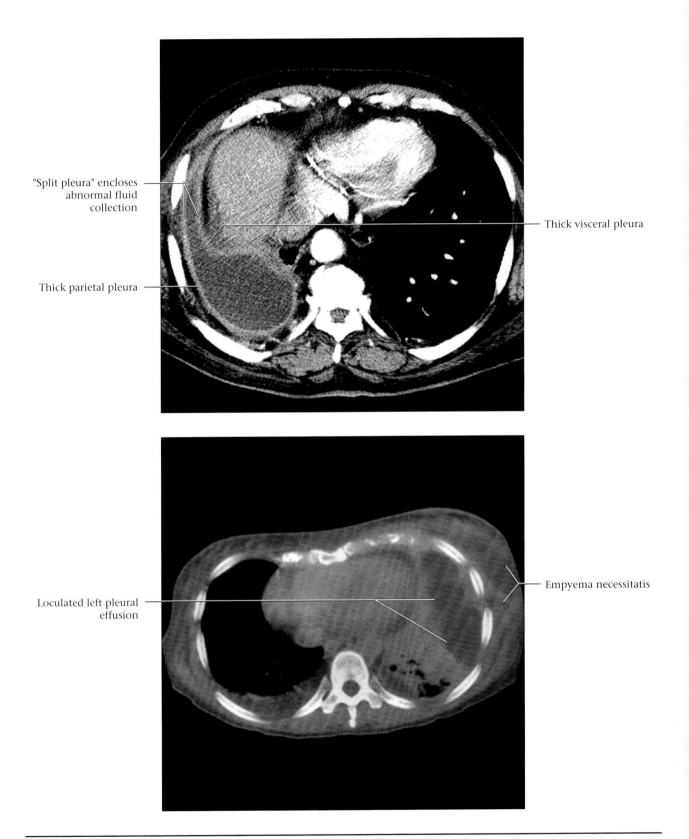

"Split pleura" encloses abnormal fluid collection

Thick visceral pleura

Thick parietal pleura

Loculated left pleural effusion

Empyema necessitatis

(Top) Contrast-enhanced chest CT (mediastinal window) of a 66 year old man with empyema demonstrates the "split pleura" sign associated with a loculated fluid collection in the posterolateral aspect of the right inferior pleural space. Enhancing smoothly thickened visceral and parietal pleurae "split" to enclose the abnormal fluid collection.
(Bottom) Chest CT (mediastinal window) of a 32 year old woman with empyema necessitatis shows a loculated left pleural effusion and pockets of fluid in the subcutaneous tissues of the adjacent chest wall.

PLEURA

RADIOGRAPHY, PLEURAL PLAQUES

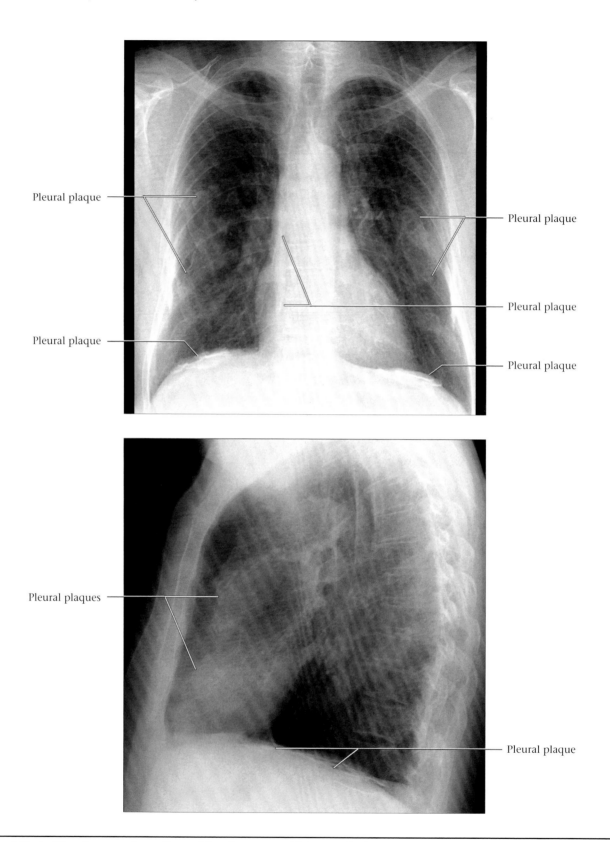

Pleural plaque

Pleural plaque

Pleural plaque

Pleural plaque

Pleural plaque

Pleural plaque

Pleural plaques

Pleural plaque

(Top) First of two images of a patient with a documented history of asbestos exposure twenty years prior to this radiographic examination. PA chest radiograph shows multiple ill-defined partially calcified plaque-like opacities overlying the 5th to 9th ribs and extending along the diaphragmatic pleurae. Some of the opacities appear to have incomplete borders. A dense vertical band of calcified pleural plaque is also shown extending along the right paravertebral region. **(Bottom)** Lateral chest radiograph demonstrates similar but less apparent opacities overlying the lungs and extending along the diaphragmatic pleurae.

PLEURA

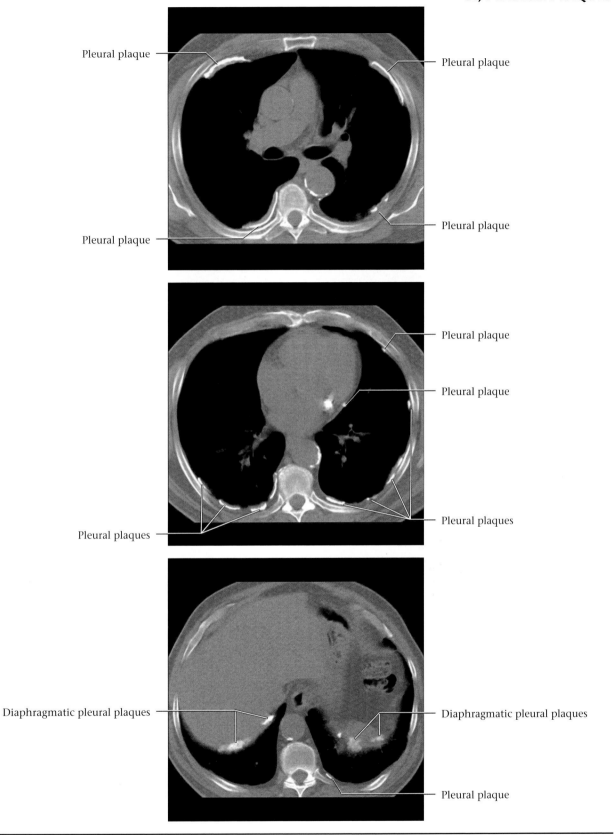

(Top) First of three axial chest CT images (mediastinal window) shows multifocal, discontinuous areas of plaque-like pleural thickening, some of which are partially calcified. Several plaques appear to extend along the inner aspect of the ribs manifesting as thickening of the costal parietal pleura. (Middle) Chest CT through the heart shows similar multifocal areas of pleural thickening that appear partially calcified and extend along the costal and mediastinal pleurae. (Bottom) Chest CT through the lung bases shows calcified pleural plaques along the diaphragmatic pleurae bilaterally.

PLEURA

RADIOGRAPHY & CT, PLEURAL THICKENING & CALCIFICATION

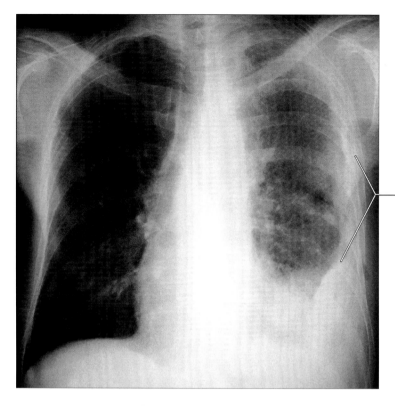

Pleural thickening and calcification

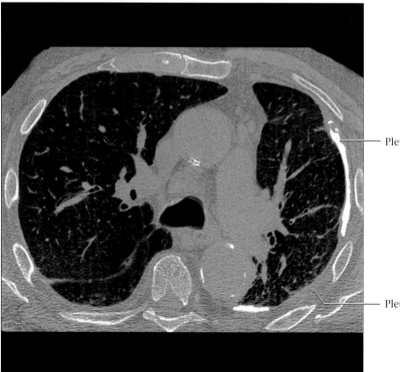

Pleural calcification

Pleural thickening

(Top) PA chest radiograph of a 64 year old man with a previous history of left empyema shows marked pleural thickening and calcification along the lower half of the left hemithorax. **(Bottom)** Chest CT (lung window) shows loss of volume in the left hemithorax and extensive pleural thickening and calcification extending along the lateral and posterior aspects of the hemithorax. The bands of pleural calcification are separated from the inner aspect of the adjacent ribs by a prominent band of pleural thickening, a distinguishing feature from calcified pleural plaques.

PLEURA

RADIOGRAPHY, FIBROTHORAX

Pleural calcification

Pleural calcification

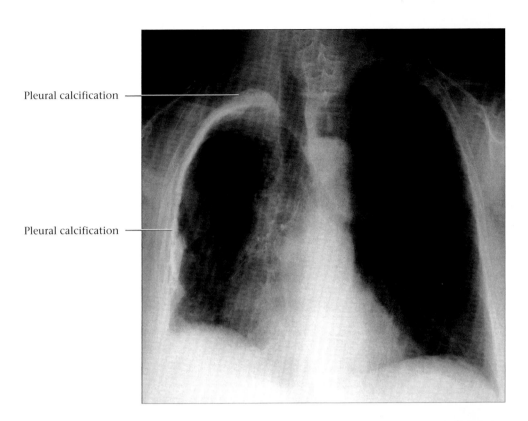

Pleural calcification

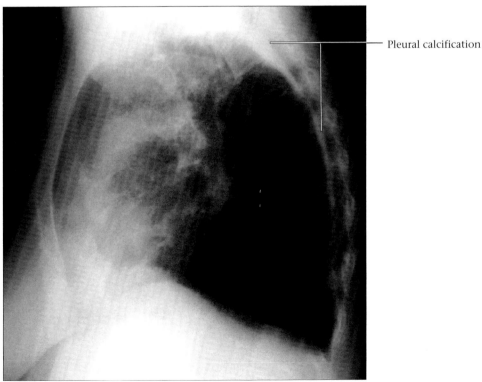

(Top) PA chest radiograph shows an extensive band of continuous pleural thickening and calcification extending along the right apical pleura and along the right lateral pleural surface. The mediastinal and diaphragmatic pleurae appear spared. **(Bottom)** Lateral chest radiograph shows the pleural thickening and calcification extending along the apical and posterior aspects of the left hemithorax.

PLEURA

MORPHOLOGY & CT, PLEURAL MASSES

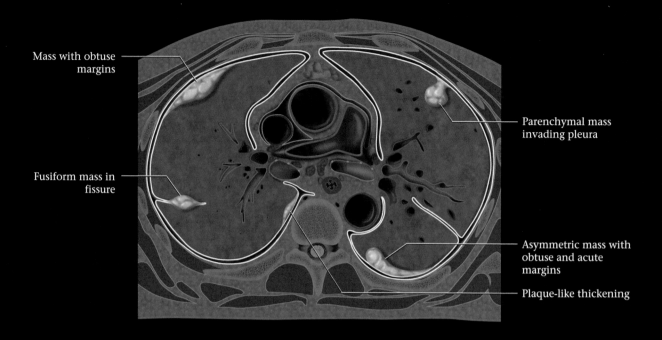

Mass with obtuse margins

Parenchymal mass invading pleura

Fusiform mass in fissure

Asymmetric mass with obtuse and acute margins

Plaque-like thickening

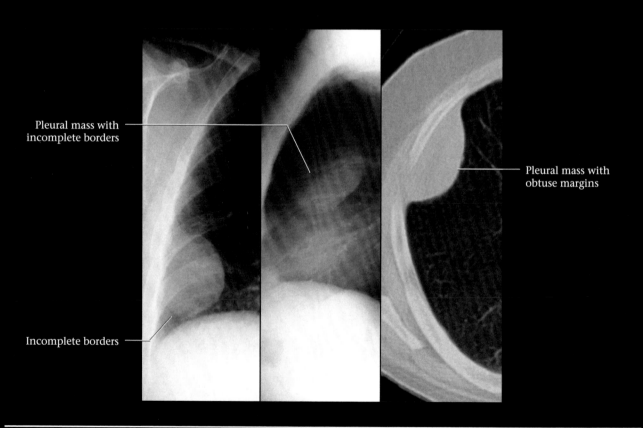

Pleural mass with incomplete borders

Pleural mass with obtuse margins

Incomplete borders

(Top) Graphic shows the variable shapes and configurations of pleural masses, including those produced by loculation of pleural fluid. Pleural masses along fissures may be fusiform, while those occurring along peripheral pleural surfaces may be symmetrically or asymmetrically lenticular with obtuse or acute angles at their interface with the adjacent pleura. Parenchymal lesions may invade adjacent pleura. (Bottom) Composite of PA and lateral coned-down chest radiographs and axial CT (lung window) through the same region shows the characteristic lentiform shape of a pleural mass with obtuse margins at the interface of the mass with adjacent pleura. As X-ray beams pass through a mass of this shape, they produce orthogonal radiographic images that often manifest as opacities that appear to have incomplete borders.

PLEURA

RADIOGRAPHY & CT, LOCALIZED FIBROUS TUMOR

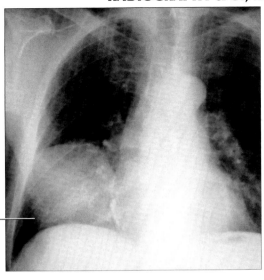

Localized fibrous tumor with incomplete inferior border

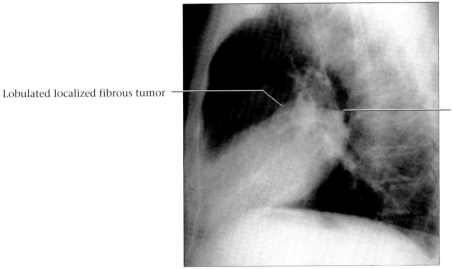

Lobulated localized fibrous tumor

Tapered posterior margin along axis of major fissure

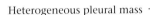
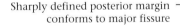
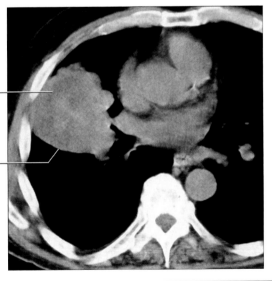

Heterogeneous pleural mass

Sharply defined posterior margin conforms to major fissure

(Top) First of three images of a 65 year old man with a localized fibrous tumor of the pleura that was discovered incidentally on chest radiography. The tumor originated within the inferior aspect of the right major fissure. PA chest radiograph shows the tumor manifesting as a lobulated soft-tissue mass with a well-defined superior border and an incompletely visualized inferolateral border. (Middle) Lateral radiograph shows the pleural tumor manifesting as a lobulated mass in the right major fissure. The posterior aspect of the tumor tapers and extends along the plane of the fissure. In this projection, the tumor borders are more uniformly visualized. (Bottom) Chest CT (mediastinal window) shows a lobulated heterogeneous pleural mass in the right major fissure.

PLEURA

RADIOGRAPHY & CT, PLEURAL METASTASES

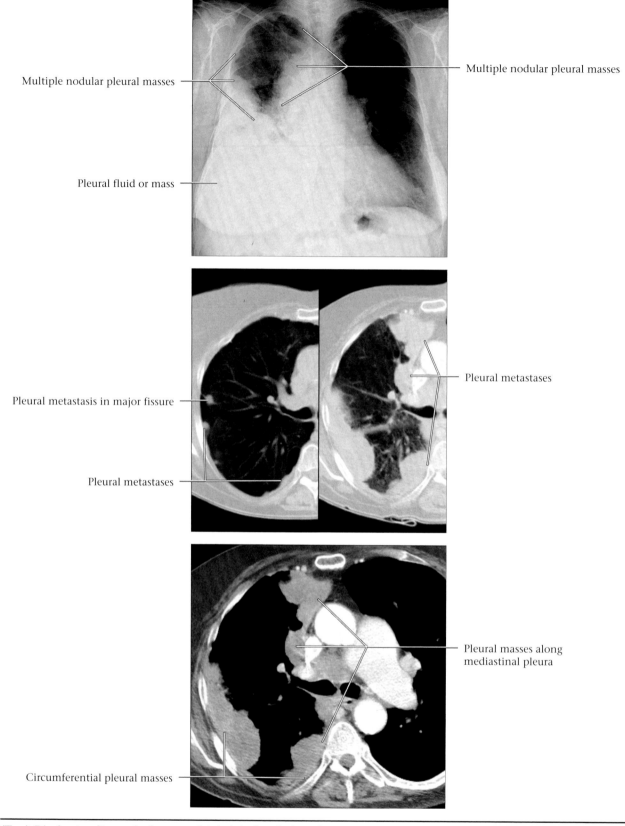

Multiple nodular pleural masses

Multiple nodular pleural masses

Pleural fluid or mass

Pleural metastasis in major fissure

Pleural metastases

Pleural metastases

Pleural masses along mediastinal pleura

Circumferential pleural masses

(Top) PA chest radiograph shows multiple lobulated pleural opacities that appear to circumferentially involve the right hemithorax and extend along the mediastinal pleural surface. (Middle) Composite of serial CT images (lung window) shows early formation of pleural metastases (left) growing along the peripheral pleural surface and within the major fissure and progression of pleural metastases six months later (right). Circumferential growth pattern and extensive involvement of mediastinal pleura are consistent with malignant pleural thickening. Additional features of malignancy include nodular growth pattern and pleural thickening > 1 cm. (Bottom) Chest CT (mediastinal window) shows extensive nodular pleural metastases > 1 cm in thickness, circumferential in distribution, and involving the mediastinal pleura.

PLEURA

RADIOGRAPHY & CT, MESOTHELIOMA

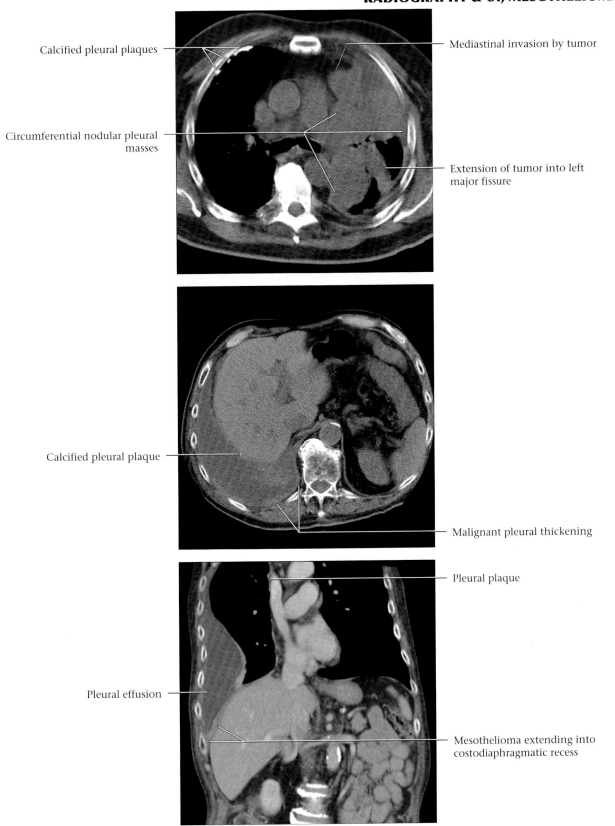

Calcified pleural plaques

Circumferential nodular pleural masses

Mediastinal invasion by tumor

Extension of tumor into left major fissure

Calcified pleural plaque

Malignant pleural thickening

Pleural plaque

Pleural effusion

Mesothelioma extending into costodiaphragmatic recess

(Top) Chest CT shows circumferential nodular pleural masses that extend into the left major fissure and invade the anterior mediastinal fat. Video-assisted thoracoscopic biopsy revealed mesothelioma. Note calcified pleural plaques, indicating prior exposure to asbestos. (Middle) First of two chest CT images of a 77 year old man with history of asbestos exposure. Axial CT image shows right pleural effusion and posteromedial pleural thickening. Note small calcified pleural plaque on the right diaphragmatic pleura. (Bottom) Coronal chest CT demonstrates pleural thickening extending into the right lateral costodiaphragmatic recess and associated pleural effusion. Subtle pleural plaque is demonstrated along the right mediastinal pleura. Video-assisted thoracoscopic biopsy revealed mesothelioma.

MEDIASTINUM

General Anatomy

Mediastinum
- Space between lungs and pleural surfaces
  - From sternum anteriorly to thoracic vertebrae posteriorly
  - From thoracic inlet superiorly to diaphragm inferiorly
- Does not include paravertebral regions

Structures
- Organs
  - **Thymus**
  - **Heart** (see "Heart" section)
- Aerodigestive tract
  - **Trachea** and **central airways** (see "Airways" section)
  - **Esophagus** (see "Esophagus" section)
- Vessels (see **Systemic Vessels** and **Pulmonary Vessels**)
  - **Systemic arteries**
    - Thoracic aorta
    - Thoracic aortic branches
  - **Systemic veins**
    - Venae cavae
    - Azygos and hemiazygos veins
  - Central pulmonary arteries and veins
- **Lymphatics, thoracic duct, lymph nodes**
- Nerves
  - **Vagus nerves (X)**
    - **Right vagus nerve** courses inferiorly along lateral trachea, behind hilum and along lateral esophagus with branches to esophagus, cardiac and pulmonary plexi
    - **Left vagus nerve** courses inferiorly along lateral aortic arch, behind hilum and along lateral esophagus with branches to esophagus, cardiac and pulmonary plexi
    - **Left recurrent laryngeal nerve**, branch of **left vagus nerve** at lateral aortic arch, courses under aortic arch, continues superiorly in a groove between the trachea and esophagus towards the neck to supply the larynx
  - **Phrenic nerves**
    - **Right phrenic nerve** is lateral to **vagus nerve**, courses along lateral aspect of right brachiocephalic vein, continues anterior to hilum along lateral pericardium
    - **Left phrenic nerve** is lateral to **vagus nerve** and proximal left brachiocephalic vein, courses along lateral proximal aortic arch, continues anterior to hilum along lateral pericardium
- Mesenchymal tissues
  - **Pericardium** (see "**Pericardium**" section)
  - Mediastinal fat

Mediastinal Compartments

General Concepts
- No true mediastinal compartments
  - No defined tissue planes compartmentalize the mediastinum
- Establishment of arbitrary mediastinal compartments

- Description of anatomic abnormalities
  - Classification of disease processes based on location
  - Differential diagnosis of mediastinal masses
- Mediastinal compartments
  - **Anatomic mediastinal compartments**
  - **Surgical mediastinal compartments**
  - **Radiologic mediastinal compartments**

Anatomic Mediastinal Compartments
- **Superior mediastinum**
  - Mediastinal contents superior to a transverse plane extending from sternal angle to T4-T5 disk
    - From manubrium sternum anteriorly to T1-T4 vertebral bodies posteriorly
  - Contents
    - **Thymus**
    - **Aortic arch**
    - **Right brachiocephalic, left common carotid, left subclavian** arteries
    - **Superior vena cava**
    - **Left superior intercostal, right and left brachiocephalic** veins
    - **Superior trachea**
    - **Superior esophagus**
    - **Phrenic, vagus, left recurrent laryngeal** nerves
    - **Superior aspect of thoracic duct**
    - **Lymph nodes**
- **Inferior mediastinum**
  - Three compartments below superior mediastinum
    - **Anterior mediastinum**
    - **Middle mediastinum**
    - **Posterior mediastinum**
  - Anterior mediastinum
    - From sternum anteriorly to pericardium posteriorly
    - Inferior **thymus**
    - Fat, nerves, lymph nodes, vessels
  - Middle mediastinum
    - Bound by **fibrous pericardium**
    - **Heart**
    - Central **systemic** and **pulmonary vessels**
    - Nerves, vessels
  - Posterior mediastinum
    - From fibrous pericardium anteriorly to thoracic vertebral bodies posteriorly
    - Inferior **esophagus**
    - Descending **aorta**
    - Portions of **azygos** system
    - **Thoracic duct, lymph nodes**
    - **Sympathetic trunks, nerves**

Radiologic Mediastinal Compartments
- **Mediastinal compartments, Felson classification**
  - Based on **left lateral chest radiograph**
  - **Includes paravertebral region**
  - **Anterior mediastinum**
    - Structures anterior to continuous line drawn along anterior trachea and posterior heart
  - **Middle mediastinum**
    - Structures anterior to imaginary line connecting points located 1 cm behind anterior margins of thoracic vertebrae, and posterior to anterior mediastinum
  - **Posterior mediastinum**

MEDIASTINUM

- Structures posterior to middle mediastinum
- **Mediastinal compartments, Fraser, Müller, Colman, Paré classification**
  - Based on **left lateral chest radiograph**
  - Localization of lesions as **predominantly within a compartment**
    - Addresses multicompartment abnormalities
  - **Anterior mediastinum**
    - Identical to anterior mediastinum of **Felson**
  - **Middle-posterior mediastinum**
    - Posterior to anterior mediastinum, anterior to thoracic vertebrae
  - **Paravertebral regions**, not in mediastinum proper
- **Mediastinal compartments, Heitzman classification**
  - **Thoracic inlet**
    - Cervicothoracic junction
    - Immediately above and below transverse plane through first rib
  - **Anterior mediastinum**
    - From thoracic inlet superiorly to diaphragm inferiorly
    - Anterior to heart, ascending aorta, superior vena cava
  - Areas posterior to the anterior mediastinum
    - **Supra-aortic area**, above aortic arch
    - **Infra-aortic area**, below aortic arch
    - **Supra-azygos area**, above azygos arch
    - **Infra-azygos area**, below azygos arch

Imaging of the Mediastinum

Radiography of the Mediastinum

- **Frontal radiography**
  - Right mediastinal contours from cephalad to caudad
    - **Superior vena cava interface, right atrium, inferior vena cava**
  - Left mediastinum from cephalad to caudad
    - **Left subclavian artery interface, aortic arch, pulmonary trunk, left atrial appendage, left ventricle**
- **Lateral radiography**
  - Anterior contours from cephalad to caudad
    - **Right ventricle, pulmonary trunk, ascending aorta**
  - Posterior contours from cephalad to caudad
    - **Aortic arch, proximal descending aorta, left atrium, left ventricle, inferior vena cava**

CT/MR of the Mediastinum

- Identification and characterization of vascular structures, organs, lymph nodes, and abnormal tissues

Mediastinal Lines, Stripes & Spaces

Mediastinal Lines

- **Anterior junction line**
  - Contact between anterior lungs just posterior to the sternum; imaging of four pleural layers
  - Radiography
    - Thin line or stripe, oblique course from lower manubrium sternum and inferiorly to the left
- **Posterior junction line** (or **stripe**)
  - Contact between posterior lungs behind esophagus and anterior to vertebrae; imaging of four pleural layers

Mediastinal Stripes

- **Right paratracheal stripe**
  - Contact between right lung and right tracheal wall above azygos arch
  - Up to 4 mm thick on radiographs of normal subjects
- **Left paratracheal stripe/interface**
  - Contact between left lung and left tracheal wall and intervening tissues
  - Thin soft tissue stripe
- **Paravertebral stripes**
  - Contact between lower lobes and paravertebral skeleton and soft tissues

Mediastinal Spaces & Recesses

- **Pretracheal space**
  - Triangular morphology
  - Anterolateral to trachea
    - Bound by aortic arch medially, mediastinal pleura laterally, superior vena cava anteriorly, trachea posteriorly
  - Contains fat, pretracheal lymph nodes
- **Prevascular space**
  - Triangular morphology
  - Anterior to aorta and superior vena cava
    - Bound by mediastinal pleurae bilaterally, sternum anteriorly, great vessels posteriorly
  - Contains thymus, lymph nodes, fat
- **Aortopulmonary window**
  - Left mediastinum lateral to trachea
    - Bound by trachea medially, mediastinal pleura laterally, aortic arch superiorly, left pulmonary artery inferiorly
  - Contains lymph nodes, fat, recurrent laryngeal nerve, ligamentum arteriosum
- **Subcarinal space**
  - Immediately below carina
    - Bound by main bronchi laterally, carina superiorly, left atrium inferiorly
  - Contains fat and lymph nodes
- **Azygoesophageal recess** (see "**Systemic Vessels**")
  - Portion of right mediastinum below tracheal carina
    - Contains azygos vein, esophagus
  - Makes contact with medial right lung
  - Concave laterally, may be convex in normal subjects with prominent azygos veins
- **Retrocrural space**
  - Medial to bilateral diaphragmatic crura
  - Adjacent to descending aorta and paravertebral region
- **Paravertebral space**
  - Not always considered anatomically part of mediastinum
  - Incorporated into mediastinal compartments by several classifications

Thymus

Anatomy

- Bilobed encapsulated organ

MEDIASTINUM

- Closely related to anterior great vessels and pericardium
- Age-related changes
  - Involution after puberty
  - Fatty infiltration after age of 40 years

Imaging
- Not visible radiographically in normal adults
- Prominent in normal infants and children
  - **Thymic sail sign**, morphologic appearance of nautical sail (5% of infants)
  - **Thymic wave sign**, indentations of normal thymus by anterior ribs
- CT
  - **Quadrilateral morphology** in **infancy and childhood**
  - **Triangular morphology** in **late childhood and adulthood**
  - Fat replacement beginning at 25 years, usually complete by age 40 years
  - Size
    - Children ≤ 5 years; average thickness **1.4 cm**
    - Patients ≤ 20 years; maximum thickness **1.8 cm**
    - Patients > 20 years; maximum thickness **1.3 cm**

Mediastinal Lymph Nodes

Rouviere Anatomic Classification
- **Parietal**, outside parietal pleura, drain chest wall
  - Internal mammary, diaphragmatic, paracardiac, intercostal
- **Visceral**, within mediastinum or hila
  - Anterior mediastinal, paratracheal, paraesophageal
  - Intrapulmonary, bronchopulmonary, tracheobronchial

Webb and Higgins Classification
- Based on common usage and visualization on cross-sectional imaging according to Webb WR, Higgins CB. Thoracic Imaging. Pulmonary and Cardiovascular Radiology. Philadelphia: Lippincott Williams & Wilkins, 2005
- **Anterior lymph nodes**
  - **Internal mammary**, parasternal locations
  - **Prevascular**, anterior to aorta/great vessels
  - **Paracardiac** (cardiophrenic angle), anterior or lateral to heart
- Tracheobronchial
  - **Paratracheal**, anterior/lateral to trachea
  - **Aortopulmonary**, aortopulmonary window, drainage of left upper lobe
  - **Peribronchial**
  - **Subcarinal**, between proximal main bronchi inferior to carina
- Posterior
  - **Paraesophageal** and **inferior pulmonary ligament**, near esophagus and descending aorta
  - **Intercostal** and **paravertebral**, paravertebral regions at intercostal spaces
  - **Retrocrural**, posterior to crura

AJCC/UICC Lymph Node Stations
- Fourteen lymph node stations (numbered 1-14)

- Mediastinal lymph nodes, N2 descriptor in lung cancer staging (nine lymph node stations)
  - Hilar and intrapulmonary lymph nodes, N1 descriptor in lung cancer staging
- R & L designations with respect to midline
- Superior mediastinal lymph nodes (1, 2, 3, 4)
  - **Highest mediastinal**, **station 1**; above horizontal line at upper left brachiocephalic vein
  - **Upper paratracheal**, **station 2**, above horizontal line tangential to upper aortic arch and below station 1
  - **Prevascular** and **retrotracheal**, **station 3**
  - **Lower paratracheal**, **station 4**
    - **Right paratracheal** lymph nodes below horizontal margin of upper aortic arch and above superior aspect of right main bronchus
    - **Left lower paratracheal** lymph nodes to left of trachea between left main bronchus at upper margin of left upper lobe bronchus and medial to ligamentum arteriosum
- **Aortic lymph nodes (stations 5, 6)**
  - **Subaortic** or **aortopulmonary**, **station 5**; lateral to ligamentum arteriosum, aorta or left pulmonary artery
  - **Para-aortic** (**ascending aortic** or **phrenic**), **station 6**; anterior and lateral to ascending aorta/arch or brachiocephalic artery below upper aortic arch
- **Inferior mediastinal lymph nodes (stations 7, 8, 9)**
  - **Subcarinal**, **station 7**; inferior to tracheal carina
  - **Paraesophageal**, **station 8**; adjacent to esophagus
  - **Pulmonary ligament**, **station 9**; within pulmonary ligament, along posterior wall of lower aspect of inferior pulmonary vein

Imaging of Mediastinal Lymph Nodes
- Round, ovoid discrete soft tissue, may exhibit fat attenuation center
- Normal short axis measurement of ≤ 1.0 cm and ≤ 1.5 cm in subcarinal region
- Enlarged lymph nodes may exhibit round/ovoid morphology or may exhibit nodal coalescence with diffuse infiltrative mediastinal soft tissue

Anatomy-Imaging Correlations

Pneumomediastinum
- Air in mediastinum, may occur spontaneously; elevated lung pressure with airway rupture, traumatic instrumentation

Mediastinal Enlargement
- **Focal masses**
  - **Primary neoplasms**, benign and malignant
  - **Congenital cysts**, typically unilocular and subcarinal
  - **Vascular lesions**, vascular enhancement, continuity with vascular lumen
  - **Glandular enlargement**, enlargement of thymus/thyroid
  - **Herniations**, visualization of abdominal fat/organs
- **Diffuse mediastinal enlargement**
  - **Lymphadenopathy** related to malignant neoplasia
  - **Lipomatosis**

MEDIASTINUM

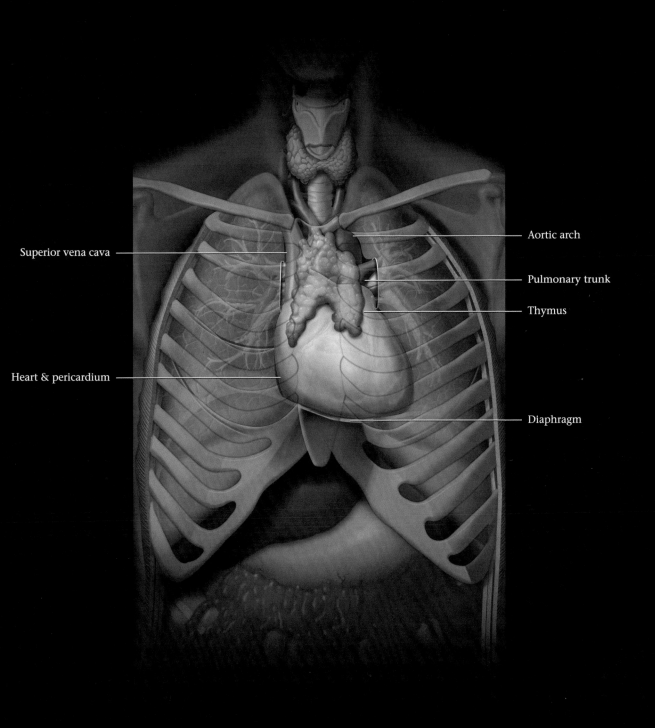

Superior vena cava

Aortic arch

Pulmonary trunk

Thymus

Heart & pericardium

Diaphragm

Graphic demonstrates the location of the mediastinum with respect to the other structures and tissues of the chest. The mediastinum is the space between the pleural spaces and lungs and contains the heart, pericardium, thymus, aerodigestive tract and the central aspects of the thoracic great vessels. The mediastinum extends from the thoracic inlet superiorly to the diaphragm inferiorly and from the sternum anteriorly to the thoracic vertebrae posteriorly.

MEDIASTINUM

CORONAL & SAGITTAL MEDIASTINAL ANATOMY

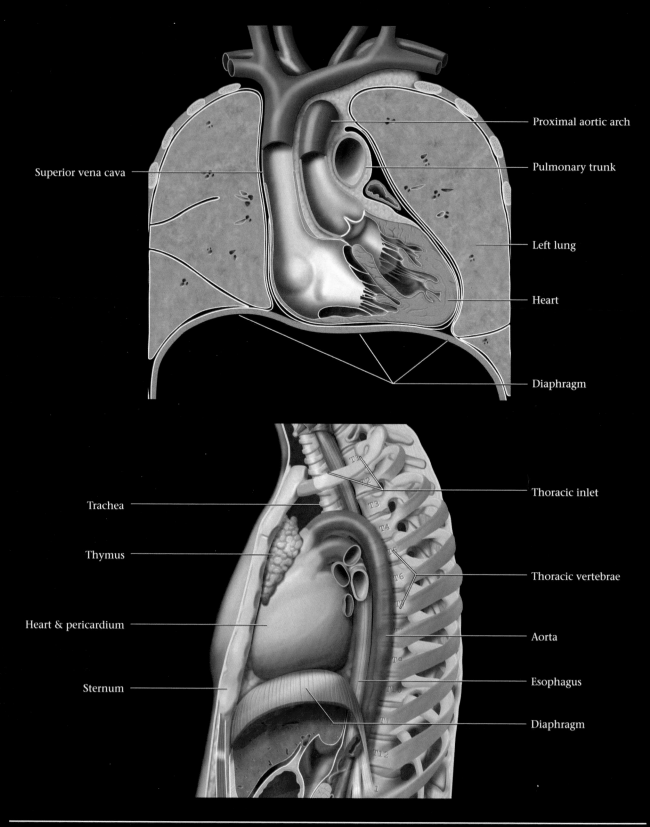

Proximal aortic arch

Pulmonary trunk

Superior vena cava

Left lung

Heart

Diaphragm

Trachea

Thoracic inlet

Thymus

Thoracic vertebrae

Heart & pericardium

Aorta

Sternum

Esophagus

Diaphragm

(Top) First of four graphics depicting the general anatomy of the mediastinum. Graphic depicting the coronal anatomy of the mid portion of the mediastinum shows that it contains the heart (seen in cross-section) and portions of the great vessels. The mediastinum is located centrally within the chest between the lungs and pleural surfaces. The inferior boundary of the mediastinum is the diaphragm. The mediastinum extends superiorly to the thoracic inlet. **(Bottom)** Graphic depicts a sagittal view of the mediastinum which extends from the sternum anteriorly to the thoracic vertebral bodies posteriorly and from the thoracic inlet superiorly to the diaphragm inferiorly. The mediastinum contains the heart, thymus, portions of the aerodigestive tract and the great vessels of the thorax. Mediastinal fat is also present in variable quantities.

MEDIASTINUM

AXIAL MEDIASTINAL ANATOMY & PARAVERTEBRAL REGION

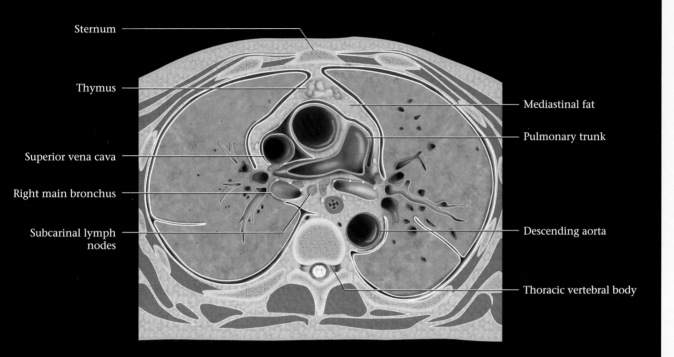

Sternum

Thymus

Superior vena cava

Right main bronchus

Subcarinal lymph nodes

Mediastinal fat

Pulmonary trunk

Descending aorta

Thoracic vertebral body

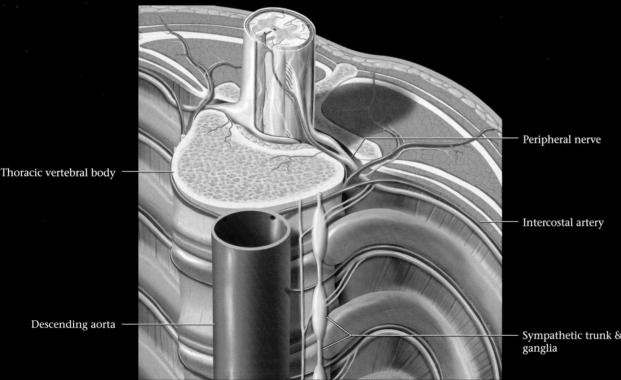

Thoracic vertebral body

Descending aorta

Peripheral nerve

Intercostal artery

Sympathetic trunk & ganglia

(Top) Graphic depicts the cross-sectional anatomy of the mediastinum at the level of the pulmonary trunk. The mediastinum is located in the middle of the thorax between the lungs and pleural surfaces. It contains several organs, vascular structures, the esophagus, the central tracheobronchial tree, lymph nodes, nerves and mediastinal fat. **(Bottom)** Graphic depicts a detail of the left paravertebral region. This area does not form part of the mediastinum proper but is often included in imaging and surgical classifications of the mediastinum and its compartments. The paravertebral region contains vascular structures, fat, lymph nodes and lymphatics and nerves. The peripheral nerves course through the paravertebral region as they exit the neural foramen. The sympathetic trunk and ganglia are oriented along the length of the paravertebral region.

MEDIASTINUM

ANATOMY, MEDIASTINAL NERVES

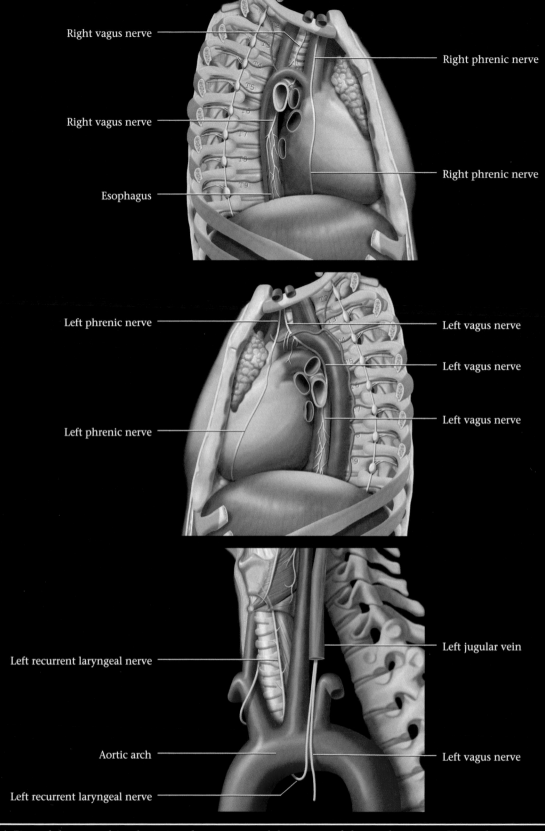

Right vagus nerve

Right vagus nerve

Esophagus

Right phrenic nerve

Right phrenic nerve

Left phrenic nerve

Left phrenic nerve

Left vagus nerve

Left vagus nerve

Left vagus nerve

Left recurrent laryngeal nerve

Left jugular vein

Aortic arch

Left vagus nerve

Left recurrent laryngeal nerve

(Top) First of three graphics depicting the anatomy of the nerves of the mediastinum. The right vagus nerve courses along the lateral trachea, and continues inferiorly posterior to the hilum and along the lateral esophagus. The right phrenic nerve courses lateral to the right brachiocephalic vein and continues inferiorly anterior to the hilum and along the pericardium. It enters the abdomen with the inferior vena cava. **(Middle)** The left vagus nerve courses along the lateral aorta and continues inferiorly posterior to the hilum along the lateral esophagus. The left phrenic nerve courses anterior to the hilum and along the pericardium and pierces the diaphragm to enter the abdomen. **(Bottom)** The left recurrent laryngeal nerve, a branch of the left vagus nerve, follows an arcuate course under the aortic arch and continues superiorly along the trachea to supply the larynx.

MEDIASTINUM

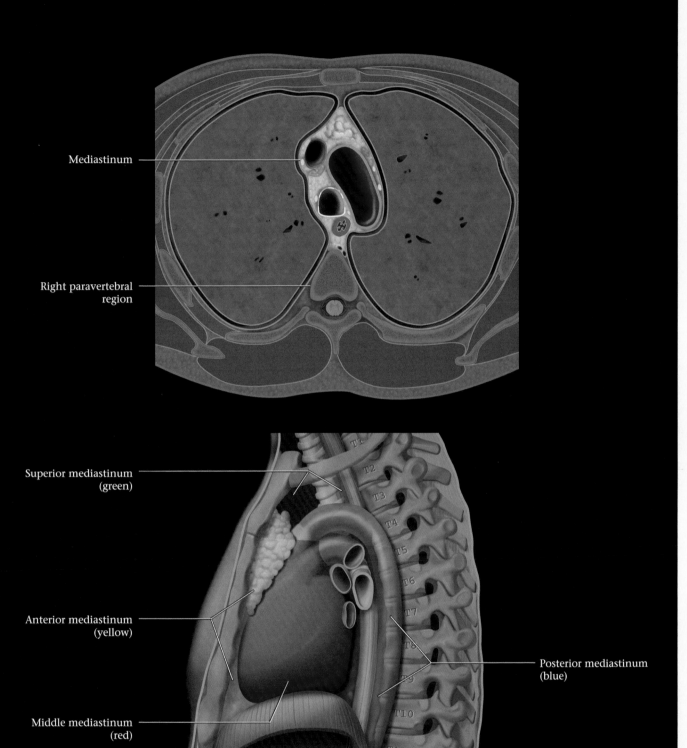

Mediastinum

Right paravertebral region

Superior mediastinum (green)

Anterior mediastinum (yellow)

Posterior mediastinum (blue)

Middle mediastinum (red)

(Top) First of two graphics depicting the anatomic mediastinal compartments. The cross-sectional anatomy of the mediastinum proper at the level of the arch is illustrated and highlighted by showing it in color. By definition, the mediastinum is the space between the pleural surfaces and the lungs bound anteriorly by the sternum and posteriorly by the vertebrae. Thus, the paravertebral regions are not included in the anatomic mediastinum although they are often included in classifications used by imagers and clinicians. (Bottom) Graphic depicts the anatomic mediastinal compartments. The superior mediastinum lies above a line drawn from the sternomanubrial junction to the T4-5 intervertebral disk. The inferior mediastinum contains anterior and posterior compartments in front and behind the heart and pericardium, and a middle compartment bound by the fibrous pericardium.

MEDIASTINUM

RADIOGRAPHIC MEDIASTINAL COMPARTMENTS, FELSON

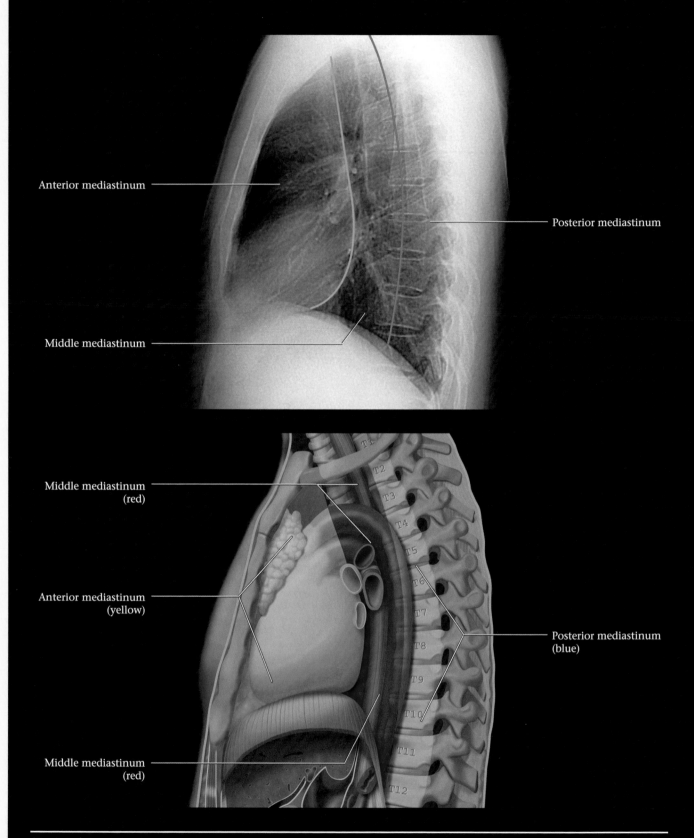

Anterior mediastinum

Posterior mediastinum

Middle mediastinum

Middle mediastinum (red)

Anterior mediastinum (yellow)

Posterior mediastinum (blue)

Middle mediastinum (red)

(Top) Left lateral chest radiograph illustrates the Felson classification of the mediastinal compartments. The anterior mediastinum is located anterior to a vertically oriented line drawn along the anterior trachea and continued along the posterior aspect of the heart. The posterior mediastinum is located behind a line drawn connecting points located 1 cm posterior to the anterior margins of the thoracic vertebral bodies. The middle mediastinum is located between the anterior and posterior compartments. This classification uses three compartments, includes the paravertebral regions and places the heart in the anterior compartment. **(Bottom)** Graphic illustrates the location of anatomic structures according to the Felson classification. The mediastinal compartments are illustrated with different colors. The posterior mediastinum includes the paravertebral region.

MEDIASTINUM

RADIOGRAPHIC MEDIASTINAL COMPARTMENTS, FRASER ET AL

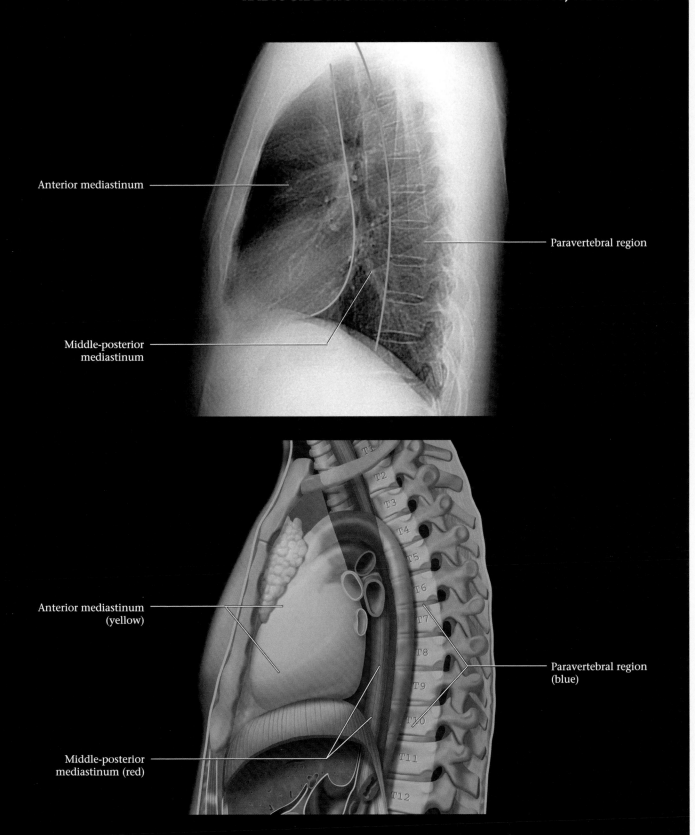

Anterior mediastinum

Paravertebral region

Middle-posterior mediastinum

Anterior mediastinum (yellow)

Paravertebral region (blue)

Middle-posterior mediastinum (red)

(Top) Left lateral chest radiograph showing the Fraser, Müller, Colman and Paré classification of the mediastinal compartments. Lesions are classified as being located predominantly within one of the compartments allowing for localization of large multicompartment lesions. The anterior mediastinum is identical to that of the Felson classification. The middle and posterior compartments are combined and placed between the anterior mediastinum and the paravertebral region. (Bottom) Graphic shows the anatomic structures of the mediastinum as they relate to the mediastinal compartments of Fraser, Müller, Colman and Paré. These authors specifically separate the paravertebral region from the traditional mediastinal compartments. It should be noted that these classifications use imaginary boundaries as there are no tissue planes that compartmentalize the mediastinum.

MEDIASTINUM

RADIOGRAPHY & CORONAL CT, NORMAL MEDIASTINUM

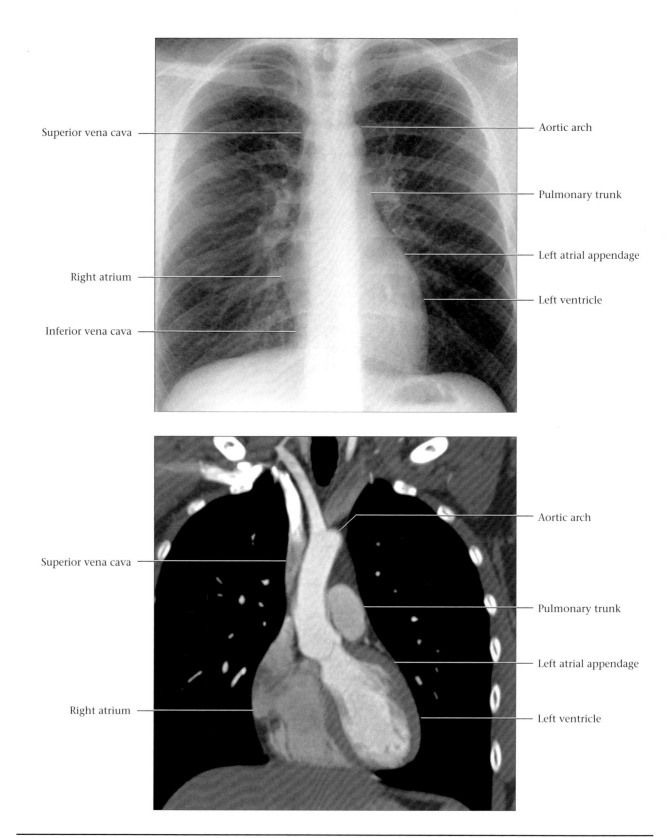

(Top) First of four normal images showing the structures that form the radiographic mediastinal contours. On PA chest radiography, the right mediastinal contour (from superior to inferior) is formed by the superior vena cava, right atrium and inferior vena cava. The right atrium forms most of the right inferior mediastinal contour. The left mediastinal contour is formed (from superior to inferior) by the aortic arch, pulmonary trunk, left atrial appendage and left ventricle. The left ventricle forms most of the left inferior mediastinal contour. **(Bottom)** Contrast-enhanced coronal chest CT (mediastinal window) shows the anatomic structures that contribute to the mediastinal contours. The superior vena cava and right atrium form the right mediastinal contour. The aortic arch, pulmonary trunk, left atrial appendage and left ventricle form the left mediastinal contour.

RADIOGRAPHY & CORONAL CT, NORMAL MEDIASTINUM

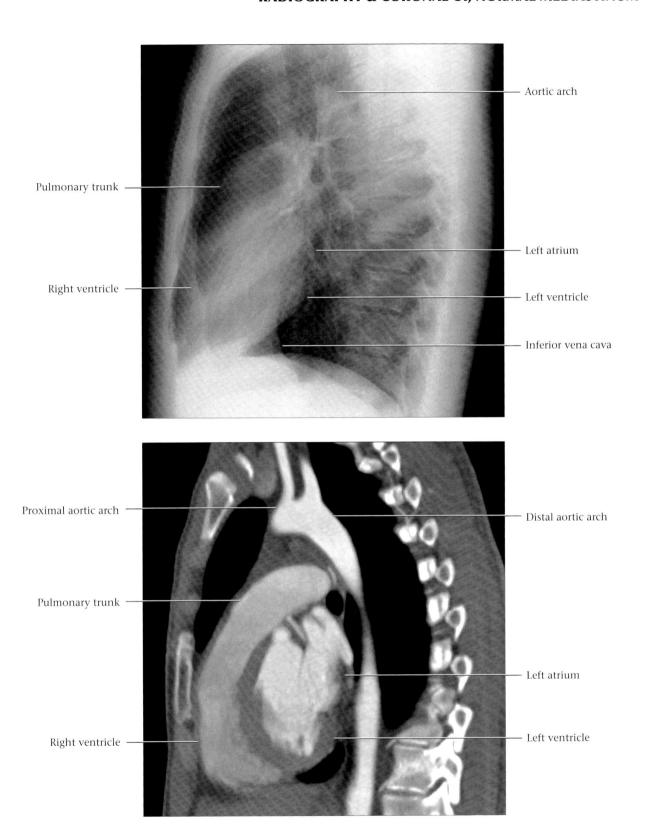

(Top) The anterior contour of the mediastinum on the left lateral chest radiograph (from inferior to superior) is formed by the right ventricle and pulmonary trunk. A portion of the proximal ascending aorta may be evident superiorly. The posterior contour (from superior to inferior) is formed by the aortic arch, left atrium, left ventricle and inferior vena cava. **(Bottom)** Sagittal contrast-enhanced chest CT (mediastinal window) shows the anatomic correlates of the mediastinal contours seen on lateral radiography. The anterior contour is formed (from inferior to superior) by the right ventricle, pulmonary trunk and proximal aortic arch. The posterior contour (from superior to inferior) is formed by the distal aortic arch, the left atrium and the left ventricle.

MEDIASTINUM

RADIOGRAPHY & CT, RIGHT & LEFT PARATRACHEAL STRIPES

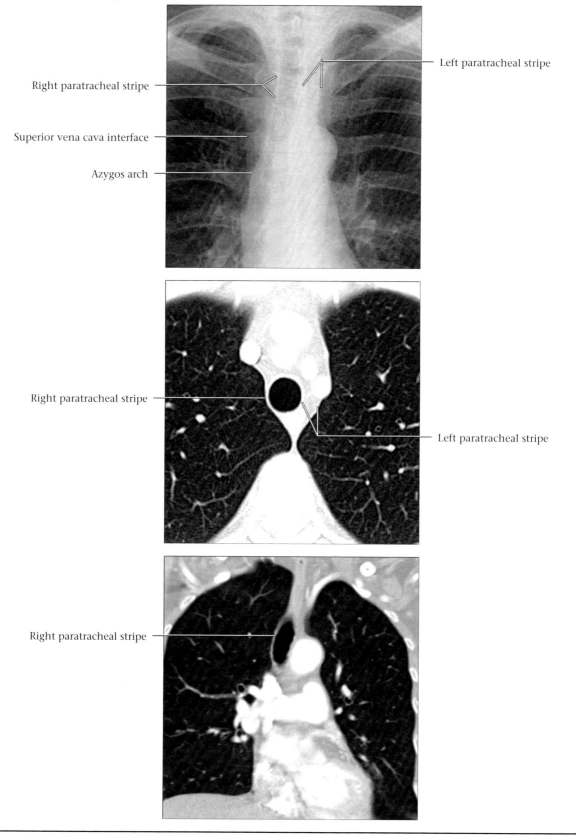

Right paratracheal stripe

Left paratracheal stripe

Superior vena cava interface

Azygos arch

Right paratracheal stripe

Left paratracheal stripe

Right paratracheal stripe

(Top) First of three images showing the paratracheal stripes. The right paratracheal stripe is a thin soft tissue line that follows the outer contour of the right intrathoracic trachea and terminates at the azygos arch. The left paratracheal stripe is of variable thickness and often includes a portion of the left subclavian artery and mediastinal fat. **(Middle)** Contrast-enhanced axial chest CT (lung window) demonstrates the anatomic correlate of the right paratracheal stripe formed as the right upper lobe comes in contact with the lateral tracheal wall. It is formed by two pleural layers, the tracheal wall and intervening fat. The left paratracheal stripe is also seen. **(Bottom)** Coronal contrast-enhanced chest CT (lung window) shows contact of the right upper lobe with the lateral wall of the trachea to form the right paratracheal stripe.

MEDIASTINUM

RADIOGRAPHY & CORONAL CT, NORMAL MEDIASTINUM

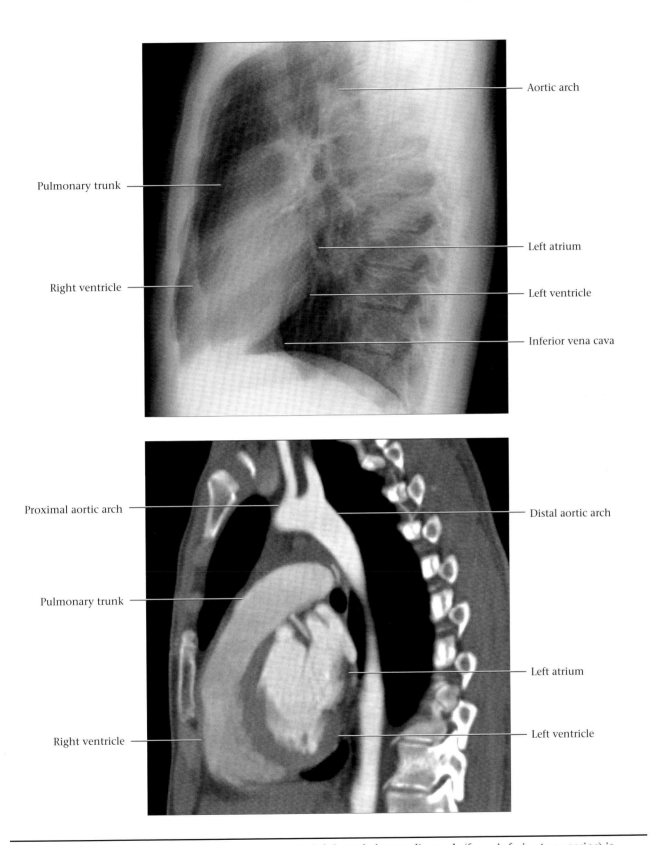

Aortic arch

Pulmonary trunk

Right ventricle

Left atrium

Left ventricle

Inferior vena cava

Proximal aortic arch

Pulmonary trunk

Right ventricle

Distal aortic arch

Left atrium

Left ventricle

(Top) The anterior contour of the mediastinum on the left lateral chest radiograph (from inferior to superior) is formed by the right ventricle and pulmonary trunk. A portion of the proximal ascending aorta may be evident superiorly. The posterior contour (from superior to inferior) is formed by the aortic arch, left atrium, left ventricle and inferior vena cava. **(Bottom)** Sagittal contrast-enhanced chest CT (mediastinal window) shows the anatomic correlates of the mediastinal contours seen on lateral radiography. The anterior contour is formed (from inferior to superior) by the right ventricle, pulmonary trunk and proximal aortic arch. The posterior contour (from superior to inferior) is formed by the distal aortic arch, the left atrium and the left ventricle.

MEDIASTINUM

RADIOGRAPHY & CT, ANTERIOR JUNCTION LINE

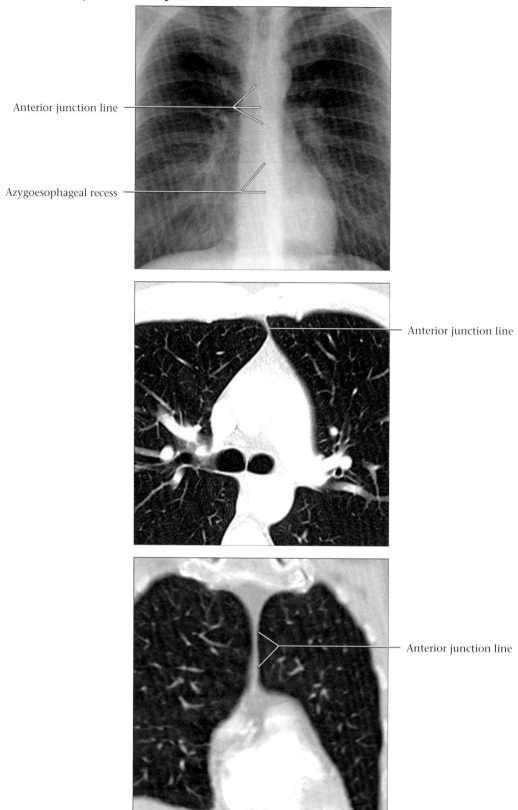

Anterior junction line

Azygoesophageal recess

Anterior junction line

Anterior junction line

(Top) First of three images illustrating the normal anterior junction line. PA chest radiograph shows the anterior junction line formed by the apposition of the anterior lungs. The line is formed by four layers of pleura, projects over the mediastinum and courses from superior to inferior from the inferior aspect of the manubrium sternum towards the left. **(Middle)** Contrast-enhanced chest CT (lung window) shows the cross-sectional anatomy of the anterior junction line. The line is formed by contact between the right and left lungs anterior to the mediastinum. **(Bottom)** Coronal chest CT (mediastinal window) shows the anterior junction line. Note the superior widening of the line (anterior triangle) formed by divergence of the pulmonary surfaces.

MEDIASTINUM

RADIOGRAPHY & CT, POSTERIOR JUNCTION LINE/STRIPE

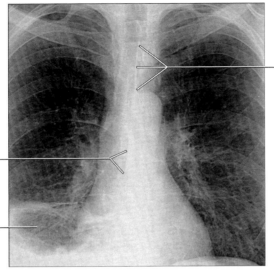

Posterior junction line

Azygoesophageal recess

Right lower lobe airspace disease

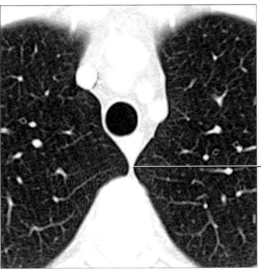

Posterior junction line

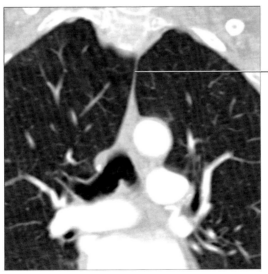

Posterior junction line

(Top) First of three images illustrating the normal posterior junction line or stripe. PA chest radiograph shows the typical appearance of the posterior junction line which represents the posterior apposition of the lung surfaces in the midline. The line terminates inferiorly at the superior aspect of the aortic arch or mid portion of the azygos arch. Note right lower lobe airspace disease related to pneumonia. **(Middle)** Axial chest CT (lung window) shows the posterior pulmonary apposition that results in the posterior junction line or stripe formed by four pleural layers and intervening mediastinal fat. **(Bottom)** Coronal chest CT (lung window) shows the apposition of the posterior right and left lungs anterior to the vertebrae forming the posterior junction line. Note that the posterior junction line terminates at the level of the aortic arch.

MEDIASTINUM

RADIOGRAPHY & CT, RIGHT & LEFT PARATRACHEAL STRIPES

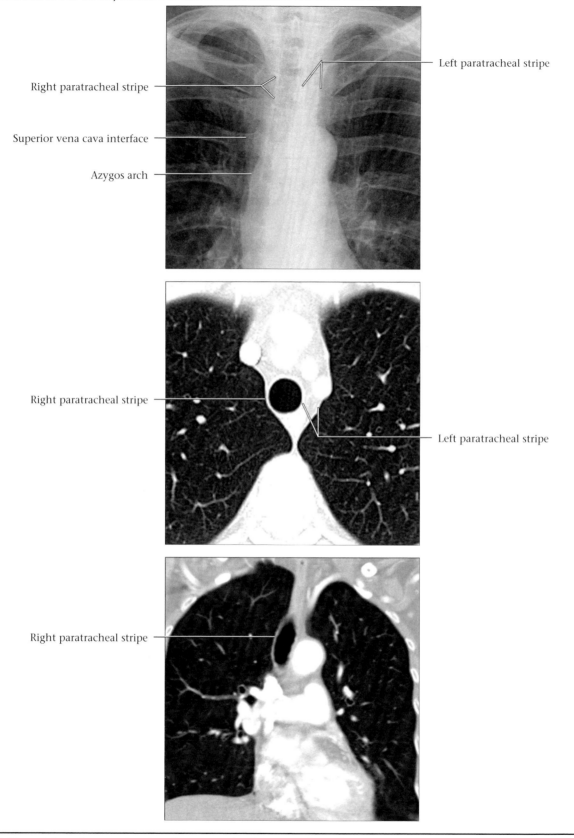

Left paratracheal stripe

Right paratracheal stripe

Superior vena cava interface

Azygos arch

Right paratracheal stripe

Left paratracheal stripe

Right paratracheal stripe

(Top) First of three images showing the paratracheal stripes. The right paratracheal stripe is a thin soft tissue line that follows the outer contour of the right intrathoracic trachea and terminates at the azygos arch. The left paratracheal stripe is of variable thickness and often includes a portion of the left subclavian artery and mediastinal fat. (Middle) Contrast-enhanced axial chest CT (lung window) demonstrates the anatomic correlate of the right paratracheal stripe formed as the right upper lobe comes in contact with the lateral tracheal wall. It is formed by two pleural layers, the tracheal wall and intervening fat. The left paratracheal stripe is also seen. (Bottom) Coronal contrast-enhanced chest CT (lung window) shows contact of the right upper lobe with the lateral wall of the trachea to form the right paratracheal stripe.

MEDIASTINUM

RADIOGRAPHY, PARAVERTEBRAL STRIPES

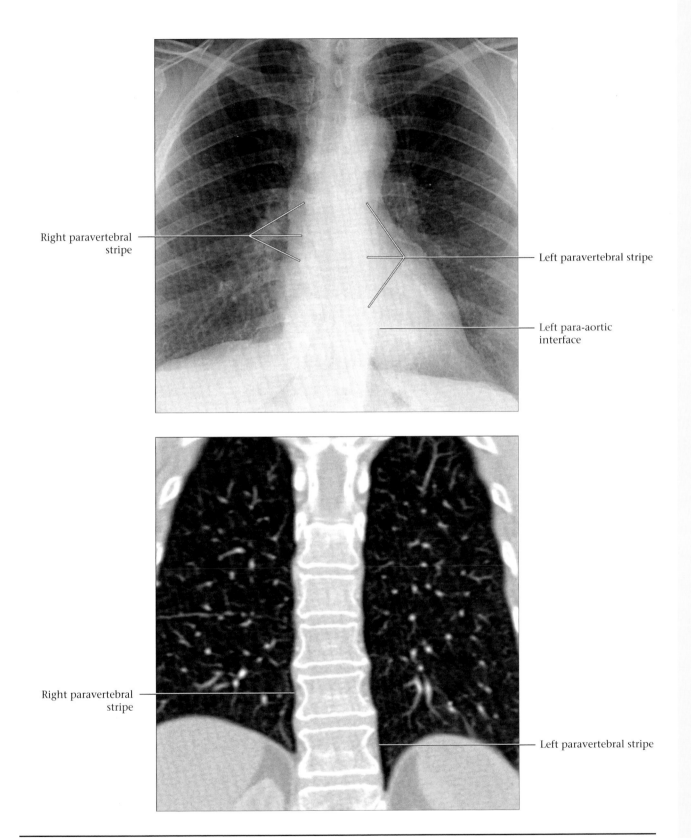

Right paravertebral stripe

Left paravertebral stripe

Left para-aortic interface

Right paravertebral stripe

Left paravertebral stripe

(Top) First of two images demonstrating the anatomy of the paravertebral stripes. PA chest radiograph shows that the left paravertebral stripe is distinct from the left para-aortic interface. It represents the apposition of the posterior lung against the paravertebral region. A portion of the right paravertebral stripe is also visualized. **(Bottom)** Contrast-enhanced coronal chest CT (lung window) shows the bilateral paravertebral stripes. They represent the points of contact between the posterior lungs and the paravertebral soft tissues.

MEDIASTINUM

AXIAL ANATOMY OF THE MEDIASTINUM

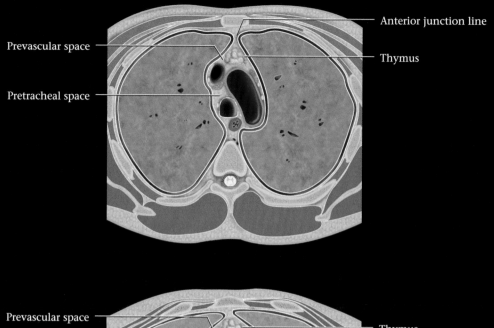

Anterior junction line

Prevascular space

Thymus

Pretracheal space

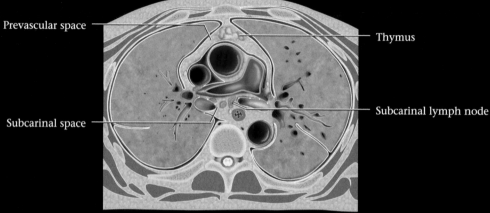

Prevascular space

Thymus

Subcarinal space

Subcarinal lymph node

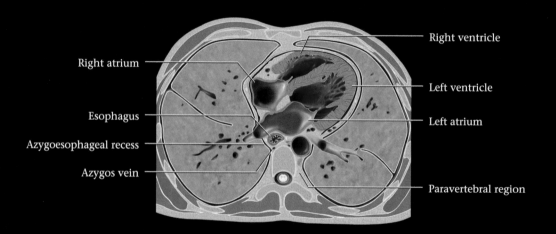

Right ventricle

Right atrium

Left ventricle

Esophagus

Left atrium

Azygoesophageal recess

Azygos vein

Paravertebral region

(Top) First of three graphics demonstrating the cross-sectional anatomy of the mediastinum and the different mediastinal spaces. Illustration of the mediastinum at the level of the aortic arch shows the anatomic correlate of the anterior junction line, the apposition of the anterior lungs in front of the mediastinum. It also shows the prevascular space occupied by the thymus and mediastinal fat. The pretracheal space is anterior to the trachea, posterior to the superior vena cava and to the left of the aortic arch. (Middle) Illustration of the mediastinum at the bifurcation of the pulmonary trunk shows the prevascular space, which contains fat and thymus and the subcarinal space which contains fat and lymph nodes. (Bottom) Illustration of the mediastinum at the level of the heart shows the azygoesophageal recess and the paravertebral regions.

MEDIASTINUM

AXIAL CT & RADIOGRAPHY, NORMAL MEDIASTINUM

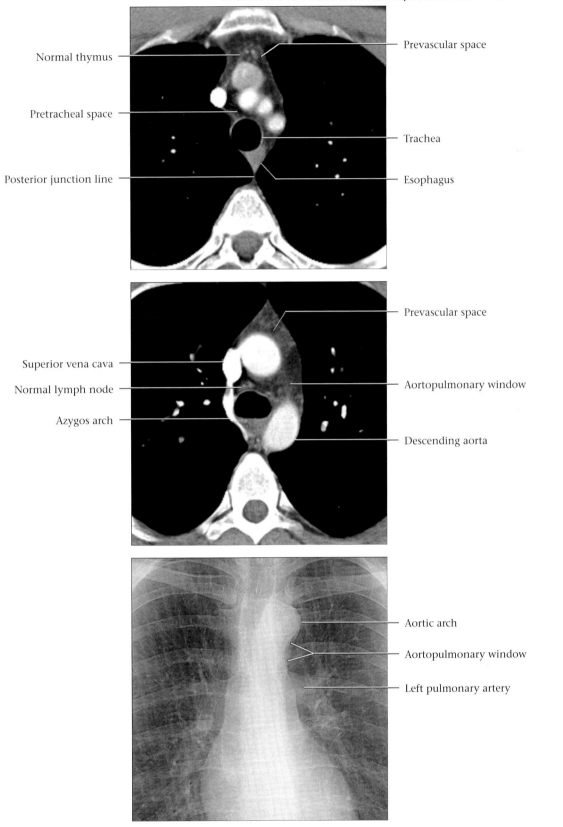

Normal thymus

Prevascular space

Pretracheal space

Trachea

Posterior junction line

Esophagus

Prevascular space

Superior vena cava

Normal lymph node

Aortopulmonary window

Azygos arch

Descending aorta

Aortic arch

Aortopulmonary window

Left pulmonary artery

(Top) First of two axial contrast-enhanced chest CT images (mediastinal window) showing the normal mediastinal spaces. The prevascular space contains fat and thymic tissue and is anterior to the great vessels. The adult normal thymus may manifest with strands of soft tissue amid mediastinal fat. The pretracheal space is anterior to the trachea and contains fat and lymph nodes. (Middle) Axial image through the azygos arch demonstrates the prevascular space anterior to the ascending aorta and the aortopulmonary window. Prevascular soft tissue strands likely relate to residual thymus. Pretracheal small nodular soft tissue foci likely represent normal mediastinal lymph nodes. (Bottom) Coned-down normal PA chest radiograph demonstrates the aortopulmonary window located between the inferior aspect of the aortic arch and the left pulmonary artery.

MEDIASTINUM

AXIAL CT, NORMAL MEDIASTINUM

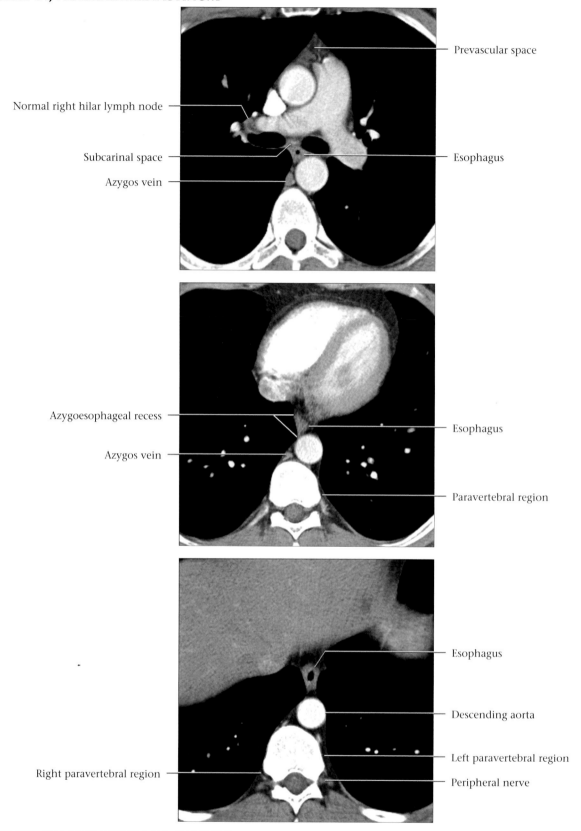

Prevascular space

Normal right hilar lymph node

Subcarinal space

Azygos vein

Esophagus

Azygoesophageal recess

Azygos vein

Esophagus

Paravertebral region

Esophagus

Descending aorta

Left paravertebral region

Right paravertebral region

Peripheral nerve

(Top) First of three normal axial contrast-enhanced chest CT images (mediastinal window) demonstrating the normal appearance of the mediastinum. Image through the pulmonary trunk shows the normal subcarinal space located immediately below the tracheal bifurcation. Soft tissue within the prevascular space represents normal thymus. **(Middle)** Axial image through the heart demonstrates the normal appearance of the azygoesophageal recess. The azygoesophageal recess is the interface produced by the contact of the right lower lobe with the retrocardiac mediastinum. The paravertebral regions are also demonstrated and normally contain paravertebral fat. **(Bottom)** Axial image through the inferior thorax demonstrates the normal paravertebral regions that contain fat and lymph nodes. The peripheral nerves and sympathetic chain are also located in the paravertebral regions.

MEDIASTINUM

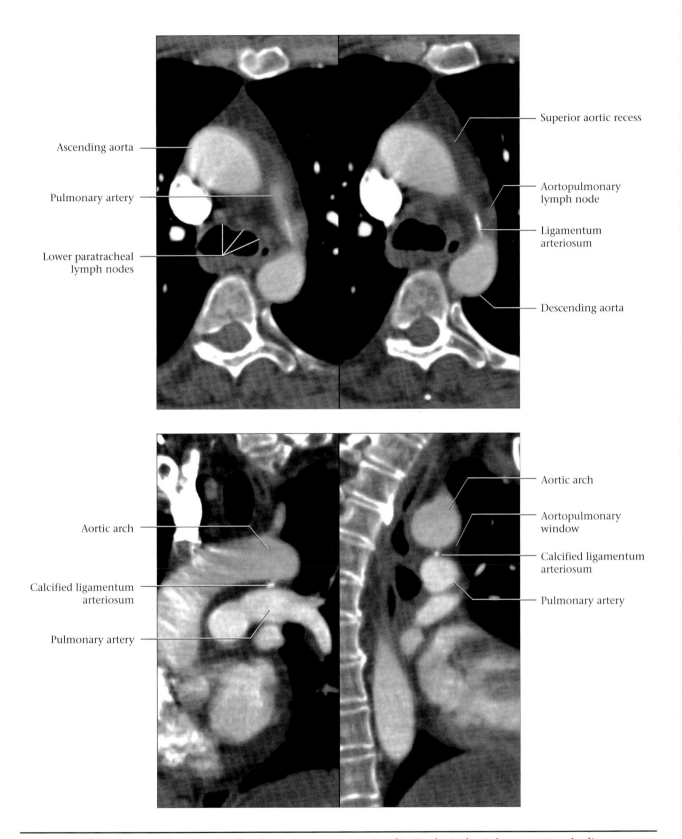

Ascending aorta

Pulmonary artery

Lower paratracheal lymph nodes

Superior aortic recess

Aortopulmonary lymph node

Ligamentum arteriosum

Descending aorta

Aortic arch

Calcified ligamentum arteriosum

Pulmonary artery

Aortic arch

Aortopulmonary window

Calcified ligamentum arteriosum

Pulmonary artery

(Top) First of two images of a normal CT pulmonary angiogram (mediastinal window) demonstrates the ligamentum arteriosum. Composite of two axial images through the aortopulmonary window shows the ligamentum arteriosum manifesting as a linear calcification that courses from the proximal descending aorta to the superior aspect of the pulmonary artery. The ligamentum arteriosum is the remnant of the ductus arteriosus which is patent during fetal life. Note fluid in the anterior portion of the superior aortic pericardial recess. Normal lymph nodes and fat are also noted in the aortopulmonary window. **(Bottom)** Composite of bilateral oblique coronal images through the ligamentum arteriosum demonstrate its anatomic location within the aortopulmonary window coursing between the inferior aspect of the aortic arch and the superior aspect of the pulmonary artery.

MEDIASTINUM

CORONAL CT, NORMAL MEDIASTINUM

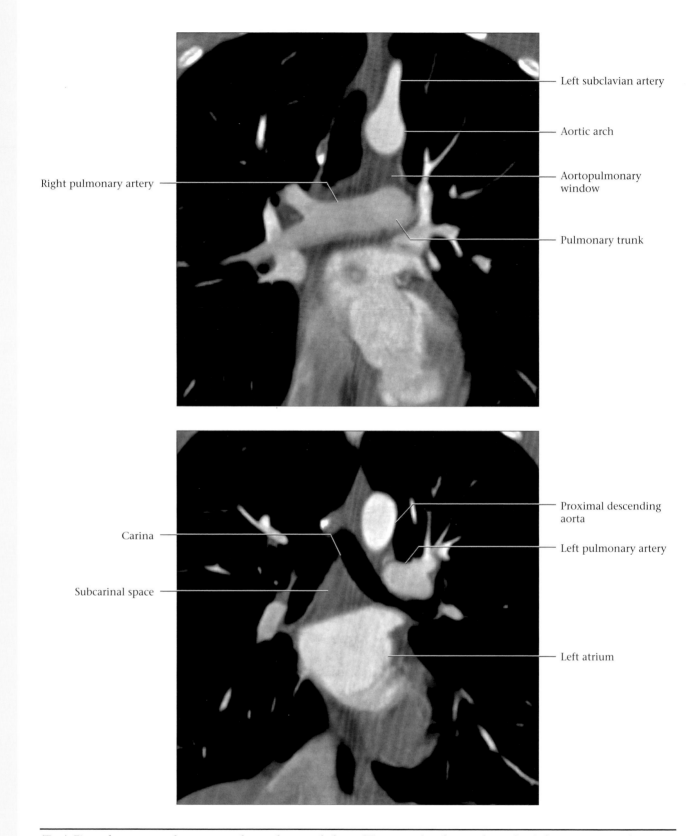

Left subclavian artery

Aortic arch

Aortopulmonary window

Pulmonary trunk

Right pulmonary artery

Carina

Subcarinal space

Proximal descending aorta

Left pulmonary artery

Left atrium

(Top) First of two normal contrast-enhanced coronal chest CT images (mediastinal window) demonstrating the anatomy of the mediastinal spaces. Image through the right pulmonary artery shows the anatomy of the aortopulmonary window situated between the inferior aspect of the aortic arch and the superior aspect of the pulmonary trunk and central pulmonary arteries. The aortopulmonary window normally contains fat and lymph nodes. **(Bottom)** Image through the carina demonstrates the anatomy of the subcarinal space, situated between the carina superiorly and the left atrium inferiorly. It typically contains mediastinal fat and lymph nodes.

MEDIASTINUM

CORONAL MR, NORMAL MEDIASTINUM

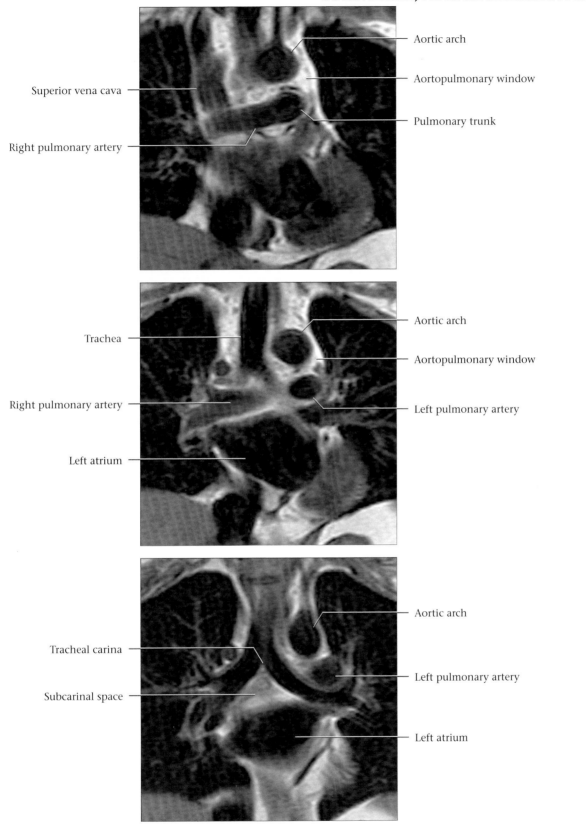

Superior vena cava — Aortic arch

Right pulmonary artery — Aortopulmonary window

— Pulmonary trunk

Trachea — Aortic arch

Right pulmonary artery — Aortopulmonary window

Left atrium — Left pulmonary artery

Tracheal carina — Aortic arch

Subcarinal space — Left pulmonary artery

— Left atrium

(Top) First of three T1-weighted coronal MR images through the mediastinum demonstrating the normal mediastinal spaces. Image through the right pulmonary artery demonstrates the aortopulmonary window located between the aortic arch superiorly and the pulmonary trunk and central pulmonary arteries inferiorly. The aortopulmonary window is filled with high signal intensity fat. (Middle) Image through the distal trachea demonstrates the posterior aspect of the aortopulmonary window. Small foci of intermediate signal intensity within the high signal mediastinal fat likely relate to normal mediastinal lymph nodes. (Bottom) Image through the carina demonstrates the normal subcarinal space located between the tracheal bifurcation superiorly and the left atrium inferiorly.

MEDIASTINUM

THYMUS

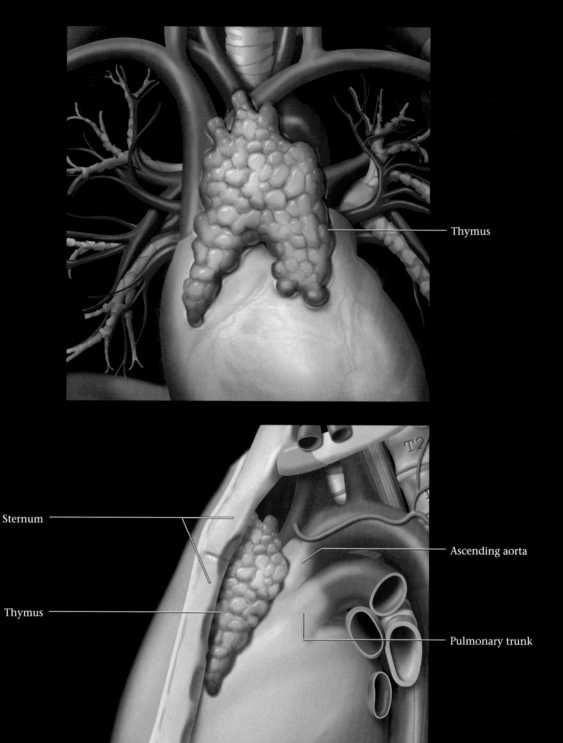

— Thymus

Sternum —

Thymus —

— Ascending aorta

— Pulmonary trunk

(Top) First of two graphics depicting the anatomy of the normal thymus. Illustration of the anterior surface of the thymus shows that it is a bilobed organ with a central isthmus. It is composed of multiple lobules covered by a thin capsule. The thymus is located immediately anterior to the superior aspect of the pericardium and the origins of the great vessels. **(Bottom)** Graphic illustrating the left lateral surface of the thymus shows its location in the prevascular anterior mediastinum. The posterior surface of the thymus is intimately related to the anterior superior aspect of the pericardium and the central great vessels. The thymus is located in the anterior mediastinum and is posterior to the sternum.

MEDIASTINUM

RADIOGRAPHY & CT, NORMAL PEDIATRIC THYMUS

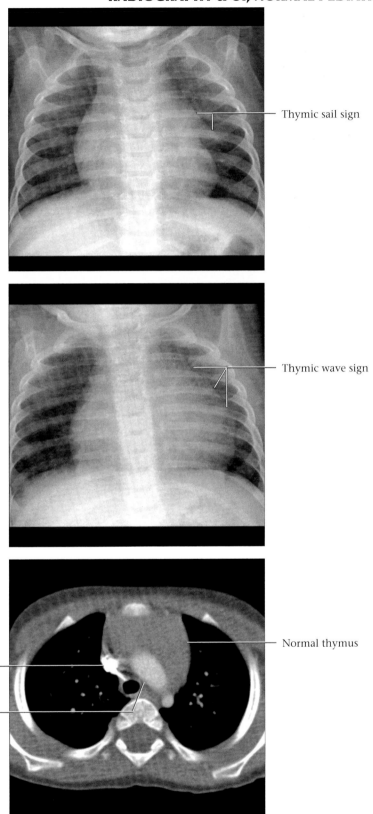

Thymic sail sign

Thymic wave sign

Normal thymus

Superior vena cava

Aortic arch

(Top) First of two chest radiographs of normal infants demonstrate variations in the appearance of the normal pediatric thymus. AP chest radiograph of a 10 month old infant illustrates the sail sign. The left thymic lobe manifests as a triangular opacity that mimics the morphology of a nautical sail. (Middle) AP chest radiograph of a 2 month old infant shows a prominent normal thymus that exhibits the thymic wave sign. The anterior ribs indent the soft prominent left thymic lobe producing an undulating wave-like contour. (Bottom) Contrast-enhanced chest CT (mediastinal window) of an 8 month old child demonstrates the appearance of the normal pediatric thymus. The anterior mediastinum is filled by homogeneous thymic soft tissue. The lateral borders of the thymus extend beyond those of the thoracic great vessels and result in a wide superior mediastinum on radiography.

MEDIASTINUM

GRAPHIC & CT, THYMIC MEASUREMENT

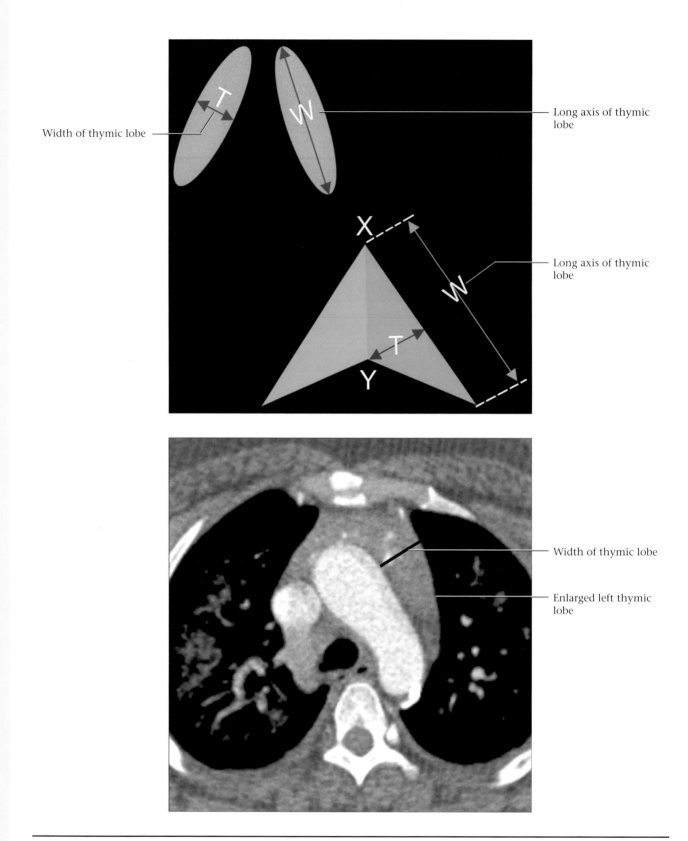

Width of thymic lobe

Long axis of thymic lobe

Long axis of thymic lobe

Width of thymic lobe

Enlarged left thymic lobe

(Top) Graphic illustrates the method for measuring the thymus. The width or thickness of the thymus (T) is measured perpendicular to the long axis (W) of each lobe. **(Bottom)** Contrast-enhanced chest CT (mediastinal window) through the thymus of a 22 year old woman with right upper lobe pneumonia shows thymic enlargement manifesting with a laterally convex enlarged left thymic lobe. Note prominent vascular structures within the thymus. The black line indicates the width or thickness of the left thymic lobe.

AXIAL CT, NORMAL THYMUS

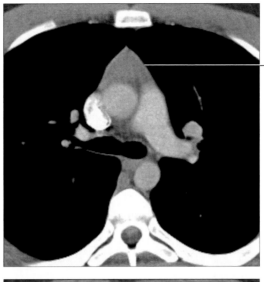

Prominent normal thymus

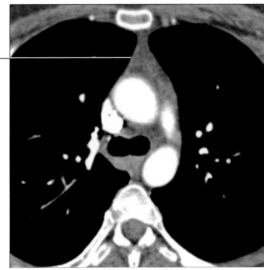

Normal thymus

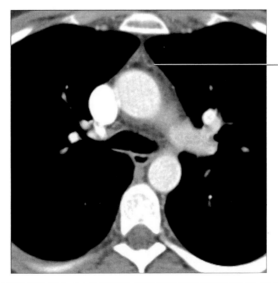

Normal thymus

(Top) First of three axial contrast-enhanced chest CT images (mediastinal window) show the normal thymus in patients of various ages. Image through the thymus of a 15 year old boy demonstrates a triangular soft tissue structure in the prevascular anterior mediastinum. Although the right thymic lobe has a laterally convex margin, the width of the thymic lobes were within normal limits for age. **(Middle)** Image through the thymus of a 20 year old woman shows a straight lateral contour of the right lobe and a mildly convex lateral contour of the left lobe. Fatty infiltration of the thymus is evident manifesting with heterogeneous attenuation in the prevascular space. **(Bottom)** Image through the thymus of a 22 year old woman shows that the thymus is small with straight lateral borders and small amounts of linear soft tissue within the mediastinal fat.

MEDIASTINUM

ANATOMY OF MEDIASTINAL LYMPH NODES

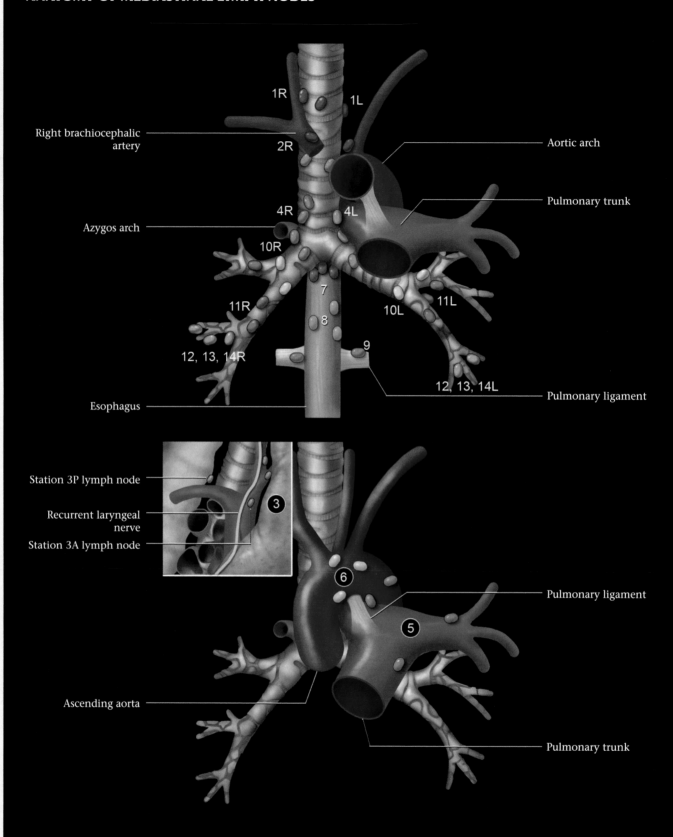

(Top) First of two graphics illustrating the regional lymph node classification for staging lung cancer according to the American Joint Committee on Cancer (AJCC) and the Union Internationale Contre le Cancer (UICC). Numbers refer to lymph node stations and L and R are used to indicate their location with respect to the midline. The following nine mediastinal lymph node stations are shown: 1) highest mediastinal; 2) upper paratracheal; 4) lower paratracheal; 5) subaortic (aortopulmonary); 6) para-aortic; 7) subcarinal; 8) paraesophageal; 9) pulmonary ligament. Lymph nodes in stations 10-14 are considered intrapulmonary. **(Bottom)** Graphic illustrates mediastinal lymph node stations 3 and 5. Station 3 denotes prevascular (3A) and retrotracheal (3P) lymph nodes. Station 5 denotes subaortic (aortopulmonary window) lymph nodes.

MEDIASTINUM

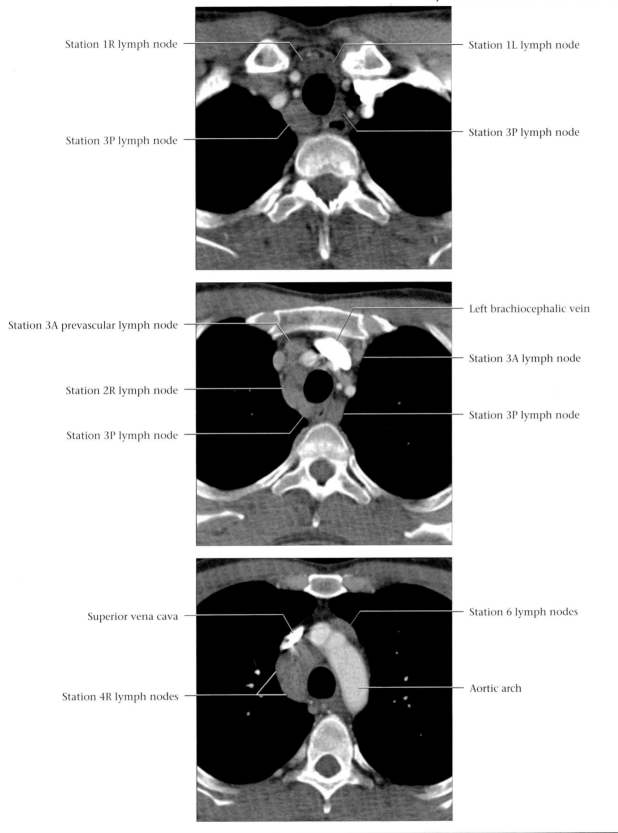

Station 1R lymph node — Station 1L lymph node

Station 3P lymph node — Station 3P lymph node

Station 3A prevascular lymph node — Left brachiocephalic vein

Station 2R lymph node — Station 3A lymph node

Station 3P lymph node — Station 3P lymph node

Superior vena cava — Station 6 lymph nodes

Station 4R lymph nodes — Aortic arch

(Top) First of nine contrast-enhanced chest CT images (mediastinal window) of a 56 year old man with non-Hodgkin lymphoma shows diffuse lymphadenopathy. Axial image through the superior mediastinum above the left brachiocephalic vein demonstrates prominent highest mediastinal (station 1) lymph nodes. There is also an enlarged right retrotracheal (3P) and a prominent left retrotracheal (3P) lymph node. **(Middle)** Axial image through the mid left brachiocephalic vein demonstrates enlargement of right upper paratracheal (station 2) lymph nodes as well as prominent retrotracheal (3P) lymph nodes. There are also prominent prevascular (station 3A) lymph nodes. **(Bottom)** Axial image through the superior aspect of the aortic arch demonstrates enlarged lower paratracheal (station 4R) lymph nodes and prominent para-aortic (station 6) lymph nodes.

MEDIASTINUM

PNEUMOMEDIASTINUM

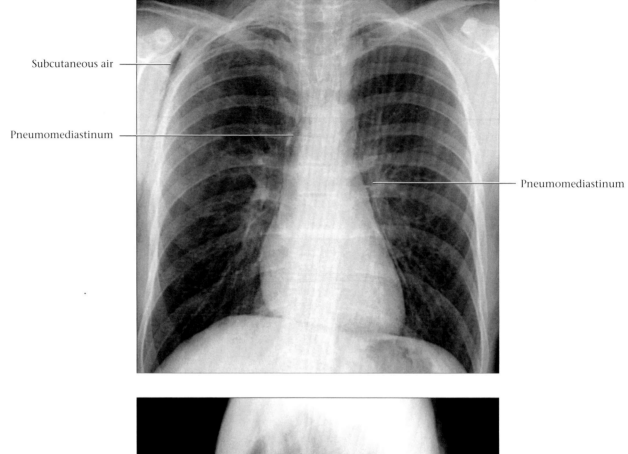

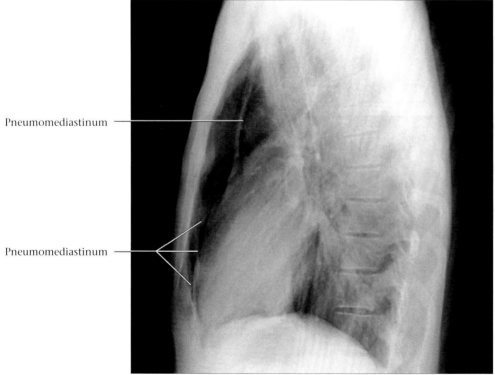

(Top) First of two images of a 19 year old man with a spontaneous pneumomediastinum and right pneumothorax shows air surrounding the heart and upper mediastinal structures. The PA chest radiograph shows subcutaneous air in the soft tissues of the neck and right axilla. The mediastinum communicates with the neck through the thoracic inlet as there are no defined tissue planes that compartmentalize the mediastinum. **(Bottom)** Left lateral chest radiograph demonstrates air in the anterior mediastinum outlining the anterior aspect of the heart and the great vessels. Spontaneous pneumomediastinum may result from an abrupt increase in intrapulmonary pressure and may occur in association with conditions such as asthma and obstructive lung disease. It may also occur as a complication of thoracic instrumentation.

MEDIASTINUM

CT, MEDIASTINAL LYMPH NODES

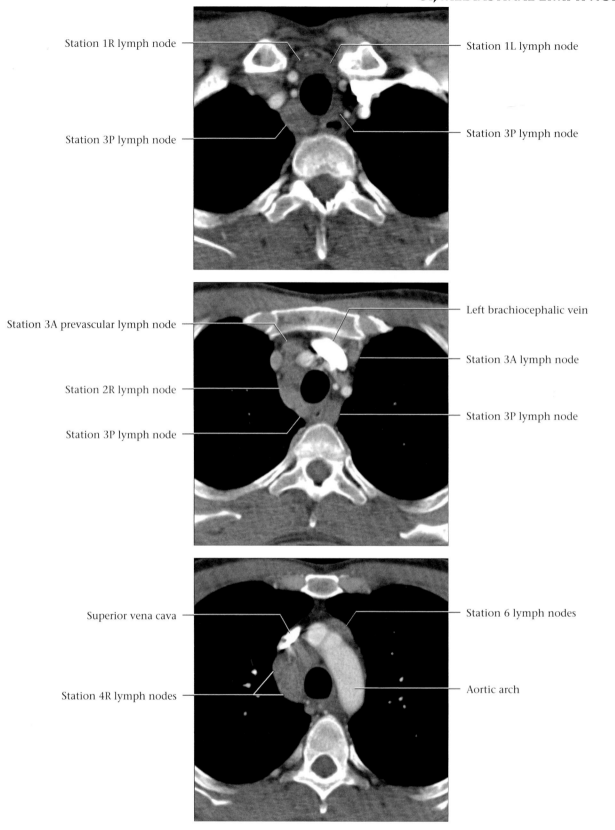

Station 1R lymph node

Station 3P lymph node

Station 1L lymph node

Station 3P lymph node

Station 3A prevascular lymph node

Station 2R lymph node

Station 3P lymph node

Left brachiocephalic vein

Station 3A lymph node

Station 3P lymph node

Superior vena cava

Station 4R lymph nodes

Station 6 lymph nodes

Aortic arch

(Top) First of nine contrast-enhanced chest CT images (mediastinal window) of a 56 year old man with non-Hodgkin lymphoma shows diffuse lymphadenopathy. Axial image through the superior mediastinum above the left brachiocephalic vein demonstrates prominent highest mediastinal (station 1) lymph nodes. There is also an enlarged right retrotracheal (3P) and a prominent left retrotracheal (3P) lymph node. **(Middle)** Axial image through the mid left brachiocephalic vein demonstrates enlargement of right upper paratracheal (station 2) lymph nodes as well as prominent retrotracheal (3P) lymph nodes. There are also prominent prevascular (station 3A) lymph nodes. **(Bottom)** Axial image through the superior aspect of the aortic arch demonstrates enlarged lower paratracheal (station 4R) lymph nodes and prominent para-aortic (station 6) lymph nodes.

MEDIASTINUM

CT, MEDIASTINAL LYMPH NODES

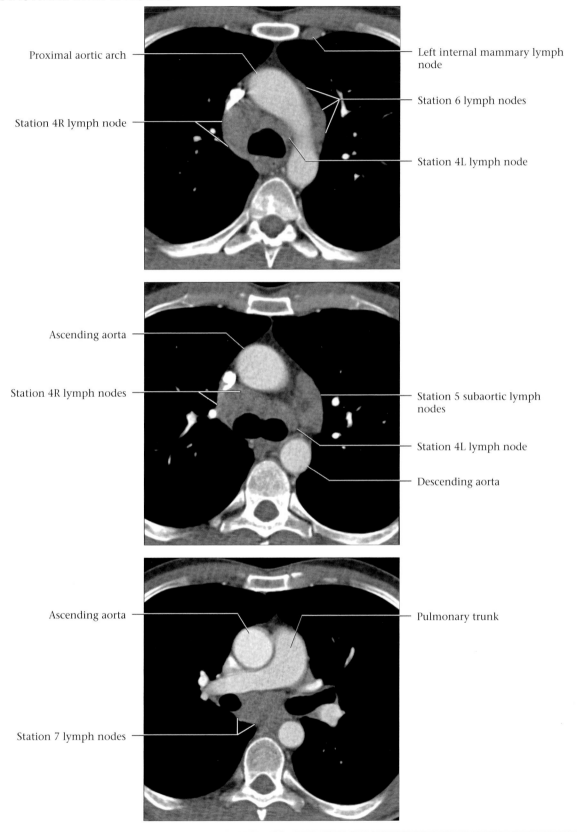

Proximal aortic arch

Left internal mammary lymph node

Station 4R lymph node

Station 6 lymph nodes

Station 4L lymph node

Ascending aorta

Station 4R lymph nodes

Station 5 subaortic lymph nodes

Station 4L lymph node

Descending aorta

Ascending aorta

Pulmonary trunk

Station 7 lymph nodes

(Top) Axial image through the inferior aspect of the aortic arch demonstrates enlargement of right and left lower paratracheal (station 4) lymph nodes as well as prominent para-aortic (station 6) lymph nodes. There is mild enlargement of a left internal mammary lymph node. (Middle) Axial image below the aortic arch demonstrates bilateral station 4 lower paratracheal lymphadenopathy. Station 5 subaortic (aortopulmonary window) lymphadenopathy is noted lateral to the expected location of the pulmonary ligament. (Bottom) Axial image obtained below the carina demonstrates abnormal soft tissue in the subcarinal region related to coalescent station 7 subcarinal lymphadenopathy.

MEDIASTINUM

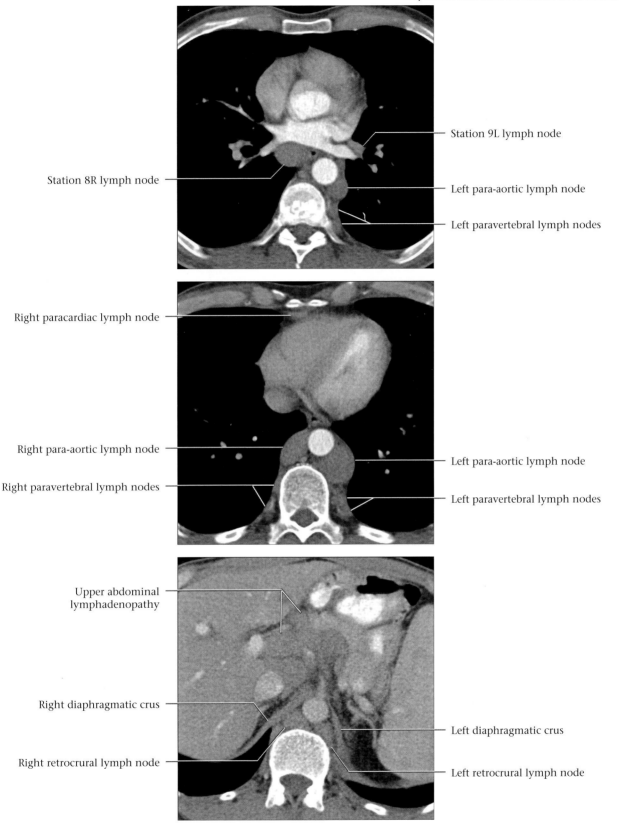

Station 9L lymph node

Station 8R lymph node

Left para-aortic lymph node

Left paravertebral lymph nodes

Right paracardiac lymph node

Right para-aortic lymph node

Left para-aortic lymph node

Right paravertebral lymph nodes

Left paravertebral lymph nodes

Upper abdominal lymphadenopathy

Right diaphragmatic crus

Left diaphragmatic crus

Right retrocrural lymph node

Left retrocrural lymph node

(Top) Axial image through the inferior aspect of the left atrium demonstrates a prominent left pulmonary ligament (station 9L) lymph node adjacent to the left inferior pulmonary vein. There is also enlargement of a right paraesophageal (station 8R) lymph node, a left para-aortic and several left paravertebral lymph nodes. (Middle) Axial image through the heart demonstrates lymphadenopathy surrounding the descending aorta. There is also lymphadenopathy in the bilateral paravertebral regions. Note the prominent right paracardiac lymph node in the right cardiophrenic angle. (Bottom) Axial image through the posterior lung bases shows lymphadenopathy in the bilateral retrocrural regions. There is also splenomegaly and upper abdominal lymphadenopathy.

MEDIASTINUM

PNEUMOMEDIASTINUM

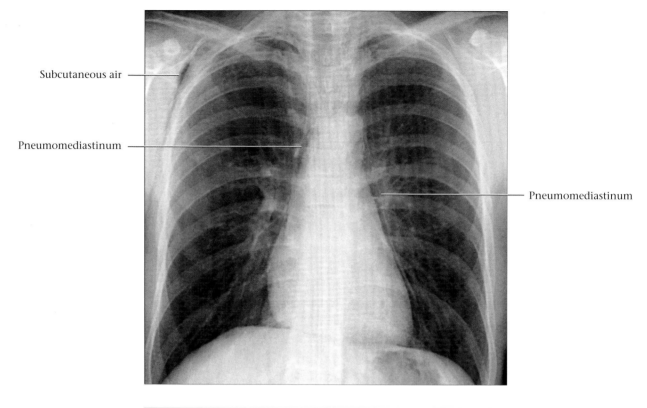

Subcutaneous air

Pneumomediastinum

Pneumomediastinum

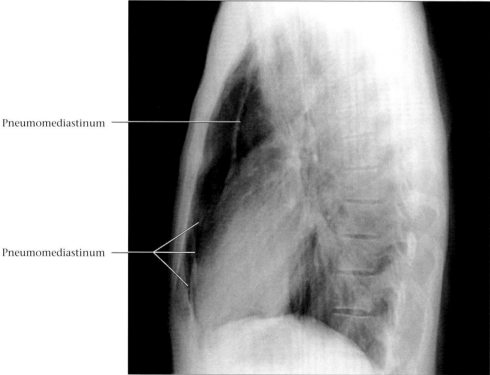

Pneumomediastinum

Pneumomediastinum

(Top) First of two images of a 19 year old man with a spontaneous pneumomediastinum and right pneumothorax shows air surrounding the heart and upper mediastinal structures. The PA chest radiograph shows subcutaneous air in the soft tissues of the neck and right axilla. The mediastinum communicates with the neck through the thoracic inlet as there are no defined tissue planes that compartmentalize the mediastinum. **(Bottom)** Left lateral chest radiograph demonstrates air in the anterior mediastinum outlining the anterior aspect of the heart and the great vessels. Spontaneous pneumomediastinum may result from an abrupt increase in intrapulmonary pressure and may occur in association with conditions such as asthma and obstructive lung disease. It may also occur as a complication of thoracic instrumentation.

MEDIASTINUM

FOCAL MEDIASTINAL ENLARGEMENT, MALIGNANT NEOPLASIA

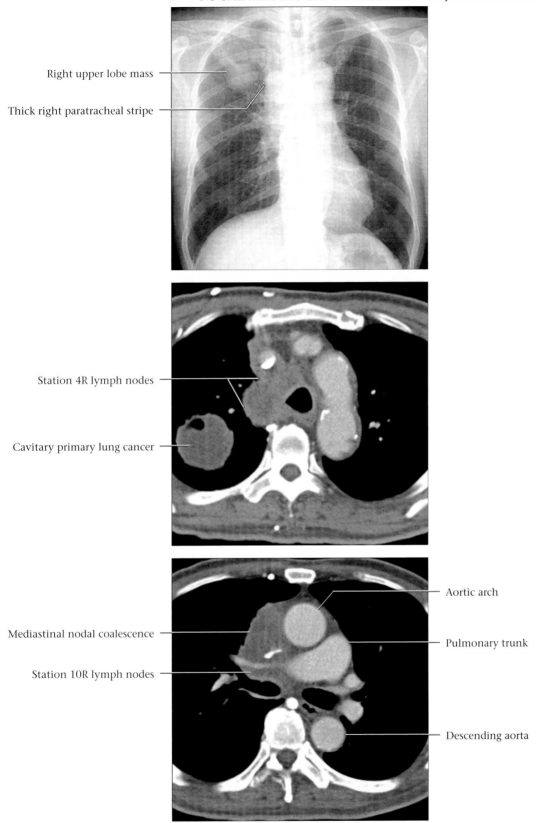

Right upper lobe mass

Thick right paratracheal stripe

Station 4R lymph nodes

Cavitary primary lung cancer

Aortic arch

Mediastinal nodal coalescence

Pulmonary trunk

Station 10R lymph nodes

Descending aorta

(Top) First of three images of a 67 year old man with advanced lung cancer. PA chest radiograph shows a right upper lobe mass and ipsilateral right mediastinal lymphadenopathy manifesting with lobular thickening of the right paratracheal stripe. (Middle) Contrast-enhanced chest CT (mediastinal window) through the aortic arch demonstrates a cavitary mass in the right upper lobe and right lower paratracheal (station 4R) lymphadenopathy. There is nodal coalescence and apparent extranodal neoplasm infiltrating the mediastinum and encasing the trachea. (Bottom) Axial image through the pulmonary trunk demonstrates the locally invasive mediastinal neoplasm encasing and nearly obstructing the superior vena cava and the right pulmonary artery. There is involvement of the right hilar (station 10R) lymph nodes.

MEDIASTINUM

DIFFUSE MEDIASTINAL ENLARGEMENT, MALIGNANT NEOPLASIA

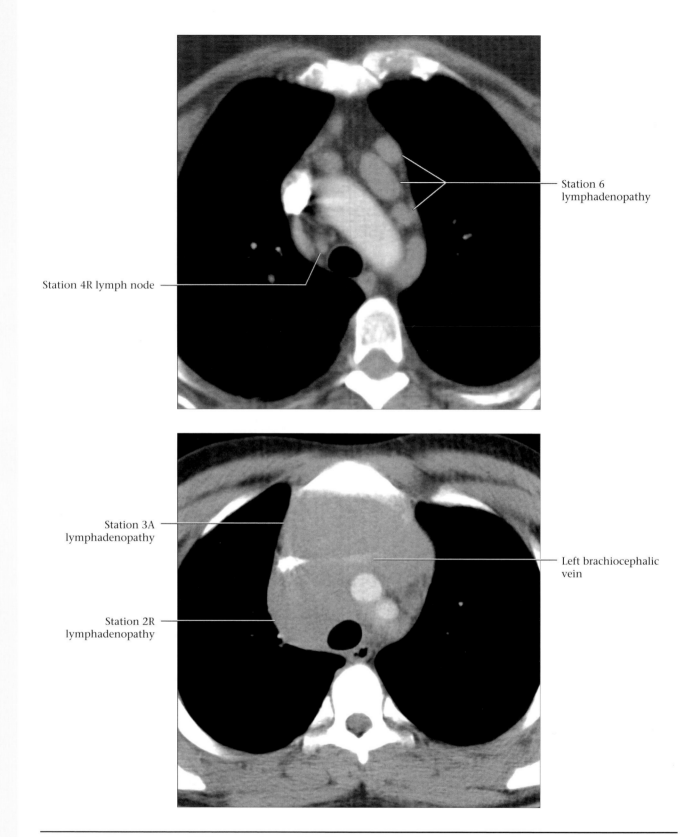

Station 6 lymphadenopathy

Station 4R lymph node

Station 3A lymphadenopathy

Station 2R lymphadenopathy

Left brachiocephalic vein

(Top) First of two images of different patients with diffuse mediastinal malignant lymphadenopathy exhibiting two different patterns of lymph node involvement. Contrast-enhanced chest CT (mediastinal window) through the aortic arch of a 62 year old woman with non-Hodgkin lymphoma demonstrates multiple discrete ovoid and rounded enlarged mediastinal lymph nodes in the para-aortic (station 6) and right lower paratracheal (station 4R) regions. **(Bottom)** Axial contrast-enhanced chest CT (mediastinal window) of a 20 year old man with Hodgkin lymphoma demonstrates diffuse mediastinal lymphadenopathy. Discrete lymph nodes are not visible. A diffuse infiltrative mediastinal soft tissue mass encases the left brachiocephalic vein and represents nodal coalescence. Involvement of at least two separate lymph node stations (2R and 3A) should suggest lymphadenopathy.

MEDIASTINUM

DIFFUSE MEDIASTINAL ENLARGEMENT, LIPOMATOSIS

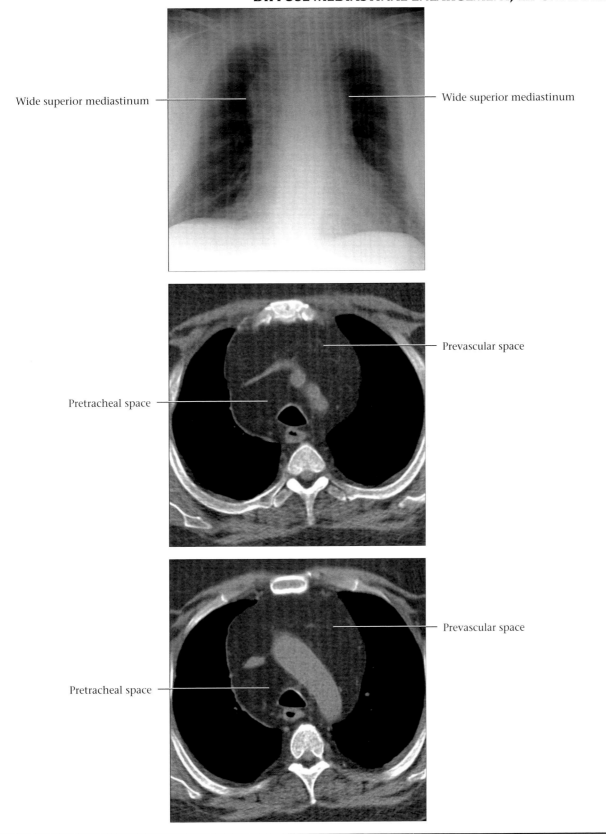

Wide superior mediastinum — Wide superior mediastinum

Prevascular space

Pretracheal space

Prevascular space

Pretracheal space

(Top) First of three images of a 41 year old man with mediastinal enlargement secondary to mediastinal lipomatosis. PA chest radiograph demonstrates diffuse bilateral mediastinal enlargement particularly affecting the superior mediastinum. (Middle) Nonenhanced chest CT (mediastinal window) demonstrates that the mediastinal enlargement is secondary to diffuse mediastinal fat deposition. Fat expands the lateral contours of the mediastinum and surrounds the vascular structures, trachea and esophagus without evidence of obstruction. (Bottom) Unenhanced chest CT (mediastinal window) through the aortic arch demonstrates diffuse mediastinal fat deposition. Mediastinal lipomatosis is the accumulation of unencapsulated non-neoplastic mediastinal fat and may result from obesity, or endogenous/exogenous hypercortisolism.

MEDIASTINUM

FOCAL MEDIASTINAL ENLARGEMENT, PRIMARY THYMIC NEOPLASM

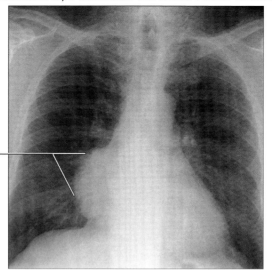

Right anterior mediastinal mass —

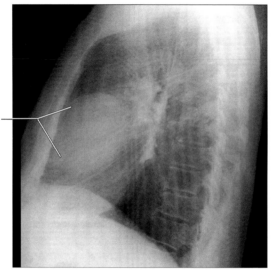

Right anterior mediastinal mass —

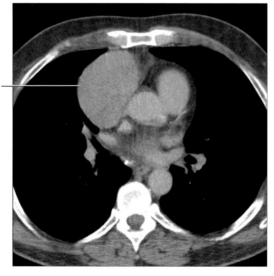

Right anterior mediastinal mass —

(Top) First of three images of an asymptomatic 63 year old man with an incidentally discovered thymoma. PA chest radiograph demonstrates a focal contour abnormality of the right inferior mediastinum obscuring the right cardiac border. (Middle) Left lateral chest radiograph demonstrates the anterior location of the mass which projects over the heart anterior to the posterior cardiac border in the radiographic anterior mediastinal compartment. (Bottom) Axial contrast-enhanced chest CT (mediastinal window) demonstrates an ovoid right anterior mediastinal soft tissue mass. A tissue plane is seen between the lesion and the adjacent vascular structures. Based on the demographic information, the focal unilateral nature of the lesion and the absence of lymphadenopathy, thymoma is the most likely diagnosis and was confirmed at surgery.

MEDIASTINUM

FOCAL MEDIASTINAL ENLARGEMENT, CONGENITAL LESION

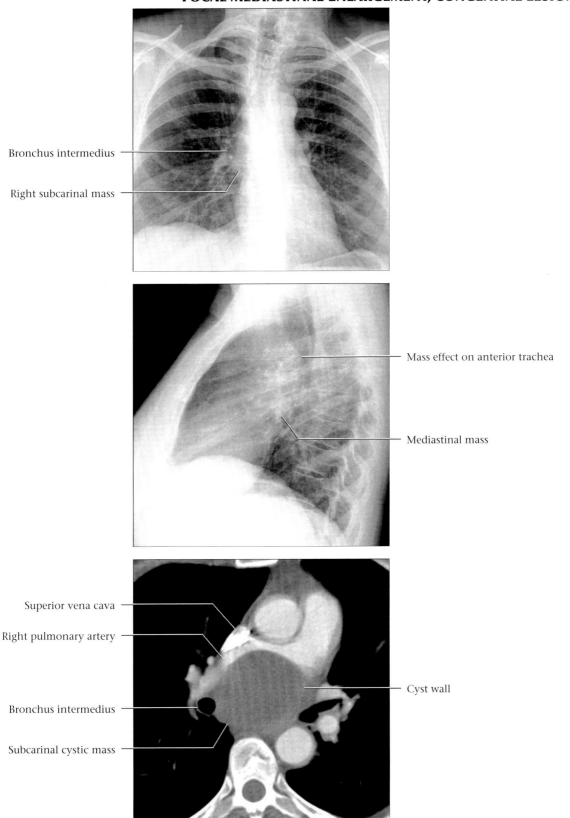

Bronchus intermedius

Right subcarinal mass

Mass effect on anterior trachea

Mediastinal mass

Superior vena cava

Right pulmonary artery

Cyst wall

Bronchus intermedius

Subcarinal cystic mass

(Top) First of three images of a 29 year old man with a bronchogenic cyst. PA chest radiograph demonstrates a soft tissue mass in the subcarinal region that produces mass effect on the medial aspect of the bronchus intermedius. **(Middle)** Left lateral chest radiograph demonstrates mass effect on the anterior aspect of the distal trachea. The mass extends into the anterior and middle-posterior radiographic mediastinal compartments. **(Bottom)** Contrast-enhanced chest CT (mediastinal window) demonstrates a large thin-walled cystic subcarinal mass which produces mass effect on the bronchus intermedius and the right pulmonary artery. The location and morphology of the lesion and its homogeneous non-enhancing water attenuation content are most consistent with congenital foregut cyst (in this case a bronchogenic cyst) confirmed at surgery.

FOCAL MEDIASTINAL ENLARGEMENT, GLANDULAR ENLARGEMENT

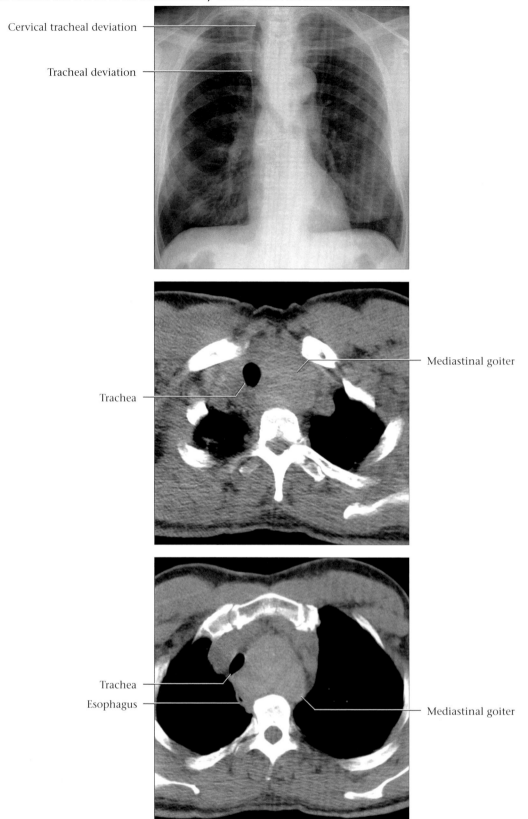

(Top) First of three images of a 70 year old man with a mediastinal goiter. PA chest radiograph demonstrates a left cervical soft tissue mass that extends inferiorly into the mediastinum. The lesion produces deviation of the trachea to the right above and below the thoracic inlet. (Middle) Unenhanced chest CT (mediastinal window) through the superior mediastinum demonstrates a polylobular soft tissue mass that deviates the trachea to the right and is continuous with the left lobe of the thyroid gland. (Bottom) Unenhanced chest CT (mediastinal window) demonstrates the intramediastinal extension of the cervical lesion which displaces the trachea and the esophagus to the left. The lesion exhibits a slightly higher attenuation than that of the adjacent soft tissues and vascular structures and subtle punctate calcifications.

MEDIASTINUM

FOCAL MEDIASTINAL ENLARGEMENT, HERNIATION

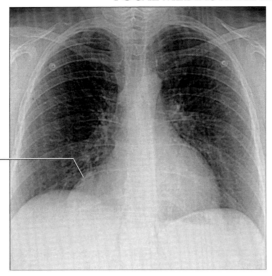

Right anterior mediastinal mass

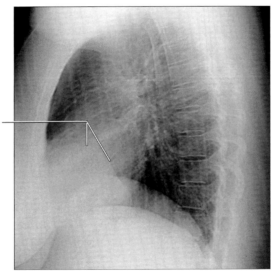

Right anterior mediastinal mass

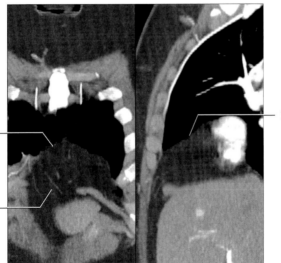

Morgagni hernia

Morgagni hernia

Right anterior diaphragmatic defect

(Top) First of three images of an asymptomatic 59 year old woman with a Morgagni hernia. PA chest radiograph demonstrates a right cardiophrenic angle anterior mediastinal mass with a well-defined rounded superior contour. The mass obscures the right cardiac border. **(Middle)** Left lateral chest radiograph shows that the lesion projects over the heart and is located in the radiographic anterior mediastinum. **(Bottom)** Composite image from a contrast-enhanced chest CT (mediastinal window) with coronal (left) and sagittal (right) reconstructions shows that the lesion represents herniation of omental fat through a diaphragmatic defect. The findings are consistent with the diagnosis of Morgagni hernia.

SYSTEMIC VESSELS

General Anatomy and Function

Anatomy
- Systemic arteries
  - **Thoracic aorta**
  - **Brachiocephalic trunk (artery)**
    - **Right common carotid artery**
    - **Right subclavian artery** (gives rise to **right vertebral artery**)
  - **Left common carotid artery**
  - **Left subclavian artery**
    - **Left vertebral artery**
- Systemic veins
  - **Right brachiocephalic vein**
  - **Left brachiocephalic vein**
  - Azygos system
    - **Azygos vein**
    - **Hemiazygos vein**
    - **Accessory hemiazygos vein**
  - **Superior vena cava**
  - **Inferior vena cava**
- Lymphatic vessels
  - **Thoracic duct**

Function
- Systemic arteries
  - Conduit and delivery of oxygenated blood from left heart to tissues
- Systemic veins
  - Conduit and delivery of deoxygenated blood from tissues to right heart

Systemic Arteries

Thoracic Aorta
- Anatomic divisions
  - **Ascending aorta**
  - **Aortic arch**
  - **Descending aorta**
- **Ascending aorta**
  - Originates at aortic orifice from **left ventricle**
  - Origin and proximal aspect within **pericardium**
  - Courses anterosuperiorly and to the right
  - Branches
    - **Coronary arteries**
  - Relationships
    - **Central location** with respect to other vascular structures
    - Anterior to left atrium, posterior to right ventricle
    - Medial to right atrium and left ventricle
- **Aortic arch**
  - Relationships
    - Ascends anterior to right pulmonary artery and tracheal carina
    - Apex on left side of distal trachea
    - Descends posterior to left hilum
  - **Ligamentum arteriosum**
    - Remnant of **ductus arteriosus** connecting superior aspect of **pulmonary trunk** to inferior aspect of **aortic arch**

- Connects pulmonary artery to aortic arch during embryonic/fetal circulation allowing blood to bypass lungs in utero; closes after birth
  - Branches
    - **Brachiocephalic artery**
    - **Left common carotid artery**
    - **Left subclavian artery**
- **Descending aorta**
  - Descends on left of midline
  - Exits thorax through **aortic hiatus** posterior to diaphragm
  - Branches
    - **Bronchial arteries**, variable number, supply right and left main bronchi
    - **Posterior intercostal arteries**
    - Pericardial, esophageal, mediastinal, superior phrenic and subcostal branches

Brachiocephalic Artery
- Relationships
  - **First branch of aortic arch**
  - Origin posterior to manubrium and left brachiocephalic vein, anterior to trachea
  - Ascends along right side of trachea toward right sternoclavicular joint where it bifurcates
- Branches
  - **Right common carotid artery**
    - Supplies right head and neck
  - **Right subclavian artery**
    - Supplies right upper extremity and upper thorax
    - Gives rise to **right vertebral artery**
  - Thyroid ima artery
    - Supplies thyroid gland

Left Common Carotid Artery
- Relationships
  - **Second branch of aortic arch**
  - Origin posterior to manubrium sternum, posterior and to the left of brachiocephalic trunk
  - Ascends anterior to left subclavian artery
  - Courses anterior and to the left of trachea

Left Subclavian Artery
- Relationships
  - **Third branch of aortic arch**
  - Ascends lateral to left aspect of trachea and left common carotid artery
  - Gives rise to **left vertebral artery**

Systemic Veins

Azygos System
- Drains posterior chest/abdominal walls and mediastinum
- May drain lower body in cases of inferior vena cava obstruction
- Azygos vein
  - Potential collateral pathway between **superior** and **inferior venae cavae** in cases of venous obstruction
  - Drains posterior chest and abdominal walls
  - Ascends on right side of anterior **T12** to **T5** vertebral bodies

SYSTEMIC VESSELS

- ○ Arches anteriorly at **T4** over **right main bronchus** to drain into posterior aspect of **superior vena cava**
- ○ Tributaries
  - **Posterior intercostal veins**; including **right superior intercostal vein** formed by second, third and fourth **intercostal veins**
  - **Hemiazygos** and **accessory hemiazygos veins**
  - Mediastinal, esophageal, pericardial and right bronchial veins
- **Hemiazygos vein**
  - ○ Ascends on left side of anterior **T12** to **T9** vertebral bodies
  - ○ Posterior to thoracic aorta as far as T9
  - ○ Crosses to the right to join azygos vein
  - ○ Tributaries
    - Inferior four or five left posterior intercostal veins
    - Esophageal and mediastinal veins
- **Accessory hemiazygos vein**
  - ○ Descends on left side of anterior **T4** to **T8** vertebral bodies
  - ○ **Frequently connects to azygos, hemiazygos** and left superior intercostal veins

Venae Cavae

- **Superior vena cava**
  - ○ Formed by anastomosis of **right** and **left brachiocephalic veins**
  - ○ Distal portion partially invested by **pericardium**
  - ○ Drains into the **right atrium**
  - ○ Tributaries
    - **Azygos vein**
- **Inferior vena cava**
  - ○ Courses through diaphragm to drain into **right atrium**; partially invested by **pericardium**

Brachiocephalic Veins

- **Right brachiocephalic vein**
  - ○ Formed by anastomosis of **right subclavian** and **right jugular veins**
  - ○ Origin posterior to medial right clavicle
  - ○ Vertical course to **superior vena cava**
  - ○ Tributaries
    - Vertebral vein
    - First posterior intercostal vein
    - Internal thoracic vein
    - Inferior thyroid and thymic veins
- **Left brachiocephalic vein**
  - ○ Formed by anastomosis of **left subclavian** and **left jugular veins**
  - ○ Origin posterior to medial left clavicle
  - ○ Crosses midline, courses to the right to anastomose with **left brachiocephalic vein** and form **superior vena cava**
  - ○ Tributaries
    - Vertebral vein
    - Left superior intercostal vein
    - Inferior thyroid vein
    - Internal thoracic vein
    - Thymic and pericardial veins

Left Superior Intercostal Vein

- Tributaries
  - ○ First two or three **left intercostal veins**
  - ○ Left bronchial veins

- ○ Left pericardiacophrenic vein
- Courses along left side of **aortic arch**
  - ○ Lateral to **left vagus nerve**
  - ○ Medial to **left phrenic nerve**
- Drains into **left brachiocephalic vein**
- May connect with **accessory hemiazygos vein**

Thoracic Lymphatics

Thoracic Duct
- Largest lymphatic channel
- Origin from **cisterna chyli**
- Ascends into thorax through **aortic hiatus**
- Crosses to the left at the T4, T5 or T6 vertebral bodies
- Drains near union of **left internal jugular** and **subclavian veins**; may drain into **left subclavian vein**
- Tributaries
  - ○ May receive **left jugular** and **left subclavian lymph trunks**
  - ○ Upper intercostal lymph trunks, posterior mediastinal lymph nodes
- Relationships
  - ○ Courses along anterior aspects of T12 to T6 vertebral bodies

Lymphatic Trunks
- Pulmonary lymphatics drain into **intrapulmonary (tracheobronchial)** and **mediastinal lymph nodes**
- Efferent lymphatic channels arise from lymph nodes, anastomose with other thoracic lymphatics
- **Right bronchomediastinal lymph trunk**
  - ○ Drains **right lung**, **left lower lobe** and mediastinum
- **Left bronchomediastinal lymph trunk**
  - ○ Drains **left upper lobe** and mediastinum

Radiography of the Great Vessels

PA Chest Radiograph
- **Superior vena cava interface**
  - ○ **Right superior mediastinum**
  - ○ Visualization of lateral border of **superior vena cava** above **azygos arch** and below thoracic inlet as it abuts mediastinal surface of **right upper lobe**
- **Azygos arch**
  - ○ Right superior mediastinum
  - ○ Ovoid opacity at **right tracheobronchial angle**
  - ○ Normal width of up to **10 mm**
- **Left subclavian artery interface**
  - ○ **Left superior mediastinum**
  - ○ Visualization of lateral border of **left subclavian artery** above **aortic arch** as it abuts mediastinal surface of left upper lobe
- **Vascular pedicle**
  - ○ Width of great vessels arising from the heart
  - ○ Measured from vertical line drawn from where **superior vena cava interface** crosses right main bronchus to point where **left subclavian artery** arises from **aortic arch**
    - Normal width of up to **58 mm**
- **Aortic arch interface**
  - ○ **Left superior mediastinum**

SYSTEMIC VESSELS

- Focal outward convexity at **left tracheobronchial angle** with mass effect on distal left tracheal wall
- **Left superior intercostal vein (aortic nipple)**
  - Left superior mediastinum
  - Rounded or triangular bulge of **aortic arch** contour; seen in < 5% of normal subjects
- **Left para-aortic interface**
  - Left mid and inferior mediastinum
  - Visualization of lateral wall of **descending aorta** from **aortic arch** to **diaphragm** as it abuts left mediastinal lung surface

Lateral Chest Radiograph

- **Ascending aorta**
  - May be visible in superior aspect of mediastinum on patients with aortic ectasia
- **Proximal descending aorta**
  - Visible in most individuals posterior to distal trachea
- **Inferior vena cava**
  - Convex, straight or concave interface posteroinferior to left ventricle

CT/MR of the Great Vessels

Supra-Aortic Mediastinum

- Great veins anterior and lateral to great arteries
- Great arteries (aortic branches) surround anterolateral trachea
- **Brachiocephalic veins**
  - **Right brachiocephalic vein**, shorter, vertical course
  - **Left brachiocephalic vein**, longer than right, horizontal or oblique course
- **Brachiocephalic artery**
  - Anterior to trachea, right of midline
- **Left common carotid artery**
  - Posterior and to the left of **brachiocephalic artery**
  - Smallest great artery at this level
- **Left subclavian artery**
  - Posterolateral or lateral to trachea

Aortic Arch Level

- **Aortic arch**
  - Proximal arch is anterior and to right of trachea
  - Courses posteriorly and to the left
  - Posterior arch is anterolateral to vertebral bodies
  - Proximal ascending aorta; average diameter of 3.6 cm (2.4-4.7 cm range)
  - Ascending aorta proximal to arch; average diameter of 3.5 cm (1.6-3.7 cm range)
- **Superior vena cava**
  - Ovoid or round morphology
  - Courses vertically anterior and to right of trachea
- Pericarinal and subcarinal region
  - **Azygos arch**
    - Courses anteriorly at **right tracheobronchial angle**
    - Drains into posterior aspect of **superior vena cava**
  - **Azygos vein**
    - Courses vertically along right anterolateral vertebral bodies
  - **Hemiazygos vein**
    - Courses vertically along left anterolateral vertebral bodies posterior to **descending aorta**

- Descending aorta
  - Courses along posterolateral aspect of the spine
  - **Mid descending aorta, 2.5 cm** diameter (1.6-3.7 cm range)
  - **Distal descending aorta, 2.4 cm** diameter (1.4-3.3 cm range)

Anatomy-Based Imaging Abnormalities

Aortic Arch Anomalies

- **Bovine arch**
  - **Left common carotid artery** originating from **brachiocephalic artery**
  - Most common great vessel anomaly, seen in up to **20% of population**
- **Aberrant right subclavian artery**
  - Seen in 0.4-2.3% of population, typically asymptomatic but may produce dyspnea/dysphagia
  - **Last aortic branch arising distal to left subclavian artery** coursing cephalad, posteriorly and to the right, usually **behind trachea and esophagus**
  - **Diverticulum of Kommerell**, focal dilatation of proximal **aberrant subclavian artery**, seen in **60% of cases**
- **Anomalous left vertebral artery**
  - Direct origin from aortic arch, seen in **10% of population**
- **Right aortic arch**
  - Seen in 0.1-0.2% of population
  - Mirror image great vessel branching associated with congenital heart disease
  - Non-mirror image great vessel branching, associated with **aberrant left subclavian artery**
- **Double aortic arch**
  - Seen in 0.05-0.3% of population, usually symptoms of stridor/dysphagia, may be asymptomatic
  - Most common complete vascular ring
  - **Right arch** gives off **right subclavian** and **right common carotid arteries**
    - Larger, extends more superiorly and posteriorly than **left arch**
  - **Left arch** gives off **left common carotid** and **left subclavian arteries**

Venous Anomalies

- **Persistent left superior vena cava**
  - Seen in 1-3% of population, usually asymptomatic
  - Arises from anastomosis of **left subclavian** and **left jugular veins**
    - Typically drains into **coronary sinus**
    - May coexist with a **right superior vena cava**, occasional venous connection between the two superior venae cavae
    - Vertical course, anomalous vessel anterior to normal **left superior pulmonary vein**
- **Azygos continuation of inferior vena cava**
  - Infrahepatic interruption of inferior vena cava with azygos continuation
  - **Enlarged azygos vein**, may mimic lymphadenopathy
  - Association with **situs ambiguus (polysplenia)**

SYSTEMIC VESSELS

OVERVIEW OF THE THORACIC SYSTEMIC VESSELS

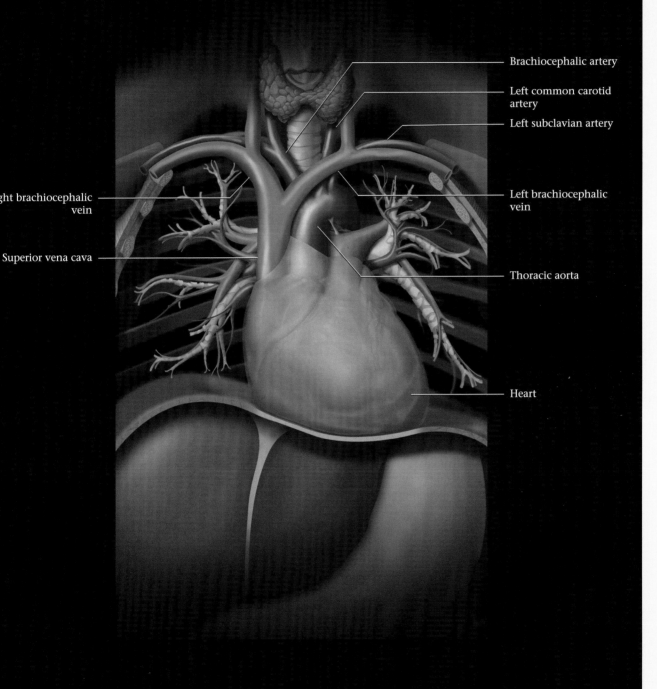

Brachiocephalic artery

Left common carotid artery

Left subclavian artery

Left brachiocephalic vein

Right brachiocephalic vein

Superior vena cava

Thoracic aorta

Heart

...phic depicts the anatomy of the principal systemic great vessels of the thorax and their relationship to the other ...racic structures. The vena cava transports de-oxygenated blood to the right heart chambers, which in turn deliver ... the alveolar-capillary interface via the pulmonary arteries. The superior vena cava is formed by the anastomosis ...the bilateral brachiocephalic veins. The thoracic aorta transports oxygenated blood from the left heart chambers to ... body. The three main branches of the thoracic aorta, the brachiocephalic, left common carotid and left ...bclavian arteries, supply the upper extremities, the thorax and the head and neck.

SYSTEMIC VESSELS

ANATOMY OF THE THORACIC SYSTEMIC VESSELS

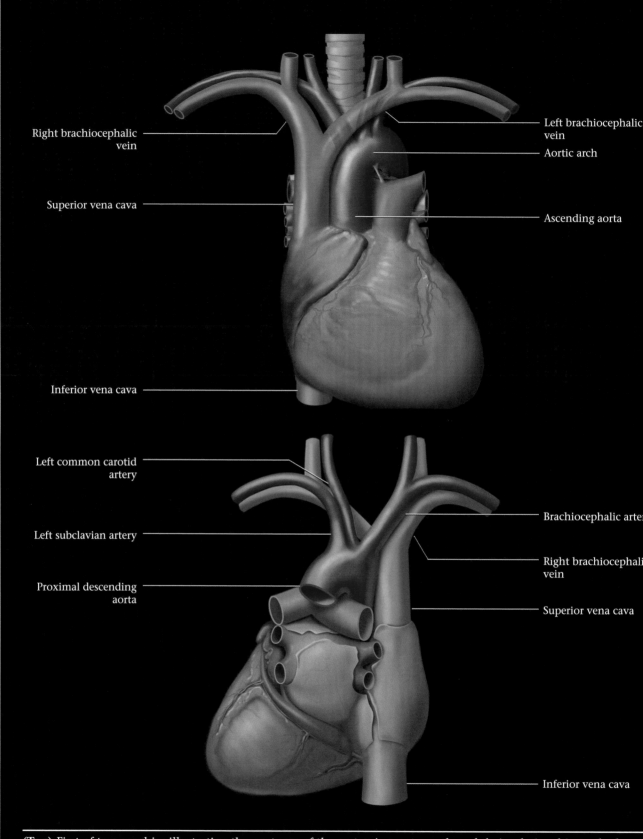

Right brachiocephalic vein

Superior vena cava

Inferior vena cava

Left brachiocephalic vein

Aortic arch

Ascending aorta

Left common carotid artery

Left subclavian artery

Proximal descending aorta

Brachiocephalic arte

Right brachiocephali vein

Superior vena cava

Inferior vena cava

(Top) First of two graphics illustrating the anatomy of the systemic great vessels and their relationship to the heart and the pulmonary vessels. Anterior view shows the superior vena cava formed by the anastomosis of the right and left brachiocephalic veins, which are located anterior to the branches of the aortic arch. The venae cavae drain into the right atrium. The proximal aorta is located centrally with respect to the surrounding vascular structures. Its ascending portion courses superiorly. The aortic arch gives off the brachiocephalic, left common carotid and left subclavian arteries in sequence. **(Bottom)** Graphic shows a posterior view of the great vessels. The superior and inferior vena cavae course into the right atrium. The branches of the aortic arch are located behind the anteriorly located great veins.

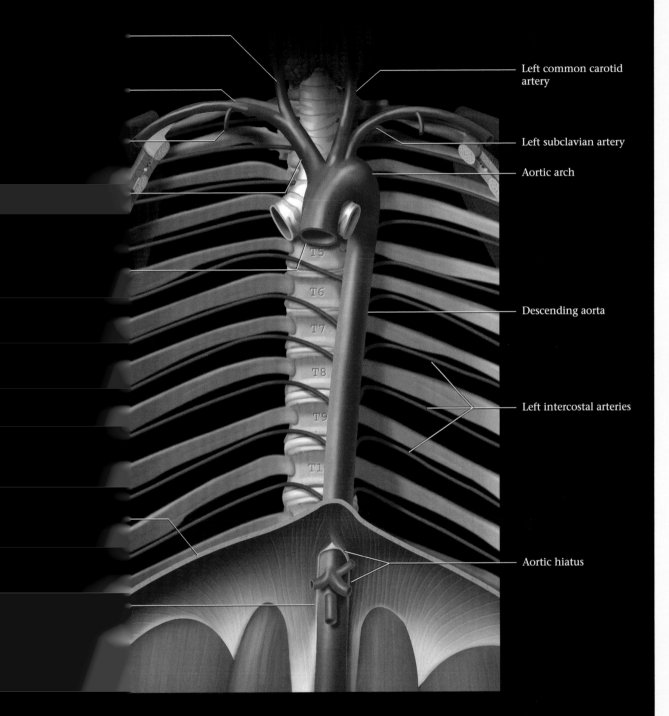

Left common carotid artery

Left subclavian artery

Aortic arch

T5

T6

T7

T8

T9

T1

Descending aorta

Left intercostal arteries

Aortic hiatus

...my of the thoracic aorta and its branches. The aorta has three major portions: ascending
...scending aorta. The ascending aorta courses superiorly and toward the left. The aortic arch
...eobronchial angle. The first branch of the aortic arch is the brachiocephalic artery followed
...tid and left subclavian arteries. These vessels supply the upper thorax, upper extremities and
...brachiocephalic artery gives rise to the right common carotid and right subclavian arteries.
...ve rise to the bilateral internal mammary arteries that supply the anterior chest wall and to

SYSTEMIC VESSELS

ANATOMY OF THE THORACIC SYSTEMIC VEINS

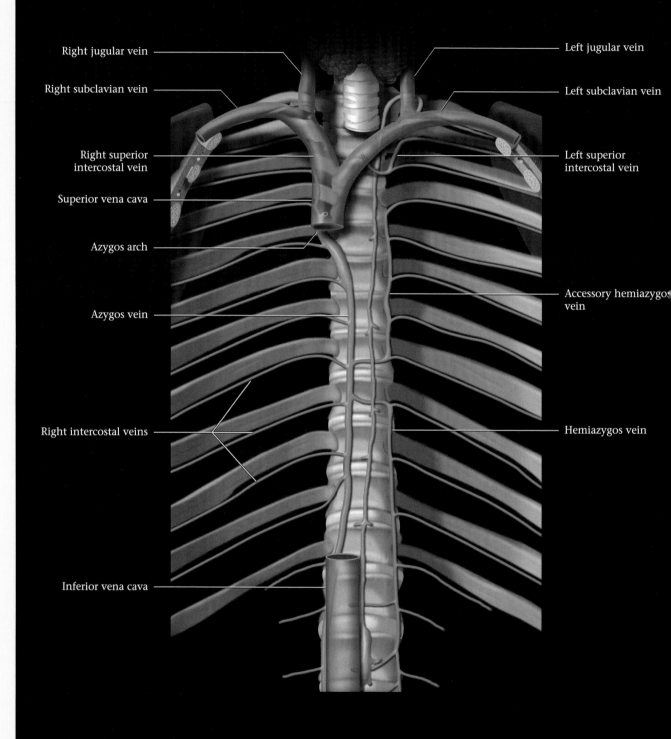

Graphic shows the anatomy of the thoracic systemic veins. The superior vena cava is formed by the anastomosis of the right and left brachiocephalic veins which in turn are formed by the anastomosis of the jugular and subclavian veins. The chest wall is drained by intercostal veins that course along the undersurfaces of the ribs and drain into the azygos vein on the right and the hemiazygos and accessory hemiazygos veins on the left. Venous anastomoses connect the azygos and hemiazygos veins. The first three left intercostal veins drain into the left superior intercostal vein that courses along the lateral aspect of the aortic arch to drain into the posterior aspect of the left brachiocephalic vein. The right superior intercostal vein, shown posterior to the superior vena cava and right brachiocephalic vein, receives the second third and fourth right intercostal veins.

SYSTEMIC VESSELS

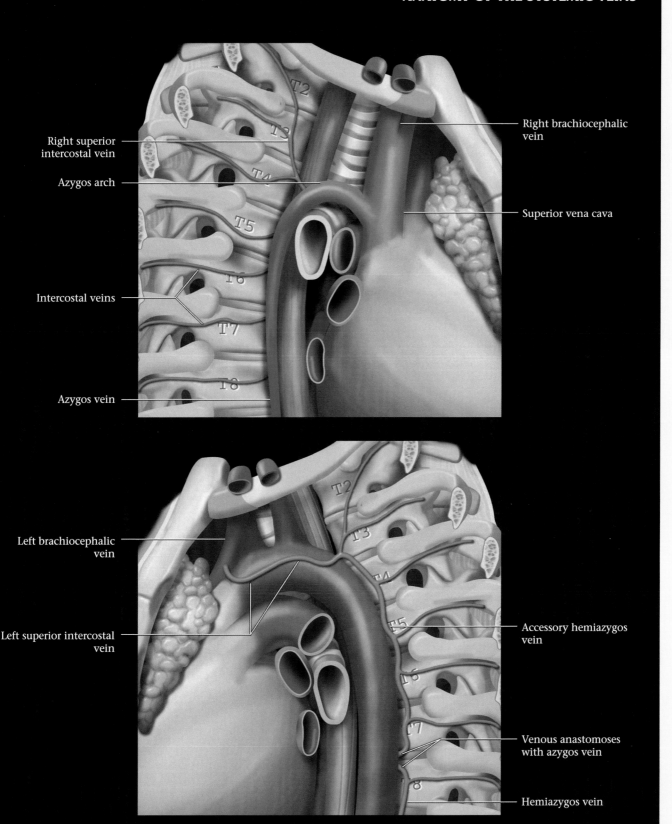

(Top) First of two graphics showing the anatomy of the azygos and hemiazygos venous systems. Illustration of the right mediastinal surface shows the intercostal veins draining into the azygos vein. The azygos arch courses over the right main bronchus to drain into the posterior aspect of the superior vena cava. The right superior intercostal vein is also shown. **(Bottom)** Illustration of the left mediastinal surface shows the intercostal veins draining into accessory hemiazygos and hemiazygos veins that communicate with the azygos vein through venous anastomoses. The left superior intercostal vein receives tributaries from the first three intercostal veins and courses along the lateral aspect of the aortic arch to drain into the left brachiocephalic vein. The left superior intercostal vein may be prominent in patients with venous obstruction and collateral flow.

SYSTEMIC VESSELS

RADIOGRAPHY, NORMAL SYSTEMIC VESSEL INTERFACES

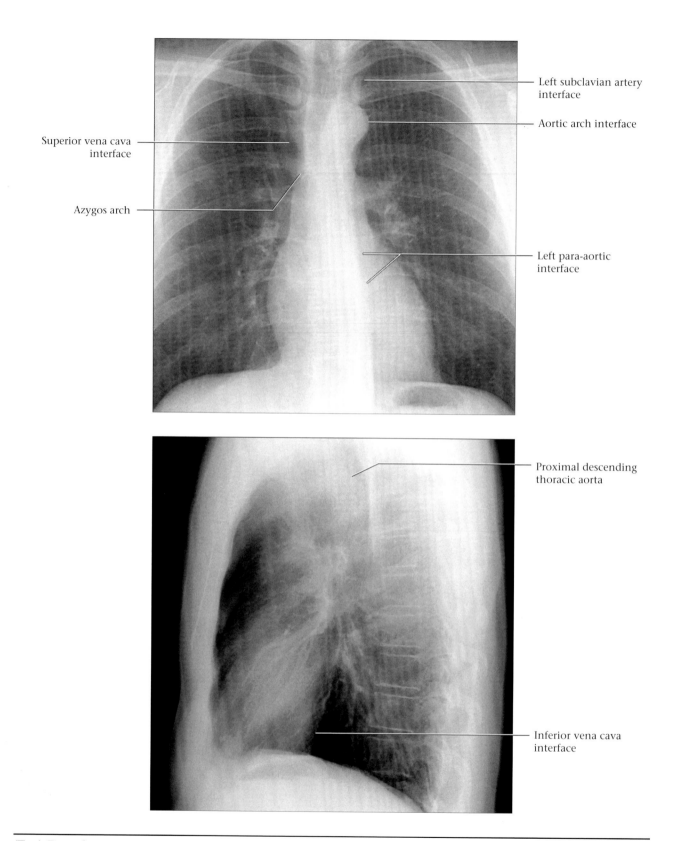

Left subclavian artery interface

Aortic arch interface

Superior vena cava interface

Azygos arch

Left para-aortic interface

Proximal descending thoracic aorta

Inferior vena cava interface

(Top) First of two normal chest radiographs of a middle-aged patient demonstrating the radiographic anatomy of the systemic great vessels. PA chest radiograph shows mild tortuosity of the thoracic aorta and a prominent aortic arch. The left subclavian artery interface is produced by contact with the adjacent mediastinal surface of the left upper lobe. The superior vena cava interface results from contact with the mediastinal surface of the right upper lobe. The left para-aortic interface is produced by contact between the left lateral descending aorta and the mediastinal surface of the left lung. **(Bottom)** Left lateral chest radiograph demonstrates the proximal aspect of the descending aorta and the inferior vena cava interface.

SYSTEMIC VESSELS

RADIOGRAPHY, NORMAL SYSTEMIC VESSEL INTERFACES

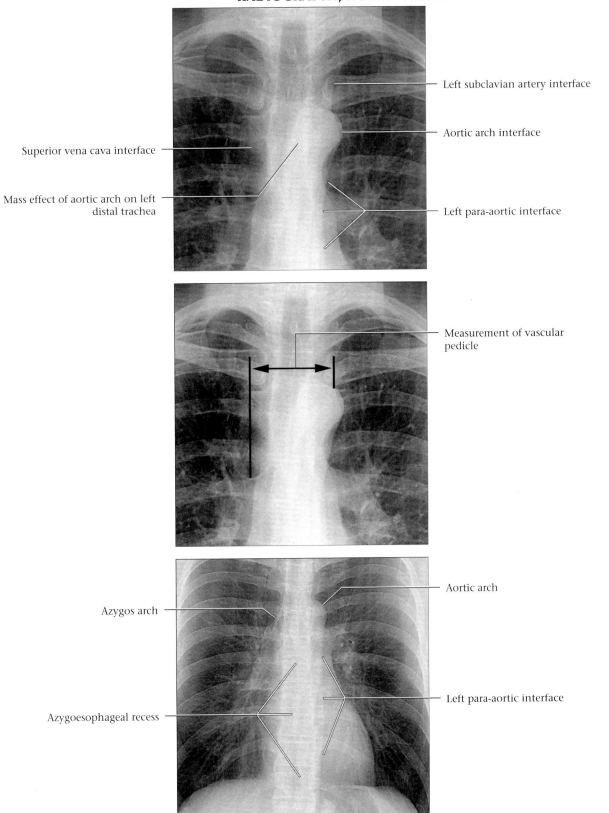

Left subclavian artery interface

Aortic arch interface

Superior vena cava interface

Mass effect of aortic arch on left distal trachea

Left para-aortic interface

Measurement of vascular pedicle

Aortic arch

Azygos arch

Left para-aortic interface

Azygoesophageal recess

(Top) Coned-down PA chest radiograph shows the superior vena cava interface and the aortic arch interface in the right and left superior mediastinum respectively. The left subclavian artery interface is seen in the left superior mediastinum where the vessel abuts the left mediastinal lung surface. (Middle) Coned-down PA chest radiograph illustrates the method for measuring the vascular pedicle, measured from a vertical line from where the superior vena cava interface crosses the right main bronchus to the point where the left subclavian artery arises from the aortic arch. (Bottom) PA chest radiograph shows the left para-aortic interface that results from contact of the vessel with the mediastinal surface of the left lung. The azygoesophageal recess results from contact of the medial right lung with the right retrocardiac mediastinum near the azygos vein and esophagus.

SYSTEMIC VESSELS

AXIAL CT, SYSTEMIC VESSELS

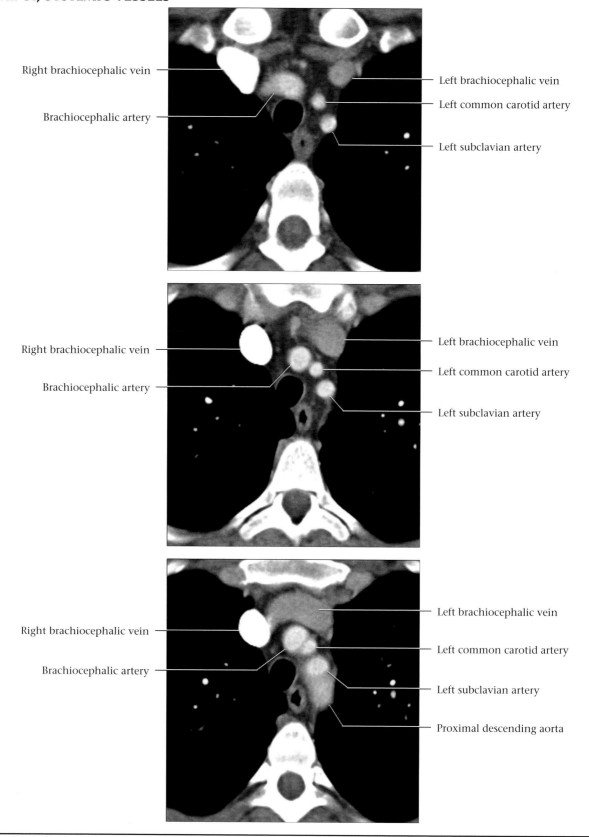

Right brachiocephalic vein

Brachiocephalic artery

Left brachiocephalic vein
Left common carotid artery

Left subclavian artery

Right brachiocephalic vein

Brachiocephalic artery

Left brachiocephalic vein

Left common carotid artery

Left subclavian artery

Right brachiocephalic vein

Brachiocephalic artery

Left brachiocephalic vein

Left common carotid artery

Left subclavian artery

Proximal descending aorta

(Top) First of nine axial contrast-enhanced chest CT images (mediastinal window) demonstrating the anatomy of the systemic great vessels. Image through the medial clavicles shows the bilateral brachiocephalic veins located anterior to the brachiocephalic, left common carotid and left subclavian arteries. **(Middle)** Image through the manubrium sternum shows the anteriorly located brachiocephalic veins. Note the oblique course of the left brachiocephalic vein compared to the vertical course of the right. The systemic arteries are located posterior to the veins. **(Bottom)** Image through the horizontal portion of the left brachiocephalic vein demonstrates its course towards the right brachiocephalic vein. The superior aspect of the aortic arch and the origins of its branches are also visualized.

SYSTEMIC VESSELS

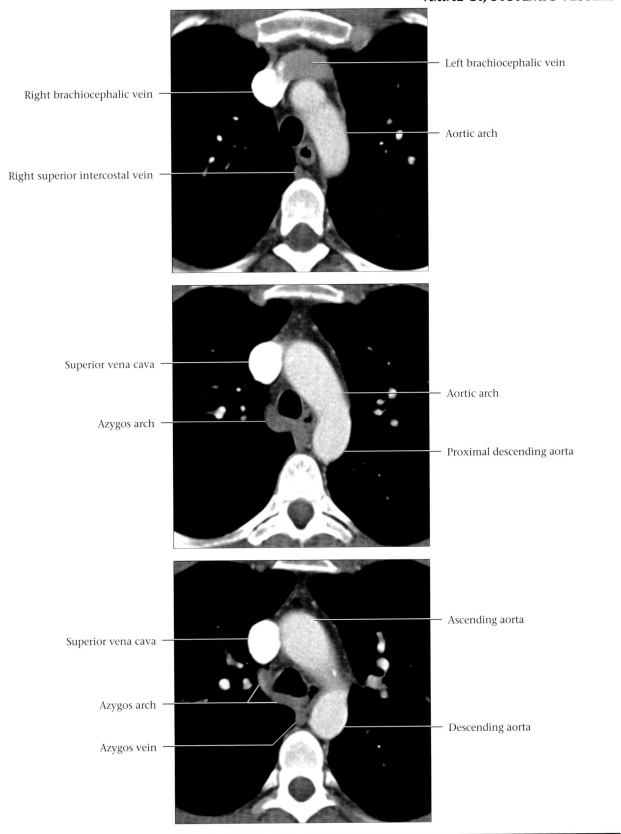

Right brachiocephalic vein

Right superior intercostal vein

Left brachiocephalic vein

Aortic arch

Superior vena cava

Azygos arch

Aortic arch

Proximal descending aorta

Superior vena cava

Azygos arch

Azygos vein

Ascending aorta

Descending aorta

(Top) Image through the aortic arch demonstrates the anastomosis of the left and right brachiocephalic veins to form the superior vena cava. The right superior intercostal vein is seen just anterior to an upper thoracic vertebral body to the right of midline. **(Middle)** Image through the mid aortic arch demonstrates the superior vena cava abutting the right upper lobe and the azygos arch which courses above the right main bronchus. The aortic arch courses over the left main bronchus. **(Bottom)** Image through the inferior portion of the aortic arch demonstrates the azygos arch which courses over the right main bronchus to drain into the posterior aspect of the superior vena cava. The ascending and descending aortas leading to and from the aortic arch respectively are also seen.

SYSTEMIC VESSELS

AXIAL CT, SYSTEMIC VESSELS

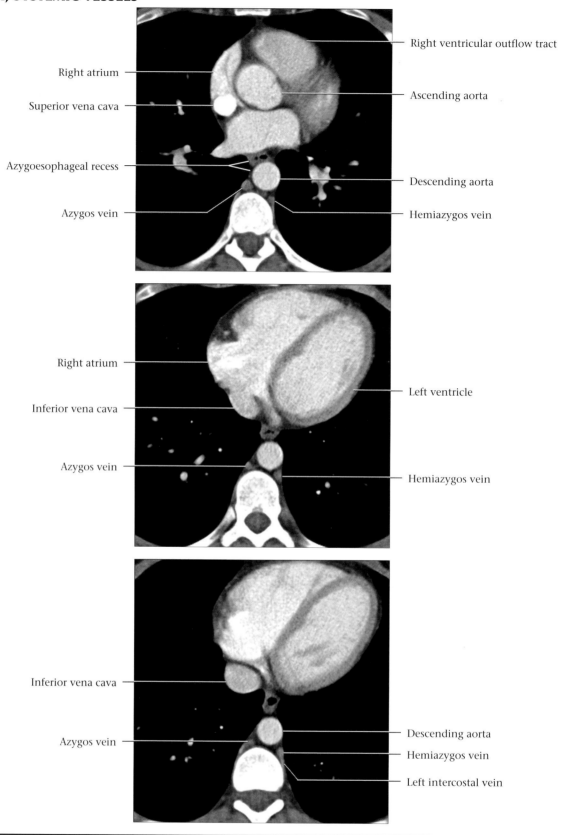

Right atrium

Superior vena cava

Azygoesophageal recess

Azygos vein

Right ventricular outflow tract

Ascending aorta

Descending aorta

Hemiazygos vein

Right atrium

Inferior vena cava

Azygos vein

Left ventricle

Hemiazygos vein

Inferior vena cava

Azygos vein

Descending aorta

Hemiazygos vein

Left intercostal vein

(Top) Image through the superior aspect of the heart demonstrates the central location of the ascending aorta with respect to the great vessels and cardiac chambers. The distal superior vena cava is seen draining into the right atrium. The azygos and hemiazygos veins are located posterior to the descending aorta on the anterior aspects of the vertebral bodies. (Middle) Image through the mid portion of the heart shows the inferior vena cava draining into the right atrium. The azygos and hemiazygos veins are seen posterior and lateral to the descending aorta. (Bottom) Axial image through sythe inferior aspect of the heart shows the inferior vena cava. Bilateral intercostal veins drain into the azygos and hemiazygos veins.

SYSTEMIC VESSELS

CORONAL CT, SYSTEMIC VESSELS

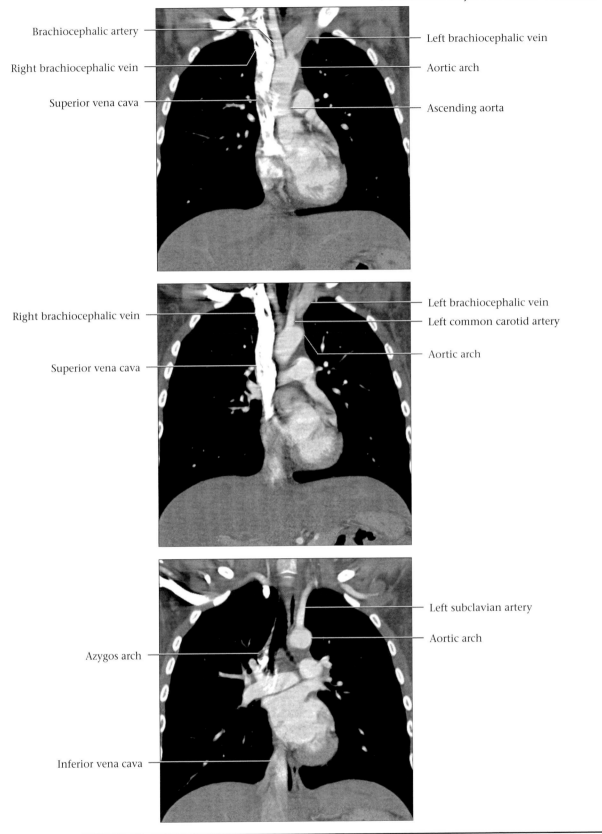

Brachiocephalic artery

Right brachiocephalic vein

Superior vena cava

Left brachiocephalic vein

Aortic arch

Ascending aorta

Right brachiocephalic vein

Superior vena cava

Left brachiocephalic vein

Left common carotid artery

Aortic arch

Azygos arch

Inferior vena cava

Left subclavian artery

Aortic arch

(Top) First of six coronal contrast-enhanced chest CT images (mediastinal window) showing the anatomy of the thoracic systemic vessels. Image through the anterior great vessels shows the anterior location of the brachiocephalic veins which anastomose to form the superior vena cava. The ascending aorta is located centrally. The aortic arch is partially visualized as is its first branch, the brachiocephalic artery. **(Middle)** Image through the mid superior vena cava shows the anatomic correlate of the superior vena cava interface seen on radiography, produced by contact of the vessel with the adjacent right lung. The left common carotid artery courses superiorly and to the left of the trachea. **(Bottom)** Image through the posterior arch shows the anatomic correlate of the aortic arch and left subclavian artery interfaces. The azygos arch and the inferior vena cava are also seen.

SYSTEMIC VESSELS

CORONAL CT, SYSTEMIC VESSELS

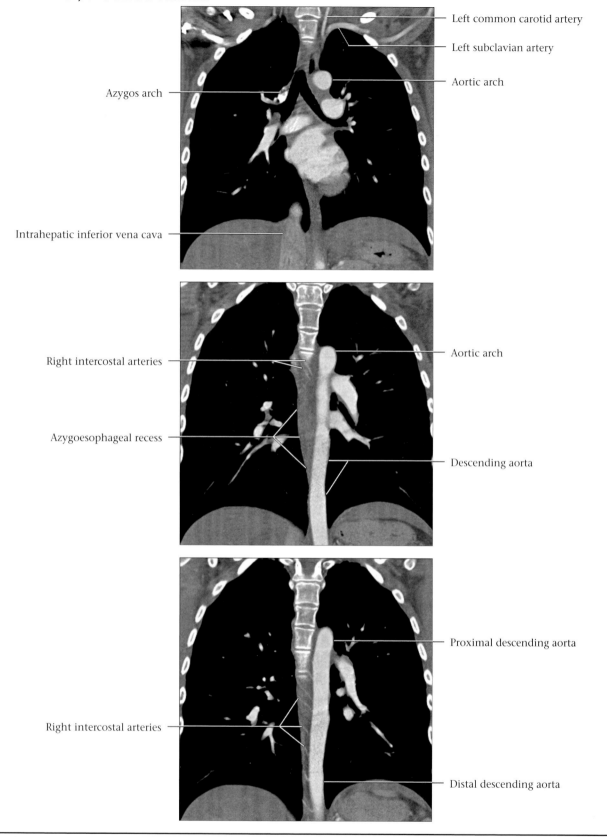

Left common carotid artery

Left subclavian artery

Aortic arch

Azygos arch

Intrahepatic inferior vena cava

Right intercostal arteries

Aortic arch

Azygoesophageal recess

Descending aorta

Right intercostal arteries

Proximal descending aorta

Distal descending aorta

(Top) Image through the carina demonstrates the dorsal aspect of the aortic arch which contacts the adjacent left lung to form the aortic arch interface. The azygos arch is located at the right tracheobronchial angle. The distal left common carotid and subclavian arteries are also imaged. **(Middle)** Image through the anterior aspect of the descending aorta shows several right intercostal arteries. The course of the unopacified azygos vein is also seen. The azygoesophageal recess seen on radiography results from contact of the right lung with the right retrocardiac mediastinum. It may exhibit a gentle lateral convexity as illustrated in this image. **(Bottom)** Image through the posterior aspect of the descending aorta demonstrates the anatomic correlate of the left para-aortic interface that results from contact of the vessel with the left mediastinal lung surface.

SYSTEMIC VESSELS

CORONAL, SAGITTAL & VOLUME RENDERED CT, SYSTEMIC VEINS

Azygos arch

Azygos vein

Azygos vein

Accessory hemiazygos vein

Anastomoses with azygos vein

Hemiazygos vein

Superior vena cava

Inferior vena cava

Azygos arch

Azygos vein

Azygos arch

Azygos vein

Anastomosis between azygos & hemiazygos veins

Descending aorta

Hemiazygos vein

(Top) First of three contrast-enhanced chest CT images (mediastinal window) demonstrating the anatomy of the systemic veins of the thorax. Coronal image through the azygos vein demonstrates a portion of the azygos arch and the course of the azygos vein in the right mediastinum. The accessory hemiazygos and hemiazygos veins are also seen. Note anastomoses of the azygos vein with the hemiazygos and accessory hemiazygos veins. (Middle) Sagittal image through the azygos vein shows the azygos arch draining into the dorsal aspect of the superior vena cava. The superior and inferior venae cavae are seen draining into the right atrium. (Bottom) Volume rendered coronal image through the azygos vein shows its vertical course in the right mediastinum and a portion of the azygos arch. The hemiazygos vein is partially obscured by the descending aorta.

SYSTEMIC VESSELS

SAGITTAL MR, THORACIC AORTA & BRANCHES

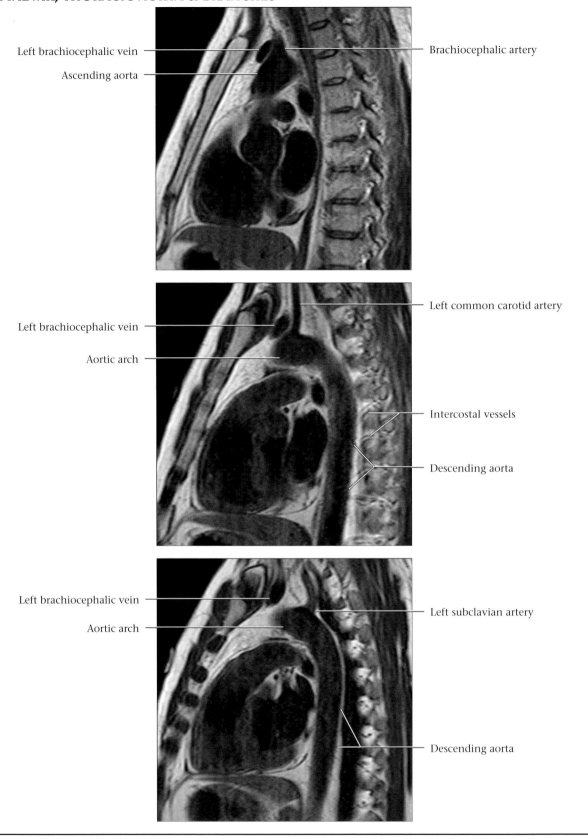

Left brachiocephalic vein

Ascending aorta

Brachiocephalic artery

Left common carotid artery

Left brachiocephalic vein

Aortic arch

Intercostal vessels

Descending aorta

Left brachiocephalic vein

Aortic arch

Left subclavian artery

Descending aorta

(Top) First of three sagittal T1-weighted magnetic resonance images through the aorta and its branches demonstrates the normal anatomy of these vessels. The distal ascending aorta and proximal arch are imaged as is the origin of the brachiocephalic artery. Note the anterior location and horizontal course of the left brachiocephalic vein imaged in cross-section. **(Middle)** Image through the mid aortic arch demonstrates the origin and course of the left common carotid artery, the second branch of the aortic arch. The descending thoracic aorta and some of its intercostal branches are seen. **(Bottom)** Image through the distal aspect of the aortic arch demonstrates the origin of the left subclavian artery, the last branch of the aortic arch. The descending aorta is also visualized.

SYSTEMIC VESSELS

CORONAL & SAGITTAL MR, AZYGOS VEIN

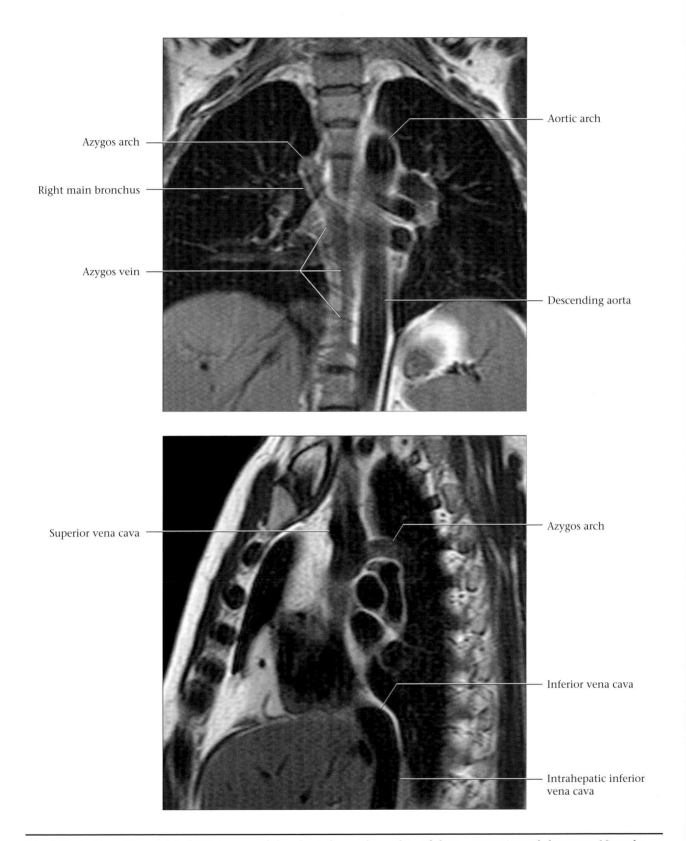

Azygos arch

Right main bronchus

Azygos vein

Aortic arch

Descending aorta

Superior vena cava

Azygos arch

Inferior vena cava

Intrahepatic inferior vena cava

(Top) First of two T1-weighted MR images of the chest shows the arches of the azygos vein and the aorta. Note the oblique vertical course of the azygos vein in the right retrocardiac mediastinum and the anatomic basis for the morphology of the azygoesophageal recess seen on radiography. The azygos arch courses over the right main bronchus. The distal descending aorta is also seen. **(Bottom)** Sagittal image through the azygos arch demonstrates its course over the right hilum to drain into the posterior aspect of the superior vena cava. The intrahepatic and intrathoracic portions of the inferior vena cava are also seen.

SYSTEMIC VESSELS

RADIOGRAPHY & CT, LEFT SUPERIOR INTERCOSTAL VEIN (AORTIC NIPPLE)

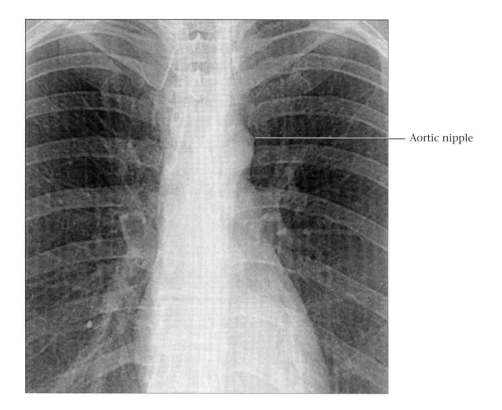

Aortic nipple

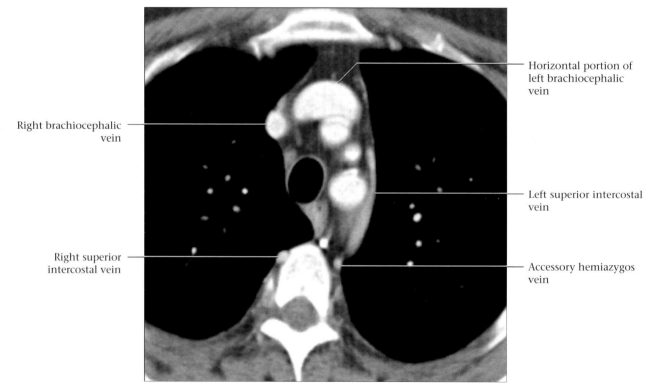

Horizontal portion of left brachiocephalic vein

Right brachiocephalic vein

Left superior intercostal vein

Right superior intercostal vein

Accessory hemiazygos vein

(**Top**) Coned-down normal PA chest radiograph demonstrates a small nodular bulge of the superolateral aspect of the aortic arch interface that corresponds to the left superior intercostal vein as it courses lateral and slightly superior to the aortic arch. This structure, also known as the aortic nipple based on its morphology, is seen in 5% of normal subjects. (**Bottom**) Contrast-enhanced chest CT (mediastinal window) of another patient demonstrates the anatomic basis for visualization of the so-called aortic nipple on radiography. The left superior intercostal vein courses along or slightly superior to the left lateral aspect of the aortic arch and may manifest as a contour irregularity of the aortic arch on radiography. The left superior intercostal vein receives the first three or four intercostal veins and usually anastomoses with the accessory hemiazygos vein.

AORTOGRAPHY

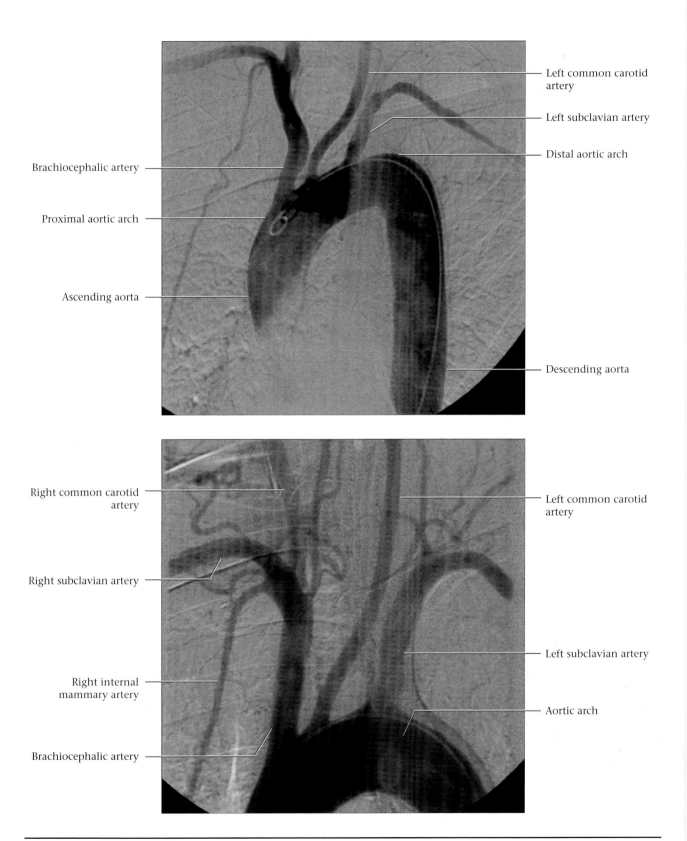

Left common carotid artery

Left subclavian artery

Distal aortic arch

Brachiocephalic artery

Proximal aortic arch

Ascending aorta

Descending aorta

Right common carotid artery

Left common carotid artery

Right subclavian artery

Left subclavian artery

Right internal mammary artery

Aortic arch

Brachiocephalic artery

(Top) Oblique thoracic aortogram demonstrates the anatomy of the aortic arch and its branches. Contrast was injected into the distal ascending aorta. The aortic arch and its branches are opacified. The first branch is the brachiocephalic artery, followed by the left symmon carotid and left subclavian arteries. The irregular contour of the descending aorta and the luminal narrowing of the left subclavian artery were secondary to atherosclerosis. **(Bottom)** Oblique thoracic aortogram demonstrates the normal branching pattern of the aortic arch. The first branch is the brachiocephalic artery which gives rise to the right subclavian and right common carotid arteries. The left common carotid and left subclavian arteries are the second and third aortic branches respectively. The right internal mammary artery, a branch of the right subclavian artery is also visualized.

SYSTEMIC VESSELS

GRAPHIC & CORONAL CT, BRONCHIAL ARTERIES

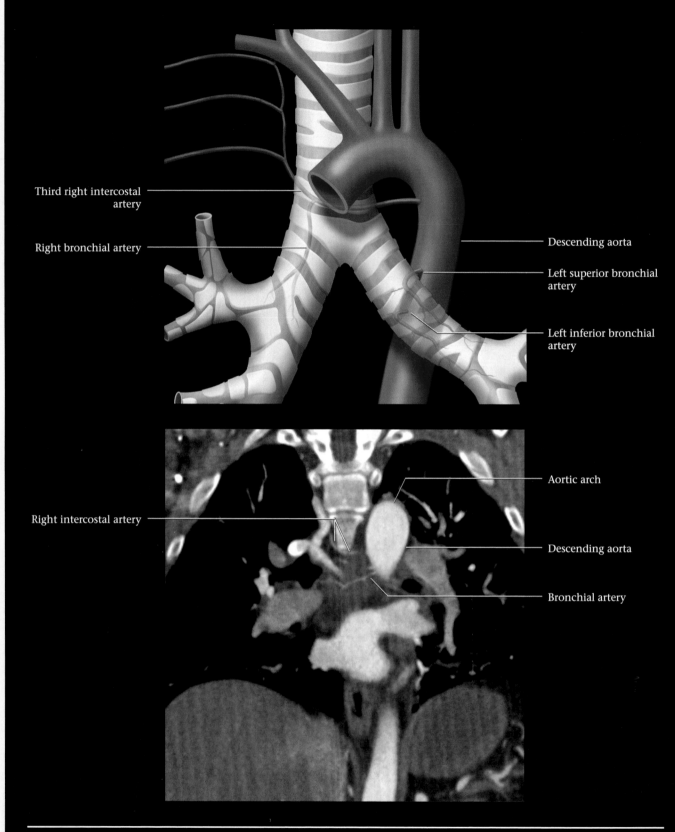

Third right intercostal artery

Right bronchial artery

Descending aorta

Left superior bronchial artery

Left inferior bronchial artery

Right intercostal artery

Aortic arch

Descending aorta

Bronchial artery

(Top) Graphic depicts a common variation of the anatomy of the bronchial arteries. In this illustration, the right bronchial artery arises from the third right intercostal artery and supplies the wall of the right main bronchus. Superior and inferior left bronchial arteries arise from the descending thoracic aorta and supply the wall of the left main bronchus. **(Bottom)** Contrast-enhanced chest CT (mediastinal window) of a 46 year old man with abdominal arterial thrombosis (not shown) demonstrates partial visualization of the bronchial arteries. Coronal image obtained posterior to the tracheal carina demonstrates several small branches of the descending thoracic aorta. One of the branches courses anteriorly to supply the right main bronchus. A right intercostal artery is also shown.

SYSTEMIC VESSELS

ANATOMIC VARIANTS OF THE BRONCHIAL ARTERIES

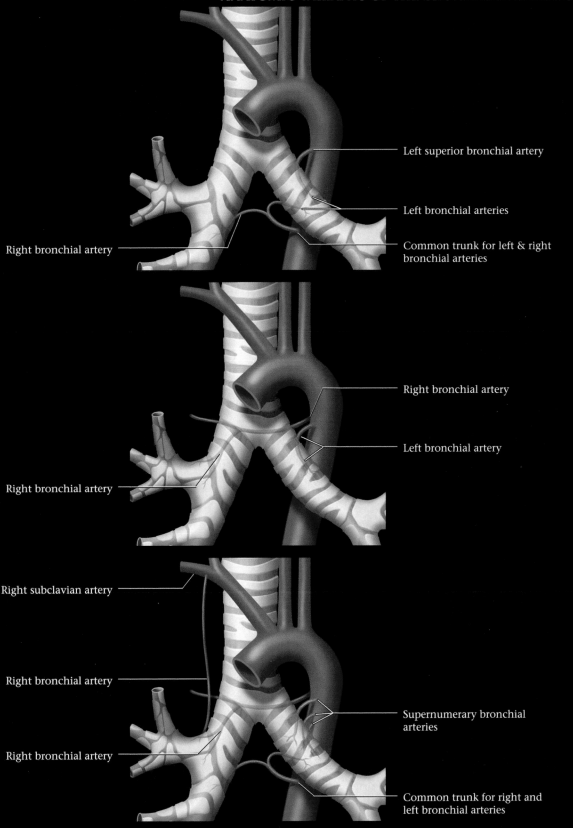

Left superior bronchial artery

Left bronchial arteries

Common trunk for left & right bronchial arteries

Right bronchial artery

Right bronchial artery

Left bronchial artery

Right bronchial artery

Right subclavian artery

Right bronchial artery

Supernumerary bronchial arteries

Right bronchial artery

Common trunk for right and left bronchial arteries

(Top) First of three graphics illustrating anatomic variations of the bronchial arteries. In this illustration the left superior bronchial artery supplies the left main bronchus. The left inferior bronchial artery also supplies the left main bronchus but gives off a right bronchial artery that supplies the right main bronchus. (Middle) Graphic shows single bronchial arteries arising from the descending aorta to supply the right and left main bronchi. (Bottom) Graphic shows several supernumerary bronchial arteries supplying the right and left main bronchi. There is also an inferior bronchial artery with branches to the right and left main bronchi and a right bronchial artery originating from the right subclavian artery.

ANATOMY OF THE THORACIC LYMPHATICS

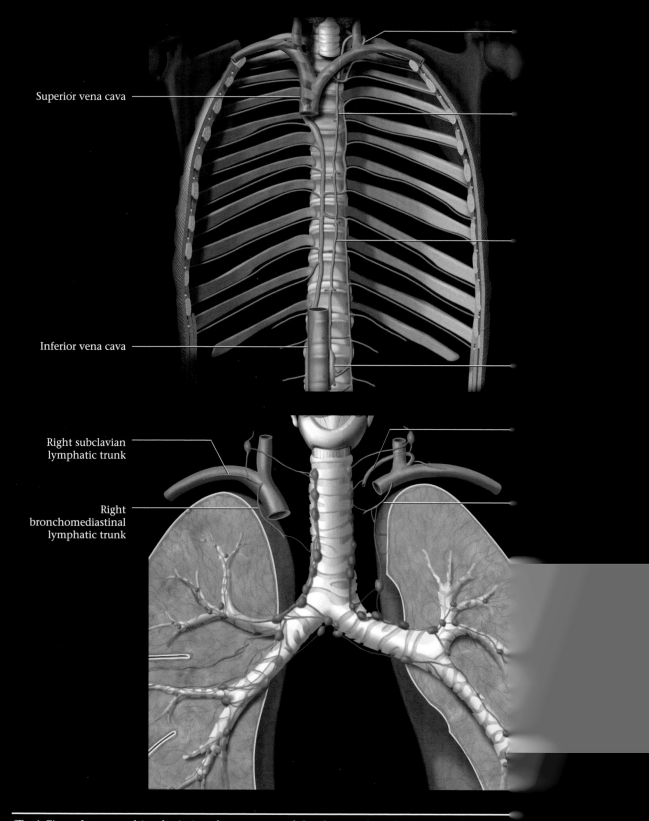

Superior vena cava

Inferior vena cava

Right subclavian
lymphatic trunk

Right
bronchomediastinal
lymphatic trunk

(Top) First of two graphics depicting the anatomy of the thoracic lymphatics. The thoracic c
cisterna chyli located at the level of the L2 vertebra. It courses superiorly and to the left of m
aspect of the spine to drain near the anastomosis of the left internal jugular and subclavian
depicts the lymphatic drainage of the thorax. The right bronchomediastinal lymphatic trun
subclavian and jugular trunks as the right lymphatic duct which drains into the proximal as
brachiocephalic vein. The thoracic duct drains into the posterior aspect of the junction of th
and subclavian veins. The left bronchomediastinal lymphatic trunk drains into the left brac

SYSTEMIC VESSELS

LYMPHANGIOGRAPHY, THORACIC DUCT

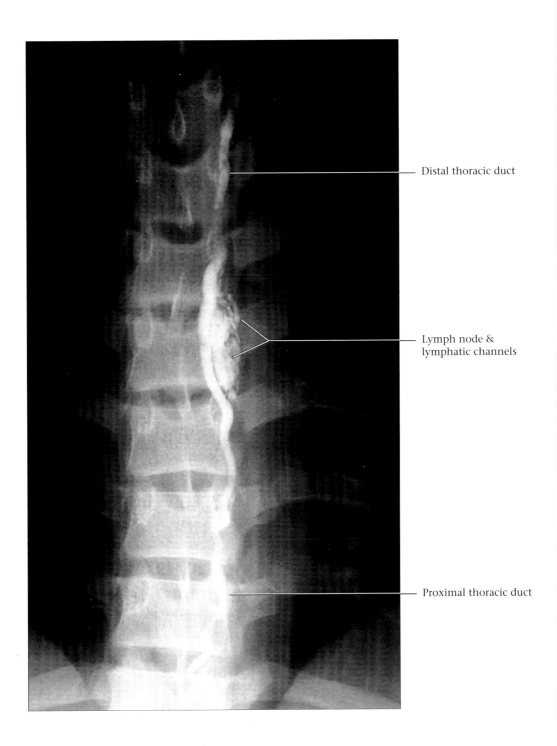

— Distal thoracic duct

Lymph node &
lymphatic channels

— Proximal thoracic duct

Frontal image from a lymphangiogram shows the proximal aspect of the thoracic duct. The variations in the caliber of the thoracic duct relate to valves within the duct lumen. The thoracic duct arises from the cisterna chyli (not shown) and courses vertically and superiorly to the left of midline anterior to the thoracic vertebrae. There is opacification of a lymph node and surrounding small lymphatic channels. Courtesy of Jud Gurney, MD, University of Nebraska Medical Center, Omaha, Nebraska.

SYSTEMIC VESSELS

LYMPHANGIOGRAPHY, THORACIC DUCT

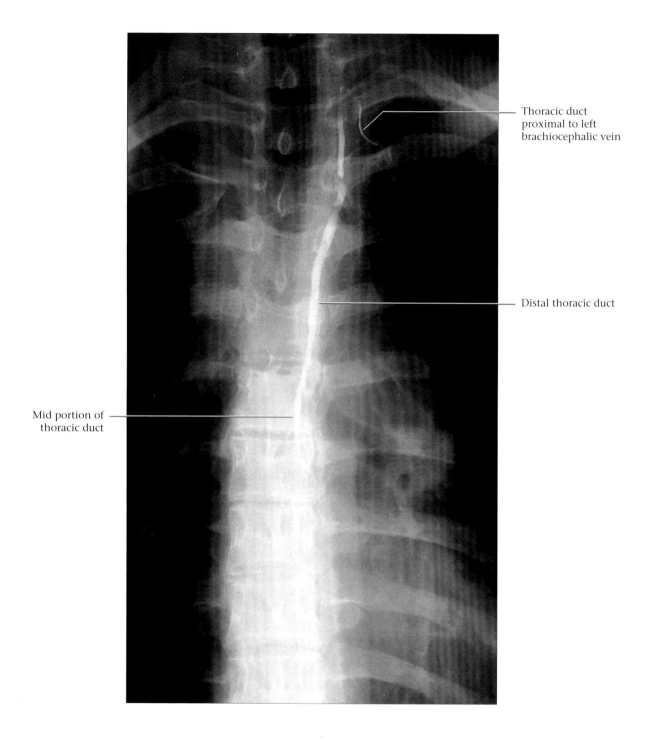

Thoracic duct proximal to left brachiocephalic vein

Distal thoracic duct

Mid portion of thoracic duct

Frontal image from a lymphangiogram demonstrates the distal aspect of the thoracic duct. The thoracic duct drains into the dorsal aspect of the proximal left brachiocephalic vein as shown. Courtesy of Jud Gurney, MD, University of Nebraska Medical Center, Omaha, Nebraska.

SYSTEMIC VESSELS

AXIAL & CORONAL CT, THORACIC DUCT & CISTERNA CHYLI

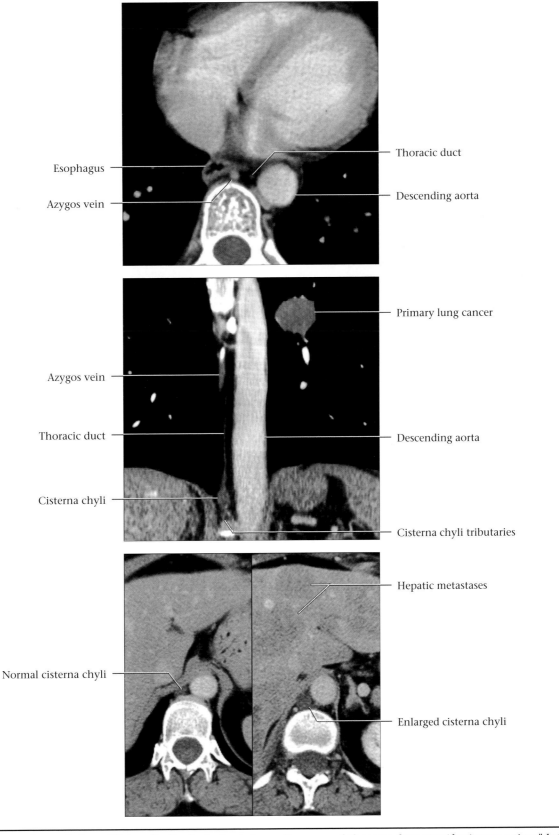

(Top) Contrast-enhanced chest CT (mediastinal window) shows the normal thoracic duct manifesting as a tiny "dot" between the azygos vein and the descending aorta. Courtesy of Elizabeth Moore, MD, University of California-Davis. (Middle) Coronal contrast-enhanced chest CT (mediastinal window) of a patient with primary lung cancer shows the normal thoracic duct arising from the cisterna chyli and coursing superiorly in the mediastinum. Courtesy of Elizabeth Moore, MD, University of California-Davis. (Bottom) Composite contrast-enhanced chest CT images (mediastinal window) showing the normal and abnormal appearances of the cisterna chyli. The abnormal cisterna chyli (right image) is enlarged secondary to obstruction related to malignancy. The normal cisterna chyli is seen in the left image. Courtesy of Elizabeth Moore, MD, University of California-Davis.

SYSTEMIC VESSELS

AORTIC ENLARGEMENT, TORTUOSITY

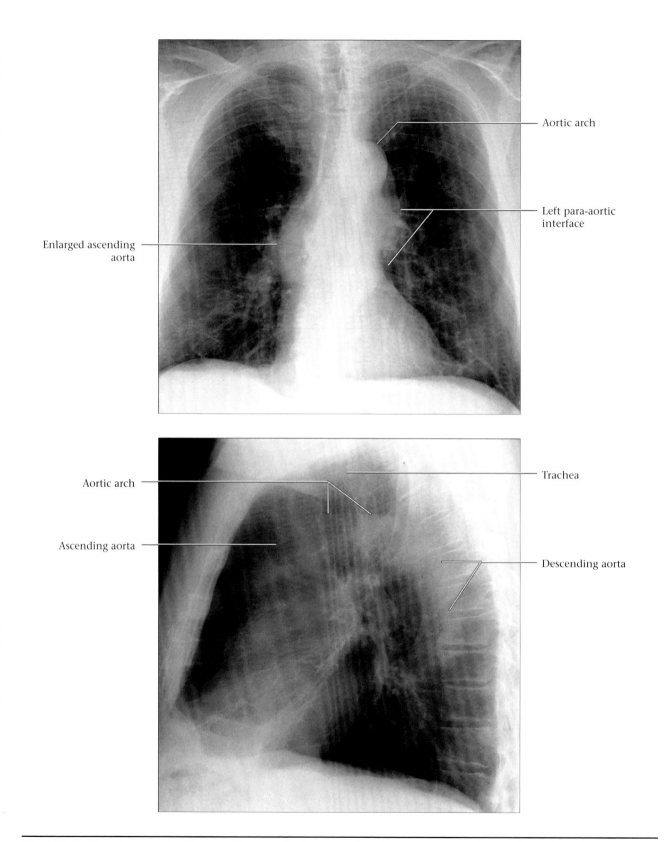

Aortic arch

Left para-aortic interface

Enlarged ascending aorta

Aortic arch

Ascending aorta

Trachea

Descending aorta

(Top) First of two images of a 63 year old man with hypertension demonstrates an abnormal ectatic and tortuous atherosclerotic aorta. PA chest radiograph shows that the ascending aorta is enlarged and produces a laterally convex interface in the right mediastinal contour. The left para-aortic interface also exhibits a laterally convex morphology. **(Bottom)** Left lateral chest radiograph shows a significant portion of the dilated tortuous thoracic aorta. With increasing aortic dilatation and tortuosity, there is visualization of a greater length of the vessel on chest radiography.

AORTIC ENLARGEMENT, ASCENDING AORTA

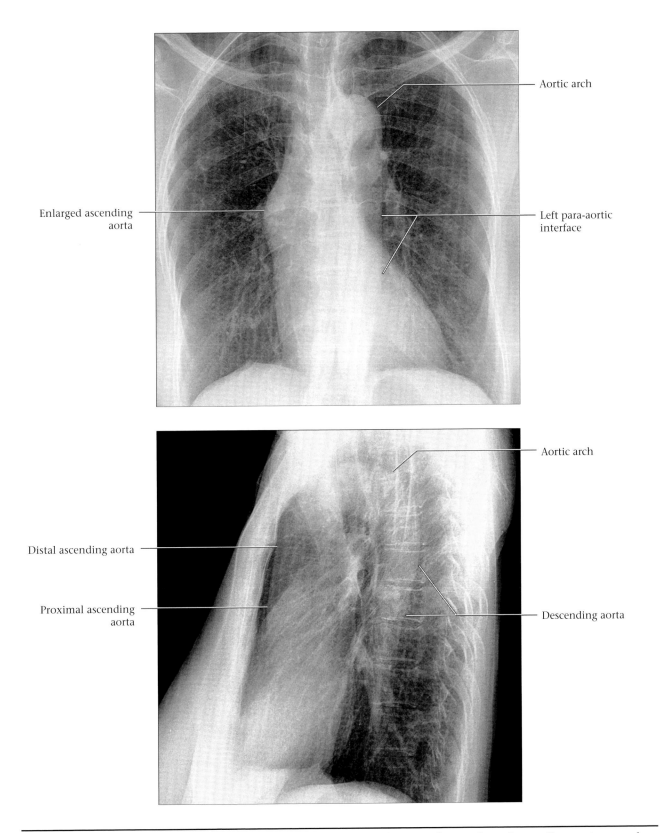

(Top) First of two images of a 28 year old woman with Marfan syndrome with an enlarged ascending aorta secondary to medial degeneration of the aorta. PA chest radiograph demonstrates an enlarged ascending aorta that produces a laterally convex interface in the mid portion of the right mediastinal border. There is also prominence and ectasia of the aortic arch and the descending aorta. **(Bottom)** Left lateral chest radiograph demonstrates a narrow AP chest diameter and marked enlargement of the ascending aorta, which is visualized almost in its entirety. Significant portions of the aortic arch and the descending aorta are also visible.

SYSTEMIC VESSELS

BOVINE ARCH, AORTOGRAPHY & CT

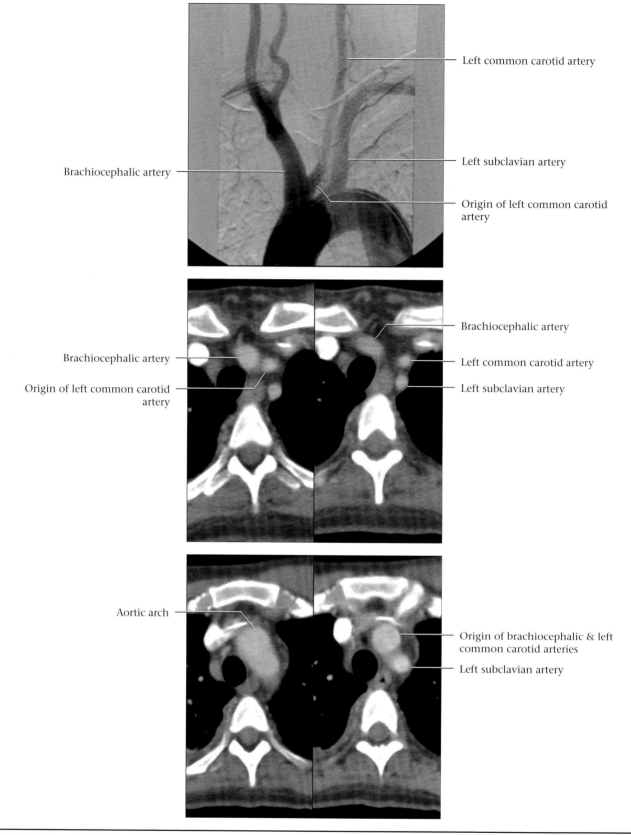

(Top) Oblique aortogram of a 59 year old patient demonstrates a common aortic arch anomaly, the bovine arch. In this anomaly the left common carotid artery arises from the proximal aspect of the brachiocephalic artery. The left subclavian artery arises independently from the aortic arch. (Middle) First of two composite axial contrast-enhanced chest CT images (mediastinal window) of a 25 year old patient with tuberculosis and a bovine arch. The left common carotid artery arises from the brachiocephalic artery. The left subclavian artery arises independently from the aortic arch. (Bottom) Images through the superior aspect of the aortic arch demonstrate that the brachiocephalic and left common carotid arteries originate from a common trunk that arises from the aortic arch. The left subclavian artery arises from the aortic arch independently.

SYSTEMIC VESSELS

ANOMALOUS LEFT VERTEBRAL ARTERY

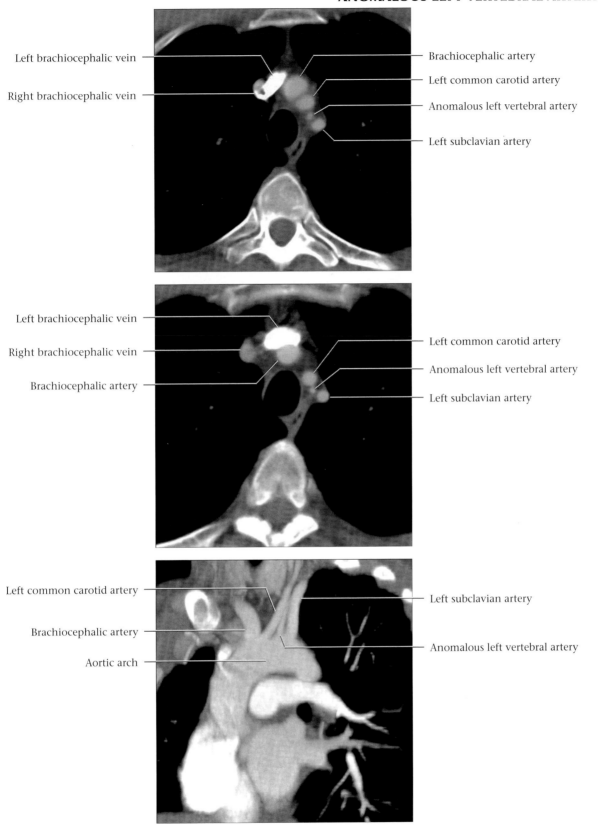

(Top) First of three contrast-enhanced chest CT images (mediastinal window) demonstrating the imaging appearance of the anomalous left vertebral artery, which arises directly from the aortic arch. The left vertebral artery typically arises from the left subclavian artery. Axial image through the origins of the aortic arch branches shows four separate vessels including an anomalous left vertebral artery located between the left common carotid and the left subclavian arteries. **(Middle)** Axial image obtained above the aortic arch shows four aortic branches including the anomalous left vertebral artery. **(Bottom)** Oblique coronal reconstruction through the aortic arch shows four aortic branches; the brachiocephalic, left common carotid, anomalous left vertebral and left subclavian arteries.

SYSTEMIC VESSELS

ABERRANT RIGHT SUBCLAVIAN ARTERY

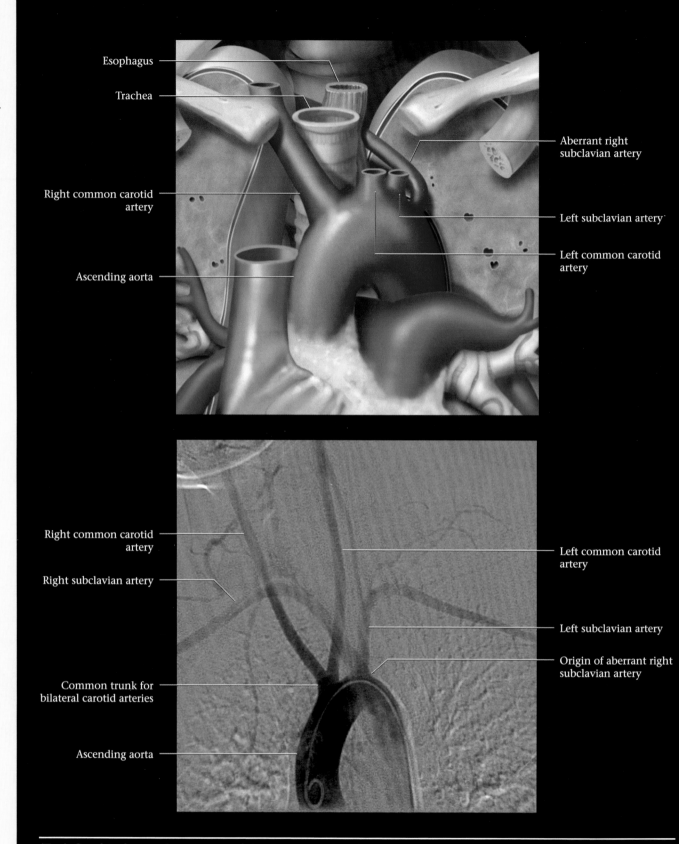

Esophagus

Trachea

Aberrant right subclavian artery

Right common carotid artery

Left subclavian artery

Left common carotid artery

Ascending aorta

Right common carotid artery

Left common carotid artery

Right subclavian artery

Left subclavian artery

Origin of aberrant right subclavian artery

Common trunk for bilateral carotid arteries

Ascending aorta

(Top) Graphic depicts the anatomy of the aberrant right subclavian artery, which arises as the last branch of the aortic arch. The anomalous vessel courses obliquely and typically behind the esophagus and trachea to supply the right upper extremity. Mass effect on the esophagus and trachea may result in symptoms. **(Bottom)** Oblique aortogram demonstrates an aberrant right subclavian artery arising as a fourth branch from the aortic arch. The superior and oblique course of the vessel towards the right upper extremity is also demonstrated. Note that the first branch of the aortic arch is an anomalous common trunk for the right and left common carotid arteries.

SYSTEMIC VESSELS

ABERRANT RIGHT SUBCLAVIAN ARTERY

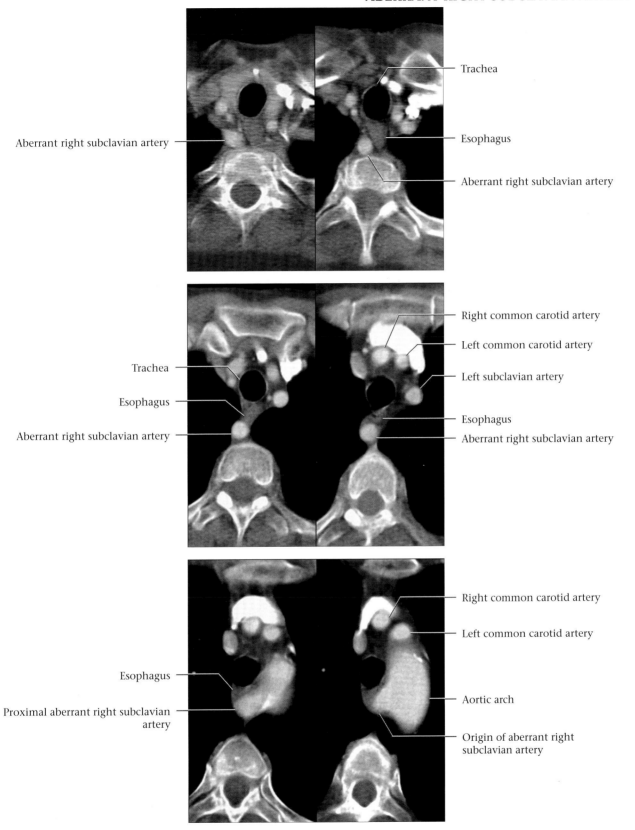

(Top) First of three composite axial contrast-enhanced chest CT images (mediastinal window) demonstrates the axial anatomy of the aberrant right subclavian artery. Images through the superior mediastinum demonstrate the abnormal posterolateral location of the distal aspect of the aberrant right subclavian artery. (Middle) Images through the superior mediastinum demonstrate the course of the aberrant right subclavian artery behind the trachea and esophagus. (Bottom) Images through the aortic arch demonstrate the anomalous right subclavian artery which arises as the last branch of the aortic arch and courses behind the trachea and esophagus to reach the right upper extremity. Dilatation of the origin of this vessel is known as the diverticulum of Kommerell.

SYSTEMIC VESSELS

ARCH ANOMALIES, RIGHT AORTIC ARCH

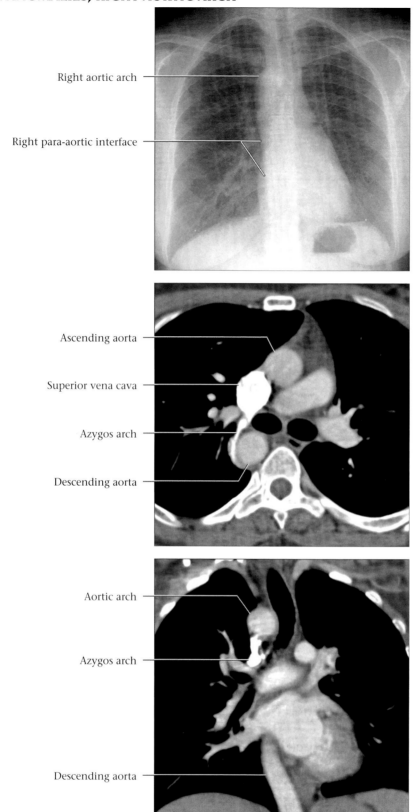

(Top) First of three images of an asymptomatic 49 year old woman with an incidentally discovered right aortic arch. The aortic arch indents the lateral wall of the distal right trachea. The aorta descends on the right side producing a right para-aortic interface. **(Middle)** Axial contrast-enhanced chest CT (mediastinal window) demonstrates the right sided location of the proximal descending aorta. Note that the azygos vein courses along the lateral aspect of the descending aorta to drain into the superior vena cava. **(Bottom)** Coronal contrast-enhanced chest CT (mediastinal window) demonstrates the right sided arch producing mass effect on the right distal trachea. The azygos arch and the right sided descending thoracic aorta are also demonstrated.

SYSTEMIC VESSELS

ARCH ANOMALIES, DOUBLE AORTIC ARCH

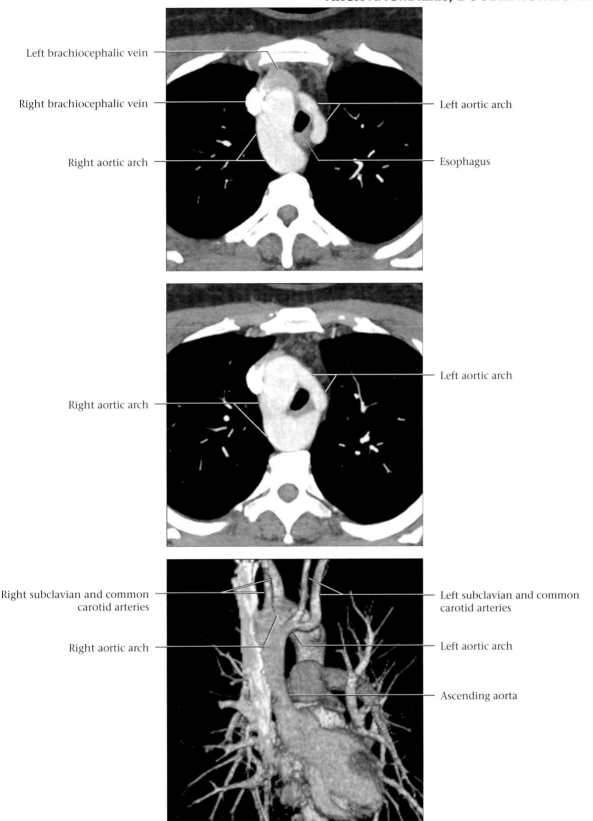

Left brachiocephalic vein

Right brachiocephalic vein

Left aortic arch

Right aortic arch

Esophagus

Right aortic arch

Left aortic arch

Right subclavian and common carotid arteries

Left subclavian and common carotid arteries

Right aortic arch

Left aortic arch

Ascending aorta

(Top) First of three contrast-enhanced chest CT images (mediastinal window) of a 50 year old woman with a double aortic arch who presented with chest pain. Axial image through the superior aspect of the left aortic arch shows that the right aortic arch is higher and larger than the left arch. This anomaly produces a complete vascular ring, and affected patients may present with stridor. **(Middle)** Axial image through the mid portion of the left aortic arch demonstrates the vascular ring that surrounds the trachea and esophagus and produces mild narrowing of the trachea. **(Bottom)** Volume rendered coronal CT image demonstrates the larger right aortic arch and the smaller left aortic arch. Note that each arch gives off separate common carotid and subclavian arteries.

SYSTEMIC VESSELS

PERSISTENT LEFT SUPERIOR VENA CAVA, NORMAL RIGHT SUPERIOR VENA CAVA

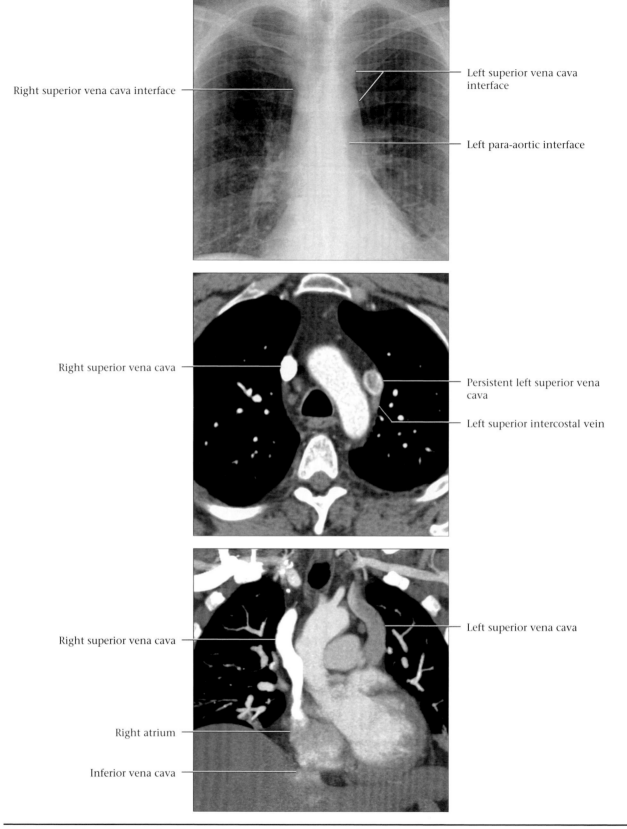

Right superior vena cava interface

Left superior vena cava interface

Left para-aortic interface

Right superior vena cava

Persistent left superior vena cava

Left superior intercostal vein

Right superior vena cava

Left superior vena cava

Right atrium

Inferior vena cava

(Top) First of three images of a 48 year old man with persistent left superior vena cava and normal right superior vena cava. PA chest radiograph shows a normal right superior vena cava interface and an unusual left superior mediastinal contour formed by a persistent left superior vena cava. The aortic arch interface is obscured but the left para-aortic interface is demonstrated. (Middle) Contrast-enhanced chest CT (mediastinal window) through the aortic arch shows the right and left superior venae cavae in cross-section. The left superior intercostal vein drains into the left superior vena cava. (Bottom) Coronal contrast-enhanced chest CT (mediastinal window) shows the anatomic correlate of the superior mediastinal interfaces seen on radiography formed by the bilateral superior venae cavae as they contact the mediastinal lung surfaces.

SYSTEMIC VESSELS

PERSISTENT LEFT SUPERIOR VENA CAVA, HYPOPLASTIC RIGHT SUPERIOR VENA CAVA

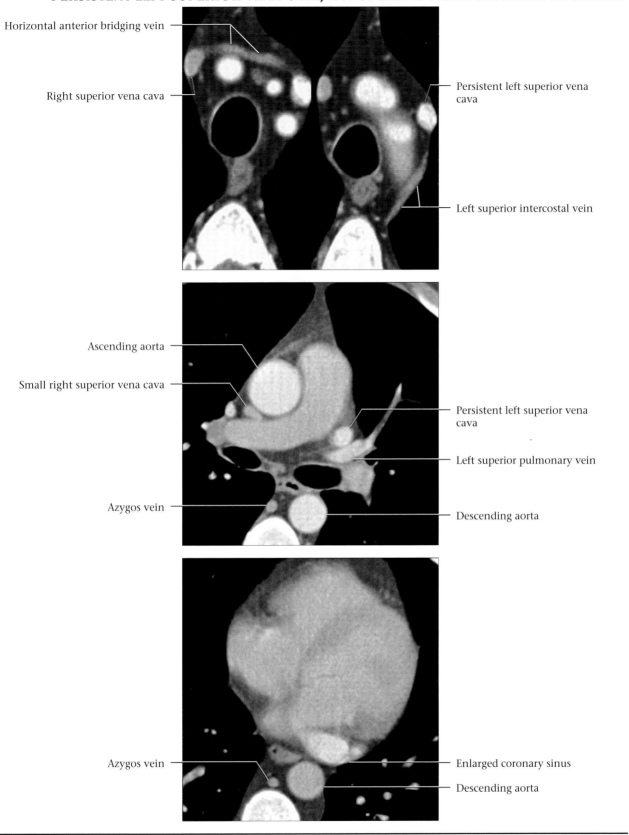

Horizontal anterior bridging vein

Right superior vena cava

Persistent left superior vena cava

Left superior intercostal vein

Ascending aorta

Small right superior vena cava

Persistent left superior vena cava

Left superior pulmonary vein

Azygos vein

Descending aorta

Azygos vein

Enlarged coronary sinus

Descending aorta

(Top) First of three axial contrast-enhanced chest CT images (mediastinal window) of a 45 year old man with persistent left superior vena cava and a hypoplastic right superior vena cava. Composite of two images through the superior mediastinum demonstrates the bilateral superior vena cavae (the right smaller than the left) connected by a bridging vein analogous to the left brachiocephalic vein. The left superior intercostal vein drains into the left superior vena cava. **(Middle)** Image through the pulmonary trunk shows a small right superior vena cava. The left superior vena cava characteristically courses inferiorly and anterior to the left superior pulmonary vein to drain into the coronary sinus. **(Bottom)** Axial image through the heart demonstrates an enlarged coronary sinus produced by the increased blood flow contributed by the persistent left superior vena cava.

SYSTEMIC VESSELS

PERSISTENT LEFT SUPERIOR VENA CAVA, ABSENT RIGHT SUPERIOR VENA CAVA

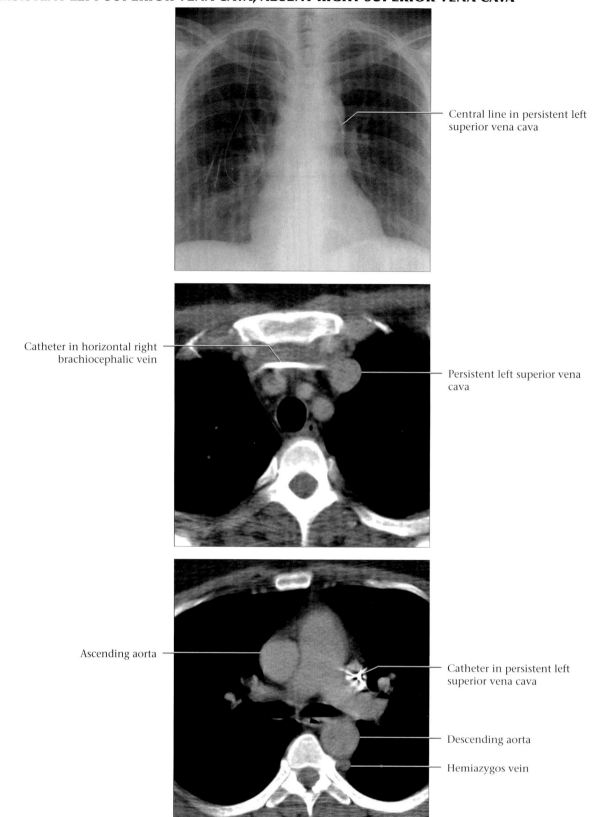

Central line in persistent left superior vena cava

Catheter in horizontal right brachiocephalic vein

Persistent left superior vena cava

Ascending aorta

Catheter in persistent left superior vena cava

Descending aorta

Hemiazygos vein

(Top) First of three images of a 51 year old woman undergoing treatment for leukemia who had an incidentally found persistent left superior vena cava. PA chest radiograph demonstrates a right internal jugular central catheter tip terminating in a left paramediastinal location instead of following the expected course into a right sided superior vena cava. **(Middle)** Unenhanced chest CT (mediastinal window) through the superior mediastinum demonstrates the endovascular catheter coursing within a horizontal anterior venous structure that anastomoses with a persistent left superior vena cava. **(Bottom)** Unenhanced chest CT (mediastinal window) through the pulmonary trunk demonstrates a catheter within a persistent left superior vena cava. The right superior vena cava was absent. A prominent hemiazygos vein is seen, but a normal right sided azygos vein was not identified.

SYSTEMIC VESSELS

AZYGOS CONTINUATION OF INFERIOR VENA CAVA

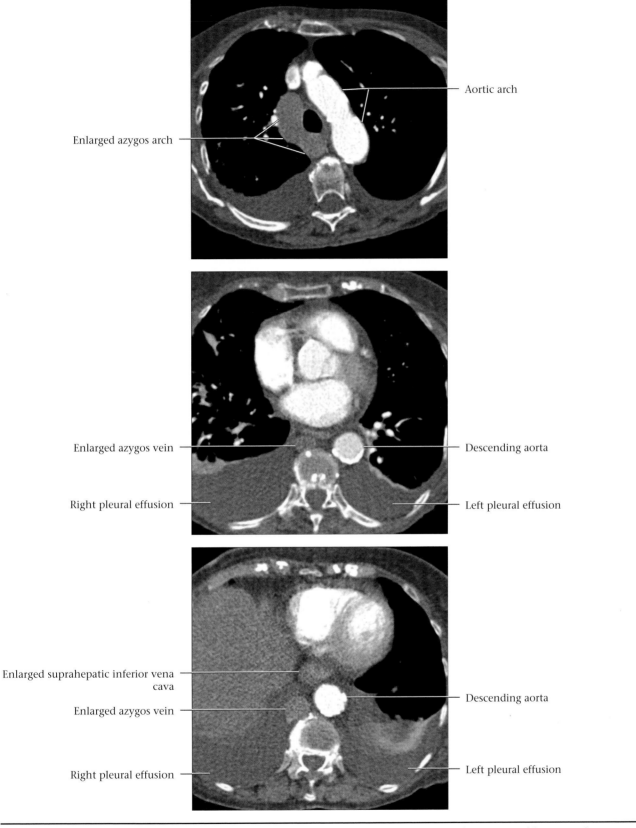

(Top) First of three axial contrast-enhanced chest CT images (mediastinal window) of a 63 year old man with azygos continuation of the inferior vena cava. Image through the aortic arch demonstrates an enlarged azygos arch. Bilateral pleural effusions are also present. (Middle) Image through the root of the aorta demonstrates bilateral pleural effusions and a prominent azygos vein. (Bottom) Image through the inferior hemithorax demonstrates enlargement of the azygos vein and the suprahepatic portion of the inferior vena cava. In this anomaly, the intrahepatic portion of the inferior vena cava is hypoplastic and the hepatic veins drain via the suprahepatic inferior vena cava. This anomaly is associated with situs ambiguous and congenital heart disease. The enlarged azygos arch may mimic lymphadenopathy on radiography.

SYSTEMIC VESSELS

HEMIAZYGOS CONTINUATION OF LEFT INFERIOR VENA CAVA, SITUS AMBIGUOUS

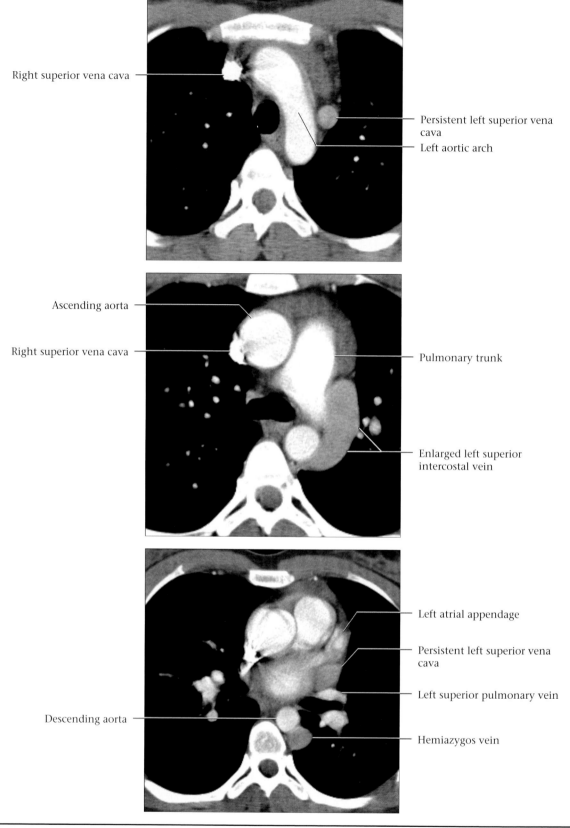

Right superior vena cava

Persistent left superior vena cava

Left aortic arch

Ascending aorta

Right superior vena cava

Pulmonary trunk

Enlarged left superior intercostal vein

Left atrial appendage

Persistent left superior vena cava

Left superior pulmonary vein

Descending aorta

Hemiazygos vein

(Top) First of six axial contrast-enhanced chest CT images (mediastinal window) of a 32 year old man with situs ambiguous, persistent left superior vena cava and hemiazygos continuation of the inferior vena cava. Image through the aortic arch demonstrates a persistent left superior vena cava. A right superior vena cava is also present. **(Middle)** Image through the pulmonary trunk demonstrates an enlarged horizontal left venous structure that likely represents an enlarged left superior intercostal vein that drains into the persistent left superior vena cava. **(Bottom)** Image through the left atrial appendage shows the persistent left superior vena cava coursing anterior to the left superior pulmonary vein to drain into the coronary sinus. The enlarged hemiazygos vein courses parallel to the descending aorta.

SYSTEMIC VESSELS

HEMIAZYGOS CONTINUATION OF LEFT INFERIOR VENA CAVA, SITUS AMBIGUOUS

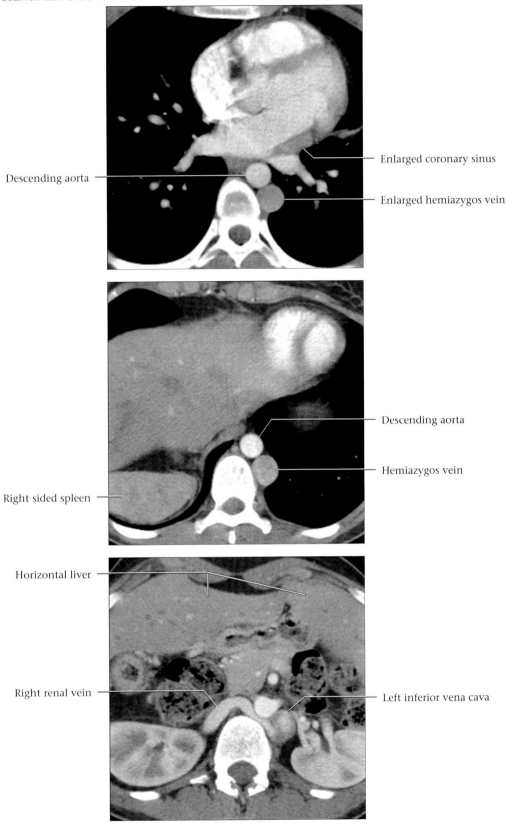

(Top) Image through the inferior pulmonary veins demonstrates enlargement of the coronary sinus. An enlarged hemiazygos vein is located posterior to the descending aorta. (Middle) Image through the inferior aspect of the thorax demonstrates findings consistent with situs ambiguous. The spleen is on the right side. The enlarged hemiazygos vein is located posterior to the descending aorta. (Bottom) Image through the upper abdomen demonstrates a horizontal liver and the right renal vein draining into a left sided inferior vena cava. In patients with this anomaly, abdominal blood reaches the right atrium by flowing from the left inferior vena cava into a dilated hemiazygos vein. The blood then flows into the left superior intercostal vein to reach a persistent left superior vena cava and finally into the coronary sinus to reach the right atrium.

HEART

General Anatomy and Function

Anatomy
- Cardiac chambers
  - **Right atrium, right ventricle, left atrium, left ventricle**
- Cardiac valves
  - **Tricuspid, pulmonic, mitral, aortic**
- Cardiac structure
  - **Epicardium**: Serous visceral pericardium
  - **Myocardium**: Specialized cardiac muscle that forms atrial and ventricular walls
  - **Endocardium**: Thin layer of cells that lines internal surfaces of cardiac chambers; participates in cardiac contraction

Function
- Pump action
  - **Delivery of de-oxygenated blood to capillary-alveolar interface**
  - **Delivery of oxygenated blood to tissues**
- Cardiac conduction system
  - **Sinoatrial (SA) node**
    - Cardiac pacemaker; atrial contraction
    - Superior end of **crista terminalis** at **superior vena cava** orifice
  - **Atrioventricular node**
    - In atrioventricular septum, near coronary sinus orifice, close to attachment of septal cusp of tricuspid valve
    - Receives impulse generated at sino-atrial node, propagates it to ventricles; produces ventricular contraction
  - **Atrioventricular bundle**
    - Continuation of atrioventricular node along interventricular septum, divides into right and left bundle branches
  - **Right bundle branch**
    - Continues along right side of interventricular septum to reach subendocardial **Purkinje fibers**
  - **Left bundle branch**
    - Continues along left side of interventricular septum to apex to reach subendocardial **Purkinje fibers**

Cardiac Shape and Orientation

Shape
- Pyramidal

Orientation
- Position analogous to pyramid on its side
- Apex oriented anteriorly, inferiorly, to the left

Cardiac Surfaces

Posterior Surface (Base)
- Quadrilateral shape
- Faces posteriorly
- Structures: **Left atrium**, small portion of **right atrium**, central **great veins**

Apex
- Faces anteriorly, inferiorly, and to the left
- Structures: Inferolateral **left ventricle**

Anterior Surface
- Faces anteriorly
- Structures: **Right ventricle**, portions of **right atrium** and **left ventricle**

Diaphragmatic Surface
- Faces inferiorly
- Rests on diaphragm
- Structures: **Left ventricle**, portion of **right ventricle**

Left Pulmonary Surface
- Faces left lung
- Structures: **Left ventricle**, portion of **left atrium**

Right Pulmonary Surface
- Faces right lung
- Structure: **Right atrium**

Cardiac Borders (Margins)

Upper Border
- Not well appreciated on imaging

Inferior (Acute) Border
- Edge between **anterior** and **diaphragmatic surfaces**
- Structures: **Right ventricle**, portion of **left ventricle**

Obtuse (Left) Border
- Between **anterior** and **left pulmonary surfaces**
- Curved morphology
- From **left atrial appendage** to apex
- Structures: **Left ventricle**, portion of **left atrial appendage**

Right Border
- Confusing terminology
- Analogous to **right pulmonary surface**

Cardiac Sulci

General Features
- Heart divided into chambers
- Internal cardiac partitions demarcate chamber boundaries
- **Sulci**: External grooves related to internal partitions

Coronary Sulcus (Atrioventricular Sulcus)
- Surrounds heart, separates atria from ventricles
- Structures: Right coronary/circumflex branch of left coronary arteries, small cardiac vein, coronary sinus

Anterior/Posterior Interventricular Sulci
- Separate ventricles
- **Anterior interventricular sulcus**
  - Anterior heart surface
  - Structures: Anterior interventricular (descending) artery, great cardiac vein
- **Posterior interventricular sulcus**
  - Diaphragmatic heart surface

HEART

○ Structures: Posterior interventricular (descending) artery, middle cardiac vein
- Anterior and posterior interventricular sulci continuous inferiorly to left of apex

Cardiac Chambers

Right Atrium

- Forms **right cardiac border** and portion of **anterior surface**
- Receives de-oxygenated blood through
  ○ **Superior vena cava:** Superior posterior right atrium
  ○ **Inferior vena cava:** Inferior posterior right atrium
  ○ **Coronary sinus:** Inferior posterior right atrium
- Blood exits through atrioventricular **tricuspid valve**
- Structures
  ○ Compartmentalized by external **sulcus terminalis** cordis
    ▪ From right of superior vena cava to right of inferior vena cava
  ○ Compartmentalized by internal **crista terminalis**
    ▪ Smooth ridge, begins at roof of atrium anterior to superior vena cava orifice, extends to anterior lip of inferior vena cava orifice
  ○ **Sinus of venae cavae**, posterior to **crista terminalis**
  ○ **Right atrium** proper
    ▪ Anterior to crista terminalis
    ▪ Wall covered by ridges called **pectinate muscles**
    ▪ **Right atrial appendage (auricle)**
  ○ Vascular orifices
    ▪ **Orifice of superior vena cava, orifices and valves of inferior vena cava and coronary sinus**
  ○ **Interatrial septum**
    ▪ **Fossa ovalis:** Depression in septum above orifice of inferior vena cava
    ▪ **Limbus fossa ovalis:** Margin of fossa ovalis
    ▪ **Fossa ovalis** marks location of primitive **foramen ovale**, which allows oxygenated blood to enter left atrium and bypass lungs in utero

Right Ventricle

- Forms **anterior cardiac surface** and small portion of **diaphragmatic surface**
- Structures
  ○ **Conus arteriosus:** Smooth walled right ventricular infundibulum or outflow tract
  ○ Right ventricular inflow tract lined by **trabeculae carneae**, form ridges and bridges
  ○ **Papillary muscles** are **trabeculae carneae** attached to ventricular surface and **chordae tendineae**, connect **chordae tendineae** to free edges of **tricuspid valve**
    ▪ **Anterior papillary muscle:** Largest, arises from anterior ventricular wall
    ▪ **Posterior papillary muscle:** Some chordae tendineae arise directly from ventricular wall
    ▪ **Septal papillary muscle:** Most inconsistent
  ○ **Septomarginal trabecula** or **moderator band**
    ▪ Forms bridge **between lower interventricular septum and base of anterior papillary muscle**

Left Atrium

- Forms **base** or **posterior cardiac surface**

- Structures
  ○ **Posterior or inflow portion:** Smooth walls, receives **pulmonary veins**
  ○ **Anterior or outflow portion:** Continuous with **left atrial appendage**, lined by **pectinate muscles**
  ○ **Interatrial septum**
    ▪ Contains **valve of foramen ovale**, prevents blood from passing from left atrium to right atrium
    ▪ **Valve of foramen ovale** may provide passage between atria during cardiac instrumentation

Left Ventricle

- Contributions to **anterior, diaphragmatic, left pulmonary cardiac surfaces**, forms **apex**
- Thickest myocardium
- Structures
  ○ Fine, delicate **trabeculae carneae**
  ○ Papillary muscles larger than in right ventricle
    ▪ **Anterior papillary muscle**
    ▪ **Posterior papillary muscle**
  ○ **Interventricular septum**
    ▪ **Thick muscular portion** forms major part of septum
    ▪ **Membranous portion**

Cardiac Skeleton

Anatomy

- **Annulus fibrosus:** Four fibrous rings between atria and ventricles
  ○ Points of origin of atrial (superior) and ventricular (inferior) myocardium
  ○ Maintains integrity of orifices
  ○ Traversed by **atrioventricular bundle**
- Surrounds atrioventricular valves and aortic/pulmonary trunk orifices
- Interconnecting fibrous tissue
  ○ **Right fibrous trigone:** Between aortic and right atrioventricular rings
  ○ **Left fibrous trigone:** Between aortic and left atrioventricular rings

Cardiac Valves

Tricuspid Valve

- Three cusps attached to fibrous ring
  ○ **Anterior, septal, posterior**
- Anatomy of right atrioventricular valve
  ○ Cusps continuous with each other at their bases, **commissures**
  ○ Free margins attached to **chordae tendineae**
  ○ **Chordae tendineae** from two papillary muscles attach to each cusp

Pulmonic Valve

- Three semilunar cusps
  ○ **Left, right, anterior**
- Anatomy of semilunar cusps
  ○ Free edges project into lumen of pulmonary trunk forming **sinuses**
  ○ Each cusp has thick central focus, **nodule of semilunar cusp**

HEART

- Each cusp has thin lateral portion, **lunule of semilunar cusp**

Mitral Valve

- Two cusps attached to fibrous ring
  - **Anterior, posterior**
- Anatomy of left atrioventricular valve
  - Cusps continuous with each other at **commissures**, **chordae tendineae** attach papillary muscles to free borders of cusps

Aortic Valve

- Three semilunar cusps
  - **Right, left, posterior (noncoronary)**
- Three sinuses
  - Right coronary artery originates from right sinus
  - Left coronary artery originates from left sinus
  - Noncoronary sinus

Imaging the Heart

Radiography

- Analysis of cardiac borders and surfaces
  - Right cardiac border: **Right atrium**
  - Left cardiac border: **Left atrial appendage and left ventricle**
  - Anterior cardiac surface: **Right ventricle**
  - Posterior cardiac surface: **Left atrium** and **left ventricle**
- Variations in cardiac morphology
  - **Infancy: Prominent cardiothymic silhouette**
  - **Childhood**, adolescence and young adulthood: **Prominent pulmonary trunk** (see "Pulmonary Vessels" section)
  - **Adulthood: Progressive left ventricular configuration** with dominant left sided structures and concavity of upper left cardiac border
- Analysis of cardiac size
  - **Cardiothoracic ratio**
    - Maximum transverse cardiac diameter to transverse thoracic diameter ≤ **0.55**
    - Influenced by rotation, lung volume, projection
  - Analysis of individual chamber enlargement
- Analysis of abnormal cardiac density/calcification

CT/MR Anatomy

- **Right atrium**
  - **Right atrial appendage** (trabeculated) anterior and superior to **right ventricle**
  - **Crista terminalis:** Vertical ridge in right atrium extending from superior to inferior venae cavae
- **Left atrium**
  - Most superior and posterior cardiac chamber
  - **Left atrial appendage** (trabeculated) anterior and superior to **left ventricle**
  - **Smooth muscle ridge** at junction of **left atrial appendage** and central **left superior pulmonary vein**
- **Interatrial septum**
  - Thin structure, difficult identification on CT; increased visibility with fat deposition
    - Fat spares **fossa ovalis** and may allow its identification

- **Right ventricle**
  - Most anterior cardiac chamber, anterior heart surface
  - Heavy trabeculations, thin wall
    - **Moderator band:** Connects anterior papillary muscle to interventricular septum near right ventricular apex, contains right bundle branch
  - **Anterior, posterior, septal papillary muscles**
- **Left ventricle**
  - Posterior and diaphragmatic cardiac surfaces
  - Thicker than right ventricle, less trabeculated
  - Anterior and posterior papillary muscles
- **Interventricular septum**
  - Thicker than interatrial septum
- **Valves**
  - Imaging in longitudinal and perpendicular planes
    - Contrast-enhanced CT and bright blood cardiac MR, thin low attenuation/signal structures
  - Assessment of function, morphology, calcification

CT/MR

- Assessment of cardiac chambers, valves, myocardium
  - Size, morphology, wall thickness, calcification, function
- **Short axis view**
  - Cross-section through short axis of left ventricular cavity and bodies of papillary muscles
- **Two chamber view**
  - Display of left atrial and ventricular chambers, evaluation of **mitral (left atrioventricular) valve**
- **Four chamber view**
  - Display of four cardiac chambers and atrioventricular valves

Anatomy-Based Cardiac and Valvular Abnormalities

Situs Abnormalities

- Indirect analysis of atrial morphology by evaluation of tracheobronchial tree
- Association with abnormal cardiac position and congenital heart disease

Cardiomegaly and Chamber Enlargement

- Increased cardiothoracic ratio
- Analysis of specific chamber enlargement

Myocardial Calcification

- Sequelae of myocardial infarction
- May be associated with ventricular aneurysm

Annular and Valvular Calcification

- **Mitral annulus calcification:** Involvement of mitral valve ring, **C- or J-shaped morphology** on radiography
- Valvular calcification
  - **Aortic stenosis: Congenital** (bicuspid or bicommissural valve), **degenerative** (fibrocalcific), **rheumatic heart disease**
  - **Mitral stenosis: Rheumatic heart disease**

HEART

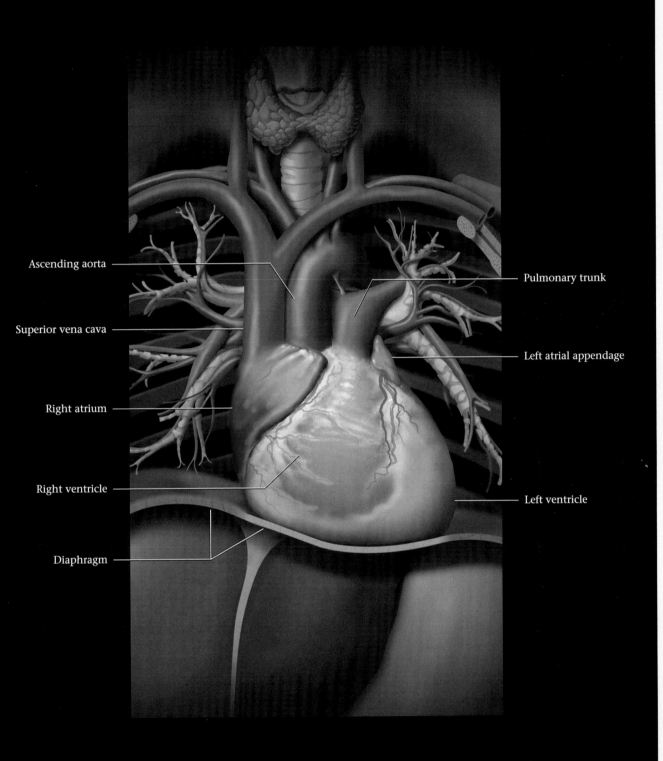

Ascending aorta

Superior vena cava

Right atrium

Right ventricle

Diaphragm

Pulmonary trunk

Left atrial appendage

Left ventricle

Graphic illustrates the location of the heart with respect to the rest of the structures and organs in the thorax. The heart is surrounded by the pericardium and has a pyramidal shape with its apex oriented inferiorly and towards the left side. The cardiac base faces posteriorly. The four heart chambers connect with the great pulmonary and systemic vessels. The heart receives blood from the systemic and pulmonary circulations via the systemic and pulmonary veins respectively. The blood is then pumped into the pulmonary circulation for delivery to the capillary-alveolar interface and into the systemic circulation for delivery to the tissues and organs of the body.

HEART

ANATOMY OF HEART SURFACES, MARGINS & SULCI

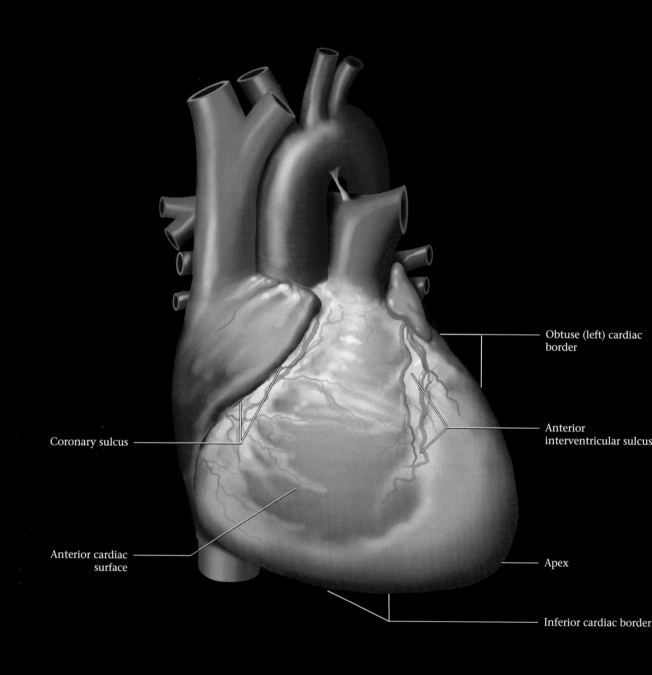

Obtuse (left) cardiac border

Anterior interventricular sulcus

Coronary sulcus

Anterior cardiac surface

Apex

Inferior cardiac border

First of three graphics depicting the surface anatomy of the heart. The heart has a pyramidal shape with a base and an apex. It has anterior, diaphragmatic, posterior and right and left pulmonary surfaces. The anterior surface is formed by the right and left ventricles with small contributions from the right atrium and left atrial appendage. The obtuse (left) cardiac border separates the anterior and left pulmonary surfaces. The inferior (acute) cardiac border separates the anterior and diaphragmatic surfaces. External sulci correspond to internal partitions that divide the heart into chambers. There are anterior and posterior interventricular sulci and a coronary sulcus. The coronary sulcus is circumferential and separates the atria from the ventricles. The anterior and posterior interventricular sulci separate the ventricles.

HEART

ANATOMY OF HEART SURFACES, MARGINS & SULCI

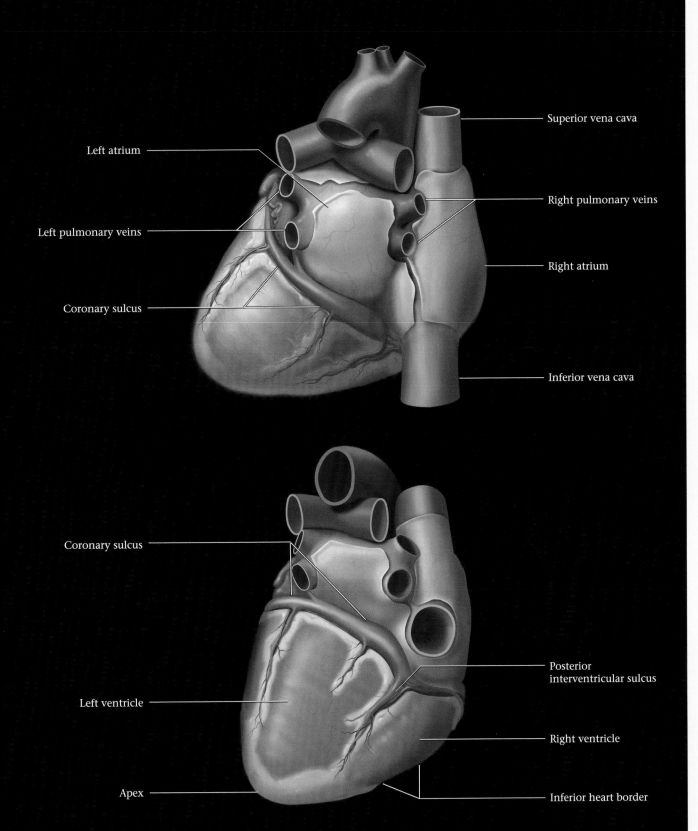

Left atrium

Superior vena cava

Left pulmonary veins

Right pulmonary veins

Coronary sulcus

Right atrium

Inferior vena cava

Coronary sulcus

Left ventricle

Posterior interventricular sulcus

Right ventricle

Apex

Inferior heart border

(Top) Graphic shows the posterior heart surface or base of the heart, which is formed by the left atrium, a small portion of the right atrium, the paired superior and inferior pulmonary veins and the superior and inferior venae cavae which fix the heart base to the pericardium. The coronary sulcus is seen at the junction of the left atrium and ventricle. **(Bottom)** Graphic shows the diaphragmatic heart surface which is formed by the right and left ventricles and is separated from the heart base by the coronary (atrioventricular) sulcus which runs along the atrioventricular groove. The inferior (acute) cardiac border separates the diaphragmatic from the anterior heart surfaces. The posterior interventricular sulcus marks the location of the interventricular septum.

HEART

RADIOGRAPHY OF THE HEART

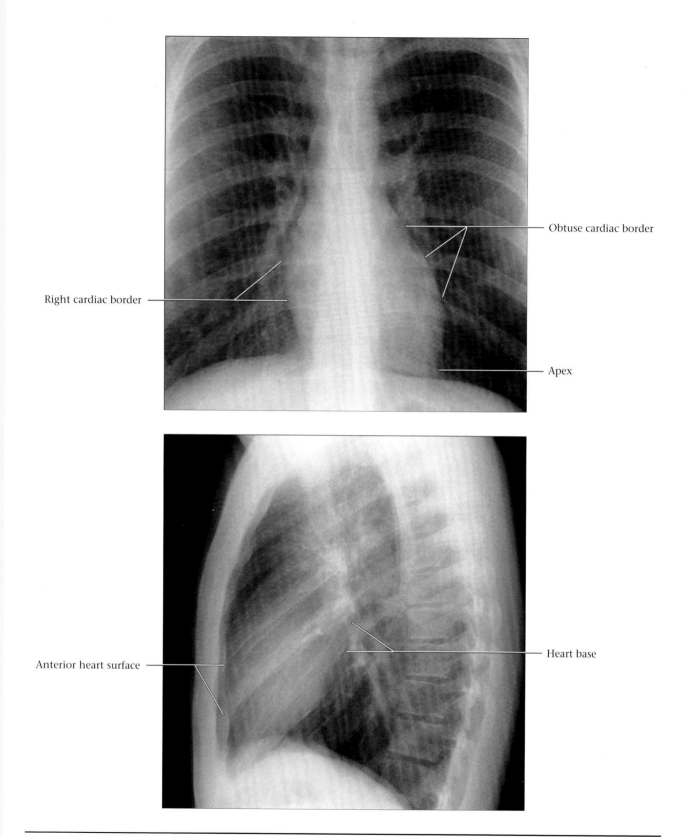

(Top) First of two normal chest radiographs illustrating the surface anatomy of the heart. PA chest radiograph shows the right and obtuse (or left) cardiac borders. The diaphragmatic cardiac surface is not visible radiographically. The right cardiac border is formed by the right atrium and is analogous to the right pulmonary cardiac surface. The left or obtuse cardiac border is formed by the left ventricle and a small portion of the left atrium, the left atrial appendage. **(Bottom)** Left lateral chest radiograph shows the anterior and posterior cardiac surfaces. The anterior surface is formed by the right ventricle. The base of the heart or posterior surface is formed by the left atrium.

HEART

CT OF HEART SURFACES, BORDERS & SULCI

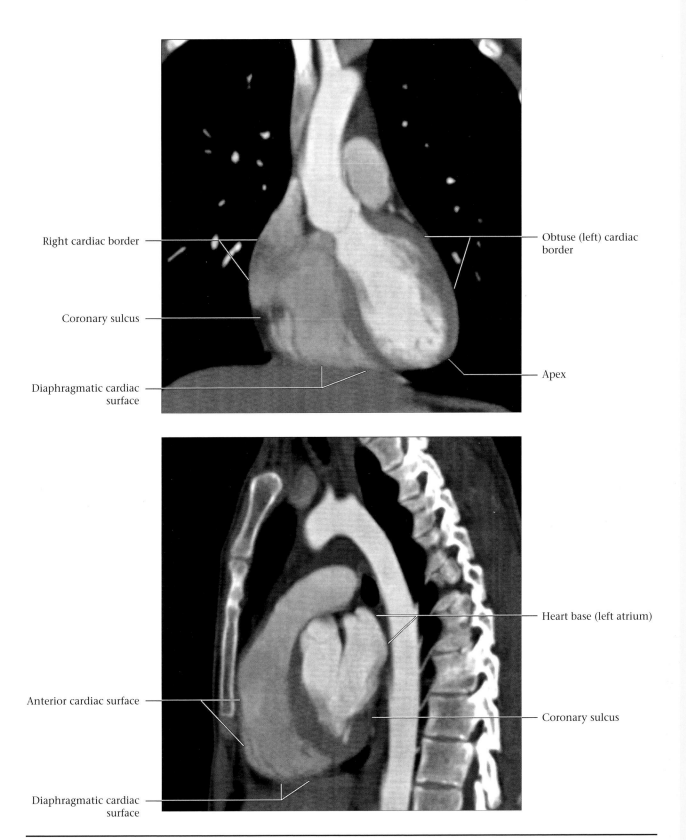

Right cardiac border

Coronary sulcus

Diaphragmatic cardiac surface

Obtuse (left) cardiac border

Apex

Anterior cardiac surface

Diaphragmatic cardiac surface

Heart base (left atrium)

Coronary sulcus

(Top) First of two normal contrast-enhanced chest CT images (mediastinal window) demonstrating the cardiac surfaces, borders and sulci. Coronal image through the aortic valve shows the right and obtuse (left) cardiac borders. The right cardiac border is analogous to the right pulmonary cardiac surface. The diaphragmatic cardiac surface is also visible. Fat is present in the coronary sulcus which demarcates the boundary between the atria and ventricles. **(Bottom)** Sagittal image demonstrates the base of the heart formed primarily by the left atrium, the diaphragmatic cardiac surface formed by the left and right ventricles and the anterior cardiac surface formed by the right ventricle. A portion of the coronary sulcus is also seen.

HEART

ANATOMY OF ANTERIOR HEART SURFACE & RIGHT ATRIUM

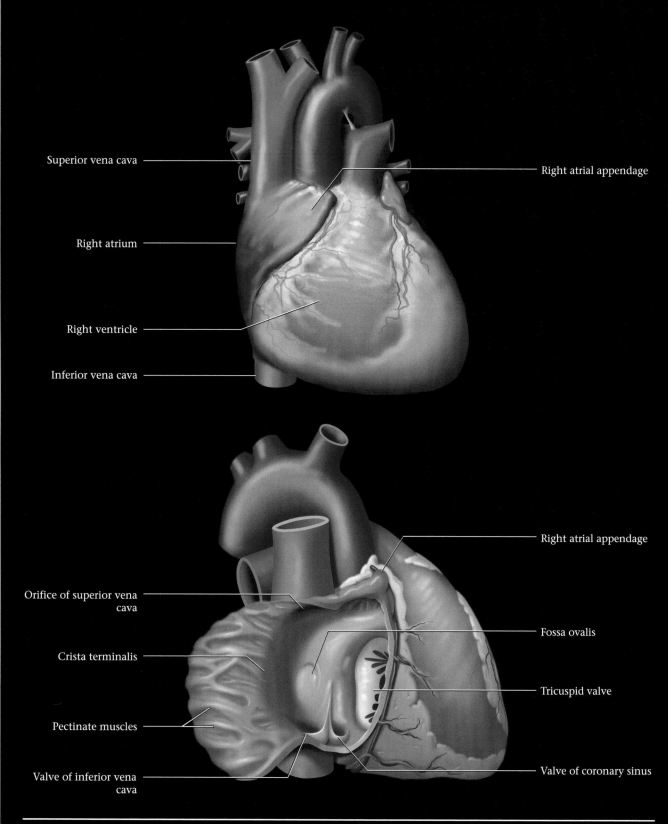

Superior vena cava

Right atrial appendage

Right atrium

Right ventricle

Inferior vena cava

Orifice of superior vena cava

Right atrial appendage

Crista terminalis

Fossa ovalis

Pectinate muscles

Tricuspid valve

Valve of inferior vena cava

Valve of coronary sinus

(Top) First of three graphics demonstrating the anatomy of the right cardiac chambers. Illustration of the anterior surface of the heart shows that it is predominantly formed by the right ventricle and portions of the right atrium and left ventricle. The right atrial appendage is also shown. **(Bottom)** Illustration of the interior of the right atrium shows trabeculated (pectinate muscles) and smooth regions separated by the crista terminalis. The posterior smooth portion receives the venae cavae (sinus of the venae cavae) and the coronary sinus. The anterior trabeculated portion is known as the right atrium proper. The interatrial septum contains the fossa ovalis, which marks the location of the embryonic foramen ovale.

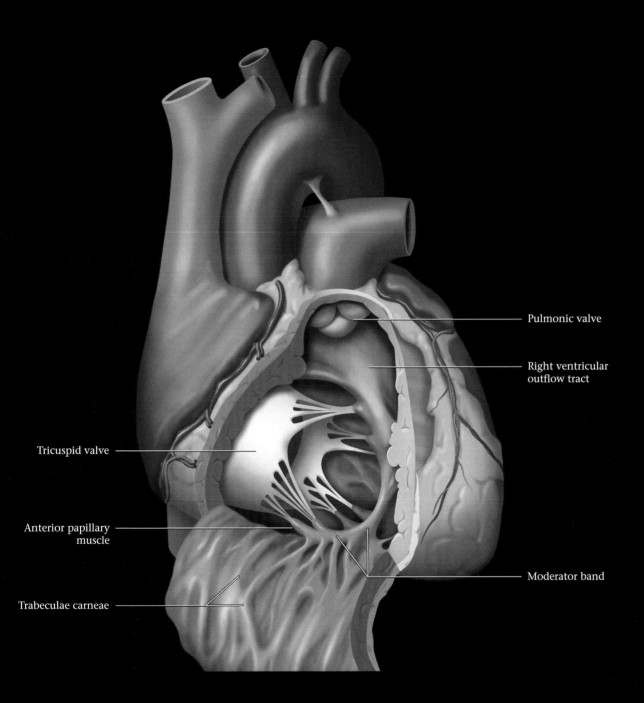

Pulmonic valve

Right ventricular outflow tract

Tricuspid valve

Anterior papillary muscle

Trabeculae carneae

Moderator band

Illustration of the interior of the right ventricle shows trabeculated and smooth areas. The proximal (inflow portion) right ventricle is characterized by the trabeculae carneae. Some of these form papillary muscles, which attach to the free edges of the tricuspid (right atrioventricular) valve cusps via chordae tendineae. There are anterior, septal and posterior papillary muscles. A thick trabecula carnea connects the interventricular septum to the anterior papillary muscle and is known as the moderator band or septomarginal trabecula. The right ventricular outflow tract leads to the pulmonic valve and is characterized by its smooth walls.

HEART

CT, RIGHT HEART CHAMBERS

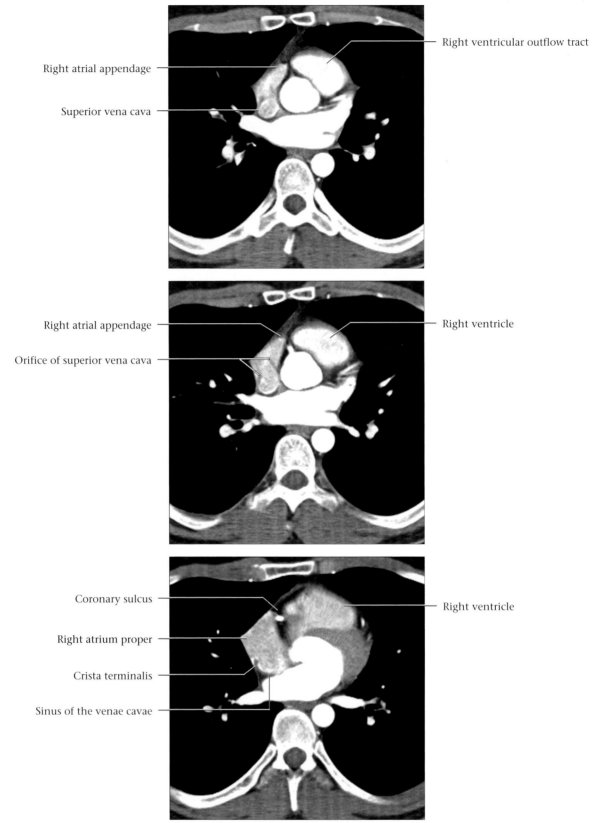

Right ventricular outflow tract

Right atrial appendage

Superior vena cava

Right atrial appendage

Orifice of superior vena cava

Right ventricle

Coronary sulcus

Right atrium proper

Crista terminalis

Sinus of the venae cavae

Right ventricle

(Top) First of six normal contrast-enhanced cardiac gated axial CT images (mediastinal window) showing the anatomy of the right heart chambers. Image through the junction of the superior vena cava and right atrium shows the anteriorly oriented triangular right atrial appendage. (Middle) Image through the upper heart shows the orifice of the superior vena cava as it enters the right atrium. The right atrium is located anterior and to the right of the left atrium and the ascending aorta. The right ventricle is located anterior and to the left of the ascending aorta. (Bottom) Image through the upper heart demonstrates the superior aspects of the right atrium and ventricle. These chambers are separated by the coronary sulcus. The crista terminalis courses between the orifices of the venae cavae and separates the atrium proper from the sinus of the venae cavae.

HEART

CT, RIGHT HEART CHAMBERS

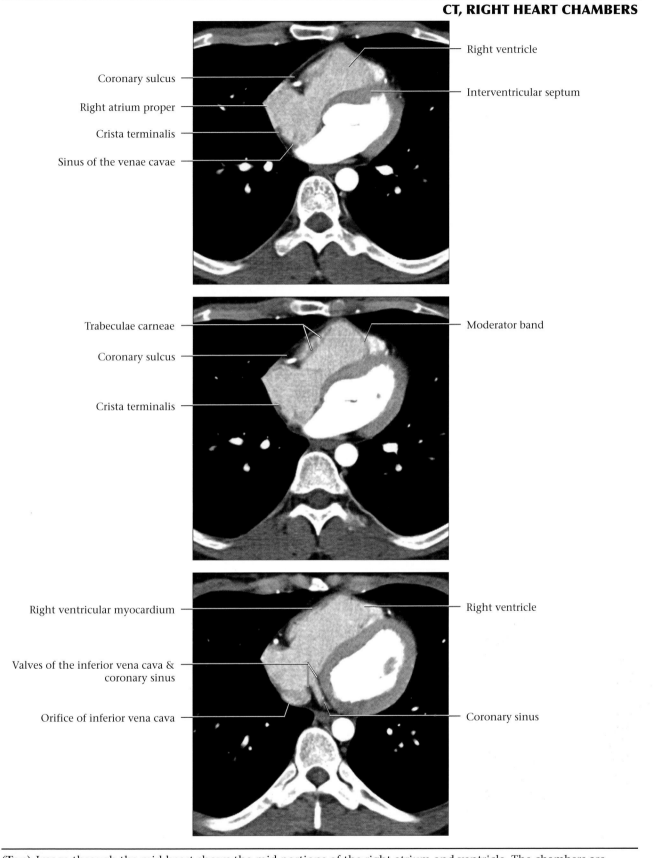

(Top) Image through the mid heart shows the mid portions of the right atrium and ventricle. The chambers are separated by the coronary sulcus. The crista terminalis is seen along the posterolateral right atrial wall. (Middle) Image through the inferior heart shows the trabeculae carneae that characterize the internal surface of the wall of the right ventricle. The septomarginal trabecula or moderator band courses from the inferior interventricular septum to the base of the anterior papillary muscle. (Bottom) Image through the inferior aspect of the heart shows the junctions of the inferior vena cava and coronary sinus with the right atrium. Note the fine trabeculations of the right ventricular myocardium produced by the trabeculae carneae. The right ventricular myocardium is very thin when compared to that of the left ventricle.

HEART

ANATOMY OF POSTERIOR HEART SURFACE & LEFT ATRIUM

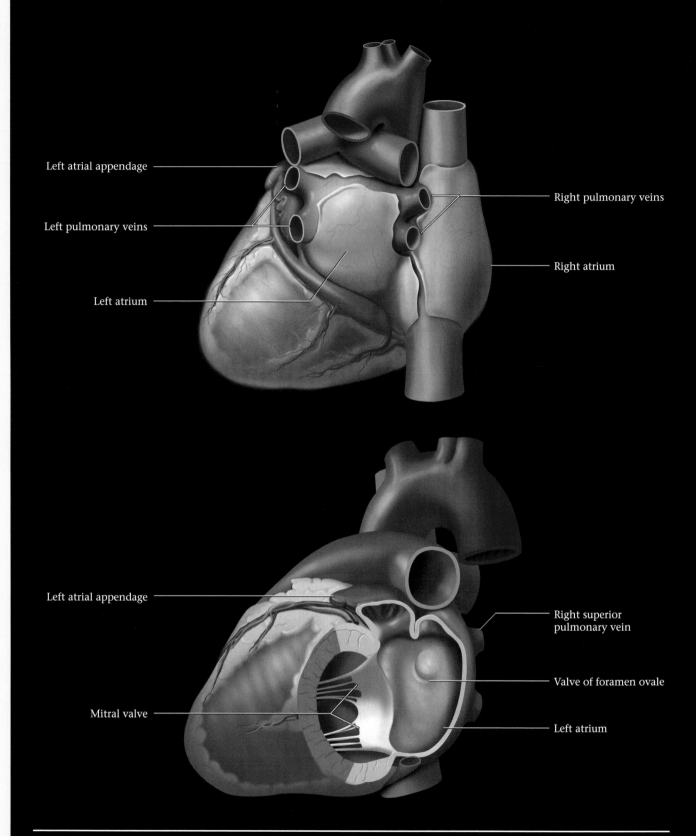

Left atrial appendage

Left pulmonary veins

Left atrium

Right pulmonary veins

Right atrium

Left atrial appendage

Mitral valve

Right superior pulmonary vein

Valve of foramen ovale

Left atrium

(Top) First of three graphics illustrating the anatomy of the left cardiac chambers. Posterior view of the heart shows the heart base formed predominantly by the left atrium and a small portion of the right atrium. The left atrium receives the paired superior and inferior pulmonary veins. **(Bottom)** Graphic shows the internal anatomy of the left atrium, which has smooth and trabeculated inner surfaces. The left atrial appendage is characterized by its trabeculated inner surface produced by the pectinate muscles. The valve of the fossa ovalis is noted on the interatrial septum and prevents passage of blood between the atria.

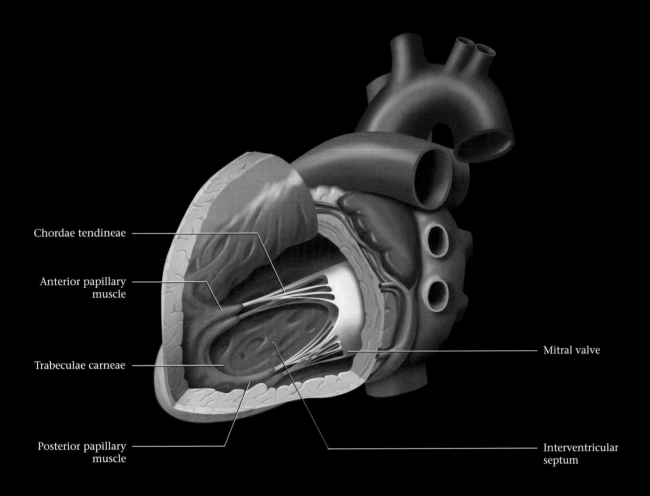

Chordae tendineae

Anterior papillary muscle

Trabeculae carneae

Posterior papillary muscle

Mitral valve

Interventricular septum

Graphic shows the internal anatomy of the left ventricle which has a thicker myocardium but thinner and more delicate trabeculae carneae than the right ventricle. The anterior and posterior papillary muscles attach to the anterior and posterior leaflets of the mitral valve respectively.

HEART

CT, LEFT HEART CHAMBERS

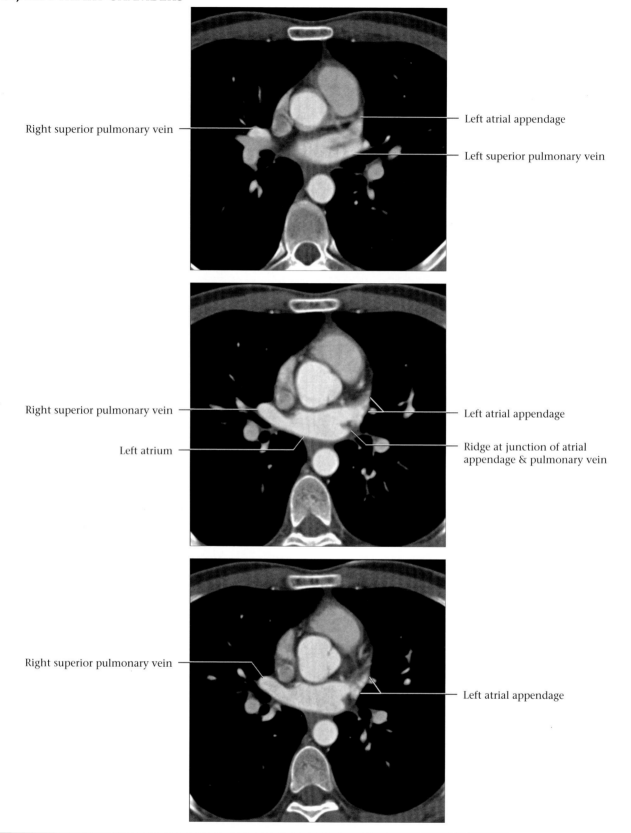

Right superior pulmonary vein — Left atrial appendage

Left superior pulmonary vein

Right superior pulmonary vein — Left atrial appendage

Left atrium — Ridge at junction of atrial appendage & pulmonary vein

Right superior pulmonary vein — Left atrial appendage

(Top) First of six contrast-enhanced axial chest CT images (mediastinal window) illustrate the anatomy of the left heart chambers. Image through the superior aspect of the left atrium demonstrates the relationship between the left atrial appendage and the left superior pulmonary vein and the smooth or nodular ridge at the junction of these two structures. (Middle) Image through the right superior pulmonary vein demonstrates the trabeculated appearance of the left atrial appendage produced by the pectinate muscles in contrast to the smooth internal wall of the left atrium proper. (Bottom) Image through the mid portion of the left atrium demonstrates the inferior aspect of the left atrial appendage and the mid portion of the right superior pulmonary vein.

HEART

CT, LEFT HEART CHAMBERS

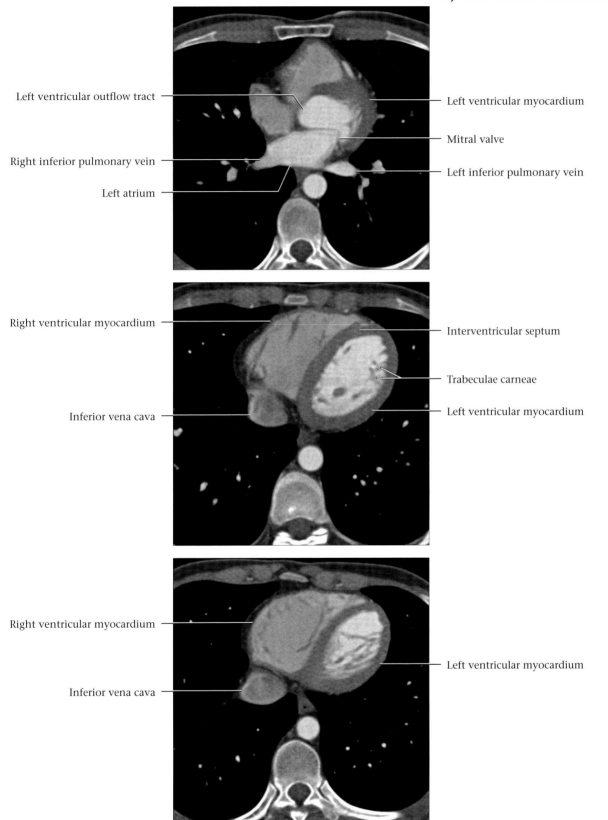

Left ventricular outflow tract — Left ventricular myocardium

— Mitral valve

Right inferior pulmonary vein — Left inferior pulmonary vein

Left atrium

Right ventricular myocardium — Interventricular septum

— Trabeculae carneae

Inferior vena cava — Left ventricular myocardium

Right ventricular myocardium

— Left ventricular myocardium

Inferior vena cava

(Top) Image through the superior aspect of the left ventricle demonstrates the thickness of the normal left ventricular wall. The trabeculae carneae produce an irregular endoluminal ventricular surface. Note the smooth appearance of the left ventricular outflow tract. (Middle) Image through the mid portion of the ventricles demonstrates internal filling defects produced by the trabeculae carneae. Compare the thickness of the left ventricular myocardium to that of the normal thinner right ventricular myocardium. (Bottom) Image through the inferior heart demonstrates the inferior portion of the left ventricle and the trabeculated appearance of its lumen. Note the trabeculated appearance of the right ventricular chamber.

HEART

CORONAL CT, NORMAL HEART

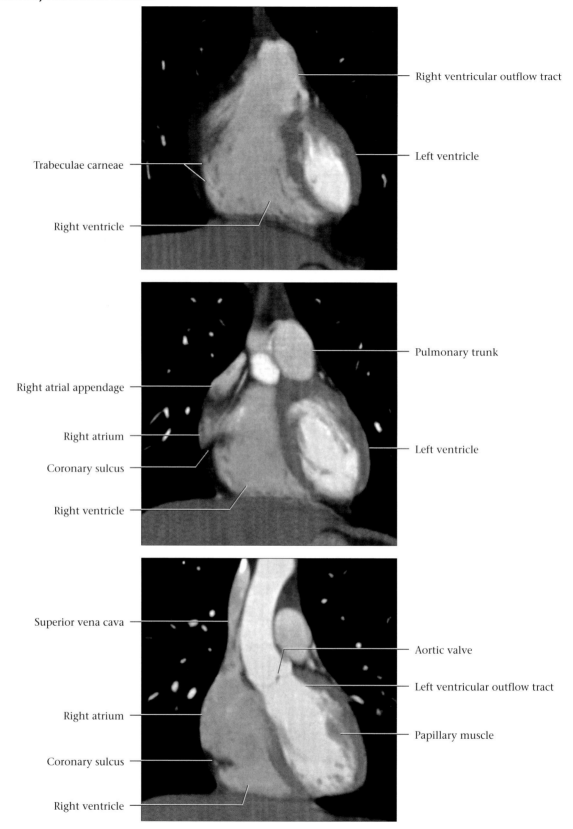

Right ventricular outflow tract

Left ventricle

Trabeculae carneae

Right ventricle

Pulmonary trunk

Right atrial appendage

Right atrium

Coronary sulcus

Left ventricle

Right ventricle

Superior vena cava

Aortic valve

Left ventricular outflow tract

Right atrium

Papillary muscle

Coronary sulcus

Right ventricle

(Top) First of six coronal contrast-enhanced chest CT images (mediastinal window) through the heart demonstrates the anteriorly located trabeculated right ventricle leading to the superiorly located and relatively smooth right ventricular outflow tract. The left ventricle forms the left cardiac border. (Middle) Image through the pulmonary trunk demonstrates the right atrial appendage. The right ventricle is anterior and to the left of the right atrium. The left ventricle forms the left heart border and has a thicker wall than that of the right ventricle. (Bottom) Image through the aortic arch shows the smooth internal wall of the left ventricular outflow tract compared to the trabeculated inner surface of left ventricle proper. The coronary sulcus separates the right atrium and right ventricle. The right atrium forms the right heart border on radiography.

HEART

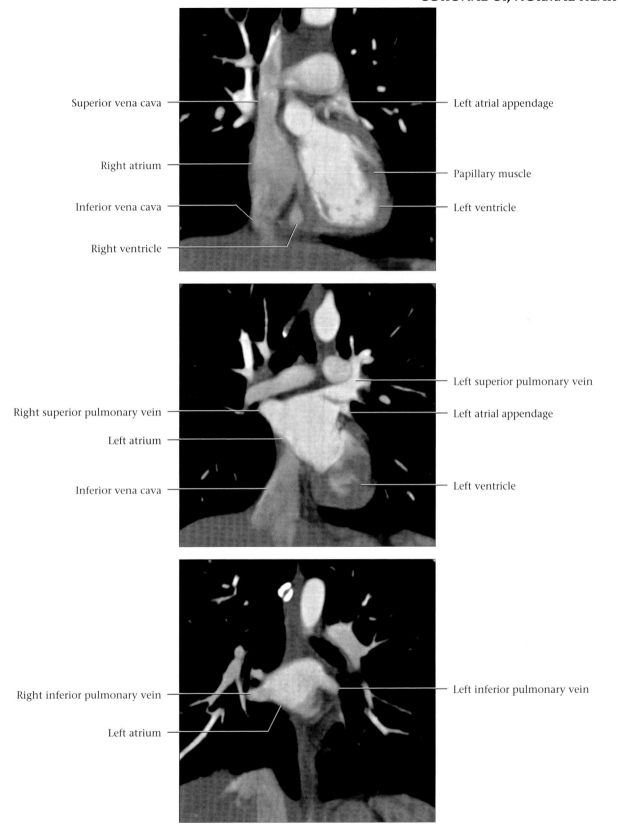

Superior vena cava — Left atrial appendage

Right atrium — Papillary muscle

Inferior vena cava — Left ventricle

Right ventricle

Right superior pulmonary vein — Left superior pulmonary vein

Left atrium — Left atrial appendage

Inferior vena cava — Left ventricle

Right inferior pulmonary vein — Left inferior pulmonary vein

Left atrium

(Top) Image through the posterior aspect of the right atrium shows its junction with the superior and inferior venae cavae. The left atrial appendage is superior to the left ventricle and forms a portion of the obtuse (left) cardiac border. A prominent papillary muscle is outlined by contrast within the left ventricle. (Middle) Image through the mid portion of the left atrium shows its junction with the bilateral superior pulmonary veins. Note the close relationship between the left superior pulmonary vein and the left atrial appendage. (Bottom) Image through the posterior aspect of the left atrium shows the bilateral inferior pulmonary veins coursing obliquely into the left atrium.

HEART

SAGITTAL CT, NORMAL HEART

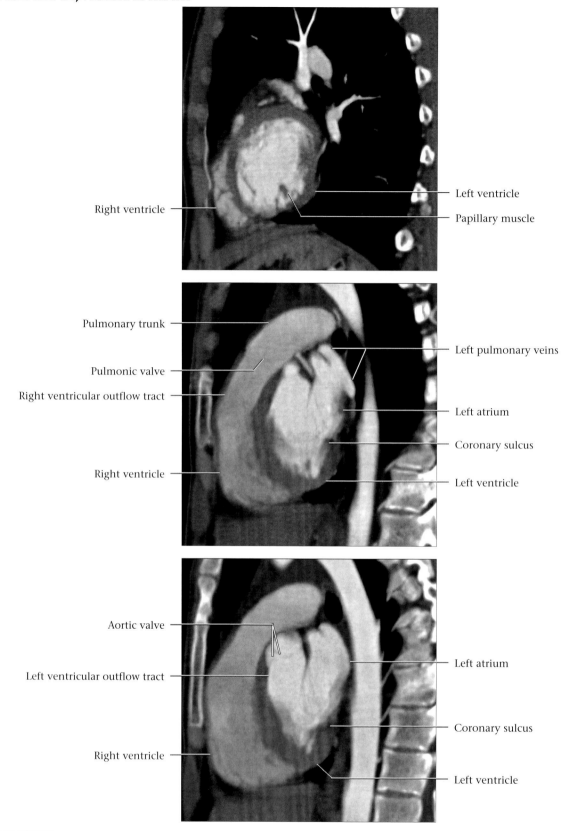

Right ventricle — Left ventricle
— Papillary muscle

Pulmonary trunk — — Left pulmonary veins
Pulmonic valve —
Right ventricular outflow tract — — Left atrium
— Coronary sulcus
Right ventricle — — Left ventricle

Aortic valve —
Left ventricular outflow tract — — Left atrium
— Coronary sulcus
Right ventricle — — Left ventricle

(Top) First of six sagittal contrast-enhanced chest CT images (mediastinal window) showing the sagittal anatomy of the heart. The images are presented from left to right. The left ventricle has a thicker myocardium when compared to the right and exhibits well-defined papillary muscles. The right ventricle forms the anterior cardiac surface. (Middle) Image through the right ventricular outflow tract shows the anterior location of the right ventricle and the posterosuperior course of the right ventricular outflow tract and pulmonary trunk. The left ventricle is posterior to the right ventricle. The left atrium is superior to the left ventricle and is separated from it by the coronary sulcus. The left pulmonary veins are seen entering the left atrium. (Bottom) Image through the mid heart shows the central location of the left ventricular outflow tract and ascending aorta.

HEART

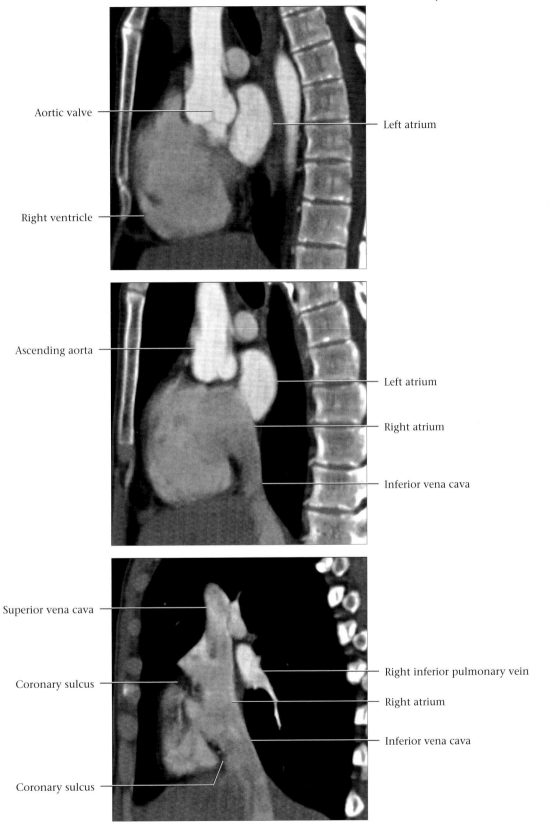

Aortic valve

Right ventricle

Left atrium

Ascending aorta

Left atrium

Right atrium

Inferior vena cava

Superior vena cava

Coronary sulcus

Coronary sulcus

Right inferior pulmonary vein

Right atrium

Inferior vena cava

(Top) Image through the aortic valve shows the anatomic location of the right ventricle, which forms the anterior cardiac surface and contributes to the diaphragmatic cardiac surface. The left atrium forms the posterior surface or base of the heart. (Middle) Image through the right heart chambers shows the posterior location of the right atrium with respect to the right ventricle and its connection with the inferior vena cava. (Bottom) Image through the right side of the heart shows the connection of the venae cavae with the right atrium. The right ventricle is located anteriorly and separated from the right atrium by the coronary sulcus.

HEART

AXIAL CT, RIGHT ATRIUM

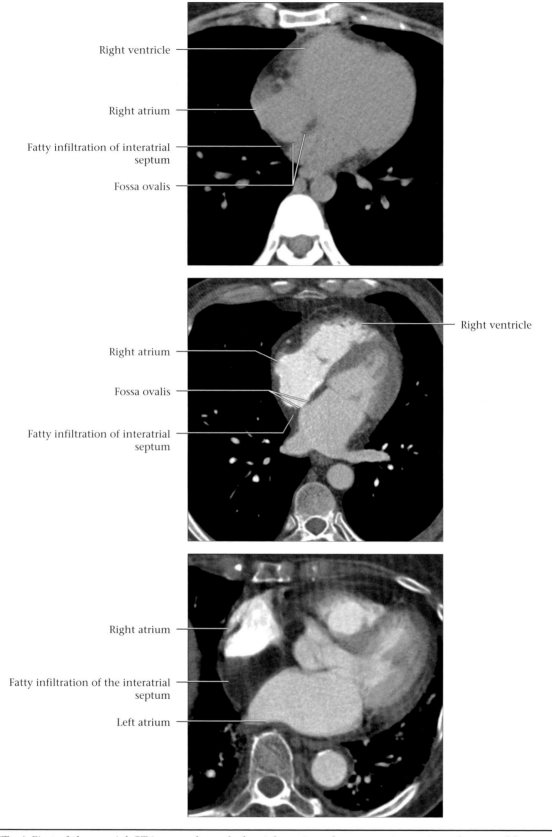

(Top) First of three axial CT images through the right atrium demonstrating various degrees of fatty infiltration of the interatrial septum. Nonenhanced chest CT (mediastinal window) demonstrates mild fatty infiltration of the interatrial septum that spares the fossa ovalis and allows its localization in the axial plane. This appearance may mimic an atrial septal defect. (Middle) Contrast-enhanced chest CT (mediastinal window) shows fatty infiltration of the interatrial septum that spares the fossa ovalis which manifests as focal thinning of the interatrial septum. (Bottom) Contrast-enhanced chest CT (mediastinal window) demonstrates prominent fatty infiltration of the interatrial septum. In this case, the area of fat replacement is mass-like and produces mass effect on the lumen of the adjacent right atrium.

HEART

CT, LEFT ATRIUM

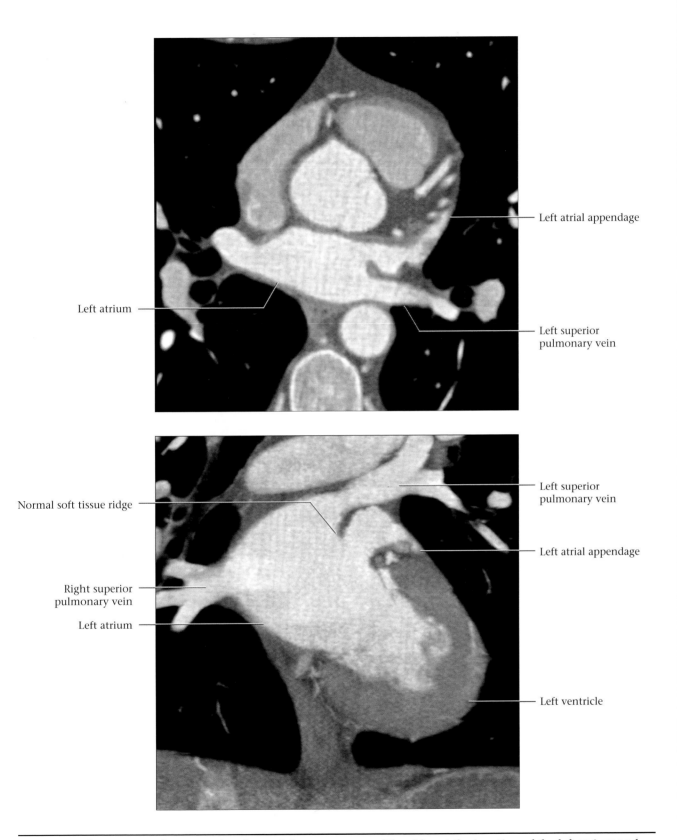

Left atrial appendage

Left atrium

Left superior
pulmonary vein

Normal soft tissue ridge

Left superior
pulmonary vein

Right superior
pulmonary vein

Left atrial appendage

Left atrium

Left ventricle

(Top) First of two images demonstrating the nodular appearance of the ridge at the junction of the left atrium and left superior pulmonary vein adjacent to the left atrial appendage. Axial image through the superior aspect of the left atrium demonstrates the constant relationship between the left superior pulmonary vein and the adjacent left atrial appendage. The left atrial appendage is always anterior and inferior to the left superior pulmonary vein. Note the nodular soft tissue ridge that protrudes into the left atrial lumen which should not be confused with thrombus or neoplasia. **(Bottom)** Coronal image through the left atrial appendage demonstrates the normal soft tissue ridge that occurs at the junction of the left atrium with the left superior pulmonary vein adjacent to the left atrial appendage.

HEART

CT, SHORT AXIS VIEW

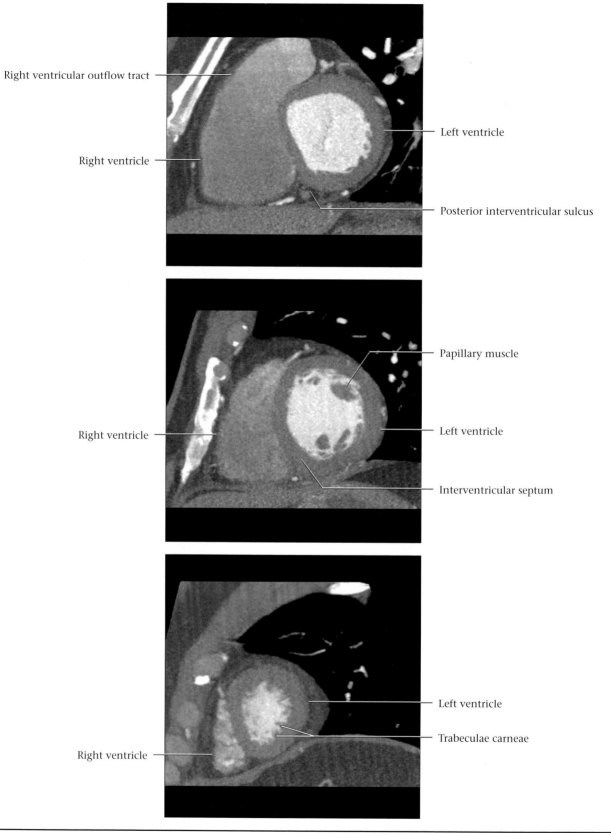

Right ventricular outflow tract

Right ventricle

Left ventricle

Posterior interventricular sulcus

Papillary muscle

Right ventricle

Left ventricle

Interventricular septum

Left ventricle

Trabeculae carneae

Right ventricle

(Top) First of three contrast-enhanced cardiac gated short axis CT images (mediastinal window) showing the ventricular chambers. The right ventricle is located anteriorly and has a thin wall. The right ventricular outflow tract courses superiorly and posteriorly to give off the pulmonary trunk. The left ventricle is posterior and has a thicker myocardium than the right ventricle. The two chambers are separated by the interventricular sulcus. **(Middle)** Image through the mid heart shows the anatomy of the left ventricular chamber. The papillary muscles manifest as filling defects within the contrast filled left ventricular lumen. **(Bottom)** Image obtained just medial to the left apex demonstrates trabeculations in both ventricular chambers produced by trabeculae carneae. The right ventricle forms the anterior heart surface.

CT, TWO CHAMBER VIEW

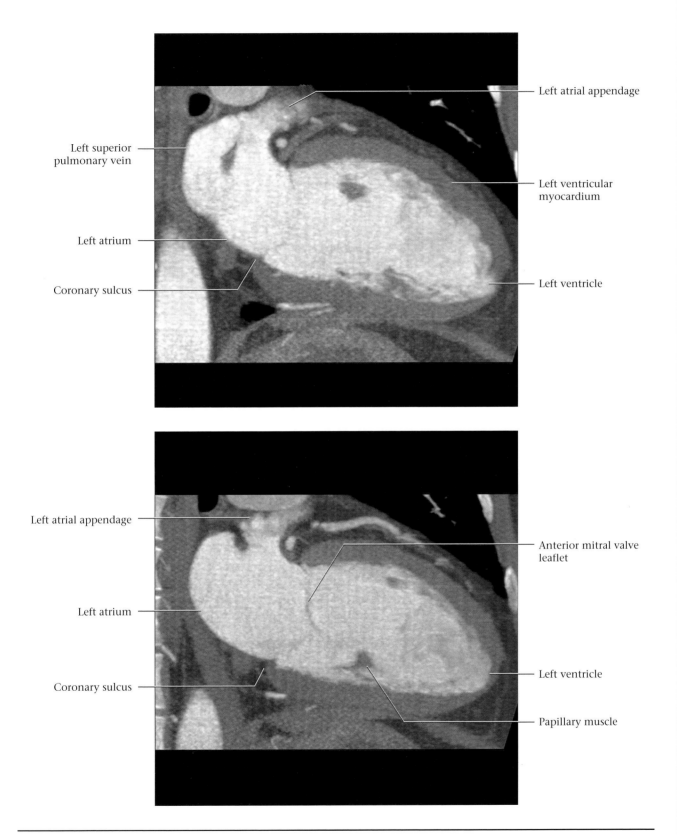

Left atrial appendage

Left superior pulmonary vein

Left ventricular myocardium

Left atrium

Coronary sulcus

Left ventricle

Left atrial appendage

Anterior mitral valve leaflet

Left atrium

Coronary sulcus

Left ventricle

Papillary muscle

(Top) First of two two-chamber contrast-enhanced gated cardiac CT images (mediastinal window) showing the anatomy of the left ventricle and left atrium. Note the intimate relationship of the left superior pulmonary vein and the left atrial appendage with an intervening nodular soft tissue ridge. The left atrial appendage exhibits a trabeculated internal surface produced by the pectinate muscles. The left ventricle, the thickness of its wall and its papillary muscles are well visualized. **(Bottom)** Image through the mitral valve obtained during systole demonstrates coaptation of the thin anterior and posterior valve cusps. The papillary muscles manifest as rounded filling defects within the contrast filled left ventricular chamber.

HEART

CT, FOUR CHAMBER VIEW

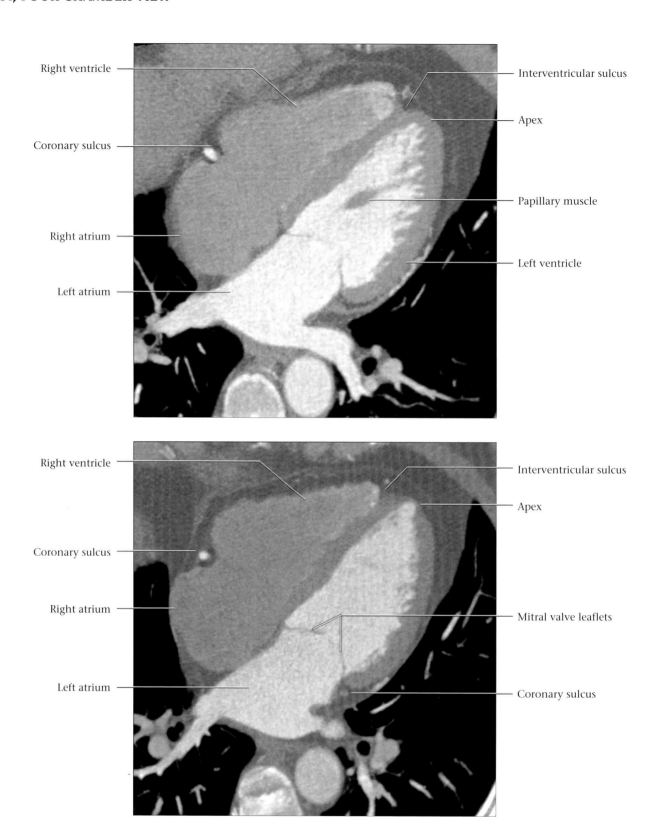

(Top) First of two contrast-enhanced gated four chamber cardiac CT images (mediastinal window) demonstrating the anatomy of the heart. This view allows simultaneous evaluation of the four cardiac chambers. The right chambers are projected anterolateral to the left heart chambers and are less opacified with contrast. The mitral valve leaflets manifest as thin linear soft tissue structures between the left atrium and left ventricle. **(Bottom)** Four-chamber gated cardiac CT image demonstrates the normal mitral valve. The four cardiac chambers and the coronary and interventricular sulci are demonstrated. The interventricular sulcus is located slightly to the right of the cardiac apex.

HEART

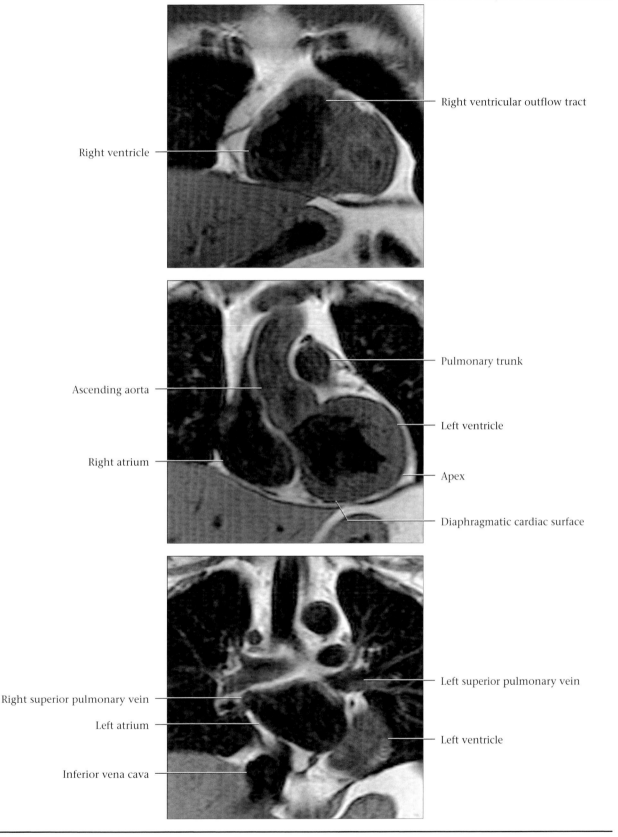

Right ventricular outflow tract

Right ventricle

Pulmonary trunk

Ascending aorta

Left ventricle

Right atrium

Apex

Diaphragmatic cardiac surface

Left superior pulmonary vein

Right superior pulmonary vein

Left atrium

Inferior vena cava

Left ventricle

(Top) First of three coronal T1-weighted magnetic resonance images of the chest showing the anatomy of the heart. Image through the anterior heart demonstrates the trabeculated wall of the right ventricle. The right ventricular outflow tract is oriented posterosuperiorly. (Middle) Image through the mid portion of the heart shows the centrally located aortic root. The right atrium forms the right cardiac border. The left ventricle forms the left or obtuse cardiac border. Note the thick left ventricular myocardium. The diaphragmatic cardiac surface is also visualized. (Bottom) Image through the posterior aspect of the heart shows the left atrium and a portion of the posterior left ventricle. The bilateral superior pulmonary veins are also imaged as is the posterior aspect of the suprahepatic inferior vena cava.

HEART

SAGITTAL MR, NORMAL HEART

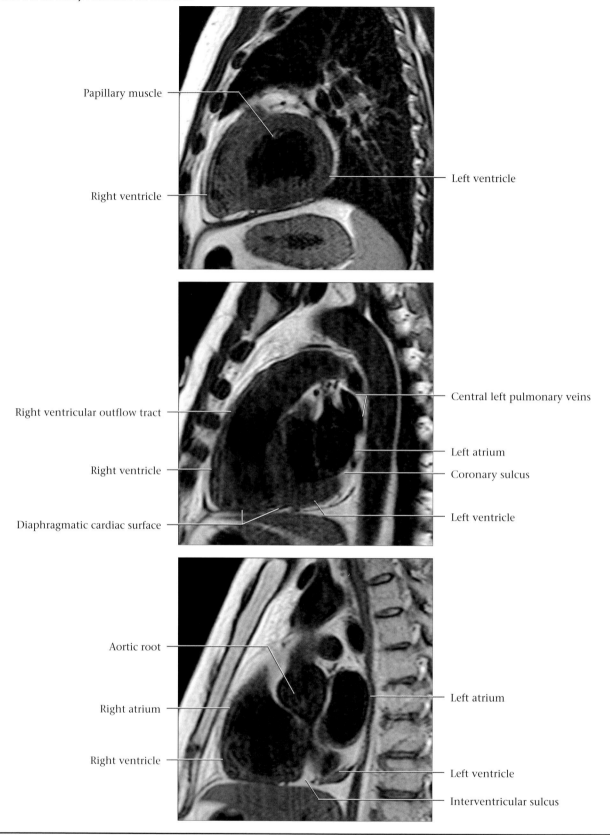

(Top) First of five sagittal T1-weighted magnetic resonance images of the chest showing the anatomy of the heart. The images are presented from left to right. Image through the ventricles demonstrates their trabeculated internal surfaces. Note the thickness of the left ventricular myocardium relative to that of the right. (Middle) Image through the pulmonary outflow tract shows the anterior location of the right ventricle, which forms the anterior cardiac surface. The left atrium is located posterior and superior to the left ventricle and forms the base of the heart. The right ventricle forms the anterior heart surface. The right and left ventricles form the diaphragmatic cardiac surface. (Bottom) Image though the root of the aorta shows its central location with respect to the vessels and the heart chambers and the anatomic relationship of the right and left atria.

HEART

SAGITTAL MR, NORMAL HEART

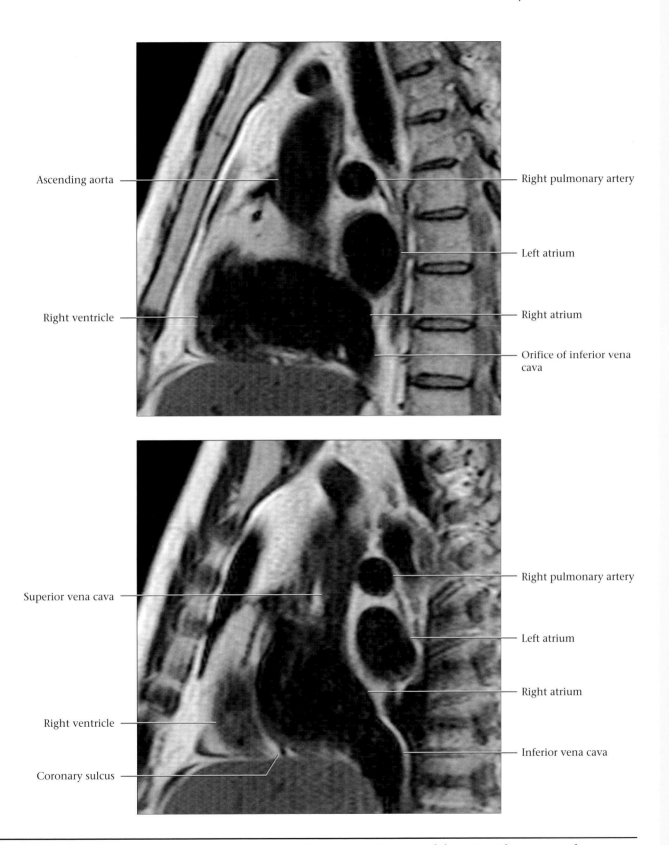

Ascending aorta — Right pulmonary artery — Left atrium — Right ventricle — Right atrium — Orifice of inferior vena cava

Superior vena cava — Right pulmonary artery — Left atrium — Right atrium — Right ventricle — Inferior vena cava — Coronary sulcus

(Top) Image through the ascending aorta demonstrates the posterior location of the atria with respect to the anteriorly located trabeculated right ventricle. The proximal ascending aorta and its root are located in the center of the heart. **(Bottom)** Image through the right atrium demonstrates its posterosuperior and posteroinferior connections with the superior and inferior venae cavae respectively. There is visualization of a small portion of the anteriorly located right ventricle. The posteriorly located left atrium, which forms a large portion of the base of the heart is also visualized. The coronary sulcus is located between the atria and ventricles.

HEART

ANATOMY OF CARDIAC SKELETON & HEART VALVES

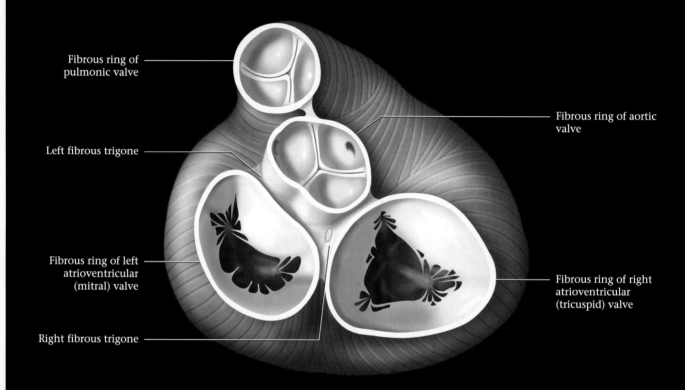

Fibrous ring of pulmonic valve · Left fibrous trigone · Fibrous ring of left atrioventricular (mitral) valve · Right fibrous trigone · Fibrous ring of aortic valve · Fibrous ring of right atrioventricular (tricuspid) valve

Graphic demonstrates the anatomy of the cardiac skeleton located between the atria and ventricles. The cardiac skeleton consists of thick fibrous connective tissue and provides support for the valve orifices and the areas of attachment for the valve cusps. In this illustration, the atria have been "removed" to expose the cardiac skeleton and heart valves seen from above. The four fibrous rings that surround the valves are known as the annulus fibrosus. The right fibrous trigone is the connective tissue bridge between the aortic valve and right atrioventricular (tricuspid) valve rings. The left fibrous trigone is the connective tissue bridge between the aortic valve and the left atrioventricular (mitral) valve rings. The yellow dot represents the atrioventricular bundle seen in cross-section as it courses caudally from the atria to the ventricles.

HEART

RADIOGRAPHY, PROSTHETIC AORTIC & MITRAL VALVES

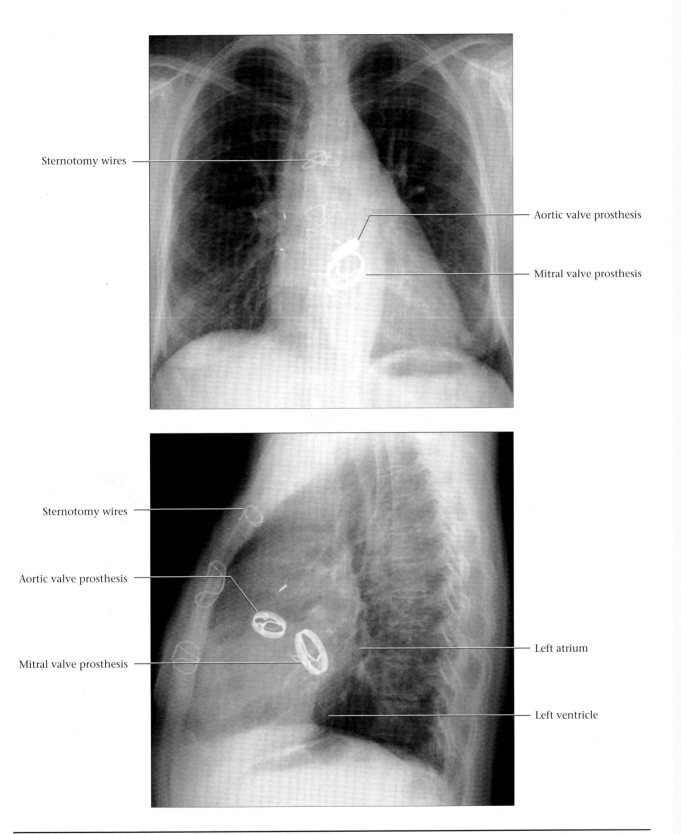

Sternotomy wires

Aortic valve prosthesis

Mitral valve prosthesis

Sternotomy wires

Aortic valve prosthesis

Mitral valve prosthesis

Left atrium

Left ventricle

(Top) First of two images of a 56 year old woman status post-aortic and mitral valve replacement for rheumatic heart disease. PA chest radiograph shows the close relationship of the aortic and mitral valves and post-surgical changes. The aortic valve prosthesis is located in the center of the heart and is oriented along the long axis of the ascending aorta. The mitral valve prosthesis is located more inferiorly and its orifice exhibits a more horizontal orientation. **(Bottom)** Left lateral chest radiograph shows the aortic valve prosthesis in the center of the heart and the more posteriorly located mitral valve prosthesis oriented along the long axis of the left atrioventricular orifice. The close relationship of these two prosthetic valves is consistent with the fact that they share a common fibrous annulus and the left fibrous trigone.

HEART

ANATOMY & CT, ATRIOVENTRICULAR VALVE

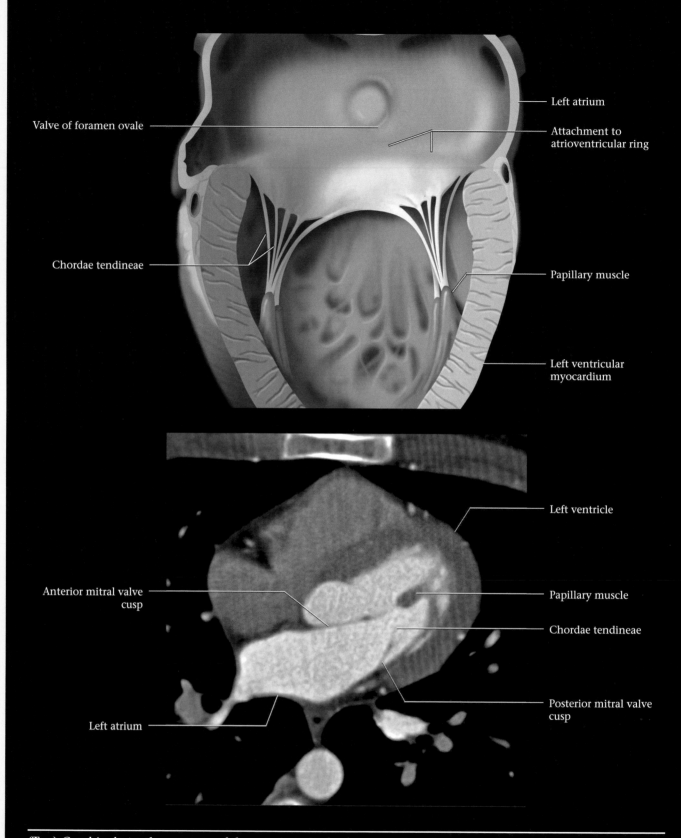

Valve of foramen ovale

Left atrium

Attachment to atrioventricular ring

Chordae tendineae

Papillary muscle

Left ventricular myocardium

Left ventricle

Anterior mitral valve cusp

Papillary muscle

Chordae tendineae

Posterior mitral valve cusp

Left atrium

(Top) Graphic shows the anatomy of the anterior mitral valve cusp. The valve cusp is flat and has a broad attachment to the fibrous atrioventricular valve ring. The free edge of the valve is attached to the tips of two sets of papillary muscles by chordae tendineae. The mitral and tricuspid valves share this morphology, but the former has two cusps and the latter has three. The valve opens during ventricular filling and its cusps protrude into the left ventricle. During ventricular systole the cusps are forced closed and are prevented from protruding into the left atrium by the chordae tendineae and papillary muscle contraction. **(Bottom)** Normal contrast-enhanced axial cardiac CT (mediastinal window) shows the mitral valve during ventricular filling. The valve cusps protrude into the ventricular lumen and are attached to the papillary muscles by thin chordae tendineae.

HEART

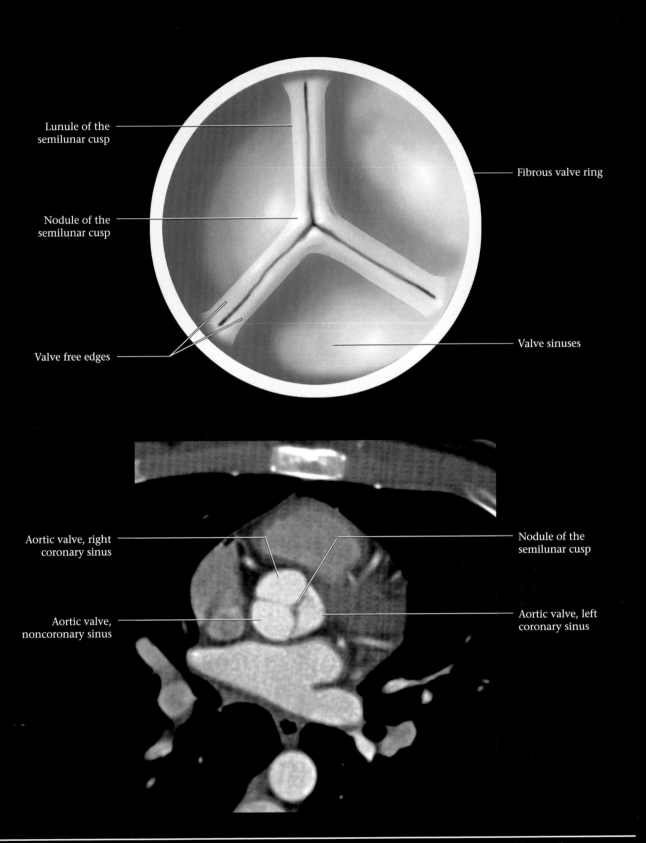

Lunule of the semilunar cusp

Fibrous valve ring

Nodule of the semilunar cusp

Valve free edges

Valve sinuses

Aortic valve, right coronary sinus

Nodule of the semilunar cusp

Aortic valve, noncoronary sinus

Aortic valve, left coronary sinus

(Top) Graphic illustrates the anatomy of the semilunar valves, the pulmonic and aortic valves. These valves are tricuspid (three cusps) and have free edges without tendinous attachments to the ventricle. The free cusp edges project into the vessel lumen during valve closure forming sinuses. Retrograde blood flow after ventricular contraction forces the valves shut. Antegrade blood flow during ventricular systole forces the valve open. The superior free edge of the valve cusp exhibits a central focus of nodular thickening, the nodule of the semilunar cusp and a thin lateral free edge, the lunule of the semilunar cusp. (Bottom) Axial contrast-enhanced gated cardiac CT (mediastinal window) shows the morphology of the aortic valve during ventricular filling. Thickened foci in the central aspects of the cusp free edges represent the nodules of the semilunar cusps.

HEART

ANATOMY OF TRICUSPID & PULMONIC VALVES

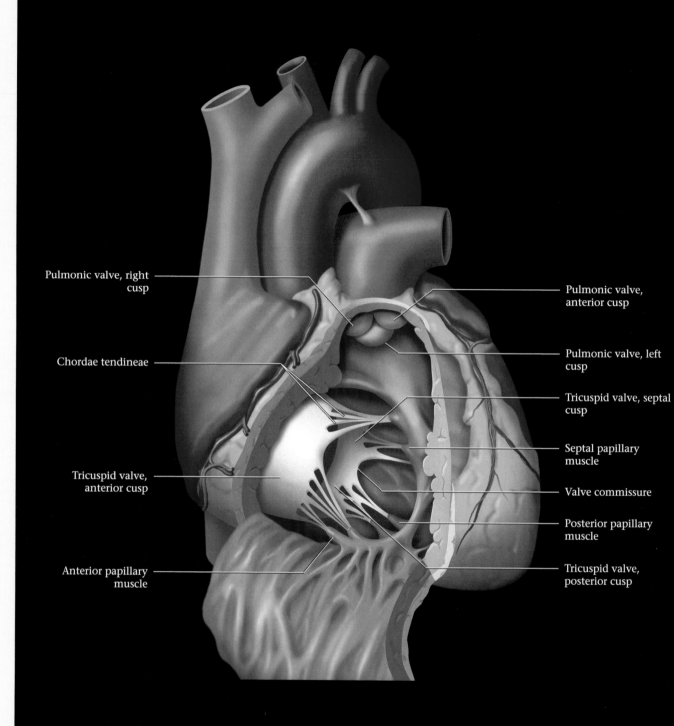

Pulmonic valve, right cusp

Chordae tendineae

Tricuspid valve, anterior cusp

Anterior papillary muscle

Pulmonic valve, anterior cusp

Pulmonic valve, left cusp

Tricuspid valve, septal cusp

Septal papillary muscle

Valve commissure

Posterior papillary muscle

Tricuspid valve, posterior cusp

Graphic illustrates the internal anatomy of the right ventricle and the anatomy of the right heart valves. The right atrioventricular valve is the tricuspid valve. It has three cusps that are attached to the fibrous valve ring and are continuous with each other at the valve commissures. The cusps are named according to their positions; anterior, septal and posterior. The free edges of the valves attach to chordae tendineae that in turn attach to the tips of papillary muscles that are also named according to their location. The pulmonic valve is a tricuspid semilunar valve located just distal to the right ventricular outflow tract. The free edges of the valve project into the pulmonary trunk forming sinuses and coapt at the nodules of the semilunar cusps. There are left, right and anterior pulmonic valve cusps.

HEART

CT, RIGHT HEART VALVES

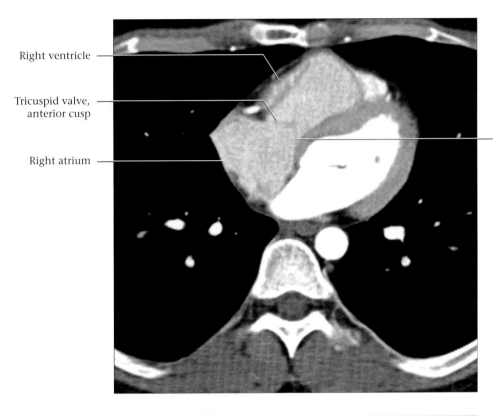

Right ventricle

Tricuspid valve, anterior cusp

Right atrium

Tricuspid valve, septal cusp

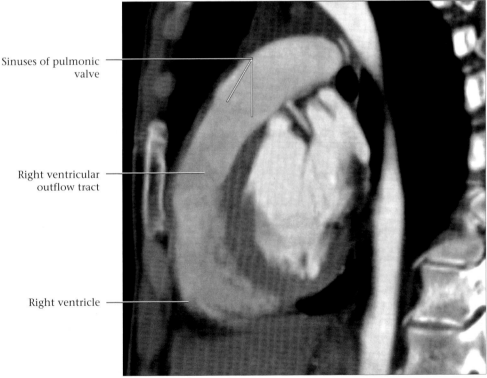

Sinuses of pulmonic valve

Right ventricular outflow tract

Right ventricle

(Top) First of two contrast-enhanced chest CT images (mediastinal window) demonstrating the anatomy and location of the right heart valves. The normal valves are thin and are difficult to visualize on conventional CT. Cardiac gated axial CT image shows the tricuspid valve imaged during ventricular systole. The coapted septal and anterior valve cusps manifest as thin soft tissue linear opacities within the contrast filled right heart chambers.
(Bottom) Sagittal image through the pulmonary trunk shows the anatomy and location of the pulmonic valve. The pulmonic valve is tricuspid and is located at the apex of the right ventricular outflow tract. This image is obtained during ventricular filling (diastole) and shows two of the three valve cusps coapted within the vessel lumen. The free valve edges protrude into the vascular lumen and form sinuses.

HEART

ANATOMY OF LEFT HEART VALVES

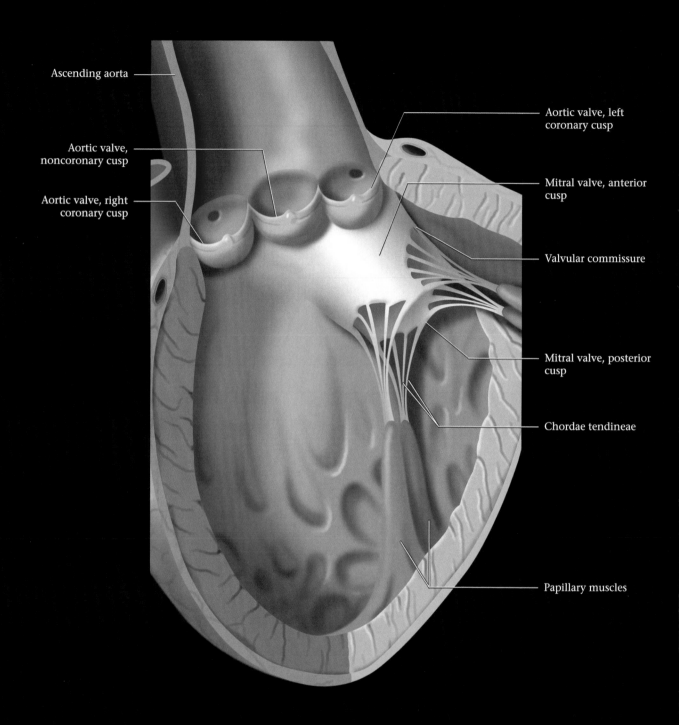

Ascending aorta

Aortic valve, noncoronary cusp

Aortic valve, right coronary cusp

Aortic valve, left coronary cusp

Mitral valve, anterior cusp

Valvular commissure

Mitral valve, posterior cusp

Chordae tendineae

Papillary muscles

Graphic depicts the close relationship between the aortic and mitral valves. These valves are supported by fibrous valve rings connected by the left fibrous trigone. Thus, the anterior cusp of the mitral valve is closely related to the left coronary cusp of the aortic valve. The aortic valve right coronary, left coronary and non-coronary cusps are shown. The semilunar cusps form sinuses during valve closure which occurs by coaptation of the free cusp edges. Each valve has a fibrous nodule on the central portion of its free edge called the nodulus arantii. The mitral valve cusps are continuous along the left atrioventricular fibrous valve ring and are connected at the valve cusp commissures. The free edges of the mitral valve cusps attach to the anterior and posterior papillary muscles via chordae tendineae.

HEART

ANATOMY & CT, LEFT HEART VALVES

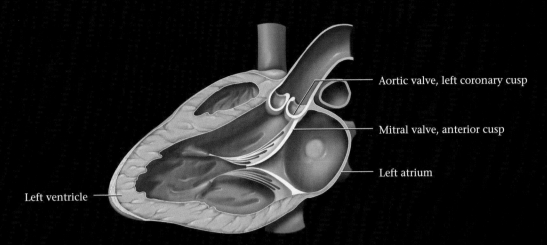

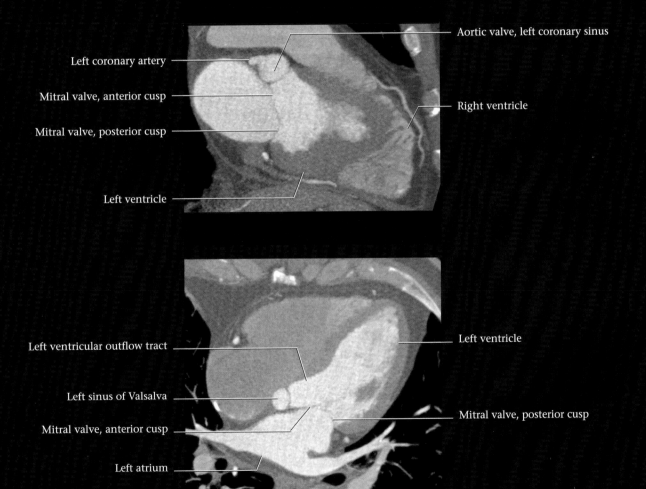

(Top) Graphic illustrates a three chamber view of the heart and the relationship between the mitral and aortic valves. The fibrous rings that support these valves share a common fibrous bridge called the left fibrous trigone. The fibrous bridge forms a connection between the anterior cusp of the mitral valve and the left coronary cusp of the aortic valve. **(Middle)** First of two contrast-enhanced gated cardiac CT images (mediastinal window) demonstrating the anatomic relationship between the aortic and mitral valves. The left coronary cusp of the aortic valve shares a common fibrous attachment with the anterior cusp of the mitral valve. **(Bottom)** Four chamber image demonstrates the close relationship between the anterior cusp of the mitral valve and the left coronary cusp of the aortic valve. The left coronary cusp is only partially visualized on this image.

HEART

CT, MITRAL VALVE

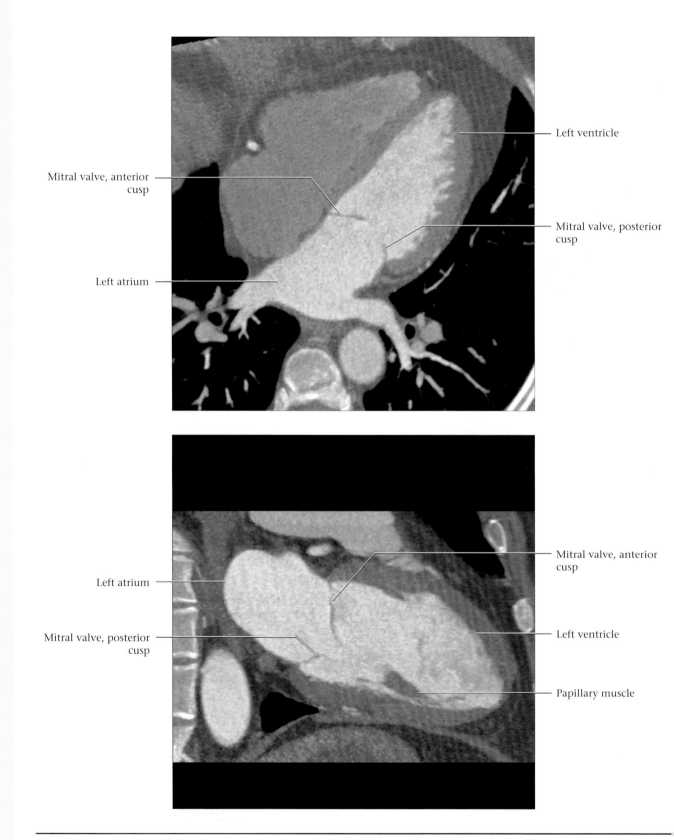

Left ventricle

Mitral valve, anterior cusp

Mitral valve, posterior cusp

Left atrium

Left atrium

Mitral valve, anterior cusp

Mitral valve, posterior cusp

Left ventricle

Papillary muscle

(Top) Contrast-enhanced four chamber gated cardiac CT (mediastinal window) demonstrates the anatomy of the mitral valve. The anterior and posterior valve cusps manifest as thin linear structures that extend across the atrioventricular orifice. While the trabeculated left ventricular wall is visible, the chordae tendineae are not visualized. (Bottom) Contrast-enhanced two chamber gated cardiac CT (mediastinal window) demonstrates the anterior and posterior leaflets of the mitral valve at the atrioventricular orifice. The posterior papillary muscle is also demonstrated.

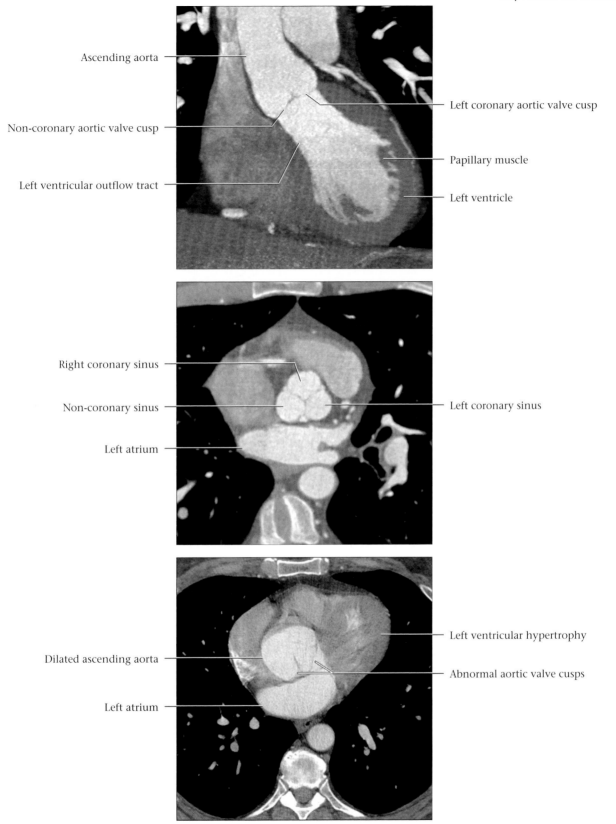

Ascending aorta

Non-coronary aortic valve cusp

Left ventricular outflow tract

Left coronary aortic valve cusp

Papillary muscle

Left ventricle

Right coronary sinus

Non-coronary sinus

Left atrium

Left coronary sinus

Dilated ascending aorta

Left atrium

Left ventricular hypertrophy

Abnormal aortic valve cusps

(Top) First of two gated contrast-enhanced cardiac CT images (mediastinal window) demonstrating the cross-sectional imaging appearance of the aortic valve. Coronal image shows the aortic valve cusps in coaptation. The valve cusps manifest as thin curvilinear soft tissue structures located at the apex of the left ventricular outflow tract. The sinuses of Valsalva are visible during diastole and are located above the valve cusps. **(Middle)** Axial image through the aortic valve in coaptation shows right coronary, left coronary and non-coronary sinuses of Valsalva bound by the aortic wall and the corresponding valve cusps. **(Bottom)** Axial image through a bicuspid or bicommissural aortic valve shows partial visualization of abnormal valve cusps. The valve was stenotic, and there was associated dilatation of the ascending aorta and left ventricular hypertrophy.

HEART

MR, VALVE FUNCTION

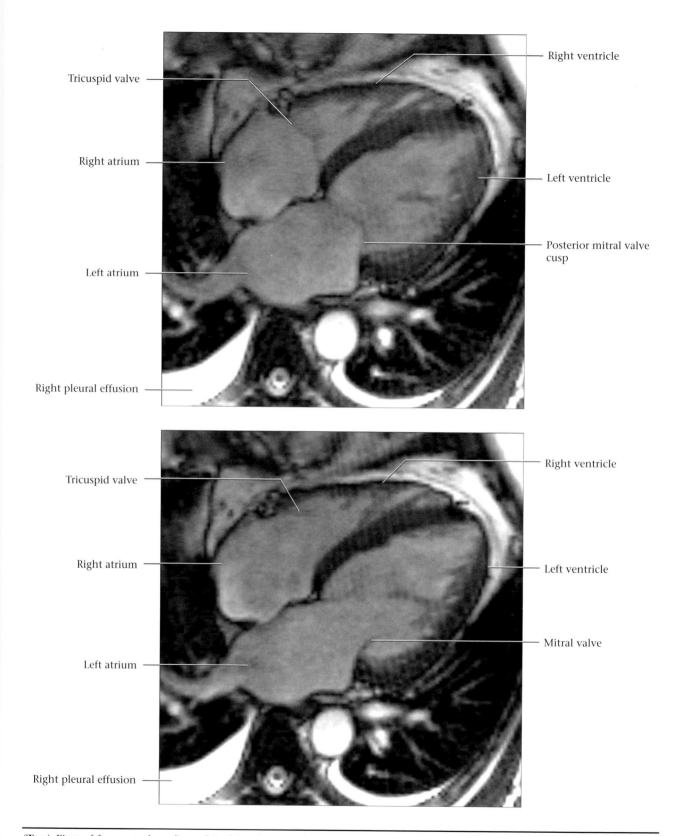

Tricuspid valve

Right atrium

Left atrium

Right pleural effusion

Right ventricle

Left ventricle

Posterior mitral valve cusp

Tricuspid valve

Right atrium

Left atrium

Right pleural effusion

Right ventricle

Left ventricle

Mitral valve

(Top) First of four gated cardiac white blood magnetic resonance images through the heart demonstrating the function of the heart valves. Four chamber view obtained during ventricular systole shows that the atrioventricular valve cusps are coapted or closed allowing blood to be pumped in an antegrade direction into the pulmonary and systemic arteries by the contracting myocardium without regurgitation or retrograde flow into the atria. **(Bottom)** Four chamber view obtained during diastole demonstrates that the cusps of the atrioventricular valves are open allowing blood to flow in an antegrade direction from the atria to fill the bilateral ventricles. The papillary muscles where the chordae tendineae attach are also visualized. There are small bilateral pleural effusions, larger on the right.

HEART

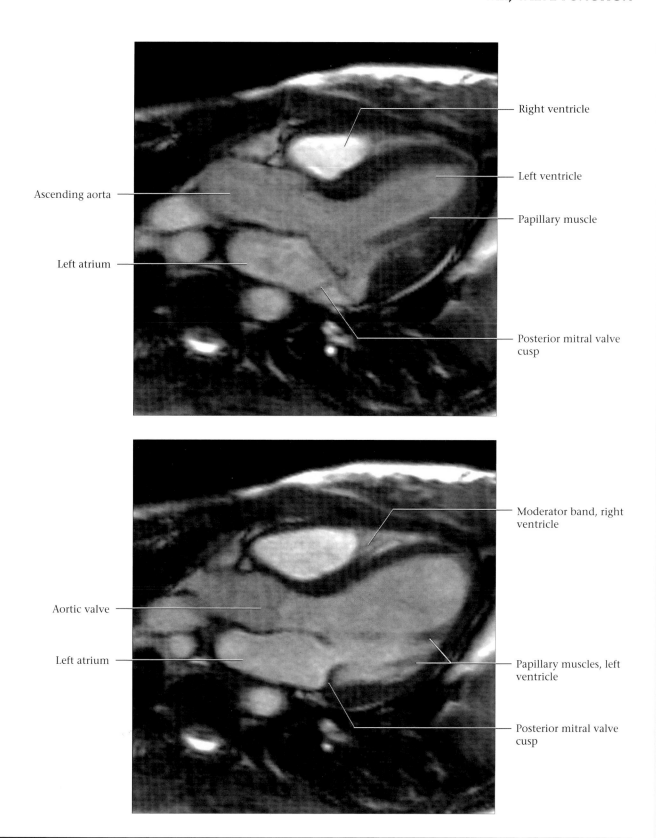

(Top) First of two gated white blood cardiac magnetic resonance images demonstrating the function of the mitral and aortic valves. Three chamber view image obtained during ventricular systole demonstrates that the aortic valve cusps are not visible at the aortic root distal to the right ventricular outflow tract indicating that the aortic valve is open to allow antegrade flow of blood into the aorta. The mitral valve cusps are closed or coapted to prevent regurgitation of ventricular blood into the left atrium. **(Bottom)** Three chamber view obtained during diastole shows that the mitral valve cusps are open to allow blood to flow into the left ventricle. The aortic valve cusps are closed preventing retrograde flow of blood from the aorta. The papillary muscles of the left ventricle and moderator band of the right ventricle are also visualized.

413

HEART

RADIOGRAPHY, NORMAL HEART

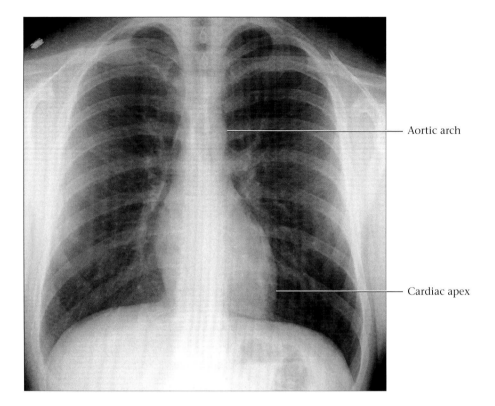

Aortic arch

Cardiac apex

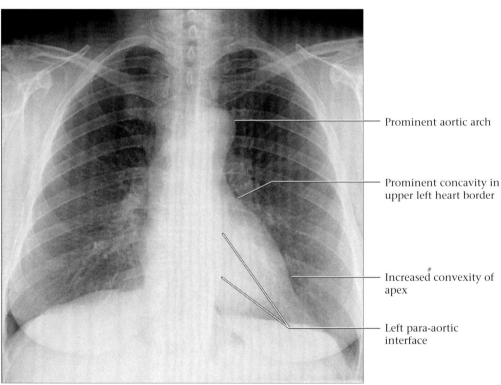

Prominent aortic arch

Prominent concavity in upper left heart border

Increased convexity of apex

Left para-aortic interface

(Top) First of two normal chest radiographs demonstrating the variability of the cardiac configuration with advancing age. PA chest radiograph of a 15 year old boy demonstrates a normal heart configuration for this age group. Patients of this age may also exhibit a prominent pulmonary trunk (see "Pulmonary Vessels" section). The aortic arch is small and the descending aorta is poorly visualized. (Bottom) PA chest radiograph of an asymptomatic 55 year old woman shows that the heart exhibits a left ventricular configuration in which the left sided structures produce the dominant radiographic findings. The pulmonary trunk is not apparent. The aortic arch is prominent, and there is a concavity in the mid left or obtuse cardiac border. The left heart border has increased convexity. The descending aorta is visible throughout its length.

HEART

ABNORMAL SITUS

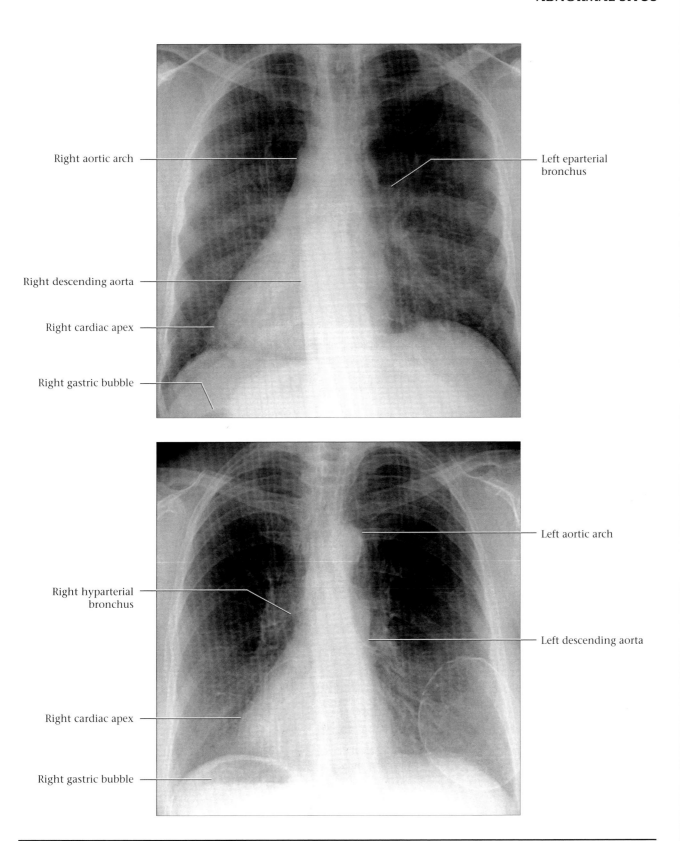

Right aortic arch

Left eparterial bronchus

Right descending aorta

Right cardiac apex

Right gastric bubble

Right hyparterial bronchus

Left aortic arch

Left descending aorta

Right cardiac apex

Right gastric bubble

(Top) PA chest radiograph of a 25 year old man with situs inversus demonstrates dextrocardia. The aortic arch, descending aorta and gastric bubble are located on the right. The diagnosis of situs inversus is supported by the presence of left eparterial and right hyparterial bronchi. Abnormal situs relates to abnormalities of atrial morphology. The most accurate radiographic indicator of atrial morphology is the configuration of the central tracheobronchial tree. **(Bottom)** PA chest radiograph of a 45 year old woman with situs ambiguous. The cardiac apex and gastric bubble are located on the right side. The aortic arch and descending aorta are located on the left side. Bilateral hyparterial bronchi are present, consistent with polysplenia or bilateral left sidedness. Bilateral chest wall round curvilinear calcifications represent partially calcified breast implants.

HEART

CARDIOMEGALY

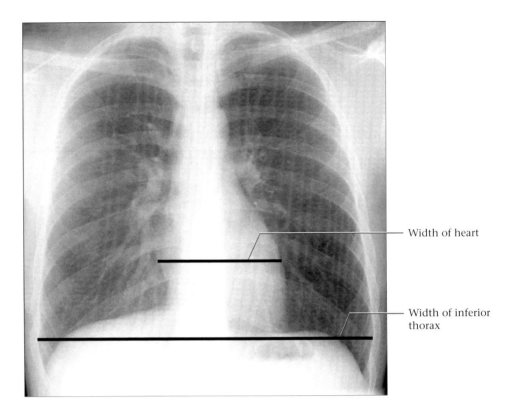

- Width of heart

- Width of inferior thorax

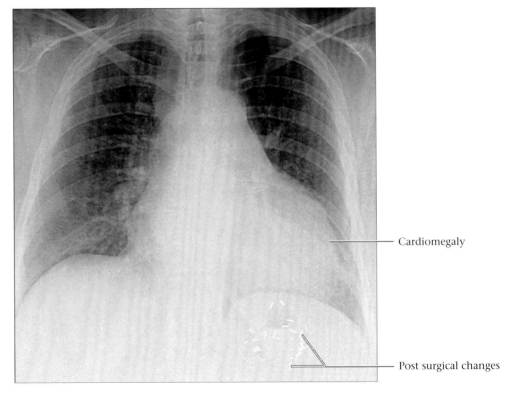

- Cardiomegaly

- Post surgical changes

(**Top**) Normal PA chest radiograph demonstrates the method for measuring the cardiothoracic ratio. The cardiothoracic ratio is the ratio of the width of the cardiac silhouette at its widest point to the width of the inferior thorax between the inner margins of the lateral ribs. The normal cardiothoracic ratio is 0.55 or less, indicating that the heart is typically a little over half as wide as the inferior thorax. (**Bottom**) PA chest radiograph of a 52 year old woman with cardiomyopathy demonstrates an abnormal cardiothoracic ratio consistent with cardiomegaly. There are post-surgical changes in the left upper quadrant.

HEART

LEFT ATRIAL ENLARGEMENT

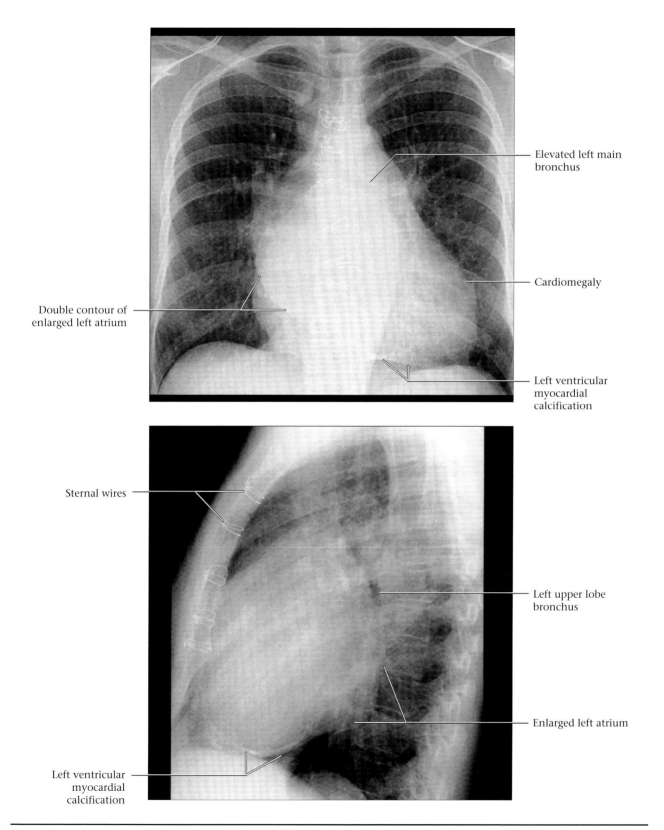

Elevated left main bronchus

Cardiomegaly

Double contour of enlarged left atrium

Left ventricular myocardial calcification

Sternal wires

Left upper lobe bronchus

Enlarged left atrium

Left ventricular myocardial calcification

(Top) First of two images of a 42 year old man with left atrial enlargement secondary to mitral stenosis. PA chest radiograph demonstrates cardiomegaly and left atrial enlargement. The latter produces a double contour superimposed on the right atrium, elevation of the left main bronchus and splaying of the carina. There are post-surgical changes of sternotomy and findings of left ventricular calcification likely related to remote myocardial infarction. There is vascular redistribution consistent with pulmonary venous hypertension. **(Bottom)** Left lateral chest radiograph demonstrates the enlarged left atrium which is easily differentiated from the left ventricle, as the latter exhibits dense mural calcification. There is posterior displacement of the left upper lobe bronchus by the enlarged left atrium. Findings of prior sternotomy are also noted.

HEART

LEFT VENTRICULAR ANEURYSM

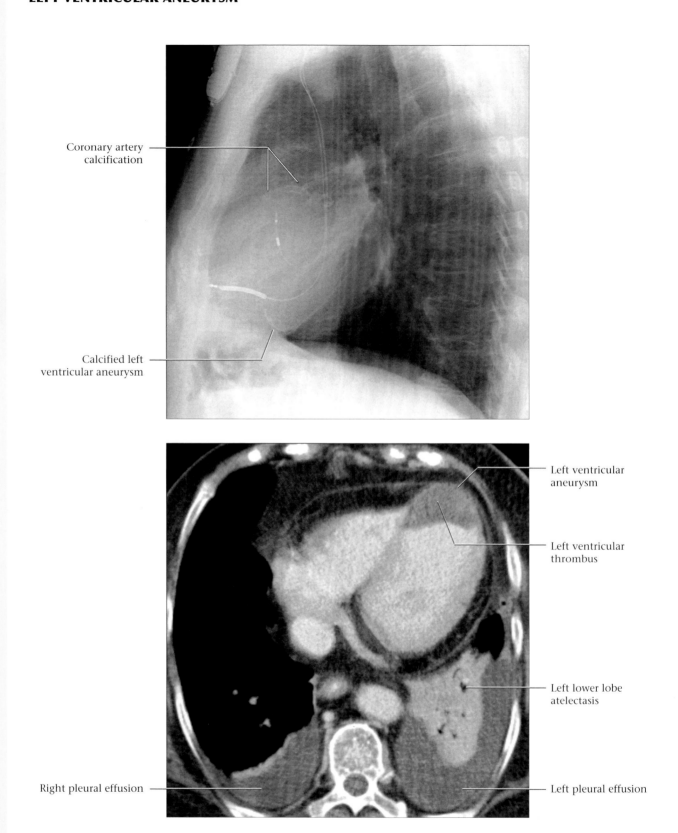

Coronary artery calcification

Calcified left ventricular aneurysm

Left ventricular aneurysm

Left ventricular thrombus

Left lower lobe atelectasis

Right pleural effusion

Left pleural effusion

(Top) Left lateral chest radiograph of a 49 year old man with coronary artery disease and a dual lead pacer/defibrillator demonstrates coronary artery calcification and an arcuate calcification projecting over the posterior inferior left ventricular wall consistent with a left ventricular aneurysm secondary to prior myocardial infarction. (Bottom) Contrast-enhanced chest CT (mediastinal window) of a 57 year old man with prior myocardial infarction and a left ventricular aneurysm shows that the heart is enlarged. The aneurysm manifests as focal thinning and outpouching of the anterior apical left ventricular myocardium with abnormal soft tissue attenuation content consistent with thrombus. There are bilateral small pleural effusions and left lower lobe relaxation atelectasis.

HEART

MITRAL ANNULUS CALCIFICATION

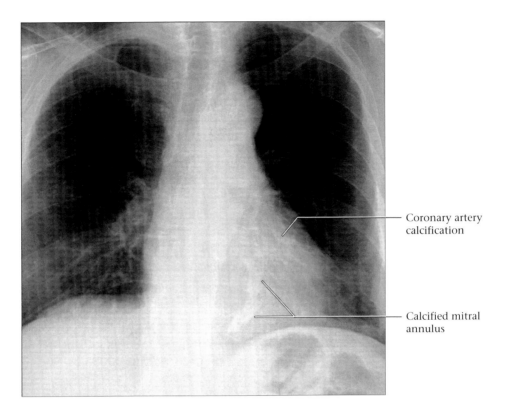

Coronary artery
calcification

Calcified mitral
annulus

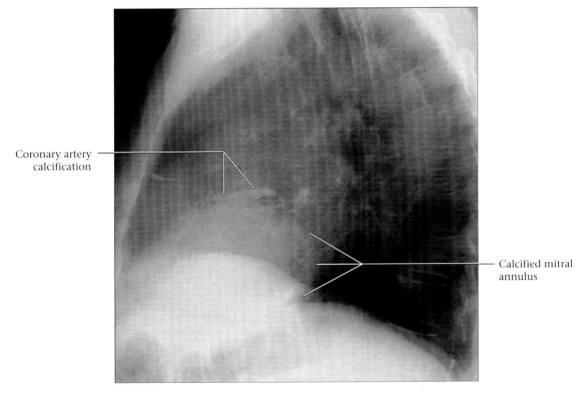

Coronary artery
calcification

Calcified mitral
annulus

(Top) First of two images of a 72 year old man with calcification of the mitral annulus. PA chest radiograph demonstrates a thick arcuate calcification projecting over the inferior aspect of the left heart in the region of the mitral valve ring. **(Bottom)** Left lateral chest radiograph demonstrates the C-shaped calcification projecting between the left atrium and left ventricle in the region of the mitral valve. The calcification conforms to the periphery of the mitral valve orifice. Calcification of the mitral annulus typically affects elderly patients, particularly women, who are often asymptomatic. Affected patients may develop valvular insufficiency or arrhythmias. The calcified mitral annulus typically manifests with dense C- or J-shaped calcification projecting over the expected location of the mitral valve ring. Note evidence of coronary artery calcification.

HEART

VALVE DISEASE, AORTIC STENOSIS

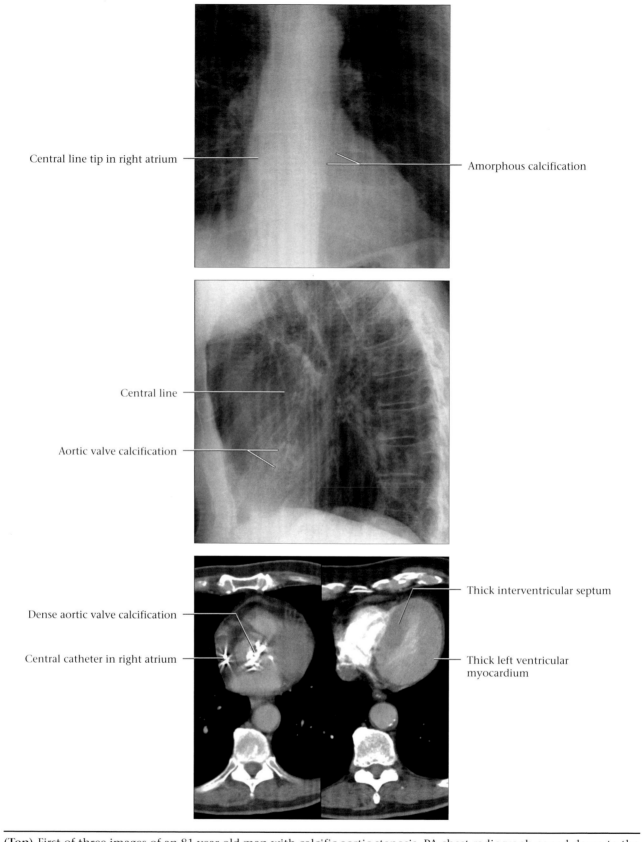

Central line tip in right atrium

Amorphous calcification

Central line

Aortic valve calcification

Dense aortic valve calcification

Central catheter in right atrium

Thick interventricular septum

Thick left ventricular myocardium

(Top) First of three images of an 81 year old man with calcific aortic stenosis. PA chest radiograph coned-down to the heart demonstrates a left ventricular cardiac configuration and a subtle focus of calcification projecting over the central portion of the heart in the expected location of the aortic valve. A right internal jugular central line terminates in the right atrium. (Middle) Left lateral chest radiograph coned-down to the heart demonstrates dense calcification in the expected location of the aortic valve. The morphology of the calcification suggests involvement of the valve cusps. (Bottom) Composite image of a contrast-enhanced chest CT (mediastinal window) shows dense calcification of the aortic valve cusps consistent with calcific aortic stenosis. Note associated thickening of the left ventricular myocardium consistent with left ventricular hypertrophy.

HEART

VALVE DISEASE, MITRAL STENOSIS

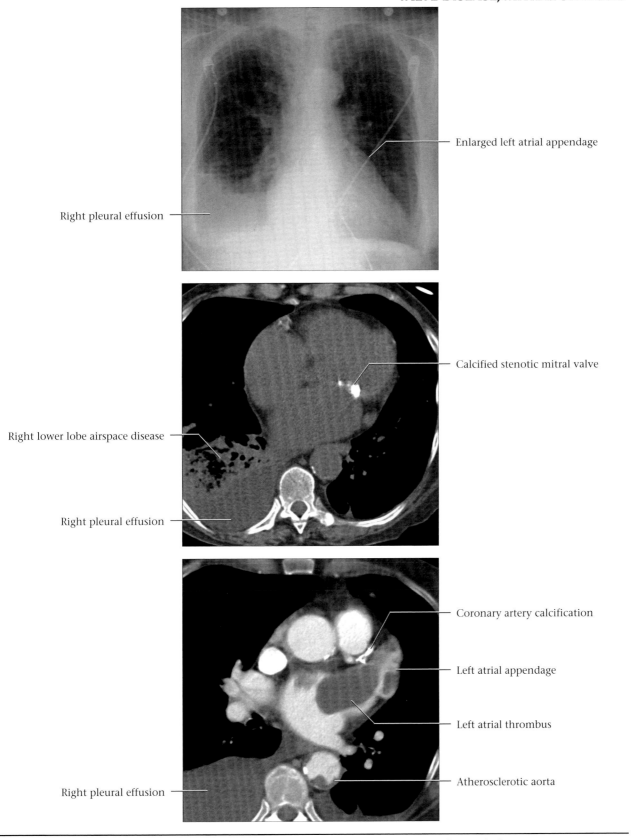

Enlarged left atrial appendage

Right pleural effusion

Calcified stenotic mitral valve

Right lower lobe airspace disease

Right pleural effusion

Coronary artery calcification

Left atrial appendage

Left atrial thrombus

Atherosclerotic aorta

Right pleural effusion

(Top) First of three images of a 72 year old woman with mitral stenosis. PA chest radiograph demonstrates cardiomegaly and a focal convexity of the superior left cardiac border representing enlargement of the left atrial appendage. The aorta is tortuous and atherosclerotic. There is a moderate right pleural effusion and mild interstitial edema. (Middle) Unenhanced chest CT (mediastinal window) through the left atrium demonstrates dense mitral valve calcification indicative of mitral stenosis. There is a right pleural effusion and right lower lobe airspace disease. (Bottom) Contrast-enhanced chest CT (mediastinal window) through the left atrium demonstrates filling defects within the atrial lumen that extend into an enlarged left atrial appendage and are consistent with atrial thrombi. Atherosclerosis and bilateral pleural effusions are also present.

CORONARY ARTERIES AND CARDIAC VEINS

Terminology

Abbreviations
- Left anterior descending artery (LAD)
- Left circumflex artery (LCX)
- Posterior descending artery (PDA)
- Right coronary artery (RCA)
- Posterolateral artery (PLA)
- Superior vena cava (SVC)

Definitions
- Coronary sulcus: Atrioventricular groove

Imaging Anatomy

Coronary Arteries
- Right and left coronary arteries, each arises from corresponding aortic coronary sinus (of Valsalva)
- Coronary artery branches generally considered end arteries
  - Myocardial segments predominately supplied by segmental coronary artery branches
  - Potential to develop collateral circulation
- **Coronary artery dominance**
  - Determined by artery(ies) supplying PDA and PLA
    - Right dominant: RCA supplies both arteries (~ 85%)
    - Left dominant: LCX supplies both arteries (~ 7.5%)
    - Co-dominant: RCA supplies PDA and LCX supplies PLA (~ 7.5%)
- **Left main coronary artery**
  - Passes leftward, posterior to pulmonary trunk and bifurcates into LAD and LCX
  - Occasionally, trifurcates into LAD, LCX and ramus intermedius
    - **Ramus intermedius:** Course similar to 1st diagonal branch of LAD to anterior left ventricle
  - May be absent: LAD and LCX arise separately from left coronary sinus
- **LAD**
  - Runs in anterior interventricular groove (sulcus) and terminates near cardiac apex
    - **Diagonal branches** to anterior free wall of left ventricle (numbered as they arise from LAD)
    - **Septal branches** to anterior interventricular septum (numbered as they arise from LAD)
- **LCX**
  - Runs in left coronary sulcus
    - **Obtuse marginal branches** to lateral left ventricle (numbered as they arise from LCX)
- **RCA**
  - Runs rightward posterior to pulmonary trunk, then downward in right coronary sulcus, toward posterior interventricular septum
  - **Conus artery**
    - First branch of RCA
    - May have separate origin directly from right coronary sinus
    - Supplies pulmonary outflow tract
  - **Sinus node artery**
    - Arises from proximal RCA in 60% of individuals

- May arise from proximal LCX
- Supplies sinoatrial node
  - Anterior branches to free wall of right ventricle
  - **Acute marginal artery**
    - Arises at junction of mid and distal RCA
    - Supplies free wall of right ventricle
  - **PDA**
    - Terminal branch of RCA
    - Runs in posterior interventricular groove
    - Can extend around apex to supply anterior interventricular septum, if LAD is small
  - **PLA**
    - Terminal branch of RCA

Coronary Veins
- Accompany coronary arteries and their branches
- **Coronary sinus**
  - Most veins of the heart drain into the coronary sinus
  - Wide venous channel in posterior part of coronary sulcus; ends in right atrium
  - **Great cardiac vein (left coronary vein)** accompanies LAD
  - **Small cardiac vein (right coronary vein)** accompanies acute marginal artery
  - **Middle cardiac vein** accompanies PDA
  - **Posterior vein of left ventricle**
  - **Oblique vein of left atrium**
    - Remnant of embryonic left SVC
    - Can persist as left SVC
- Other cardiac veins do not end in coronary sinus; drain directly in right atrium
  - Anterior cardiac veins
  - Smallest cardiac veins

Anatomy-Based Imaging Issues

Imaging Recommendations
- Catheter angiography remains gold standard for coronary artery imaging
  - Main advantage is ability to perform coronary interventions if arterial stenosis is detected
- CT coronary angiography is gaining popularity as an excellent non-invasive technique for coronary artery imaging
  - High sensitivity, specificity, accuracy and negative predictive value for coronary artery disease
  - Specially suited for coronary artery anomalies
    - Multiplanar capabilities
- Myocardial segmentation
  - Standard 17 segments model has been adopted for left ventricular wall
    - Used to assess myocardial perfusion, left ventricular function and coronary anatomy
- Coronary artery anomalies
  - ~ 1% of coronary angiograms
  - Types of coronary artery anomalies
    - High takeoff
    - Multiple ostia
    - Single coronary artery
    - Origin from opposite or noncoronary sinus
    - Origin from pulmonary artery

CORONARY ARTERIES AND CARDIAC VEINS

ANTERIOR VIEW OF THE CORONARY ARTERIES

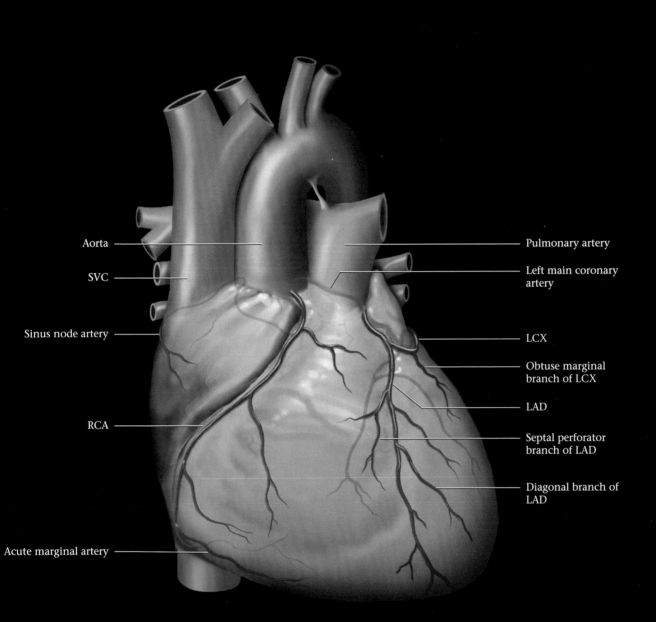

Aorta

SVC

Sinus node artery

RCA

Acute marginal artery

Pulmonary artery

Left main coronary artery

LCX

Obtuse marginal branch of LCX

LAD

Septal perforator branch of LAD

Diagonal branch of LAD

Graphic illustrates branches of the coronary arteries. The left main coronary artery divides into the LAD and the LCX. The LAD runs in the anterior interventricular groove and gives off septal perforator branches to the interventricular septum and diagonal branches to the free wall of the left ventricle. The LCX gives off obtuse marginal branches to the lateral wall of the left ventricle. The RCA runs in the right coronary sulcus and gives off the conus artery, sinus node artery (in 60% of the population), anterior branches to the free wall of the right ventricle and the acute marginal artery. It then curves around the inferior cardiac border and divides into the PDA and posterolateral ventricular artery (in a right dominant coronary circulation).

CORONARY ARTERIES AND CARDIAC VEINS

POSTERIOR VIEW OF THE CORONARY ARTERIES

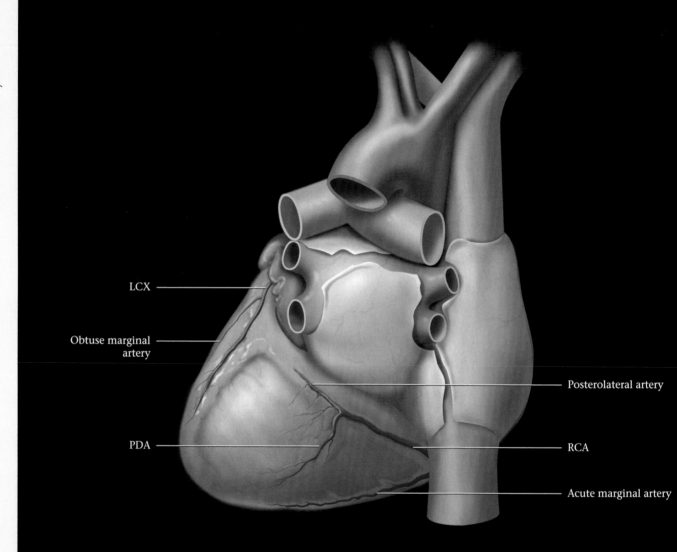

LCX

Obtuse marginal
artery

Posterolateral artery

PDA

RCA

Acute marginal artery

Illustration of the coronary artery anatomy, viewed from the posterior aspect of the heart, in a right dominant coronary circulation. The RCA runs in the right coronary sulcus and divides into two terminal branches: PDA and posterolateral artery. The PDA runs in the posterior interventricular groove. The LCX is seen along the left cardiac border and ends as an obtuse marginal branch. The coronary circulation is classified as right dominant if the RCA supplies the PDA and at least one branch of the posterolateral artery. It is classified as left dominant if the LCX supplies both arteries (PDA, PLA). It is co-dominant if the RCA supplies the PDA and the LCX supplies the posterolateral branch(es).

CORONARY ARTERIES AND CARDIAC VEINS

LEFT VENTRICULAR SEGMENTATION

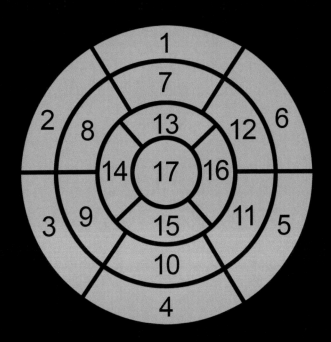

1. Basal anterior
2. Basal anteroseptal
3. Basal inferoseptal
4. Basal inferior
5. Basal inferolateral
6. Basal anterolateral
7. Mid anterior
8. Mid anteroseptal
9. Mid inferoseptal
10. Mid inferior
11. Mid inferolateral
12. Mid anterolateral
13. Apical anterior
14. Apical septal
15. Apical inferior
16. Apical lateral
17. Apex

Standardized, 17 myocardial segments were adopted by the Cardiac Imaging Committee of the Council on Clinical Cardiology of the American Heart Association, for tomographic imaging of the left ventricle. The names for the myocardial segments define the location relative to both the long and short axis of the left ventricle. Basal, mid-cavity and apical designations localize the segments along the long axis of the left ventricle. With regard to the circumferential location on the bull's-eye view, the basal (segments 1-6) and mid-cavity (segments 7-12) sections are divided into 6 segments of 60° each. The apical section (segments 13-16) is divided into 4 segments of 90° each. The cardiac apex is segment 17. The attachment of the right ventricular wall to the left ventricle is used to separate the septum from the left ventricular anterior and inferior free walls.

CORONARY ARTERIES AND CARDIAC VEINS

CORONARY ARTERY TERRITORIES

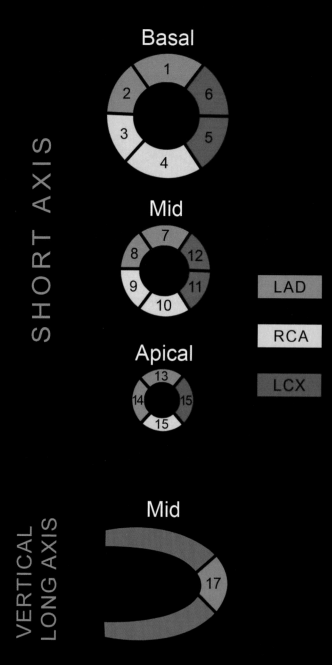

Graphic illustrations of the left ventricular myocardial segments and the distribution of coronary blood flow to these segments. Segmentation of left ventricular myocardium is used to assess myocardial perfusion, left ventricular function and coronary anatomy. Myocardial perfusion and function can be assessed using nuclear medicine cardiac SPECT and cardiac MR.

CORONARY ARTERIES AND CARDIAC VEINS

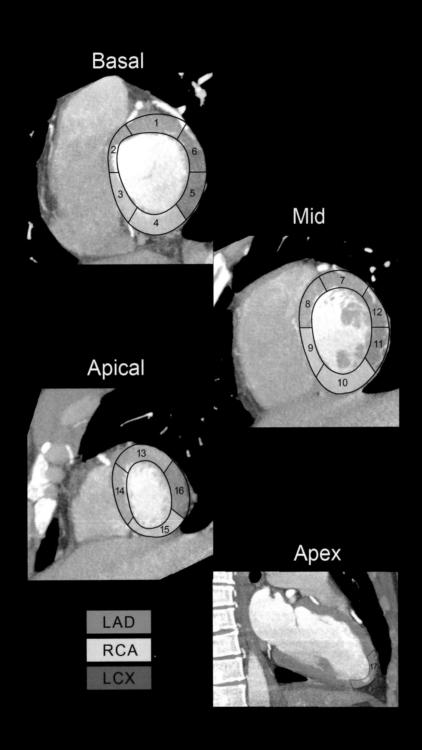

The first three images are short axis CECT views of the left ventricular wall at the basal, mid and apical levels. The fourth image is a vertical long axis image, obtained from the same data set, reformatted to show the apex. Different colors are assigned to show the vascular territories of the coronary arteries. The LAD supplies the anterior septum, the anterior wall, and in most cases, the apex. On a short axis image, it usually supplies from 9 to 1 o'clock at the basal and mid ventricular levels. The LCX supplies the lateral wall, usually from 2 to 4 o'clock . The RCA supplies the inferior wall segments and the posterior septum, usually from 5 to 8 o'clock. It should be emphasized, however, that great variation in the distribution of coronary blood flow is observed in clinical practice.

CORONARY ARTERIES AND CARDIAC VEINS

CATHETER CORONARY ANGIOGRAPHY

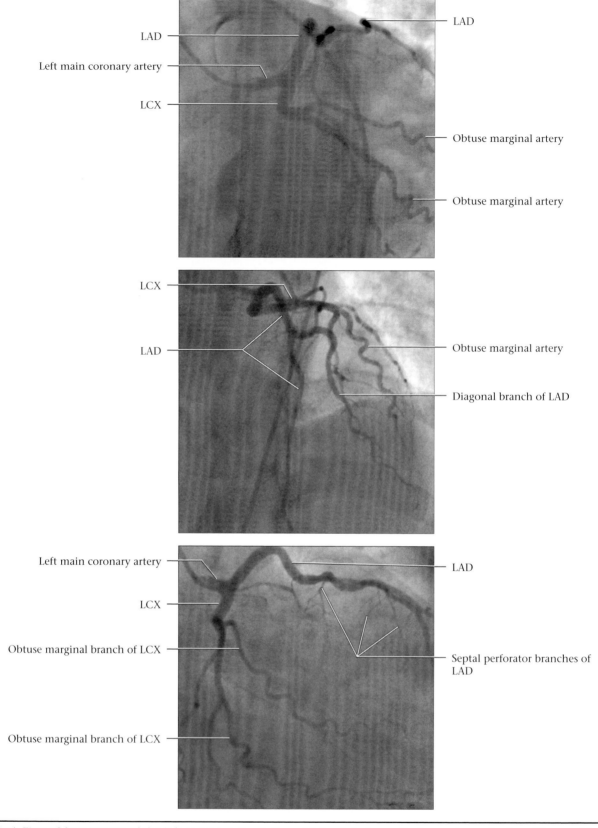

LAD

LAD

Left main coronary artery

LCX

Obtuse marginal artery

Obtuse marginal artery

LCX

LAD

Obtuse marginal artery

Diagonal branch of LAD

Left main coronary artery

LAD

LCX

Obtuse marginal branch of LCX

Septal perforator branches of LAD

Obtuse marginal branch of LCX

(Top) First of four images of the left coronary circulation obtained during catheter angiography in a 48 year old patient who presented with chest pain. Because of the overlap between the branches of the coronary arteries, multiple radiographic projections are obtained to show different segments in greater detail. The first image is a LAO caudal view showing the bifurcation of the left main coronary artery into the LAD and LCX. The LAD is foreshortened on this projection, while the LCX with its obtuse marginal branches is well seen. (Middle) LAO cranial projection shows the LAD and its diagonal branch. It is difficult to separate the LCX and its obtuse marginal branches on this projection. (Bottom) RAO caudal view shows the origin of the LAD and LCX from the left main coronary artery. The diagonal branch of LAD is projecting over the LAD. Note the septal perforator branches of LAD.

CORONARY ARTERIES AND CARDIAC VEINS

CATHETER CORONARY ANGIOGRAPHY

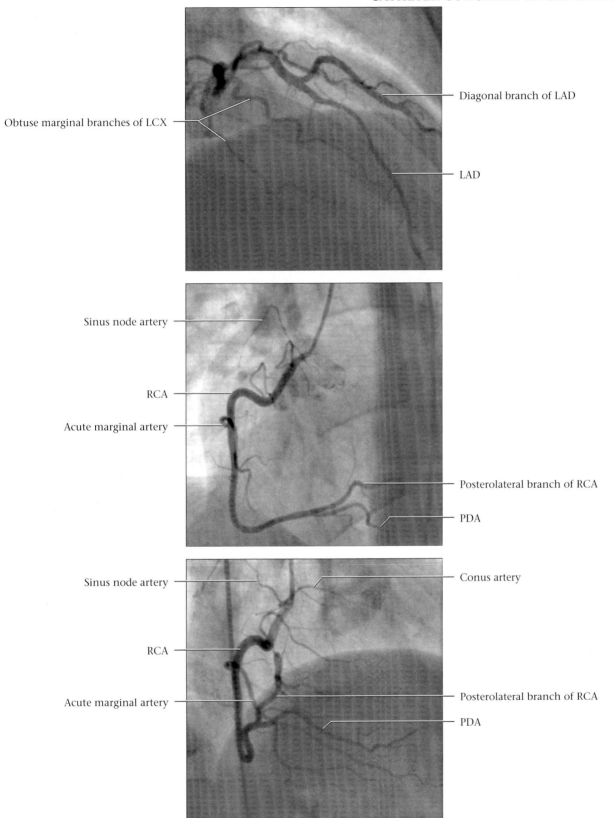

Diagonal branch of LAD

LAD

Obtuse marginal branches of LCX

Sinus node artery

RCA

Acute marginal artery

Posterolateral branch of RCA

PDA

Sinus node artery

Conus artery

RCA

Acute marginal artery

Posterolateral branch of RCA

PDA

(Top) RAO cranial projection separates the LAD from its diagonal branch. The LCX is not well seen, but its obtuse marginal branches are well delineated. **(Middle)** First of two images obtained during injection of the RCA. LAO cranial view shows the branches of the RCA and its bifurcation into the PDA and the posterolateral artery. The acute marginal artery is superimposed on the RCA on this projection. **(Bottom)** RAO cranial projection shows the branches of the RCA. The conus artery is usually the first branch and supplies the pulmonary outflow tract. The acute marginal artery is separated on this projection from the RCA.

CORONARY ARTERIES AND CARDIAC VEINS

3D VOLUME RENDERED IMAGES OF THE CORONARY ARTERIES

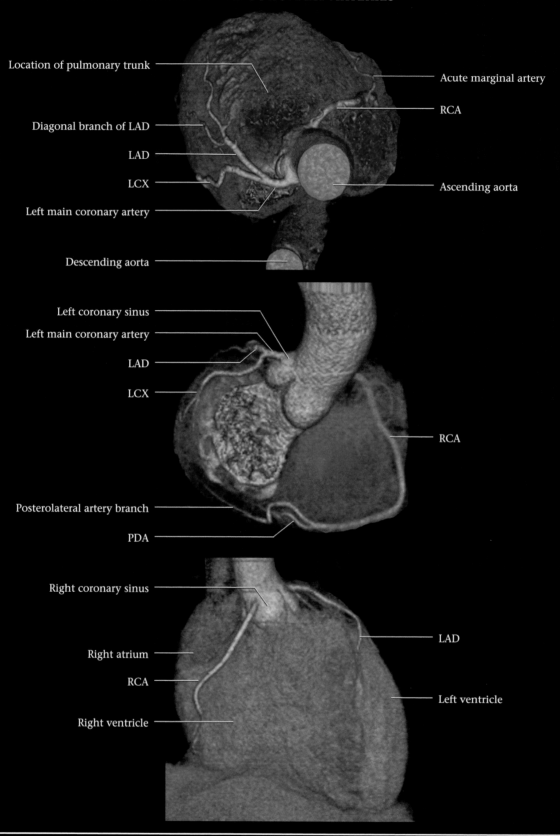

Location of pulmonary trunk

Acute marginal artery

RCA

Diagonal branch of LAD

LAD

LCX

Left main coronary artery

Ascending aorta

Descending aorta

Left coronary sinus

Left main coronary artery

LAD

LCX

RCA

Posterolateral artery branch

PDA

Right coronary sinus

LAD

Right atrium

RCA

Left ventricle

Right ventricle

(Top) First of three volume rendered images of the coronary arteries. In this image viewed from above (pulmonary trunk digitally removed), the origins of the coronary arteries are shown. The right coronary artery arises from the right coronary sinus. The short left main coronary artery arises from the left coronary sinus and divides into the LAD, which runs in the anterior interventricular groove, and the LCX, which runs in the left coronary sulcus. (Middle) Posterior oblique volume rendered image shows the RCA and LCX forming a circle as each runs in its respective coronary sulcus. (Bottom) A frontal oblique image shows the origin of the RCA from the right coronary sinus. The RCA passes to the right of the pulmonary artery (removed during image post processing) to reach the right coronary sulcus (atrioventricular groove).

CORONARY ARTERIES AND CARDIAC VEINS

RIGHT DOMINANT CORONARY CIRCULATION

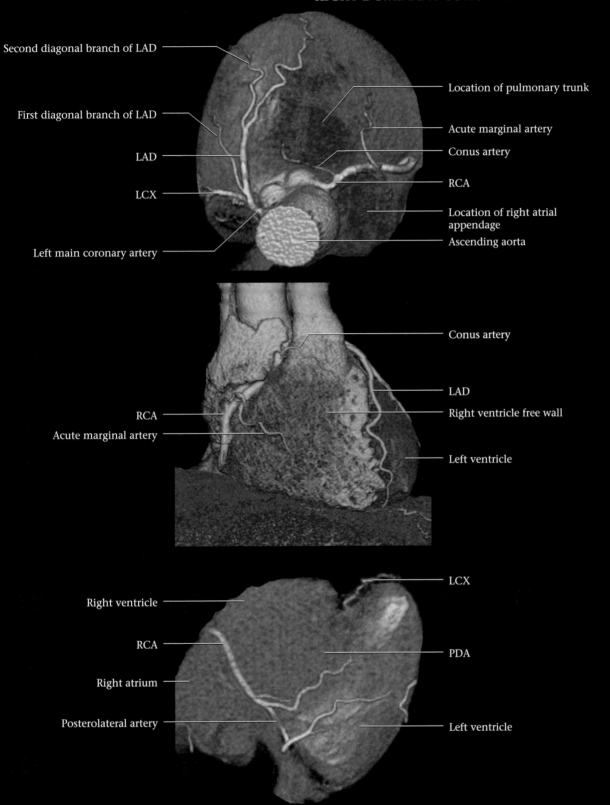

Second diagonal branch of LAD

First diagonal branch of LAD

LAD

LCX

Left main coronary artery

Location of pulmonary trunk

Acute marginal artery

Conus artery

RCA

Location of right atrial appendage

Ascending aorta

Conus artery

RCA

Acute marginal artery

LAD

Right ventricle free wall

Left ventricle

Right ventricle

RCA

Right atrium

Posterolateral artery

LCX

PDA

Left ventricle

(Top) The first of three volume rendered images in a patient with right dominant coronary circulation shows the conus artery, usually the 1st branch of the RCA, which supplies the pulmonary outflow tract. The acute marginal artery arises at the junction between the mid and distal parts of the RCA and supplies the anterior wall of the right ventricle. (Middle) Frontal image shows the conus and acute marginal arteries. During its course in the coronary sulcus, the RCA also gives off multiple branches to the right ventricular free wall. (Bottom) Axial image through the base of the heart shows the two terminal branches of the RCA in a right dominant coronary circulation (85% of population). The posterolateral artery supplies the posterolateral wall of the left ventricle, while the PDA diverges to run in the posterior interventricular groove.

CORONARY ARTERIES AND CARDIAC VEINS

LEFT DOMINANT CORONARY CIRCULATION

Ascending aorta

Pulmonary trunk

RCA

Conus artery

LAD

Left main coronary artery

LCX

LAD

Obtuse marginal branch of LCX

Diagonal branch of LAD

Diagonal branch of LAD

Posterior interventricular groove

Cardiac apex

LAD

Right coronary sulcus

PDA

LCX

(Top) First of three volume rendered images in a patient with left dominant coronary circulation. Frontal oblique image shows a common origin of the RCA and conus artery from the the right coronary sinus. The RCA is small and ends before reaching the posterior interventricular septum. (Middle) Frontal oblique image shows the branches of the left coronary artery. The LAD is large and wraps around the cardiac apex. The LCX is also large and runs in the left coronary sulcus to reach the posterior interventricular groove. (Bottom) A diaphragmatic view of the heart shows the LAD wrapping around to supply the cardiac apex and anterior portion of interventricular septum. The LCX supplies a small PDA. Note the absence of the RCA in the right coronary sulcus.

CORONARY ARTERIES AND CARDIAC VEINS

MAXIMUM INTENSITY PROJECTION (MIP) OF CORONARY ARTERIES

(Top) First of three maximum intensity projection (MIP) images depicting the origins of both coronary arteries. The RCA arises from the right coronary sinus, passes to the right behind the pulmonary outflow tract, to reach the right coronary sulcus. The short stem left main coronary artery divides into the LAD and LCX. (Middle) Axial oblique MIP image of the left coronary system, in another patient with mild coronary artery disease, shows the LAD in the anterior interventricular groove and the LCX in the left coronary sulcus. Note the mild calcification of the LAD. The obliquity of the plane of reconstruction makes the left coronary sinus appear aneurysmal and masks the left coronary artery origin. (Bottom) Coronal oblique thin MIP image of the same patient delineates the course of the LAD in the anterior interventricular groove and again shows calcifications of the vessel wall.

CORONARY ARTERIES AND CARDIAC VEINS

MAXIMUM INTENSITY PROJECTION (MIP) OF CORONARY ARTERIES

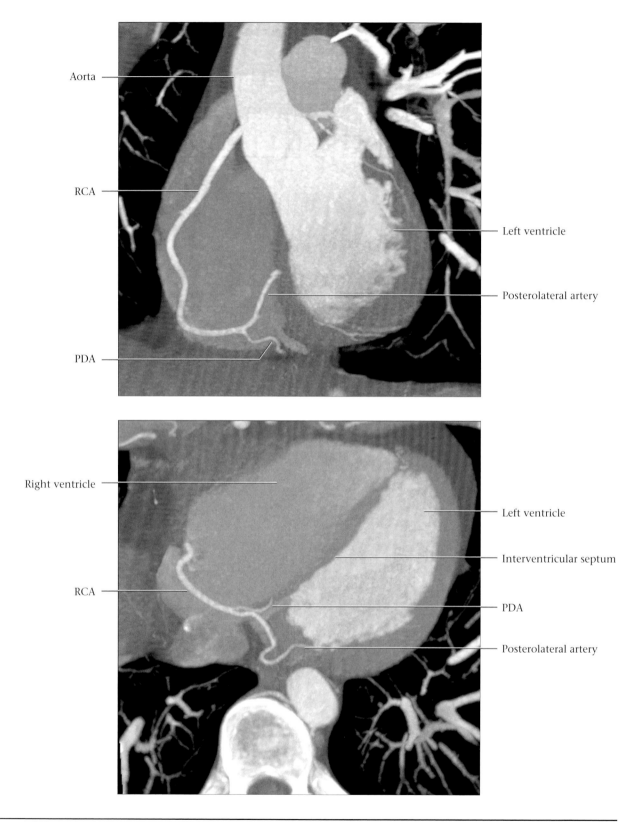

(Top) Coronal oblique MIP image shows the vertical course of the RCA within the right coronary sulcus and its two terminal branches: PDA and posterolateral ventricular artery. This is the usual branching pattern in a right dominant coronary artery circulation. The coronary circulation is right dominant if the RCA supplies the PDA and at least a posterolateral ventricular branch. (Bottom) Axial MIP image, through the base of the heart, shows the horizontal course of the RCA as it courses to the posterior interventricular septum, before branching into the PDA and posterolateral ventricular artery. The PDA runs in the posterior interventricular groove. MIP images are useful to delineate the course of an artery, but should not be used alone to diagnose arterial stenosis, because areas of narrowing can be masked by contrast in the plane of reconstruction.

CORONARY ARTERIES AND CARDIAC VEINS

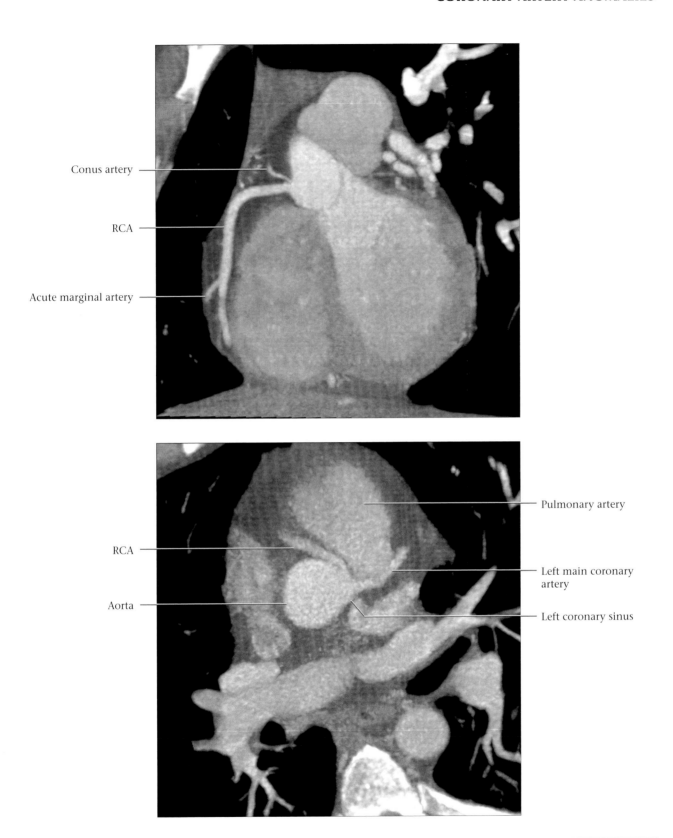

Conus artery

RCA

Acute marginal artery

RCA

Aorta

Pulmonary artery

Left main coronary artery

Left coronary sinus

(Top) Coronal oblique maximum intensity projection (MIP) image in a patient with a separate ostium of the conus artery, which is arising directly from the right coronary sinus rather than from the RCA. **(Bottom)** Axial oblique MIP image in a different patient shows the RCA arising from the left coronary sinus and passing between the aorta and the pulmonary trunk. This interarterial RCA position has been noted in approximately 0.1% of patients undergoing catheter coronary angiography. It is associated with sudden death in about 30% of patients and may relate to compression of the right coronary artery between the pulmonary artery and the aorta, especially during exercise when dilatation of the aorta occurs. Because of its multiplanar capabilities, coronary CTA is especially well-suited for the evaluation of congenital anomalies and variants of the coronary circulation.

CORONARY ARTERIES AND CARDIAC VEINS

SINGLE CORONARY ARTERY FROM THE RIGHT CORONARY SINUS

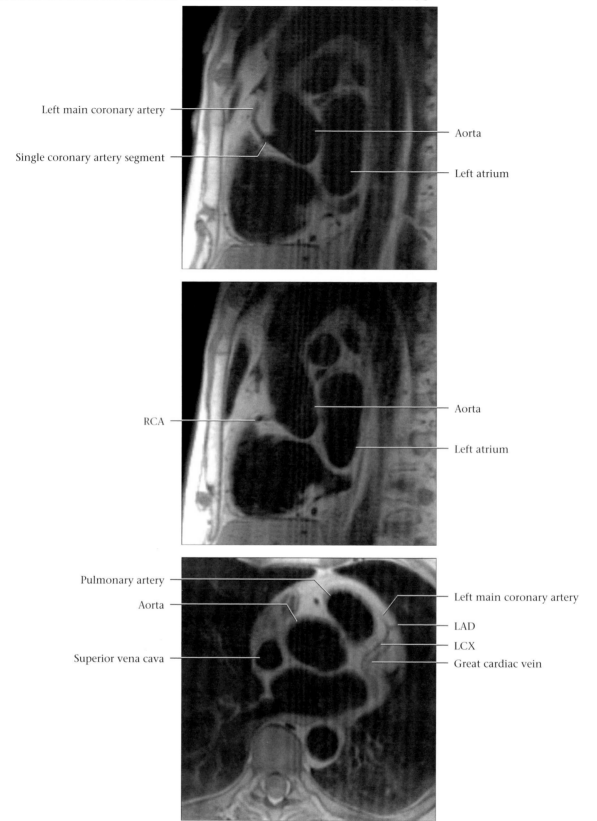

(Top) First of three double IR MR images in a 70 year old patient with chest pain. A sagittal image through the root of the aorta shows a single coronary artery segment arising from the right coronary sinus. The left main coronary artery arises from the common trunk and is directed upward. (Middle) A sagittal image shows the right coronary artery which has a normal course. (Bottom) An axial image shows the left main coronary artery, after looping anterior to the pulmonary trunk, dividing into the LAD and LCX. The LAD descends in the anterior interventricular groove while the LCX, which has a longer course, runs in the upper part of the anterior interventricular groove (normally where the LAD runs) and then curves to assume its normal course in the left coronary sulcus.

SINGLE RIGHT CORONARY ARTERY

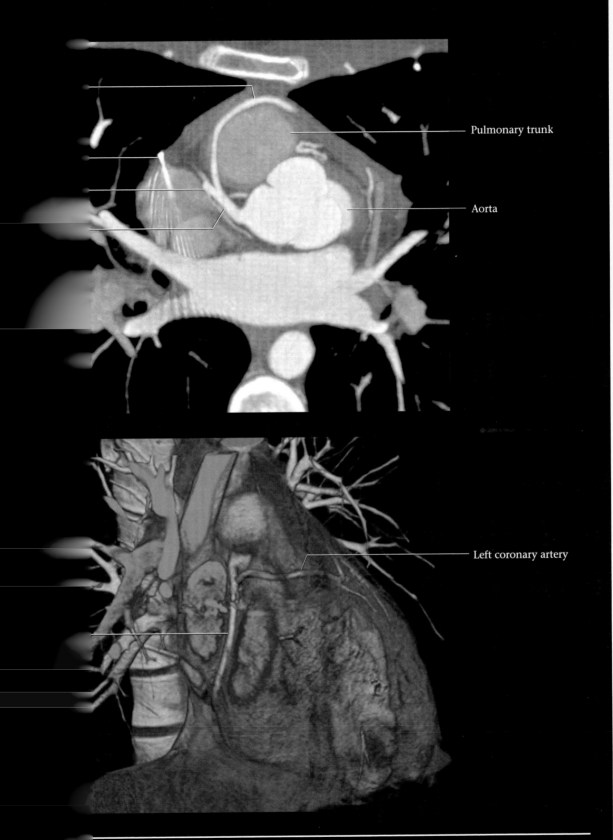

Pulmonary trunk

Aorta

Left coronary artery

tient with D-transposition of the great vessels who underwent arterial switch procedure as
thick MIP image showing a single coronary artery arising from the right coronary sinus.
nto a left coronary artery and an RCA proper, which continues in the expected course of
left coronary artery loops in front of the pulmonary trunk in this patient. A single RCA,
nary artery passing in front of the pulmonary trunk, occurs in about 10% of patients with
essels. Note the location of the pulmonary trunk to the right and anterior to the aorta.
d image in the same patient shows the anterior course of the left coronary artery, anterior

CORONARY ARTERIES AND CARDIAC VEINS

ANTERIOR VIEW OF CORONARY VEINS

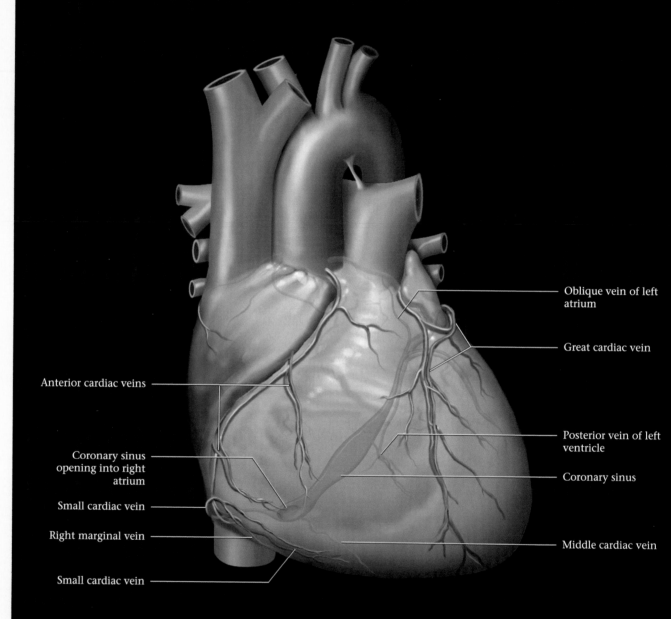

Oblique vein of left atrium

Great cardiac vein

Anterior cardiac veins

Posterior vein of left ventricle

Coronary sinus opening into right atrium

Coronary sinus

Small cardiac vein

Right marginal vein

Middle cardiac vein

Small cardiac vein

Graphic illustrates the venous drainage of the heart. The great cardiac vein starts at the apex, runs in the anterior interventricular groove, curves to the left in the coronary sulcus to open at the left end of coronary sinus. The oblique vein of left atrium runs obliquely on the posterior aspect of the left atrium to merge with the greater cardiac vein. The small cardiac vein runs in the coronary sulcus to open at the right end of the sinus. The middle cardiac vein starts at the apex, runs in the posterior interventricular groove and opens in the right aspect of the coronary sinus. The posterior vein of left ventricle runs on the diaphragmatic surface of left ventricle to reach the sinus. The anterior cardiac veins (3 or 4) open directly into the right atrium. The right marginal vein may join the small cardiac vein or drain directly into the right atrium.

CORONARY SINUS

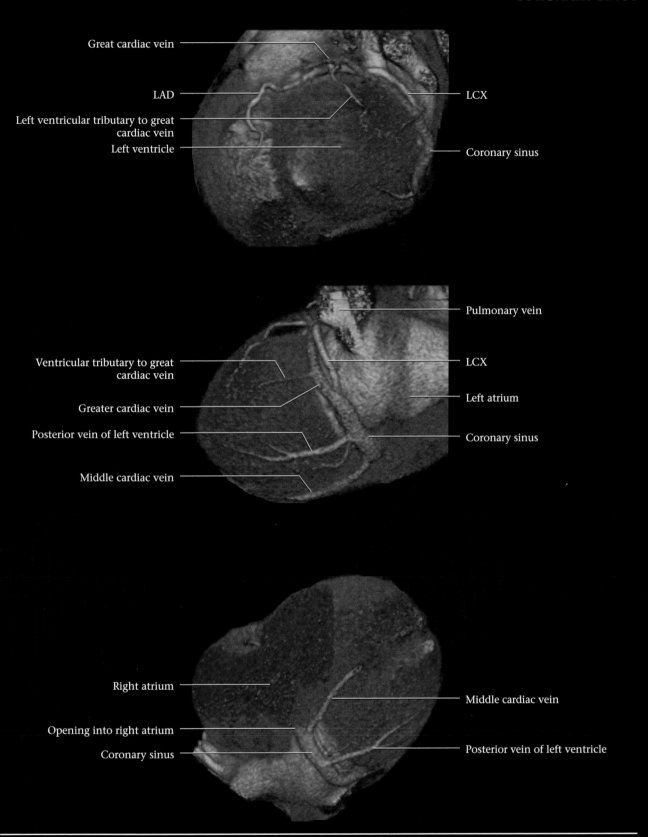

Top image labels:
Great cardiac vein
LAD
Left ventricular tributary to great cardiac vein
Left ventricle
LCX
Coronary sinus

Middle image labels:
Ventricular tributary to great cardiac vein
Greater cardiac vein
Posterior vein of left ventricle
Middle cardiac vein
Pulmonary vein
LCX
Left atrium
Coronary sinus

Bottom image labels:
Right atrium
Opening into right atrium
Coronary sinus
Middle cardiac vein
Posterior vein of left ventricle

(Top) Three different volume rendered images in a patient undergoing coronary CTA show the coronary sinus venous system. The left lateral view shows the great cardiac vein as it accompanies the LAD in the anterior interventricular groove, then as it curves in arte the left coronary sinus to accompany the LCX. The confluence of the great cardiac vein with the oblique vein of the left atrium (not seen on the image) marks the start of the coronary sinus. Multiple left ventricular veins drain into the great cardiac vein. **(Middle)** Posterior view of the coronary sinus shows its major tributaries: The great cardiac vein, the middle cardiac vein and the posterior vein of the left ventricle. **(Bottom)** Diaphragmatic view of the coronary sinus shows it entering into the right atrium. The middle cardiac vein accompanies the PDA in the posterior interventricular groove.

CORONARY ARTERIES AND CARDIAC VEINS

DOUBLE SVC

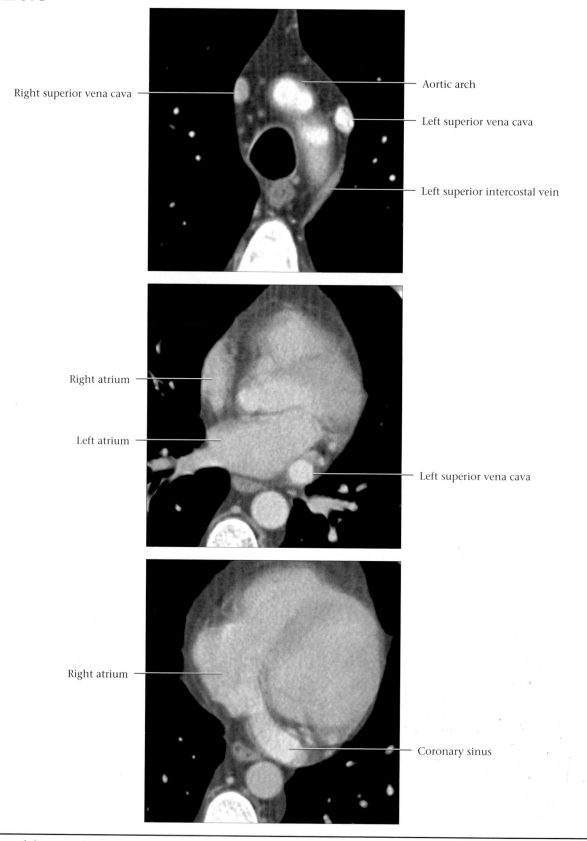

(Top) First of three axial CECT images in a patient with double SVC. Axial image at the level of the top of the aortic arch shows an enhancing tubular structure to the left of the aortic arch. This represents the continuation the left brachiocephalic vein into a left-sided SVC. (Middle) Axial image at the level of the top of the right atrium shows the right SVC entering the right atrium. The left superior vena cava lies posterolateral to the left atrial wall. (Bottom) Axial image at the level of the base of the heart shows the left SVC terminating in the coronary sinus, which is slightly dilated. The coronary sinus drains into the right atrium. The left SVC is an embryonic structure that can persist in adult life as a single left or double SVC (0.3% of normal adults and in 4.5% in patients with congenital heart disease).

CORONARY ARTERIES AND CARDIAC VEINS

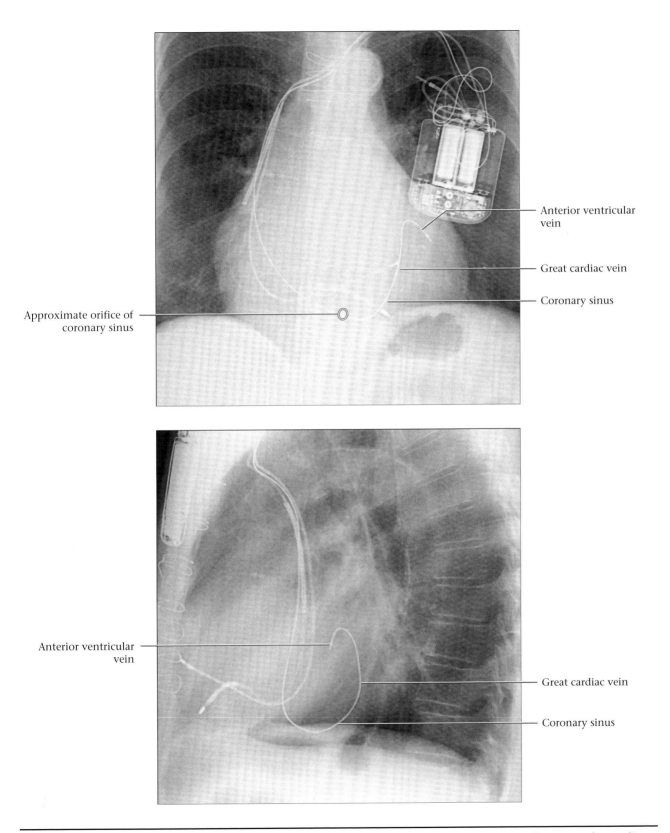

Anterior ventricular vein

Great cardiac vein

Coronary sinus

Approximate orifice of coronary sinus

Anterior ventricular vein

Great cardiac vein

Coronary sinus

(Top) First of two chest radiographs of a patient with a dilated cardiomyopathy and biventricular pacing for cardiac resynchronization therapy. This PA radiograph shows a transvenous left ventricular pacing lead extending from the right atrium retrograde into the coronary arinus, through the greater cardiac vein, and into an anterior ventricular vein. The coronary sinus lead shows the oblique orientation of the coronary sinus in the coronary sulcus. **(Bottom)** Lateral radiograph shows the location and orientation of the coronary sinus on a lateral radiograph. Prolonged conduction in patients with heart failure leads to asynchronous contraction of the ventricles and decreased cardiac output. Biventricular pacing results in synchronization of ventricular contraction and improved cardiac output. Stimulation of the left ventricle is achieved through the coronary sinus lead.

PERICARDIUM

Anatomy of the Pericardium

General Concepts

- **Pericardium, sac-like membrane** that surrounds **heart** and **proximal great vessels**
- Located in **anatomic middle mediastinum**
- Function
  ○ Protects heart
  ○ Maintains heart in normal midline position
  ○ Limits heart distention and pericardial fluid volume
  ○ **Pericardial space**
    ▪ Permits cardiac motion and changes in morphology
  ○ **Pericardial fluid**
    ▪ Provides **lubrication** during cardiac motion
    ▪ **15-50 mL** of serous fluid in normal subjects

Fibrous Pericardium

- Cone-shaped sac-like tough connective tissue layer
  ○ Surrounds **heart**, but is not attached to it
  ○ Lined internally by **serous parietal pericardium**
  ○ Continuous with **great vessel adventitia**
  ○ Continuous with **pretracheal fascia**
- Defines outer boundaries of **anatomic middle mediastinum**
- Attachments
  ○ Base attached to **central tendinous portion of diaphragm**
    ▪ **Pericardiophrenic ligament**
  ○ Anterior surface attached to anterior chest wall (posterior aspect of **sternum**)
    ▪ **Superior sternopericardial ligaments**
    ▪ **Inferior sternopericardial ligaments**
- Conduit for **neurovascular structures**
  ○ **Phrenic nerves**
  ○ **Pericardiacophrenic vessels**

Serous Pericardium

- Closed sac-like membrane that surrounds the **heart** within the **fibrous pericardium**
- **Continuous serosal layer** with **parietal** and **visceral** components
  ○ Lined by **mesothelial cells**
- **Parietal pericardium**
  ○ **Lines internal surface of fibrous pericardium**
- **Visceral pericardium**
  ○ **Adherent to heart**
    ▪ Also known as **epicardium**
    ▪ Covers the **subepicardial fat**

Pericardial Reflections

- **Superior reflection** surrounds
  ○ **Ascending aorta**
  ○ **Pulmonary trunk**
- **Posterior reflection** surrounds
  ○ **Superior vena cava**
  ○ **Inferior vena cava**
  ○ **Pulmonary veins**

Pericardial Innervation

- **Vagus nerves**
- **Sympathetic trunks**
- **Phrenic nerves** (C3, C4, C5)
  ○ Somatic innervation of **parietal pericardium**
  ○ Dermatomes of supraclavicular region; referred pain to shoulder in cases of pericardial inflammation

Pericardial Vessels

- Arterial supply
  ○ **Internal thoracic arteries**
    ▪ **Pericardiacophrenic arteries**
    ▪ **Musculophrenic arteries**
  ○ **Thoracic aorta**
    ▪ **Superior phrenic arteries**
    ▪ **Coronary arteries**
- Venous drainage
  ○ **Azygos system**
  ○ **Internal thoracic veins**
    ▪ **Pericardiacophrenic veins**

Pericardial Space & Pericardial Recesses

General Concepts

- Serosal pericardial reflections arranged around two tubes
  ○ One tube encloses **aorta** and **pulmonary trunk**
  ○ One tube encloses **superior** and **inferior venae cavae** and **pulmonary veins**
- **Transverse sinus**
  ○ Passage between the two tubes
- **Oblique sinus**
  ○ Posterior pericardial extension behind **left atrium**
- **No communication between transverse and oblique sinuses**
  ○ Separated by two pericardial reflections

Transverse Sinus

- General
  ○ **Horizontal orientation**
  ○ Posterior to **ascending aorta** and **pulmonary trunk**
  ○ Superior to **left atrium**
  ○ Superior and anterior to **oblique sinus**
  ○ May mimic aortic dissection or lymphadenopathy
- **Superior aortic recess**
  ○ **Superior extent of transverse sinus**
  ○ Partially surrounds **ascending aorta**
  ○ Abuts aorta without intervening fat tissue plane
  ○ **Posterior portion**
    ▪ Also known as **superior pericardial recess/sinus**
    ▪ **Crescent-shaped** fluid collection abutting **posterior wall of ascending aorta**
    ▪ May extend cephalad into **right paratracheal region**
    ▪ May mimic lymphadenopathy
  ○ **Anterior portion**
    ▪ **Triangular-shaped** fluid with beak-like extension between **ascending aorta** and **pulmonary trunk**
    ▪ May mimic aortic dissection
  ○ **Right lateral portion**
    ▪ Fluid extending between **ascending aorta** and **superior vena cava**
- **Inferior aortic recess**
  ○ Inferior extension of **transverse sinus**
  ○ **Crescent-shaped fluid** between **right lateral ascending** aorta and **right atrium**

PERICARDIUM

■ Posterior to aorta, anterior to left atrium
- **Right and left pulmonic recesses**
  - ○ **Lateral extensions of transverse sinus**
  - ○ **Right pulmonic recess**
    - ■ Inferior to proximal **right pulmonary artery**
  - ○ **Left pulmonic recess**
    - ■ Inferior to **left pulmonary artery**, superior to **left superior pulmonary vein**

Pericardial Cavity

- Some recesses arise from the pericardial cavity proper
- **Postcaval recess**
  - ○ Small fluid collection along posterolateral aspect of **superior vena cava**
- **Right and left pulmonary venous recesses**
  - ○ Small fluid collections along **lateral heart borders**
  - ○ Between **superior** and **inferior pulmonary veins**
  - ○ Left identified more frequently than right on CT
  - ○ May mimic lymphadenopathy

Oblique Sinus

- **Inferior to transverse sinus**
  - ○ Separated from **transverse sinus** by double pericardial reflection
  - ○ **No communication between transverse and oblique sinuses**
- Superior and posterior to **left atrium**
- Posterior to **right pulmonary artery**, medial to **bronchus intermedius**
  - ○ Sometimes called **posterior pericardial recess**
- May mimic esophageal pathology or foregut cyst

Imaging the Normal Pericardium

General Concepts

- Typically imperceptible on radiography
- **Echocardiography**, modality of choice for initial evaluation
  - ○ Assessment of pericardial effusion and tamponade
  - ○ Inability to assess entire pericardium or detect pericardial thickening

Cross-sectional Imaging (CT/MR)

- Normal thickness of **1-2 mm**
  - ○ Combined thicknesses of **fibrous pericardium** and **serous parietal/visceral pericardium**
  - ○ **Serous visceral pericardium** (epicardium) closely adherent to heart surface
- Most visible anterior to right ventricle
  - ○ Outlined by **subepicardial** and **mediastinal fat**
- Visualization/identification of **pericardial sinuses** and **recesses**
  - ○ May mimic lymphadenopathy, dissection
- MR
  - ○ Pericardial visualization in **80% of normal subjects**
  - ○ Normal pericardium exhibits low signal on T1- and T2-weighted SE images
  - ○ Outlined by bright signal mediastinal and subepicardial fat
  - ○ **Increasing thickness near diaphragm; ligamentous insertions**

Anatomy Related Imaging Abnormalities

Congenital Absence of Pericardium

- **Complete absence of pericardium**
- **Partial absence of pericardium**, more common than complete absence, usually affects left pericardium
  - ○ Association with left atrial herniation
  - ○ Potentially life-threatening condition
- Imaging
  - ○ Cardiac displacement to the left and posterior cardiac rotation with complete absence
  - ○ Interposition of lung between ascending aorta and pulmonary trunk on CT/MR

Pericardial Cyst

- Developmental anomaly characterized by non-communicating outpouching of **parietal pericardium**
- Typically located in **anterior cardiophrenic angles (70% right, 20% left)**
- Imaging
  - ○ Smooth, round, ovoid or tear drop shaped mass abutting the heart
  - ○ Homogeneous fluid attenuation/signal
  - ○ Thin/imperceptible wall
  - ○ No contrast-enhancement

Pericardial Effusion

- Abnormal amount of fluid in pericardium
  - ○ Capacity for accumulation of **300 mL of fluid**
- Imaging
  - ○ "**Water bottle**" morphology of **cardiopericardial silhouette**
  - ○ **Epicardial (subepicardial) fat pad sign**, water density band (**> 4 mm**) **between subepicardial and substernal fat stripes**
  - ○ Homogeneous water attenuation/signal on CT/MR in uncomplicated effusion
  - ○ Hemopericardium
    - ■ High attenuation
    - ■ High signal on T1-weighted MR; low signal on gradient-echo cine images

Pericardial Thickening

- **Thickness > 4 mm**
- Difficult distinction from small pericardial effusion on CT
- **Constrictive pericarditis**
  - ○ Symptomatic patients with ventricular dysfunction
  - ○ Thick fibrotic pericardium limits ventricular expansion
  - ○ Etiologies: Radiation, cardiac surgery, infection, neoplasia, connective tissue disorders
  - ○ Imaging
    - ■ Pericardial thickening/calcification/adhesions
    - ■ Tubular deformity of ventricles (particularly right ventricle) with decreased volume
    - ■ Flat or sigmoid interventricular septum
    - ■ Dilatation of atria, coronary sinus and systemic veins

PERICARDIUM

OVERVIEW OF THE PERICARDIUM

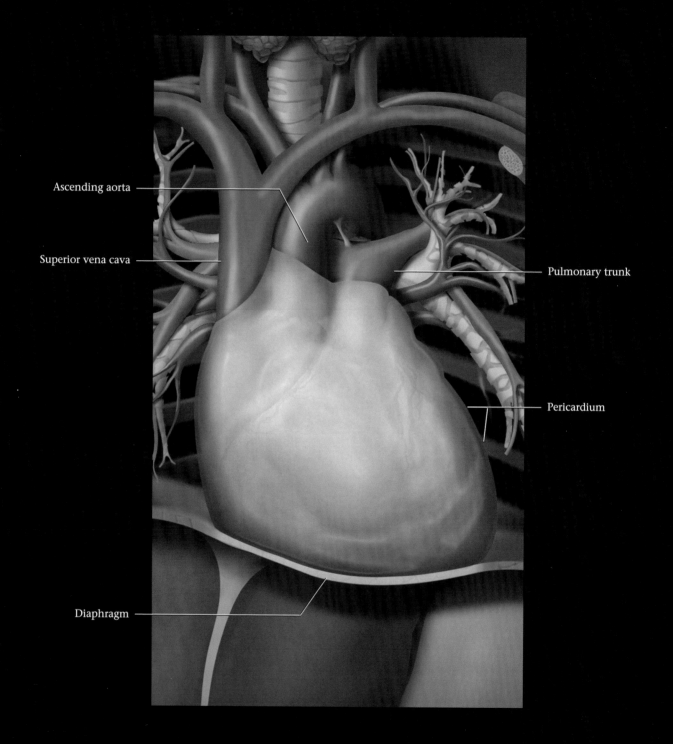

Ascending aorta

Superior vena cava

Pulmonary trunk

Pericardium

Diaphragm

The pericardium is a sac-like membrane that surrounds the heart and the origins of the great vessels. It has a conical shape with the apex of the cone oriented inferiorly and to the left. The pericardium normally contains 15-50 mL of serous fluid that provides lubrication of its apposing serous surfaces during cardiac motion. Although the heart can move relatively freely and change its morphology within the pericardial cavity, the pericardium poses some restrictions on cardiac motion and pericardial fluid volume.

PERICARDIUM

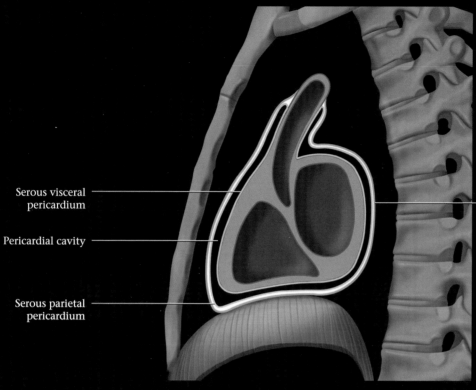

Serous visceral pericardium

Pericardial cavity

Serous parietal pericardium

Fibrous pericardium

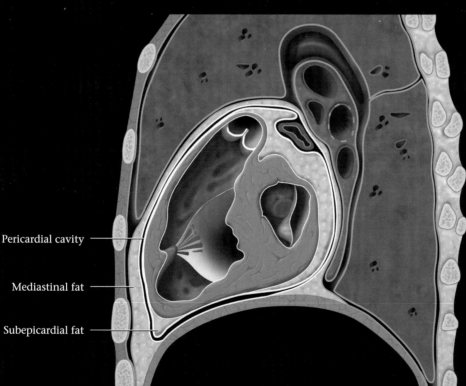

Pericardial cavity

Mediastinal fat

Subepicardial fat

(Top) Graphic shows the anatomy of the pericardial layers. The fibrous pericardium (green) is composed of tough connective tissue, is continuous with the proximal great vessel adventitia and forms the boundaries of the anatomic middle mediastinum. The serous pericardium (blue) surrounds the heart with two continuous thin layers lined by mesothelial cells. The serous parietal pericardium lines the internal surface of the fibrous pericardium. The serous visceral pericardium (epicardium) lines the heart. Between the two serous layers is a potential space that contains a small amount of fluid. **(Bottom)** Graphic shows the pericardial cavity and the thin pericardial layers. Visualization of the pericardium on cross-sectional imaging is enhanced by subepicardial fat deep to the serous visceral layer and mediastinal fat surrounding the fibrous and serous parietal pericardial layers.

PERICARDIUM

ANATOMY OF THE PERICARDIUM

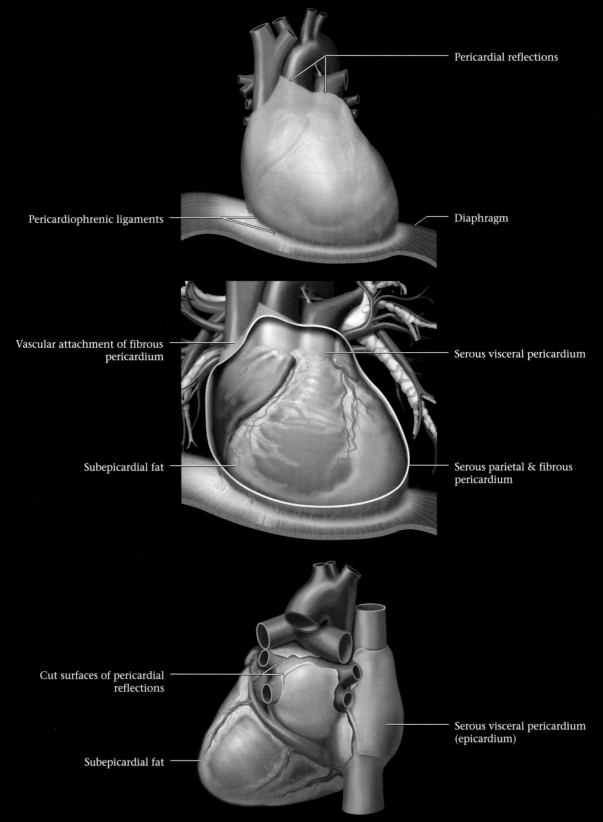

Pericardial reflections

Pericardiophrenic ligaments

Diaphragm

Vascular attachment of fibrous pericardium

Serous visceral pericardium

Subepicardial fat

Serous parietal & fibrous pericardium

Cut surfaces of pericardial reflections

Serous visceral pericardium (epicardium)

Subepicardial fat

(Top) Graphic shows the surface anatomy of the fibrous pericardium that forms the boundaries of the anatomic middle mediastinum. The base of the pericardium is attached to the diaphragm by the pericardiophrenic ligaments and to the chest wall by the sternopericardial ligaments (not shown). These attachments anchor the pericardium and prevent excessive cardiac motion. **(Middle)** Graphic shows the pericardial cavity seen by "cutting away" the anterior (fibrous and serous parietal) pericardium. The fibrous pericardium is continuous with the great vessel adventitia and is lined by the serous parietal pericardium, which is continuous with the serous visceral pericardium (epicardium) that covers the heart and subepicardial fat. **(Bottom)** Graphic shows that the fibrous/parietal pericardium has been removed to reveal the posterior visceral serous pericardium and its reflections.

PERICARDIUM

ANATOMY OF THE PERICARDIAL RECESSES

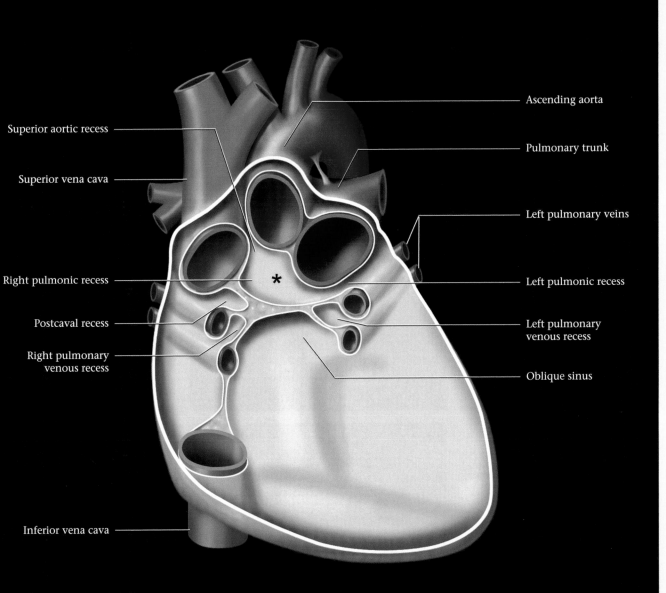

Superior aortic recess

Superior vena cava

Right pulmonic recess

Postcaval recess

Right pulmonary venous recess

Inferior vena cava

Ascending aorta

Pulmonary trunk

Left pulmonary veins

Left pulmonic recess

Left pulmonary venous recess

Oblique sinus

*

Graphic depicts the pericardial sinuses and recesses. The anterior pericardium and heart have been removed. Two tubes, one surrounding the ascending aorta and pulmonary trunk and the other surrounding the superior and inferior venae cavae and the pulmonary veins are separated by the transverse sinus (*). The transverse and oblique sinuses are separated by a pericardial reflection. The superior aortic, right pulmonic and left pulmonic recesses arise from the transverse sinus. The oblique sinus is located above and behind the left atrium. The postcaval, left and right pulmonary venous recesses arise from the pericardial cavity proper.

PERICARDIUM

AXIAL CT, NORMAL PERICARDIUM

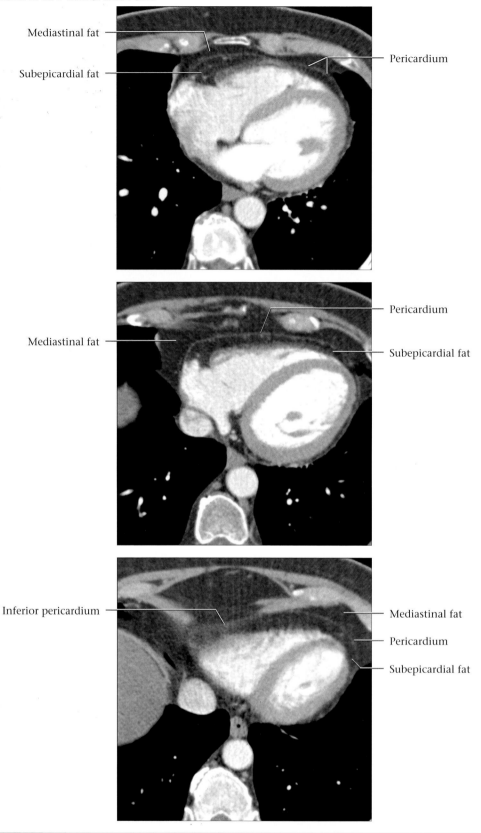

(Top) First of three contrast-enhanced axial cardiac gated CT images (mediastinal window) through the heart showing the appearance of the normal pericardium. Image at the level of the mitral valve shows the anterior pericardium manifesting as a thin soft tissue line outlined by subepicardial fat posteriorly and mediastinal fat anteriorly. The thin line represents the combined thicknesses of the fibrous pericardium and the serous parietal and visceral pericardium. (Middle) Image through the orifice of the coronary sinus demonstrates the anterior pericardium. The normal thickness of the pericardium is less than 2 mm in most cases, but can normally reach up to 4 mm. (Bottom) Image through the inferior aspect of the heart demonstrates the normal pericardium. Note the apparent increased thickness of the inferior pericardium.

PERICARDIUM

CORONAL & SAGITTAL CT, NORMAL PERICARDIUM

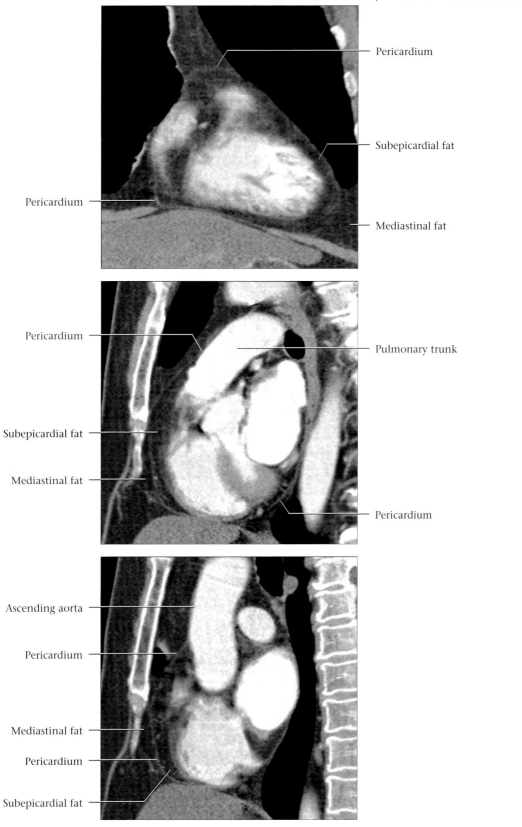

Pericardium

Subepicardial fat

Mediastinal fat

Pericardium

Pericardium

Pulmonary trunk

Subepicardial fat

Mediastinal fat

Pericardium

Ascending aorta

Pericardium

Mediastinal fat

Pericardium

Subepicardial fat

(Top) First of three contrast-enhanced cardiac gated CT images (mediastinal window) showing the normal pericardium. Coronal image through the anterior heart shows the normal pericardium manifesting as a thin soft tissue line. The superior pericardium manifests as an ill-defined soft tissue band. (Middle) Sagittal image through the pulmonary trunk shows the anterior and posterior pericardium. The normal pericardium is usually not visible over the atria and left ventricle. Note the superior pericardial reflection at the pulmonary trunk where the fibrous pericardium is continuous with the vascular adventitia. (Bottom) Sagittal image through the ascending aorta demonstrates the superior pericardial reflection. The superior pericardium surrounds the central great vessels and is continuous with the vascular adventitia of the ascending aorta.

PERICARDIUM

AXIAL & CORONAL MR, NORMAL PERICARDIUM

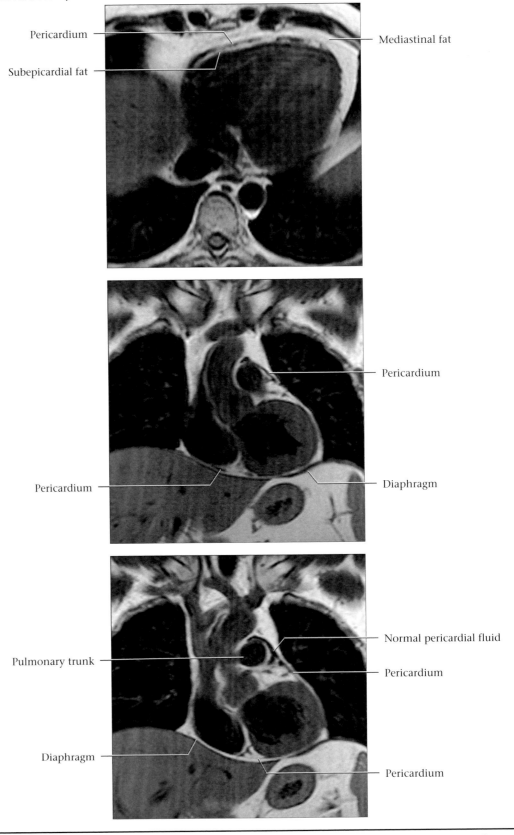

Pericardium — Mediastinal fat

Subepicardial fat —

— Pericardium

Pericardium — — Diaphragm

Pulmonary trunk — — Normal pericardial fluid

— Pericardium

Diaphragm — — Pericardium

(Top) First of six normal double inversion recovery MR images through the mediastinum. Axial image through the inferior aspect of the heart shows the normal pericardium manifesting as a thin low signal line outlined by high signal subepicardial and mediastinal fat. The pericardium is typically best visualized along its anterior surface on CT and MR imaging. (Middle) Coronal image through the aortic root shows the superior pericardial reflection that surrounds the pulmonary trunk. (Bottom) Coronal image through the proximal aortic arch shows the thin low signal pericordium accentuated by surrounding fat. The superior pericardial reflection is visible over the pulmonary trunk and contains a small amount of fluid located within the left pulmonic and superior aortic pericardial recesses of the transverse sinus.

PERICARDIUM

SAGITTAL MR, NORMAL PERICARDIUM

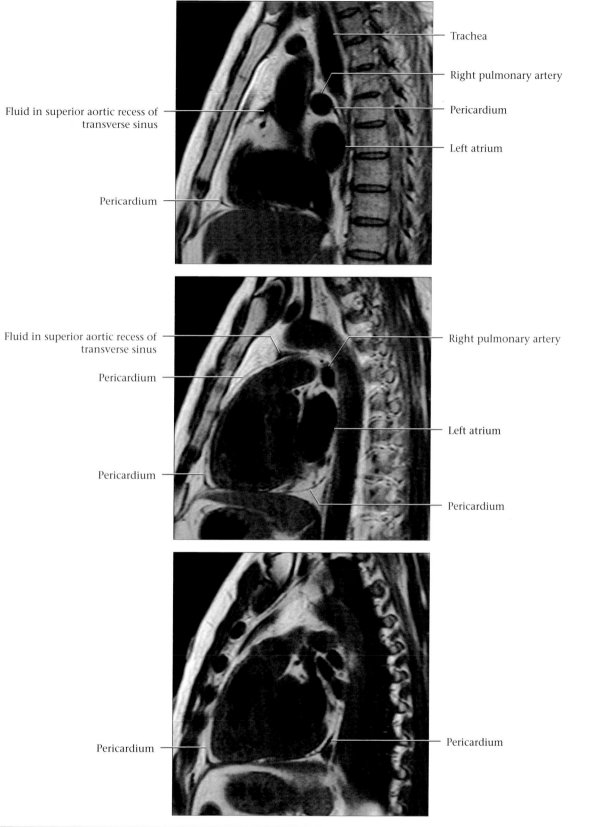

Trachea

Right pulmonary artery

Pericardium

Left atrium

Fluid in superior aortic recess of transverse sinus

Pericardium

Fluid in superior aortic recess of transverse sinus

Pericardium

Right pulmonary artery

Left atrium

Pericardium

Pericardium

Pericardium

Pericardium

(Top) Sagittal image through the ascending aorta shows the normal anterior inferior pericardium. The superior pericardial reflection is also noted as is fluid in the superior aortic recess of the transverse sinus. Note the pericardial reflection over the right pulmonary artery. (Middle) Sagittal image through the pulmonary trunk shows the anterior and posterior aspects of the normal pericardium. The pericardium is not visible adjacent to the left atrium. There is a small amount of fluid in the anterior portion of the superior aortic recess of the transverse sinus. (Bottom) Sagittal image through the left lateral aspect of the pulmonary trunk demonstrates partial visualization of the normal pericardium. In this case, the posterior pericardium over the left ventricle is well visualized.

PERICARDIUM

AXIAL CT, PERICARDIAL RECESSES

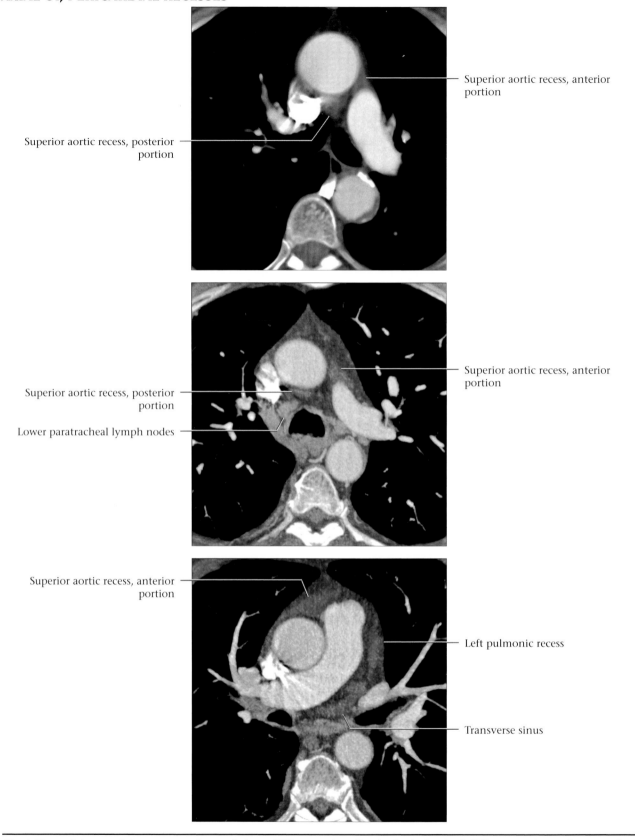

Superior aortic recess, anterior portion

Superior aortic recess, posterior portion

Superior aortic recess, anterior portion

Superior aortic recess, posterior portion

Lower paratracheal lymph nodes

Superior aortic recess, anterior portion

Left pulmonic recess

Transverse sinus

(Top) First of three axial contrast-enhanced chest CT images (mediastinal window) of different patients showing the recesses of the pericardium. The superior aortic recess (an extension of the transverse sinus) has anterior, posterior and lateral portions. The anterior portion is triangular and projects between the ascending aorta and pulmonary trunk. The posterior portion is crescentic in shape and is located posterior to the ascending aorta. **(Middle)** Axial image through the carina shows the cleft-like anterior and crescentic posterior portions of the superior aortic recess. Pericardial recesses are distinguished from lymph nodes based on location, morphology and attenuation. **(Bottom)** Image through the right pulmonary artery shows the anterior portion of the superior aortic recess and the left pulmonic recess. These recesses are extensions of the transverse sinus.

PERICARDIUM

AXIAL & CORONAL CT, PERICARDIAL RECESSES

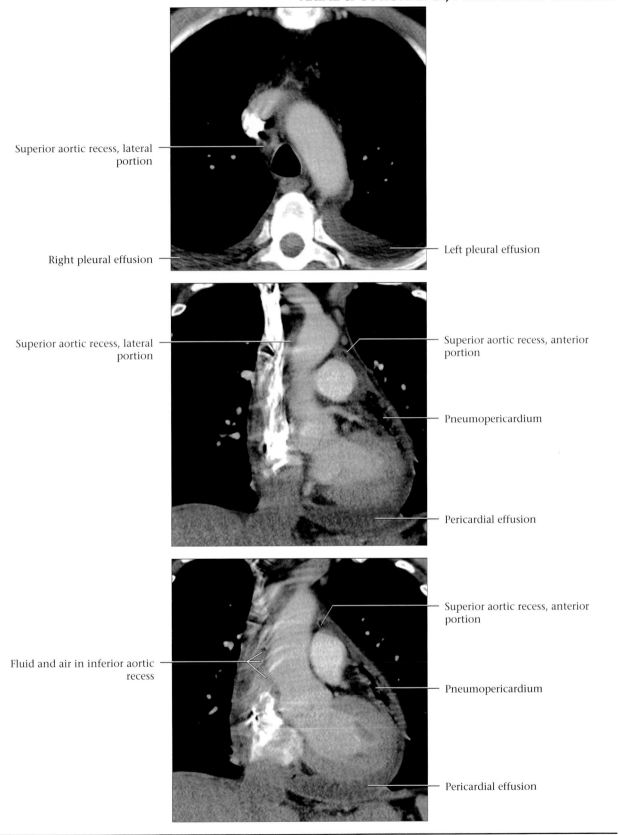

Superior aortic recess, lateral portion

Right pleural effusion

Left pleural effusion

Superior aortic recess, lateral portion

Superior aortic recess, anterior portion

Pneumopericardium

Pericardial effusion

Fluid and air in inferior aortic recess

Superior aortic recess, anterior portion

Pneumopericardium

Pericardial effusion

(Top) First of three contrast-enhanced chest CT images (mediastinal window) of a 42 year old man who sustained penetrating chest trauma complicated by pericardial infection. Axial image through the aortic arch demonstrates fluid in the lateral portion of the superior aortic recess. Bilateral pleural effusions are also present. (Middle) Coronal image through the anterior portion of the aortic root, shows fluid in the lateral portion of the superior aortic recess. Note pericardial effusion, pericardial enhancement and pneumopericardium. Fluid and air are also noted in the anterior portion of the superior aortic recess. (Bottom) Coronal image through the aortic root shows a complicated pericardial effusion and pneumopericardium. Fluid and air are seen in the inferior aortic recess which extends between the ascending aorta and the right atrium.

PERICARDIUM

AXIAL CT, PERICARDIAL RECESSES

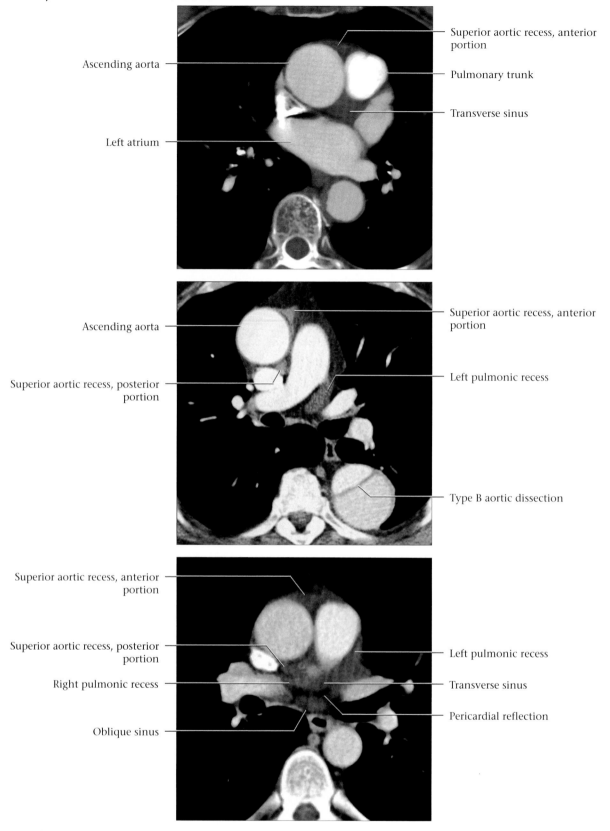

(Top) First of three axial contrast-enhanced chest CT images (mediastinal window) of different patients show the transverse sinus of the pericardium and its recesses. Image through the left atrium shows the transverse sinus of the pericardium. **(Middle)** Image through the pulmonary trunk shows the anterior and posterior portions of the superior aortic recess of the transverse sinus. The left pulmonic recess of the transverse sinus is also noted. Note chronic type B aortic dissection. **(Bottom)** Image through the pulmonary trunk shows the transverse and oblique sinuses of the pericardium. These sinuses do not communicate with each other and are separated by a pericardial reflection manifesting as a tissue plane. The recesses of the transverse sinus (superior aortic, left pulmonic and right pulmonic) are also shown.

PERICARDIUM

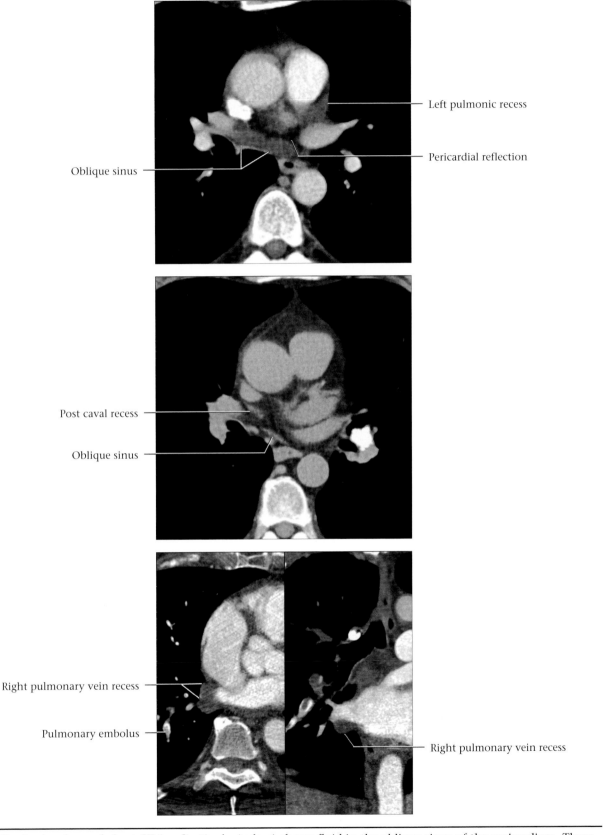

Left pulmonic recess

Pericardial reflection

Oblique sinus

Post caval recess

Oblique sinus

Right pulmonary vein recess

Pulmonary embolus

Right pulmonary vein recess

(Top) Contrast-enhanced chest CT (mediastinal window) shows fluid in the oblique sinus of the pericardium. There is also fluid in the left pulmonic recess of the transverse sinus. The transverse and oblique sinuses do not communicate with each other and are separated by a pericardial reflection. (Middle) Unenhanced axial image (mediastinal window) through the pulmonary trunk shows a small amount of fluid in the postcaval pericardial recess and in the oblique sinus. The postcaval recess arises from the pericardial cavity proper. A densely calcified granuloma in seen the left hilum. (Bottom) Composite of axial and coronal contrast-enhanced chest CT images (mediastinal window) of a patient with pulmonary emboli shows the right pulmonary venous recess adjacent to the right inferior pulmonary vein. Fluid in the pulmonary venous recesses may mimic lymphadenopathy.

PERICARDIUM

ABSENCE OF PERICARDIUM

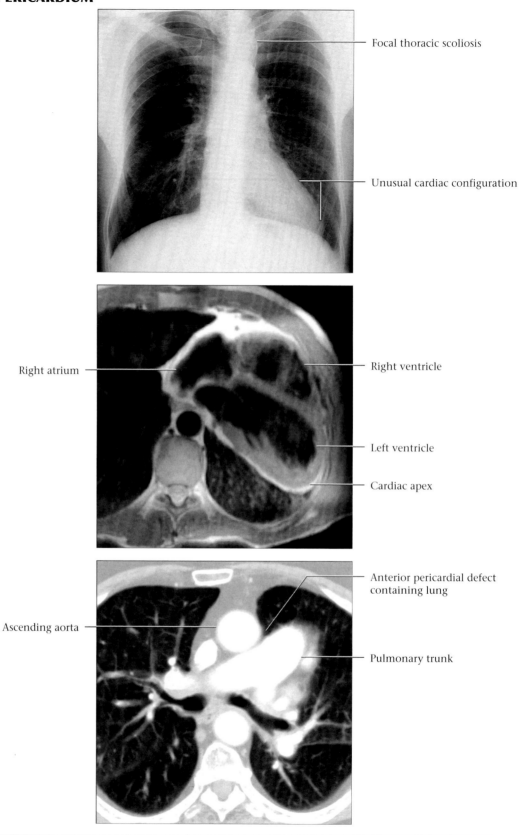

Focal thoracic scoliosis

Unusual cardiac configuration

Right atrium

Right ventricle

Left ventricle

Cardiac apex

Ascending aorta

Anterior pericardial defect containing lung

Pulmonary trunk

(Top) First of two images of an asymptomatic 22 year old man with congenital absence of the pericardium. PA chest radiograph shows upper thoracic scoliosis and an unusual configuration of the heart characterized by an elongate morphology and an inferior orientation of its long axis. **(Middle)** Axial double IR magnetic resonance image of the chest shows displacement of the heart to the left and posterior orientation of the cardiac apex consistent with absence of the pericardium. **(Bottom)** Contrast-enhanced chest CT (lung window) of an asymptomatic 84 year old man evaluated because of an abnormal cardiac configuration seen on chest radiography (not shown) shows interposition of lung between the ascending aorta and pulmonary trunk in the expected location of the anterior portion of the superior aortic recess indicating absence of the pericardium in this area.

PERICARDIUM

PERICARDIAL CYST

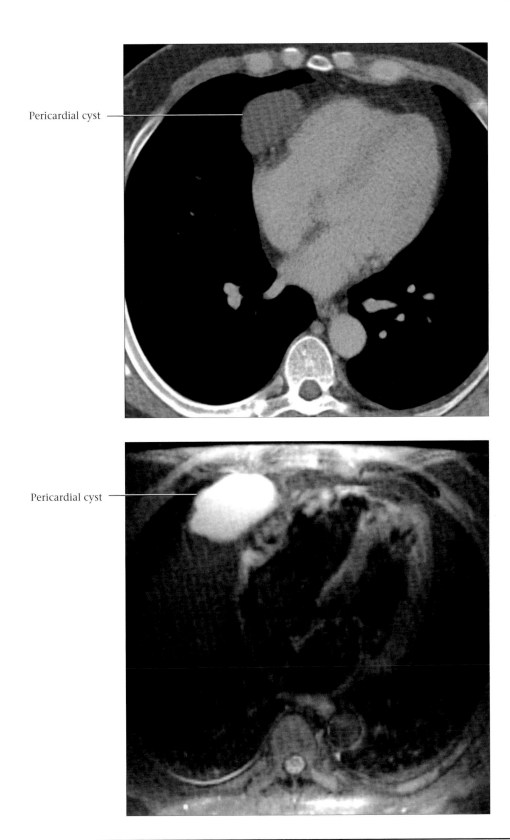

Pericardial cyst

Pericardial cyst

(Top) First of two images of an asymptomatic 53 year old man with an incidentally discovered pericardial cyst. Unenhanced chest CT (mediastinal window) demonstrates an ovoid water attenuation lesion located in the right cardiophrenic angle and abutting the right anterior pericardial surface. (Bottom) Axial T2-weighted magnetic resonance image through the lesion demonstrates that it has a slightly lobular posterolateral contour and homogeneous internal high signal. No foci of mural thickening or internal septations were identified.

PERICARDIUM

PERICARDIAL EFFUSION

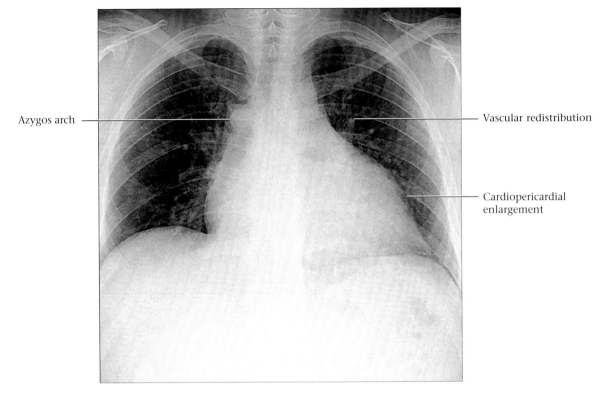

Azygos arch

Vascular redistribution

Cardiopericardial enlargement

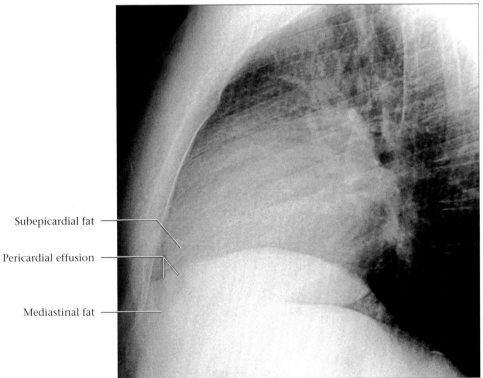

Subepicardial fat

Pericardial effusion

Mediastinal fat

(Top) First of two images of a 45 year old man with a pericardial effusion who presented with mild dyspnea and chest pain. PA chest radiograph demonstrates cardiomegaly. The cardiopericardial silhouette exhibits a globular or so-called "water bottle" morphology. There is mild vascular redistribution and enlargement of the azygos vein suggesting biventricular dysfunction. **(Bottom)** Left lateral chest radiograph demonstrates cardiomegaly. The epicardial fat sign, characterized by visualization of a water density band that measures over 4 mm in thickness, is demonstrated. The water density band represents anterior pericardial fluid outlined posteriorly by subepicardial fat and anteriorly by mediastinal fat.

PERICARDIUM

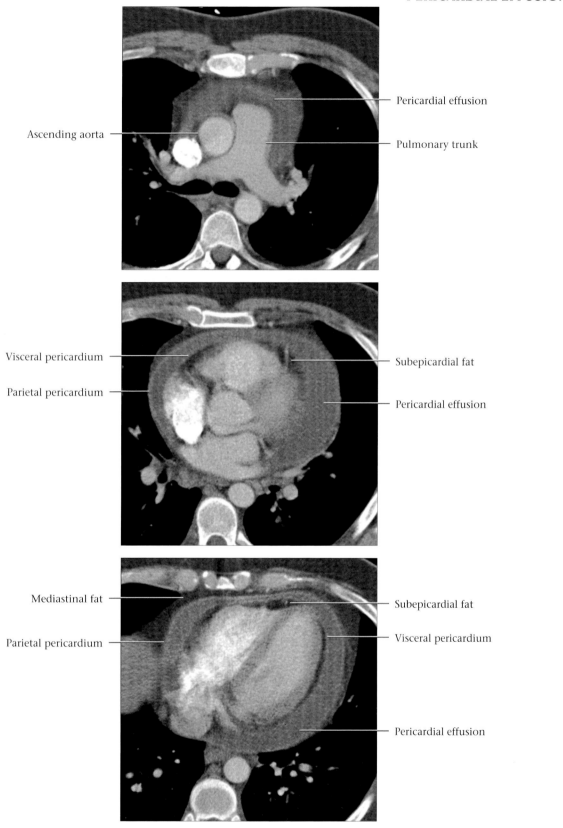

Pericardial effusion

Ascending aorta

Pulmonary trunk

Visceral pericardium

Subepicardial fat

Parietal pericardium

Pericardial effusion

Mediastinal fat

Subepicardial fat

Parietal pericardium

Visceral pericardium

Pericardial effusion

(Top) First of three axial contrast-enhanced chest CT images (mediastinal window) of a 36 year old man who presented with pericardial effusion secondary to viral pericarditis. Image through the pulmonary trunk shows fluid surrounding the ascending aorta and pulmonary trunk in the expected location of the pericardial cavity. (Middle) Image through the aortic root shows a moderate pericardial effusion surrounding the heart. There is enhancement of the serous visceral and parietal pericardial layers likely related to inflammation. (Bottom) Image through the inferior aspect of the heart demonstrates low attenuation pericardial fluid and enhancement of the serous visceral pericardium (epicardium) that covers the heart and the underlying subepicardial fat. The serous parietal pericardium also exhibits contrast-enhancement consistent with pericardial inflammation.

PERICARDIUM

PERICARDIAL THICKENING & CALCIFICATION

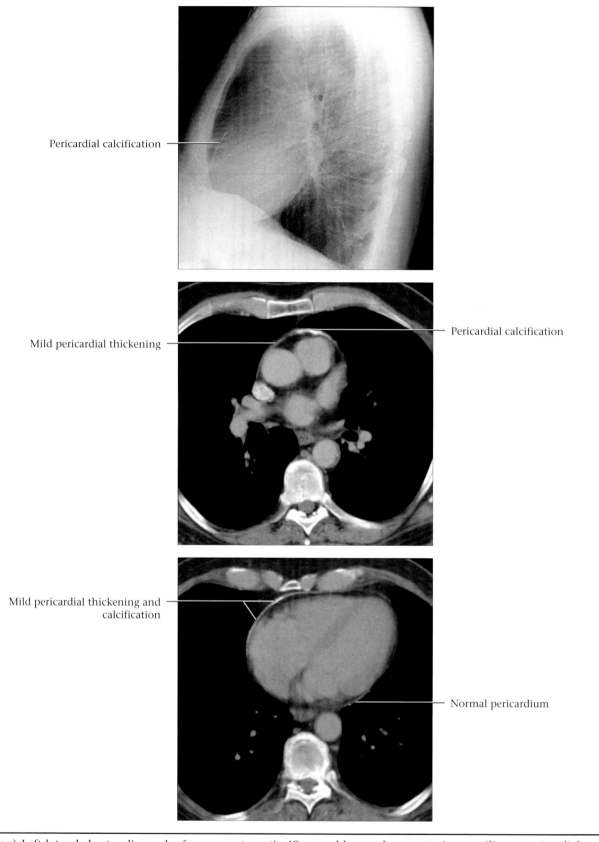

Pericardial calcification

Mild pericardial thickening

Pericardial calcification

Mild pericardial thickening and calcification

Normal pericardium

(Top) Left lateral chest radiograph of an asymptomatic 49 year old man shows anterior curvilinear pericardial calcification. The heart size, pulmonary vascularity and pleural surfaces are normal. (Middle) First of two axial contrast-enhanced chest CT images (mediastinal window) of a 60 year old man with incidentally discovered pericardial calcification. Image through the right ventricular outflow tract demonstrates mild thickening and partial calcification of the anterosuperior pericardium. (Bottom) Image through the mid aspect of the heart demonstrates mild thickening of the anterior pericardium with focal calcification. There is no associated pericardial effusion or morphologic abnormality of the underlying cardiac chambers. Pericardial calcification is typically secondary to prior injury, infection or connective tissue disease but may also be idiopathic.

PERICARDIUM

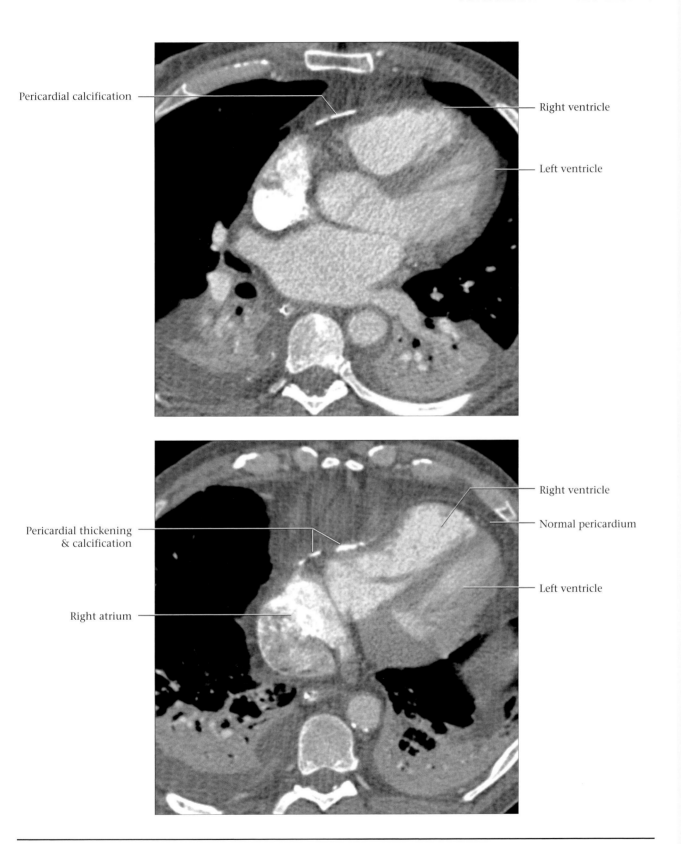

Pericardial calcification

Right ventricle

Left ventricle

Pericardial thickening & calcification

Right ventricle

Normal pericardium

Right atrium

Left ventricle

(Top) First of two axial images from a contrast-enhanced chest CT (mediastinal window) of a 67 year old man with diastolic ventricular dysfunction secondary to constrictive pericarditis. Image through the aortic root demonstrates focal linear calcification of the anterior aspect of the pericardium, bilateral pleural effusions and bilateral lower lobe relaxation atelectasis. **(Bottom)** Image through the inferior heart shows discontinuous linear calcification of the anterior pericardium associated with mass effect on the right ventricle, enlargement of the right atrium and coronary sinus, bibasilar atelectasis and pleural effusions. The tubular configuration of the right ventricle is consistent with the diagnosis of constrictive pericarditis, and the presence of pericardial calcification allows differentiation of this condition from restrictive cardiomyopathy.

CHEST WALL

General Anatomy and Function

Chest Wall Anatomy
- Skin, subcutaneous fat
- Blood vessels, lymphatics, nerves
- Bone, cartilage
- Muscles
- Endothoracic fascia, fibroelastic connective tissue between inner aspect of chest wall and costal pleura

Function
- **Musculoskeletal cage:** Surrounds cardiorespiratory system; effects respiration by expanding and contracting during ventilation

Surface Landmarks
- **Suprasternal (jugular) notch:** At superior manubrium of sternum; between sternal ends of clavicles
- **Sternal angle:** Landmark for internal thoracic anatomy; **anterior projection** at level of costal cartilage of 2nd rib
- **Costal margin:** Inferior margins of lowest ribs and costal cartilages

Skeletal Structures

Thoracic Vertebrae
- Twelve vertebrae (**T1-T12**); normal kyphotic curve
- Articular facets for ribs on vertebrae and transverse processes (except T11-T12)
- Broad laminae and spinous processes (projecting downward) overlap with those of vertebra beneath

Shoulder Girdle
- **Three synovial articulations** between clavicle, scapula and proximal humerus
  - Acromioclavicular, sternoclavicular, glenohumeral joints
- **One functional articulation** (scapulothoracic "joint")
  - Mobile scapula suspended on rib cage by muscles

Sternum
- Flat, broad bone forms anterior thoracic wall; three parts (**manubrium, body, xiphoid process**)
- **Manubrium** forms superior part of sternum
- **Body** articulates with manubrium superiorly, xiphoid process inferiorly, bilateral costal cartilages of 2nd-7th ribs
- **Xiphoid process** variable size, shape, ossification; articulates with body of sternum superiorly

Clavicle
- Slender, s-shaped bone; connects sternum to scapula

Scapula
- Large, triangular flat bone; parallel to upper posterior thorax; extends from 2nd-7th ribs bilaterally
- **Glenoid fossa** at glenohumeral joint

Ribs
- 12 pairs, symmetrically arrayed; numbered in accordance with attached vertebral body
- **True ribs** (1-7) attach to sternum by costal cartilages (synovial joints)

- **False ribs** (8-10) articulate by costal cartilages with costal cartilage of 7th rib
- **Floating ribs** (11-12) do not articulate with sternum or rib costal cartilages; short costal cartilages terminate in abdominal wall muscle
- **Head** articulates with demifacets of two adjacent vertebral bodies; **neck** located between head and tubercle of each rib; **tubercle** articulates with vertebral transverse process
- **Body:** Longest part of each rib
- **Angle:** Most posterior part
- **Costal groove** on inner surface of inferior border; accommodates intercostal neurovascular bundle

Muscles

Pectoral
- **Pectoralis major:** Largest muscle in breast and pectoral region; originates from anterior chest wall, sternum, and clavicle; adducts, flexes and medially rotates arm
- **Pectoralis minor:** Deep to pectoralis major; originates from chest wall, inserts onto coracoid process of scapula; stabilizes scapula

Intercostal
- **External:** Contained within 11 intercostal spaces; extend from tubercle of ribs to costochondral junction
- **Internal:** Middle layer; occupy 11 intercostal spaces; extend from border of sternum to angle of ribs
- **Innermost:** Form inner layer of chest wall muscles with **subcostales** and **transversus thoracis muscles**

Serratus Anterior
- Thin muscular sheet; overlies lateral thoracic cage and intercostal muscles; arises from upper eight ribs; wraps around rib cage; inserts along medial border of anterior surface of scapula

Back Muscles
- **Superficial extrinsic muscles** (connect upper limbs to trunk; limb movement); **trapezius, latissimus dorsi, levator scapulae, rhomboids**
- **Intermediate extrinsic muscles** (superficial respiratory muscles); **serratus posterior**
- **Deep intrinsic muscles** (postvertebral muscles; control posture, vertebral and head movement); **splenius muscle, erector spinae muscles, deep transversospinales muscles**

Vessels

Arteries
- **Internal thoracic (internal mammary):** Branch of subclavian artery; descends posterior to first six costal cartilages; supplies upper anterior chest wall
  - Supplies **anterior intercostal arteries** to first six intercostal spaces

CHEST WALL

Veins
- **Azygos vein** receives drainage from **posterior intercostal veins**, **hemi-azygos** and accessory **hemi-azygos veins**

Lymphatics
- Chest wall drainage through **thoracic duct** (right upper limb, right face and neck drained by **right lymphatic duct**)

Soft Tissues

Skin and Subcutaneous Tissues
- **Nipple:** Superficial to 4th intercostal space (males and prepuberal females)

Nerves
- Anterior rami of thoracic spinal nerves (T1-T11) supply skin, tissues of chest wall; form intercostal nerves
- **Intercostal nerves** run in costal groove, between internal and innermost intercostal muscles
- **Brachial plexus:** Branching network of nerve roots, trunks, divisions, cords and branches
  - Spinal roots form three trunks; behind clavicle, each dividing into anterior and posterior divisions

Anatomic Regions

Thoracic Inlet
- Opening at superior end of thoracic rib cage; conduit for cervical structures to enter thorax
- Bounded by T1 vertebral body, right and left 1st ribs and their costal cartilages, and manubrium of sternum

Thoracic Outlet
- Opening at inferior end of thoracic rib cage; conduit for thoracic structures to exit thorax
- Bounded by T12 vertebral body, right and left 12th ribs, costal cartilages of 7th-12th ribs, xiphisternal joint

Supraclavicular Region
- Supraclavicular lymph nodes in and around carotid sheath
- Lymph drainage of breast superiorly to supraclavicular and inferior deep nodes, laterally to axillary nodes, medially to parasternal (internal mammary) and mediastinal nodes, inferiorly to diaphragmatic nodes

Axilla
- Pyramidal-shaped space between lateral chest and upper arm; bounded by pectoralis muscles (anteriorly), subscapularis, latissimus dorsi and teres major muscles (posteriorly), convergence of axillary fold muscles (laterally), and clavicle, scapula and outer border of first rib (apex)
- Axillary lymph nodes drain breast, thoracoabdominal wall above umbilicus, and upper arm

Breast and Pectoral Region
- Anterior and superior part of chest; muscles and fascia assist movement of upper limb; mammary glands

Imaging

Radiography
- Limited capabilities; may detect congenital deformities, soft-tissue masses, bone destruction

Computed Tomography
- Helical CT and multiplanar reformations optimal for visualization of osseous and soft-tissue lesions

Magnetic Resonance Imaging
- Multiplanar capabilities and advanced pulse sequences optimal for chest wall tumor evaluation

Imaging Anatomic Correlations

Congenital and Developmental Abnormalities
- **Pectus excavatum** (syn. funnel chest): Abnormal growth of costal cartilages; sternal depression/rotation; compression/obscuration of right heart border on PA radiograph
- **Pectus carinatum** (syn. pigeon breast): Abnormal growth of costal cartilage; sternal protrusion
- **Cervical rib:** Supernumerary rib, usually arising from seventh cervical vertebra
- **Poland syndrome:** Uncommon; partial or total absence of pectoralis major muscle; associated malformations of ipsilateral ribs (2-5) and clavicle; congenital absence of ipsilateral breast tissue

Inflammatory and Infectious Disease
- Primary chest wall infection rare; associated with immune suppression, diabetes mellitus, trauma
- Heroin addicts prone to septic arthritis of sternoclavicular and sternochondral joints
- Secondary involvement more common: From pulmonary infection (tuberculous, fungal) or pleural empyema (empyema necessitatis)

Neoplasia
- Benign
  - **Lipoma:** Contiguous with fat in chest wall; CT numbers diagnostic
  - **Smooth pressure erosion** of bone implies slow growth (e.g., neurofibroma)
- Malignant
  - **Chondrosarcoma:** Rib (11%), commonly anterior rib near costochondral junction; lytic, expanded, often thick sclerotic border; chondroid calcification (60-75%)
  - **Myeloma:** Commonly manifests as rib destruction with associated soft-tissue mass
  - **Metastatic disease:** Destruction of ribs, thoracic vertebrae, scapulae, clavicles, sternum

CHEST WALL

CHEST WALL OVERVIEW

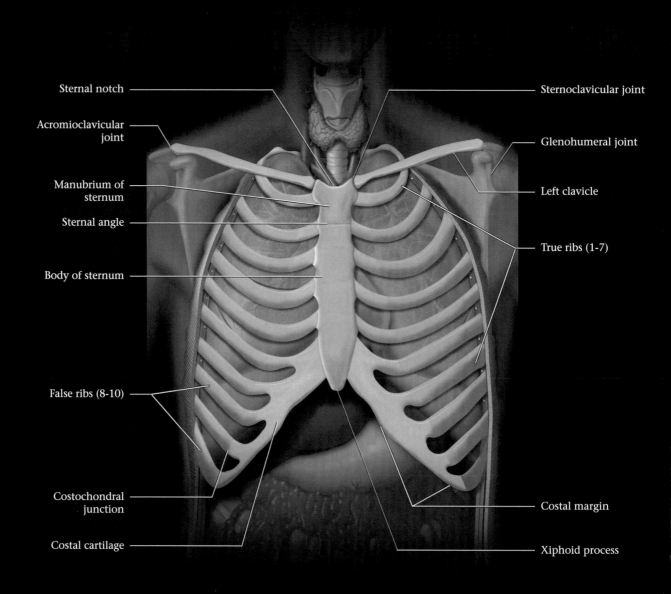

Sternal notch

Acromioclavicular joint

Manubrium of sternum

Sternal angle

Body of sternum

False ribs (8-10)

Costochondral junction

Costal cartilage

Sternoclavicular joint

Glenohumeral joint

Left clavicle

True ribs (1-7)

Costal margin

Xiphoid process

Graphic depicts the chest wall structures, forming a musculoskeletal thoracic cage that surrounds the cardiorespiratory organs and effects respiration by expanding and contracting during ventilation.

CHEST WALL

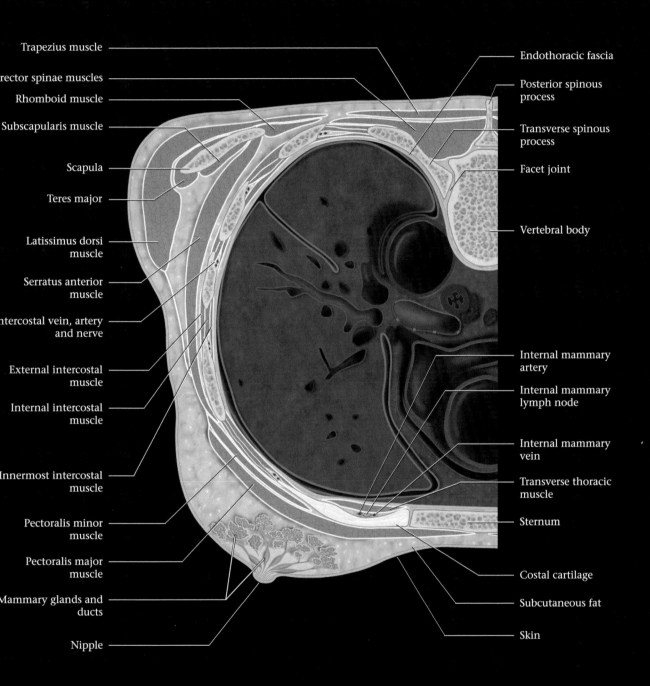

Trapezius muscle

Erector spinae muscles

Rhomboid muscle

Subscapularis muscle

Scapula

Teres major

Latissimus dorsi muscle

Serratus anterior muscle

Intercostal vein, artery and nerve

External intercostal muscle

Internal intercostal muscle

Innermost intercostal muscle

Pectoralis minor muscle

Pectoralis major muscle

Mammary glands and ducts

Nipple

Endothoracic fascia

Posterior spinous process

Transverse spinous process

Facet joint

Vertebral body

Internal mammary artery

Internal mammary lymph node

Internal mammary vein

Transverse thoracic muscle

Sternum

Costal cartilage

Subcutaneous fat

Skin

Graphic depicts the chest wall layers as visualized in the axial plane including skin, subcutaneous fat, blood vessels, lymphatics, and musculoskeletal structures. The innermost layer, the endothoracic fascia, is a fibroelastic connective tissue layer between the inner aspect of the chest wall and the pleura.

CHEST WALL

THORACIC INLET, SUPRACLAVICULAR AND AXILLARY REGIONS

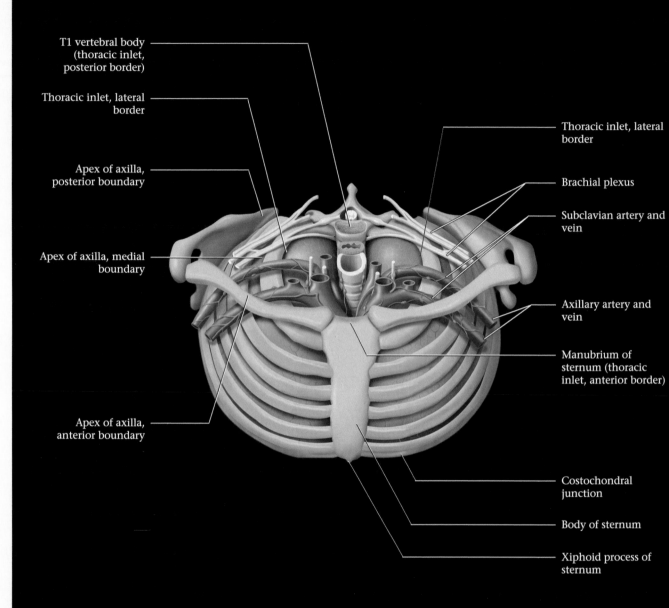

T1 vertebral body
(thoracic inlet,
posterior border)

Thoracic inlet, lateral
border

Apex of axilla,
posterior boundary

Apex of axilla, medial
boundary

Apex of axilla,
anterior boundary

Thoracic inlet, lateral
border

Brachial plexus

Subclavian artery and
vein

Axillary artery and
vein

Manubrium of
sternum (thoracic
inlet, anterior border)

Costochondral
junction

Body of sternum

Xiphoid process of
sternum

Graphic depicts the thoracic inlet, supraclavicular structures, and the axillary regions. The thoracic inlet is bounded by the T1 vertebral body, the right and left first ribs and their costal cartilages, and the manubrium of the sternum. The apex of the axillary region is bounded by the clavicle, scapula, and outer border of the first rib. Vascular structures allow blood flow to enter and exit the thorax through the thoracic inlet and join with brachial plexus components to supply the thorax and upper limbs.

CHEST WALL

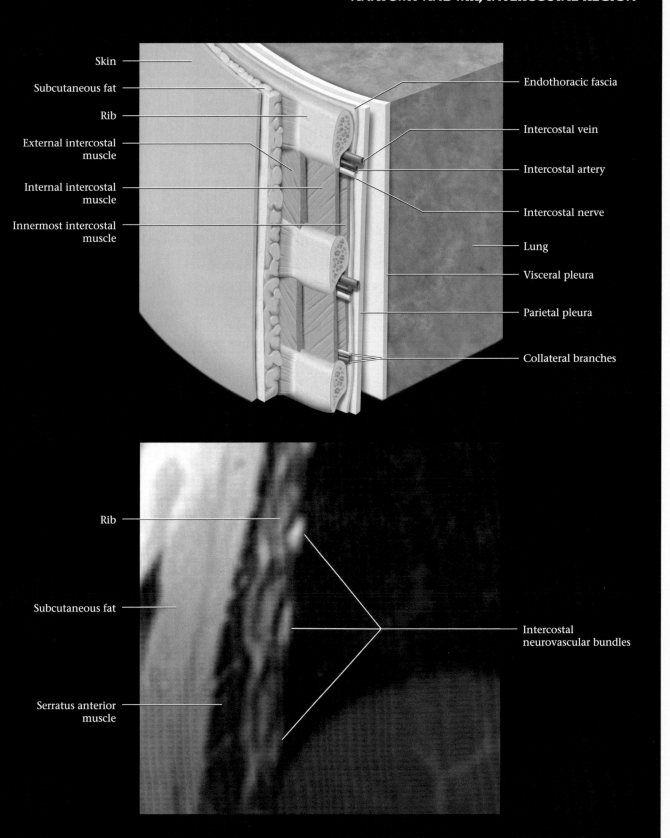

(Top) Graphic demonstrates details of the intercostal region, showing three layers of intercostal muscles (external, internal and innermost) between the ribs. The costal groove along the inferomedial aspect of each rib accommodates the intercostal neurovascular bundle (vein, artery and nerve). Small collateral branches of the major intercostal vessels and nerves may be present above the body of the subjacent rib. The endothoracic fascia forms a connective tissue layer between the inner aspect of the chest wall and the costal parietal pleura. (Bottom) Detail of a coronal MR section through the right lower chest wall demonstrates the intercostal neurovascular bundle as an ovoid area of increased signal intensity.

CHEST WALL

AXIAL CT, NORMAL CHEST WALL

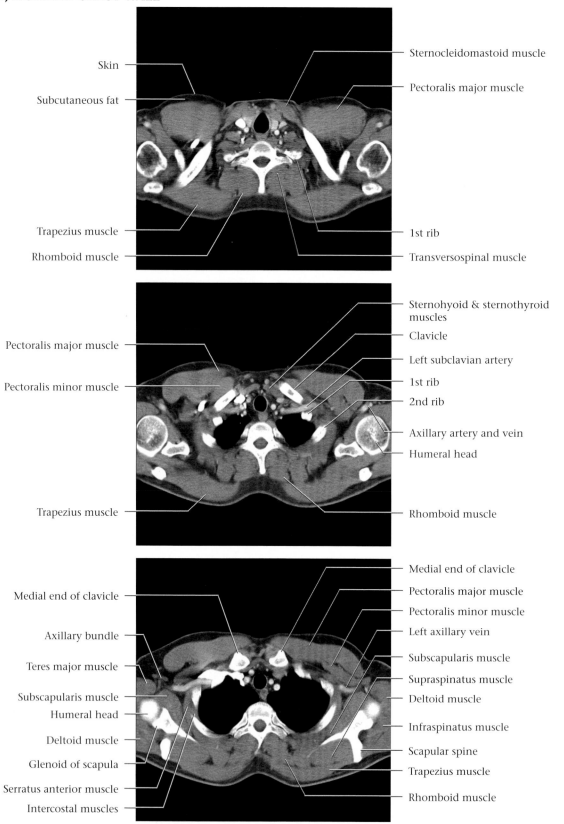

Skin

Subcutaneous fat

Sternocleidomastoid muscle

Pectoralis major muscle

Trapezius muscle

Rhomboid muscle

1st rib

Transversospinal muscle

Pectoralis major muscle

Pectoralis minor muscle

Trapezius muscle

Sternohyoid & sternothyroid muscles

Clavicle

Left subclavian artery

1st rib

2nd rib

Axillary artery and vein

Humeral head

Rhomboid muscle

Medial end of clavicle

Axillary bundle

Teres major muscle

Subscapularis muscle

Humeral head

Deltoid muscle

Glenoid of scapula

Serratus anterior muscle

Intercostal muscles

Medial end of clavicle

Pectoralis major muscle

Pectoralis minor muscle

Left axillary vein

Subscapularis muscle

Supraspinatus muscle

Deltoid muscle

Infraspinatus muscle

Scapular spine

Trapezius muscle

Rhomboid muscle

(Top) First of six axial contrast-enhanced CT images (mediastinal window) demonstrating normal chest wall structures. The first image demonstrates chest wall muscles in the supraclavicular region. **(Middle)** CT image through the lung apices includes normal subclavian and axillary vessels. **(Bottom)** CT image at the level of the medial clavicles demonstrates muscles related to the scapula.

CHEST WALL

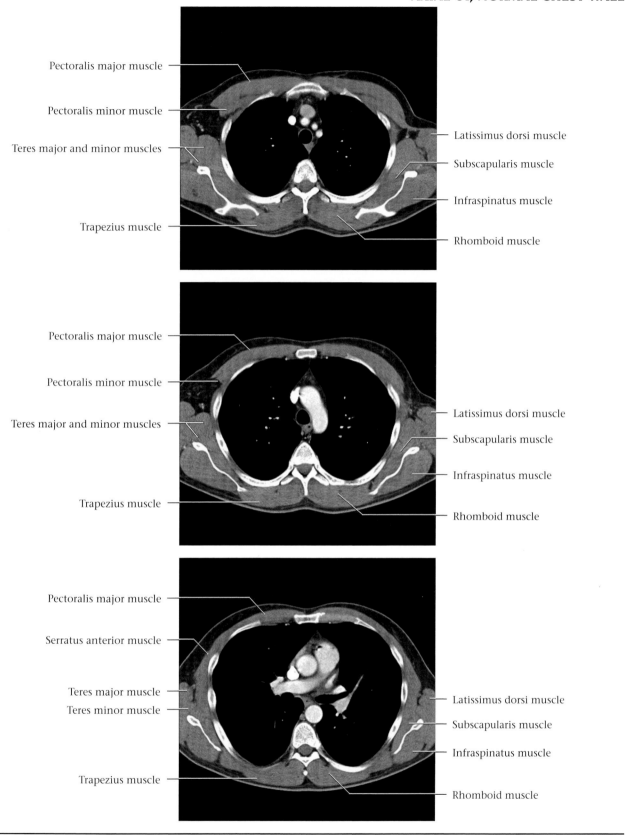

Pectoralis major muscle

Pectoralis minor muscle

Teres major and minor muscles

Trapezius muscle

Latissimus dorsi muscle

Subscapularis muscle

Infraspinatus muscle

Rhomboid muscle

Pectoralis major muscle

Pectoralis minor muscle

Teres major and minor muscles

Trapezius muscle

Latissimus dorsi muscle

Subscapularis muscle

Infraspinatus muscle

Rhomboid muscle

Pectoralis major muscle

Serratus anterior muscle

Teres major muscle
Teres minor muscle

Trapezius muscle

Latissimus dorsi muscle

Subscapularis muscle

Infraspinatus muscle

Rhomboid muscle

(Top) CT image through the level of the aortic arch branches. **(Middle)** CT image at the level of the aortic arch. **(Bottom)** CT image through the subcarinal region.

CHEST WALL

AXIAL MR, NORMAL CHEST WALL

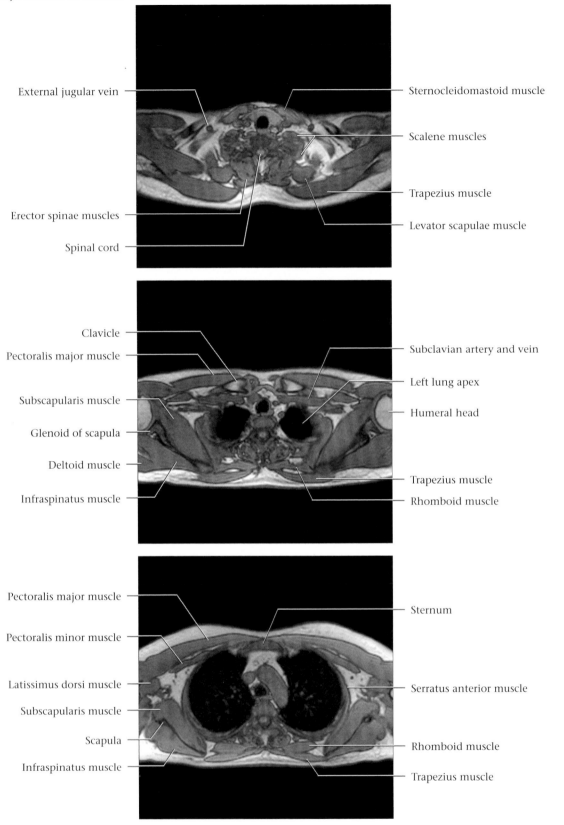

External jugular vein

Sternocleidomastoid muscle

Scalene muscles

Trapezius muscle

Levator scapulae muscle

Erector spinae muscles

Spinal cord

Clavicle

Pectoralis major muscle

Subclavian artery and vein

Left lung apex

Subscapularis muscle

Humeral head

Glenoid of scapula

Deltoid muscle

Infraspinatus muscle

Trapezius muscle

Rhomboid muscle

Pectoralis major muscle

Pectoralis minor muscle

Sternum

Latissimus dorsi muscle

Serratus anterior muscle

Subscapularis muscle

Scapula

Rhomboid muscle

Infraspinatus muscle

Trapezius muscle

(Top) First of six axial T1-weighted MR images demonstrating normal chest wall structures. The first section is through the supraclavicular region. (Middle) Axial MR image through the lung apices. (Bottom) Axial MR image at the level of the aortic arch.

CHEST WALL

AXIAL MR, NORMAL CHEST WALL

Pectoralis major muscle — Sternum
Pectoralis minor muscle
Latissimus dorsi muscle — Serratus anterior muscle
Subscapularis muscle
Scapula — Rhomboid muscle
Infraspinatus muscle — Trapezius muscle

Sternum
Pectoralis major muscle
Pectoralis minor muscle
Serratus anterior muscle
Subscapularis muscle
Scapula — Rhomboid muscle
Infraspinatus muscle — Trapezius muscle

Pectoralis major muscle
Serratus anterior muscle
Latissimus dorsi muscle
Infraspinatus muscle — Trapezius muscle
Serratus anterior muscle — Transversospinalis muscle

(Top) Axial MR image at the level of the aortico-pulmonary window. **(Middle)** Axial MR image through the pulmonary arteries. **(Bottom)** Axial MR image through the lower lobes and inferior pulmonary veins.

CHEST WALL

CORONAL CT, NORMAL CHEST WALL

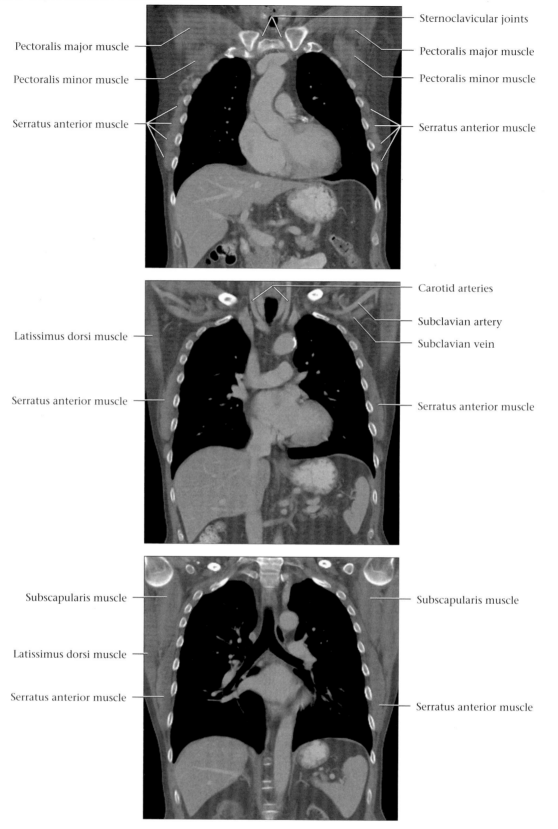

Pectoralis major muscle

Pectoralis minor muscle

Serratus anterior muscle

Sternoclavicular joints

Pectoralis major muscle

Pectoralis minor muscle

Serratus anterior muscle

Latissimus dorsi muscle

Serratus anterior muscle

Carotid arteries

Subclavian artery

Subclavian vein

Serratus anterior muscle

Subscapularis muscle

Latissimus dorsi muscle

Serratus anterior muscle

Subscapularis muscle

Serratus anterior muscle

(Top) First of six coronal contrast-enhanced chest CT images (bone window) shown from anterior to posterior demonstrate normal chest wall muscles. The first section is through the level of the sternoclavicular joints. (Middle) Coronal CT section through the level of the pulmonary arteries. (Bottom) Coronal CT section through the level of the carina.

CHEST WALL

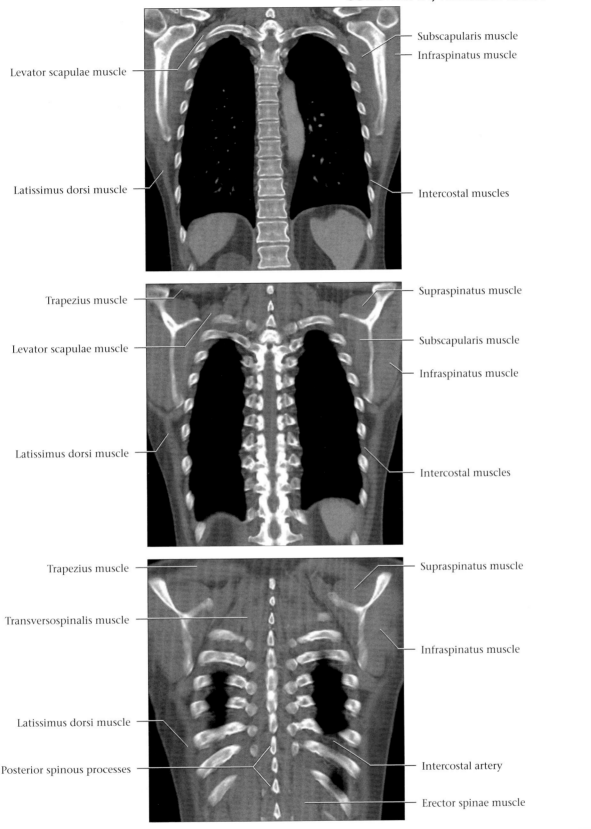

Levator scapulae muscle

Latissimus dorsi muscle

Subscapularis muscle

Infraspinatus muscle

Intercostal muscles

Trapezius muscle

Levator scapulae muscle

Latissimus dorsi muscle

Supraspinatus muscle

Subscapularis muscle

Infraspinatus muscle

Intercostal muscles

Trapezius muscle

Transversospinalis muscle

Latissimus dorsi muscle

Posterior spinous processes

Supraspinatus muscle

Infraspinatus muscle

Intercostal artery

Erector spinae muscle

(Top) Coronal CT section through the level of the descending thoracic aorta. (Middle) Coronal CT section through the level of the thoracic spinal canal. (Bottom) Coronal CT section through the level of the posterior ribs and posterior spinous processes.

CHEST WALL

CORONAL MR, NORMAL CHEST WALL

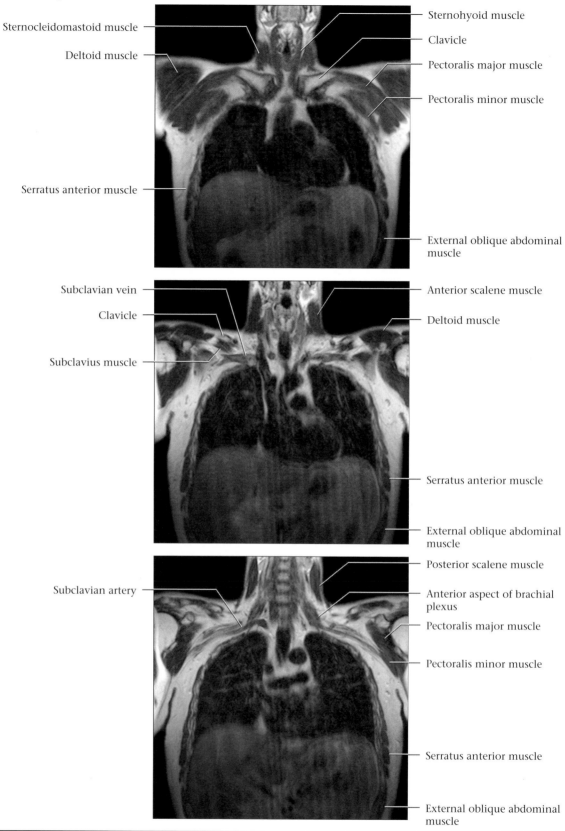

Sternocleidomastoid muscle

Deltoid muscle

Serratus anterior muscle

Sternohyoid muscle

Clavicle

Pectoralis major muscle

Pectoralis minor muscle

External oblique abdominal muscle

Subclavian vein

Clavicle

Subclavius muscle

Anterior scalene muscle

Deltoid muscle

Serratus anterior muscle

External oblique abdominal muscle

Subclavian artery

Posterior scalene muscle

Anterior aspect of brachial plexus

Pectoralis major muscle

Pectoralis minor muscle

Serratus anterior muscle

External oblique abdominal muscle

(Top) First of six coronal T1-weighted MR images demonstrating normal chest wall structures (shown from anterior to posterior). The first section is through the medial clavicles. **(Middle)** Coronal MR section through the level of the subclavian veins. **(Bottom)** Coronal MR section through the level of the subclavian arteries and anterior aspect of the brachial plexus.

CHEST WALL

CORONAL MR, NORMAL CHEST WALL

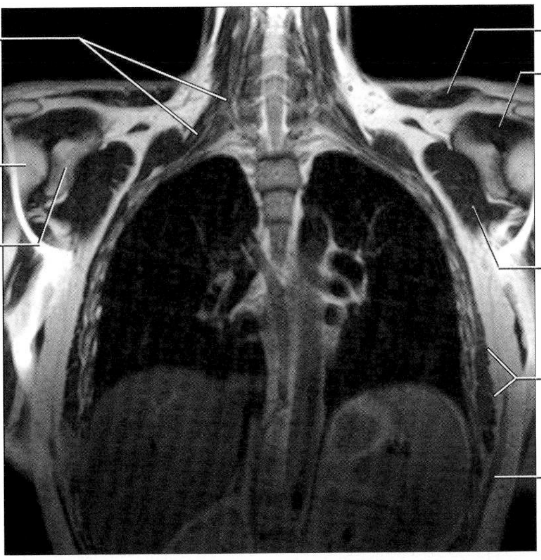

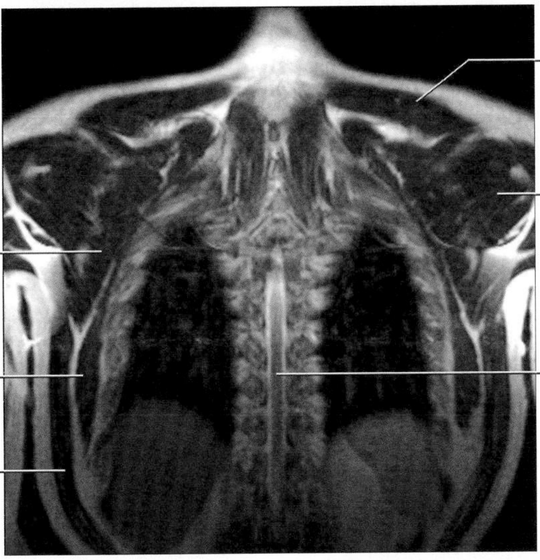

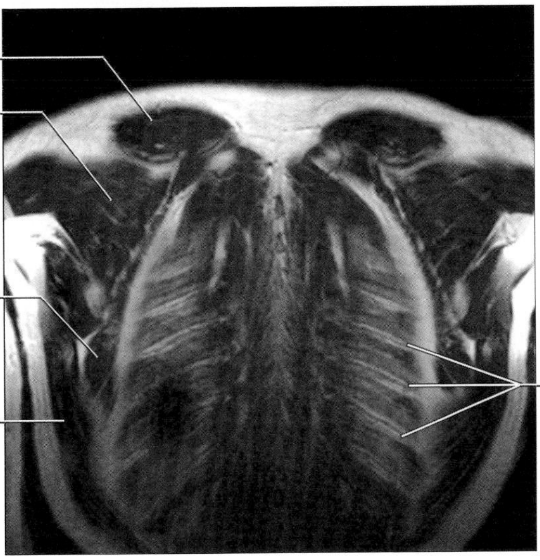

Brachial plexus — Trapezius muscle

Supraspinatus muscle

Humeral head — Subscapularis muscle

Glenoid of scapula — Serratus anterior muscles

Latissimus dorsi muscle

Subscapularis muscle — Trapezius muscle

Infraspinatus muscle

Serratus anterior muscle — Spinal cord

Latissimus dorsi muscle

Trapezius muscle — Intercostal neurovascular bundles

Rhomboid muscle

Serratus anterior muscle

Latissimus dorsi muscle

(**Top**) Coronal MR section through the brachial plexus and prevertebral structures. (**Middle**) Coronal MR section through the level of the thoracic spinal canal. (**Bottom**) Coronal MR section through the level of the posterior ribs.

CHEST WALL

RADIOGRAPHY AND CT, STERNUM

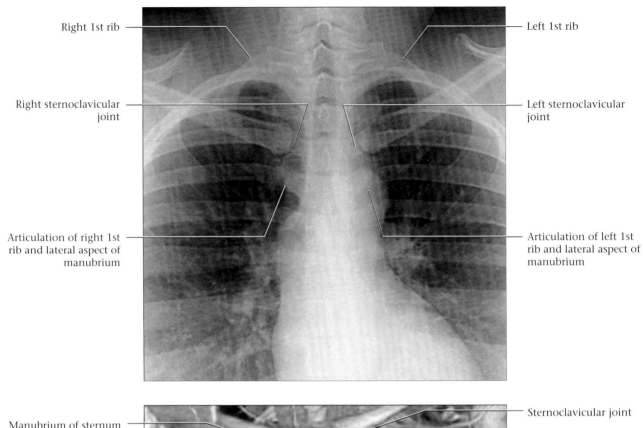

Right 1st rib

Right sternoclavicular joint

Articulation of right 1st rib and lateral aspect of manubrium

Left 1st rib

Left sternoclavicular joint

Articulation of left 1st rib and lateral aspect of manubrium

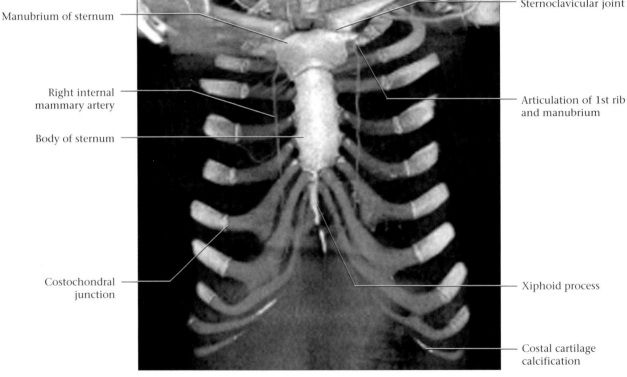

Manubrium of sternum

Right internal mammary artery

Body of sternum

Costochondral junction

Sternoclavicular joint

Articulation of 1st rib and manubrium

Xiphoid process

Costal cartilage calcification

(Top) Normal coned-down PA chest radiograph demonstrates partial visualization of the manubrium of the sternum, the sternoclavicular joints, and the characteristic course of the 1st ribs and their articulations with the lateral aspects of the manubrium. (Bottom) Contrast-enhanced chest CT (3D rendering) of a normal 20 year old man demonstrates the manubrium, body, and xiphoid process of the sternum. The xiphoid process is slender and elongated, a variation of normal anatomy. There is faint calcification of the 9th and 10th costal cartilages. The internal mammary arteries are visualized bilaterally.

CHEST WALL

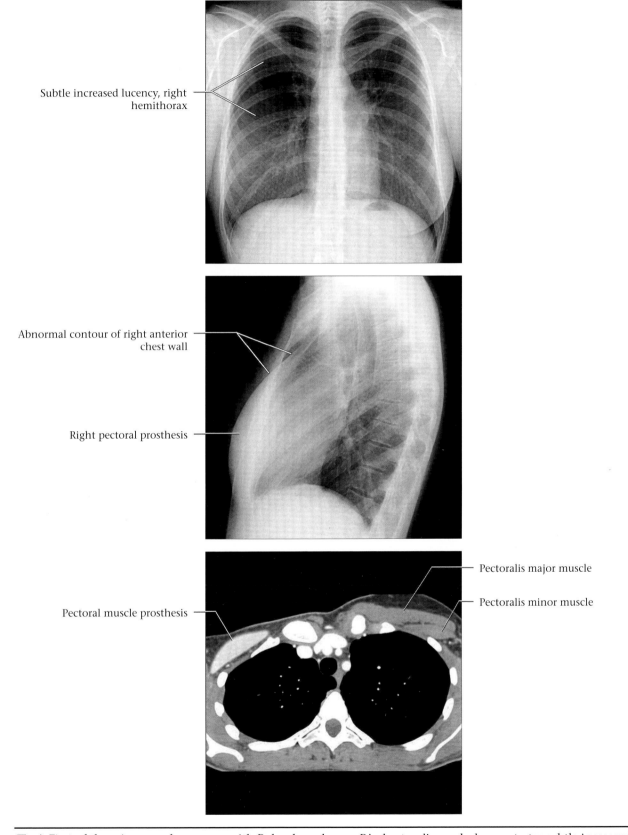

Subtle increased lucency, right hemithorax

Abnormal contour of right anterior chest wall

Right pectoral prosthesis

Pectoral muscle prosthesis

Pectoralis major muscle

Pectoralis minor muscle

(Top) First of three images of a woman with Poland syndrome. PA chest radiograph demonstrates subtle increased lucency of the right hemithorax and asymmetry of the breast soft tissue density. **(Middle)** Lateral chest radiograph demonstrates asymmetry of chest wall soft-tissues manifesting as an abnormal contour coursing across the anterior chest wall. The abnormal contour reflects the lack of pectoralis major musculature in the right upper thorax. Increased density inferiorly represents a prosthesis inserted to compensate for the lack of musculature in the right anterior chest wall. **(Bottom)** Contrast-enhanced chest CT demonstrates a pectoral muscle prosthesis in the subcutaneous tissues of the right anterior chest wall. There is congenital absence of the right pectoralis major and pectoralis minor muscles. Courtesy of Jerry Speckman, MD, University of Florida.

CHEST WALL

RADIOGRAPHY, PECTUS EXCAVATUM

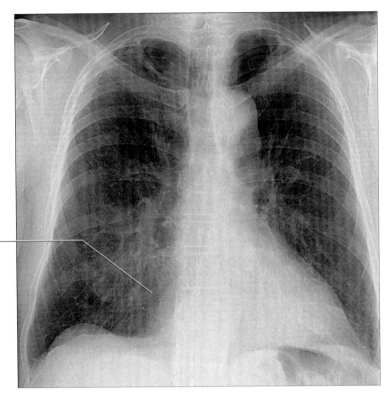

Indistinct right heart border

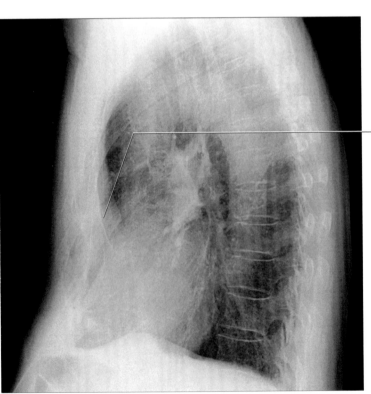

Sternum displaced posteriorly

(Top) First of four images of a patient with pectus excavatum deformity. PA chest radiograph demonstrates an indistinct right heart border and exaggerated vertical course of the anterior portions of the ribs. **(Bottom)** Lateral chest radiograph demonstrates posterior displacement of the sternum with resultant narrowing of the anteroposterior distance between the sternum and thoracic vertebrae.

CHEST WALL

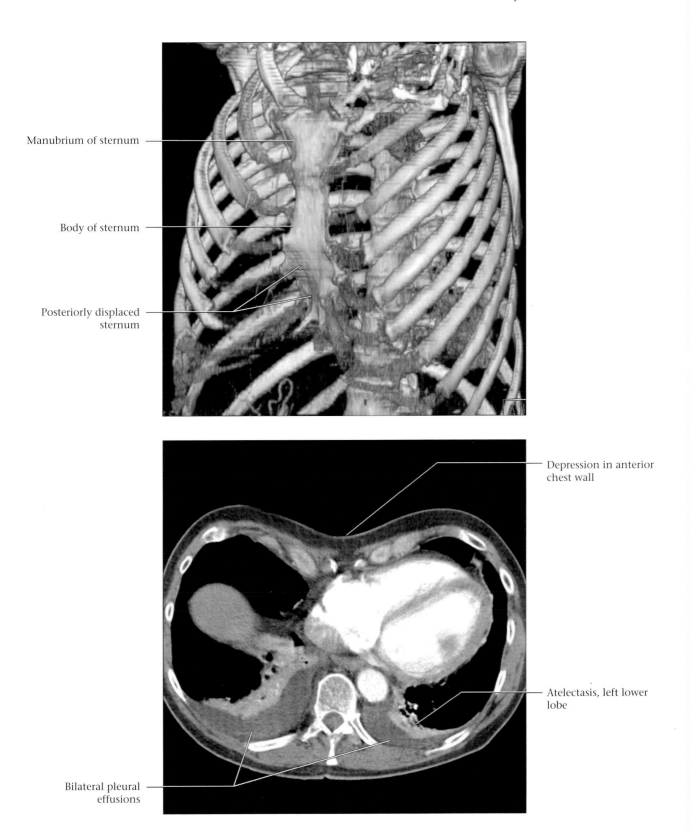

Manubrium of sternum

Body of sternum

Posteriorly displaced sternum

Depression in anterior chest wall

Atelectasis, left lower lobe

Bilateral pleural effusions

(Top) 3D reformatted chest CT image of rotated thorax demonstrates pectus excavatum with posterior displacement of the mid-to-inferior body of the sternum. **(Bottom)** Contrast-enhanced chest CT (mediastinal window) demonstrates posterior displacement of the lower sternum and associated depression of the anterior chest wall.

CHEST WALL

RADIOGRAPHY, PECTUS CARINATUM

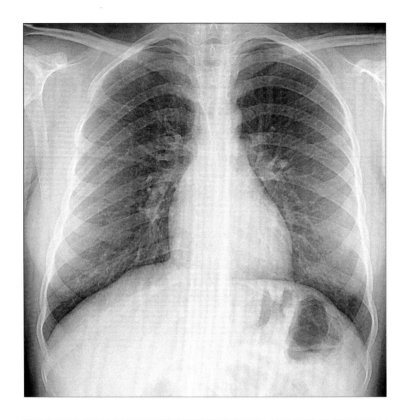

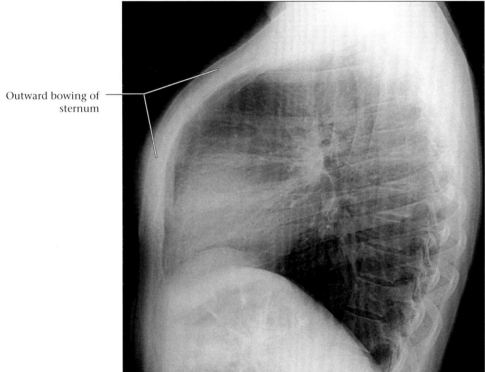

Outward bowing of
sternum

(Top) First of two chest radiographs of a patient with pectus carinatum. PA radiograph appears normal. (Bottom) Lateral radiograph demonstrates outward bowing of the sternum and adjacent costochondral elements. There is increased distance between the upper sternum and thoracic vertebrae.

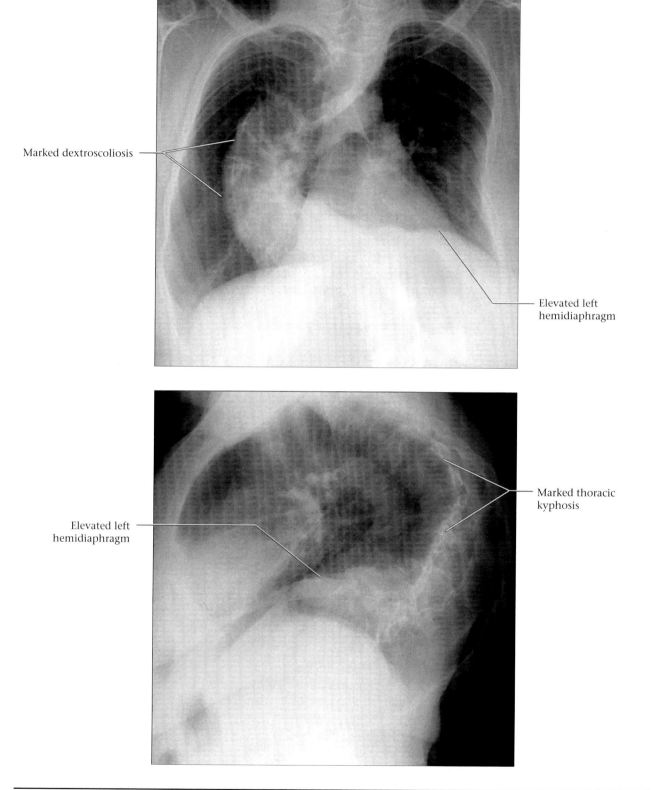

Marked dextroscoliosis

Elevated left hemidiaphragm

Elevated left hemidiaphragm

Marked thoracic kyphosis

(**Top**) First of two chest radiographs demonstrating marked kyphoscoliosis. PA radiograph demonstrates marked dextroscoliosis and associated loss of volume in the left hemithorax on the concave aspect of the thoracic spinal deformity manifested by elevation of the left hemidiaphragm. (**Bottom**) Lateral radiograph demonstrates marked kyphotic deformity of the thoracic spine and elevation of the left hemidiaphragm.

CHEST WALL

RADIOGRAPHY, CERVICAL RIBS AND POST-TRAUMATIC DEFORMITY

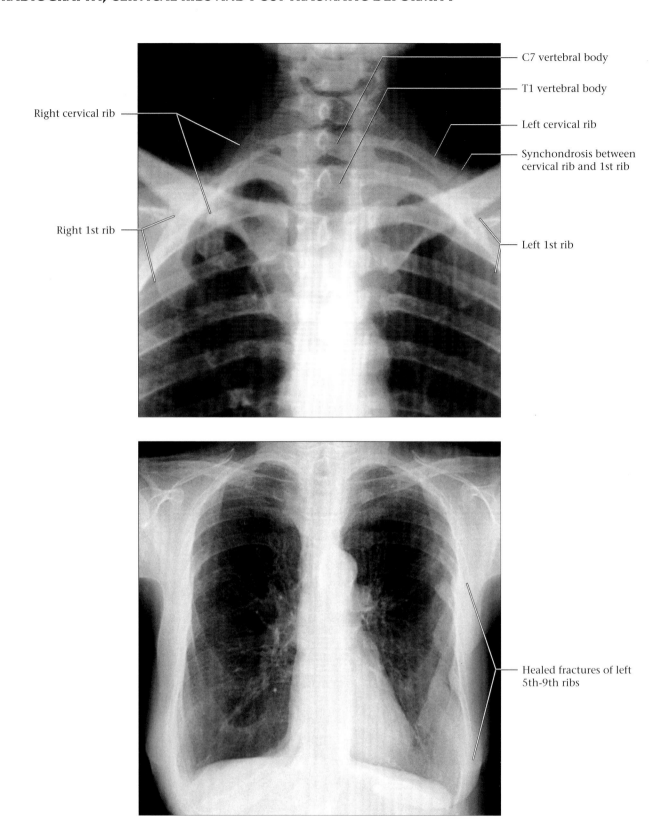

Right cervical rib

Right 1st rib

C7 vertebral body

T1 vertebral body

Left cervical rib

Synchondrosis between cervical rib and 1st rib

Left 1st rib

Healed fractures of left 5th-9th ribs

(Top) Coned-down PA chest radiograph demonstrates bilateral cervical ribs arising from the C7 vertebral body. The distal aspect of the left cervical rib forms a synchondrosis with the mid-portion of the left 1st rib. **(Bottom)** PA chest radiograph of a patient who sustained trauma and multiple left rib fractures 10 years prior to this examination demonstrates deformity of the left lateral chest wall. Multiple healed rib fractures are shown, involving the left 5th through 9th ribs. Associated mild pleural thickening manifests as hazy opacity overlying the left lateral hemithorax.

CHEST WALL

RADIOGRAPHY AND CT, COSTAL CARTILAGE CALCIFICATION

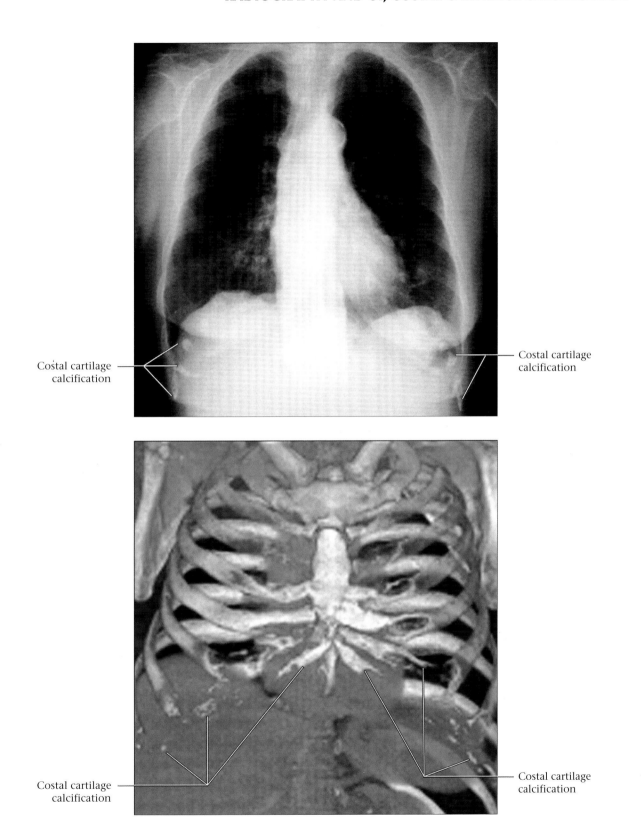

Costal cartilage calcification

Costal cartilage calcification

Costal cartilage calcification

Costal cartilage calcification

(Top) PA chest radiograph of a 77 year old woman demonstrates focal and band-like calcification of the costal cartilages of the 7th through 11th ribs. (Bottom) 3D reformatted chest image of an elderly female demonstrates bilateral costal cartilage calcification.

CHEST WALL

RADIOGRAPHY AND CT, PSEUDONODULE

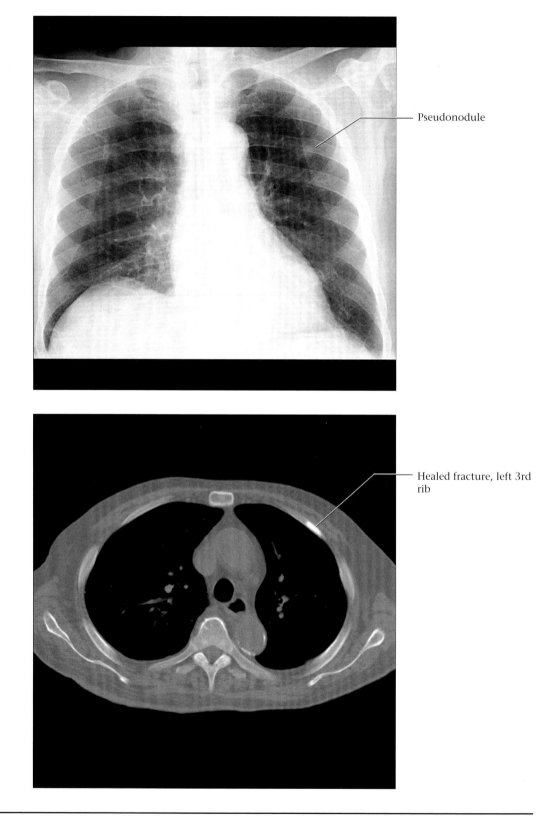

Pseudonodule

Healed fracture, left 3rd rib

(Top) PA chest radiograph demonstrates a focal area of increased opacity overlying the anterior aspect of the left 3rd rib, suggesting the presence of a solitary pulmonary nodule (so-called pseudonodule). **(Bottom)** Chest CT (bone window) demonstrates a healed fracture of the anterior aspect of the left third rib manifesting as a focal area of sclerotic change that correlates with the suspicious abnormality on the chest radiograph. On chest radiographs, chest wall abnormalities may mimic the presence of underlying pulmonary pathology.

CHEST WALL

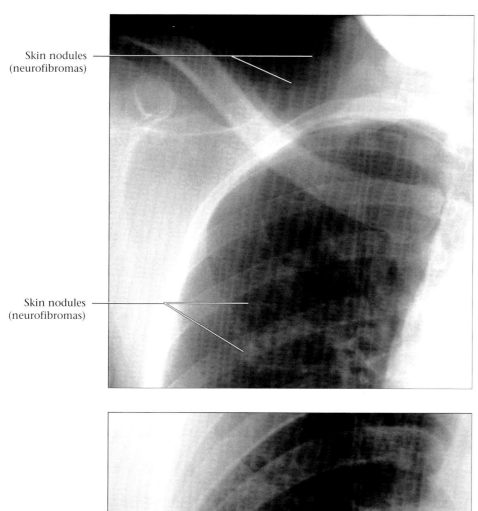

Skin nodules
(neurofibromas)

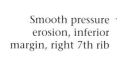

Skin nodules
(neurofibromas)

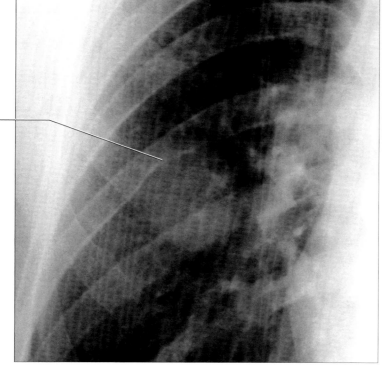

Smooth pressure
erosion, inferior
margin, right 7th rib

(**Top**) Coned-down chest radiograph of a patient with cutaneous neurofibromatosis demonstrates multiple nodular opacities overlying the right lung and visible on the skin in the supraclavicular region. Chest wall nodules such as neurofibromas, may overly lung parenchyma and mimic the presence of pulmonary nodules. (**Bottom**) Coned-down chest radiograph of a patient with neurofibromatosis demonstrates a neurofibroma in the right posterior chest wall producing smooth pressure erosion along the undersurface of the right 7th rib. Pressure erosion along an inferior rib margin and the presence of an associated soft-tissue mass suggests the presence of a slowly growing lesion, such as a neurofibroma, originating in the intercostal neurovascular bundle. Incomplete bonder visualization and associated pressure erosion suggests the diagnosis of a neurogenic neoplasm.

CHEST WALL

RADIOGRAPHY AND CT, EXTRAMEDULLARY HEMATOPOIESIS

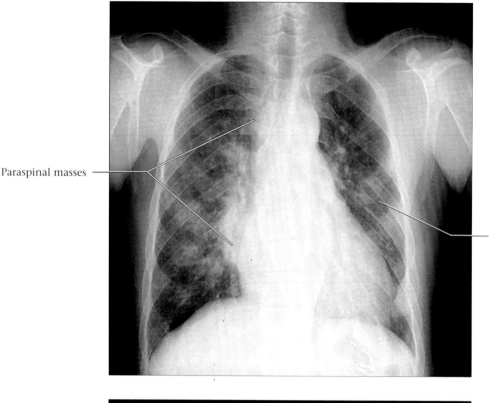

Paraspinal masses ——

—— Expanded anterior rib

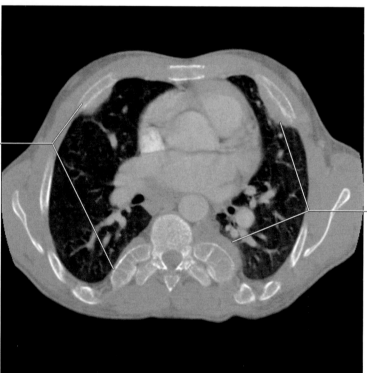

Marrow expansion, rib
and transverse process ——

—— Soft tissue masses
adjacent to areas of
marrow expansion

(Top) First of two images of a 24 year old man with thalassemia major and profound hemolytic anemia. PA chest radiograph demonstrates expansion of ribs and other osseous erythroid bone marrow spaces and coarsened trabeculation. Bilateral paraspinal soft tissue masses are also present. (Bottom) Contrast-enhanced chest CT (bone window) demonstrates marrow expansion of skeletal structures and adjacent soft tissue masses representing extramedullary hematopoiesis.

CHEST WALL

CT, CHEST WALL INFECTION

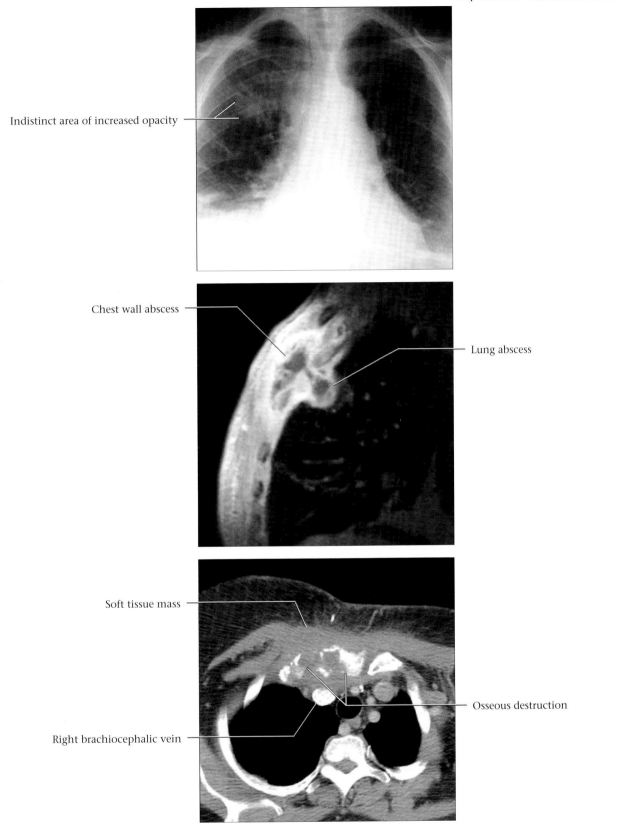

Indistinct area of increased opacity

Chest wall abscess

Lung abscess

Soft tissue mass

Osseous destruction

Right brachiocephalic vein

(Top) First of two images of a 54 year old diabetic man with a tender, palpable mass in the right anterior chest wall. PA chest radiograph demonstrates an indistinct area of increased density overlying the right upper chest wall. **(Middle)** Sagittal MR demonstrates a lung abscess extending into the adjacent anterior chest wall, manifesting as a heterogeneous mass with an irregular central area of low signal intensity. Culture of an aspirated specimen revealed Streptococcus pneumoniae. **(Bottom)** Contrast-enhanced chest CT of a 34 year old heroin addict demonstrates infection of the right sternoclavicular joint manifesting as osseous destruction and soft tissue mass obscuring tissue planes and displacing the right subclavian vein posteriorly. Cultures revealed Staphylococcus aureus. Courtesy of Elizabeth Moore, MD, University of California-Davis.

CT, FIBROUS DYSPLASIA AND CHEST WALL LIPOMA

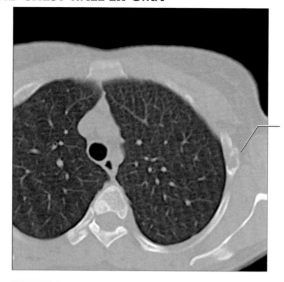

— Fibrous dysplasia, left 4th rib

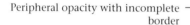

Peripheral opacity with incomplete border

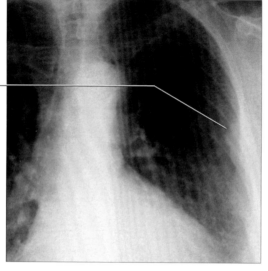

Chest wall lipoma

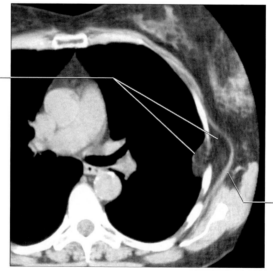

— Displaced serratus anterior muscle

(Top) Chest CT (bone window) demonstrates fibrous dysplasia involving the lateral aspect of the left 4th rib, manifesting as irregular fusiform enlargement and deformity with cortical thickening. **(Middle)** First of two images of a 57 year-old man with a chest wall lipoma, manifesting on a coned-down PA chest radiograph as a focal peripheral opacity in the left hemithorax. The opacity has an incomplete border, a finding consistent with an extraparenchymal lesion occurring in the pleura or chest wall. **(Bottom)** Contrast-enhanced chest CT (mediastinal window) demonstrates a chest wall lipoma manifesting as a fat attenuation lesion producing focal mass effect within the chest wall and protruding into the thoracic cavity. The lipoma displaces the serratus anterior muscle laterally.

CHEST WALL

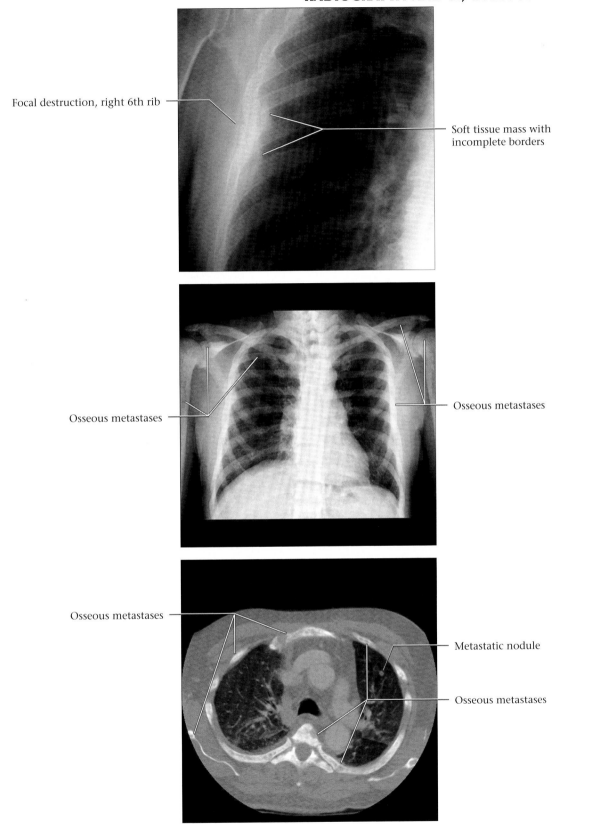

Focal destruction, right 6th rib

Soft tissue mass with incomplete borders

Osseous metastases

Osseous metastases

Osseous metastases

Metastatic nodule

Osseous metastases

(Top) Coned-down PA chest radiograph demonstrates focal destruction of the lateral aspect of the right 6th rib with an associated soft tissue mass that manifests with incomplete borders. Biopsy revealed metastatic renal cell carcinoma. **(Middle)** First of two images of a 53 year old man with metastatic breast cancer. PA chest radiograph demonstrates diffuse osseous metastases manifesting as sclerotic and lytic lesions involving the spine, ribs, clavicles, scapulae and both humeri. **(Bottom)** Contrast-enhanced chest CT (bone window) demonstrates sclerotic and lytic metastases involving the thoracic spine, ribs, sternum and scapulae. A metastatic nodule is demonstrated in the left upper lobe.

CHEST WALL

RADIOGRAPHY, METASTATIC BREAST CANCER

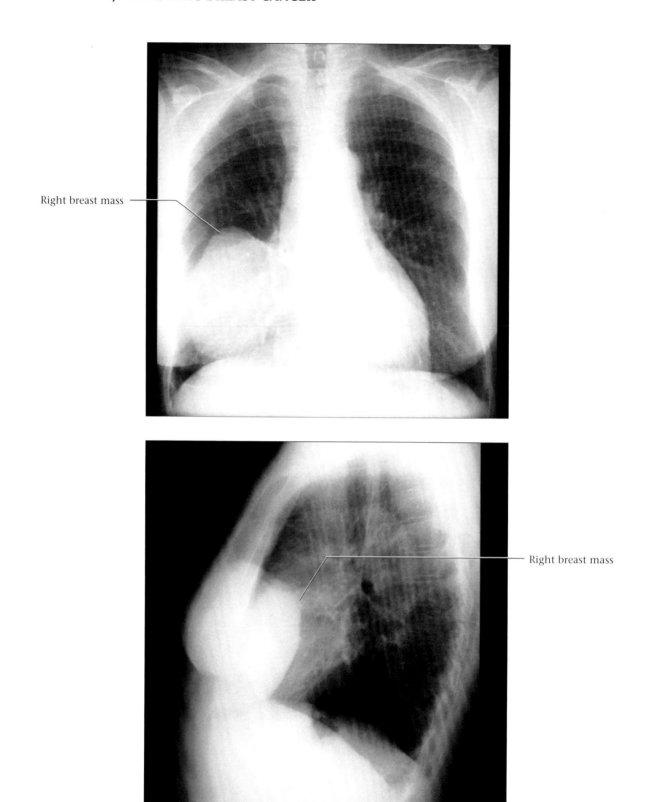

Right breast mass

Right breast mass

(Top) First of three images of a 47 year old woman with metastatic breast cancer. PA chest radiograph demonstrates a smoothly bordered mass that appears associated with the medial aspect of the right breast. (Bottom) Lateral radiograph confirms its association with the right breast but the underlying anterior chest wall is obscured.

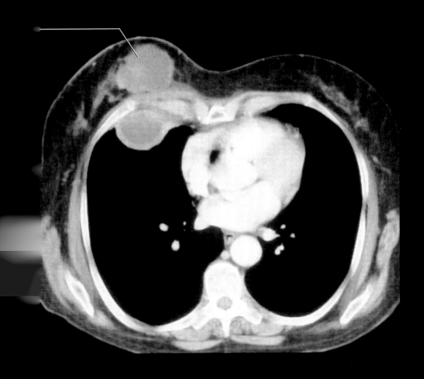

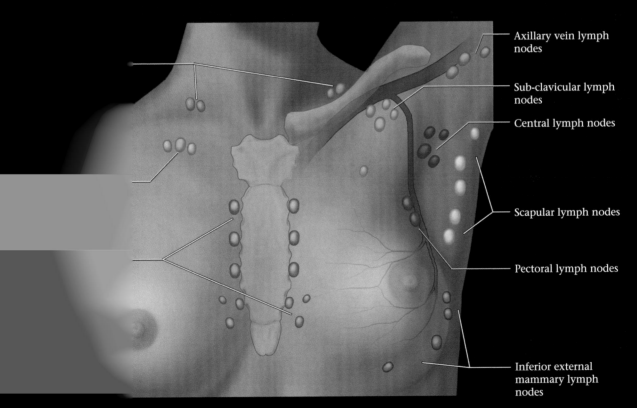

Axillary vein lymph
nodes

Sub-clavicular lymph
nodes

Central lymph nodes

Scapular lymph nodes

Pectoral lymph nodes

Inferior external
mammary lymph
nodes

chest CT (mediastinal window) demonstrates a heterogeneous mass within the right breast djacent anterior chest wall and internal mammary lymph nodes. Biopsy revealed invasive uperficial lymphatic vessels of the thoracic wall converge on the axillary nodes. Axillary atics from the breast, the upper limb, and the thoracoabdominal wall above the umbilicus. node chains course along each internal mammary artery and drain afferents from the rior abdominal wall, the superior hepatic surface, and deeper parts of the anterior thoracic atics join with tracheobronchial and brachiocephalic nodes to form the

CHEST WALL

CT, LYMPHOMA

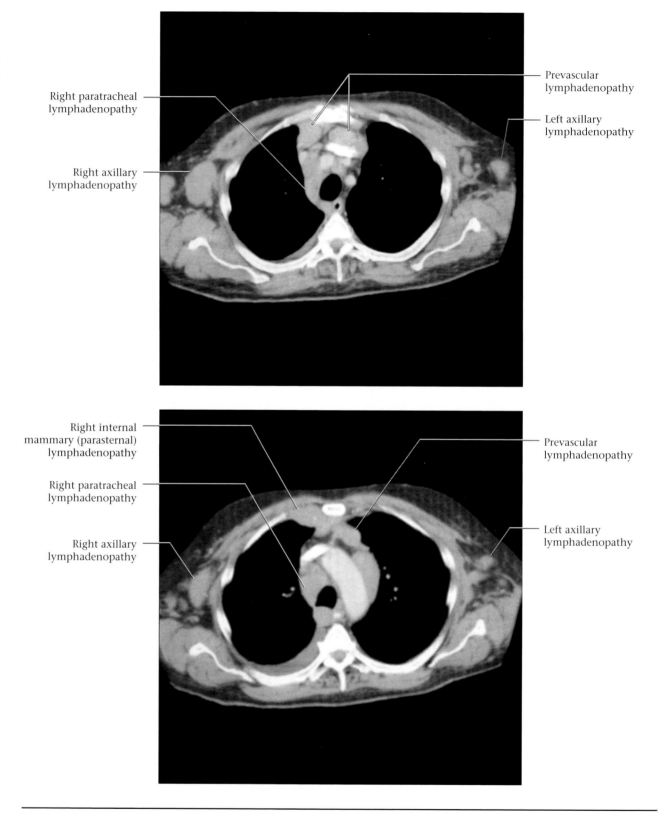

Right paratracheal lymphadenopathy

Right axillary lymphadenopathy

Prevascular lymphadenopathy

Left axillary lymphadenopathy

Right internal mammary (parasternal) lymphadenopathy

Right paratracheal lymphadenopathy

Right axillary lymphadenopathy

Prevascular lymphadenopathy

Left axillary lymphadenopathy

(Top) First of two contrast-enhanced chest CT images (mediastinal window) of a patient with lymphoma demonstrates bilateral axillary, prevascular and right paratracheal lymphadenopathy. **(Bottom)** At the level of the aortic arch, CT demonstrates bilateral axillary, right internal mammary, prevascular, and right paratracheal lymphadenopathy and a small right pleural effusion.

CHEST WALL

CT AND RADIOGRAPHY, CHONDROSARCOMA AND CHEST WALL METASTASIS

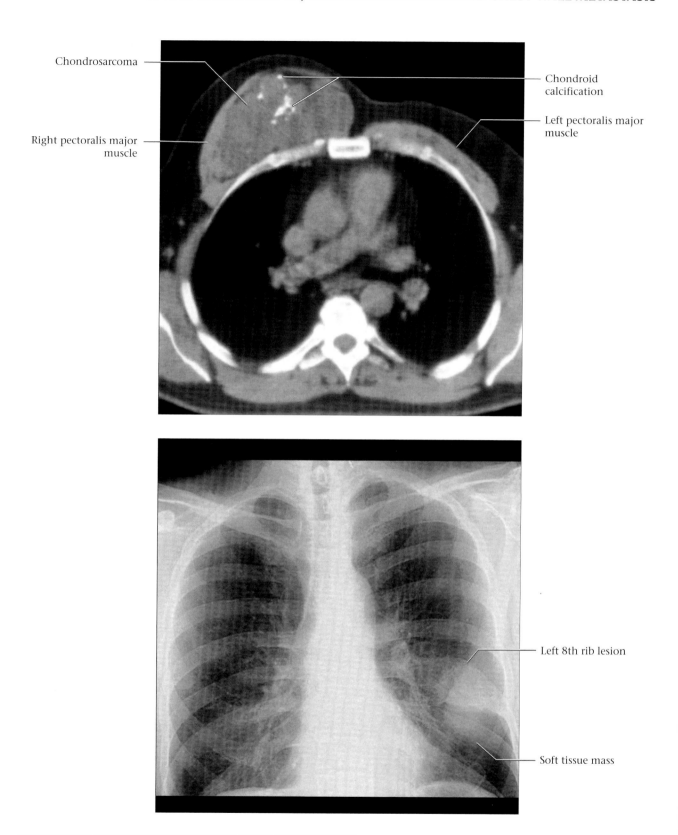

Chondrosarcoma

Chondroid calcification

Right pectoralis major muscle

Left pectoralis major muscle

Left 8th rib lesion

Soft tissue mass

(Top) Contrast-enhanced chest CT (mediastinal window) of a 43 year old man with chondrosarcoma demonstrates a large heterogeneous mass with chondroid calcification projecting from the anterior chest wall and right costochondral region and elevating the right pectoralis major muscle. **(Bottom)** PA chest radiograph in a 47-year old man with metastatic renal cell carcinoma. There is an expansile, lytic lesion in the posterior aspect of the left 8th rib. An associated soft-tissue mass shows incomplete borders, a finding consistent with a chest wall mass.

PART II
Abdomen

Embryology of the Abdomen

Abdominal Wall

Diaphragm

Peritoneal Cavity

Vessels, Lymphatic System and Nerves

Esophagus

Gastroduodenal

Small Intestine

Colon

Spleen

Liver

Biliary System

Pancreas

Retroperitoneum

Adrenal

Kidney

Ureter and Bladder

18 DAY EMBRYO (LATERAL)

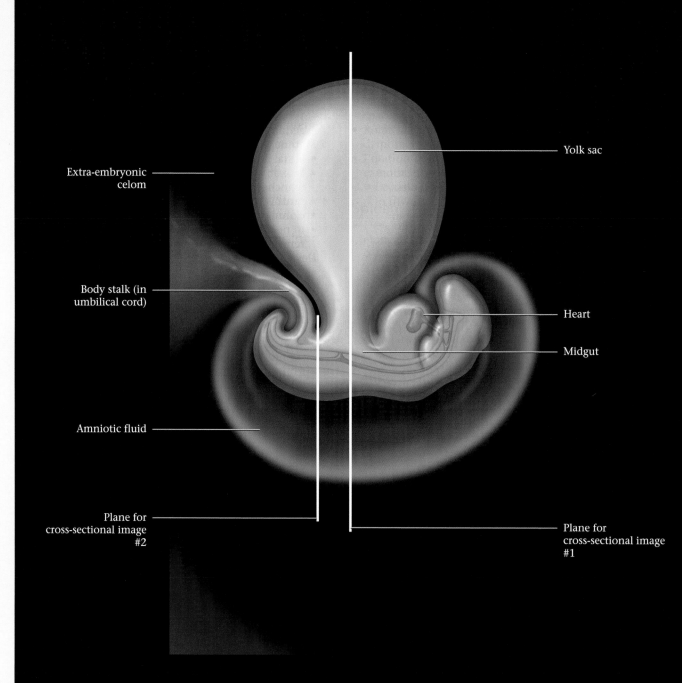

Extra-embryonic celom

Body stalk (in umbilical cord)

Amniotic fluid

Plane for cross-sectional image #2

Yolk sac

Heart

Midgut

Plane for cross-sectional image #1

Lateral illustration of an 18 day embryo. The roof of the yolk sac becomes incorporated in the form of a tube, the primitive gut. The cranial end of the tube becomes the foregut and the caudal end, the hindgut.

PART II
Abdomen

Embryology of the Abdomen

Abdominal Wall

Diaphragm

Peritoneal Cavity

Vessels, Lymphatic System and Nerves

Esophagus

Gastroduodenal

Small Intestine

Colon

Spleen

Liver

Biliary System

Pancreas

Retroperitoneum

Adrenal

Kidney

Ureter and Bladder

EMBRYOLOGY OF THE ABDOMEN

Gross Anatomy

Early Embryologic Events

- Yolk sac provides nutrition to early embryo
  - Broad opening into primitive gut
  - **Yolk stalk** is connection between yolk sac and gut
    - Becomes progressively longer and thinner as fetus develops
    - Connects distal midgut to umbilical cord
    - In neonate, atrophies and disappears (failure to regress completely may result in **Meckel diverticulum**, blind outpouching from distal ileum
  - Gut is suspended from anterior and posterior abdominal walls by **ventral** and **dorsal mesenteries**
    - Mesenteries separate to enclose developing alimentary tube
- In early fetal life, important viscera develop in mesentery of caudal part of foregut
  - Fetal stomach is suspended by 2 mesogastria
    - **Dorsal mesogastrium**: Site for developing spleen, body-tail of pancreas
    - **Ventral mesogastrium**: Site for developing liver, bile ducts, head of pancreas
- Ventral "bud" migrates clockwise around duodenum and subsequently merges with dorsal bud to join pancreatic and biliary tree within pancreatic head
- Dorsal part of ventral mesogastrium becomes **lesser omentum**
  - In adult, lesser omentum includes the **gastrohepatic ligament** and **hepatoduodenal ligament**
    - Gastrohepatic ligament carries left gastric artery and vein, celiac nodes
    - Hepatoduodenal ligament carries portal vein, hepatic artery, bile duct and hepatic/celiac nodes

Fetal Vessels

- Major fetal arteries course anteriorly through dorsal mesenteries from the aorta to supply gut and intramesenteric viscera
- **Umbilical vein**
  - Carries oxygenated blood from placenta to fetus
  - Major source of blood flow to fetal liver
  - Enters liver through ventral part of ventral mesentery, which becomes **falciform ligament** in adults
  - Obliterated umbilical vein becomes **ligamentum teres**
- **Vitelline veins**
  - Paired vessels that carry blood from yolk sac to fetus in 1st few weeks of gestation
  - Give rise to venous plexus within liver
    - Precursor to hepatic and portal veins and sinusoids
  - Proximal extrahepatic veins evolve into **portal venous system**
    - Carries blood (and nutrients) from gut to liver
  - Proximal vitelline veins are precursors to **hepatic veins**
    - Carry blood from liver to heart via inferior vena cave (IVC)
- **Ductus venosus**
  - Derived from left umbilical vein (after right vein has atrophied)
  - Acts as a bypass of the liver to carry umbilical vein blood primarily to IVC and heart
  - In neonate, atrophies to become **ligamentum venosum** (on posterior surface of liver near porta hepatis)
- **Portal sinus**
  - In fetus, diverts some oxygenated blood from umbilical vein to liver parenchyma

Liver

- Arises from ventral bud of foregut
- Rapid growth is main factor in distortion of peritoneal spaces and mesentery
- Rotates counterclockwise and attaches to right side of diaphragm at bare area
- Rotation of liver results in **right peritoneal space** extending to the left, posterior to stomach
  - Becomes **lesser sac (omental bursa)**

Spleen

- Develops within dorsal mesogastrium, which elongates to form **gastrosplenic ligament**
  - Carries **short gastric vessels** and forms left anterior wall of **lesser sac (omental bursa)**
  - Elongated caudal parts of gastrosplenic ligament hang down like a drape from stomach
    - Forms **greater omentum** and **gastrocolic ligament**
  - Greater omentum and gastrocolic ligament carry **gastroepiploic (gastro-omental) vessels**

Pancreas

- Develops within dorsal part of **dorsal mesentery**, which usually fuses with posterior abdominal wall
  - Leaves only a short **splenorenal ligament**
    - Carries **splenic vessels** and tail of pancreas
    - Forms left posterior wall of **lesser sac**
- Pancreas becomes a retroperitoneal organ

Small and Large Intestine

- **Duodenum**
  - In fetus, is "intraperitoneal", has a mesoduodenum
    - Ventral pancreas also lies in mesoduodenum
  - Becomes retroperitoneal organ when ascending mesocolon fuses to posterior abdominal wall, "trapping" duodenum and pancreas in retroperitoneum
- **Small intestine**
  - Develops within dorsal mesentery which elongates and persists into adulthood as small bowel mesentery
    - Carries superior mesenteric vessels
- **Large intestine (colon)**
  - Develops as a straight tube within dorsal mesentery
- Small and large intestine elongate greatly and herniate out through fetal umbilicus
- Bowel returns to fetal abdomen after counterclockwise rotation around the axis of superior mesenteric vessels
  - Degree of rotation is variable according to segment of bowel
    - Transverse colon 90°
    - Ascending colon 180°

EMBRYOLOGY OF THE ABDOMEN

- ▪ Small intestine 270°
- **Ascending** and **descending colon** usually lose their mesentery and become retroperitoneal structures in adult
  - ○ Common variant: Ascending colon that is mobile due to a persistent mesocolon (predisposes to twist & obstruction of colon, "cecal volvulus")
- Mesentery for transverse colon persists (**transverse mesocolon**)
  - ○ Attaches to posterior abdominal wall anterior to pancreas and duodenum
  - ○ Root of **transverse mesocolon** divides peritoneal cavity onto **supramesocolic** and **inframesocolic** components
    - ▪ These spaces communicate only laterally via **paracolic gutters** (recesses)

Peritoneal Spaces

- **Ventral mesentery** resorbs to allow communication between right and left peritoneal cavity in adults
- Variations in complex rotation, fusion and growth of mesenteric viscera result in common variations in peritoneal and retroperitoneal spaces in adults
- All **peritoneal recesses** potentially communicate
  - ○ Adhesions between peritoneal surfaces may seal off loculated collections of fluid

Abdominal Viscera

- Intraperitoneal contents of abdomen derive from
  - ○ Alimentary tube
    - ▪ **Foregut** (esophagus, stomach, duodenum); supplied by branches of **celiac artery**
    - ▪ **Midgut** (small intestine, colon up to splenic flexure); supplied by **superior mesenteric artery** (SMA)
    - ▪ **Hindgut** (descending and sigmoid colon, rectum); supplied by **inferior mesenteric artery** (IMA)
  - ○ Supporting mesentery
  - ○ Intramesenteric viscera
    - ▪ Develop from buds ("diverticula") of ventral or dorsal foregut

Extraperitoneal Spaces

- Includes all structures lying between **posterior parietal peritoneum** and **transversalis fascia**
- Components: **Abdominal retroperitoneum** and **pelvic extraperitoneum** (perivesical and prevesical spaces)
  - ○ **Prevesical space** surrounds perirectal and perivesical spaces
    - ▪ Continuous with **presacral space** and **retroperitoneum**
- **Abdominal retroperitoneum** consists of **anterior** and **posterior pararenal** and **perirenal spaces**
  - ○ These potentially communicate with each other, especially via **interfascial planes** and **perirenal septa**
  - ○ Communication with intraperitoneal structures
    - ▪ Bowel via **subperitoneal space** between leaves of **small bowel mesentery** and **transverse mesocolon**
    - ▪ Viscera via ligaments (e.g., **gastrohepatic ligament** → liver; spleen via **gastrosplenic** and **splenorenal ligaments**)

Development of Genitourinary (GU) System

- Urinary system in early fetus
  - ○ Goes through stages of development similar to those found in more "primitive" animals (e.g., invertebrates, amphibians)
    - ▪ In human fetus, **pronephron** degenerates and is replaces by **mesonephron**
    - ▪ Mesonephron degenerates and is replaced by **metanephron** which develops into permanent kidney
    - ▪ Degeneration proceeds from top to bottom (cephalad to caudal); caudal end of mesonephric duct persists and differentiates into **Müllerian** and **Wolffian ducts** (primordial forms of internal genitalia)
  - ○ **Metanephric duct (ureteric bud)**
    - ▪ Distal end enters urinary bladder, becomes **ureter**
    - ▪ Proximal end extends into early kidney and branches to form **calices** and **collecting ducts**
  - ○ **Allantois (urachus)**
    - ▪ Connects fetal bladder to umbilical cord
    - ▪ In neonate, atrophies to become **urachal remnant (median umbilical ligament)**
  - ○ Development and "ascent" of kidneys
    - ▪ Early fetus, kidneys lie low in pelvis, close together, renal hila facing anteriorly
    - ▪ Fetal kidneys comprised of contiguous lobules (which remain unfused in some animals; may persist as "fetal lobation" in humans)
    - ▪ Fetal kidneys successively "recruit" arterial blood supply from iliac arteries and aorta
    - ▪ Common anomalies: Renal ectopia, usually accompanied by low position, abnormal rotation, multiple anomalous blood supply; renal fusion anomalies (e.g., horseshoe kidney, crossed fused ectopia)

Genital Tract Development in Fetus

- Male fetus
  - ○ Müllerian ducts mostly disappear
  - ○ Wolffian duct gives rise to epididymis, ductus deferens, seminal vesicle and ejaculatory tract
  - ○ Urogenital sinus evolves into urethra and bladder
- Female fetus
  - ○ Lower Müllerian ducts unite to form **uterovaginal canal**
  - ○ Unfused Müllerian ducts become **fallopian tubes**
  - ○ Invagination of perineum forms distal **vagina**
- Common congenital anomalies
  - ○ Reflect errors of insertion, differentiation, development of portions of GU system
  - ○ Often occur in combinations on same (ipsilateral) side
    - ▪ Examples: Renal agenesis + absence of seminal vesicle
  - ○ Duplicated ureter may empty into vagina
  - ○ Distal portions of GI and GU system may retain communication, like fetal **cloaca**
  - ○ Rectum and/or vagina may fail to open onto the perineum (e.g., **imperforate anus**)
  - ○ **Ambiguous genitalia**, failure of progressive fetal differentiation may result in perineal structures with features of both male and female genitalia

18 DAY EMBRYO (LATERAL)

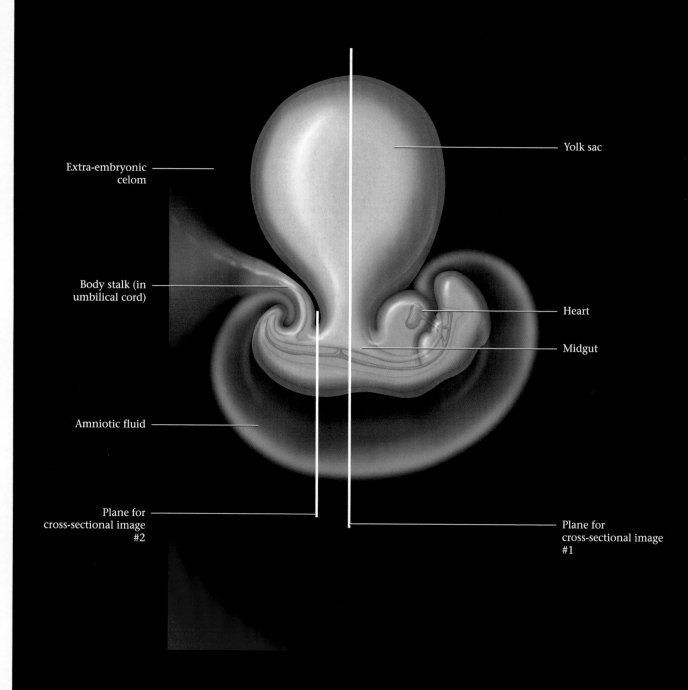

Extra-embryonic celom

Body stalk (in umbilical cord)

Amniotic fluid

Plane for cross-sectional image #2

Yolk sac

Heart

Midgut

Plane for cross-sectional image #1

Lateral illustration of an 18 day embryo. The roof of the yolk sac becomes incorporated in the form of a tube, the primitive gut. The cranial end of the tube becomes the foregut and the caudal end, the hindgut.

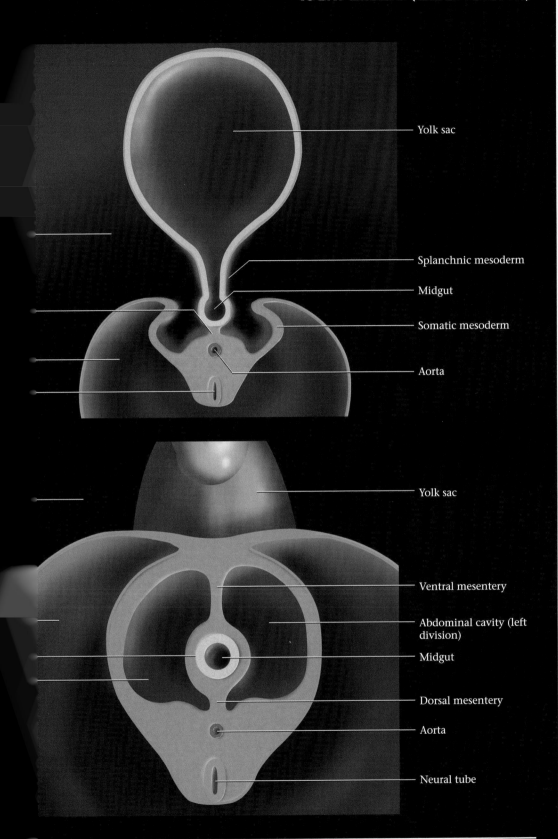

Yolk sac

Splanchnic mesoderm

Midgut

Somatic mesoderm

Aorta

Yolk sac

Ventral mesentery

Abdominal cavity (left division)

Midgut

Dorsal mesentery

Aorta

Neural tube

stration along plane #1 indicated on the lateral 18 day embryo. The midgut has a wide
yolk sac at this phase. **(Bottom)** Cross-sectional illustration along plane #2 indicated on the

4 WEEK EMBRYO (LATERAL)

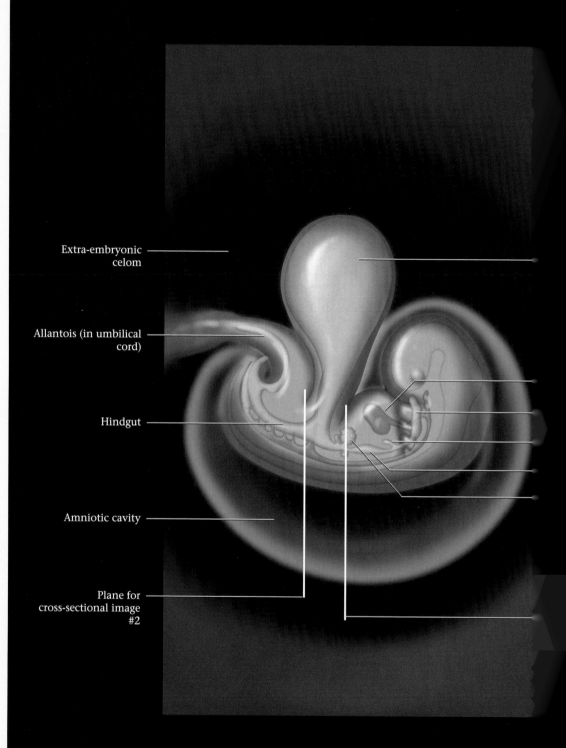

Extra-embryonic
celom

Allantois (in umbilical
cord)

Hindgut

Amniotic cavity

Plane for
cross-sectional image
#2

Lateral illustration of a 4 week embryo. The pharynx and lung bud arise from the foregut, alc
The allantois connects the body stalk to the hindgut. The yolk sac communicates broadly wit
Errors in development include communication between the foregut branches, such as a track

4 WEEK EMBRYO (CROSS-SECTION)

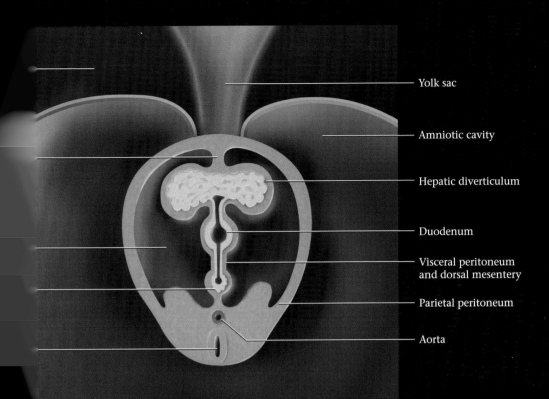

- Yolk sac
- Amniotic cavity
- Hepatic diverticulum
- Duodenum
- Visceral peritoneum and dorsal mesentery
- Parietal peritoneum
- Aorta

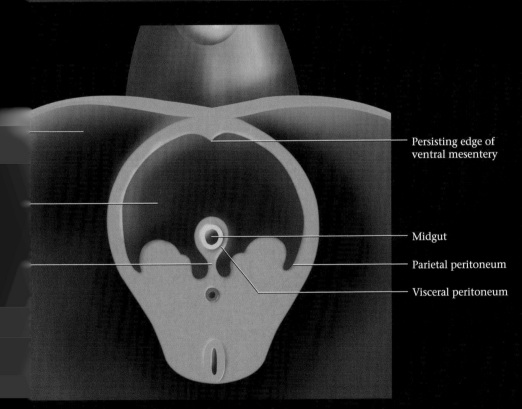

- Persisting edge of ventral mesentery
- Midgut
- Parietal peritoneum
- Visceral peritoneum

...stration along plane #1 indicated on the lateral 4 week embryo. The liver arises from a ..., while the pancreas arises from the dorsal mesentery. **(Bottom)** Cross-sectional illustration ...on the lateral 4 week embryo. The ventral mesentery begins to disintegrate to allow ...right and left sides of the abdominal cavity.

EMBRYOLOGY OF THE ABDOMEN

GI TRACT DEVELOPMENT (5 WEEKS)

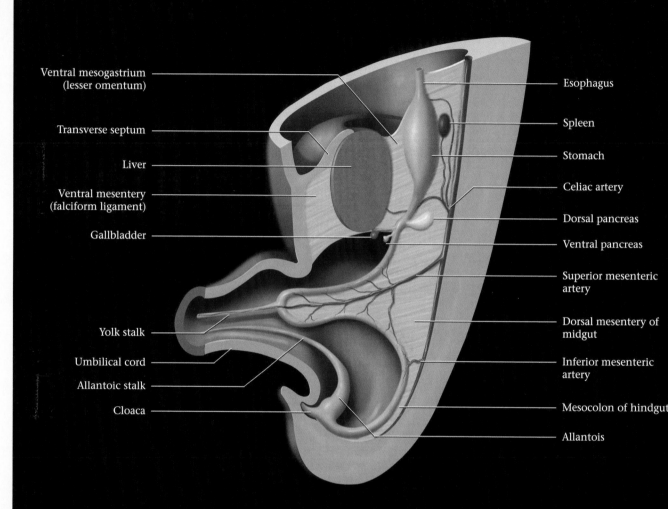

Ventral mesogastrium (lesser omentum)

Transverse septum

Liver

Ventral mesentery (falciform ligament)

Gallbladder

Yolk stalk

Umbilical cord

Allantoic stalk

Cloaca

Esophagus

Spleen

Stomach

Celiac artery

Dorsal pancreas

Ventral pancreas

Superior mesenteric artery

Dorsal mesentery of midgut

Inferior mesenteric artery

Mesocolon of hindgut

Allantois

The transverse septum grows as a shelf from the anterior body wall, becoming the ventral part of the diaphragm. The esophagus and stomach begin to develop as distinct structures. During a period of its development, the esophageal lumen is occluded and it shares a foregut origin with the trachea. Errors in abdevelopment may result in esophageal atresia or tracheo-esophageal fistula. The primary gut begins to elongate along with its dorsal mesentery. The hepatic diverticulum gives rise to the biliary tree and ventral pancreas. The arterial supply to the gut is already defined: Celiac artery (foregut); superior mesenteric artery (midgut); and inferior mesenteric artery (hindgut).

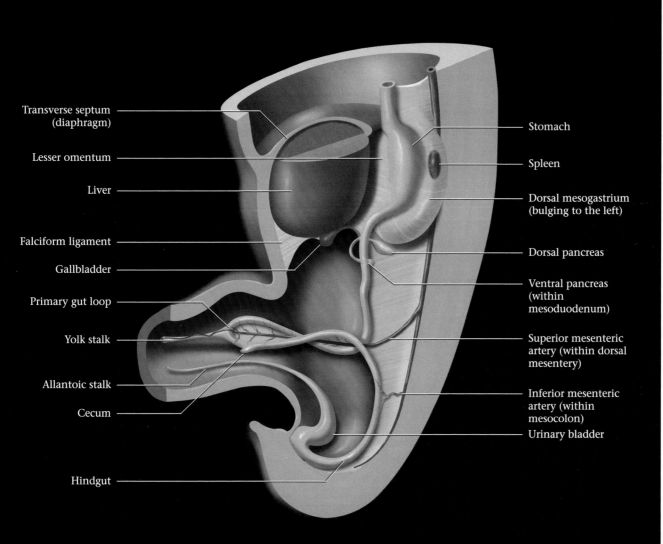

Transverse septum (diaphragm)

Lesser omentum

Liver

Falciform ligament

Gallbladder

Primary gut loop

Yolk stalk

Allantoic stalk

Cecum

Hindgut

Stomach

Spleen

Dorsal mesogastrium (bulging to the left)

Dorsal pancreas

Ventral pancreas (within mesoduodenum)

Superior mesenteric artery (within dorsal mesentery)

Inferior mesenteric artery (within mesocolon)

Urinary bladder

The liver expands within the ventral mesentery, which later disintegrates, leaving only the falciform ligament and the lesser omentum. The common bile duct, portal vein and hepatic artery traverse the caudal part of the lesser omentum. The primary gut elongates and herniates out into the umbilical cord. The primitive gut and urinary system terminate in the cloaca and connect to the umbilical cord via the yolk stalk and allantois, respectively.

EMBRYOLOGY OF THE ABDOMEN

GI TRACT DEVELOPMENT (8 WEEKS)

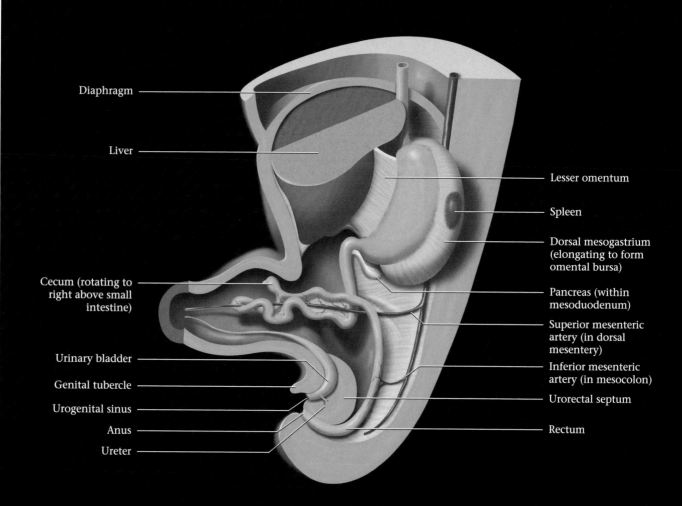

Diaphragm

Liver

Cecum (rotating to right above small intestine)

Urinary bladder

Genital tubercle

Urogenital sinus

Anus

Ureter

Lesser omentum

Spleen

Dorsal mesogastrium (elongating to form omental bursa)

Pancreas (within mesoduodenum)

Superior mesenteric artery (in dorsal mesentery)

Inferior mesenteric artery (in mesocolon)

Urorectal septum

Rectum

The diaphragm is nearly complete. The liver continues its rapid enlargement. Only the caudal part of the ventral mesentery remains (falciform ligament) allowing the more cephalad portions of the peritoneal cavity to communicate. The dorsal mesogastrium elongates considerably, forming the left and caudal portions of the lesser sac. The gut continues to elongate and rotates counterclockwise around the superior mesenteric artery within the dorsal mesentery. The urogenital sinus has separated from the rectum and anus. Common developmental errors include midgut malrotation, persistent omphalocele and imperforate anus.

EMBRYOLOGY OF THE ABDOMEN

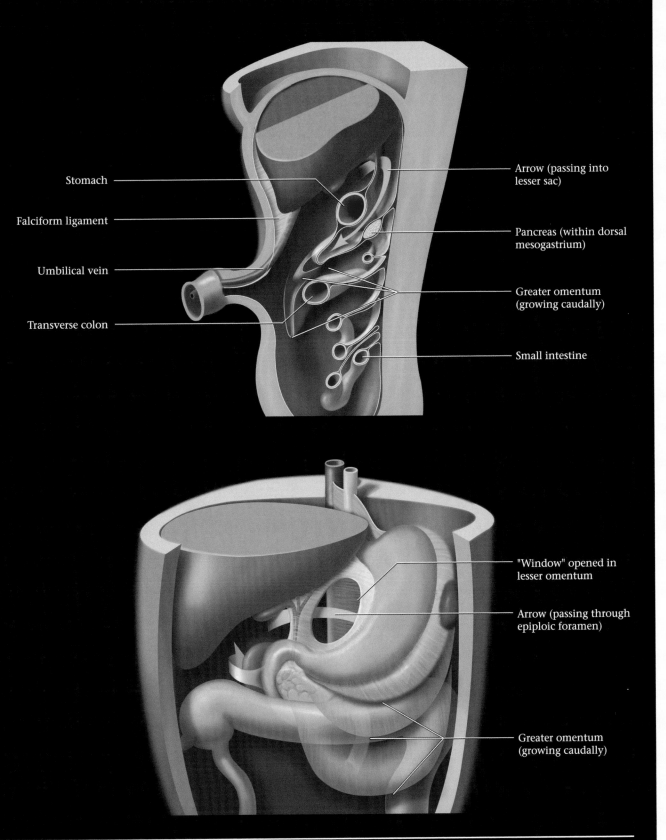

Stomach

Falciform ligament

Umbilical vein

Transverse colon

Arrow (passing into lesser sac)

Pancreas (within dorsal mesogastrium)

Greater omentum (growing caudally)

Small intestine

"Window" opened in lesser omentum

Arrow (passing through epiploic foramen)

Greater omentum (growing caudally)

(**Top**) The umbilical vein enters the liver along the caudal (free) edge of the falciform ligament. The duodenum and pancreas are "intraperitoneal" at this point. The leaves of the greater omentum elongate to the left and caudally, expanding the volume of eme lesser sac and beginning to cover the transverse colon and small intestine. (**Bottom**) The greater peritoneal cavity and lesser sac communicate through the epiploic foramen.

EMBRYOLOGY OF THE ABDOMEN

DEVELOPMENT OF GI TRACT (10 WEEK FETUS)

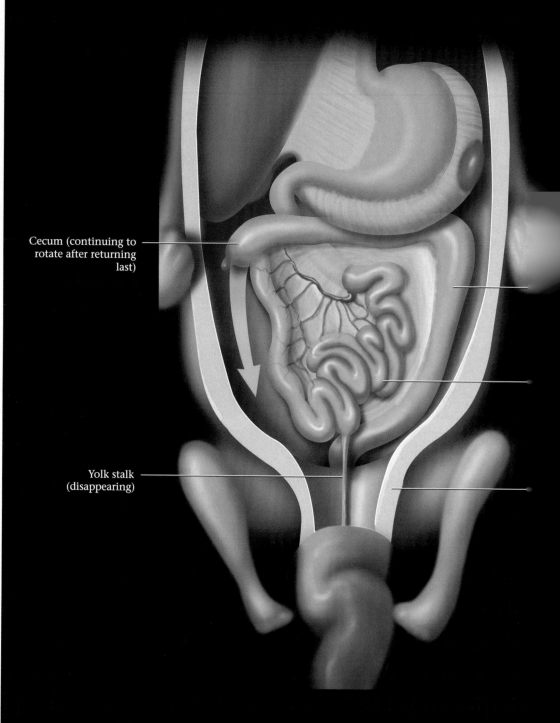

Cecum (continuing to rotate after returning last)

Yolk stalk (disappearing)

The small intestine has returned to the abdomen, having previously elongated and herniated cord. The yolk stalk (vitelline duct) is disintegrating, having connected the yolk sac to the pr of the distal small intestine. The cecum is the last part of the gut to return and continues to r counterclockwise direction until reaching its adult position in the right lower quadrant. The superficial to the intestine. Errors in development include persistence of a part of the yolk sta diverticulum) and errors of bowel rotation and mesenteric fusion.

EMBRYOLOGY OF THE ABDOMEN

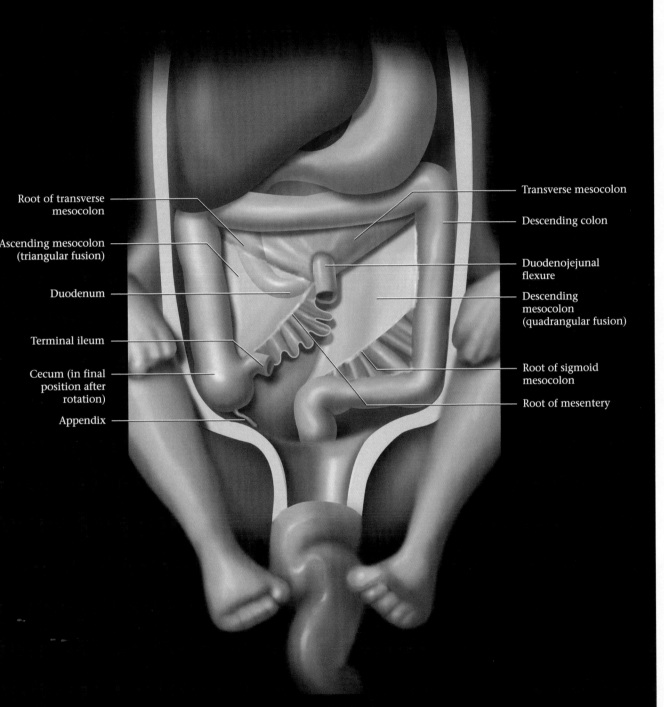

Root of transverse mesocolon

Ascending mesocolon (triangular fusion)

Duodenum

Terminal ileum

Cecum (in final position after rotation)

Appendix

Transverse mesocolon

Descending colon

Duodenojejunal flexure

Descending mesocolon (quadrangular fusion)

Root of sigmoid mesocolon

Root of mesentery

By 4 to 5 months of gestation, the ascending and descending colon are fixed in a retroperitoneal location by fusion of their mesocolons to the posterior abdominal wall. The fusion of the ascending mesocolon covers the duodenum and pancreas, resulting in their retroperitoneal location. The transverse and sigmoid colon remain intraperitoneal, suspended on a mesentery. The root of the small bowel mesentery is fused to the posterior abdominal wall but the intestine is suspended on a long, fan-shaped mesentery.

EMBRYOLOGY OF THE ABDOMEN

DEVELOPMENT OF HEPATIC VEINS (4-6 WEEK FETUS)

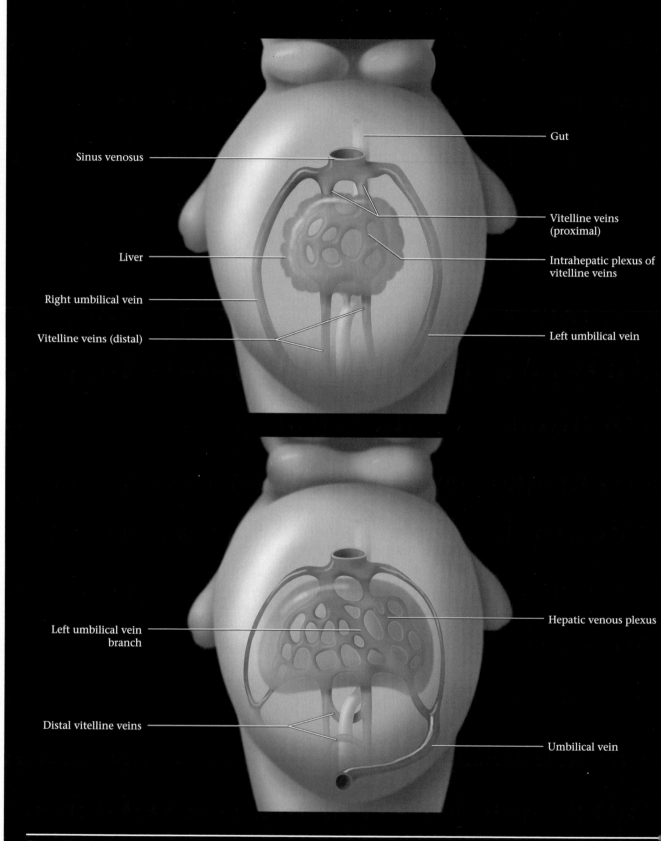

Gut

Sinus venosus

Vitelline veins (proximal)

Liver

Intrahepatic plexus of vitelline veins

Right umbilical vein

Vitelline veins (distal)

Left umbilical vein

Left umbilical vein branch

Hepatic venous plexus

Distal vitelline veins

Umbilical vein

(Top) The vitelline veins return blood from the yolk sac and branch out within the liver to form the hepatic sinusoids and venous system. They unite again to form the proximal vitelline veins which join with the (initially) paired umbilical veins to enter the sinus venosus of the heart. **(Bottom)** Graphic shows the entire right umbilical vein and much of the left atrophy. The left umbilical vein sends a large branch to the liver which anastomoses with the plexus derived from the vitelline veins. The extrahepatic (distal) vitelline veins form around the gut, as precursor to the portal venous system.

EMBRYOLOGY OF THE ABDOMEN

DEVELOPMENT OF HEPATIC VEINS (8-12 WEEK FETUS)

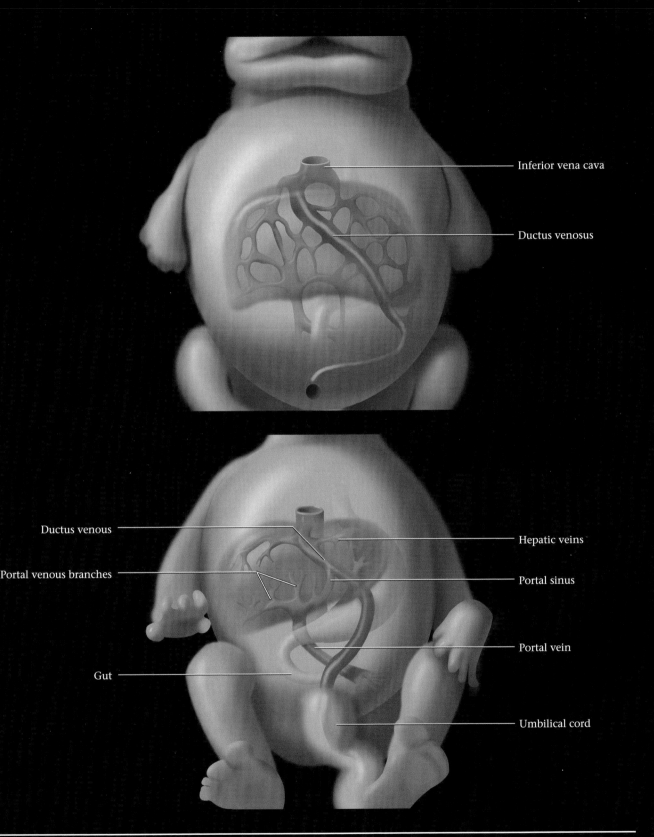

(**Top**) The entire right umbilical vein and much of the left have disappeared. The left hepatic branch of the umbilical vein has become the ductus venosus, which bypasses the liver to deliver oxygenated blood from the placenta directly to the heart. (**Bottom**) The portal sinus diverts some oxygenated blood to the liver. The proximal parts of the vitelline veins have become the hepatic veins, returning blood from the liver to the heart. The distal parts have developed into the portal venous system, returning blood from the gut to the liver sinusoids.

EMBRYOLOGY OF THE ABDOMEN

PRENATAL ABDOMINAL CIRCULATION

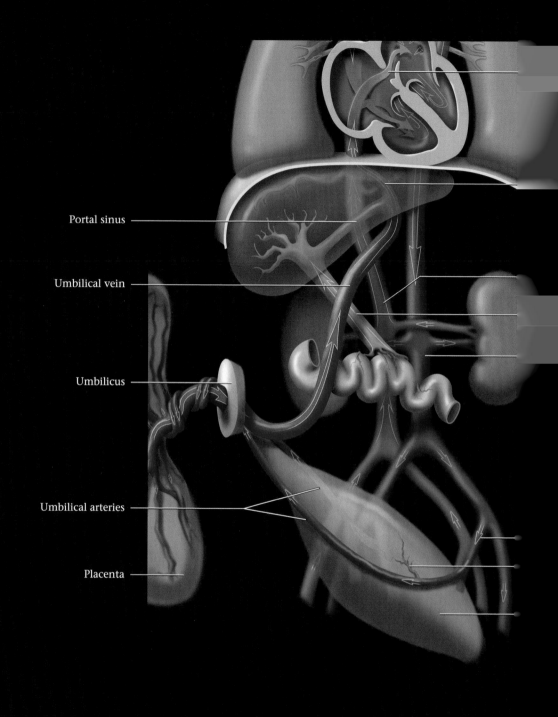

Portal sinus

Umbilical vein

Umbilicus

Umbilical arteries

Placenta

A simplified view of fetal circulation, not drawn to scale. The placenta sends oxygenated blo
fetus via the umbilical vein. Some oxygenated blood perfuses the liver via reflux through the
bypasses the liver via the ductus venosus which empties into the inferior vena cava. The pat
oxygenated blood to pass from the right atrium into the left atrium. The portal vein returns
to the liver, and the aorta carries moderately oxygenated blood to the entire body and retur
via the umbilical arteries, branches of the internal iliac arteries. The fetal bladder is large an

EMBRYOLOGY OF THE ABDOMEN

POST NATAL CIRCULATION

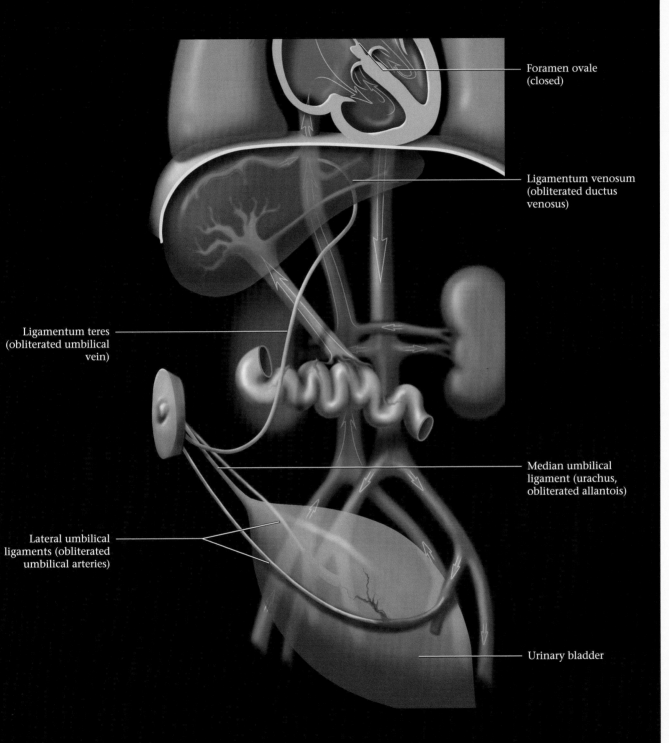

Foramen ovale
(closed)

Ligamentum venosum
(obliterated ductus
venosus)

Ligamentum teres
(obliterated umbilical
vein)

Median umbilical
ligament (urachus,
obliterated allantois)

Lateral umbilical
ligaments (obliterated
umbilical arteries)

Urinary bladder

After birth, the umbilical vein is obliterated, becoming the ligamentum teres in the free edge of the falciform ligament. The ductus venosus also closes, to become the ligamentum venosum. The foramen ovale closes as the lungs now return oxygen-rich blood to the left atrium and aorta. The umbilical arteries atrophy to become the lateral umbilical ligaments. The allantois that connected the urinary bladder to the umbilicus closes to become the median umbilical ligament. Failure of this tract to close results in a urachal cyst or diverticulum.

EMBRYOLOGY OF THE ABDOMEN

PERITONEAL REFLECTIONS IN PARACOLIC "GUTTERS"

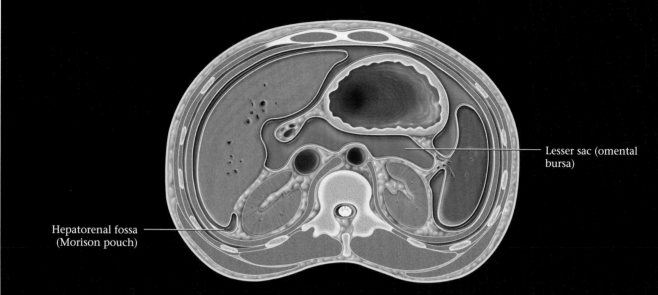

Lesser sac (omental bursa)

Hepatorenal fossa (Morison pouch)

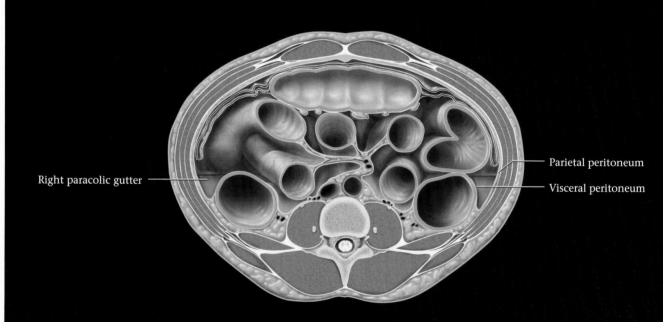

Parietal peritoneum

Visceral peritoneum

Right paracolic gutter

(Top) Graphic of axial section through the upper abdomen shows ascites (fluid, green) within the subphrenic spaces bilaterally and lesser sac. The hepatorenal fossa (Morison pouch) is the most dependent peritoneal recess in the upper abdomen. **(Bottom)** The paracolic gutters are the main conduit for fluid between the upper (supramesocolic) and lower (inframesocolic) parts of the peritoneal cavity.

EMBRYOLOGY OF THE ABDOMEN

SAGITTAL SECTION OF MESENTERIES & PERITONEAL CAVITY

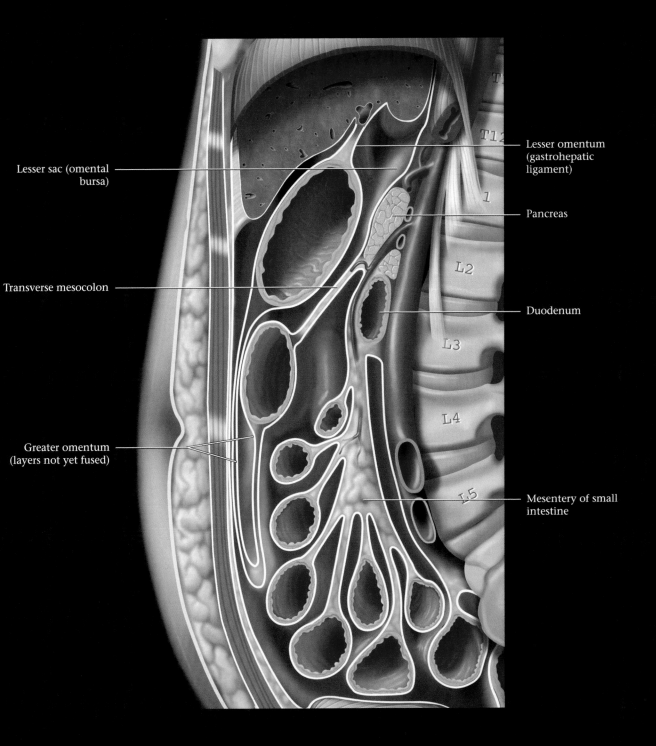

Lesser sac (omental bursa)

Lesser omentum (gastrohepatic ligament)

Pancreas

Transverse mesocolon

Duodenum

Greater omentum (layers not yet fused)

Mesentery of small intestine

The peritoneal cavity is artificially distended, as if insufflated with air. The peritoneum is represented by a white line covering the entire cavity, lining the inner abdominal wall (parietal peritoneum) & the surface of abdominal organs (visceral peritoneum or serosa). Organs are considered intraperitoneal if they are mostly covered with peritoneum (e.g., intestine) or retroperitoneal if they have no or only partial peritoneal covering. Intraperitoneal and retroperitoneal compartments communicate via the "subperitoneal" space, between the leaves of the mesenteries. Note how bleeding or inflammation originating in the (retroperitoneal) pancreas can easily spread through the mesocolon & mesentery to affect the bowel. The greater omentum is depicted as a 4-layered fold of peritoneum, although these layers usually fuse together below the transverse colon.

EMBRYOLOGY OF THE ABDOMEN

PERITONEAL REFLECTIONS & SPACES

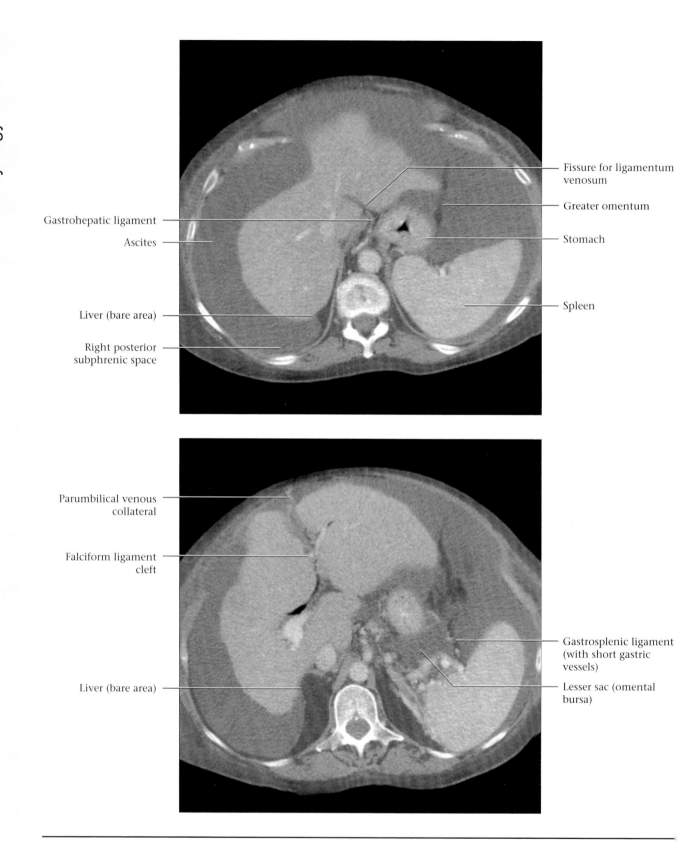

(Top) First of eight axial CT sections of a 60 year old man with cirrhosis and ascites. The ascites distends the peritoneal cavity and outlines the mesenteries and ligaments. Note the bare area, the nonperitonealized attachment of the liver to the diaphragm, where ascites is excluded. Most mesenteries, omenta and ligaments contain enough fat to allow them to be identified. (Bottom) Parumbilical venous collaterals have formed in the falciform ligament due to portal hypertension, re-establishing a fetal site of collateral circulation.

EMBRYOLOGY OF THE ABDOMEN

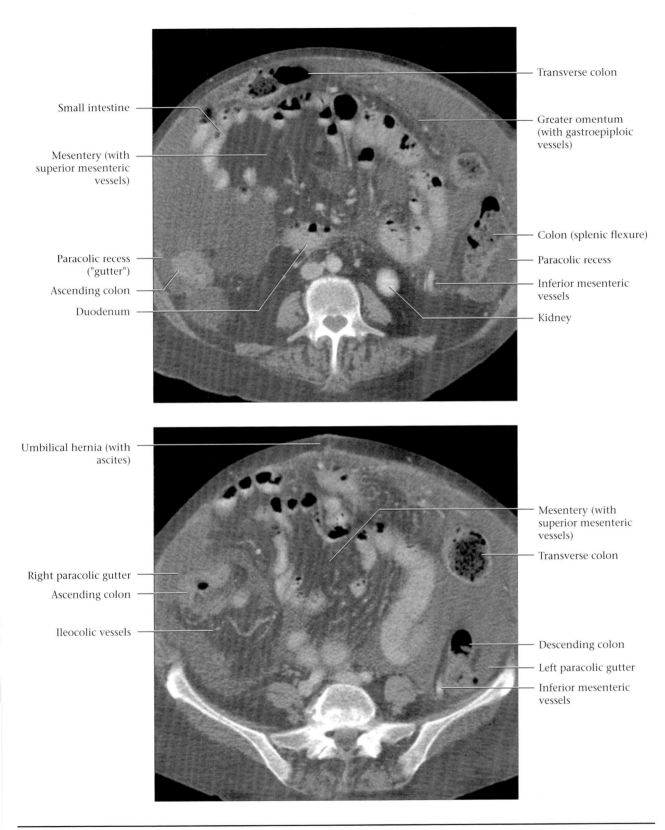

Small intestine

Mesentery (with superior mesenteric vessels)

Paracolic recess ("gutter")

Ascending colon

Duodenum

Transverse colon

Greater omentum (with gastroepiploic vessels)

Colon (splenic flexure)

Paracolic recess

Inferior mesenteric vessels

Kidney

Umbilical hernia (with ascites)

Right paracolic gutter

Ascending colon

Ileocolic vessels

Mesentery (with superior mesenteric vessels)

Transverse colon

Descending colon

Left paracolic gutter

Inferior mesenteric vessels

(Top) The vessels to the intraperitoneal organs are carried through the various peritoneal reflections (mesenteries, omenta and ligaments). Vessels to the retroperitoneal organs, including the ascending and descending colon, do not traverse mesenteries. **(Bottom)** The upper and lower portions of the peritoneal cavity "communicate" via the left and right paracolic recesses ("gutters"), which are formed by reflections of the peritoneum covering the colon and the inside of the antero-lateral abdominal wall.

EMBRYOLOGY OF THE ABDOMEN

MESENTERIES & PERITONEAL SPACES

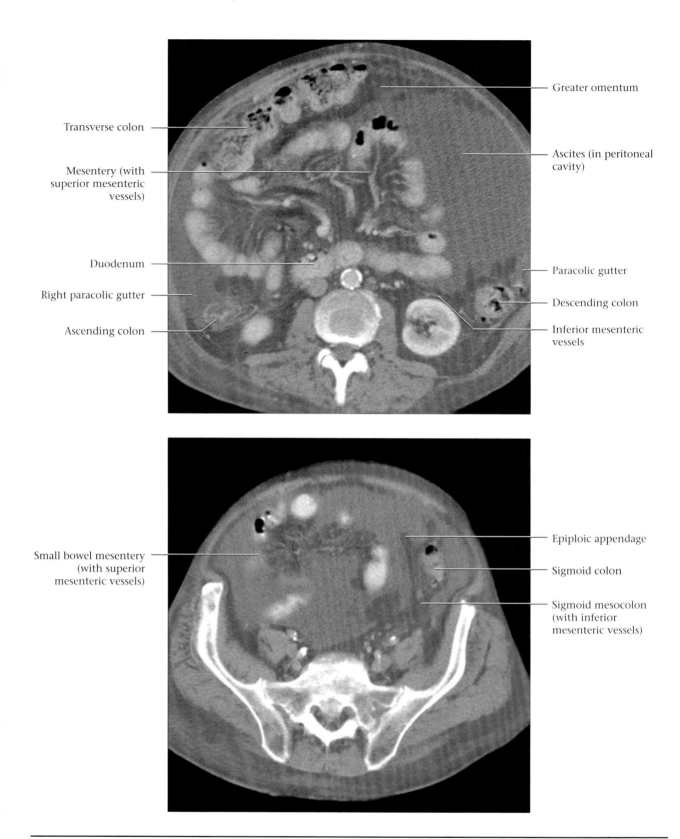

Greater omentum

Transverse colon

Mesentery (with superior mesenteric vessels)

Ascites (in peritoneal cavity)

Duodenum

Right paracolic gutter

Ascending colon

Paracolic gutter

Descending colon

Inferior mesenteric vessels

Small bowel mesentery (with superior mesenteric vessels)

Epiploic appendage

Sigmoid colon

Sigmoid mesocolon (with inferior mesenteric vessels)

(Top) First of five axial CT sections of a 50 year old man with cirrhosis and ascites. The relationship between the intraperitoneal and retroperitoneal organs is evident in this patient with ascites. The vessels, nerves and lymphatics travel through the retroperitoneum and, for the intraperitoneal organs, extend out through the fibro-fatty tissue in the mesenteries, between layers of visceral peritoneum. **(Bottom)** In this and the previous images, note the paracolic gutters, formed by reflections of peritoneum over the ascending and descending colon.

EMBRYOLOGY OF THE ABDOMEN

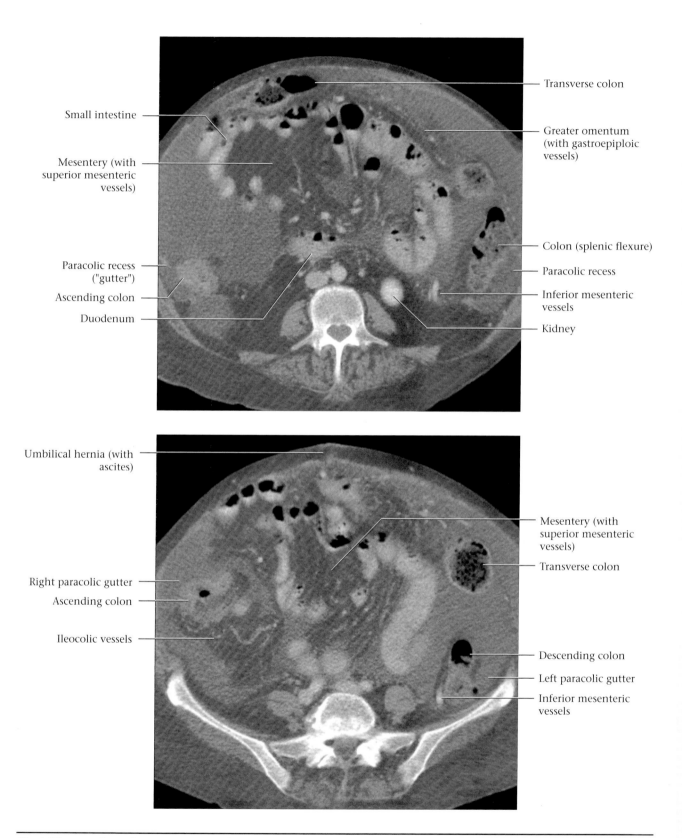

(Top) The vessels to the intraperitoneal organs are carried through the various peritoneal reflections (mesenteries, omenta and ligaments). Vessels to the retroperitoneal organs, including the ascending and descending colon, do not traverse mesenteries. (Bottom) The upper and lower portions of the peritoneal cavity "communicate" via the left and right paracolic recesses ("gutters"), which are formed by reflections of the peritoneum covering the colon and the inside of the antero-lateral abdominal wall.

EMBRYOLOGY OF THE ABDOMEN

PERITONEAL REFLECTIONS & SPACES

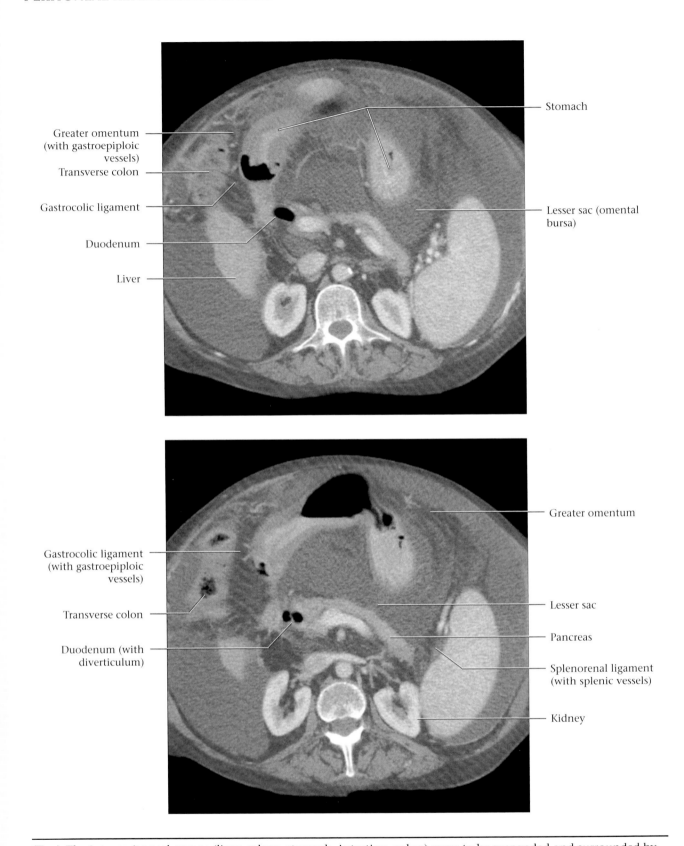

(Top) The intraperitoneal organs (liver, spleen, stomach, intestine, colon) seem to be suspended and surrounded by ascites (intraperitoneal fluid), while the retroperitoneal pancreas, duodenum and kidneys are not. (Bottom) The margins of the lesser sac include the stomach, caudate lobe of the liver, gastrosplenic and splenorenal ligaments, pancreas and the lesser omentum (gastrohepatic and hepatoduodenal ligaments).

EMBRYOLOGY OF THE ABDOMEN

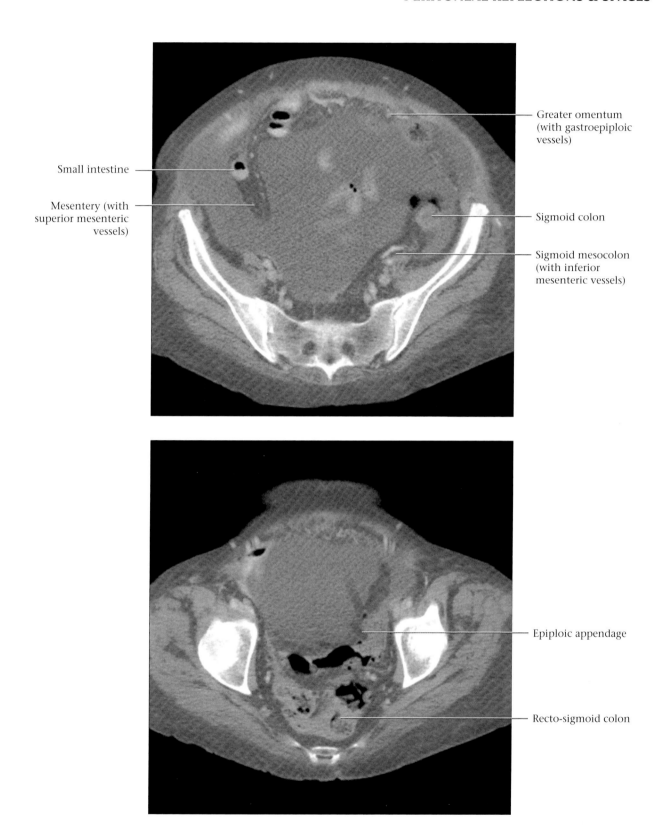

Greater omentum (with gastroepiploic vessels)

Small intestine

Mesentery (with superior mesenteric vessels)

Sigmoid colon

Sigmoid mesocolon (with inferior mesenteric vessels)

Epiploic appendage

Recto-sigmoid colon

(Top) The sigmoid colon is "intraperitoneal", suspended on the sigmoid mesocolon through which the inferior mesenteric vessels run. **(Bottom)** Ascites outlines fatty epiploic appendages which are prominent in the sigmoid colon. The rectum lies in the pelvic extraperitoneal space and is not surrounded by ascites.

EMBRYOLOGY OF THE ABDOMEN

MESENTERIES & PERITONEAL SPACES

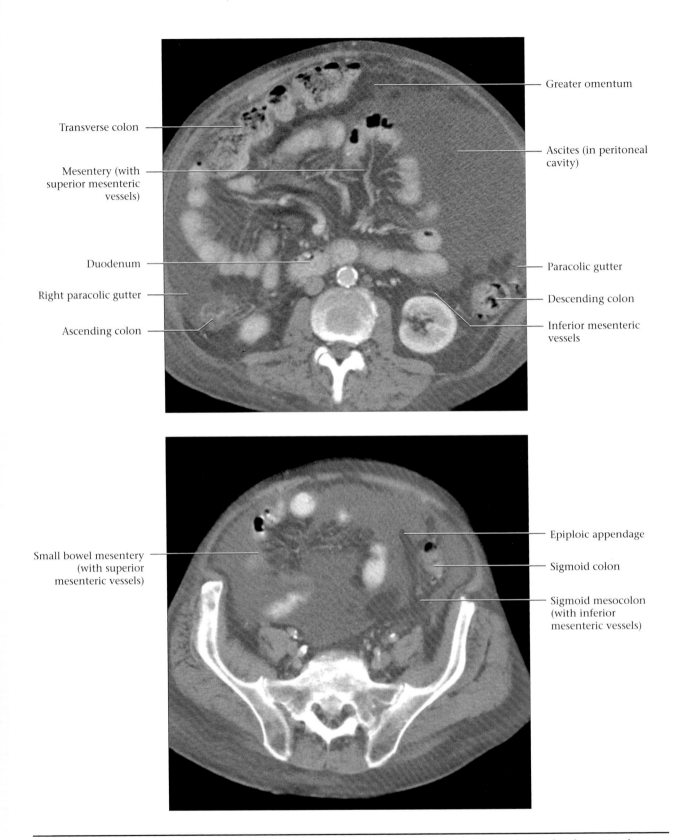

(Top) First of five axial CT sections of a 50 year old man with cirrhosis and ascites. The relationship between the intraperitoneal and retroperitoneal organs is evident in this patient with ascites. The vessels, nerves and lymphatics travel through the retroperitoneum and, for the intraperitoneal organs, extend out through the fibro-fatty tissue in the mesenteries, between layers of visceral peritoneum. **(Bottom)** In this and the previous images, note the paracolic gutters, formed by reflections of peritoneum over the ascending and descending colon.

EMBRYOLOGY OF THE ABDOMEN

Lateral umbilical ligament

Sigmoid colon

Inferior mesenteric vessels

Inferior epigastric vessels

Perivesical fat

Ascites

Lateral umbilical ligaments

Urinary bladder

External iliac vessels

Internal iliac vessels

Inferior epigastric vessels

Urinary bladder

Rectovesical space (with ascites)

Rectum

(Top) Ascites surrounds the intraperitoneal intestine and sigmoid colon. (Middle) Ascites outlines the lateral umbilical ligaments (remnants of the umbilical arteries). The main vessels and nerves supplying the antero-lateral abdominal wall travel between muscle layers or between the peritoneum and the transversalis fascia, such as the inferior epigastric vessels, which arise from the external iliac vessels in the pelvis. (Bottom) The rectovesical space is the most dependent recess of the peritoneal cavity.

EMBRYOLOGY OF THE ABDOMEN

RETROPERITONEAL SPACES & PLANES

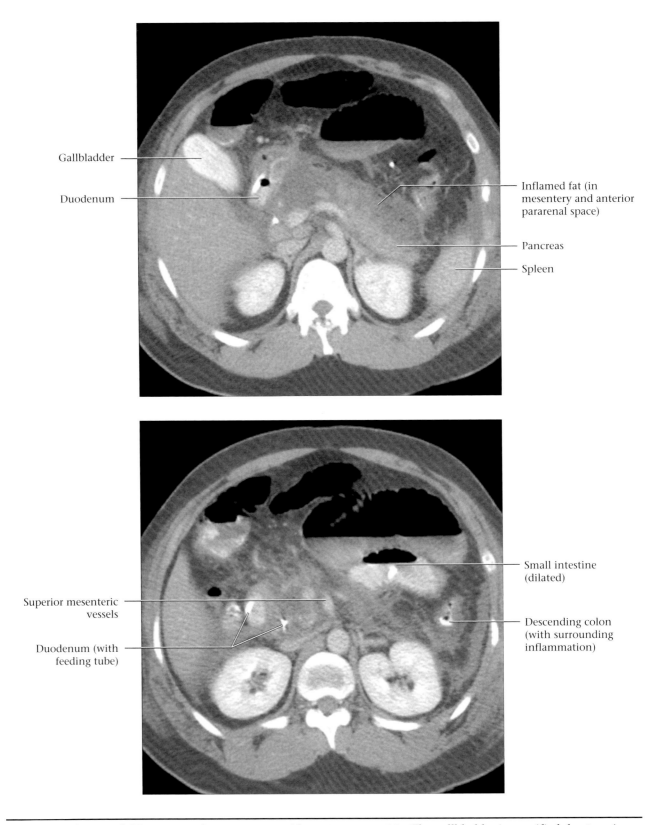

Gallbladder

Duodenum

Inflamed fat (in mesentery and anterior pararenal space)

Pancreas

Spleen

Superior mesenteric vessels

Duodenum (with feeding tube)

Small intestine (dilated)

Descending colon (with surrounding inflammation)

(Top) First of six axial CT sections of a young man with acute pancreatitis. The gallbladder is opacified due to prior administration of contrast material. The pancreas is enlarged and enhances heterogeneously due to acute pancreatitis. Inflammation spreads ventrally into the mesentery and laterally throughout the anterior pararenal space, which is bordered by the peritoneum in front and the perirenal fascia behind. **(Bottom)** Mesenteric involvement is evident by infiltration of the fat surrounding the superior mesenteric vessels. Organs sharing the anterior pararenal space with the pancreas, namely the duodenum, ascending and descending colon, are similarly involved.

RETROPERITONEAL SPACES & PLANES

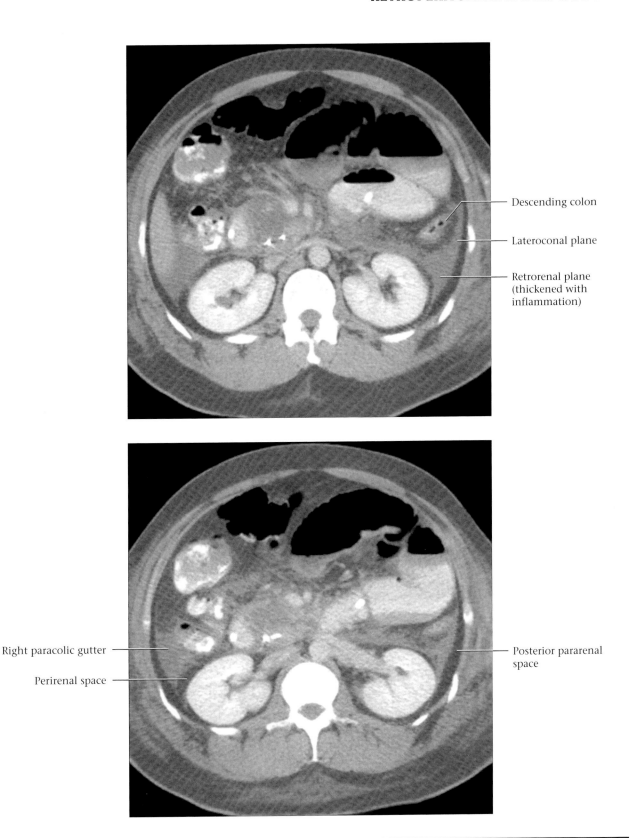

Descending colon

Lateroconal plane

Retrorenal plane (thickened with inflammation)

Right paracolic gutter

Perirenal space

Posterior pararenal space

(Top) The inflammatory process splits apart and thickens the double-layered renal and lateroconal fascia to reveal retrorenal and lateroconal planes. (Bottom) The perirenal and posterior pararenal spaces remain uninvolved as the renal and lateroconal fascia have blocked further spread of inflammation. Abtraperitoneal fluid (ascites) in the right paracolic gutter is adjacent to, and difficult to distinguish from, inflammation in the right anterior pararenal space, which surrounds the ascending colon. Inflammation has breached the posterior parietal peritoneum to cause the ascites.

EMBRYOLOGY OF THE ABDOMEN

RETROPERITONEAL SPACES & PLANES

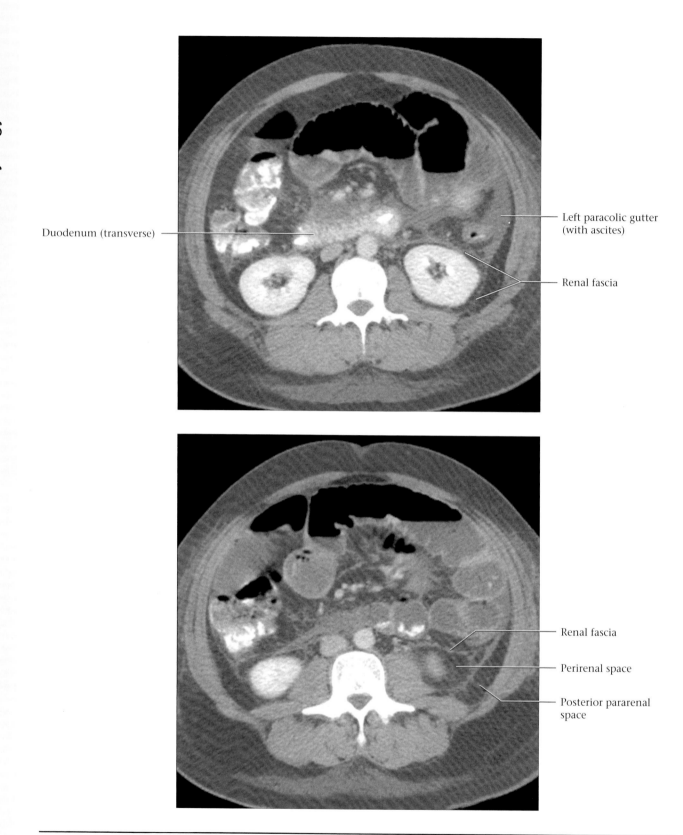

Duodenum (transverse)

Left paracolic gutter (with ascites)

Renal fascia

Renal fascia

Perirenal space

Posterior pararenal space

(Top) Ascites in the left paracolic gutter lies in the recess lateral to the colon. The space behind the colon and the thickening of the perirenal fascia are representative of the retroperitoneal (anterior pararenal space) inflammation. **(Bottom)** On more caudal section, just above the iliac wing, the leaves of renal fascia approach each other. Caudal to this point, there is only a single abdominal retroperitoneal space which communicates with the pelvic extraperitoneal spaces (pre- and perivesical).

EMBRYOLOGY OF THE ABDOMEN

COMMUNICATION AMONG EXTRAPERITONEAL SPACES

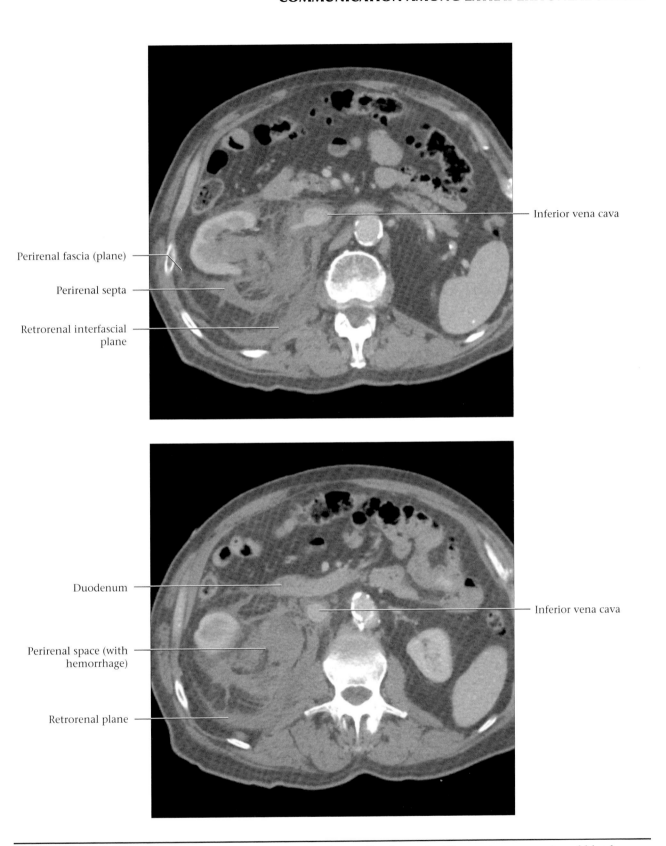

(Top) First of six axial CT sections of an elderly man (on Coumadin therapy) with spontaneous perirenal bleed. Blood spreads through perirenal space along the perirenal septa to "decompress" into the retrorenal interfascial plane. **(Bottom)** The perirenal space does not extend to the midline, but the interfascial planes do, allowing hemorrhage to surround the IVC.

COMMUNICATION AMONG EXTRAPERITONEAL SPACES

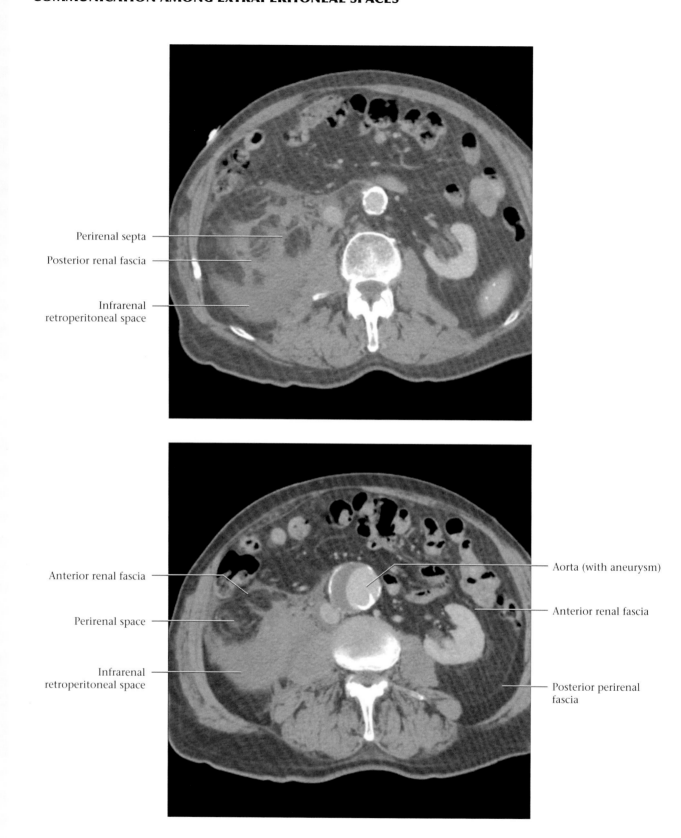

Perirenal septa

Posterior renal fascia

Infrarenal
retroperitoneal space

Anterior renal fascia

Perirenal space

Infrarenal
retroperitoneal space

Aorta (with aneurysm)

Anterior renal fascia

Posterior perirenal
fascia

(Top) The thickened perirenal septa and retrorenal interfascial planes are well-defined. The perirenal space decreases in diameter caudally as the leaves of the renal (Gerota) fascia approach each other. **(Bottom)** An aortic aneurysm is noted, but is not the source of the hemorrhage. Caudal to the perirenal space there is only a single infrarenal retroperitoneal space.

COMMUNICATION AMONG EXTRAPERITONEAL SPACES

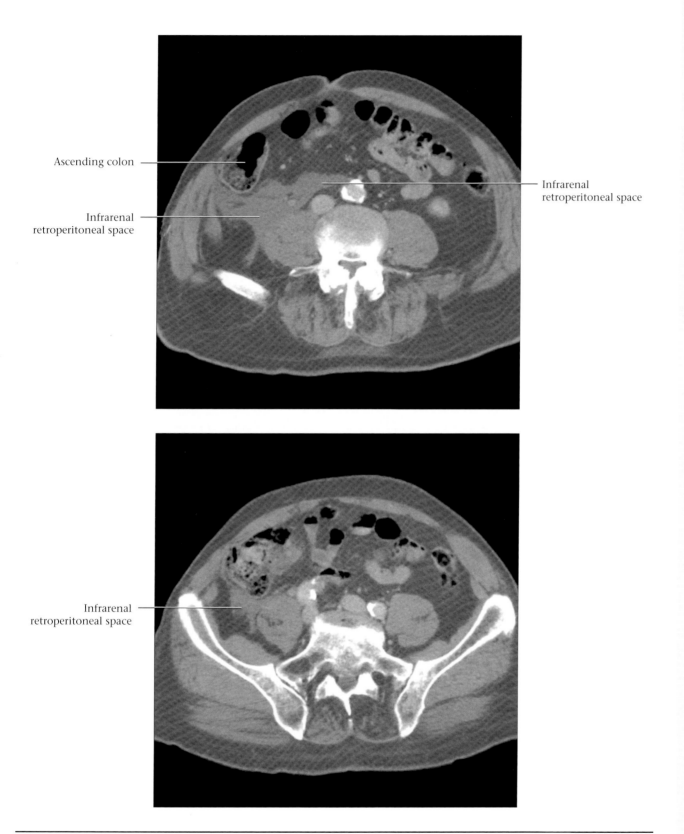

Ascending colon

Infrarenal retroperitoneal space

Infrarenal retroperitoneal space

Infrarenal retroperitoneal space

(Top) The infrarenal retroperitoneal space is contiguous with the psoas muscle and communicates across the midline. **(Bottom)** The infrarenal retroperitoneal space communicates caudally with the extraperitoneal pelvic spaces.

EMBRYOLOGY OF THE ABDOMEN

DEVELOPMENT OF GU TRACT

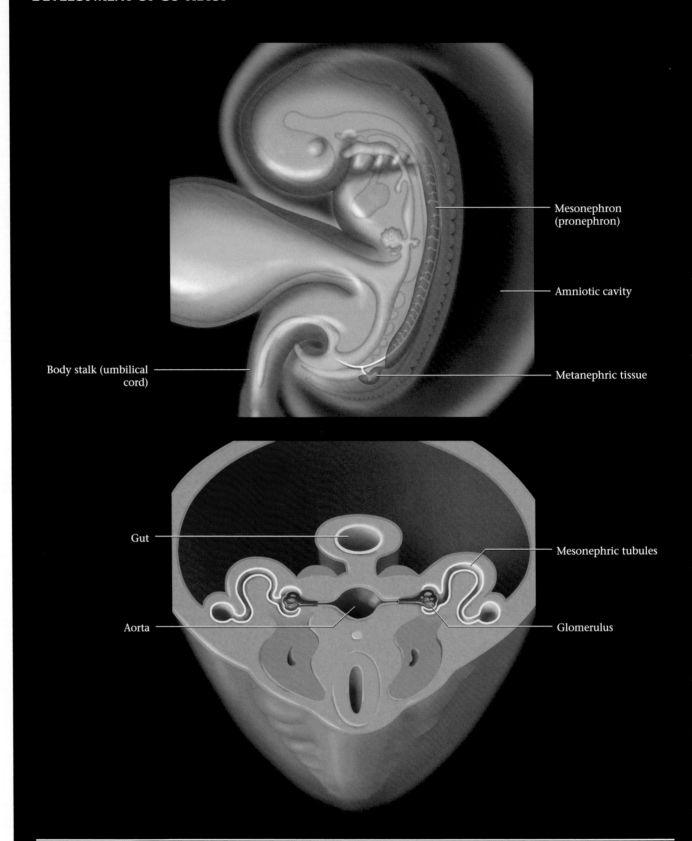

Mesonephron
(pronephron)

Amniotic cavity

Body stalk (umbilical
cord)

Metanephric tissue

Gut

Mesonephric tubules

Aorta

Glomerulus

(Top) The primitive genitourinary system develops in parallel with the gastrointestinal tract. The pronephron is a transient development in vertebrate animals and degenerates to be replaced by the mesonephron. The mesonephron also degenerates (in mammals) and is replaced by the metanephron, which will be the permanent kidney. **(Bottom)** By the 4th fetal week, the mesonephric tubules and duct are formed. Branched vessels from the aorta reach the blind ends of the tubules to form glomeruli. Although these achieve excretory function in the human embryo, they degenerate from the cranial toward the caudal end. The caudal end of the mesonephric duct persists and differentiates into the Müllerian and Wolffian ducts, which later give rise to the internal genitalia.

DEVELOPMENT OF GU TRACT (5 WEEK FETUS)

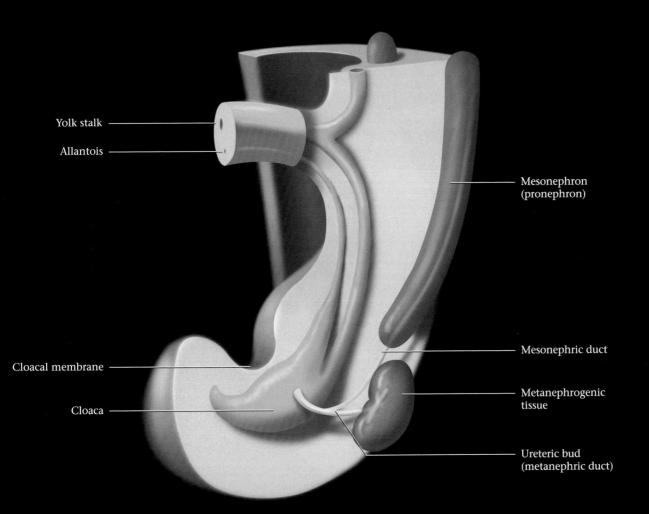

Yolk stalk

Allantois

Mesonephron
(pronephron)

Cloacal membrane

Mesonephric duct

Cloaca

Metanephrogenic
tissue

Ureteric bud
(metanephric duct)

he metanephric duct (ureteric bud) has grown out of the mesonephric duct near its termination in the cloaca, and
as extended into the metanephrogenic tissue (kidney). Within the kidney, the ureteric bud branches and expands
o form calices and these arborize to form successive generations of collecting ducts. At the 5th fetal week, the
indgut and developing urinary tract both terminate in the blind-ending cloaca.

EMBRYOLOGY OF THE ABDOMEN

URINARY BLADDER DEVELOPMENT

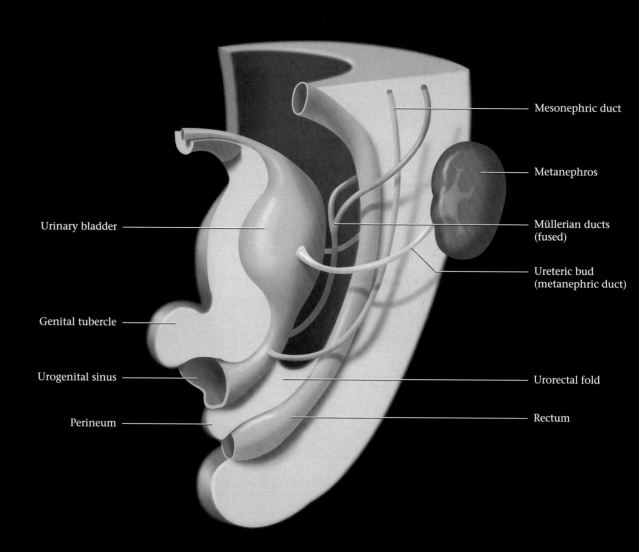

Mesonephric duct

Metanephros

Müllerian ducts (fused)

Ureteric bud (metanephric duct)

Urorectal fold

Rectum

Urinary bladder

Genital tubercle

Urogenital sinus

Perineum

The development of the genital, urinary and gastrointestinal tracts are closely related. The urorectal fold migrates caudally to separate the rectum posteriorly from the urogenital sinus anteriorly. The cloacal membrane has broken down and the rectum and urogenital sinus open onto the perineum. The metanephros (kidney) has migrated cranially. The mesonephric and metanephric ducts have shifted, with the former now entering the future urethra and the latter entering the bladder. At this stage, the male and female fetuses are indistinguishable. The mesonephros degenerates and the mesonephric duct differentiates into Müllerian and Wolffian ducts which are the primordial forms of the internal genitalia.

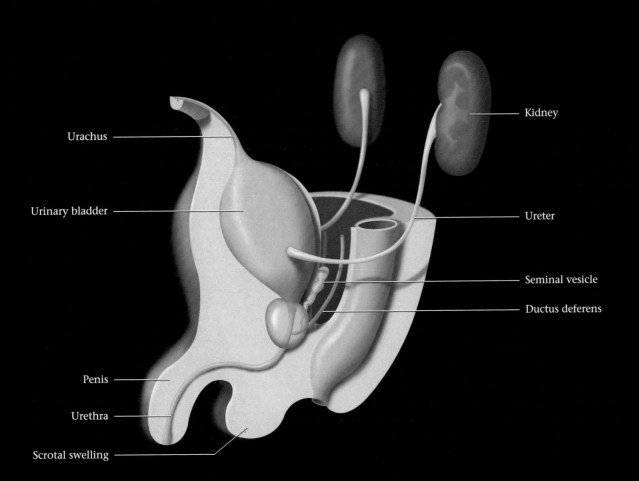

Urachus

Urinary bladder

Penis

Urethra

Scrotal swelling

Kidney

Ureter

Seminal vesicle

Ductus deferens

In the male fetus, the Müllerian ducts mostly disappear while the Wolffian duct develops and differentiates due to the influence of testosterone secreted by the ipsilateral testis. During the 4th month of gestation, the caudal end of the Wolffian duct gives rise to the epididymis, ductus deferens, seminal vesicle and ejaculatory duct. The urogenital sinus evolves into the bladder and urethra. In both male and female, the allantois has degenerated into the urachus which usually obliterates in postnatal life to become the median umbilical ligament.

EMBRYOLOGY OF THE ABDOMEN

DEVELOPMENT OF GU TRACT (20 WEEK FEMALE FETUS)

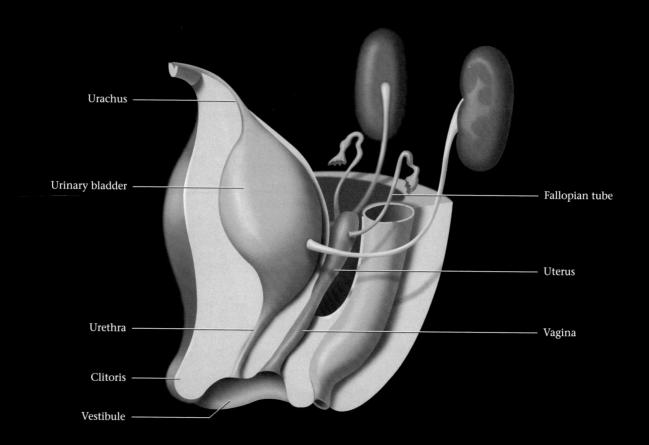

Urachus

Urinary bladder

Urethra

Clitoris

Vestibule

Fallopian tube

Uterus

Vagina

In the female fetus, the lower Müllerian ducts unite to form a uterovaginal canal. The unfused portions of the ducts give rise to the fallopian tubes. The distal part of the vagina forms from invagination of a solid mass of cells between the uterovaginal canal and the urogenital sinus. Other parts of the urogenital sinus form the bladder, urethra and vestibule. Accessory glands derived from the urethra are inconspicuous in most females as urethral and periurethral glands, while these develop into the prostate gland in males.

EMBRYOLOGY OF THE ABDOMEN

KIDNEY ASCENT & ROTATION (6 WEEKS)

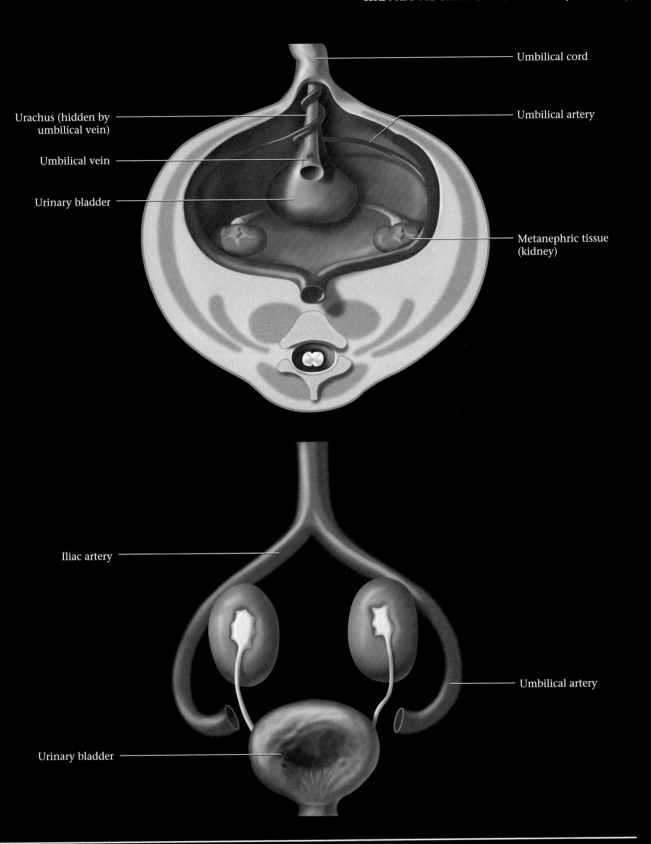

Umbilical cord

Umbilical artery

Urachus (hidden by umbilical vein)

Umbilical vein

Urinary bladder

Metanephric tissue (kidney)

Iliac artery

Umbilical artery

Urinary bladder

(Top) The early metanephros (kidneys) lie close together in the pelvis, and may even touch each other. (This may lead to various anomalies of fusion and ectopic location). **(Bottom)** The fetal kidneys "face forward".

EMBRYOLOGY OF THE ABDOMEN

KIDNEY ASCENT & ROTATION (7 WEEKS)

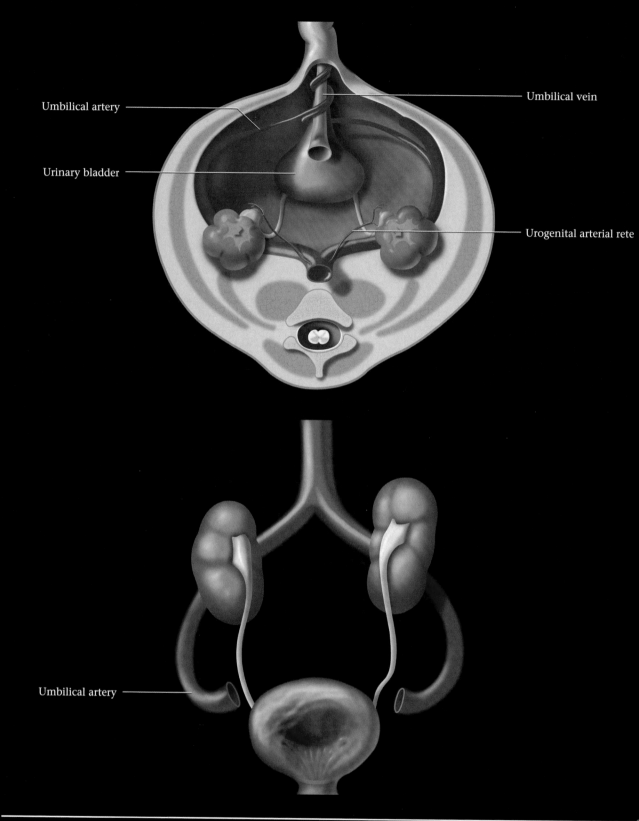

Umbilical artery

Urinary bladder

Umbilical vein

Urogenital arterial rete

Umbilical artery

(Top) The early metanephros (kidney) lies below the aortic bifurcation. Arterial supply is from multiple branches of the aorta, each part of a plexus called the urogenital arterial rete. As the kidneys "ascend" with fetal growth, usually only one artery remains to supply each kidney. **(Bottom)** At this stage of development, the fetal kidneys "face forward". If the fetal kidney fails to ascend normally (remains "ectopic"), it is likely to retain a multiple arterial supply and fail to rotate medially.

EMBRYOLOGY OF THE ABDOMEN

KIDNEY ASCENT & ROTATION (9 WEEKS)

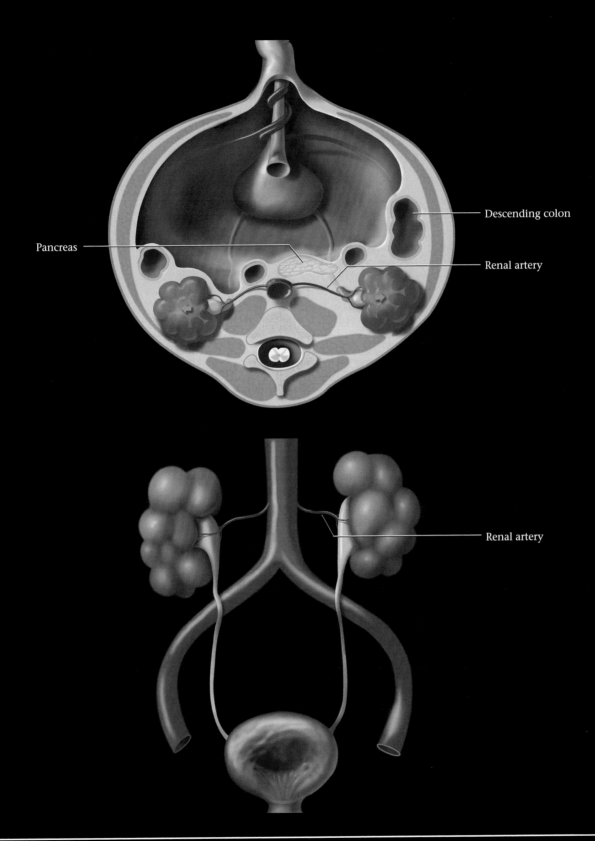

Pancreas

Descending colon

Renal artery

Renal artery

(Top) By the 9th fetal week, the kidneys have occupied their retroperitoneal location (along with the pancreas and duodenum). Each kidney is usually supplied by a single arterial branch of the aorta. (Bottom) The kidneys now lie at about the level of the 3rd lumbar vertebra and have rotated along their longitudinal axis so that the renal hila face medially. Fetal lobation remains a distinctive feature, reflecting the lobular origin of the primitive kidney.

ABDOMINAL WALL

Terminology

Definitions
- Abdomen is region between **diaphragm** and pelvis

Gross Anatomy

Anatomic Boundaries
- Anterior abdominal wall bounded superiorly by xiphoid process and costal cartilages of 7th-10th ribs
- Anterior wall bounded inferiorly by **iliac crest**, iliac spine, **inguinal ligament** and **pubis**
- Inguinal ligament is inferior edge of the aponeurosis of the external oblique muscle

Muscles of Anterior Abdominal Wall
- Consist of three flat muscles (external, internal oblique and transverse abdominal), and one strap-like muscle (rectus)
- Combination of muscles and **aponeuroses** (sheet-like tendons) act as a corset to confine and protect abdominal viscera
- **Linea alba** is a fibrous raphe stretching from xiphoid to pubis
  - Forms central anterior attachment for abdominal wall muscles
  - Formed by interlacing fibers of aponeuroses of the oblique and transverse abdominal muscles
  - **Rectus sheath** is also formed by these aponeuroses as they surround the rectus muscle
- **External oblique muscle**
  - Largest and most superficial of the 3 flat abdominal muscles
  - Origin: External surfaces of ribs 5-12
  - Insertion: Linea alba, iliac crest, pubis via a broad aponeurosis
- **Internal oblique muscle**
  - Middle of the 3 flat abdominal muscles
  - Runs at right angles to external oblique
  - Origin: Posterior layer of **thoracolumbar fascia**, iliac crest and inguinal ligament
  - Insertion: Ribs 10-12 posteriorly, linea alba via a broad aponeurosis, pubis
- **Transverse abdominal muscle**
  - Innermost of the 3 flat abdominal muscles
  - Origin: Lowest six costal cartilages, thoracolumbar fascia, iliac crest, inguinal ligament
  - Insertion: Linea alba via broad aponeurosis, pubis
- **Rectus abdominal muscle**
  - Origin: Pubic symphysis and pubic crest
  - Insertion: Xiphoid process and costal cartilages 5-7
  - Rectus sheath: Strong fibrous compartment that envelops each rectus muscle
  - Rectus sheath contains **superior** and **inferior epigastric vessels**
- Actions of anterior abdominal wall muscles
  - Support and protect abdominal viscera
  - Help flex and twist trunk, maintain posture
  - Increase intra-abdominal pressure for defecation, micturition and childbirth
  - Stabilize the pelvis during walking, sitting up
- **Transversalis fascia**
  - Lies deep to the abdominal wall muscles and lines entire abdominal wall
  - Is separated from **parietal peritoneum** by layer of **extraperitoneal fat**

Muscles of Posterior Abdominal Wall
- Consist of psoas (major and minor), iliacus and quadratus lumborum
- **Psoas**: Long thick, fusiform muscle lying lateral to vertebral column
  - Origin: Transverse processes and bodies of vertebrae T12-L5
  - Insertion: Lesser trochanter of femur (passing behind inguinal ligament)
  - Action: Flexes thigh at hip joint; bends vertebral column laterally
- **Iliacus**: Large triangular sheet of muscle lying along lateral side of psoas
  - Origin: Superior part of iliac fossa
  - Insertion: Lesser trochanter of femur (after joining with the psoas tendon)
  - Action: "Iliopsoas muscle" flexes the thigh
- **Quadratus lumborum**: Thick sheet of muscle lying adjacent to transverse processes of lumbar vertebrae
  - Origin: Iliac crest and transverse processes of lumbar vertebrae
  - Insertion: 12th rib
  - Actions: Stabilizes position of thorax and pelvis during respiration, walking
    - Bends trunk to side

Clinical Implications

Clinical Importance
- **Rectus** and iliopsoas muscle compartments are common sites for **spontaneous bleeding** in patients with coagulopathy
  - Rectus sheath is incomplete caudally; bleeding → into extraperitoneal pelvis
- Obesity and lack of exercise result in atrophy of abdominal wall muscles
  - **Pannus** (panniculus): Lax abdominal wall and excess subcutaneous fat; may simulate a ventral hernia clinically and on imaging
  - Results in dysfunction affecting micturition, defecation, etc.
  - Results in common occurrence of abdominal **wall hernias**, especially following abdominal surgery ("incisional hernia")
- Congenital points of weakness in aponeuroses predispose to other common external hernias
  - **Ventral hernia**: Through congenital defect in aponeuroses forming the linea alba, in the midline
  - **Spigelian hernia**: Lateral to the rectus muscle below umbilicus through defect in aponeurosis of internal oblique and transverse abdominal muscles
    - External oblique aponeurosis is often intact; hernia sac may be intermuscular
  - **Lumbar hernia**
    - At congenital point of deficiency just above iliac crest = **inferior lumbar triangle (of Petit)**

ABDOMINAL WALL

POSTERIOR ABDOMINAL WALL MUSCLES

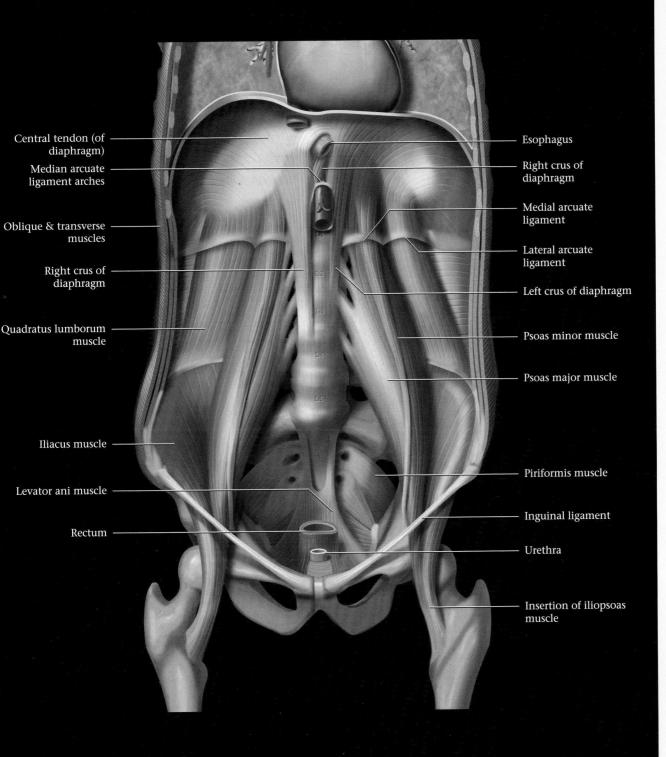

Central tendon (of diaphragm)

Median arcuate ligament arches

Oblique & transverse muscles

Right crus of diaphragm

Quadratus lumborum muscle

Iliacus muscle

Levator ani muscle

Rectum

Esophagus

Right crus of diaphragm

Medial arcuate ligament

Lateral arcuate ligament

Left crus of diaphragm

Psoas minor muscle

Psoas major muscle

Piriformis muscle

Inguinal ligament

Urethra

Insertion of iliopsoas muscle

Lumbar vertebrae are covered and attached by the anterior longitudinal ligament, and the diaphragmatic crura are closely attached to it, as are the origins of the psoas muscles, which also arise from the transverse processes. Iliacus muscle arises from the iliac fossa of pelvis and inserts into the tendon of the psoas major, constituting iliopsoas muscle, which inserts into the lesser trochanter. Quadratus lumborum arises from the iliac crest and inserts into the 12th rib and transverse processes of the lumbar vertebrae. Diaphragm and transverse abdominal fibers interlace. Psoas and quadratus lumborum pass behind diaphragm under medial and lateral arcuate ligaments.

ABDOMINAL WALL

ANTERIOR WALL MUSCLES

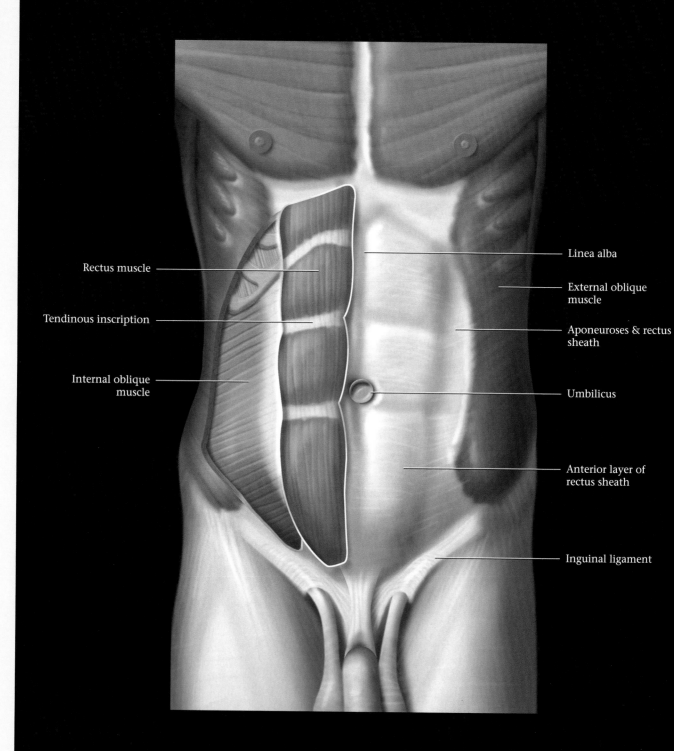

Rectus muscle

Tendinous inscription

Internal oblique muscle

Linea alba

External oblique muscle

Aponeuroses & rectus sheath

Umbilicus

Anterior layer of rectus sheath

Inguinal ligament

The aponeuroses of the internal and external oblique and transverse abdominal muscles are two-layered and interweave with each other, covering the rectus muscle, constituting the rectus sheath and linea alba. About midway between the umbilicus and symphysis, the posterior rectus sheath ends and the transversalis fascia is the only structure between the rectus muscle and parietal peritoneum.

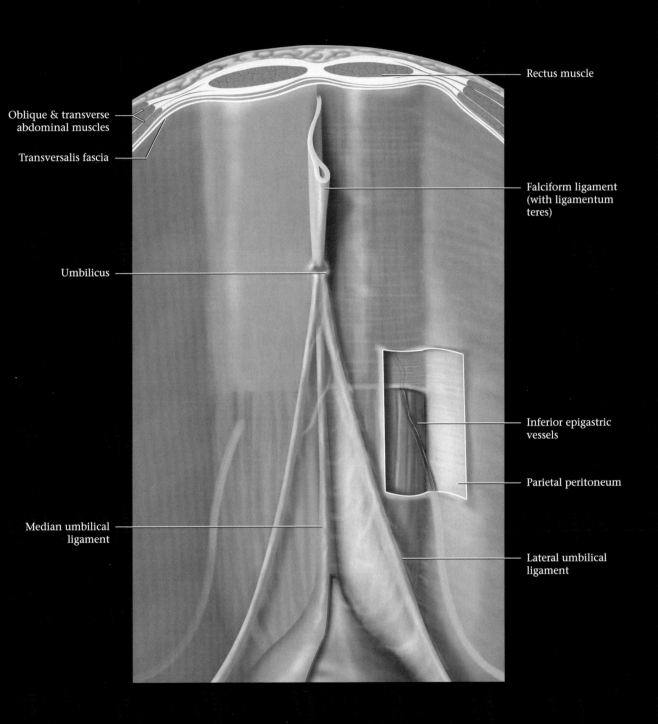

Rectus muscle

Oblique & transverse abdominal muscles

Transversalis fascia

Falciform ligament (with ligamentum teres)

Umbilicus

Inferior epigastric vessels

Parietal peritoneum

Median umbilical ligament

Lateral umbilical ligament

Graphic view of anterior abdominal wall from inside. The umbilical ligaments are remnants of the fetal umbilical arteries and allantois (urachus). The falciform ligament is the remnant of the umbilical vein. All of these converge at the umbilicus. Transversalis fascia lines muscular wall of abdomen. Epigastric vessels lie between transversalis fascia and parietal peritoneum.

ABDOMINAL WALL

THORACOLUMBAR FASCIA

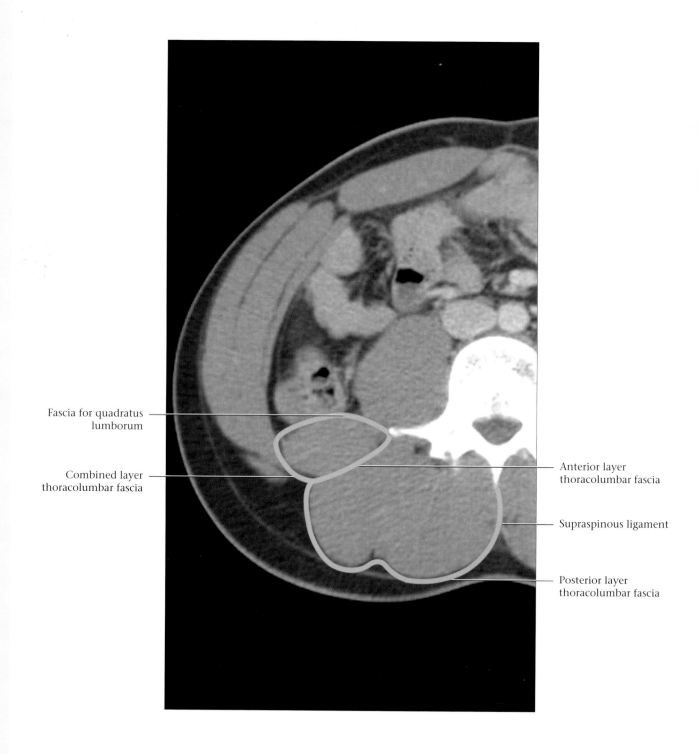

Fascia for quadratus lumborum

Combined layer thoracolumbar fascia

Anterior layer thoracolumbar fascia

Supraspinous ligament

Posterior layer thoracolumbar fascia

The thoracolumbar (lumbodorsal) fascia is a strong fibrous sheath that encloses the quadratus lumborum and erector spinae muscles. The aponeuroses of the transverse abdominal and internal oblique muscles attach to the combined or posterior layer of the thoracolumbar fascia.

ABDOMINAL WALL

ABDOMINAL WALL MUSCLES

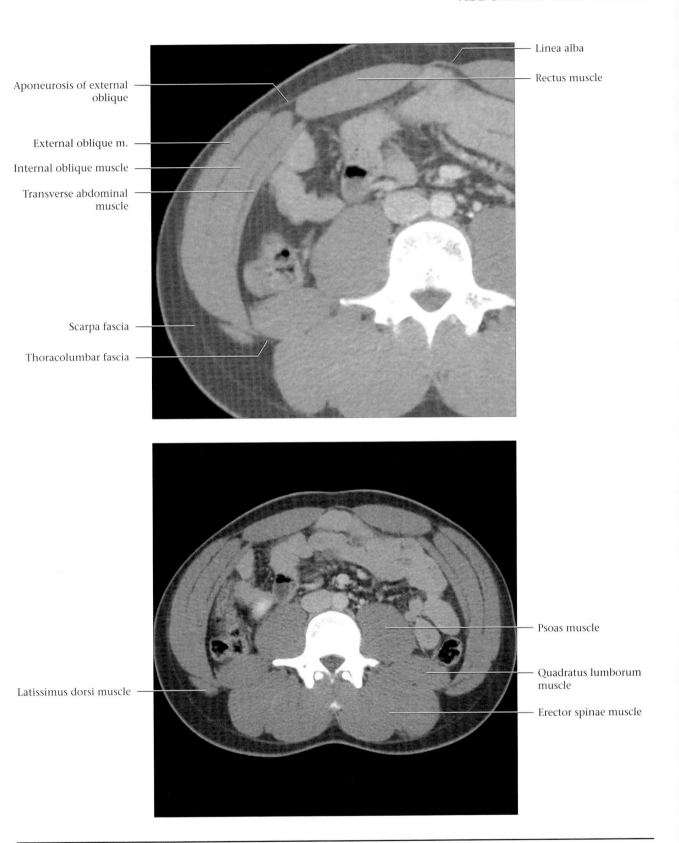

Aponeurosis of external oblique

External oblique m.

Internal oblique muscle

Transverse abdominal muscle

Scarpa fascia

Thoracolumbar fascia

Linea alba

Rectus muscle

Latissimus dorsi muscle

Psoas muscle

Quadratus lumborum muscle

Erector spinae muscle

(Top) First of two axial CT sections in a muscular young man. Note that the aponeuroses of the oblique and transverse abdominal muscles surround the rectus muscle as the rectus sheath, and then continue to form and insert upon the linea alba. **(Bottom)** Aponeuroses of oblique and transverse abdominal muscles blend with and attach to the thoracolumbar fascia which surrounds the paraspinal and quadratus lumborum muscles.

ABDOMINAL WALL

ABDOMINAL WALL MUSCLES

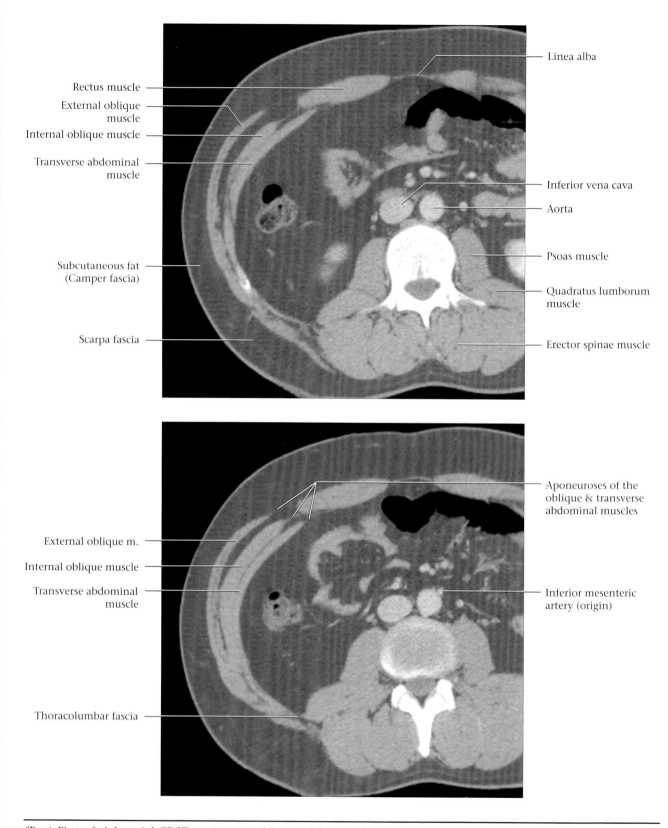

Rectus muscle

External oblique muscle

Internal oblique muscle

Transverse abdominal muscle

Subcutaneous fat (Camper fascia)

Scarpa fascia

Linea alba

Inferior vena cava

Aorta

Psoas muscle

Quadratus lumborum muscle

Erector spinae muscle

External oblique m.

Internal oblique muscle

Transverse abdominal muscle

Thoracolumbar fascia

Aponeuroses of the oblique & transverse abdominal muscles

Inferior mesenteric artery (origin)

(Top) First of eight axial CECT sections in a 29 year old man. The rectus sheath is formed by aponeuroses of oblique and transverse abdominal muscles which also form the linea alba, the central anterior attachment for anterior muscles. Subcutaneous tissue has 2 layers, superficial fatty layer (Camper fascia) and deep membranous layer (Scarpa fascia) that continue down to the perineum. **(Bottom)** Thoracolumbar fascia surrounds the quadratus lumborum and paraspinal muscles, forms important posterior attachment for abdominal wall muscles. Aponeuroses are the flat tendons that extend from the muscles.

ABDOMINAL WALL

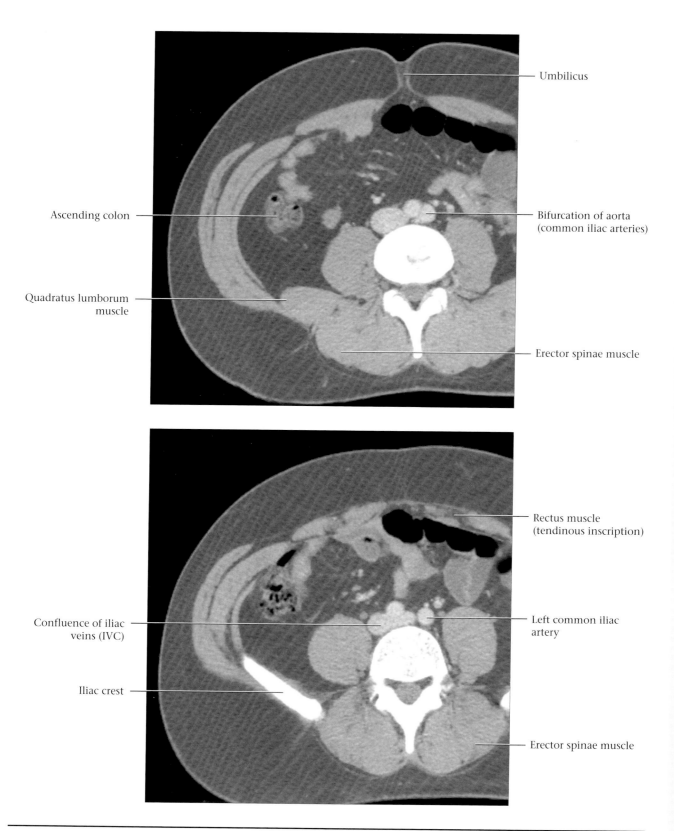

Umbilicus

Ascending colon

Bifurcation of aorta (common iliac arteries)

Quadratus lumborum muscle

Erector spinae muscle

Rectus muscle (tendinous inscription)

Confluence of iliac veins (IVC)

Left common iliac artery

Iliac crest

Erector spinae muscle

(Top) The origins of the anterior abdominal wall muscles include the iliac crest and thoracolumbar fascia inferiorly. The transversalis fascia lies deep to abdominal wall muscles and lines the entire wall, but is usually not detectible on imaging studies. (Bottom) Muscle attachments to iliac crest are evident.

ABDOMINAL WALL

ABDOMINAL WALL MUSCLES

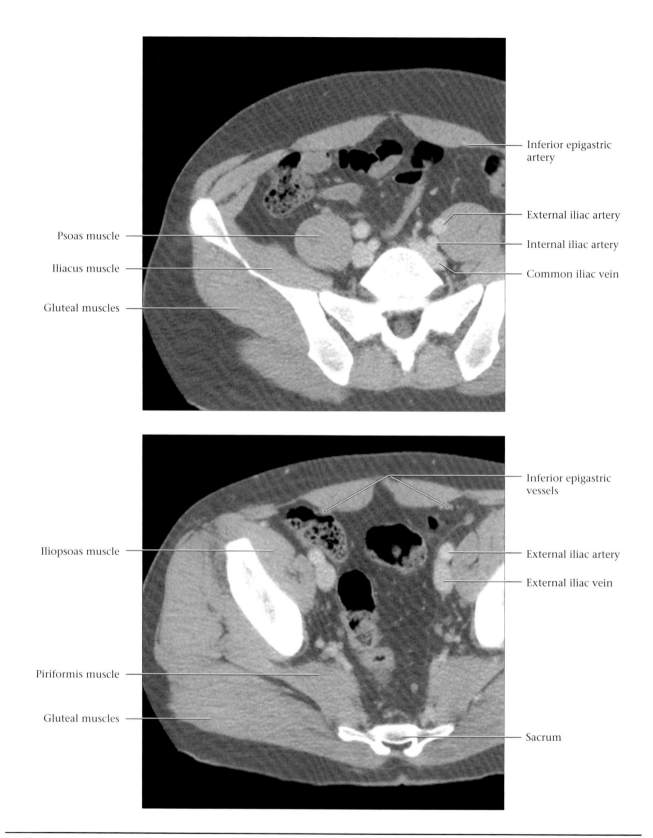

Inferior epigastric artery

Psoas muscle

Iliacus muscle

Gluteal muscles

External iliac artery

Internal iliac artery

Common iliac vein

Inferior epigastric vessels

Iliopsoas muscle

Piriformis muscle

Gluteal muscles

External iliac artery

External iliac vein

Sacrum

(Top) The inferior epigastric arteries and veins course along the underside of the rectus muscles and arise from the external iliac vessels, low in pelvis. **(Bottom)** The external iliac vessels run along surface of iliopsoas muscles.

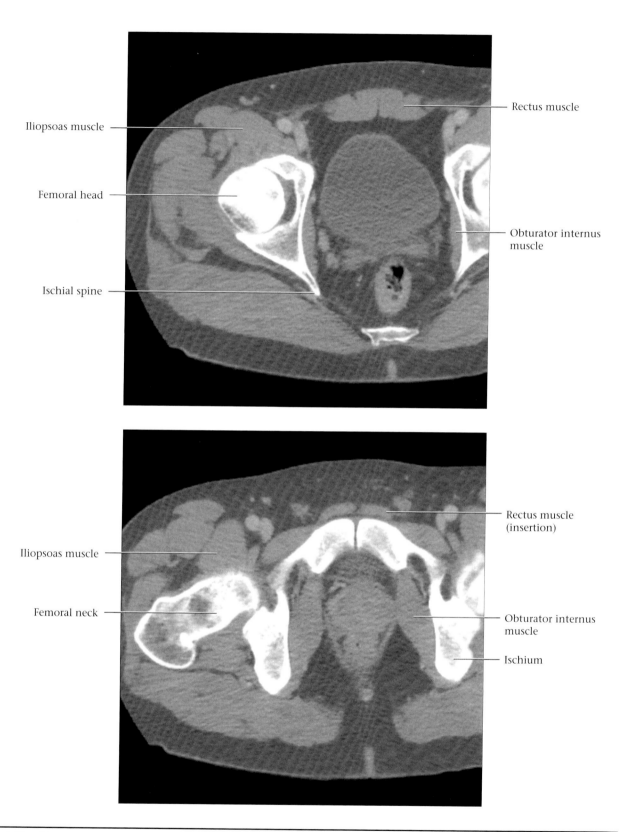

Iliopsoas muscle

Femoral head

Ischial spine

Rectus muscle

Obturator internus muscle

Iliopsoas muscle

Femoral neck

Rectus muscle (insertion)

Obturator internus muscle

Ischium

(Top) The iliopsoas muscle leaves the abdomen passing under inguinal ligament. **(Bottom)** Iliopsoas muscle passes anterior to femoral head and neck to insert on lesser trochanter of femur. The rectus muscle inserts on the pubis.

ABDOMINAL WALL

ABDOMINAL WALL, MUSCLES & VESSELS

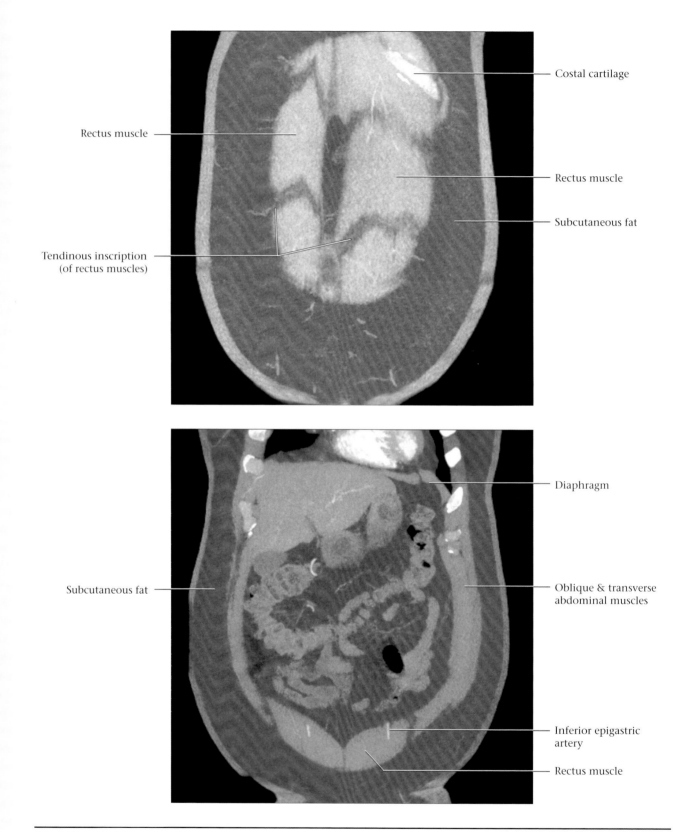

Costal cartilage

Rectus muscle

Rectus muscle

Subcutaneous fat

Tendinous inscription
(of rectus muscles)

Diaphragm

Subcutaneous fat

Oblique & transverse
abdominal muscles

Inferior epigastric
artery

Rectus muscle

(**Top**) First of eight coronal images in a 54 year old man. Rectus muscles arise from pubis and insert into xiphoid process and costal cartilages 5 to 7. Cephalad attachments of oblique and transverse abdominal muscles include the lower ribs and costal cartilages. (**Bottom**) Rectus sheath contains the superior and inferior epigastric arteries, which anastomose with each other near level of umbilicus.

ABDOMINAL WALL

ABDOMINAL WALL, MUSCLES & VESSELS

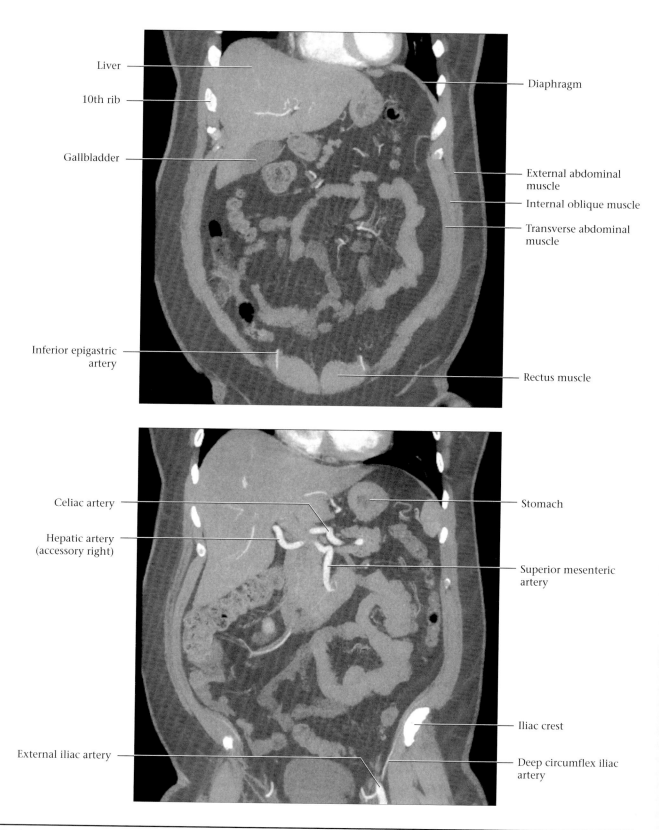

Liver

10th rib

Gallbladder

Inferior epigastric artery

Diaphragm

External abdominal muscle

Internal oblique muscle

Transverse abdominal muscle

Rectus muscle

Celiac artery

Hepatic artery (accessory right)

External iliac artery

Stomach

Superior mesenteric artery

Iliac crest

Deep circumflex iliac artery

(Top) Attachment of the oblique and transverse abdominal muscles to the lower ribs is evident. **(Bottom)** Caudal attachment of the oblique and transverse abdominal muscles to the iliac crest.

ABDOMINAL WALL

ABDOMINAL WALL, MUSCLES & VESSELS

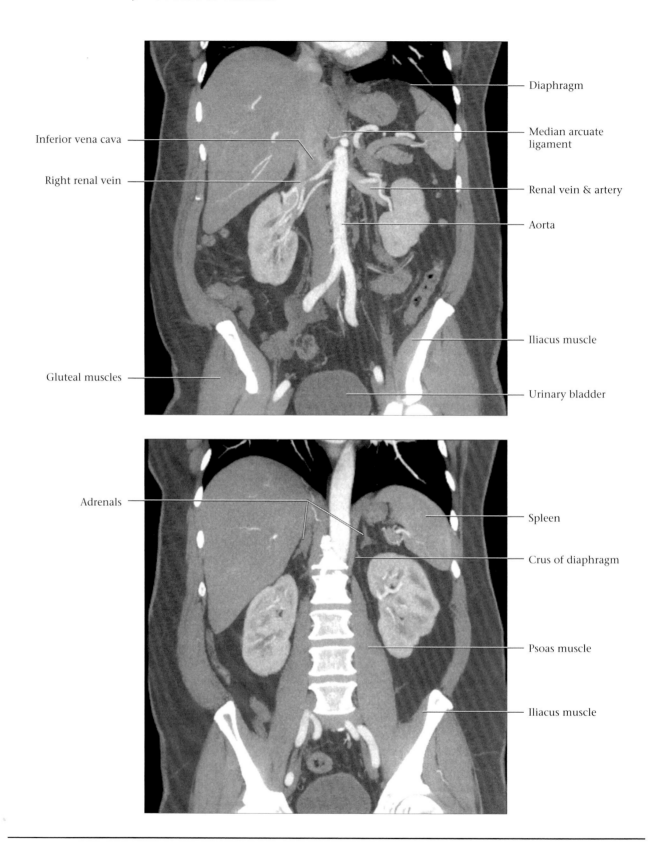

Inferior vena cava

Right renal vein

Gluteal muscles

Diaphragm

Median arcuate ligament

Renal vein & artery

Aorta

Iliacus muscle

Urinary bladder

Adrenals

Spleen

Crus of diaphragm

Psoas muscle

Iliacus muscle

(Top) Aorta enters the abdomen behind the median arcuate ligament, the junction of the diaphragmatic crura. Adrenals lie just lateral to crura. **(Bottom)** Psoas muscle arises from transverse processes and bodies of lumbar vertebrae. After joining iliacus muscle in the pelvis, it passes beneath inguinal ligament to enter thigh and insert on lesser trochanter of femur.

ABDOMINAL WALL

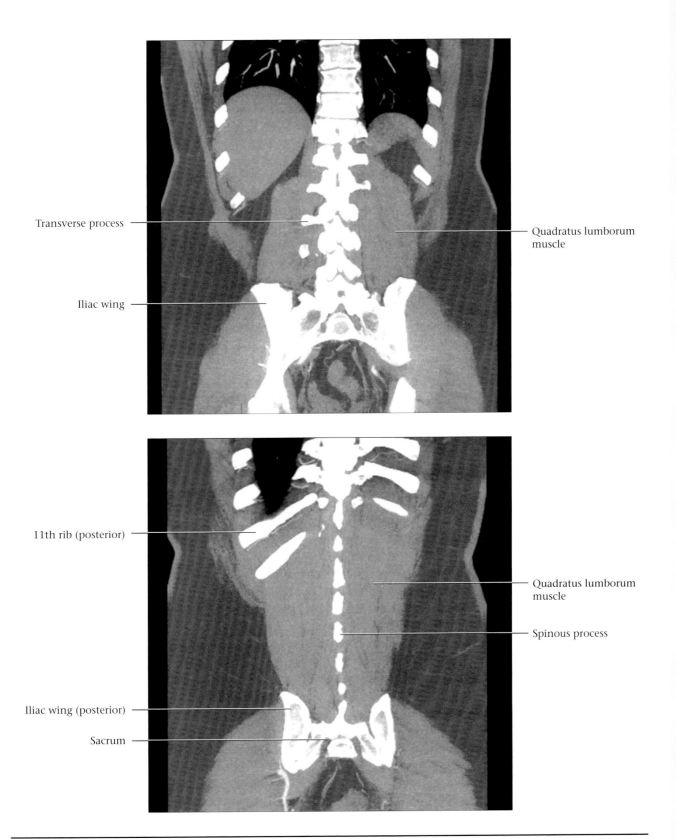

Transverse process

Quadratus lumborum muscle

Iliac wing

11th rib (posterior)

Quadratus lumborum muscle

Spinous process

Iliac wing (posterior)

Sacrum

(Top) Quadratus lumborum muscle arises from the iliac crest, iliolumbar ligament and transverse processes of lumbar vertebrae. (Bottom) Quadratus lumborum passes behind the diaphragm, under the lateral lumbocostal arch (not evident on imaging studies).

ABDOMINAL WALL

ABDOMINAL WALL MUSCLES

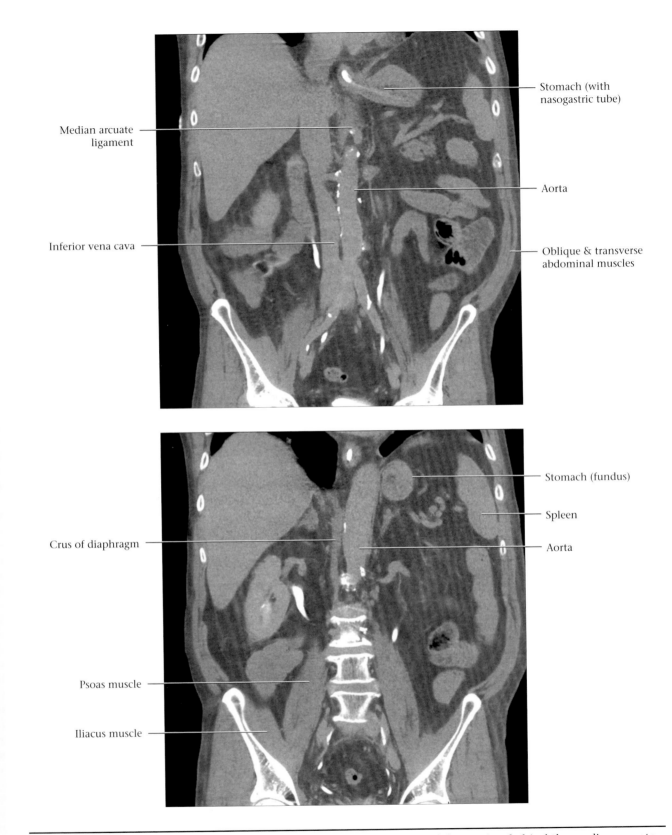

Stomach (with nasogastric tube)

Median arcuate ligament

Aorta

Inferior vena cava

Oblique & transverse abdominal muscles

Crus of diaphragm

Stomach (fundus)

Spleen

Aorta

Psoas muscle

Iliacus muscle

(Top) First of eight coronal CT sections in a 71 year old man. Aorta enters abdomen just behind the median arcuate ligament which connects the crura of the diaphragm. **(Bottom)** Oblique and transverse abdominal muscles stabilize the trunk by attaching to the lower ribs and the iliac crest and inguinal ligament.

ABDOMINAL WALL

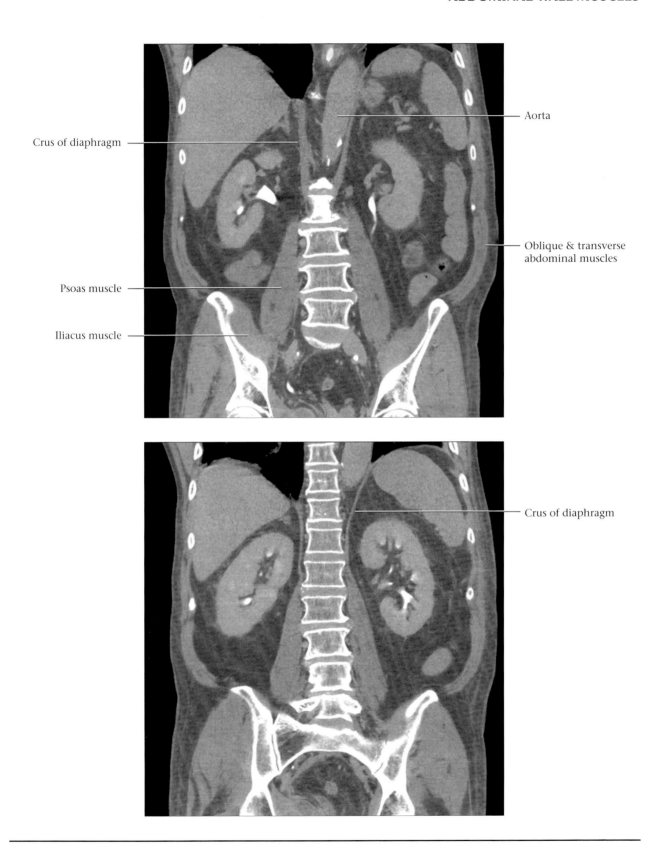

Crus of diaphragm

Aorta

Psoas muscle

Oblique & transverse abdominal muscles

Iliacus muscle

Crus of diaphragm

(Top) Iliacus muscle fills much of the iliac fossa and forms the lateral wall of the abdomino-pelvic cavity. **(Bottom)** Inferior attachments of the diaphragmatic crura and the origins of psoas muscle include upper lumbar vertebrae and the anterior longitudinal ligament which covers them.

ABDOMINAL WALL

ABDOMINAL WALL MUSCLES

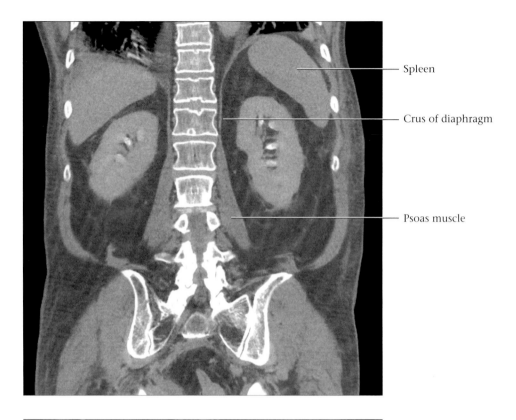

- Spleen
- Crus of diaphragm
- Psoas muscle

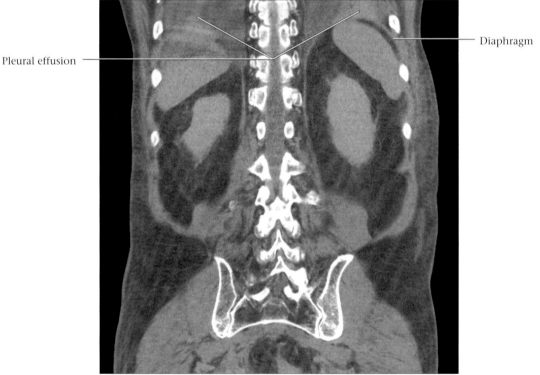

- Diaphragm
- Pleural effusion

(Top) Abdominal wall muscles are thin and lax in this elderly man. **(Bottom)** Note the pleural effusion above the diaphragm.

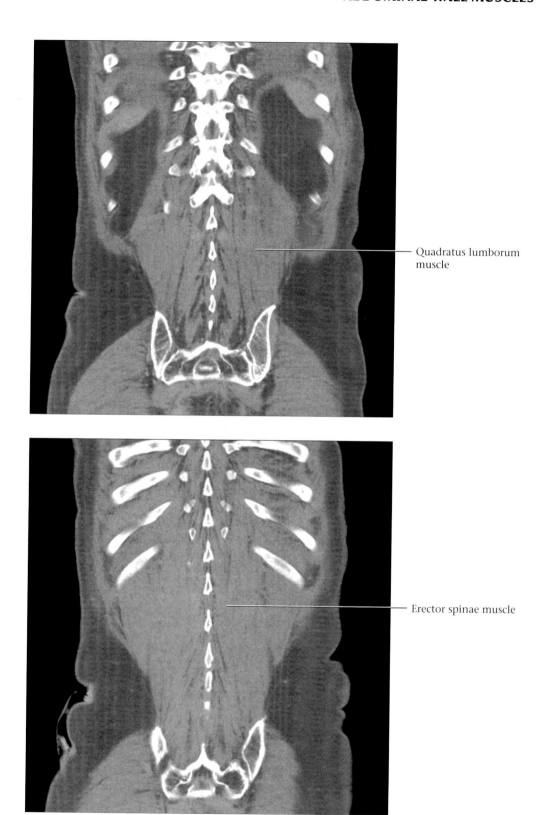

Quadratus lumborum muscle

Erector spinae muscle

(Top) Quadratus lumborum muscle stabilizes the spine and pelvis, connecting 12th rib to transverse processes of lumbar vertebrae and to the iliac crest and iliolumbar ligament. **(Bottom)** More posteriorly, erector spinae muscles stabilize the spine.

ABDOMINAL WALL

RECTUS HEMORRHAGE INTO PERIVESICAL SPACE

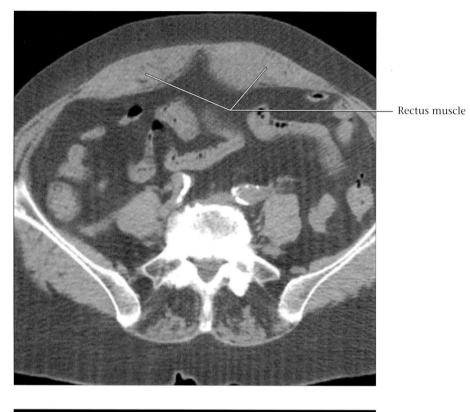

Rectus muscle

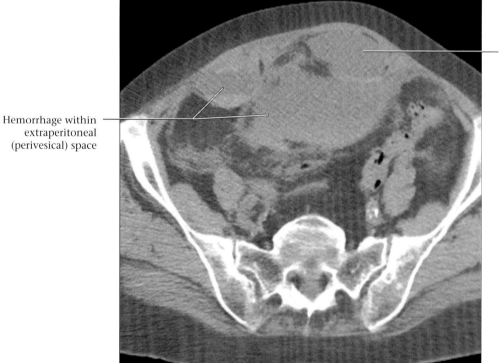

Hemorrhage within rectus muscle

Hemorrhage within extraperitoneal (perivesical) space

(Top) First of five axial CT images depicting a spontaneous abdominal wall and extraperitoneal hemorrhage in an elderly woman receiving anticoagulant medication. The rectus muscles are enlarged due to hemorrhage within the rectus sheath. (Bottom) Hemorrhage has "leaked" through the incomplete posterior layer of the rectus sheath to extend into the extraperitoneal pelvis. Note the cellular-fluid levels within the hemorrhage, called the "hematocrit sign", indicative of a coagulopathic hemorrhage.

ABDOMINAL WALL

RECTUS HEMORRHAGE INTO PERIVESICAL SPACE

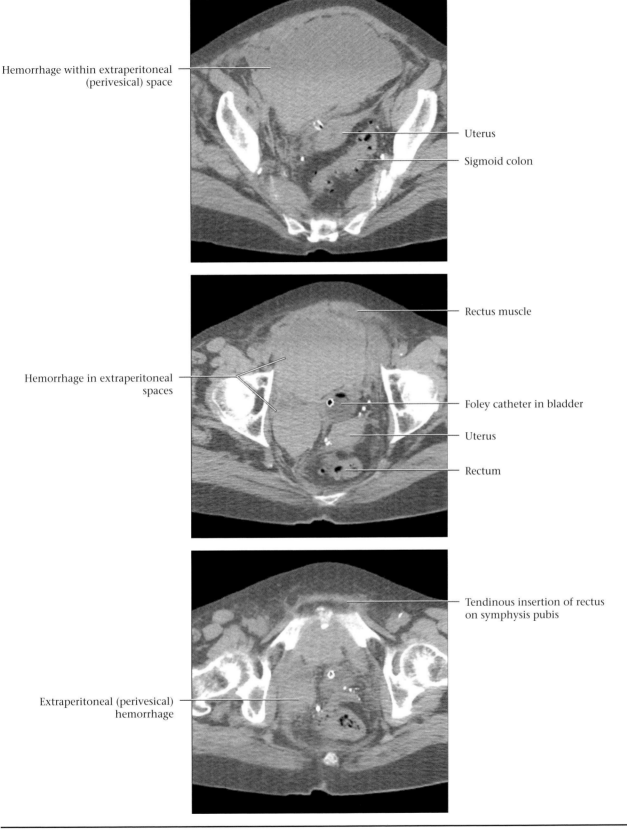

Hemorrhage within extraperitoneal (perivesical) space

Uterus

Sigmoid colon

Rectus muscle

Hemorrhage in extraperitoneal spaces

Foley catheter in bladder

Uterus

Rectum

Tendinous insertion of rectus on symphysis pubis

Extraperitoneal (perivesical) hemorrhage

(Top) Note the large abdominal extraperitoneal hemorrhage, with the "hematocrit sign". **(Middle)** The abdominal extraperitoneal spaces communicate caudally with the pelvic extraperitoneal spaces, including perivesical space. **(Bottom)** The pelvic hemorrhage displaces the uterus, bladder and rectum.

PANNUS SIMULATING VENTRAL HERNIA

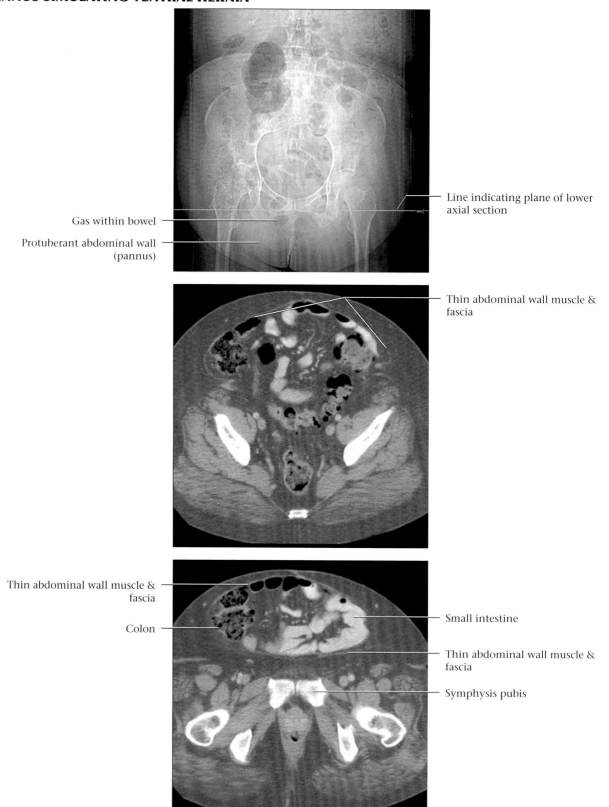

Line indicating plane of lower axial section

Gas within bowel

Protuberant abdominal wall (pannus)

Thin abdominal wall muscle & fascia

Thin abdominal wall muscle & fascia

Colon

Small intestine

Thin abdominal wall muscle & fascia

Symphysis pubis

(Top) Elderly woman with a protuberant abdomen simulating a ventral hernia. Frontal computed radiograph shows obese abdomen and bowel gas below level of symphysis pubis. **(Middle)** First of two axial CT sections in the same patient as previous image shows the thin abdominal wall is stretched and elongated, allowing anterior and caudal protrusion of abdominal contents (pannus). **(Bottom)** This image shows bowel in pannus below the symphysis pubis.

ABDOMINAL WALL

VENTRAL HERNIA, INCARCERATED CAUSING BOWEL OBSTRUCTION

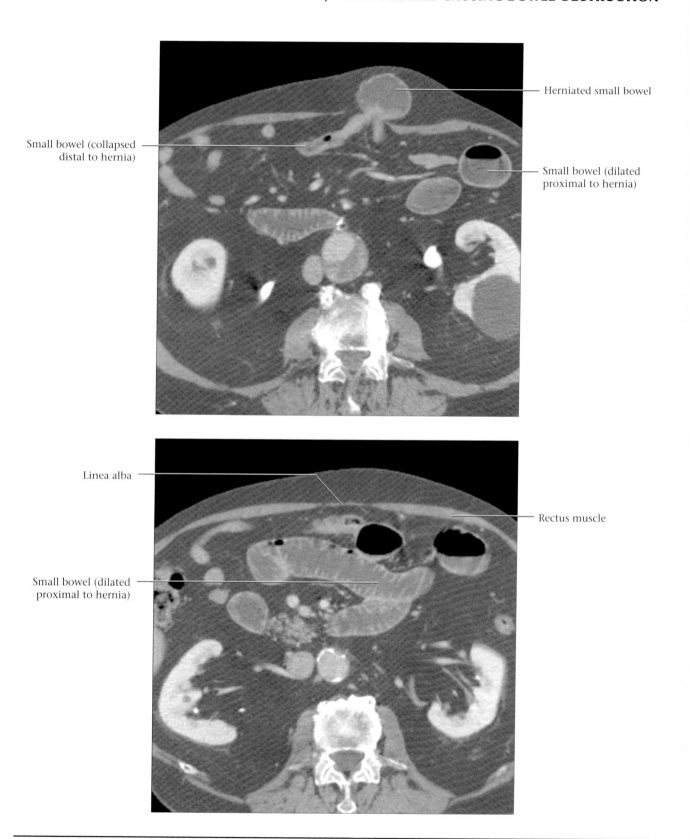

Herniated small bowel

Small bowel (collapsed distal to hernia)

Small bowel (dilated proximal to hernia)

Linea alba

Rectus muscle

Small bowel (dilated proximal to hernia)

(Top) First of two axial CT images shows a segment of small intestine herniated through a defect in the linea alba. The hernia is "incarcerated" (nonreducible). **(Bottom)** Small intestine is dilated upstream from the ventral hernia and collapsed downstream, indicating that the hernia is causing bowel obstruction.

ABDOMINAL WALL

INCISIONAL HERNIA CONTAINING COLON

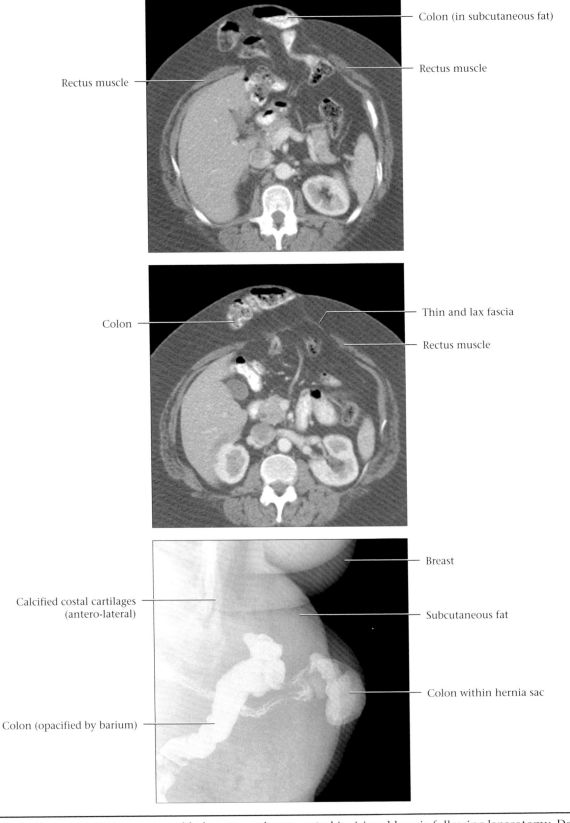

Colon (in subcutaneous fat)

Rectus muscle

Rectus muscle

Colon

Thin and lax fascia

Rectus muscle

Breast

Calcified costal cartilages (antero-lateral)

Subcutaneous fat

Colon within hernia sac

Colon (opacified by barium)

(Top) First of two axial CT images in a elderly woman shows ventral incisional hernia following laparotomy. Defect in anterior abdominal wall (through the linea alba) allows herniation of colon and omental fat. **(Middle)** Rectus muscles, linea alba and aponeuroses are thin and stretched. **(Bottom)** Lateral view of barium enema in the same patient as previous two images. Colon is herniated into the subcutaneous fat, with no overlying muscle.

ABDOMINAL WALL

INGUINAL HERNIA CAUSING SMALL BOWEL OBSTRUCTION

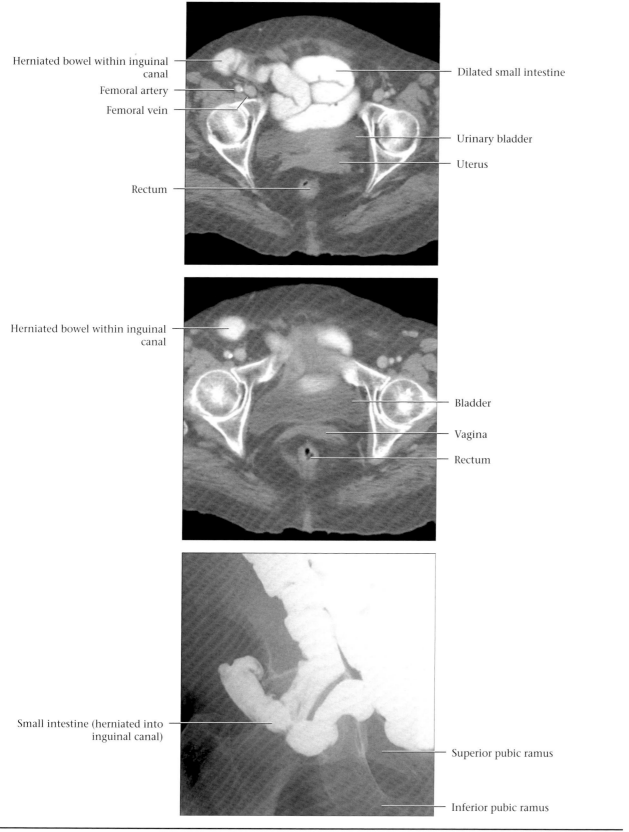

Herniated bowel within inguinal canal

Femoral artery

Femoral vein

Rectum

Dilated small intestine

Urinary bladder

Uterus

Herniated bowel within inguinal canal

Bladder

Vagina

Rectum

Small intestine (herniated into inguinal canal)

Superior pubic ramus

Inferior pubic ramus

(Top) First of two axial CT images in a elderly woman with inguinal hernia causing small bowel obstruction. Note the dilated small intestine and collapsed rectum. **(Middle)** A segment of small intestine has herniated into the inguinal canal and is causing the bowel obstruction. **(Bottom)** Barium small bowel follow through in the same patient as previous two images shows a portion of dilated small bowel is trapped within the inguinal canal, causing the bowel obstruction.

ABDOMINAL WALL

SPIGELIAN HERNIA CAUSING COLONIC OBSTRUCTION

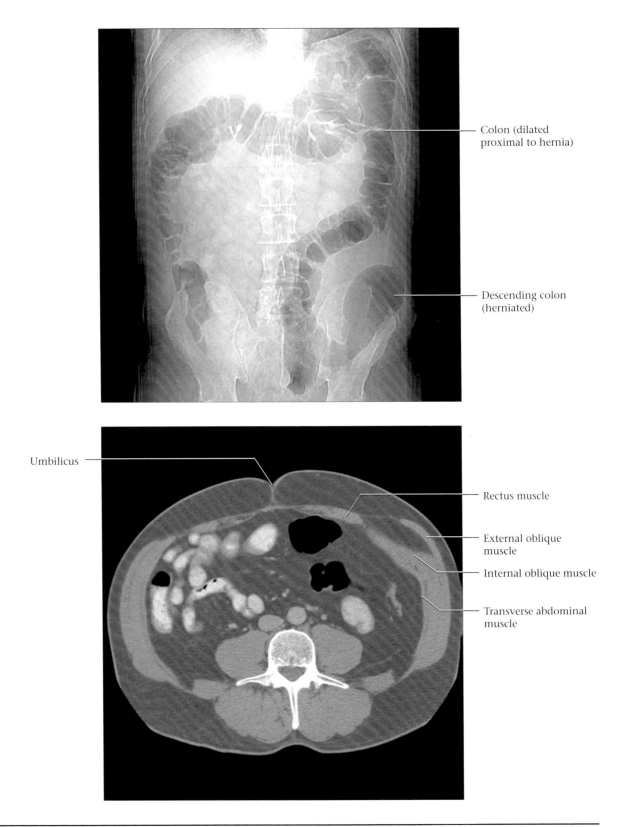

Colon (dilated proximal to hernia)

Descending colon (herniated)

Umbilicus

Rectus muscle

External oblique muscle

Internal oblique muscle

Transverse abdominal muscle

(**Top**) Supine radiograph shows dilated colon and abrupt angulation and herniation of the descending colon in a 59 year old man. (**Bottom**) First of four axial CT sections in same patient as previous image.

ABDOMINAL WALL

SPIGELIAN HERNIA CAUSING COLONIC OBSTRUCTION

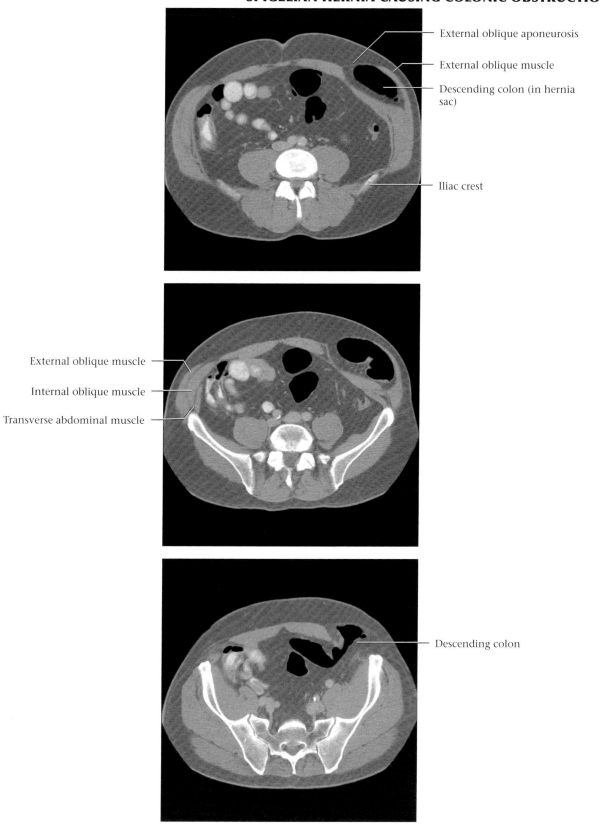

External oblique aponeurosis

External oblique muscle

Descending colon (in hernia sac)

Iliac crest

External oblique muscle

Internal oblique muscle

Transverse abdominal muscle

Descending colon

(Top) Descending colon has herniated into the subcutaneous fat and is covered only by external oblique muscle and aponeurosis. **(Middle)** Compare with the intact muscles of the right anterior abdominal wall. **(Bottom)** Colon herniates through a defect in the aponeurosis of the internal oblique and transverse abdominal muscles.

ABDOMINAL WALL

LUMBAR HERNIA

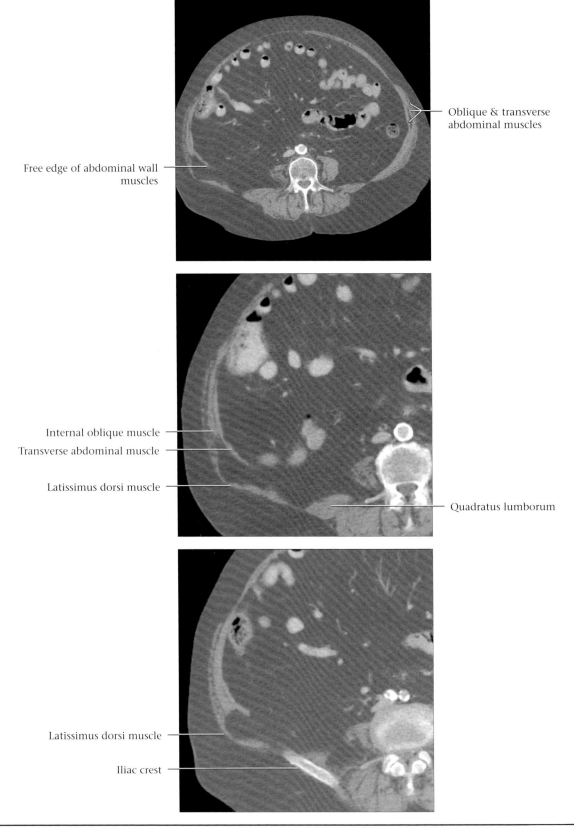

Oblique & transverse abdominal muscles

Free edge of abdominal wall muscles

Internal oblique muscle

Transverse abdominal muscle

Latissimus dorsi muscle

Quadratus lumborum

Latissimus dorsi muscle

Iliac crest

(Top) First of three axial CT sections in a elderly man with a bulge near his iliac crest. The abdomen has excessive fat and thin abdominal wall muscles. Abdominal fat bulges out through inferior lumbar triangle. **(Middle)** There is a defect in abdominal wall (aponeuroses of oblique and transverse abdominal muscles) covered only by latissimus dorsi muscle. **(Bottom)** The oblique and transverse abdominal muscles fail to attach to iliac crest and thoracolumbar fascia, resulting in a lumbar hernia.

ABDOMINAL WALL

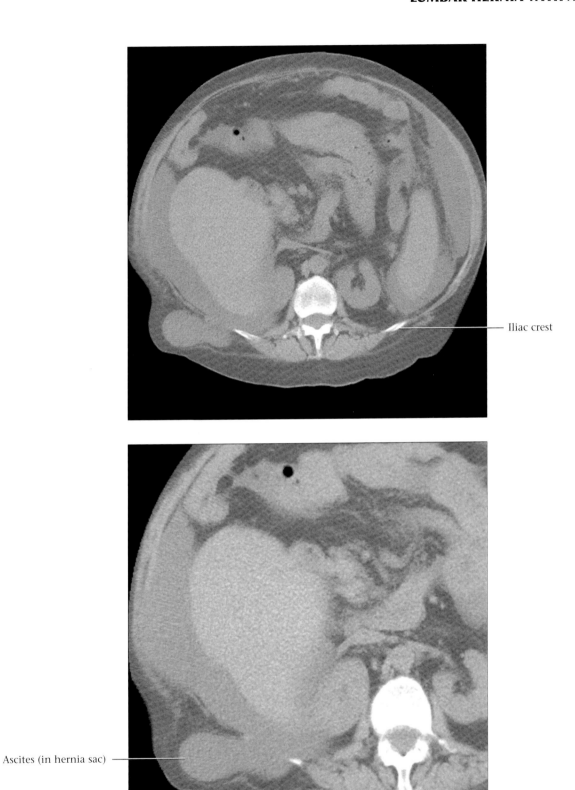

Iliac crest

Ascites (in hernia sac)

(Top) First of two axial CT images shows lumbar hernia with ascites in a 58 year old woman. The abdominal wall muscles are very thin and weak. **(Bottom)** Parietal peritoneum and ascites have herniated through a defect in the aponeuroses of the internal oblique and transverse abdominal muscles.

DIAPHRAGM

Gross Anatomy

Diaphragm Components

- Muscular portions originate from thoracolumbar abdominal wall and converge medially as an aponeurosis (central tendon)
  - **Central tendon** is fused to the fibrous pericardium, but has no osseous attachment
- Origins
  - Anterior: **Xiphoid process**
  - Anterolateral: Ribs & costal cartilage margins 7-12
    - Interdigitate with transverse abdominal muscle
  - Posterolateral: Lumbar vertebrae via the crura and arcuate ligaments
    - **Crura of diaphragm** blend with anterior longitudinal ligament of the vertebral column
    - Right crus is longer than left, extends down to L3 vertebra (left to L2)
    - Fibers of right crus surround esophageal hiatus
  - **Arcuate ligaments** are three, give rise to diaphragm posteriorly
    - **Median arcuate ligament** unites both crura
    - Median arcuate ligament passes over anterior surface of aorta (and can compress the celiac artery in some individuals)
    - **Medial arcuate ligaments** attach to thoracolumbar fascia over the psoas muscles
    - **Lateral arcuate ligaments** attach to thoracolumbar fascia over quadratus lumborum muscles
    - **Vertebrocostal triangle** is a thin membrane that may result from failure of the arcuate ligament to reach the 12th rib
- Apertures of diaphragm
  - **Vena caval foramen** is in the right side of the central tendon
    - Usually located at T8 vertebral level
    - May also transmit the right phrenic nerve
  - **Esophageal hiatus** is just left of midline and passes through the right crus of diaphragm
    - Usually at the level of T10 vertebra
    - Also transmits **vagus nerves** and esophageal branches of **left gastric vessels**
  - **Aortic hiatus**
    - Actually passes posterior to the diaphragm and the median arcuate ligament (**retrocrural space**)
    - Also transmits **thoracic duct** and **azygous and hemiazygous veins**, individual lymph nodes, sympathetic trunk
- Actions of diaphragm
  - Chief muscle of respiration
  - Diaphragm descends to increase thoracic volume and decrease intra-thoracic pressure
  - Helps circulation of blood by creating reciprocal increases/decreases in thoracic/abdominal pressure
  - Helps raise intra-abdominal pressure for defecation, micturition and childbirth

Anatomy-Based Imaging Issues

Imaging Recommendations

- Diaphragm is difficult to demonstrate on transverse CT or MR
  - Coronal or sagittal plane images show the diaphragm better
  - Sonography shows diaphragm as echogenic line
- **Diaphragmatic insertions** on the thoracoabdominal wall may take the form of thin "slips" of muscle and tendon, rather than smooth sheet of tissue
  - On axial CT and MR sections these can be mistaken for nodular tumor implants on the peritoneum
  - Keys to recognition are continuity on sequential axial sections and viewing sagittal or coronal sections

Clinical Implications

Clinical Importance

- **Peridiaphragmatic fluid collections** are very common with important clinical implications
  - Pleural effusions lie above or "outside the confines" of the diaphragm
  - Ascites (or a subphrenic abscess) lies below or "within the confines" of the diaphragm
- **Elevation** of one **hemidiaphragm** is common
  - May be caused by abdominal mass displacement
  - May be due to paralysis
  - Phrenic nerve is the sole motor supply to the diaphragm and can be injured by trauma, thoracic surgery or thoracic malignancy
  - Paralysis results in permanent elevation and paradoxical movement of the hemidiaphragm on forced inspiration
  - May be due to congenital thinning (**eventration**)
    - Left > right
- Diaphragm is not always impermeable
  - Ascites, pleural effusion, tumor, pus, extraluminal air may pass from the abdomen into the thorax (and vice versa)
  - **Defects in diaphragm** increase with age and emphysema
- Congenital defects in diaphragm are common
  - Left posterolateral defect at **vertebrocostal triangle** is known as **Bochdalek hernia** (abdominal fat, gut or viscera may herniate into chest)
  - Eventration of diaphragm is thinning or absence of a part of the diaphragm
    - Left > central tendon > right
  - Anterior paramedian defect at **sternocostal hiatus** is known as **Morgagni hernia**
    - Right > left
- Acquired hernias are common
  - **Hiatal hernia**: Widening of the esophageal hiatus, allowing part of the stomach to herniate into the chest
- **Traumatic rupture**: Relatively uncommon, resulting from blunt or penetrating trauma
  - More than 90% are left-sided, through apex or posterior portion

DIAPHRAGM

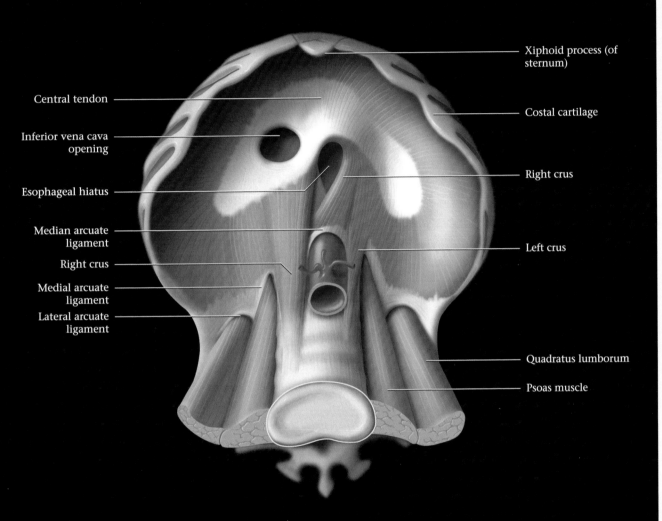

Central tendon

Inferior vena cava opening

Esophageal hiatus

Median arcuate ligament

Right crus

Medial arcuate ligament

Lateral arcuate ligament

Xiphoid process (of sternum)

Costal cartilage

Right crus

Left crus

Quadratus lumborum

Psoas muscle

Graphic view of abdominal surface of diaphragm. Note origins of the diaphragm from the sternum, costal cartilages and lumbar vertebrae and insertion into the trefoil-shaped central tendon, the fibrous aponeurosis of diaphragmatic muscle fibers. Inferior vena cava (IVC) hiatus is through the central tendon. The esophageal hiatus is surrounded by the right crus. The median arcuate ligament unites the crura and passes over the aorta just above the celiac axis. The right crus is longer and thicker than the left, and both insert into the anterior longitudinal ligament of the lumbar spine. The psoas passes behind the medial arcuate ligament, and the quadratus lumborum behind the lateral arcuate ligament.

DIAPHRAGM

NORMAL AXIAL CT SECTIONS, DIAPHRAGM & CRURA

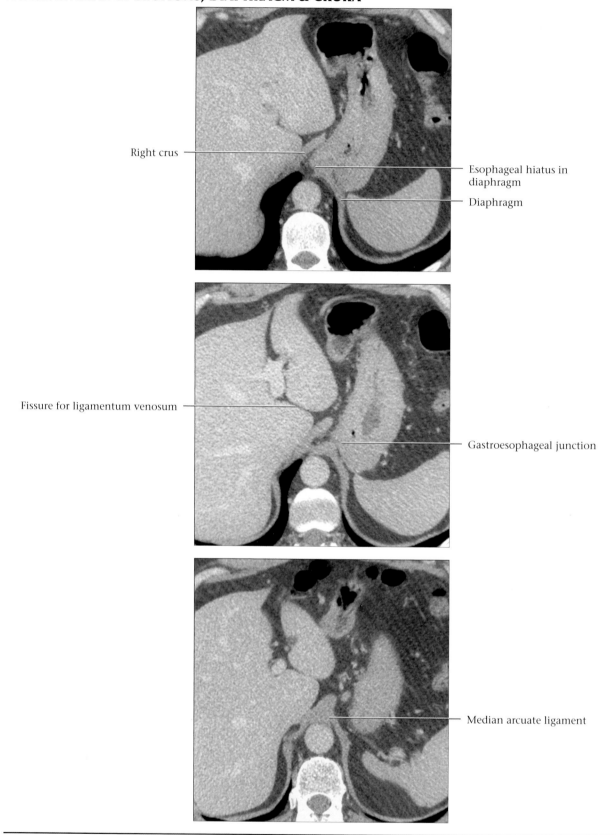

Right crus — Esophageal hiatus in diaphragm — Diaphragm

Fissure for ligamentum venosum — Gastroesophageal junction

Median arcuate ligament

(**Top**) First of six axial CT sections shows the esophagus entering the abdomen through a decussation (crossing) of fibers of the right crus. (**Middle**) The gastroesophageal junction lies just caudal to the esophageal hiatus at the level of the fissure for the ligamentum venosum. (**Bottom**) The musculotendinous arch of the median arcuate ligament joins the two crura.

DIAPHRAGM

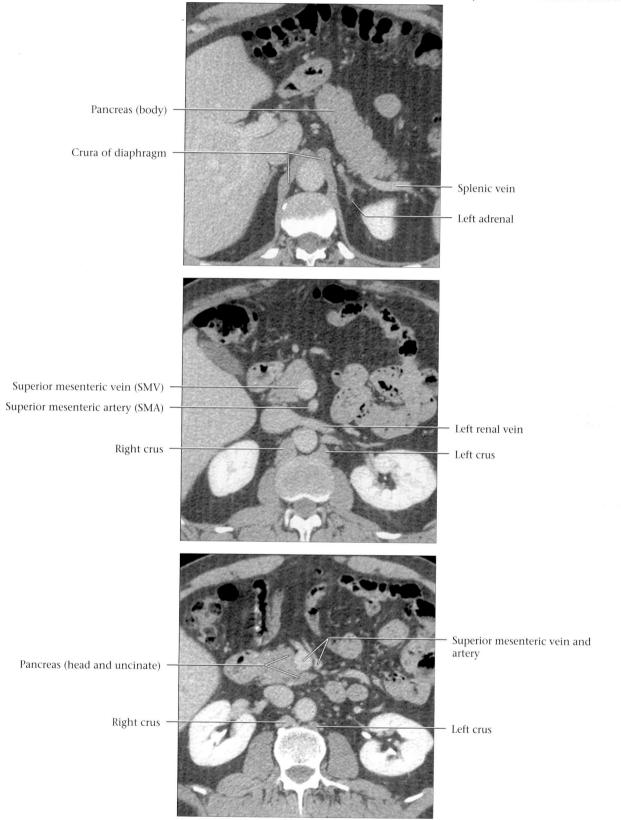

Pancreas (body)

Crura of diaphragm

Splenic vein

Left adrenal

Superior mesenteric vein (SMV)

Superior mesenteric artery (SMA)

Right crus

Left renal vein

Left crus

Pancreas (head and uncinate)

Superior mesenteric vein and artery

Right crus

Left crus

(Top) The crura may appear somewhat nodular. The adrenals lie just lateral to the crura. **(Middle)** The right crus is usually thicker and longer than the left, inserting lower along the lumbar spine (at L3 level). **(Bottom)** On axial CT sections the crus may be mistaken for an enlarged periaortic lymph node.

DIAPHRAGM

AORTIC & ESOPHAGEAL OPENINGS

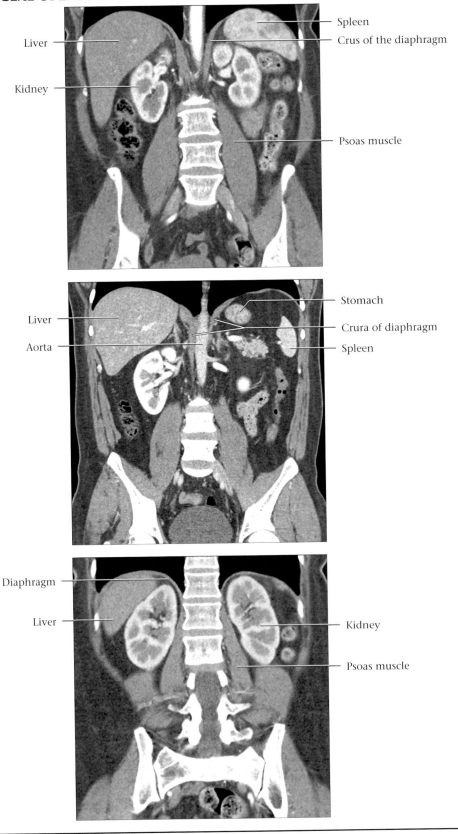

(Top) First of three coronal CT sections shows aorta entering abdomen between and behind the crura. Psoas enters abdomen behind medial arcuate ligament, which is difficult to display on imaging. **(Middle)** The diaphragm is a smooth sheet of muscle in this patient. **(Bottom)** Most dorsal section shows diaphragmatic origins on lower ribs and costal cartilages.

DIAPHRAGM

AORTIC & ESOPHAGEAL OPENINGS

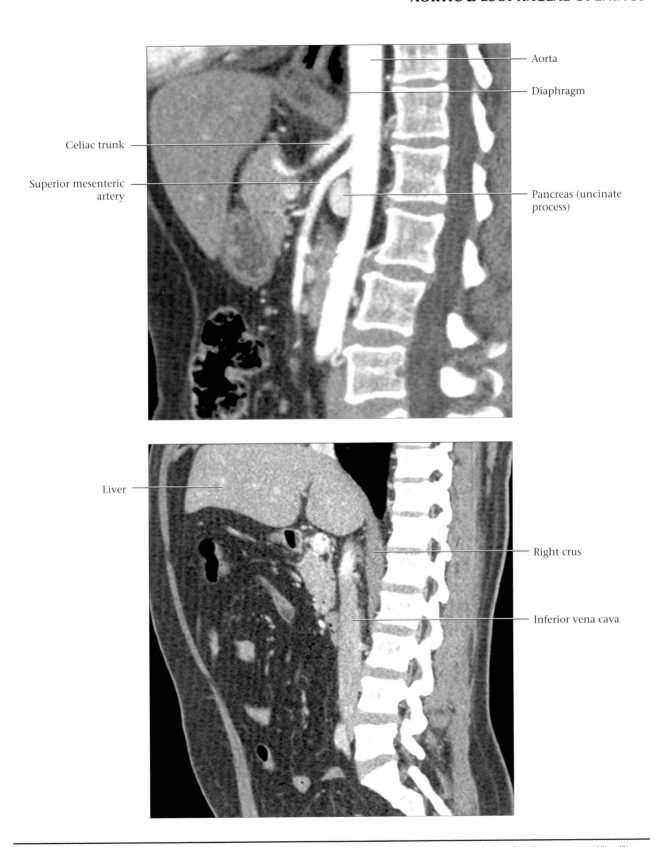

(Top) First of two sagittal CT sections showing the aorta entering the abdomen behind the diaphragm, specifically, the median arcuate ligament. Note the normal origin of celiac trunk from the proximal abdominal aorta. (Bottom) Sagittal section to the right of the previous image shows the inferior vena cava approaching its diaphragmatic hiatus. The right crus originates along the lumbar vertebrae.

DIAPHRAGM

CORONAL & AXIAL CT, DIAPHRAGM

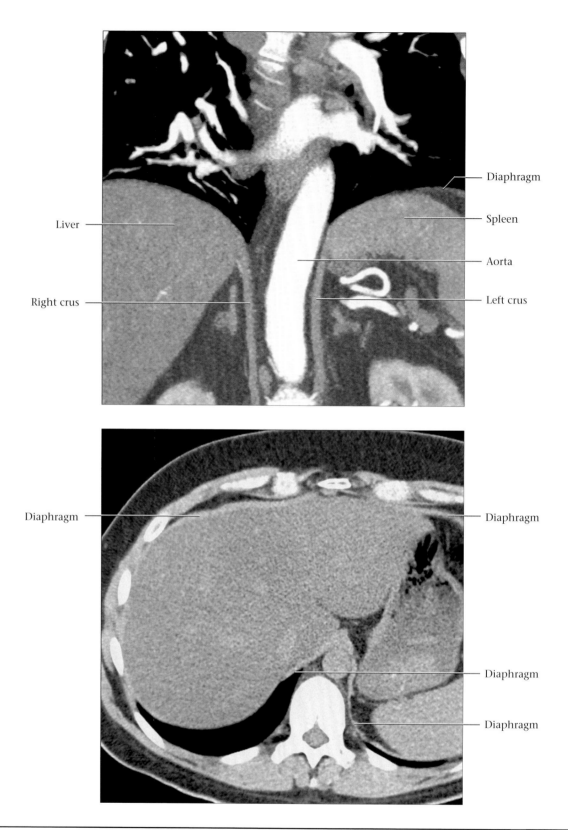

Liver

Diaphragm

Spleen

Aorta

Right crus

Left crus

Diaphragm

Diaphragm

Diaphragm

Diaphragm

(Top) Coronal CT section. The diaphragm is a smooth sheet of tissue that abuts the liver and spleen and is often hard to distinguish on imaging because it is of similar attenuation (density) as these organs. **(Bottom)** Axial CT section. Because of steatosis, the liver is of low density and diaphragm is seen as a distinct "white" curvilinear structure.

DIAPHRAGM

NORMAL DIAPHRAGM, DEMONSTRATION OF CRURA & GE JUNCTION

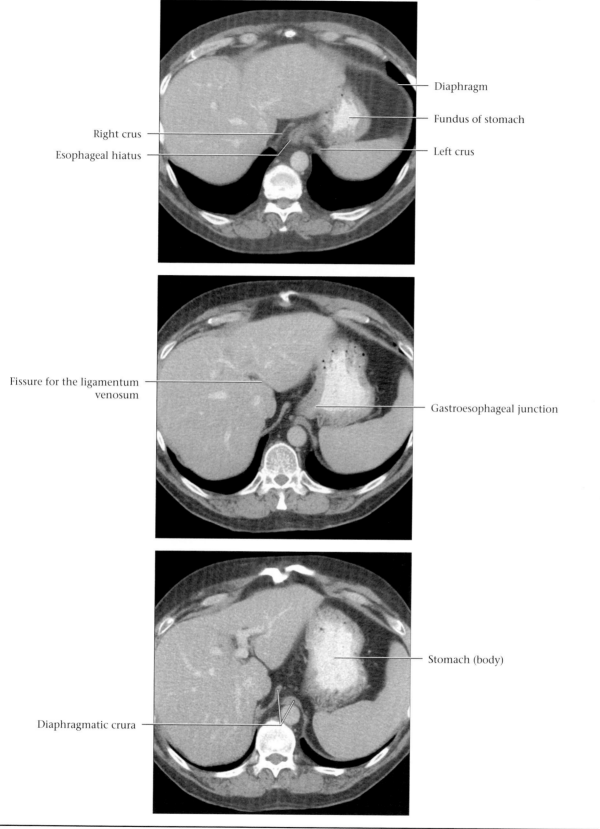

(Top) First of three axial CT sections shows the esophagus entering the abdomen through its diaphragmatic hiatus, surrounded by the right crus of diaphragm. Compression of the esophagus by the crus contributes to lower esophageal sphincter function. **(Middle)** The gastroesophageal (GE) junction is normally at about the same transverse plane as the fissure for the ligamentum venosum of the liver. **(Bottom)** Caudal to the esophagus hiatus, the crura join at the median arcuate ligament (just below this section).

DIAPHRAGM

DIAPHRAGM & GE JUNCTION IN MULTIPLE PLANES

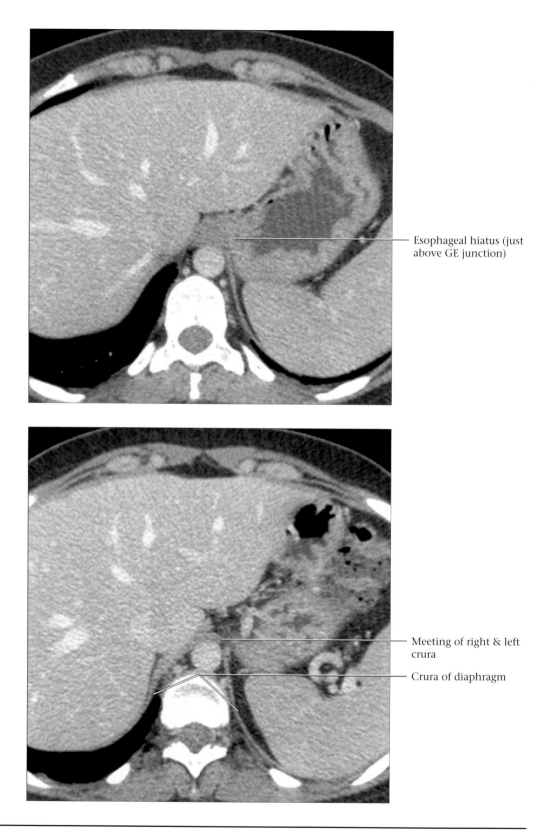

Esophageal hiatus (just above GE junction)

Meeting of right & left crura

Crura of diaphragm

(Top) First of four CT sections of a young man. The gastroesophageal junction is usually seen as a prominent soft tissue thickening, comprised of the muscular walls and submucosa of the esophagus and stomach. **(Bottom)** Axial CT section just below the esophageal hiatus. The right and left crura join at the midline just in front of the aorta.

DIAPHRAGM

DIAPHRAGM & GE JUNCTION IN MULTIPLE PLANES

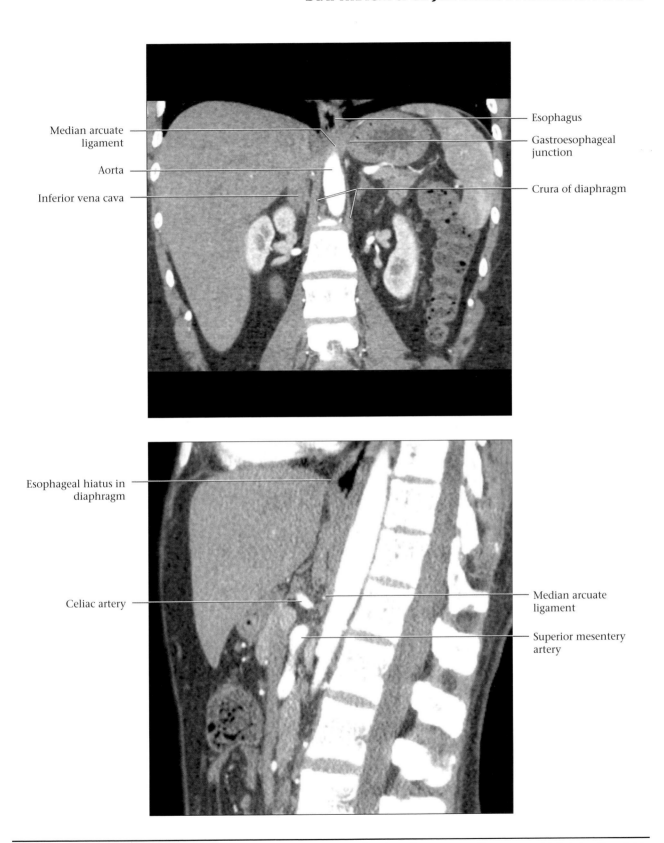

Median arcuate ligament

Aorta

Inferior vena cava

Esophagus

Gastroesophageal junction

Crura of diaphragm

Esophageal hiatus in diaphragm

Celiac artery

Median arcuate ligament

Superior mesentery artery

(Top) Coronal CT section shows aorta entering abdomen just behind median arcuate ligament, which joins the right and left crura. **(Bottom)** Sagittal CT section. The esophageal hiatus is usually just left and ventral to the aortic hiatus, but is also considerably more cephalic. The aortic "hiatus" is marked by the median arcuate ligament and its impression on the celiac trunk.

DIAPHRAGM

DIAPHRAGMATIC OPENINGS & MEDIAN ARCUATE LIGAMENT

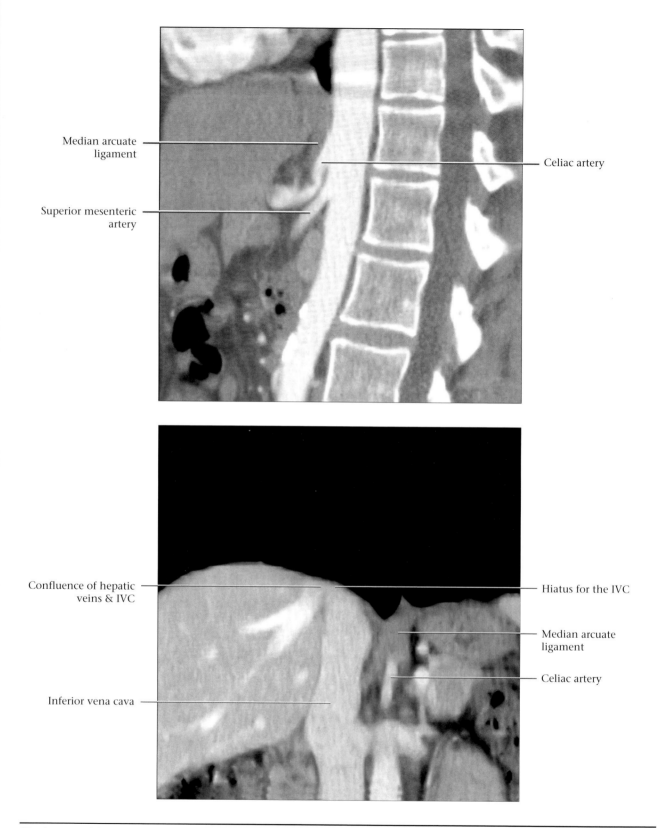

(Top) First of four CT sections of young woman with abdominal pain. Sagittal CT section shows extrinsic indentation of the celiac artery by the median arcuate ligament. **(Bottom)** Coronal CT section shows celiac artery and the tendinous arch of the median arcuate ligament, which impinges upon it.

DIAPHRAGM

DIAPHRAGMATIC OPENINGS & MEDIAN ARCUATE LIGAMENT

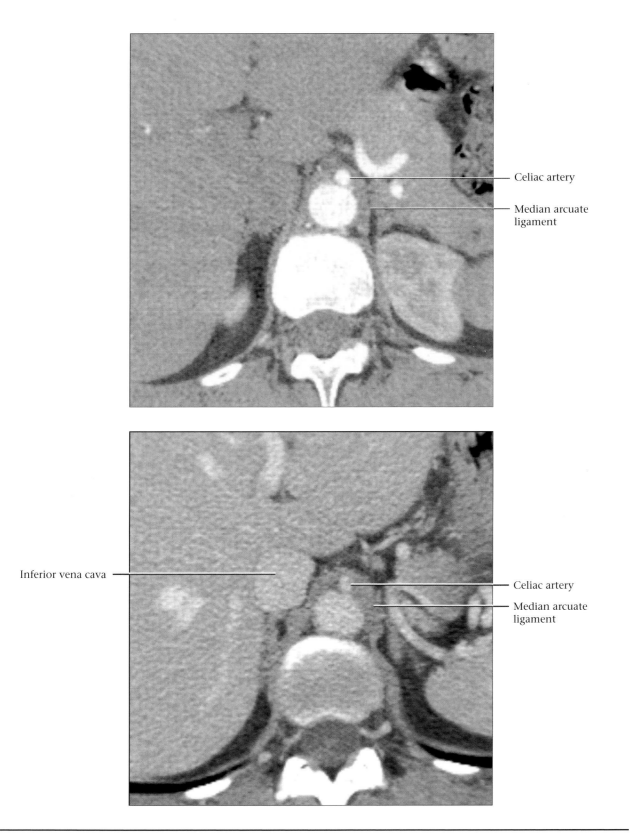

Celiac artery

Median arcuate ligament

Inferior vena cava

Celiac artery

Median arcuate ligament

(Top) Arterial phase, axial CT shows compression of the proximal celiac artery against the aorta. **(Bottom)** Median arcuate ligament is seen as a musculotendinous arch closely applied to the aorta and celiac artery.

DIAPHRAGM

SAGITTAL CT, MEDIAN ARCUATE LIGAMENT

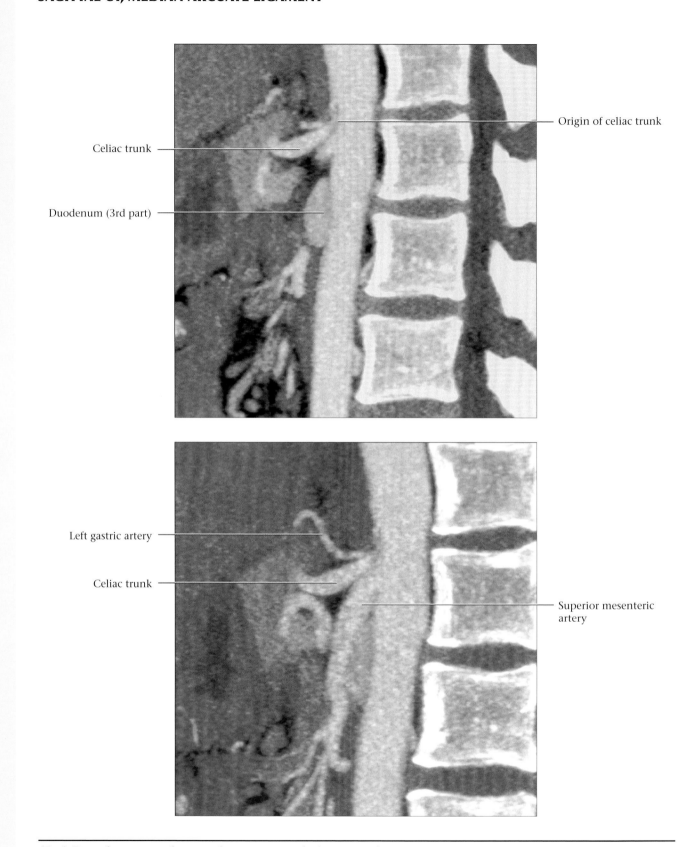

Celiac trunk

Duodenum (3rd part)

Origin of celiac trunk

Left gastric artery

Celiac trunk

Superior mesenteric artery

(**Top**) First of two sagittal views of contrast-opacified arteries of a 30 year old man shows sharply angulated and narrowed origin of the celiac trunk at its origin from the aorta. (The left gastric artery has a separate origin in this patient and is also acutely angled and compressed). (**Bottom**) Post-stenotic dilation of the celiac trunk is present and the proximal celiac artery is compressed against the superior mesenteric artery. Findings are characteristic of compression of the celiac trunk by the median arcuate ligament.

DIAPHRAGM

DIAPHRAGM WITH LOOSE CRUS & HIATAL HERNIA

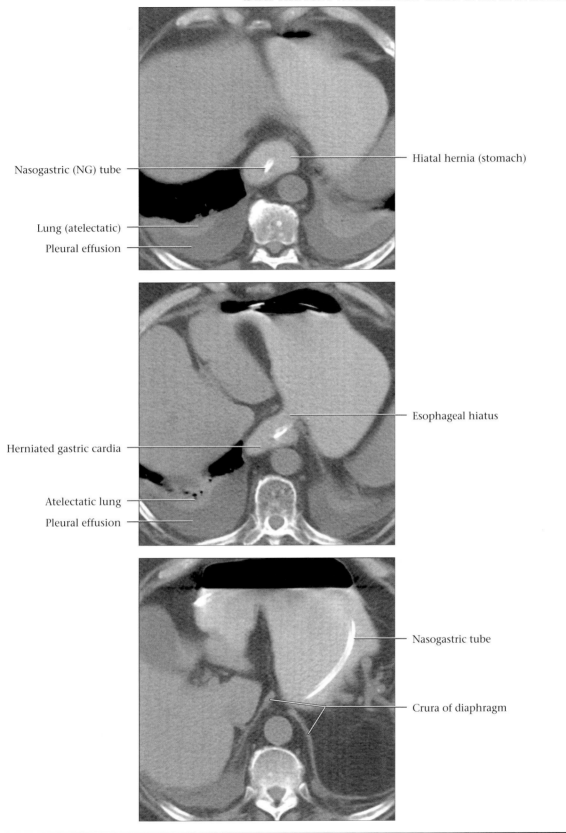

Nasogastric (NG) tube

Lung (atelectatic)

Pleural effusion

Hiatal hernia (stomach)

Esophageal hiatus

Herniated gastric cardia

Atelectatic lung

Pleural effusion

Nasogastric tube

Crura of diaphragm

(Top) First of three axial CT sections in a elderly woman with gastro-esophageal reflux. The gastric cardia has herniated into the mediastinum. **(Middle)** The esophageal hiatus is patulous, and the distal esophagus is not compressed (as it should be) by the right crus. This allows the stomach to herniate, and gastric contents to reflux up into the esophagus. **(Bottom)** The crura are thin and spaced apart, instead of having joined together in the midline at this level.

DIAPHRAGM

DIAPHRAGM WITH PROMINENT SLIPS

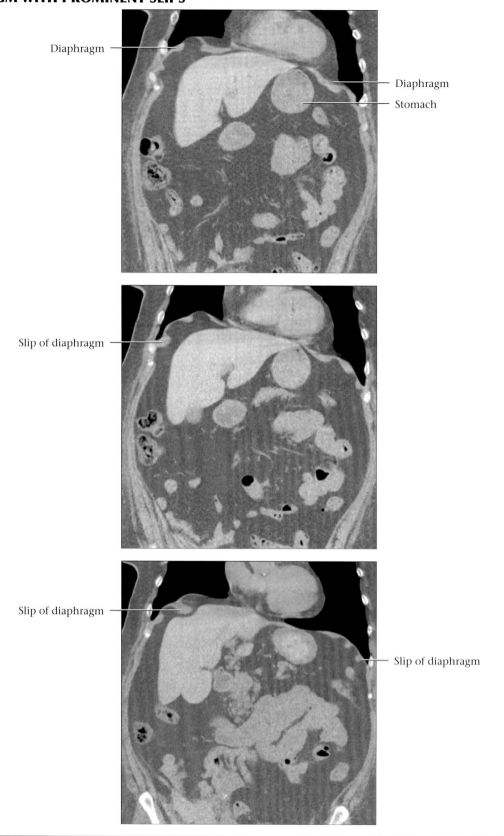

(Top) First of three coronal sections in a elderly woman. Instead of being a smooth sheet of muscle, the diaphragm may have finger-like "slips" of muscle fibers that extend toward points of attachment along the chest wall. (Middle) On individual sections, the "slips" may appear as nodular "lesions", but can be followed as long thin structures on contiguous sections. (Bottom) One slip of diaphragm indents the superior surface of the liver. Note the nodular appearance of the left hemidiaphragm on this section.

DIAPHRAGM

DIAPHRAGM WITH PROMINENT SLIPS

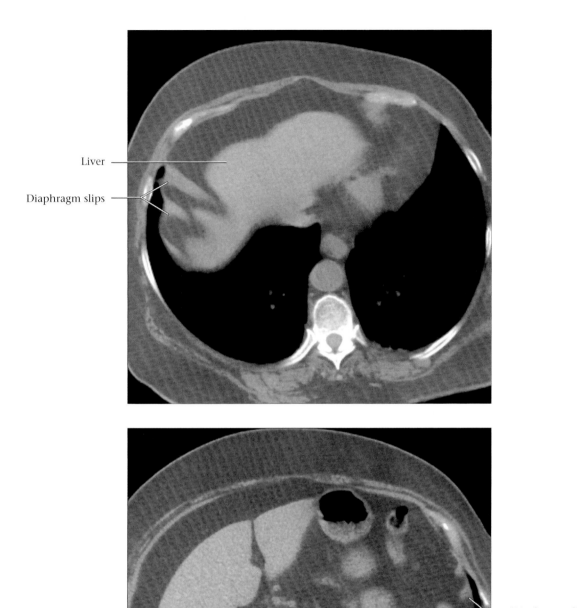

Liver

Diaphragm slips

Diaphragm slips

(Top) First of two axial CT sections in same patient as previous three images. The finger-like "slips" of diaphragm may indent the surface of the liver or spleen; they are outlined by subdiaphragmatic fat. **(Bottom)** On individual CT sections, the slips may appear as nodular lesions but can be recognized as long thin structures on contiguous sections that extend to the chest wall.

DIAPHRAGM

DIAPHRAGM SEPARATING PLEURAL & PERITONEAL FLUID COLLECTIONS

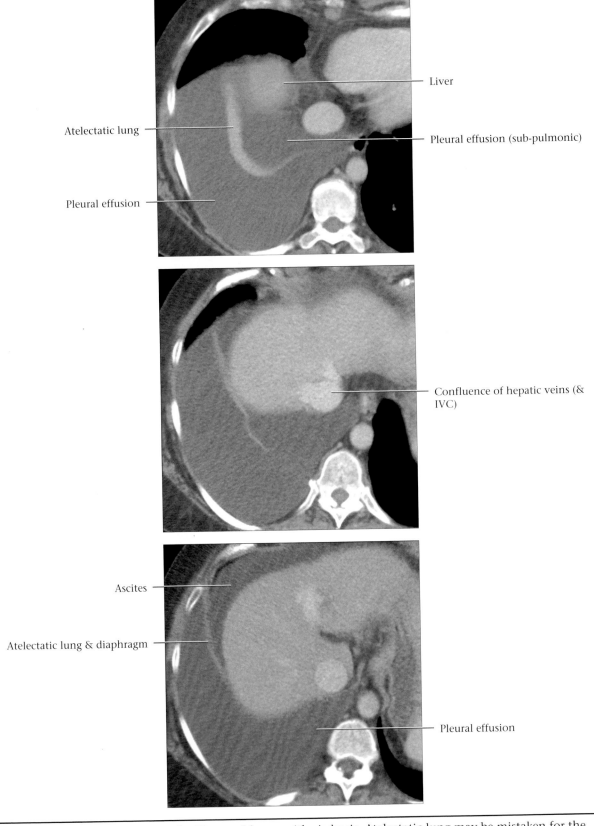

Liver

Atelectatic lung

Pleural effusion (sub-pulmonic)

Pleural effusion

Confluence of hepatic veins (& IVC)

Ascites

Atelectatic lung & diaphragm

Pleural effusion

(Top) First of five axial CT sections of a 45 year old man with cirrhosis. Atelectatic lung may be mistaken for the diaphragm, but it is surrounded by a subpulmonic pleural effusion. **(Middle)** Atelectatic lung and diaphragm are held close together by the inferior pulmonary ligament. **(Bottom)** Note the "fuzzy" interface between the pleural effusion and the surface of the liver, while ascites has a sharp interface, since it lies immediately next to the liver, not separated by the diaphragm.

DIAPHRAGM

DIAPHRAGM SEPARATING PLEURAL & PERITONEAL FLUID COLLECTIONS

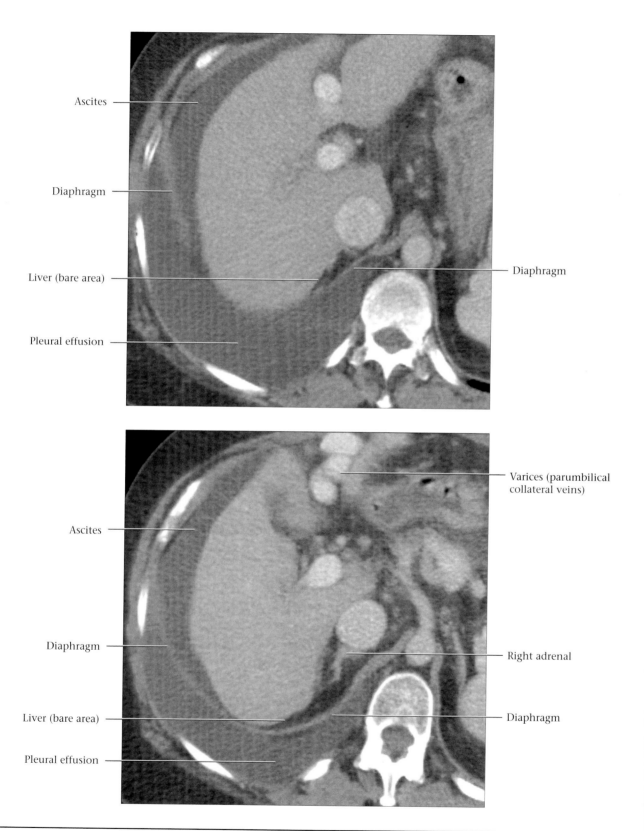

(Top) Ascites and other abdominal contents are suspended away from the postero-lateral chest wall by the diaphragm. (Bottom) The diaphragm separates the thorax from the abdomen. Pleural fluid lies above and "outside the confines of" the diaphragm, while ascites lies below and within the confines of the diaphragm. Ascites cannot contact the "bare" (nonperitonealized) surface of the liver.

DIAPHRAGM

ELEVATED HEMIDIAPHRAGM, PHRENIC NERVE INJURY

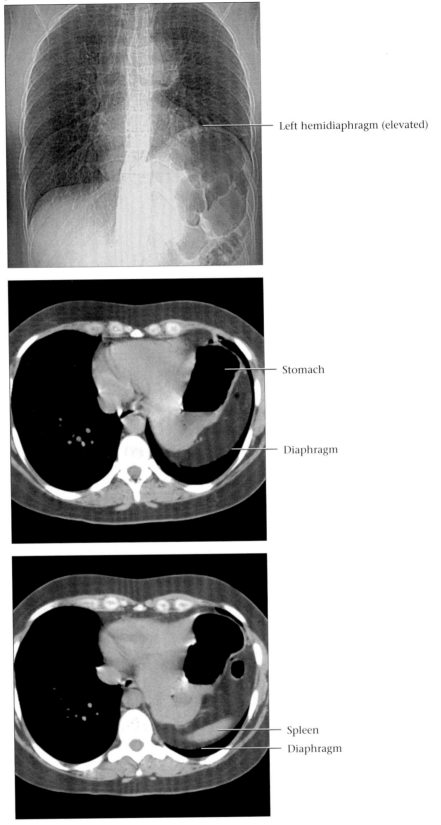

Left hemidiaphragm (elevated)

Stomach

Diaphragm

Spleen

Diaphragm

(Top) Frontal radiograph shows marked elevation of the left hemidiaphragm. **(Middle)** The diaphragm is very thin and is difficult to see as a distinct structure. **(Bottom)** An intact hemidiaphragm is indicated by the smooth contour and by "suspension" of the spleen and abdominal fat away from the chest wall.

DIAPHRAGM

CORONAL & SAGITTAL CT, EVENTRATION OF DIAPHRAGM

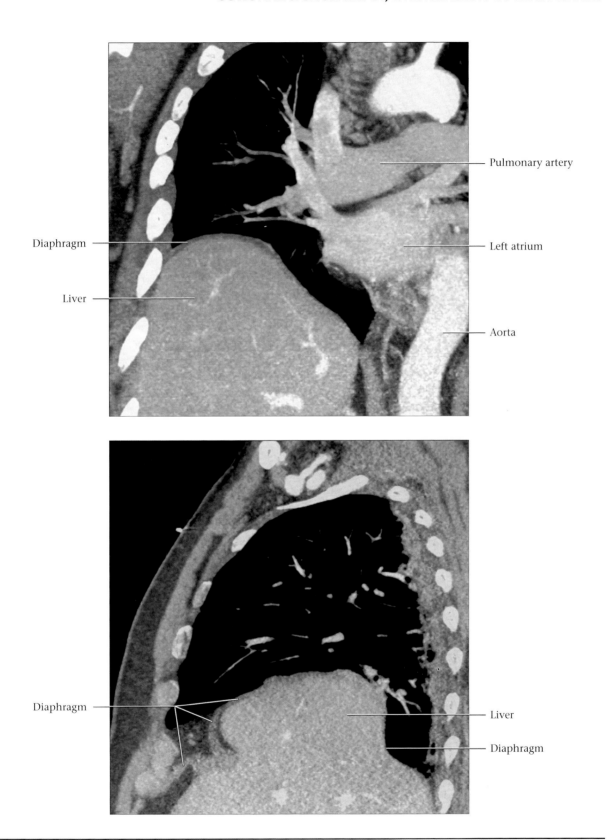

Labels in image: Pulmonary artery, Diaphragm, Left atrium, Liver, Aorta, Diaphragm, Liver, Diaphragm

(Top) Coronal CT view shows a supero-lateral bulge of the liver "dome". **(Bottom)** Sagittal CT view shows the liver bulge, characteristic of eventration (congenital thinning) of the diaphragm, usually an asymptomatic condition.

DIAPHRAGM

BOCHDALEK HERNIA

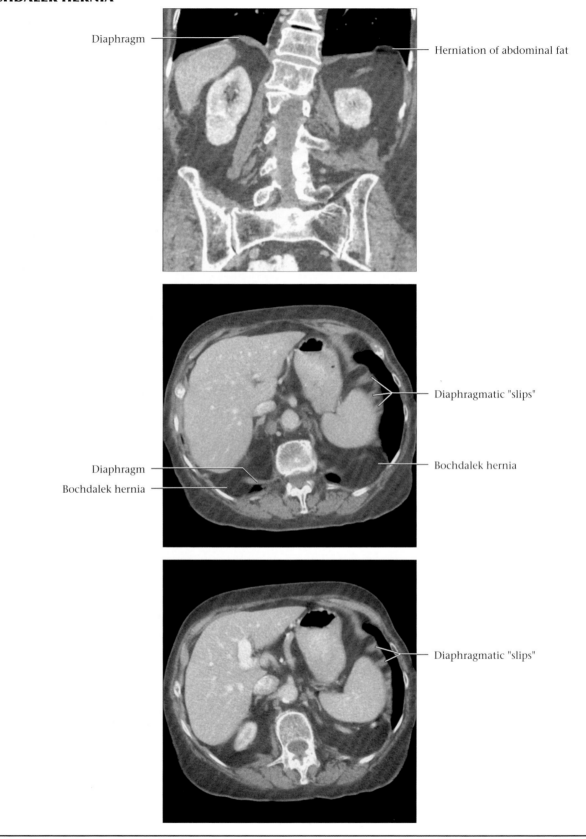

(Top) Coronal CT section in an 88 year old male with bilateral Bochdalek hernias shows thin diaphragm with focal marked thinning or absence of left hemidiaphragm, allowing abdominal fat to herniate into the thorax. **(Middle)** First of two axial CT sections shows discontinuity of the diaphragm posterolaterally with focal herniation of fat into thorax; bilateral Bochdalek hernias. **(Bottom)** Most caudal CT section shows diaphragmatic "slips".

DIAPHRAGM

LARGE HIATAL & MORGAGNI HERNIAS

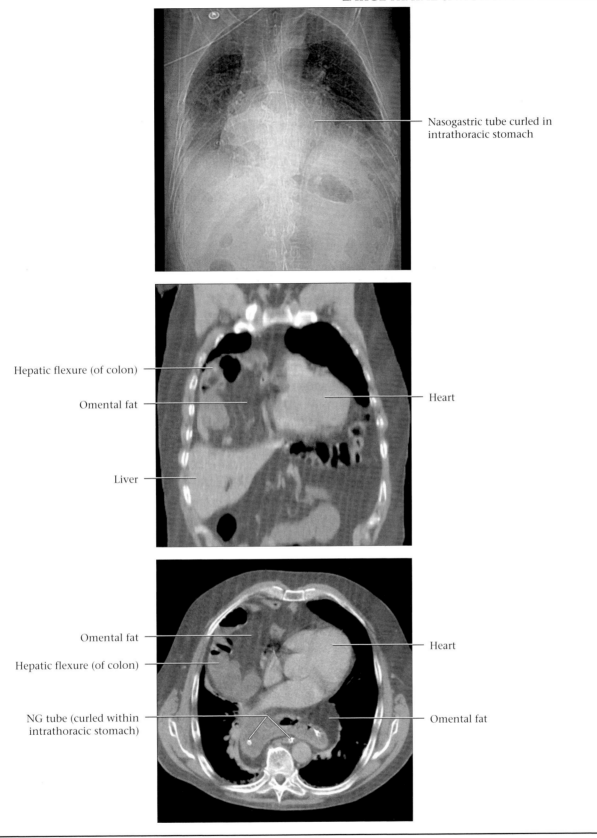

Nasogastric tube curled in intrathoracic stomach

Hepatic flexure (of colon)

Omental fat

Heart

Liver

Omental fat

Hepatic flexure (of colon)

Heart

NG tube (curled within intrathoracic stomach)

Omental fat

(Top) Frontal radiograph of a 71 year old man shows herniation of the entire stomach into the chest through a widened esophageal hiatus (type IV paraesophageal hernia). (Middle) Coronal CT section shows a large segment of colon and omental fat within the right hemithorax adjacent to the heart. It has herniated through a large anterior defect on the diaphragm, a Morgagni hernia. (Bottom) Axial CT section shows the intrathoracic stomach in a large paraesophageal hernia, and the antero-medial defect (Morgagni hernia) that allows the herniation of omental fat and colon.

DIAPHRAGM

TRAUMATIC DIAPHRAGMATIC RUPTURE

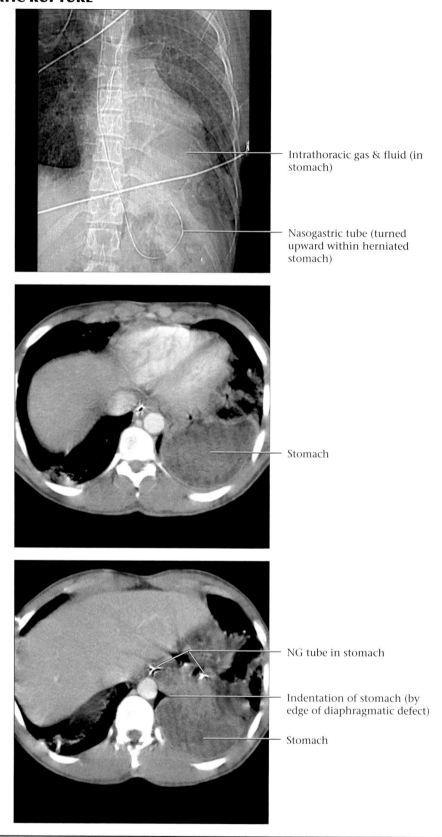

Intrathoracic gas & fluid (in stomach)

Nasogastric tube (turned upward within herniated stomach)

Stomach

NG tube in stomach

Indentation of stomach (by edge of diaphragmatic defect)

Stomach

(Top) First of five images of a 18 year old male with a traumatic rupture of the diaphragm. Frontal chest film shows intrathoracic gas and fluid, and an upward deviation of the tip of the nasogastric tube. The left hemidiaphragm is poorly-defined. (Middle) The stomach has herniated into the left hemithorax through a diaphragmatic defect, and has "fallen" against the posterior chest wall. This is an example of the "fallen viscus" sign of diaphragmatic rupture. The intact diaphragm suspends abdominal contents away from the postero-lateral chest wall. (Bottom) The medial surface of the stomach is indented by the intact margin of the left hemidiaphragm.

DIAPHRAGM

TRAUMATIC DIAPHRAGMATIC RUPTURE

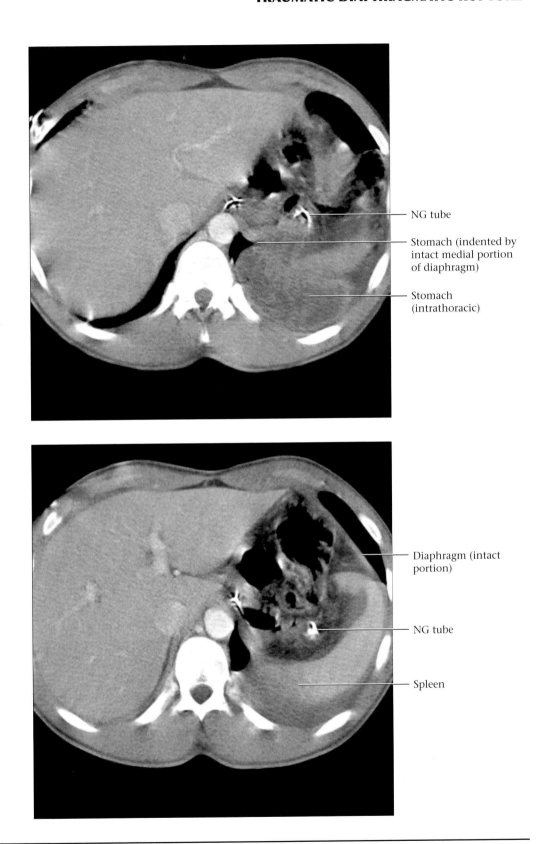

NG tube

Stomach (indented by intact medial portion of diaphragm)

Stomach (intrathoracic)

Diaphragm (intact portion)

NG tube

Spleen

(Top) The herniated portion of the stomach lies "fallen" against the posterior chest wall. **(Bottom)** The medial part of the spleen is heterogeneous due to a parenchymal laceration and hematoma.

PERITONEAL CAVITY

Terminology

Definitions

- **Peritoneal cavity: Potential space** in abdomen between visceral and parietal peritoneum, usually containing only small amount of peritoneal fluid (for lubrication)
- **Abdominal cavity:** Not synonymous with peritoneal cavity
  - Contains all of abdominal viscera (intra- and retroperitoneal)
  - Limited by abdominal wall muscles, diaphragm and (arbitrarily) by pelvic brim

Gross Anatomy

Divisions

- **Greater sac** of peritoneal cavity
- **Lesser sac (omental bursa)**
  - Communicates with greater sac via **epiploic foramen** (of **Winslow**)
  - Bounded in front by caudate lobe, stomach and greater omentum; in back by pancreas, left adrenal and kidney; to the left by **splenorenal** and **gastrosplenic ligaments**; to the right by epiploic foramen and lesser omentum

Peritoneum

- Thin serous membrane consisting of a single layer of squamous epithelium **(mesothelium)**
  - **Parietal peritoneum** lines abdominal wall; contains nerves to adjacent abdominal wall and is pain sensitive (with sharp localization)
  - **Visceral peritoneum (serosa)** lines abdominal organs; sensitive to pain due to stretching of bowel or mesentery (with poor localization)

Mesentery

- Double layer of peritoneum that encloses an organ and connects it to abdominal wall
- Covered on both sides by mesothelium and has a core of loose connective tissue containing fat, lymph nodes, blood vessels and nerves passing to and from viscera
- Most mobile parts of intestine have mesentery, while ascending and descending colon are considered retroperitoneal (covered only by peritoneum on their anterior surface)
- **Root of mesentery** is its attached border with posterior abdominal wall
- Root of small bowel mesentery is ≈ 15 cm in length and passes from left side of L2 vertebra downward and to the right; contains **superior mesenteric vessels**, nerves and lymphatics
- **Transverse mesocolon** crosses almost horizontally in front of pancreas, duodenum and right kidney

Omentum

- Multi-layered fold of peritoneum that extends from stomach to adjacent organs
- **Lesser omentum** joins lesser curve of stomach and proximal duodenum to liver

- **Hepatogastric** and **hepatoduodenal ligament** components contain **common bile duct, hepatic** and **gastric vessels** and **portal vein**
- **Greater omentum**
  - 4 layered fold of peritoneum hanging from greater curve of the stomach like an apron, covering transverse colon and much of the small intestine
    - Contains variable amounts of fat and abundant lymph nodes
    - Mobile and can fill gaps between viscera
    - Acts as barrier to generalized spread of intraperitoneal infection or tumor

Ligaments

- All double layered folds of peritoneum other than mesentery and omentum are peritoneal ligaments
- Connect one viscus to another (e.g., **splenorenal ligament**) or a viscus to abdominal wall (e.g., **falciform ligament**)
- Contain blood vessels or remnants of fetal vessels

Folds

- Reflections of peritoneum with defined borders, often lifting peritoneum off abdominal wall (e.g., **median umbilical fold** covers **urachus** and extends from dome of urinary bladder to umbilicus)

Peritoneal Recesses

- Dependent pouches formed by reflections of peritoneum
- Because of clinical relevance, often have eponyms [e.g., **Morison pouch** for **posterior subhepatic (hepatorenal) recess; pouch of Douglas** for **rectouterine recess**]

Anatomy-Based Imaging Issues

Imaging Pitfalls

- Peritoneal cavity and its various mesenteries and recesses are usually not apparent on imaging studies unless distended or outlined by intraperitoneal fluid or air

Clinical Implications

Clinical Importance

- Peritoneum that is evident on imaging is **thickened** due to inflammation or tumor
  - Nodular thickening is usually due to malignancy
- Peritoneal recesses are common sites for accumulation of **peritoneal fluid (ascites), pus** or **peritoneal tumor** implants
- Recesses all potentially communicate with each other but become functionally isolated by processes that cause adherence between layers of peritoneum (e.g., an abscess)
  - **Phrenicocolic ligament** limits spread of fluid from left subphrenic space to left paracolic gutter

PERITONEAL CAVITY

LATERAL VIEW OF MESENTERIES & PERITONEAL CAVITY

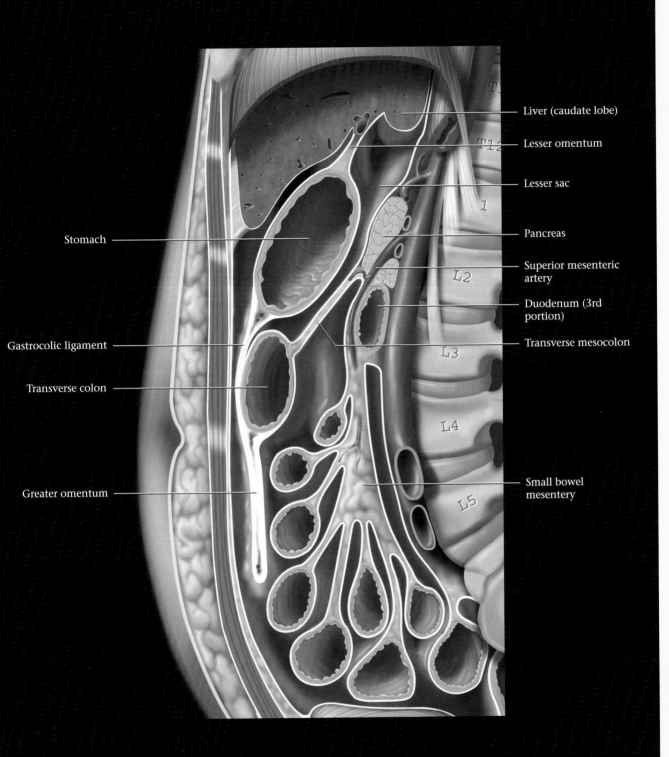

Liver (caudate lobe)

Lesser omentum

Lesser sac

Pancreas

Superior mesenteric artery

Duodenum (3rd portion)

Transverse mesocolon

Small bowel mesentery

Stomach

Gastrocolic ligament

Transverse colon

Greater omentum

Sagittal section of the abdomen showing the peritoneal cavity artificially distended, as with air. Note the margins of the lesser sac in this plane, including caudate lobe of liver, stomach and gastrocolic ligament anteriorly, and pancreas posteriorly. The hepatogastric ligament is part of the lesser omentum, and carries hepatic artery and portal vein to the liver. The mesenteries are multi-layered folds of peritoneum that enclose a layer of fat, and convey blood vessels, nerves, and lymphatics to the intraperitoneal abdominal viscera. The greater omentum is a 4 layered fold of peritoneum that extends down from the stomach, covering much of the colon and small intestine. The layers are generally fused together caudal to the transverse colon. The gastrocolic ligament is part of the greater omentum.

PERITONEAL CAVITY

LESSER SAC & PERITONEAL RECESSES

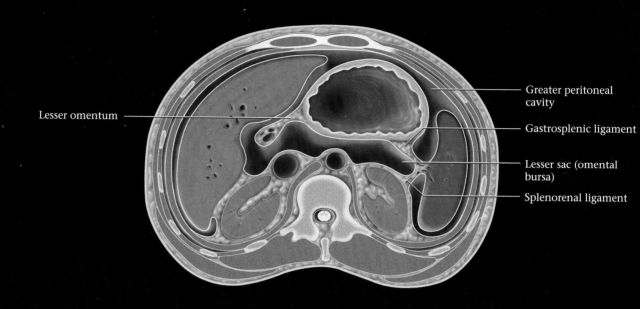

Lesser omentum

Greater peritoneal cavity

Gastrosplenic ligament

Lesser sac (omental bursa)

Splenorenal ligament

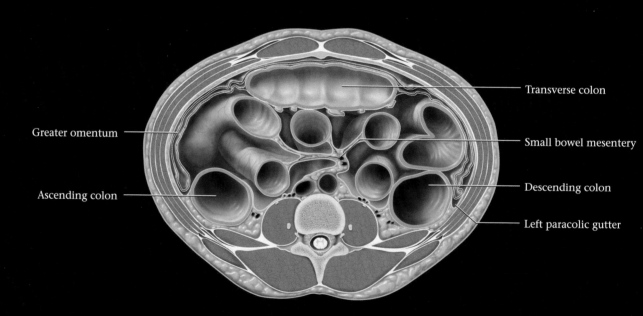

Greater omentum

Ascending colon

Transverse colon

Small bowel mesentery

Descending colon

Left paracolic gutter

(Top) The borders of the lesser sac (omental bursa) include the lesser omentum, which conveys the common bile duct, hepatic and gastric vessels. The left borders include the gastrosplenic ligament (with short gastric vessels) and the splenorenal ligament (with splenic vessels). **(Bottom)** The paracolic gutters are formed by reflections of peritoneum covering the ascending and descending colon and the lateral abdominal wall. Note the innumerable potential peritoneal recesses lying between the bowel loops and their mesenteric leaves. The greater omentum covers much of the bowel like an apron.

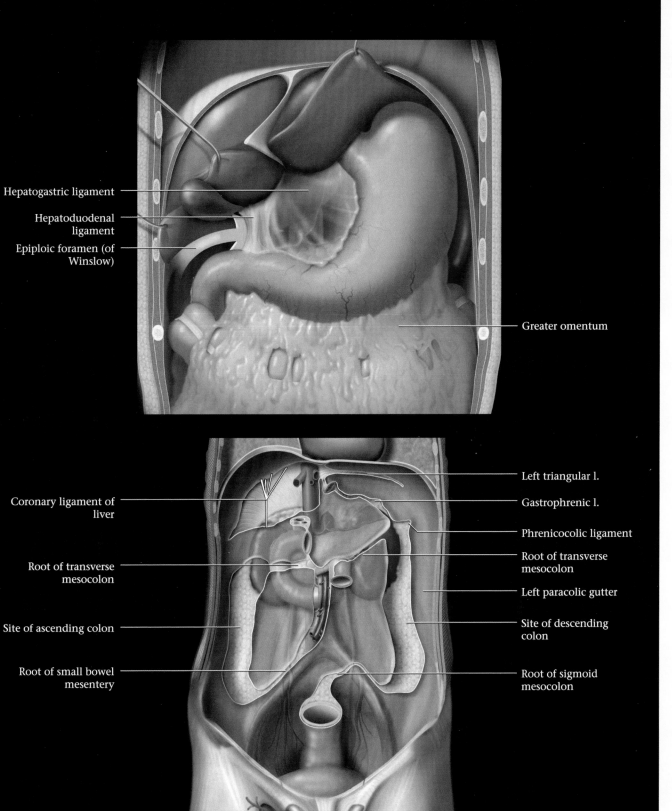

Hepatogastric ligament

Hepatoduodenal ligament

Epiploic foramen (of Winslow)

Greater omentum

Coronary ligament of liver

Root of transverse mesocolon

Site of ascending colon

Root of small bowel mesentery

Left triangular l.

Gastrophrenic l.

Phrenicocolic ligament

Root of transverse mesocolon

Left paracolic gutter

Site of descending colon

Root of sigmoid mesocolon

(Top) The liver has been retracted upward. The lesser omentum is comprised of the hepatoduodenal and hepatogastric ligaments, forms part of the anterior wall of the lesser sac, and conveys the common bile duct, hepatic and gastric vessels, and the portal vein. The aorta and celiac artery can be seen through the lesser omentum, as they lie just posterior to the lesser sac. **(Bottom)** Frontal view of abdomen with all of the intraperitoneal organs removed. The root of the transverse mesocolon divides the peritoneal cavity into supramesocolic and inframesocolic spaces that communicate only along the paracolic gutters. The coronary and triangular ligaments suspend the liver from the diaphragm. The superior mesenteric vessels traverse the small bowel mesentery whose root crosses obliquely from the upper left to the lower right posterior abdominal wall.

PERITONEAL CAVITY

PERITONEAL SPACES & REFLECTIONS

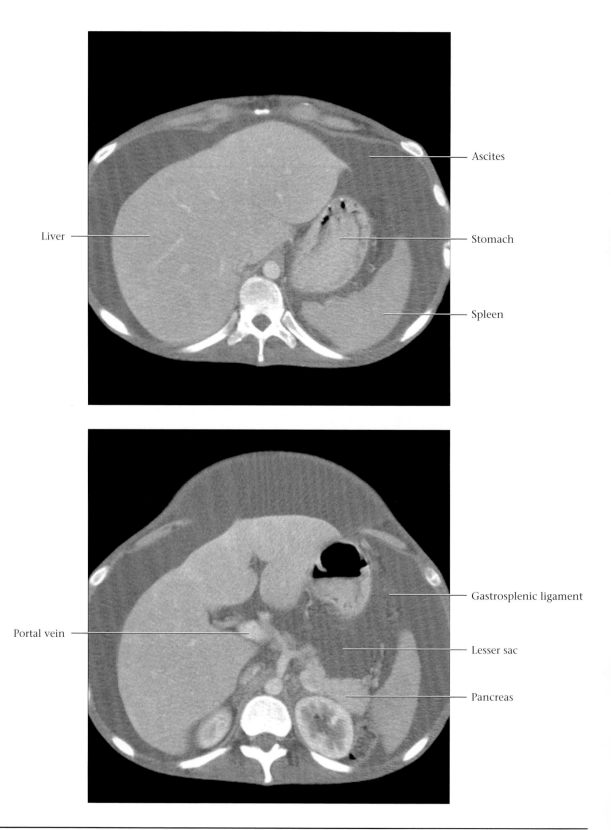

Ascites

Liver

Stomach

Spleen

Portal vein

Gastrosplenic ligament

Lesser sac

Pancreas

(Top) First of four axial CT sections of a middle-aged man with cirrhosis. Ascites distends the peritoneal cavity, allowing visualization of recesses and peritoneal reflections not normally seen. **(Bottom)** The lesser sac and greater peritoneal cavity are distended with ascites. The gastrosplenic ligament and pancreas border the lesser sac, as does the lesser omentum whose position is marked by the portal vein and celiac trunk.

PERITONEAL SPACES & REFLECTIONS

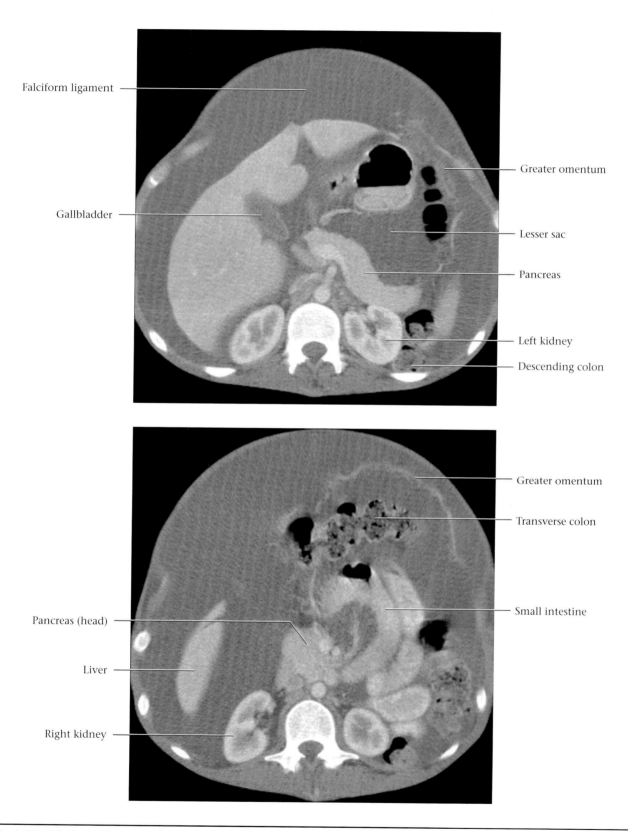

(Top) The falciform ligament suspends the liver from the anterior abdominal wall. The greater omentum lies between the bowel and the anterior abdominal wall. **(Bottom)** The intraperitoneal organs, such as the liver, transverse colon and small bowel are suspended within the ascites, while the position of the retroperitoneal organs, such as the kidneys and pancreas, is unaffected.

PERITONEAL CAVITY

PERITONEAL SPACES & MESENTERIES

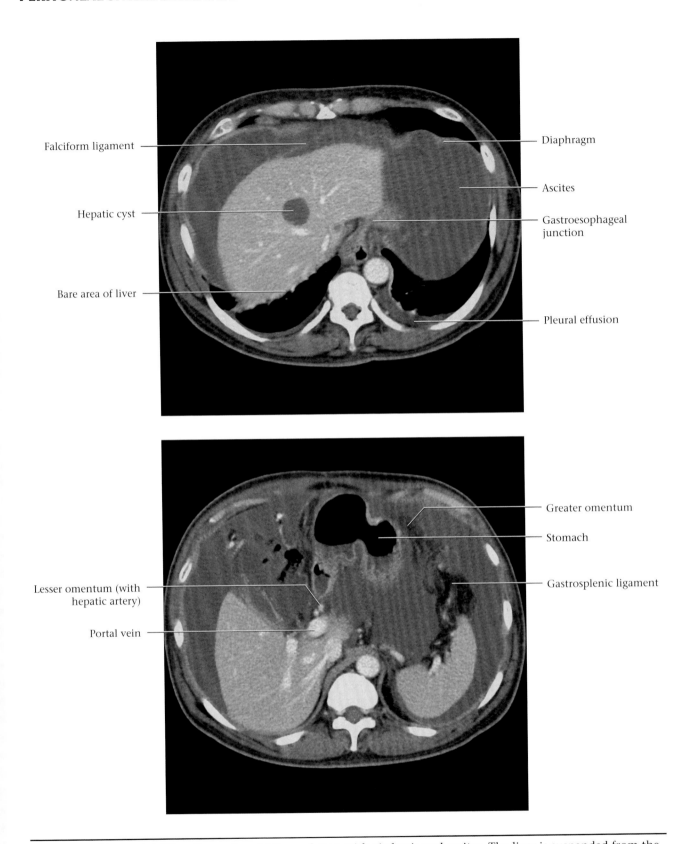

Falciform ligament

Hepatic cyst

Bare area of liver

Diaphragm

Ascites

Gastroesophageal junction

Pleural effusion

Lesser omentum (with hepatic artery)

Portal vein

Greater omentum

Stomach

Gastrosplenic ligament

(**Top**) First of four axial CT sections of a middle-aged man with cirrhosis and ascites. The liver is suspended from the anterior abdominal wall by the falciform ligament, and from the diaphragm by the coronary ligament, between the leaves of which lies the bare area of the liver. (**Bottom**) The lesser omentum and gastrosplenic ligament comprise two of the walls of the lesser sac.

PERITONEAL CAVITY

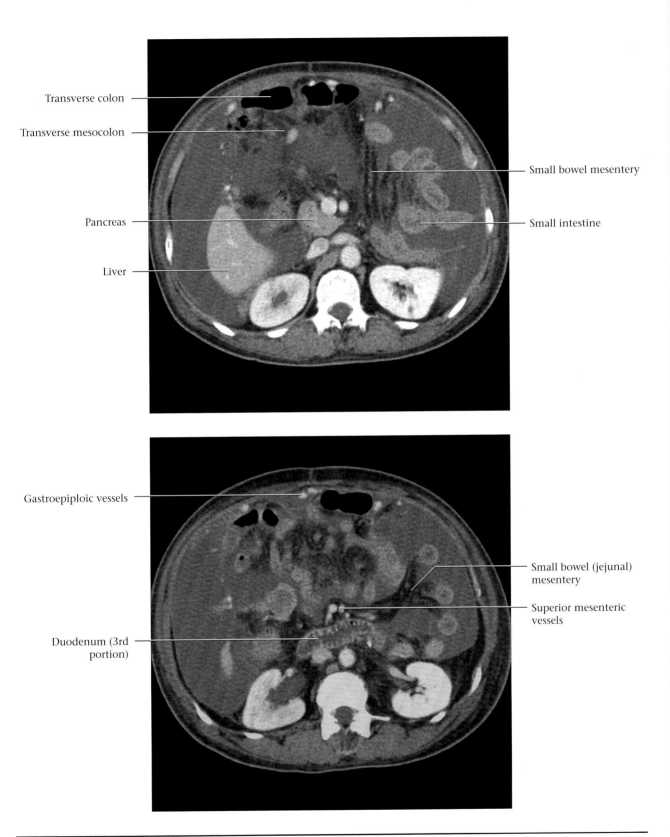

Transverse colon

Transverse mesocolon

Pancreas

Liver

Small bowel mesentery

Small intestine

Gastroepiploic vessels

Small bowel (jejunal) mesentery

Superior mesenteric vessels

Duodenum (3rd portion)

(Top) The mesenteries are easily identified by their content of fat (dark in attenuation) and blood vessels. Retroperitoneal organs, such as the pancreas and kidneys remain in normal position surrounded by retroperitoneal fat that conveys their blood supply. **(Bottom)** Note the retroperitoneal position of the duodenum. The third portion of duodenum crosses behind the superior mesenteric vessels, which supply the small intestine. The branches of the mesenteric vessels lie within the leaves of the mesentery, surrounded by fat.

DISTENDED PERITONEAL CAVITY

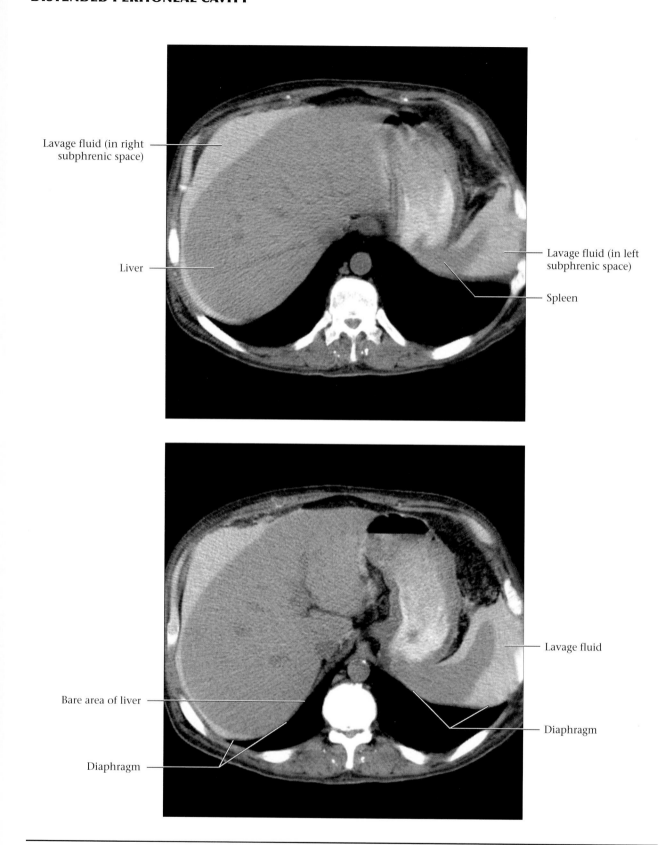

(**Top**) First of seven axial CT sections of an elderly man with renal failure treated with peritoneal dialysis. Contrast medium was added to the dialysate to identify potential sites of loculated fluid, and accounts for the "white" appearance of the fluid. The lavage fluid appears relatively dense due to the added contrast medium. Note the intraperitoneal fluid collecting in the subphrenic spaces. (**Bottom**) Note how the diaphragm suspends the liver and spleen away from the chest wall. The bare area of the liver is in direct contact with the diaphragm, but not with the peritoneal cavity; thus, the lavage fluid is not in contact with the bare area.

PERITONEAL CAVITY

DISTENDED PERITONEAL CAVITY

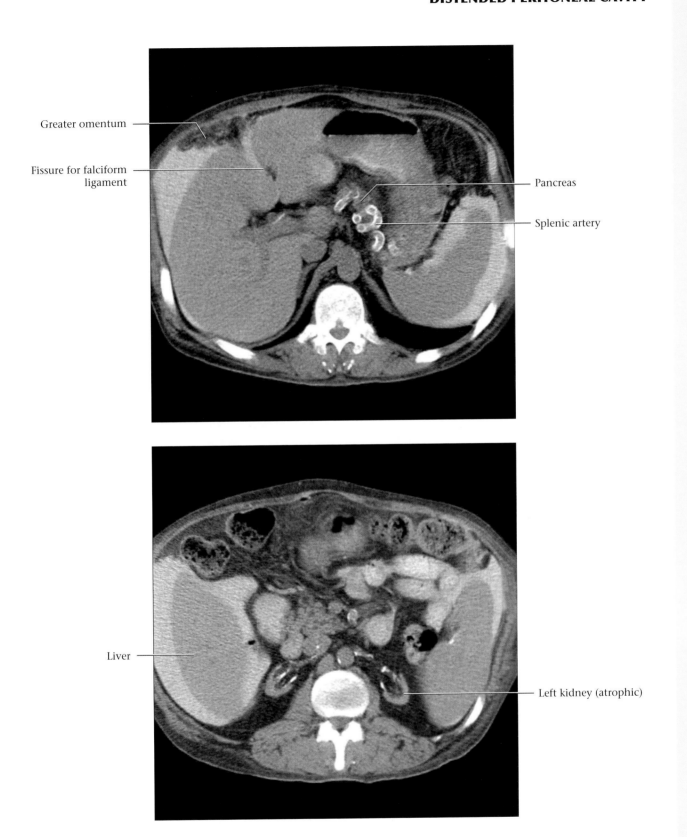

Greater omentum

Fissure for falciform ligament

Pancreas

Splenic artery

Liver

Left kidney (atrophic)

(Top) Fluid invaginates into the fissure for the falciform ligament. Note that there is no fluid within the lesser sac. As a general rule, unless the ascites is tense or of a "local" source (such as a perforated gastric ulcer or pancreatitis), it remains confined to the greater peritoneal cavity, and does not pass through the epiploic foramen. Note the tortuous splenic artery, a typical finding in patients with atherosclerosis. The greater omentum "floats" on top of the ascites; note its fat density with small vessels, its normal appearance. **(Bottom)** Note the small kidneys, reflecting chronic renal failure.

PERITONEAL CAVITY

DISTENDED PERITONEAL CAVITY

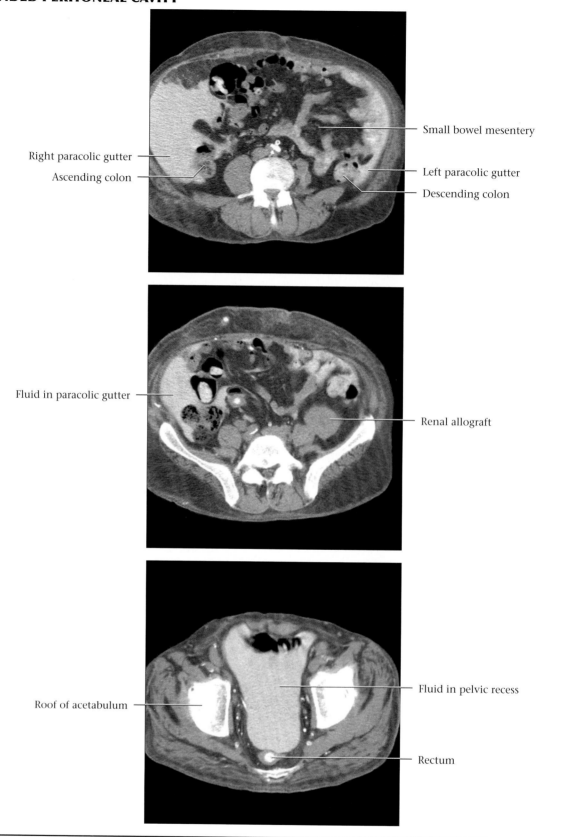

Small bowel mesentery

Right paracolic gutter

Ascending colon

Left paracolic gutter

Descending colon

Fluid in paracolic gutter

Renal allograft

Fluid in pelvic recess

Roof of acetabulum

Rectum

(Top) The peritoneal fluid is mostly confined to the paracolic gutters at this level. (Middle) The peritoneal fluid is somewhat loculated, which is typical in the setting of chronic peritoneal dialysis, which results in inflammation and scarring of the peritoneum over time. Note the transplanted kidney in the left iliac fossa, which had stopped functioning due to rejection. (Bottom) The most dependent recess of the peritoneal cavity is in the pelvis, which is distended by dialysis fluid in this patient.

PERITONEAL CAVITY

MESENTERIES OUTLINED BY ASCITES

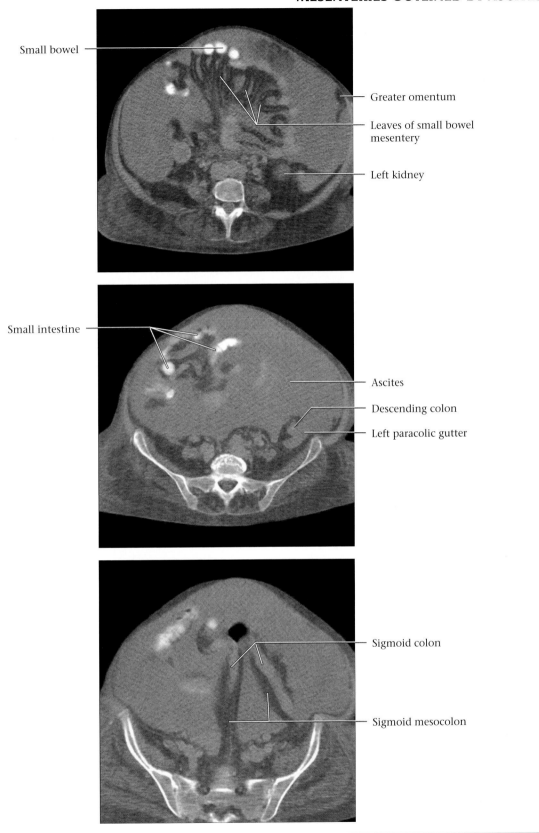

Small bowel — (Top image)

Greater omentum

Leaves of small bowel mesentery

Left kidney

Small intestine — (Middle image)

Ascites

Descending colon

Left paracolic gutter

Sigmoid colon — (Bottom image)

Sigmoid mesocolon

(Top) First of three axial CT images in a patient with ascites due to cirrhosis. The leaves of the small bowel mesentery are separated and accentuated by ascites. Each "leaf" of mesentery carries blood vessels, nerves, and lymphatics to a bowel segment. **(Middle)** Ascites distends the abdomen to the point of being "tense" (firm to palpation). Retroperitoneal fat-containing spaces are unaffected. Ascites is present in the left paracolic gutter, the intraperitoneal recess lateral to the descending colon. **(Bottom)** The sigmoid colon and its mesentery are well-defined by the ascites.

PERITONEAL CAVITY

PERITONEAL RECESSES (MORISON & DOUGLAS)

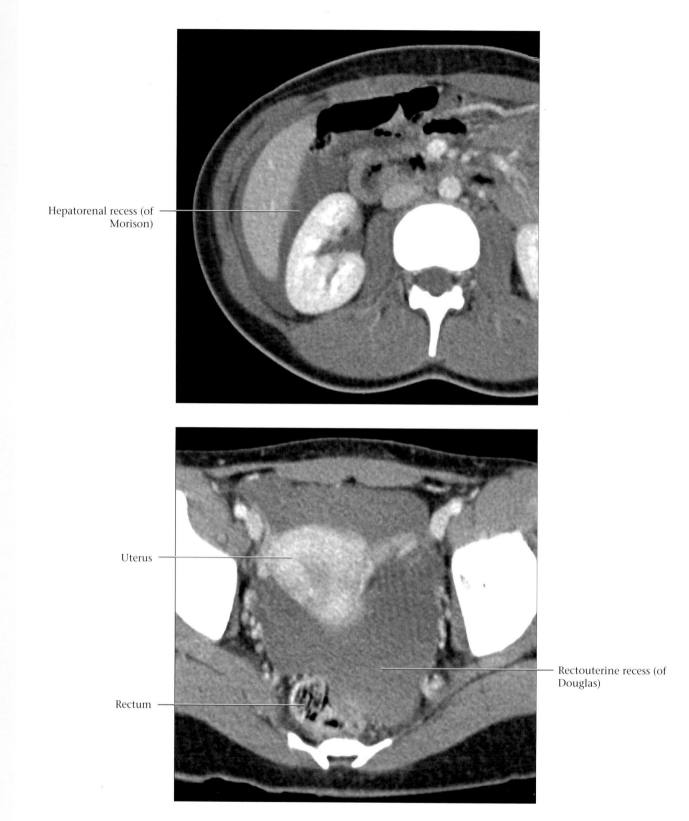

Hepatorenal recess (of Morison)

Uterus

Rectum

Rectouterine recess (of Douglas)

(Top) First of two axial CT sections. The most dependent peritoneal recess in the upper abdomen is the hepatorenal recess, also known as the posterior subhepatic space, and as Morison pouch. It communicates superiorly with the right subphrenic space and inferiorly with the right paracolic gutter. (Bottom) The pouch of Douglas, also known as the rectouterine recess, is the most dependent recess of the entire peritoneal cavity in either the upright or supine position, and is a common site for inflammatory, neoplastic or traumatic fluid collections.

PERITONEAL CAVITY

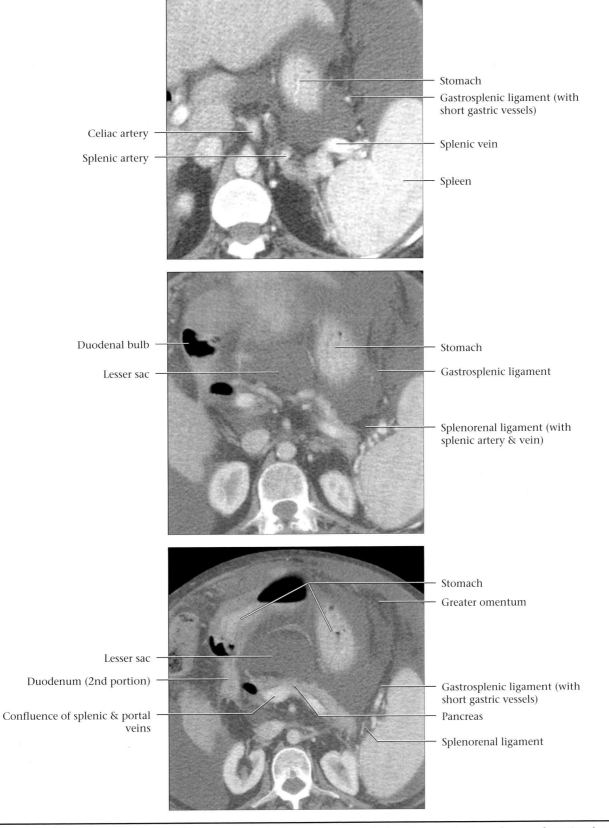

Celiac artery

Splenic artery

Stomach

Gastrosplenic ligament (with short gastric vessels)

Splenic vein

Spleen

Duodenal bulb

Lesser sac

Stomach

Gastrosplenic ligament

Splenorenal ligament (with splenic artery & vein)

Lesser sac

Duodenum (2nd portion)

Confluence of splenic & portal veins

Stomach

Greater omentum

Gastrosplenic ligament (with short gastric vessels)

Pancreas

Splenorenal ligament

(**Top**) First of three axial CT sections. The gastrosplenic ligament connects the stomach to the spleen and carries the short gastric vessels. Abdominal "ligaments" are double-layered folds of peritoneum that connect one viscus to another. They contain fat and transmit the vessels, nerves and lymphatics between the retroperitoneum and the abdominal viscera. (**Middle**) The gastrosplenic and splenorenal ligaments form the left anterior and posterior walls of the lesser sac, respectively. (**Bottom**) Note the structures abutting the lesser sac, including the stomach anteriorly and the pancreas posteriorly.

PERITONEAL CAVITY

UMBILICAL LIGAMENTS, DELINEATED BY ASCITES

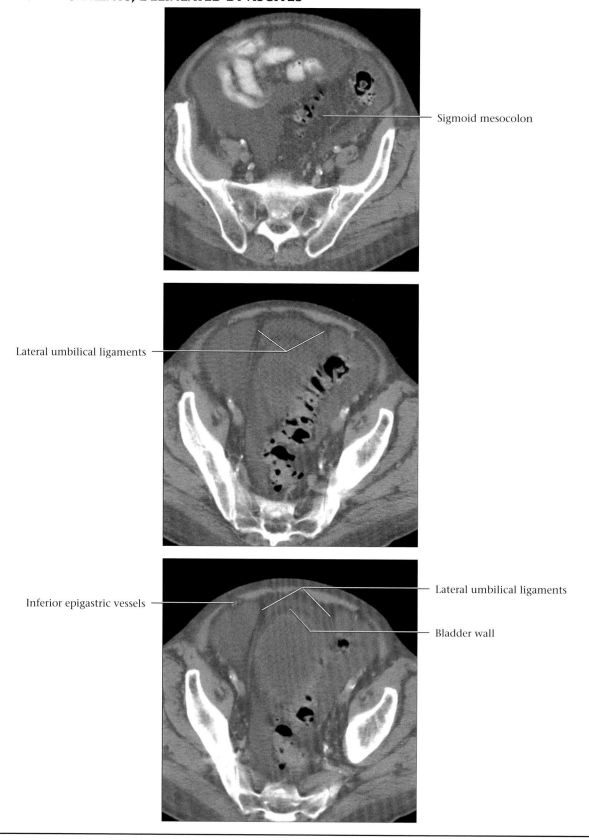

Sigmoid mesocolon

Lateral umbilical ligaments

Inferior epigastric vessels

Lateral umbilical ligaments

Bladder wall

(Top) First of three axial CT sections. Ascites outlines the sigmoid mesocolon and small bowel loops. (Middle) The umbilical ligaments are outlined by ascites. These are the remnants of the fetal umbilical arteries that had connected the internal iliac arteries to the umbilical cord. The peritoneal reflections covering these ligaments are the lateral umbilical folds. (Bottom) The ascites is not loculated, but normal structures, such as the umbilical ligaments and the wall of the urinary bladder, may be mistaken for septations within the fluid collection.

PERITONEAL CAVITY

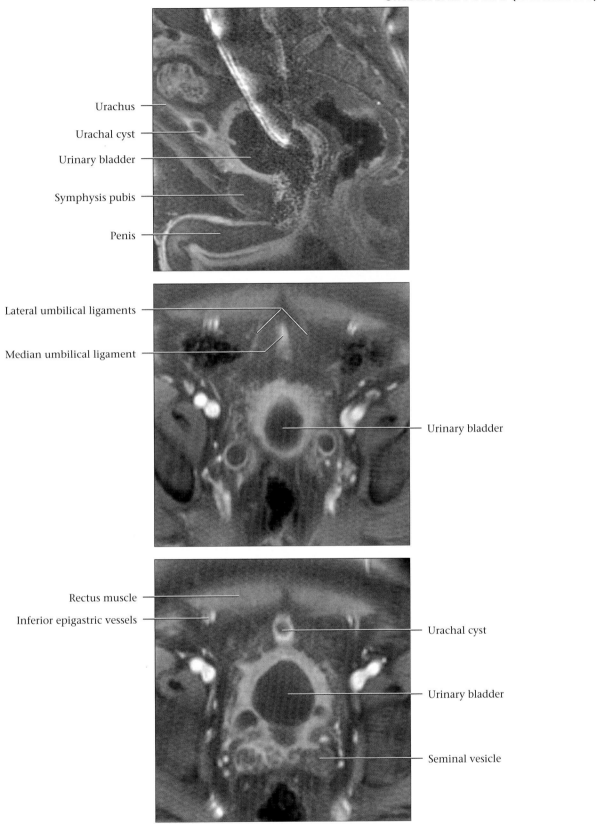

Urachus

Urachal cyst

Urinary bladder

Symphysis pubis

Penis

Lateral umbilical ligaments

Median umbilical ligament

Urinary bladder

Rectus muscle

Inferior epigastric vessels

Urachal cyst

Urinary bladder

Seminal vesicle

(Top) Sagittal MR section of the pelvis shows a linear structure extending from the umbilicus to the dome of the urinary bladder, the urachus (median umbilical ligament). This is the fibrous remnant of the allantois and should be completely obliterated after birth. In some individuals, parts of the tract may remain patent, leading to a urachal diverticulum or a urachal cyst, as in this person. (Middle) The median and lateral umbilical ligaments are evident in this individual on an axial MR section. Recall that these are covered with peritoneal reflections, called the median and lateral umbilical folds, respectively. (Bottom) The urachal cyst is evident within the median umbilical fold, on axial MR section. The bright signal around the cyst indicates inflammation (infection) of the cyst, which brought the patient to clinical attention.

PERITONEAL CAVITY

LOCULATED ASCITES

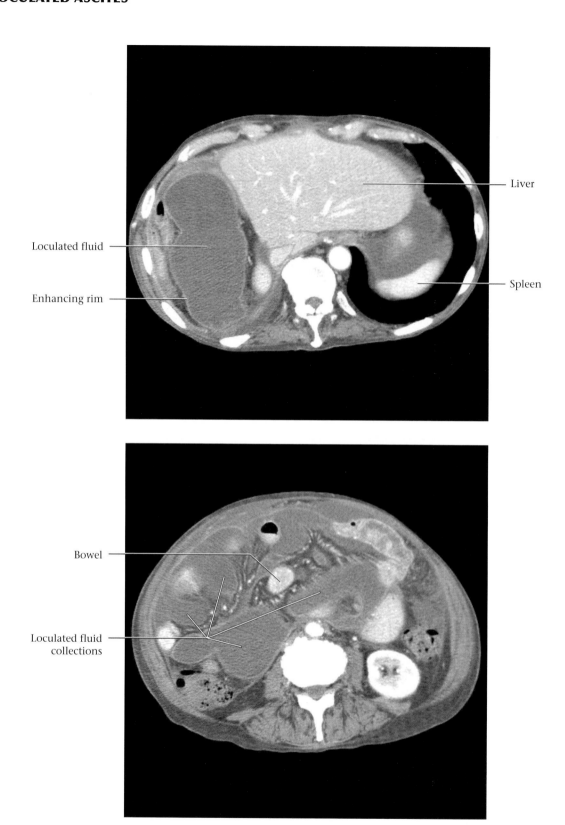

(Top) First of two axial CT sections in a patient with abdominal pain and fever following resection of the right lobe of the liver. Section through upper abdomen shows a large, loculated fluid collection in the right subphrenic space, with a contrast-enhancing rim or capsule. (Bottom) Lower in the abdomen there are numerous, noncommunicating, loculated collections of fluid, all of which have distinct, enhancing walls. These were aspirated under CT guidance and found to contain bilious fluid. Bile leaking into the peritoneal cavity from the cut surface of the liver had induced an intense peritonitis, accounting for adherence and thickening of peritoneal surfaces.

PERITONEAL CAVITY

BACTERIAL PERITONITIS WITH ASCITES & THICKENED PERITONEUM

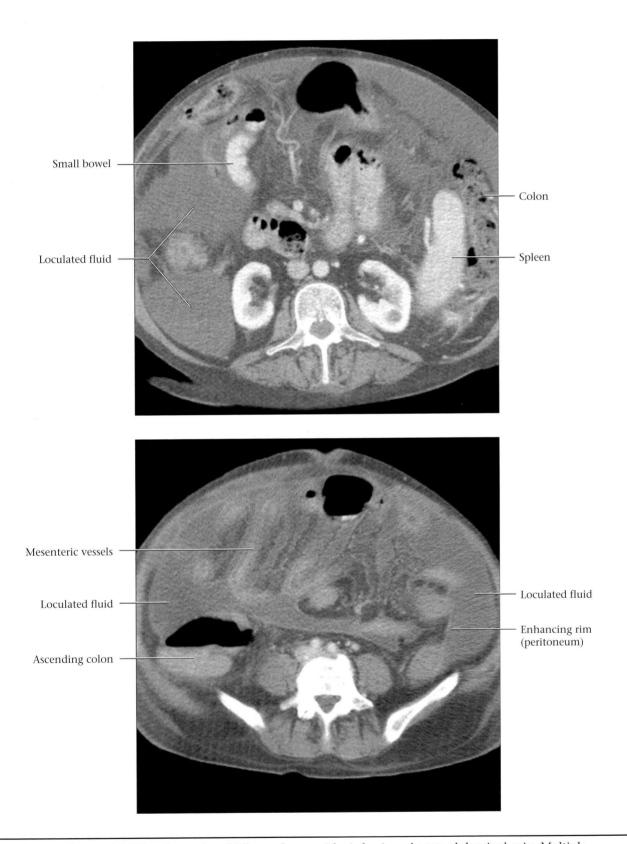

Small bowel

Loculated fluid

Colon

Spleen

Mesenteric vessels

Loculated fluid

Loculated fluid

Enhancing rim (peritoneum)

Ascending colon

(Top) First of two axial CT sections of a middle-aged man with cirrhosis and acute abdominal pain. Multiple loculated intraperitoneal fluid collections are noted. Ultrasound-guided aspiration yielded infected ascites, characteristic of "spontaneous bacterial peritonitis". **(Bottom)** Each leaf of small bowel mesentery is "stiff" in appearance, with straightening of the mesenteric blood vessels, and is coated with thickened, contrast-enhanced peritoneum. The parietal peritoneum is also thickened and contrast-enhanced, causing each loculated collection of fluid to have a capsule or rim. Adherence between the inflamed peritoneal surfaces accounts for the loculation of the fluid.

PERITONEAL CAVITY

FIBROSING PERITONITIS DUE TO PERITONEAL DIALYSIS

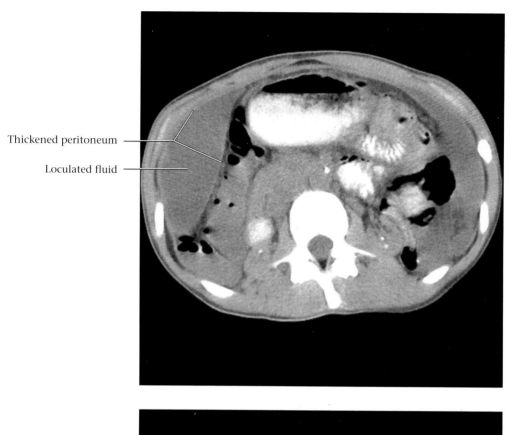

Thickened peritoneum

Loculated fluid

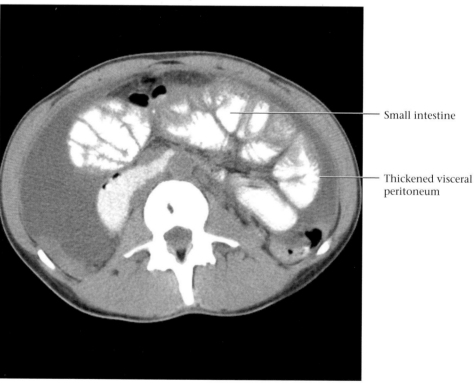

Small intestine

Thickened visceral peritoneum

(Top) First of four images of a young woman with chronic renal failure being treated with peritoneal dialysis. Axial CT section shows loculated intraperitoneal fluid with a thickened capsule of inflamed peritoneum. (Bottom) The small bowel appears to be encased in a "cocoon" of thickened visceral caviteum (serosa) that compresses the bowel loops together in a rounded mass.

PERITONEAL CAVITY

FIBROSING PERITONITIS DUE TO PERITONEAL DIALYSIS

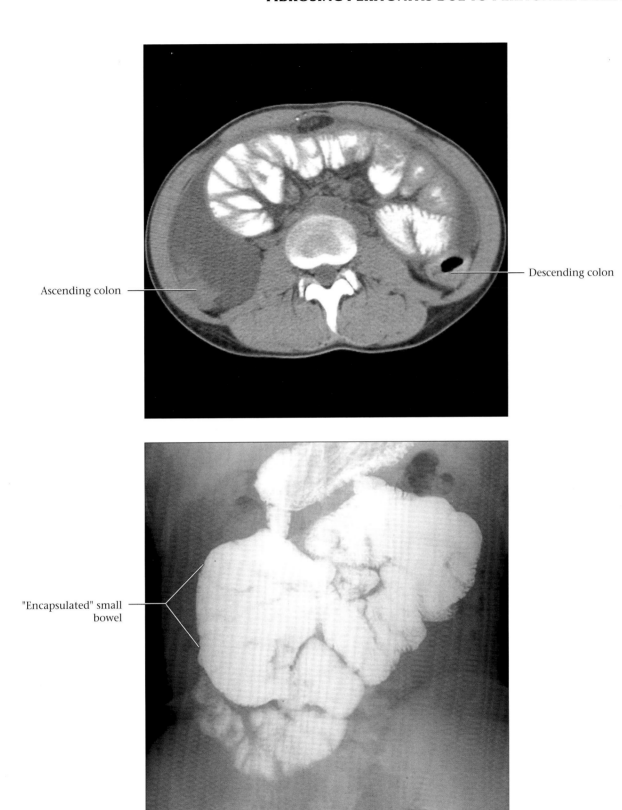

Ascending colon

Descending colon

"Encapsulated" small bowel

(Top) Note the encapsulated appearance of the small bowel. The lumen of the bowel is also moderately dilated. The ascending and descending colon are uninvolved, as they lie retroperitoneally. **(Bottom)** Abdominal radiograph taken 2 hours after ingestion of barium shows slow transit of the barium and dilated small bowel. The small bowel loops are also crowded together and fixed in position, instead of being freely mobile on their mesentery, as normal. This is an example of severe fibrosing peritonitis, a rare complication of peritoneal dialysis.

PERITONEAL CAVITY

MALIGNANT ASCITES, PERITONEAL METASTASES

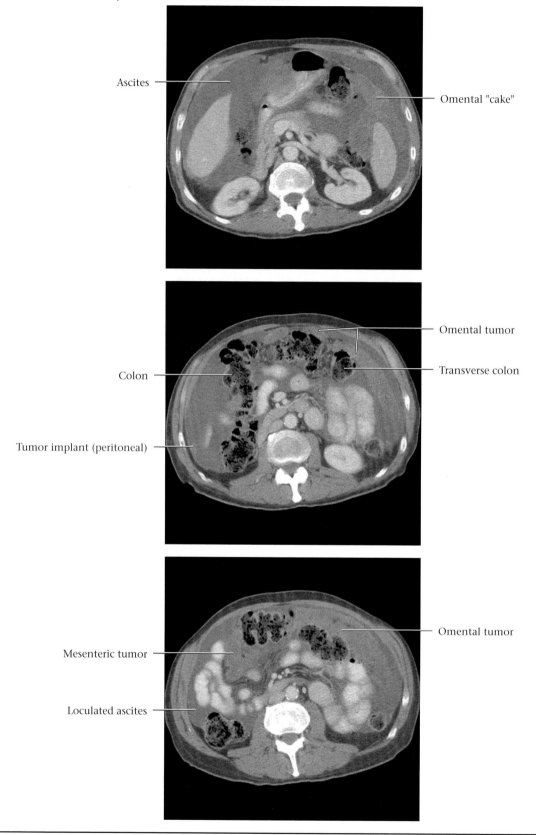

Ascites

Omental "cake"

Omental tumor

Colon

Transverse colon

Tumor implant (peritoneal)

Mesenteric tumor

Omental tumor

Loculated ascites

(Top) First of three axial CT sections of a middle-aged man with colon cancer and a distended abdomen. CT shows a solid mantle of tissue overlying the colon. This is called an "omental cake", and is virtually diagnostic of malignant peritoneal implants. **(Middle)** A nodular implant on the parietal peritoneal surface is also characteristic of peritoneal malignancy. Recall that the omentum lies superficial to the colon and small bowel, while the mesentery lies between the retroperitoneum and the "inside" of the bowel. **(Bottom)** Omental and mesenteric soft tissue density tumor deposits are evident, indicating widespread intraperitoneal spread from the primary colon carcinoma.

NODULAR OMENTAL METASTASES

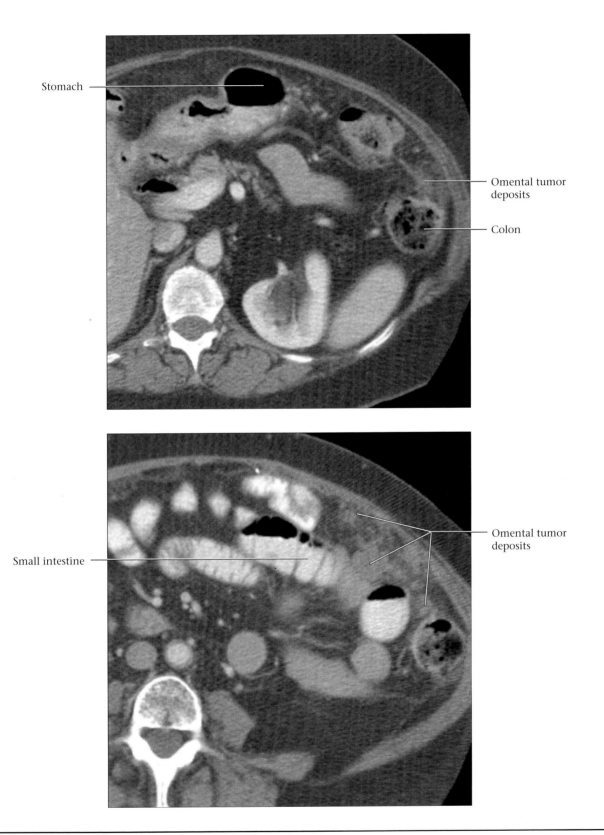

Stomach

Omental tumor deposits

Colon

Small intestine

Omental tumor deposits

(Top) First of two axial CT sections of a middle-aged woman with ovarian carcinoma. Subtle soft tissue density nodules are present in the omental fat overlying the colon and small bowel. These are characteristic of peritoneal tumor deposits. **(Bottom)** The nodular tumor deposits in the omentum are more evident on this CT section. Peritoneal spread of tumor is often, but not always, accompanied by malignant ascites, which is absent in this case.

PERITONEAL CAVITY

PERITONEAL TUMOR & OMENTAL METASTASES

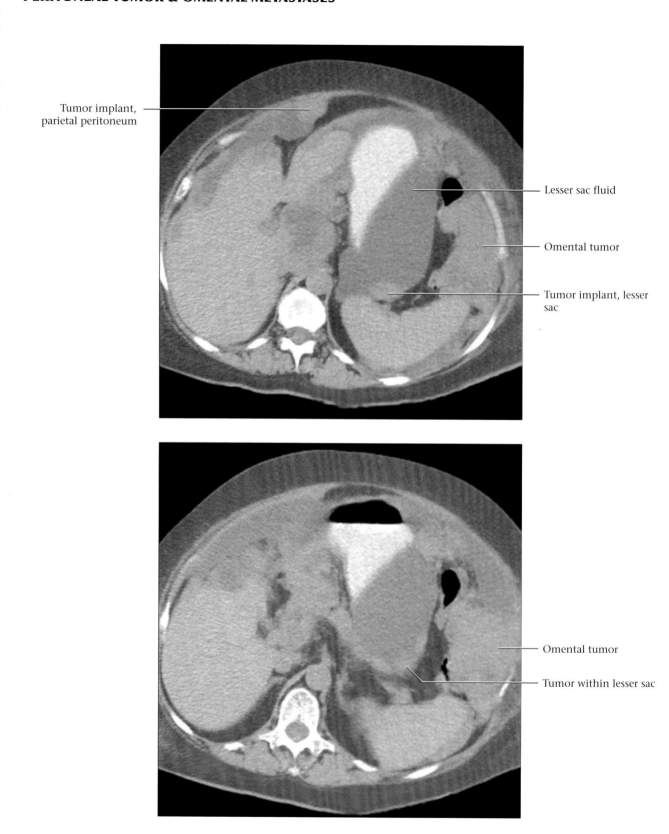

Tumor implant, parietal peritoneum

Lesser sac fluid

Omental tumor

Tumor implant, lesser sac

Omental tumor

Tumor within lesser sac

(Top) First of four axial CT sections of a patient with peritoneal carcinomatosis. Nodular soft tissue density tumor implants are present within the lesser sac and along the parietal peritoneum. A mass of tumor is noted in the omentum, a so-called "omental cake". (Bottom) Loculated fluid within the lesser sac is suggestive of infectious peritonitis or, as in this patient, peritoneal carcinomatosis.

PERITONEAL TUMOR & OMENTAL METASTASES

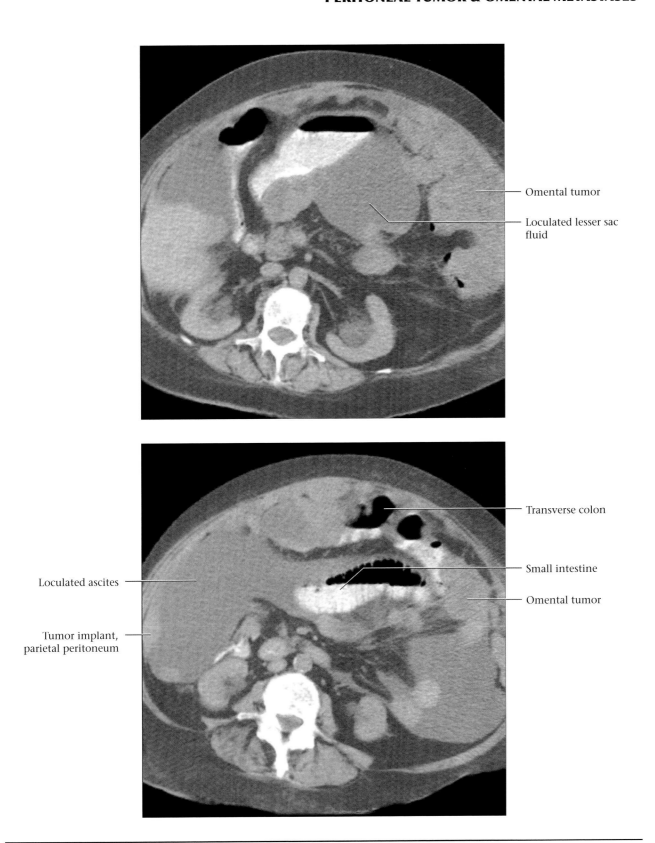

Omental tumor

Loculated lesser sac fluid

Transverse colon

Small intestine

Omental tumor

Loculated ascites

Tumor implant, parietal peritoneum

(Top) Recall that the omentum should appear as a mostly fatty "apron" of tissue lying over the surface of the bowel and colon. An extensive soft tissue mass, as in this patient, is indicative of malignancy. (Bottom) Loculated ascites is caused by adhesions (usually from prior surgery), peritonitis, or peritoneal carcinomatosis.

PSEUDOMYXOMA PERITONEI, APPENDICEAL CARCINOMA

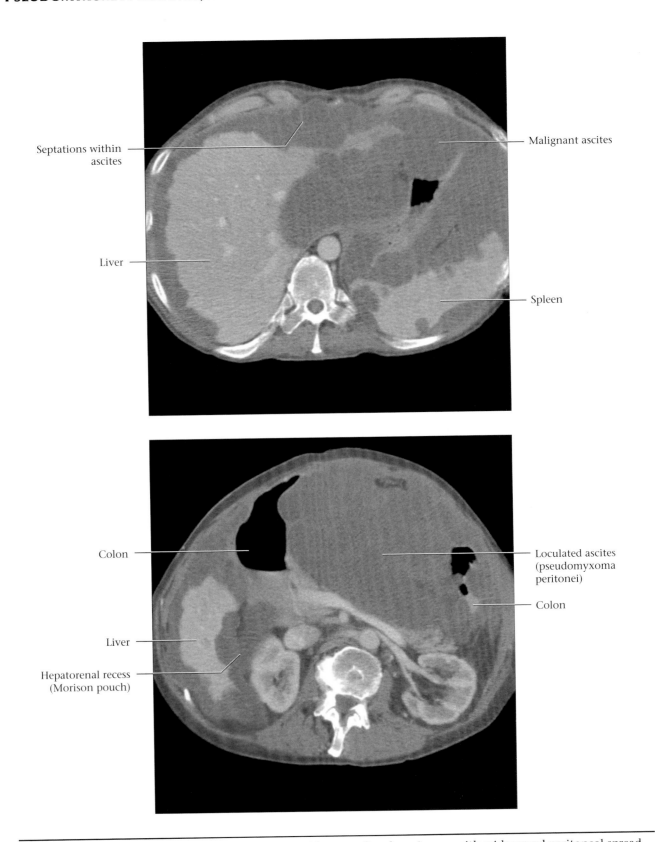

(Top) First of two axial CT sections of a young man with appendiceal carcinoma with widespread peritoneal spread. Note the "scalloped" surface of the liver and spleen, and the complex, septated appearance of the ascites. These findings are characteristic of pseudomyxoma peritonei, in which peritoneal metastases from a mucin-secreting tumor, such as appendiceal carcinoma, result in profuse accumulation of gelatinous material within the peritoneal cavity. The loculations and quantity of the material produce the typical mass effect, or indentations, on abdominal viscera and often result in bowel obstruction. **(Bottom)** Note the complex, septated appearance of the "ascites", which is actually semi-solid gelatinous material. The surface of the liver is markedly distorted, while the kidneys are unaffected, due to their retroperitoneal location.

PERITONEAL CAVITY

PERITONEAL & OVARIAN METASTASES, GASTRIC CARCINOMA

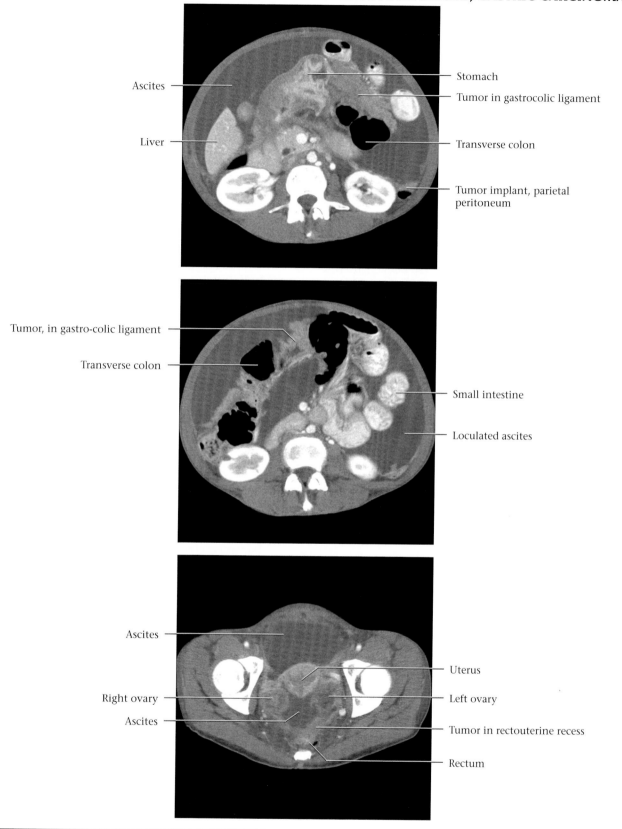

Ascites

Liver

Stomach

Tumor in gastrocolic ligament

Transverse colon

Tumor implant, parietal peritoneum

Tumor, in gastro-colic ligament

Transverse colon

Small intestine

Loculated ascites

Ascites

Right ovary

Ascites

Uterus

Left ovary

Tumor in rectouterine recess

Rectum

(Top) First of three axial CT sections in a woman with gastric carcinoma, metastatic to her peritoneum and ovaries. The tumor encases and distorts the stomach, and spreads along the gastro-colic ligament into the transverse colon. Loculated ascites and parietal peritoneal tumor implants are noted. **(Middle)** Extensive tumor is present along the transverse colon and the parietal peritoneum. Small bowel lumen is "dense" due to oral - enteric contrast medium. **(Bottom)** Loculated ascites and peritoneal tumor are present in the dependent recesses of the pelvis, including the rectouterine recess (pouch of Douglas). Both ovaries are enlarged by cystic-solid masses, due to metastatic spread of tumor to the ovaries. Metastases to the ovaries from a gastric carcinoma are referred to as Krukenberg metastases, after the pathologist who first identified this phenomenon.

VESSELS, LYMPHATIC SYSTEM AND NERVES

Terminology

Abbreviations

- Inferior vena cava (IVC)
- Superior mesenteric artery (SMA)
- Superior mesenteric vein (SMV)
- Superior vena cava (SVC)
- Inferior mesenteric artery (IMA)
- Inferior mesenteric vein (IMV)

Gross Anatomy

Overview

- **Abdominal aorta**
  - Enters abdomen at the T12 level, bifurcates at L4
  - Gives rise to arteries in 3 vascular planes
    - **Anterior midline plane**: Unpaired visceral arteries to alimentary tract; **celiac artery**, **SMA** and **IMA**
    - **Lateral plane**: Paired visceral arteries to urogenital and endocrine organs; **renal**, **adrenal** and **gonadal arteries** (testicular or ovarian)
    - **Posterolateral plane**: Paired parietal arteries to diaphragm and body wall; **subcostal**, **inferior phrenic**, **lumbar arteries**
- **Inferior vena cava**
  - Returns poorly oxygenated blood to heart from lower extremities, abdominal wall, back and abdominal-pelvic viscera
  - Blood from alimentary tract passes through portal venous system before entering IVC through **hepatic veins**
  - Begins at L5 level with union of **common iliac veins**
  - Leaves abdomen via IVC hiatus in diaphragm at T8 level
  - IVC tributaries correspond to paired visceral and parietal branches of aorta
    - **Right adrenal vein**, left and **right renal veins**, **right gonadal vein**
    - **Left adrenal** and **gonadal veins** drain into left renal vein → IVC
    - Paired parietal branches = inferior phrenic, L3 and L4 veins
  - IVC and SVC are connected through **azygous** and **ascending lumbar veins**
    - These are important collateral pathways when SVC or IVC flow is obstructed or slowed
    - Additional collateral pathways include epidural venous plexus and **epigastric veins** (anterior abdominal wall)
  - IVC development has complex embryology
    - **Various anomalies** are common (up to 10% of population), especially at and below the level of renal veins
    - All are variations of persistence/regression of embryologic sub- and supracardinal veins
- **Lymphatics of posterior abdominal wall**
  - Major lymphatic vessels and nodal chains lie along major blood vessels (aorta, IVC, iliac) and have same names (e.g., common iliac nodes)

- Lymph from alimentary tract, liver, spleen and pancreas passes along celiac, superior mesenteric chains to nodes with similar names (e.g., **celiac nodes**)
  - Efferent vessels from alimentary nodes form **intestinal lymphatic trunks**
  - **Cisterna chyli** (**chyle cistern**): Formed by confluence of intestinal lymphatic trunks and **right and left lumbar lymphatic trunks** (which receive lymph from nonalimentary viscera, abdominal wall and lower extremities); may be discrete sac or plexiform convergence
- **Thoracic duct**: Inferior extent is chyle cistern at the L1-2 level
  - Formed by the convergence of main lymphatic ducts of abdomen
  - Ascends through **aortic hiatus** in diaphragm to enter posterior mediastinum
  - Ends by entering junction of **left subclavian** and **internal jugular veins**
- Lymphatic system drains surplus fluid from extracellular spaces and returns it to bloodstream
  - Has important function in defense against infection, inflammation and tumor via lymphoid tissue that is present in lymph nodes, wall of gut, spleen and thymus
  - Absorbs and transports dietary lipids from intestine to thoracic duct and bloodstream
- **Major nerves**
  - Nerves of anterolateral abdominal wall come from anterior rami of spinal nerves T7-L1
    - **Dermatomes** (areas of sensory innervation) resemble oblique stripes around trunk following slope of ribs, beginning posteriorly over intervertebral foramen from which spinal nerve exits
    - Nerves run in **neurovascular plane** between transverse abdominal and internal oblique muscles; supply muscles and skin
  - Nerves of posterior abdominal wall
    - Sensory and motor fibers come from anterior and posterior rami of spinal nerves T12 and L1-5 (**lumbar plexus**); lie deep to **psoas muscle**
  - Innervation of abdominal viscera
    - **Sympathetic innervation**, from **lower thoracic** and **abdominopelvic splanchnic nerves** from spinal cord levels T5-L3; via para-aortic prevertebral ganglia (innervates blood vessels of abdominal viscera; inhibitory to parasympathetic innervation)
    - **Parasympathetic**, from **vagus nerve** (esophagus through transverse colon) and **pelvic splanchnic nerve** (descending colon to rectum)
    - **Intrinsic parasympathetic ganglia** within muscular wall of stomach and gut, called **myenteric plexus (of Auerbach)**; promotes peristalsis and secretion (though secretion is largely controlled hormonally)
    - **Sensory innervation of viscera**, pain sensation carried by fibers accompanying sympathetic nerves; reflex afferent innervation accompanies **vagus** (parasympathetic) nerves

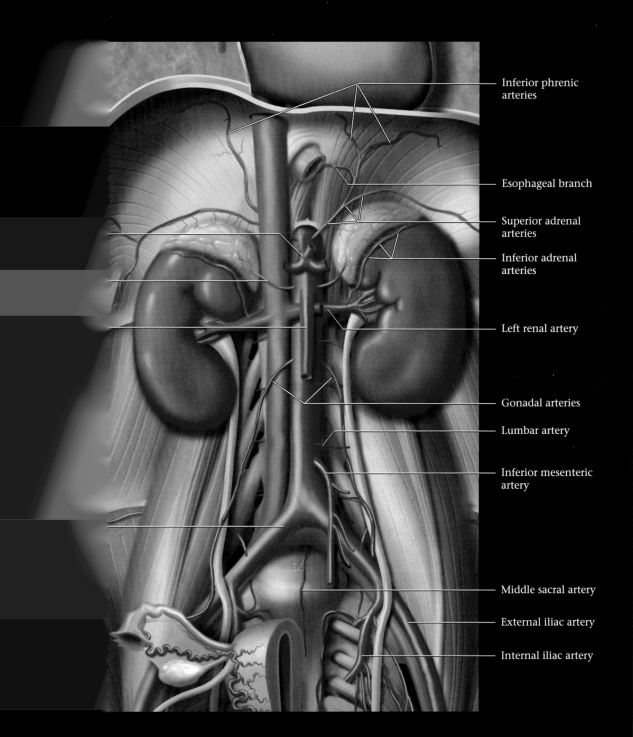

Inferior phrenic arteries

Esophageal branch

Superior adrenal arteries

Inferior adrenal arteries

Left renal artery

Gonadal arteries

Lumbar artery

Inferior mesenteric artery

Middle sacral artery

External iliac artery

Internal iliac artery

gut arise as unpaired vessels from the aortic midline plane and include the celiac, superior
rteries. Branches to the urogenital and endocrine organs arise as paired vessels in the lateral
nal, adrenal, and gonadal (testicular or ovarian) arteries. The diaphragm and posterior
ied by paired branches in the posterolateral plane, including the inferior phrenic and
s, only one of which is labeled in this graphic). The anterior abdominal wall is supplied by
d deep circumflex iliac arteries, both branches of the external iliac artery. The inferior
periorly to run in the rectus sheath, where it anastomoses with the superior epigastric artery,

VESSELS, LYMPHATIC SYSTEM AND NERVES

CT ANGIOGRAM, NORMAL AORTIC BRANCHES

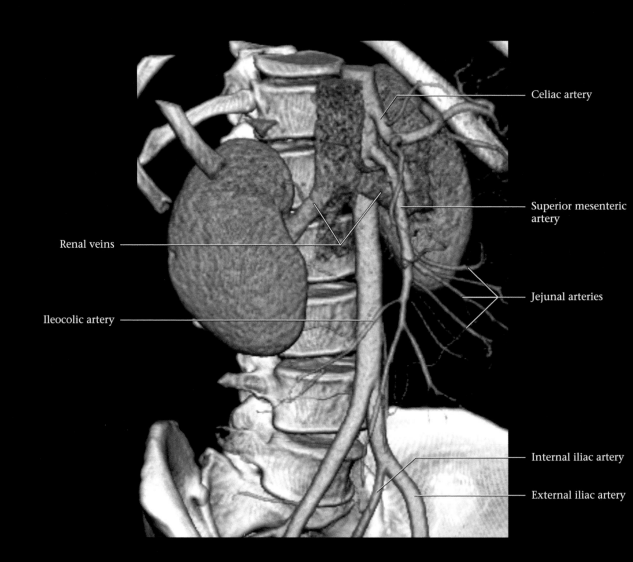

Renal veins

Ileocolic artery

Celiac artery

Superior mesenteric artery

Jejunal arteries

Internal iliac artery

External iliac artery

Volume rendered CT angiogram shows the aorta and some of its major abdominal branches. This image was obtained in the late arterial phase of imaging, resulting in some opacification of the renal veins and the supra-renal inferior vena cava. The infra-renal Inferior vena cava is not yet opacified because the circulation to the lower abdominal organs and legs is not as abundant nor rapid as it is to the kidneys.

NORMAL CATHETER AORTOGRAM

Renal arteries

Superior mesenteric artery (& branches)

Lumbar arteries

Jejunal branches of superior mesenteric artery

Inferior mesenteric artery

Common iliac arteries

Lumbar arteries

Kidney

Right common iliac artery

Internal iliac arteries

Middle sacral artery

External iliac artery

(Top) First of three images from a catheter aortogram shows many of the major branches, overlapped to a degree due to the nonselective (upper aortic) injection and the nontomographic nature of the radiograph. **(Middle)** The four paired lumbar arteries are well shown, arising from the posterolateral abdominal aorta. A fifth lumbar artery may arise from the middle sacral or internal iliac artery. **(Bottom)** The last branches of the abdominal aorta are the middle sacral and common iliac arteries. The latter branch into the external and internal iliac arteries. The internal iliac (hypogastric) artery supplies all the pelvic viscera and muscles, while the external iliac supplies the anterior abdominal wall (through the deep circumflex iliac and inferior epigastric arteries) before leaving the abdomen (behind the inguinal ligament) to supply the lower extremity.

II

VESSELS, LYMPHATIC SYSTEM AND NERVES

AXIAL CT, NORMAL VESSELS

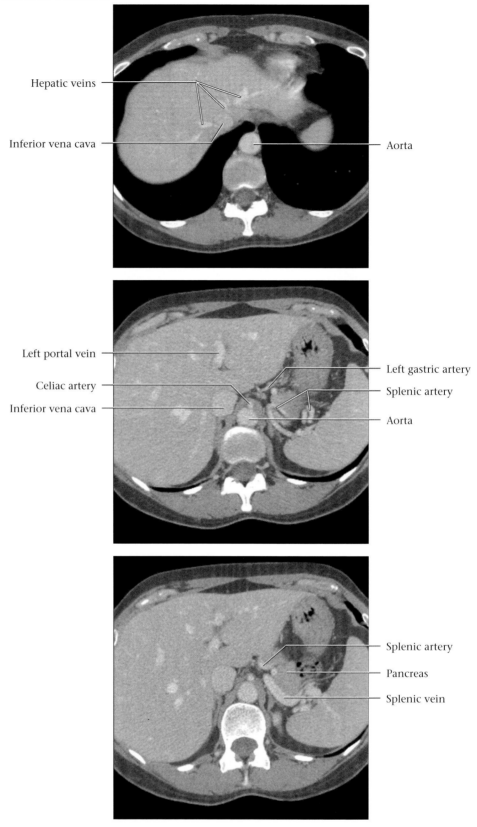

Hepatic veins

Inferior vena cava

Aorta

Left portal vein

Celiac artery

Inferior vena cava

Left gastric artery

Splenic artery

Aorta

Splenic artery

Pancreas

Splenic vein

(Top) First of twelve axial CT sections. The hepatic veins (usually 3 major branches) join the inferior vena cava just below the diaphragm. **(Middle)** The celiac artery is the first (most cephalic) midline branch of the abdominal aorta. Its three major branches are the left gastric, splenic and common hepatic arteries. **(Bottom)** The splenic vein and artery run along the body of the pancreas. The artery is more tortuous (curved) than the vein, and curves into and out of the plane of axial sections, while the splenic vein usually lies in a straight horizontal plane.

VESSELS, LYMPHATIC SYSTEM AND NERVES

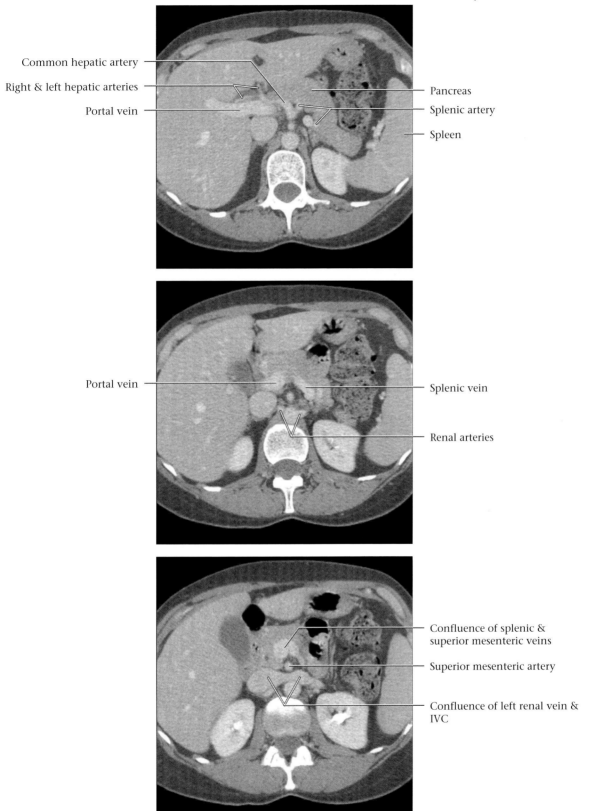

Common hepatic artery

Right & left hepatic arteries

Portal vein

Pancreas

Splenic artery

Spleen

Portal vein

Splenic vein

Renal arteries

Confluence of splenic & superior mesenteric veins

Superior mesenteric artery

Confluence of left renal vein & IVC

(Top) The main branches of the celiac axis (with many variations) are the common hepatic, left gastric, and splenic arteries. The hepatic artery is smaller than, and lies ventral to the portal vein at the porta hepatis. (Middle) The splenic and superior mesenteric veins join to form the portal vein. The renal arteries are the first major paired lateral branches of the abdominal aorta. The inferior phrenic arteries are the first paired lateral branches, but are much smaller, less apparent on imaging, and of less clinical importance. (Bottom) The left renal vein usually crosses in front of the aorta and behind the superior mesenteric artery to join the inferior vena cava.

VESSELS, LYMPHATIC SYSTEM AND NERVES

AXIAL CT, NORMAL VESSELS

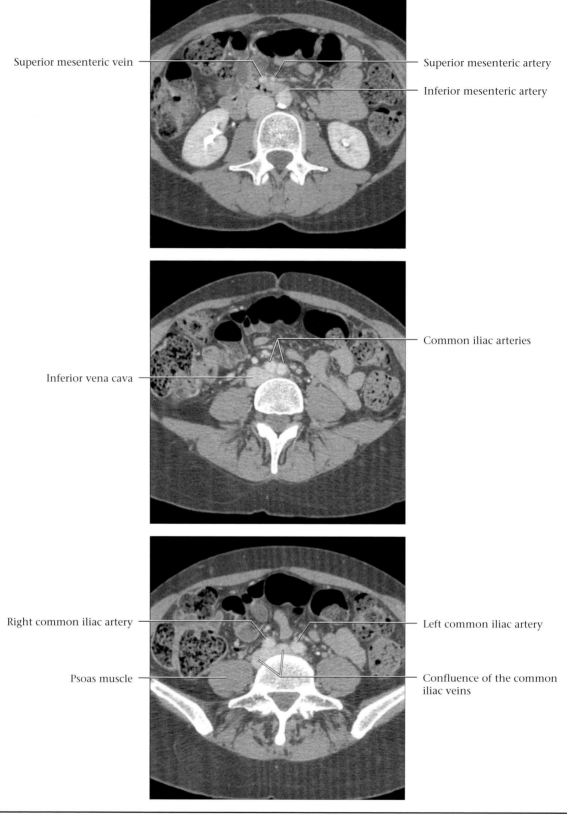

Superior mesenteric vein

Superior mesenteric artery

Inferior mesenteric artery

Common iliac arteries

Inferior vena cava

Right common iliac artery

Left common iliac artery

Psoas muscle

Confluence of the common iliac veins

(Top) The superior mesenteric artery usually lies to the left of and is smaller than the superior mesenteric vein. The inferior mesenteric artery arises from the aorta just above the aortic bifurcation, and supplies the left side of the colon. **(Middle)** The aorta bifurcates into the common iliac arteries at the level of the 4th lumbar vertebra, about 2 cm higher (more cephalic) than the confluence of the common iliac veins, which join to form the inferior vena cava. **(Bottom)** The confluence of the common iliac veins appears as a "peanut" lying behind the right common iliac artery.

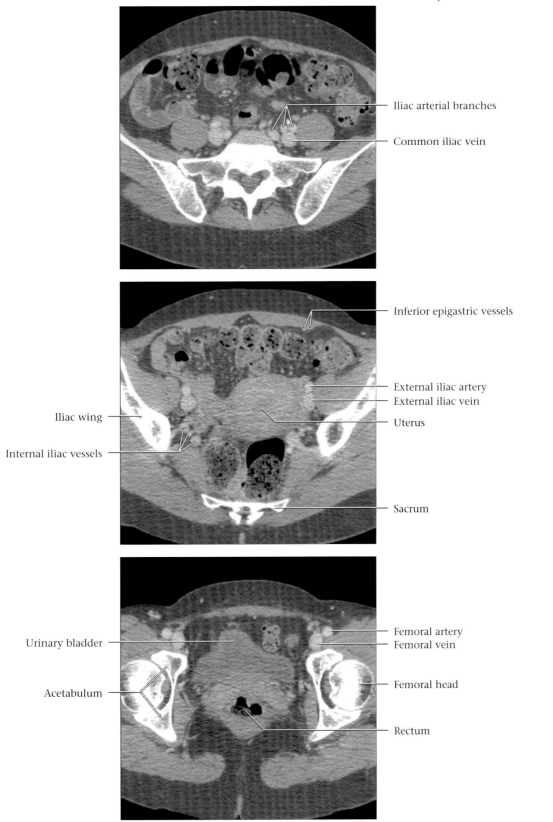

(Top) The internal iliac artery gives off numerous small branches to pelvic muscles and viscera. (Middle) The major pelvic branches of the external iliac artery are the inferior epigastric and deep circumflex iliac arteries, which feed the anterior abdominal wall muscles from below, and freely anastomose with branches of the superior epigastric and musculophrenic arteries. These are the terminal branches of the internal mammary (thoracic) artery, and constitute important collateral pathways in the event of occlusion of the iliac arteries (a relatively common result of atherosclerosis). (Bottom) As the external iliac artery passes under the inguinal ligament it becomes the femoral artery, which supplies the lower extremity as well as branches to the anterior abdominal wall and external genitalia. The femoral artery lies lateral to the vein and is smaller in diameter.

CTA, NORMAL CELIAC & SMA

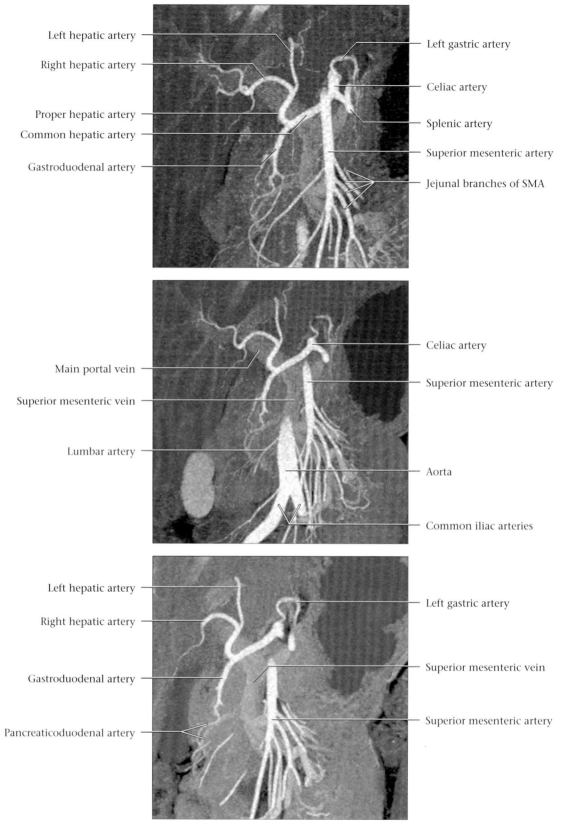

Left hepatic artery

Right hepatic artery

Proper hepatic artery

Common hepatic artery

Gastroduodenal artery

Left gastric artery

Celiac artery

Splenic artery

Superior mesenteric artery

Jejunal branches of SMA

Main portal vein

Superior mesenteric vein

Lumbar artery

Celiac artery

Superior mesenteric artery

Aorta

Common iliac arteries

Left hepatic artery

Right hepatic artery

Gastroduodenal artery

Pancreaticoduodenal artery

Left gastric artery

Superior mesenteric vein

Superior mesenteric artery

(Top) First of three CT images. Maximum intensity image (MIP) in the coronal plane shows the overlapping branches of the celiac and superior mesenteric arteries. An arbitrarily set thickness of the plane of reconstruction results in some peripheral portions of the SMA and splenic artery being excluded from the image. **(Middle)** A more ventral plane of coronal section shows peripheral branches of the SMA, and also some of the distal aorta and common iliac arteries. The portal vein and its major branches are seen faintly, as these CT images were acquired in the predominantly arterial phase after IV administration of contrast medium. **(Bottom)** A more ventral coronal section shows additional branches of the SMA and celiac artery.

Left hepatic artery

Left gastric artery

Gastroduodenal artery

Splenic artery

Catheter

Right hepatic artery

Superior mesenteric artery

Replaced left hepatic artery

Replaced right hepatic artery

Left renal arteries

(Top) First of three images showing variations of the origin of the hepatic arteries. Catheter arteriogram with injection of the celiac trunk shows a normal splenic artery, a large left gastric artery that gives off the left hepatic artery, and the gastroduodenal artery arising directly from the celiac trunk. **(Middle)** Catheter injection of the SMA shows the right hepatic artery arising from the SMA. **(Bottom)** CT Arteriogram, volume-rendered in the coronal plane, shows "replacement" (aberrant origin) of the left and right hepatic arteries. Also noted are three separate left renal arteries.

VARIATION, HEPATIC ARTERIES

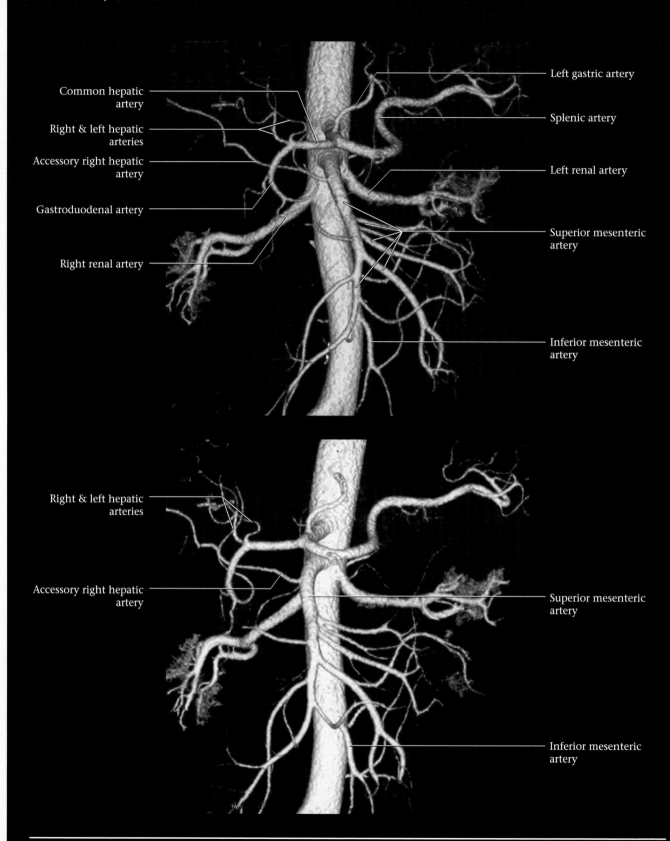

Common hepatic artery

Right & left hepatic arteries

Accessory right hepatic artery

Gastroduodenal artery

Right renal artery

Left gastric artery

Splenic artery

Left renal artery

Superior mesenteric artery

Inferior mesenteric artery

Right & left hepatic arteries

Accessory right hepatic artery

Superior mesenteric artery

Inferior mesenteric artery

(Top) First of two views of a CT arteriogram (volume-rendered, shaded surface display). Note the conventional origins of all the major abdominal aortic visceral branches. The right hepatic artery, arising from the proper hepatic branch of the celiac artery, is smaller lyhan usual because there ys an accessory right hepatic nertery arising from the superior mesenteric artery, a common variant. **(Bottom)** Oblique view of CTA clearly shows the origin of the accessory right hepatic artery from the superior mesenteric artery.

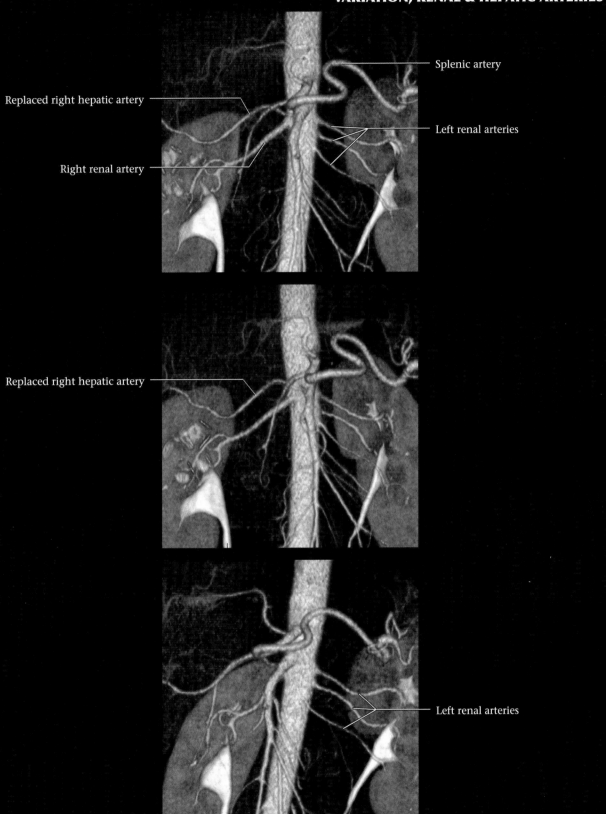

(Top) First of three images of a CT arteriogram, volume-rendered. There are three left renal arteries, each having a separate origin from the aorta. A single right renal artery is present. The right hepatic artery arises from the superior mesenteric artery, rather than the celiac artery, a common variation called a "replaced" hepatic artery. *(Middle)* In this obliquity it is easier to recognize the replaced hepatic artery, but more difficult to distinguish the multiple left renal arteries from branches of the superior mesenteric artery. *(Bottom)* The three left renal arteries are best shown in this obliquity.

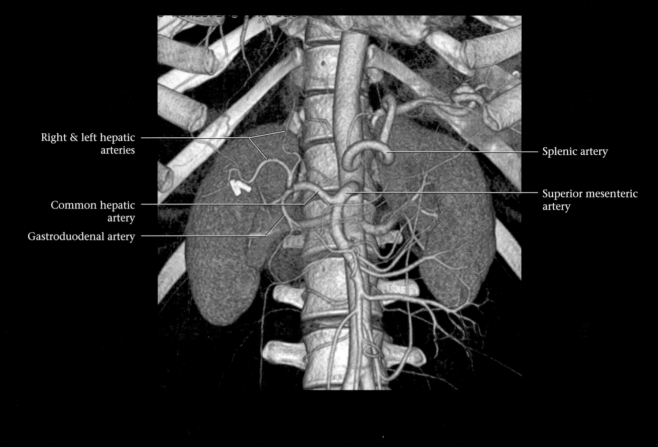

Right & left hepatic arteries

Common hepatic artery

Gastroduodenal artery

Splenic artery

Superior mesenteric artery

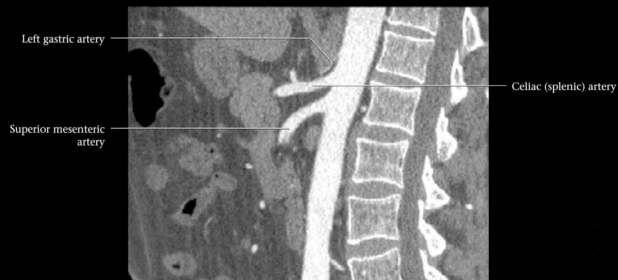

Left gastric artery

Superior mesenteric artery

Celiac (splenic) artery

(Top) Coronal volume-rendered image shows the entire common hepatic artery arising from the superior mesenteric artery. The left gastric artery also has a separate origin from the aorta, though difficult to perceive on this image. The "celiac trunk" in this patient consists lynly of the splenic artery. **(Bottom)** Sagittal MIP image in the midline shows the small left gastric artery with its separate origin from the aorta. The celiac trunk, essentially the splenic artery in this variation, and the origin of the superior mesenteric artery are shown.

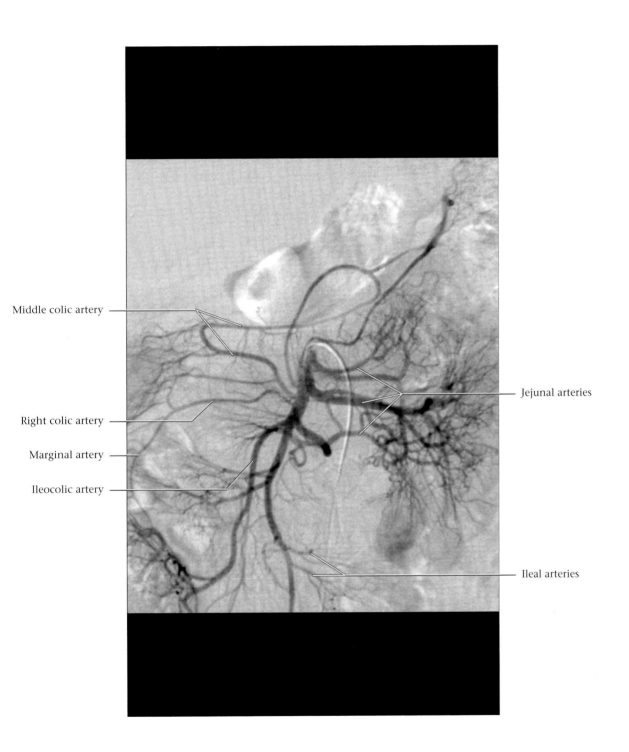

Middle colic artery

Right colic artery

Marginal artery

Ileocolic artery

Jejunal arteries

Ileal arteries

atheter injection of the superior mesenteric artery shows opacification of all the arterial branches that supply the ntire small intestine, the appendix, cecum, ascending and transverse colon. The marginal artery has a course parallel o the entire length of the colon and anastomoses with the marginal artery on the left, which is supplied by branches f the inferior mesenteric artery. This is an important collateral pathway that can supply flow to parts of the colon at would otherwise be made ischemic due to occlusion of the main trunk or branches of the SMA or IMA.

CORONAL ABDOMINAL VEINS

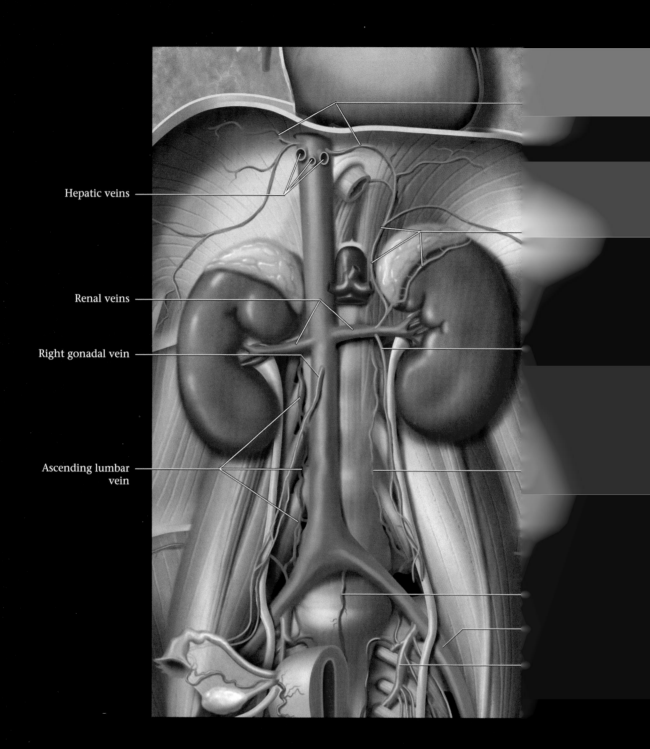

Hepatic veins

Renal veins

Right gonadal vein

Ascending lumbar vein

The inferior vena cava begins at the L5 level with the confluence of the common iliac veins, the result of the confluence of the internal and external iliac veins. Note the ascending lumb anastomose freely between the IVC, the azygous and hemiazygous and the renal veins. These pathway for collateral flow in the event of obstruction of the IVC or one of its major tributar an important role in spread of tumor and infection from the pelvis and spine to the thorax, The right renal vein rarely receives tributaries, while the left receives the gonadal, adrenal, ar adrenal vein also anastomoses with the inferior phrenic vein. The hepatic veins return blood

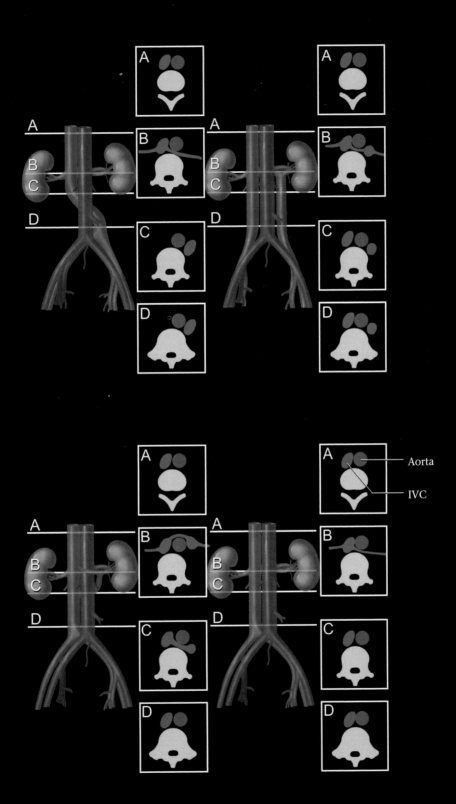

(Top) Four graphics illustrate common variations of the IVC. The labeled lines on the frontal graphics correspond to the levels of the axial sections. The left graphic shows transposition of the IVC, in which the infrarenal portion of the IVC lies predominantly to the left side of the aorta. A more symmon anomaly is shown on right graphic, a "duplication" of the IVC in which the left common iliac vein continues in a cephalad direction without crossing over to join the right iliac vein. Instead, it joins the left renal vein, and then crosses over to the right. The suprarenal IVC has a conventional course and appearance. **(Bottom)** The left graphic shows a circumaortic left renal vein, with the smaller, more cephalic vein passing in front of the aorta & the larger vein passing behind & caudal. The right graphic shows a completely retroaortic renal vein.

VARIATION, LEFT-SIDED IVC (TRANSPOSITION)

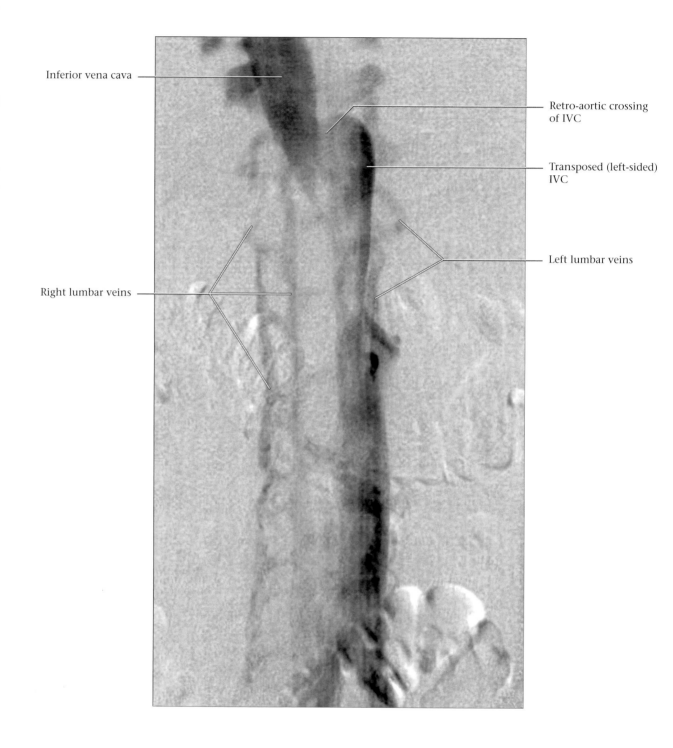

Inferior vena cava

Retro-aortic crossing of IVC

Transposed (left-sided) IVC

Left lumbar veins

Right lumbar veins

First of three images from a catheter injection of the inferior vena cava shows the vena cava lying to the left of midline, an anomalous position. In the mid abdomen it crosses over to the right side behind the aorta, which results in compression of the inferior vena cava. The luminal narrowing results in increased flow through collateral venous channels, including the lumbar veins.

VESSELS, LYMPHATIC SYSTEM AND NERVES

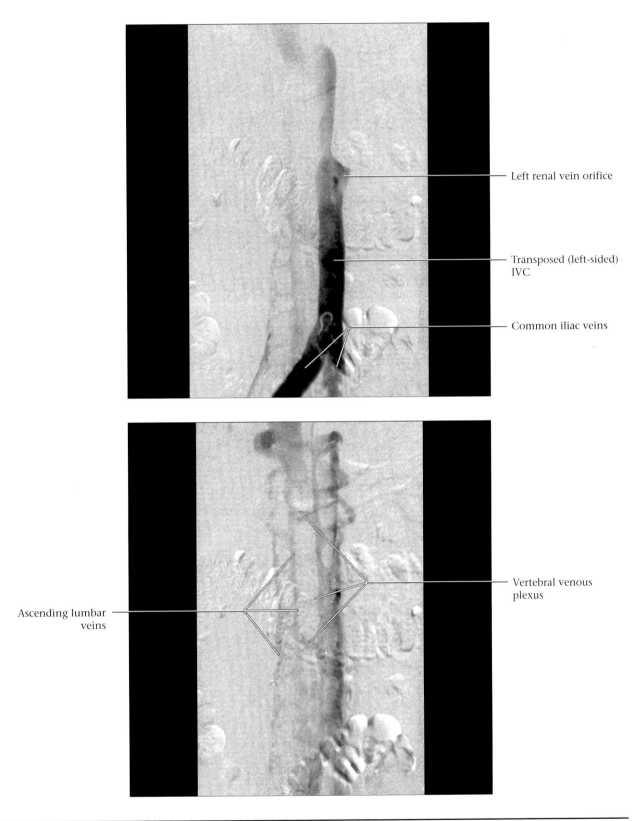

Left renal vein orifice

Transposed (left-sided) IVC

Common iliac veins

Ascending lumbar veins

Vertebral venous plexus

(**Top**) This image shows the common iliac veins and some retrograde opacification of the orifice of the left renal vein. (**Bottom**) A later film from the same study shows that contrast material has cleared from most of the inferior vena cava, while the collateral veins of the vertebral plexus and ascending lumbar veins remain opacified. Note the numerous connections between the venous plexus which surrounds the vertebrae and the lumbar veins.

VARIATION, DUPLICATED IVC

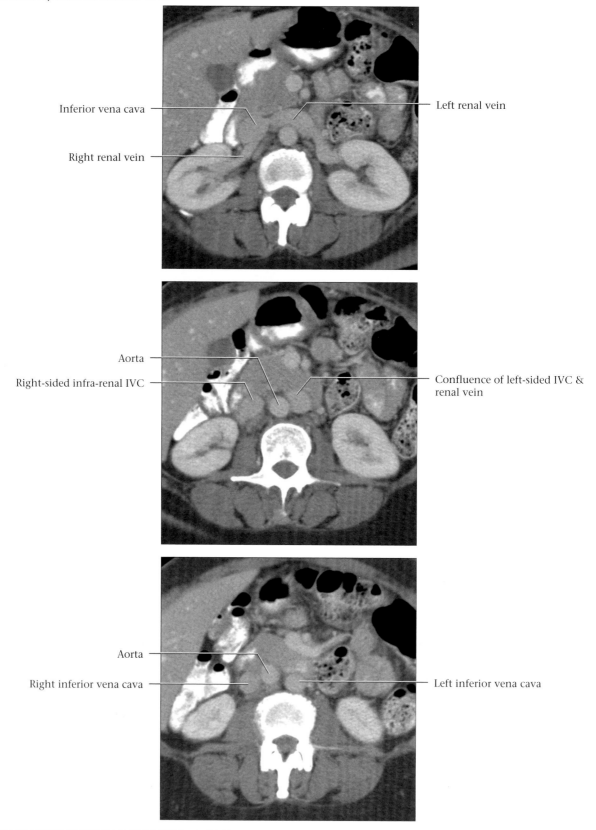

(Top) First of six axial CT sections showing a duplicated inferior vena cava. At this level the left renal vein has received the duplicated infra-renal inferior vena cava and is emptying into the inferior vena cava. Note the much larger diameter of the left renal vein as a result of this anomaly. **(Middle)** At this more caudal level the infra-renal left-sided inferior vena cava has joined the left renal vein. **(Bottom)** More caudal section shows two venous structures of similar size running a parallel course on either side of the aorta.

VESSELS, LYMPHATIC SYSTEM AND NERVES

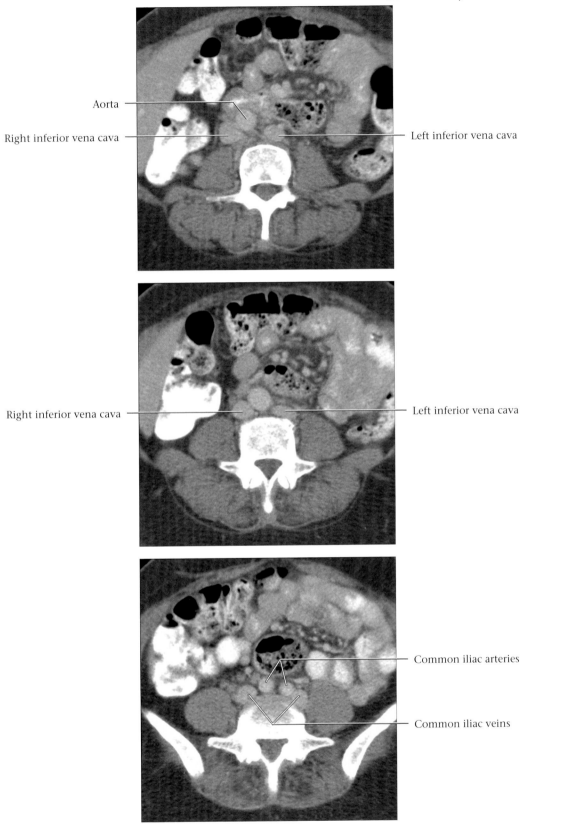

Aorta

Right inferior vena cava

Left inferior vena cava

Right inferior vena cava

Left inferior vena cava

Common iliac arteries

Common iliac veins

(Top) More caudal section shows duplication of the infra-renal inferior vena cava. **(Middle)** At this more caudal section the common iliac veins would normally have joined to form the inferior vena cava. Instead, there is a continuation of the left common iliac vein as it courses in a cephalad path. **(Bottom)** At this more caudal level, the position and appearance of the common iliac veins are normal.

VARIATION, IVC DUPLICATION

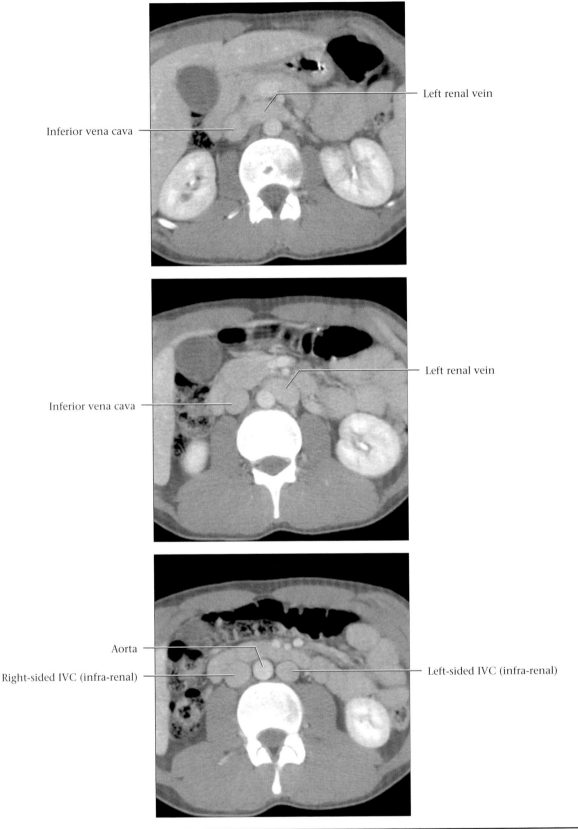

(Top) First of five axial CT sections shows an enlarged left renal vein joining the inferior vena cava. From this level cephalad, the inferior vena cava had a normal caliber and course, lying in its usual site to the right of the aorta. (Middle) More caudal section shows the infrarenal duplicated inferior vena cava joining the left renal vein. (Bottom) Caudal section below the kidneys shows both the left and right-sided inferior vena cava. Failure to recognize this as a cylindrical structure in continuity with the common iliac vein caudally and the left renal vein cephalically might lead to a mistaken diagnosis of a para-aortic mass, such as lymphadenopathy.

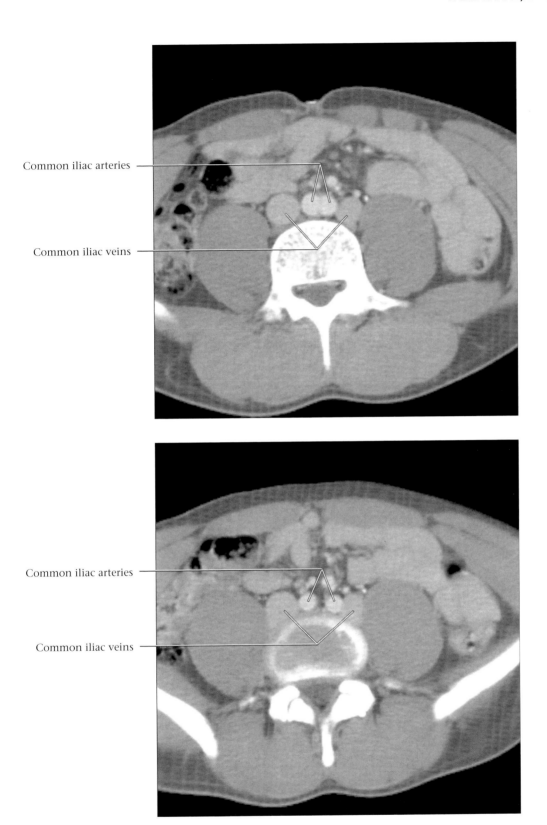

Common iliac arteries

Common iliac veins

Common iliac arteries

Common iliac veins

(Top) More caudal section shows the bifurcation of the aorta into the common iliac arteries. At this level the left common iliac vein would normally have crossed over to join the right common iliac vein to form the inferior vena cava. **(Bottom)** More caudal section shows a normal appearance and location of the common iliac veins.

VARIATION, CIRCUMAORTIC RENAL VEIN

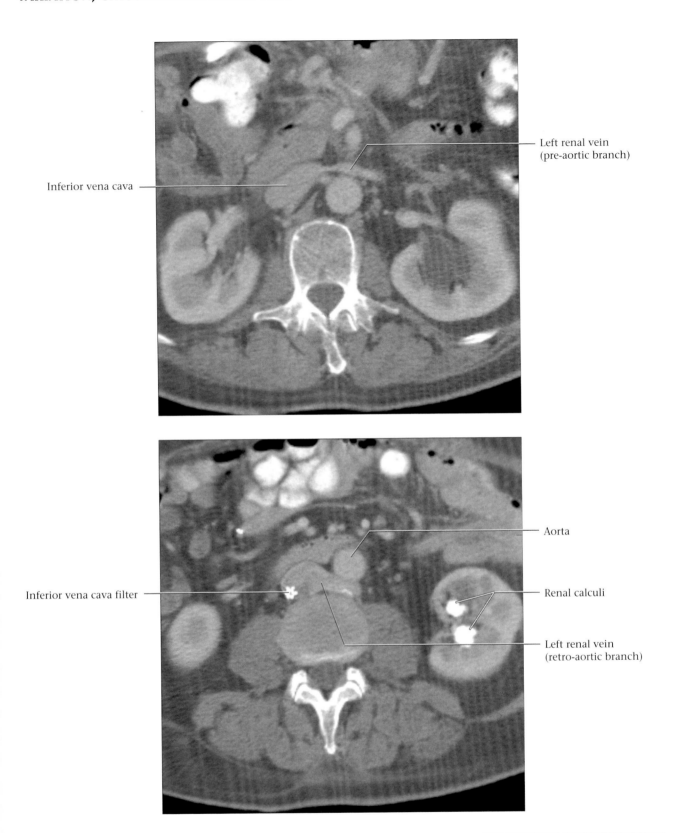

(Top) First of four images in a patient with a circumaortic left renal vein. Variations of the left renal vein are much more common than those affecting the right vein. One common anomaly is a circumaortic left renal vein, in which the pre-aortic branch passes, as usual, between the aorta and the superior mesenteric vessels. The pre-aortic branch is smaller and more cephalad in position than the retro-aortic component. (Bottom) The retro-aortic branch of the left renal vein is usually larger and lies about one vertebral body lower (more caudal) than the pre-aortic branch. This anomaly is of importance if surgery of the left kidney or aorta is being considered, or if interventions on the inferior vena cava are implemented (such as placement of an inferior vena cava filter in this patient with lower extremity venous thromboses).

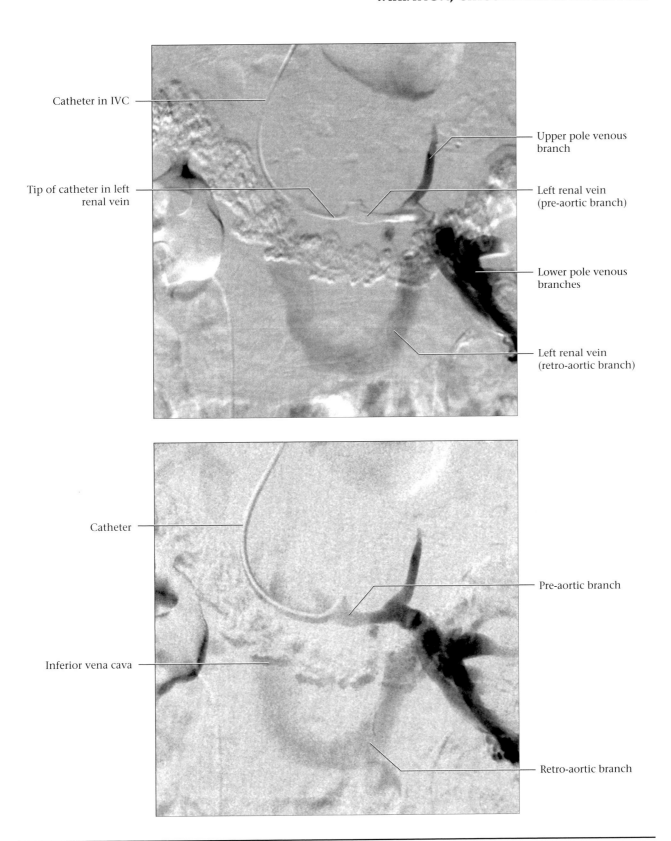

Catheter in IVC

Tip of catheter in left renal vein

Upper pole venous branch

Left renal vein (pre-aortic branch)

Lower pole venous branches

Left renal vein (retro-aortic branch)

Catheter

Inferior vena cava

Pre-aortic branch

Retro-aortic branch

(Top) In anticipation of placing an inferior vena cava filter, a catheter was introduced into the inferior vena cava from an arm vein. The tip of the catheter is seen curving to the left and entering a renal vein branch that represents the pre-aortic branch seen on the CT scan. Note its small size synd cephalic position relative to the retro-aortic branch, which is also opacified by injection of contrast material through the catheter tip. **(Bottom)** The pre- and retro-aortic branches of the circumaortic left renal vein communicate with each other and drain separately into the inferior vena cava.

VESSELS, LYMPHATIC SYSTEM AND NERVES

VARIATION, IVC & POLYSPLENIA

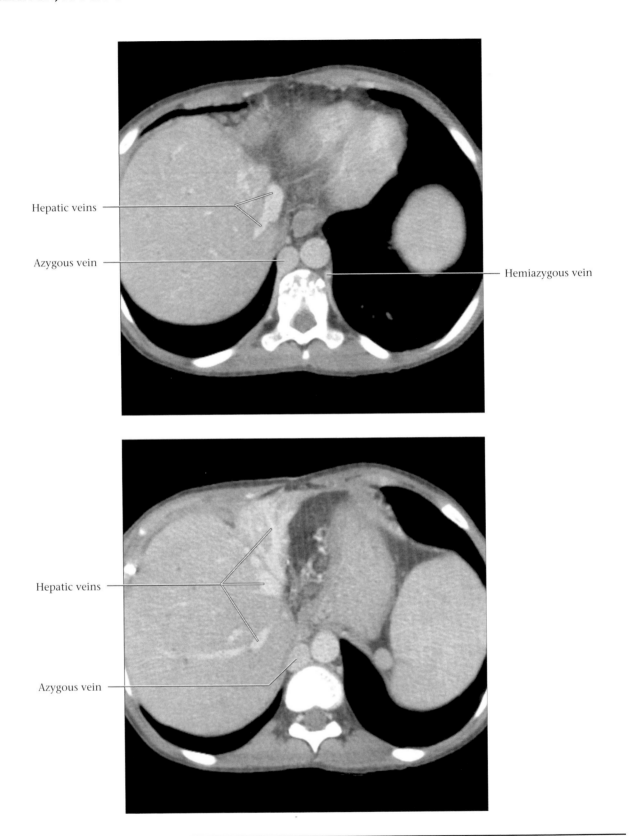

Hepatic veins

Azygous vein

Hemiazygous vein

Hepatic veins

Azygous vein

(Top) First of five CT images in a patient with polysplenia syndrome shows an enlarged azygous vein, which serves as the primary route of venous drainage of the abdomen and lower extremities in this condition. The inferior vena cava is absent between the level of the renal veins and the hepatic veins, which drain directly into the right atrium. (Bottom) More caudal image shows a dysmorphic liver and the first of multiple splenic masses.

II

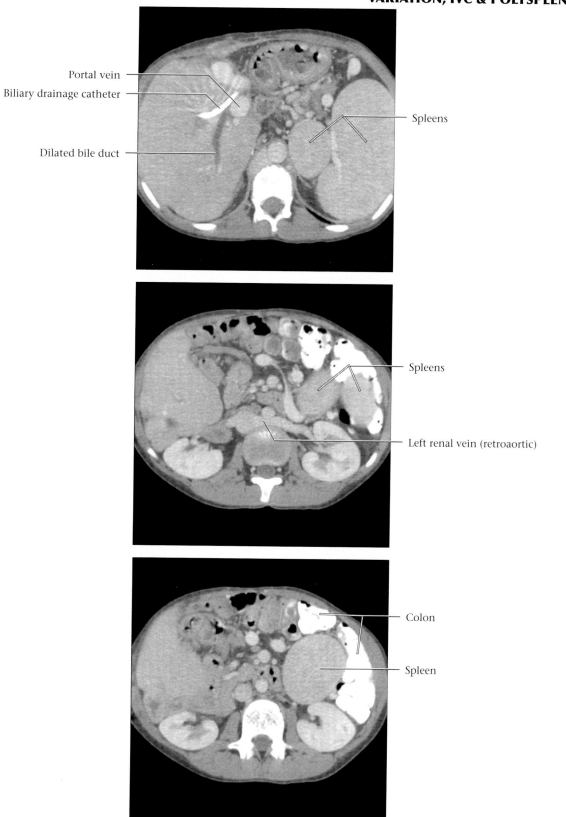

(Top) More caudal section shows absence of the retrohepatic inferior vena cava. Dilation of the intrahepatic bile ducts is noted, along with a biliary drainage stent. Multiple splenic masses are noted; in this syndrome, these may number from 2-16. **(Middle)** An associated vascular anomaly is a retroaortic left renal vein. Above this level the inferior vena cava is absent, and the azygous/hemiazygous and other collateral veins must return blood to the heart. **(Bottom)** More caudal section shows all of the colon lying on the left side of the abdomen, while all of the small bowel lies to the right. Various bowel anomalies, including malrotation, duplication, and atresia are associated with the polysplenia syndrome.

VARIATION, POLYSPLENIA WITH ANOMALIES OF IVC & SVC

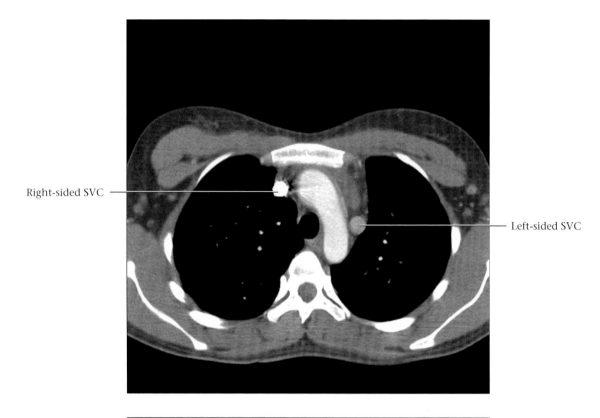

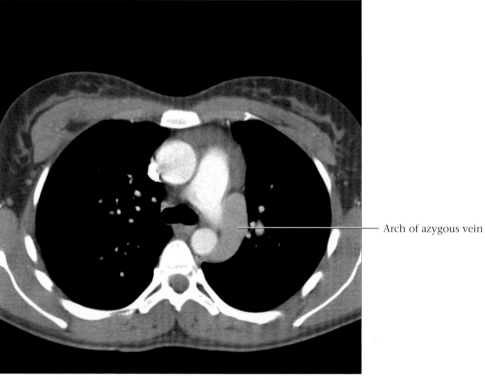

(Top) First of eight CT sections in a patient with polysplenia syndrome and associated vascular anomalies shows duplication of the superior vena cava. (Bottom) The arch of the dilated azygous vein is seen in this more caudal section as it enters the back of the superior vena cava. Normally the azygous would enter into the superior vena cava to the right of midline; this is part of the situs anomalies in this syndrome.

VESSELS, LYMPHATIC SYSTEM AND NERVES

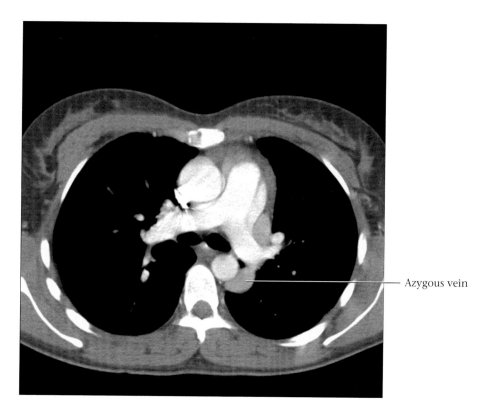

Azygous vein

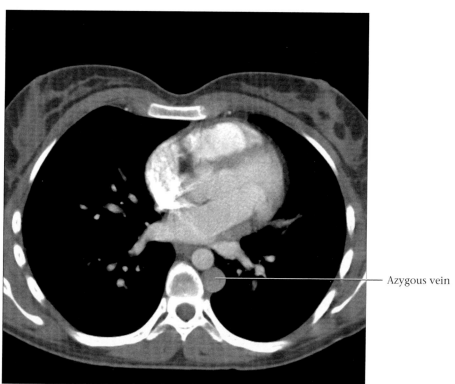

Azygous vein

(Top) The azygous vein is in an anomalous left-sided position and is dilated due to interruption of the supra-renal inferior vena cava. This condition is referred to as "azygous continuation of the inferior vena cava". (Bottom) The heart appears normal in this patient. 65% of patients with polysplenia syndrome have an absent supra-renal inferior vena cava with azygous continuation.

VESSELS, LYMPHATIC SYSTEM AND NERVES

VARIATION: SVC, IVC & POLYSPLENIA

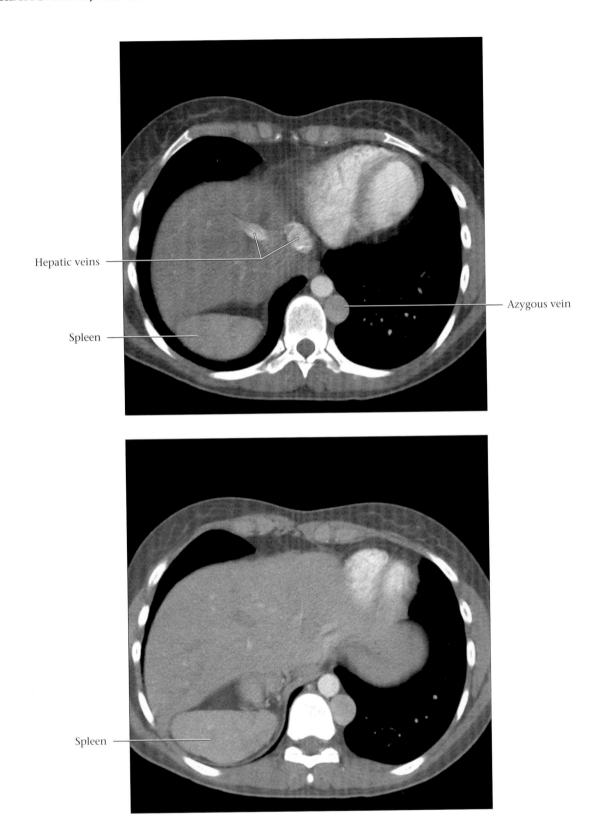

Hepatic veins

Spleen

Azygous vein

Spleen

(Top) The hepatic veins empty directly into the right atrium. One of several splenic masses is seen, lying on the right side of the abdomen instead of the normal left side. **(Bottom)** More caudal section shows situs ambiguous (rather than simple situs inversus, or a mirror-image arrangement of the abdominal viscera).

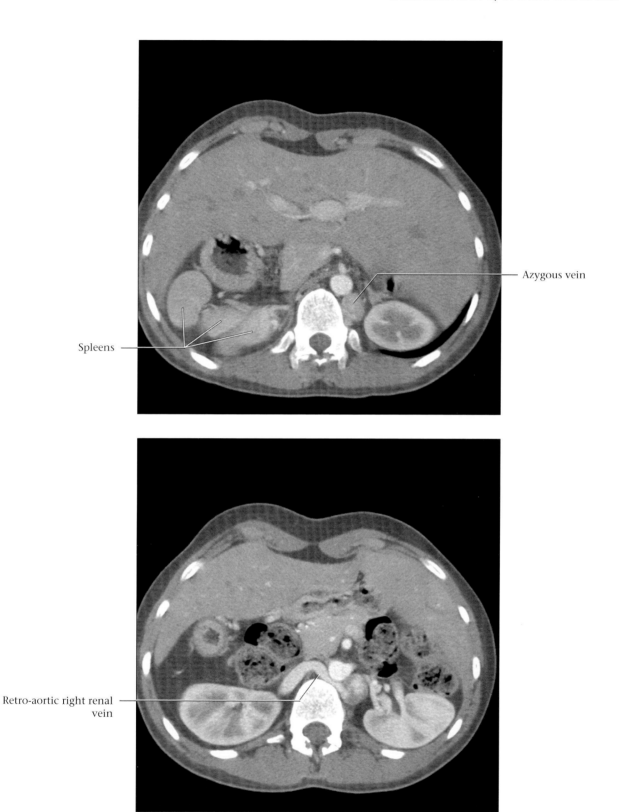

Azygous vein

Spleens

Retro-aortic right renal vein

(Top) Multiple spleens are noted. The liver is more symmetric and midline than normal, part of the situs ambiguous pattern. **(Bottom)** A retroaortic renal vein is noted. Due to the presence of the infrarenal inferior vena cava on the left side of the abdomen, it is the right renal vein which is retro-aortic in this patient.

VESSELS, LYMPHATIC SYSTEM AND NERVES

VARIATION, HEPATIC VEINS

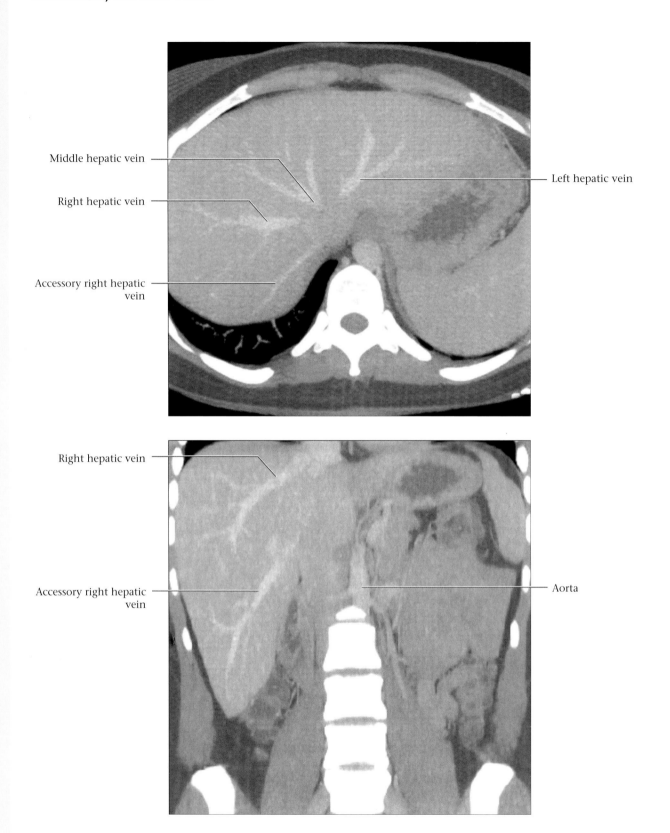

(Top) First of four CT sections shows variation in hepatic venous drainage into the inferior vena cava. Thick axial reconstructed CT section shows the three major hepatic veins (left, middle, and right) in addition to an accessory right hepatic vein which has a separate entry into the inferior syena cava. **(Bottom)** Coronal CT section shows the long axes of the right and accessory right hepatic veins which have separate orifices in the inferior vena cava. Venous anomalies, such as these, are important to recognize if hepatic surgery (e.g., partial hepatectomy) is being considered.

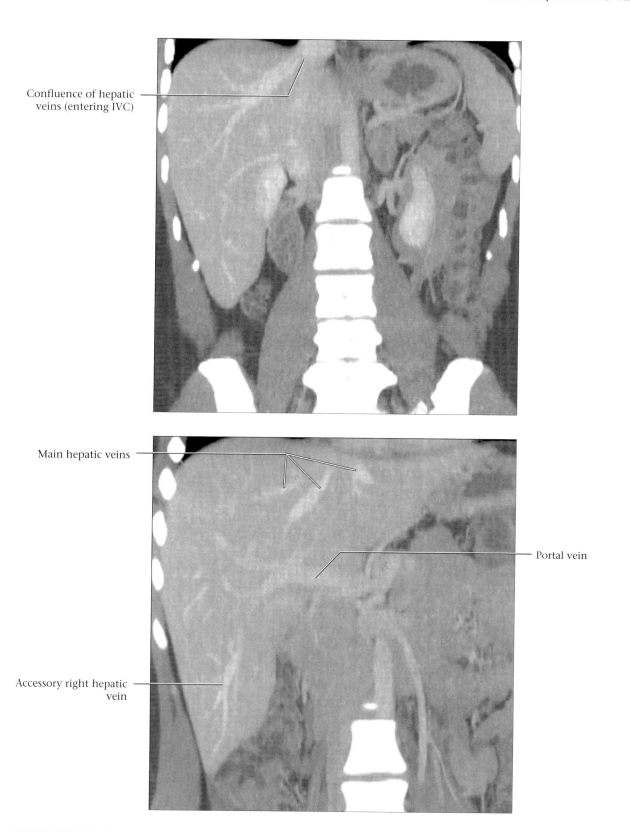

Confluence of hepatic veins (entering IVC)

Main hepatic veins

Portal vein

Accessory right hepatic vein

(Top) The three major hepatic veins enter the inferior vena cava just below the diaphragm. They may have three separate orifices or may join together before entering the inferior vena cava. Commonly, the left and middle hepatic veins join and empty through a single lyrifice. **(Bottom)** No single plane of section is sufficient to show the entire course of vessels, though 3 dimensional surface renderings are often helpful, particularly for visualization of arteries, as these can be rendered quite dense and apparent with the IV administration of a bolus of contrast medium. This MIP image in the coronal plane shows the portal and hepatic veins well.

VESSELS, LYMPHATIC SYSTEM AND NERVES

VARIATION, INTERRUPTED IVC

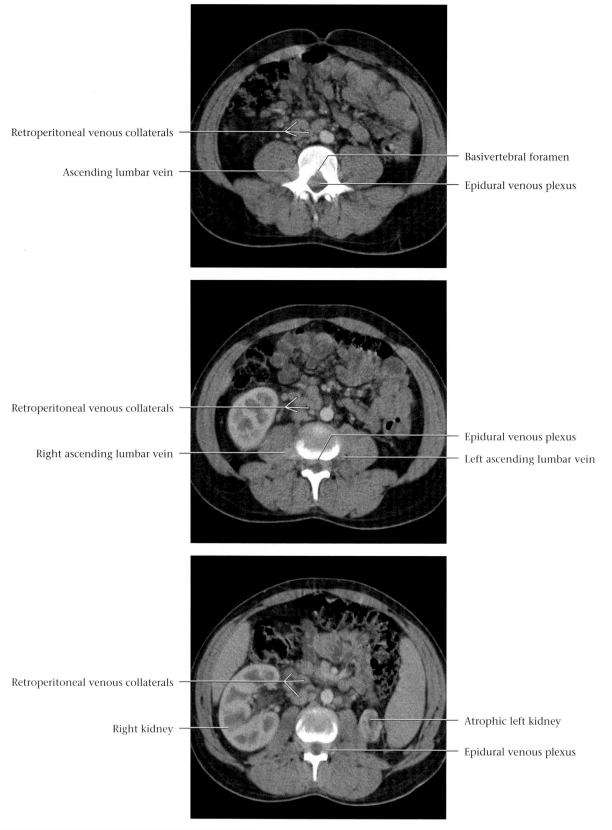

Retroperitoneal venous collaterals

Ascending lumbar vein

Basivertebral foramen

Epidural venous plexus

Retroperitoneal venous collaterals

Right ascending lumbar vein

Epidural venous plexus

Left ascending lumbar vein

Retroperitoneal venous collaterals

Right kidney

Atrophic left kidney

Epidural venous plexus

(Top) First of five axial CT images in a 15 year old male with interruption of the infrarenal inferior vena cava. The inferior vena cava is absent and is replaced by multiple retroperitoneal venous collaterals. Note the widened basivertebral foramen due to dilatation of the basivertebral vein connecting the dilated epidural plexus to the ascending lumbar veins on both sides of the lumbar vertebral bodies. **(Middle)** The left lumbar vein joins a medial root from the left renal vein to form the hemiazygos vein whereas the right ascending lumbar vein joins a medial root from the inferior vena cava to form the azygos vein. Note the dilated ascending lumbar veins. **(Bottom)** Note the extensive retroperitoneal venous collaterals replacing the absent inferior vena cava. Incidental note of atrophic left kidney with compensatory hypertrophy of the right kidney.

VARIATION, INTERRUPTED IVC

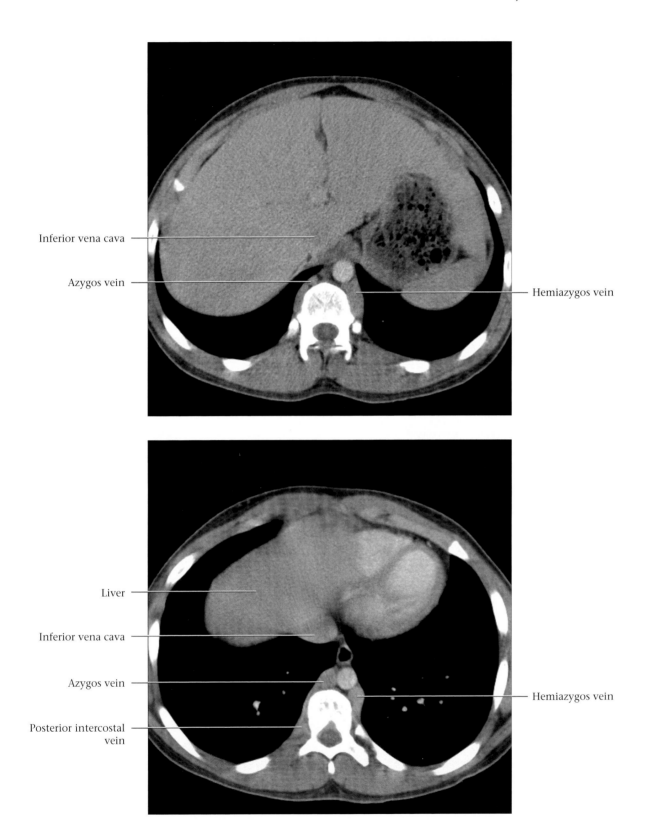

Inferior vena cava

Azygos vein

Hemiazygos vein

Liver

Inferior vena cava

Azygos vein

Hemiazygos vein

Posterior intercostal vein

(Top) The hemiazygos vein crosses the midline at T8 to drain into the azygos vein which drains into the superior vena cava. This is a crucial pathway for drainage of the lower part of the body in patients with inferior vena cava obstruction. Note dilatation of both lyme azygos and hemiazygos sveins carrying blood from nrhe lower part of the body to drain into the superior vena cava. **(Bottom)** The thoracic epidural venous plexus drains into the azygos and hemiazygos veins via the posterior intercostal veins. Note the dilated right posterior intercostal vein on this image.

VESSELS, LYMPHATIC SYSTEM AND NERVES

CORONAL LYMPH NODES

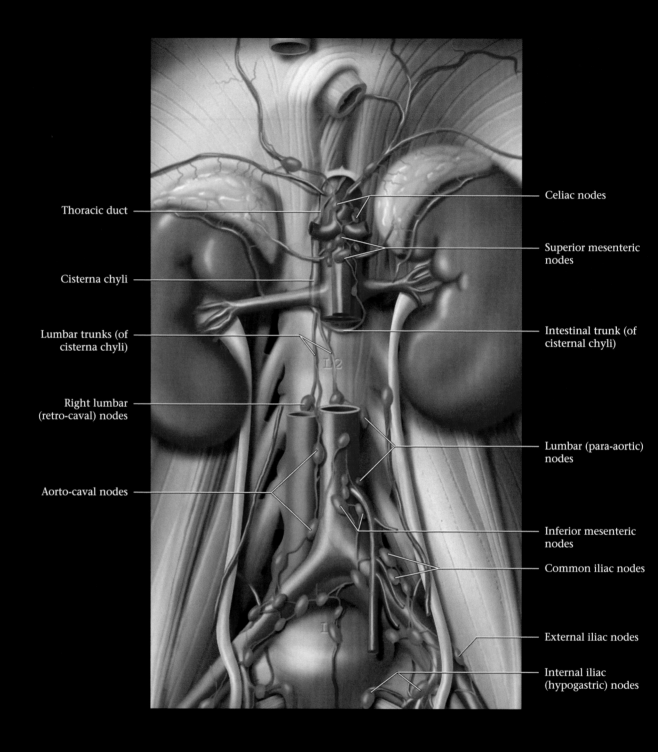

Thoracic duct

Cisterna chyli

Lumbar trunks (of cisterna chyli)

Right lumbar (retro-caval) nodes

Aorto-caval nodes

Celiac nodes

Superior mesenteric nodes

Intestinal trunk (of cisternal chyli)

Lumbar (para-aortic) nodes

Inferior mesenteric nodes

Common iliac nodes

External iliac nodes

Internal iliac (hypogastric) nodes

The major lymphatics and lymph nodes of the abdomen are located along, and share the same name as the major blood vessels, such as the external iliac nodes, celiac and superior mesenteric nodes. The para-aortic and para-caval nodes are also referred to as the lumbar nodes and receive afferents from the lower abdominal viscera, abdominal wall and lower extremities; they are frequently involved in inflammatory and neoplastic processes. The lumbar trunks join with an intestinal trunk (at about the L1 level) to form the cisterna chyli, which may be a discrete sac or a plexiform convergence. The cisterna chyli and other major lymphatic trunks join to form the thoracic duct which passes through the aortic hiatus to enter the mediastinum. After picking up additional lymphatic trunks within the thorax, the thoracic duct empties into the left subclavian or innominate vein.

VESSELS, LYMPHATIC SYSTEM AND NERVES

NORMAL LYMPHANGIOGRAM

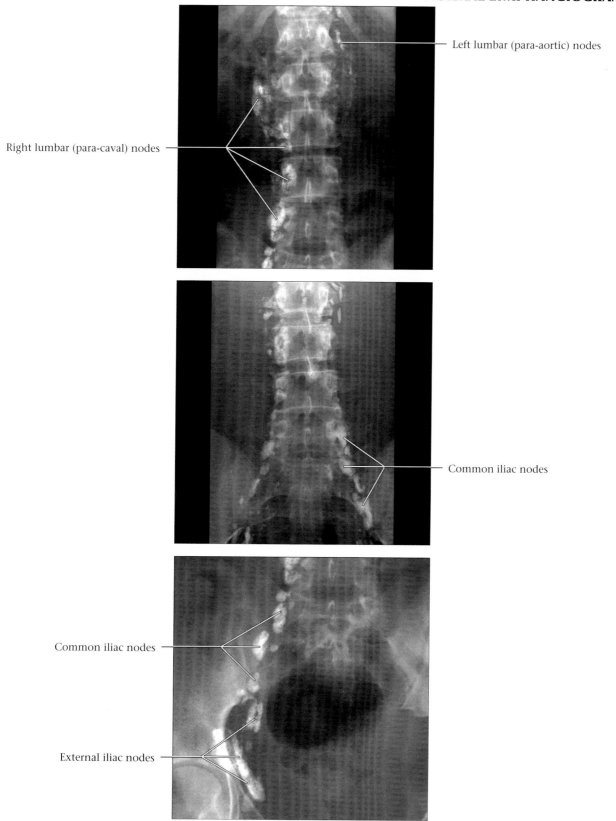

Left lumbar (para-aortic) nodes

Right lumbar (para-caval) nodes

Common iliac nodes

Common iliac nodes

External iliac nodes

(Top) First of three images from a lymphangiogram, in which iodinated oil is slowly infused into the lymphatics of the foot to produce opacification of the lymph channels and nodes. Note the sub-centimeter (short axis) diameter of these normal retroperitoneal lymph nodes. (Middle) Lymphatic channels and lymph nodes parallel the course of major blood vessels and share similar names, such as these common iliac nodes. (Bottom) With the availability of CT, MR and PET (positron emission tomography), lymphangiograms are performed much less frequently than in the past.

LYMPHADENOPATHY DUE TO LYMPHOMA

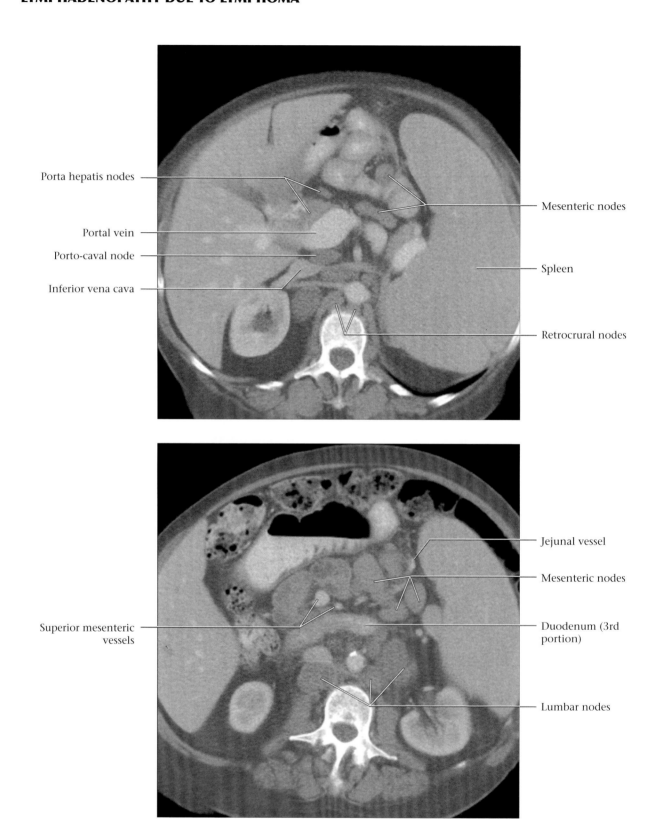

Porta hepatis nodes

Portal vein

Porto-caval node

Inferior vena cava

Mesenteric nodes

Spleen

Retrocrural nodes

Jejunal vessel

Mesenteric nodes

Duodenum (3rd portion)

Superior mesenteric vessels

Lumbar nodes

(**Top**) First of four CT sections of a 50 year old woman with non-Hodgkin lymphoma shows splenomegaly and marked enlargement of multiple upper abdominal lymph nodes. The use of intravenous and oral contrast opacifies the blood vessels and bowel, respectively, facilitating identification of the nodes. Note enlargement of the retrocrural nodes that accompany the aorta as it passes behind the diaphragm as it enters the thorax. (**Bottom**) The lumbar nodes are often referred to as para- or retro-aortic (or -caval), indicating their position relative to the great vessels. Note the ventral displacement of the duodenum by the large retroperitoneal nodes, and the mesenteric vessels surrounded or "sandwiched" by mesenteric nodes.

VESSELS, LYMPHATIC SYSTEM AND NERVES

LYMPHADENOPATHY DUE TO LYMPHOMA

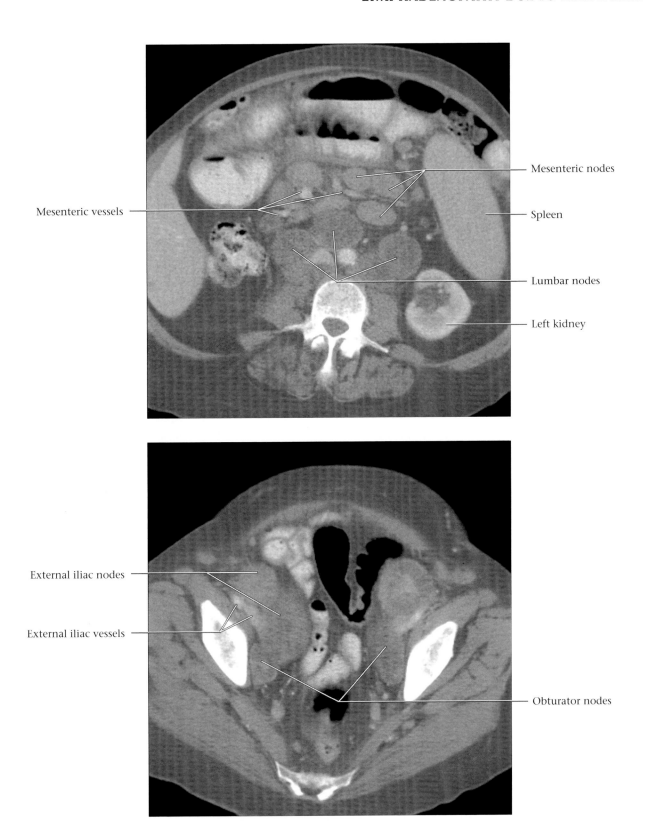

Mesenteric vessels — Mesenteric nodes — Spleen — Lumbar nodes — Left kidney

External iliac nodes — External iliac vessels — Obturator nodes

(Top) Normal abdominal lymph nodes are usually less than one cm in diameter. Size alone is not always a reliable criterion for diagnosing malignant nodal involvement, as benign processes, including infection and inflammation (e.g., mononucleosis or sarcoidosis) can result in similar nodal enlargement. Conversely, nodes containing malignant deposits are not always enlarged. Note that some of the enlarged lumbar nodes are quite low in attenuation (density), probably due to partial necrosis. (Bottom) The major lymphatic channels and nodes follow the major blood vessels and have similar names.

AUTONOMIC NERVES & GANGLIA OF THE ABDOMEN

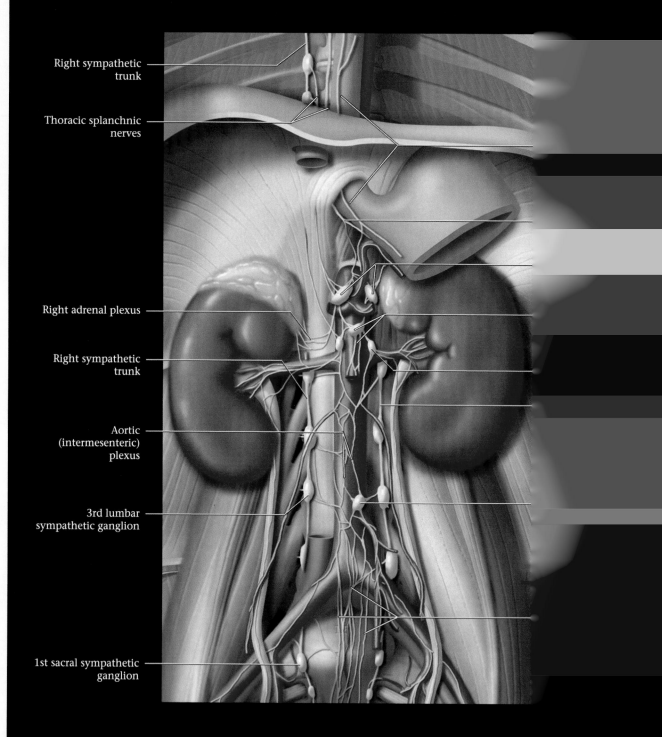

Right sympathetic trunk

Thoracic splanchnic nerves

Right adrenal plexus

Right sympathetic trunk

Aortic (intermesenteric) plexus

3rd lumbar sympathetic ganglion

1st sacral sympathetic ganglion

Autonomic innervation of the abdominal viscera comes from several splanchnic nerves and vagus (CN10), which deliver presynaptic sympathetic and parasympathetic fibers (respective and its sympathetic ganglia. Periarterial extensions of these plexuses deliver postsynaptic syn parasympathetic fibers to the abdominal viscera, where intrinsic parasympathetic ganglia occ are mixed, sharing sympathetic, parasympathetic, and visceral afferent fibers. Thoracic splan main source of presynaptic sympathetic fibers to the abdominal viscera. The cell bodies of th sympathetic neurons constitute the prevertebral ganglia that cluster around the roots of the abdominal aorta, including the celiac, aortorenal, superior and inferior mesenteric ganglia.

NEURAL INVASION BY PANCREATIC CANCER

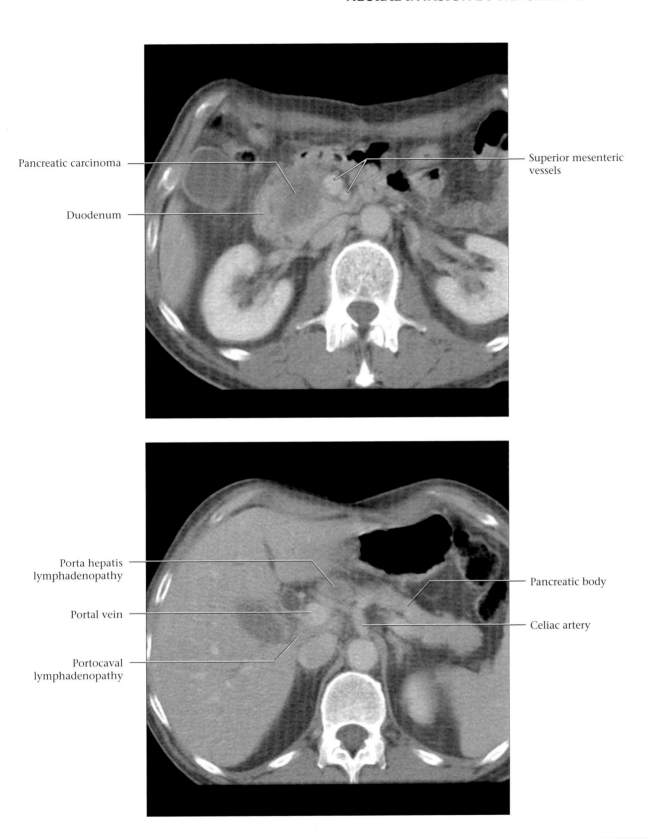

Pancreatic carcinoma

Superior mesenteric vessels

Duodenum

Porta hepatis lymphadenopathy

Pancreatic body

Portal vein

Celiac artery

Portocaval lymphadenopathy

(Top) First of two CT images in a patient with intractable abdominal pain shows a mass in the head of the pancreas, representing carcinoma. The fat planes around the superior mesenteric vessels are infiltrated with tumor. Recall that the celiac and superior mesenteric ganglia lie in this area. Invasion of these structures is common in patients with pancreatic carcinoma and is a major cause of morbidity and mortality, as these neural and vascular structures cannot be removed surgically without sacrificing the entire bowel. **(Bottom)** A more cephalic section shows tumor infiltrating and enlarging multiple regional lymph nodes. Individual abdominal nerves and ganglia are rarely visible on cross-sectional imaging. Neural pathology may be inferred by imaging evidence of a mass and clinical signs and symptoms compatible with adjacent nerve involvement.

II

ESOPHAGUS

Terminology

Abbreviations
- Gastroesophageal reflux disease (GERD)

Definitions
- **A ring**: Sporadically imaged indentation of esophageal lumen at cephalic end of lower esophageal sphincter
- **B ring**: Transverse mucosal fold marking esophagogastric junction, often corresponding to mucosal junction between squamous and columnar epithelium

Gross Anatomy

Overview
- Esophagus is fibromuscular tube about 25 cm long that extends from pharynx to stomach
  - Enters thorax at about T1 level; occupies posterior mediastinum
  - Enters abdomen through **esophageal hiatus** in diaphragm through right crus, at about T10
- Physiologic areas of narrowing or constriction
  - At its origin by **cricopharyngeus muscle** (upper esophageal sphincter)
  - By **arch of aorta** (left anterolateral surface of esophagus)
  - By **left main bronchus**
  - By **diaphragm** (and mucosal, B ring at gastroesophageal junction about 40 cm from incisor teeth)
- **Mural anatomy**
  - Has internal circular and external longitudinal **layers of muscle**
    - Superior third of esophagus consists of voluntary, striated muscle; lower $\frac{1}{3}$ = smooth muscle; middle $\frac{1}{3}$ = both types
  - Lacks serosal lining
  - Lined by stratified squamous epithelium
- **Gastroesophageal junction (GEJ)**
  - Marked on mucosal surface by **Z line**: Demarcates end of smooth, pearly pink esophageal mucosa beginning of reddish, textured gastric columnar mucosa
  - GEJ attached to liver at fissure for ligamentum venosum by **gastrohepatic ligament**
  - GEJ often appears thickened on axial imaging (may simulate a tumor)
- Attached to diaphragm by **phrenicoesophageal ligament** (collagenous band, tends to weaken & elongate with age, may lead to hiatal hernia)
- **Vessels, nerves, lymphatics**
  - Esophageal arteries (from aorta) in thorax
  - Left gastric (from celiac) and inferior phrenic arteries in abdomen
  - Venous drainage through azygous system (systemic) and left gastric (to portal venous)
  - Innervation: Right and left **vagus nerves**; sympathetic trunk
  - Lymphatic drainage
    - Lower $\frac{1}{3}$ → left gastric and celiac nodes
    - Upper $\frac{2}{3}$ → posterior mediastinal nodes

Imaging Anatomy

Internal Structures-Critical Contents
- Pharynx
  - **Nasopharynx**
    - From base of skull to top of soft palate
  - Oro (**mesopharynx**)
    - From soft palate to hyoid bone
  - Hypo (**laryngopharynx**)
    - From hyoid to bottom of cricopharyngeus muscle
- Upper esophageal sphincter
  - At pharyngoesophageal junction
  - Formed primarily by cricopharyngeus muscle
- **Lower esophageal sphincter**
  - Defined by manometric evidence of high resting tone or pressure
  - Essentially synonymous with "esophageal vestibule" or "**phrenic ampulla**"
  - Occasionally recognized radiographically as a 2-4 cm long luminal dilation between esophageal A and B rings

Anatomy-Based Imaging Issues

Imaging Recommendations
- Best means of evaluating mucosal disease (inflammation, superficial tumor): Double contrast barium esophagram and endoscopy
- Best test for GERD: Esophagram and pH testing by esophageal probe or capsule
- Best test for stricture: Single contrast esophagram
- Best test for mass lesion: Esophagram and endoscopy
- Best test for depth of tumor invasion: Endoscopic sonography
- Best test for staging esophageal cancer: Combined PET-CT (positron emission & computed tomography)

Clinical Implications

Clinical Importance
- **Hiatal hernia** and GERD are extremely common and usually occur together
  - Hiatal hernia results in loss of the constriction & angulation of the esophagus by the crus of diaphragm (part of the lower esophageal sphincter)
  - Reflux often causes spasm of esophageal longitudinal muscles, resulting in shortening of esophagus and more herniation
- **Esophageal varices** are common
  - Submucosal veins drain into systemic & portal venous system and constitute potential collateral pathway
  - Usual form is "uphill varices" due to portal hypertension (cirrhosis) causing hepatofugal flow (away from liver) through varicose collaterals around esophagus
  - "Downhill varices" result from obstruction of superior vena cava → esophageal varices → inferior vena cava and portal vein

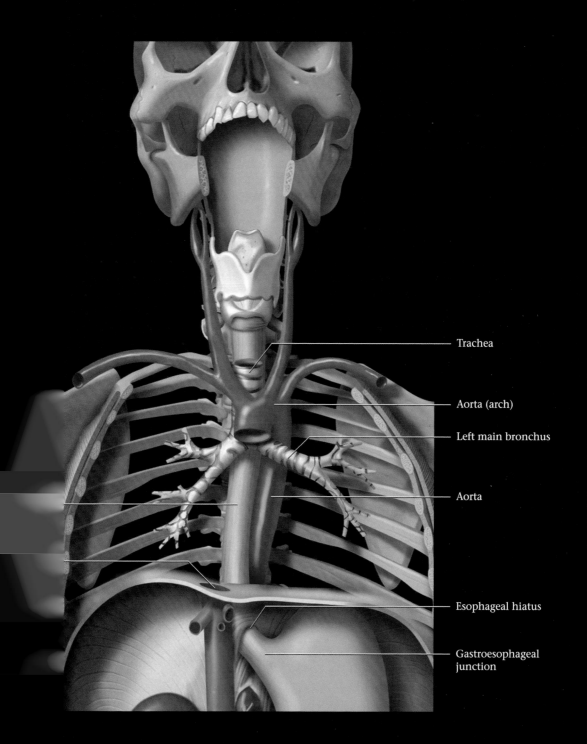

Trachea

Aorta (arch)

Left main bronchus

Aorta

Esophageal hiatus

Gastroesophageal
junction

thorax at about T1 level behind and slightly to the left of the trachea. It is usually indented
urface by the arch of the aorta and the left main bronchus. The esophagus is closely applied
ts course, and may be pushed or pulled by aortic abnormalities, such as aneurysm or ectasia.
abdomen at about the T10 level, between fibers of the right crus of diaphragm. The
re caudal than the hiatus for the inferior vena cava, and cephalad to the aortic hiatus

ESOPHAGUS SAGITTAL RELATIONS

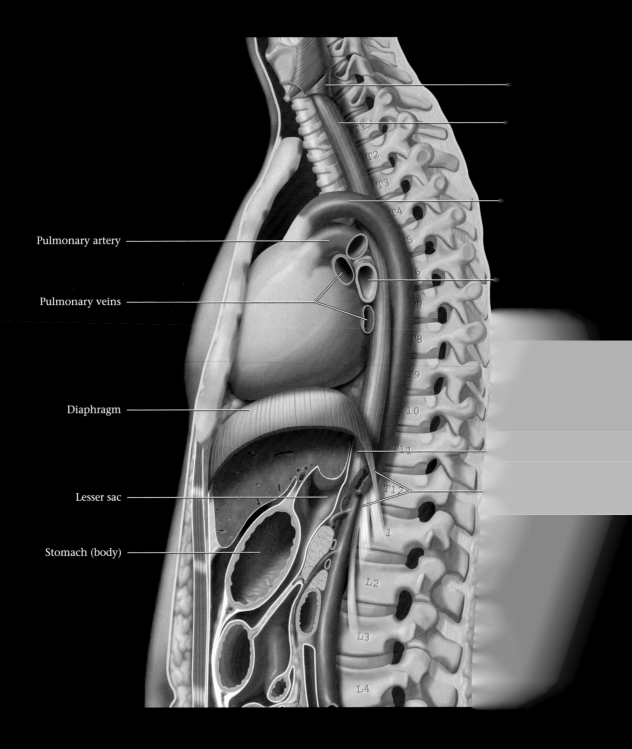

Pulmonary artery

Pulmonary veins

Diaphragm

Lesser sac

Stomach (body)

T1
T2
T3
T4
5
6
7
T8
T9
T10
T11
T12
1
L2
L3
L4

The esophagus is about 25 cm long and extends from the level of the cricopharynge
the gastroesophageal junction (at about the T10-11 level). Note the relationship bet
structures, including the heart, which may indent or displace the esophageal lumer

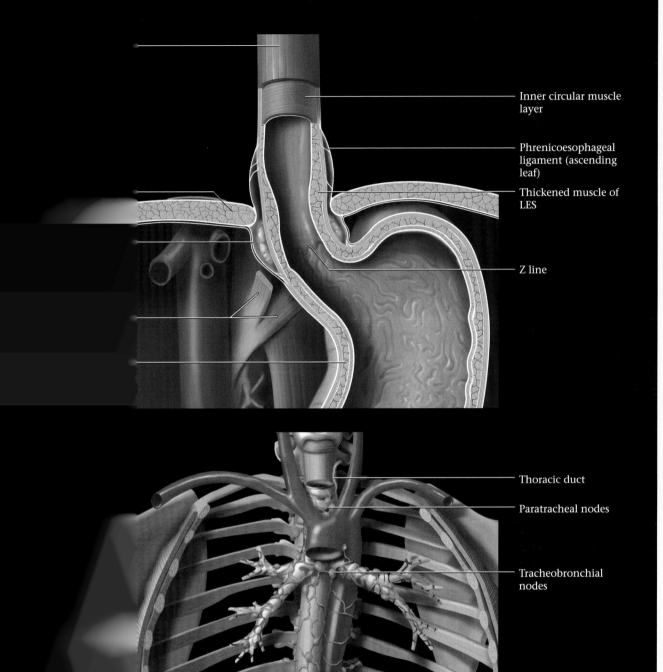

Inner circular muscle layer

Phrenicoesophageal ligament (ascending leaf)

Thickened muscle of LES

Z line

Thoracic duct

Paratracheal nodes

Tracheobronchial nodes

Diaphragmatic nodes

Left gastric nodes

l musculature consists of an inner circular layer and an outer longitudinal layer. In the
ageal sphincter (LES), the muscle layers are thickened. This, along with diaphragmatic
lation of the esophagus as it passes into the abdomen and enters the stomach, helps to
ontents. The Z line marks the junction of the esophageal and gastric mucosa. **(Bottom)**
the upper part of the esophagus is usually to the paratracheal and posterior mediastinal
ophagus drains to the diaphragmatic, celiac and left gastric nodes; however, there is
tracheobronchial nodes lie near the carina and may be responsible for the formation of
they become fibrosed, usually as a result of tuberculosis or histoplasmosis

ESOPHAGUS

NORMAL IMPRESSIONS ON ESOPHAGUS

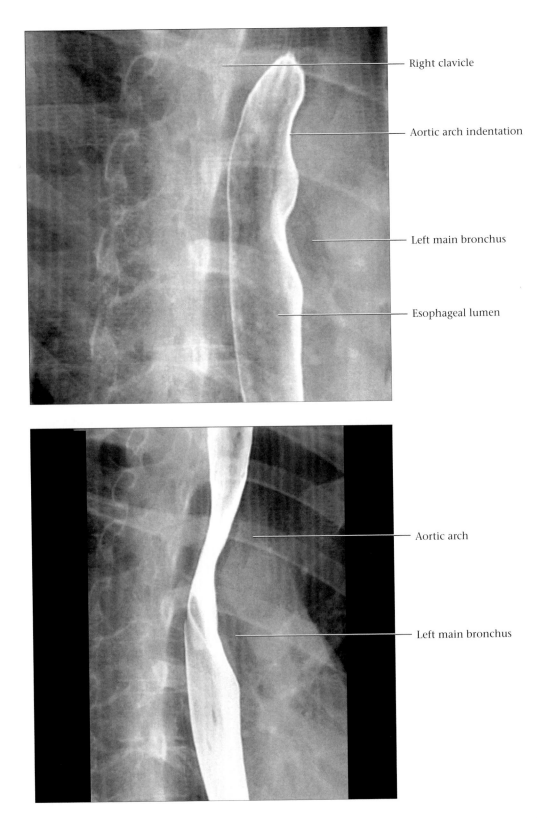

Right clavicle

Aortic arch indentation

Left main bronchus

Esophageal lumen

Aortic arch

Left main bronchus

(Top) First of two films from a barium esophagram with air contrast (lumen distended by gas from ingested gas granules and water). The esophagus is normal and has a featureless smooth mucosal surface. The left anterior wall of the esophagus is indented by two adjacent structures, the arch of the aorta and the left main bronchus. **(Bottom)** The esophageal lumen appears narrowed between the aortic arch and the left main bronchus, but this is a normal finding. The bronchus is identified as the air-filled tubular structure next to the esophagus.

ESOPHAGUS

BARIUM ESOPHAGRAM, ESOPHAGEAL A & B RINGS

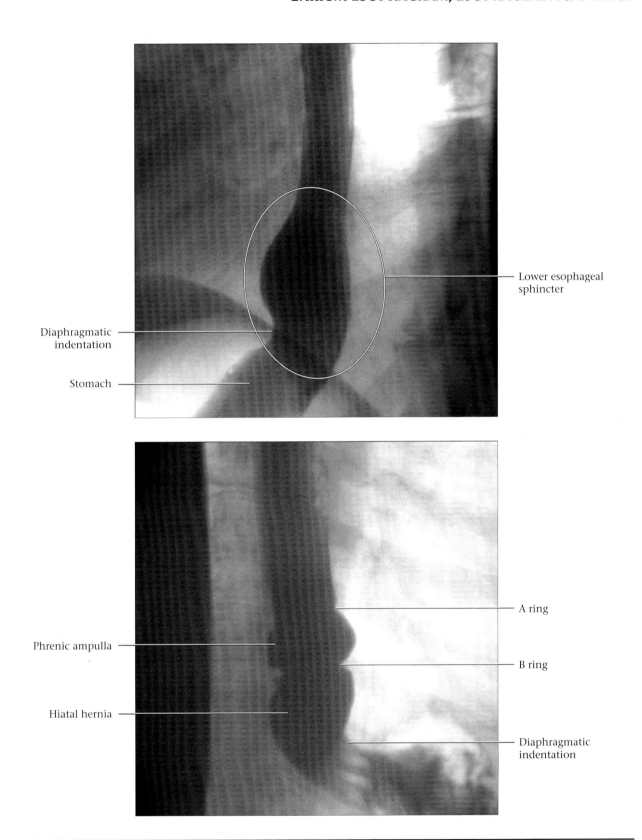

Lower esophageal sphincter

Diaphragmatic indentation

Stomach

Phrenic ampulla

A ring

B ring

Hiatal hernia

Diaphragmatic indentation

(Top) Two films from a single contrast barium esophagram. This image shows a smooth dilation of the distal few centimeters of the esophageal lumen, often referred to as the phrenic ampulla or esophageal vestibule. This is the anatomic correlate to the LES, which is defined manometrically as the zone of increased resting tone or pressure within the esophagus. The LES contributes to the anti-reflux valve effect at the gastroesophageal junction. **(Bottom)** Same patient as previous image with film taken during abdominal straining (Valsalva maneuver). A small hiatal hernia is demonstrated. The A and B rings of the esophagus are well-defined, and mark the upper and lower limits of the lower esophageal sphincter, respectively. The B ring marks the gastroesophageal junction, which is above the diaphragm in this patient, indicating a hiatal hernia.

ESOPHAGUS

NORMAL GASTROESOPHAGEAL JUNCTION

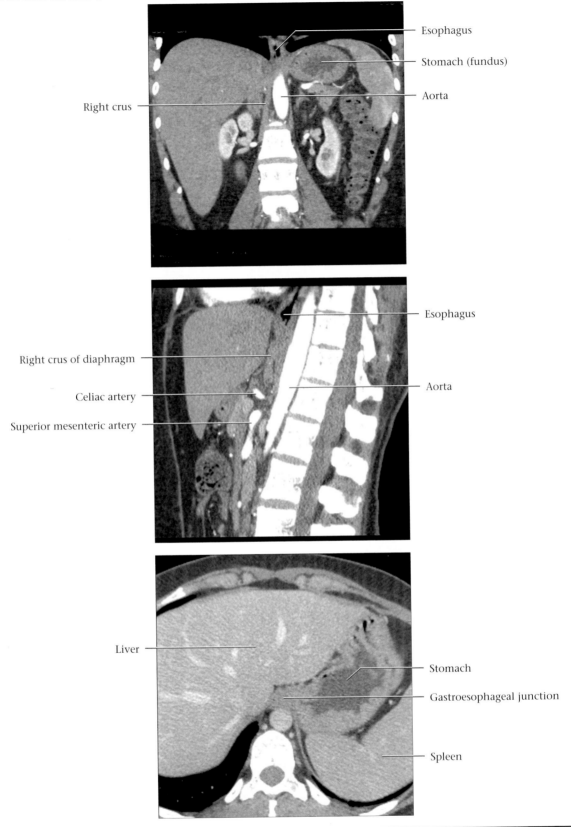

(Top) First of three CT sections through the upper abdomen. Coronal CT section shows the esophagus and aorta entering the abdomen. The esophagus enters at about the T10 vertebral level between fibers of the right crus of diaphragm. The aorta enters at about the T12 level behind the median arcuate ligament of the diaphragm. **(Middle)** Sagittal CT section in the midline shows the esophagus and aorta entering the abdomen. Only portions of the celiac and superior mesenteric arteries are seen in this section, but the origin of the celiac is usually just caudal to the median arcuate ligament, which marks the entry of the aorta into the abdomen. **(Bottom)** The gastroesophageal junction usually lies at the same level as the fissure for the ligamentum venosum in the liver and commonly appears thickened relative to the walls of the distal esophagus or proximal stomach.

ESOPHAGUS

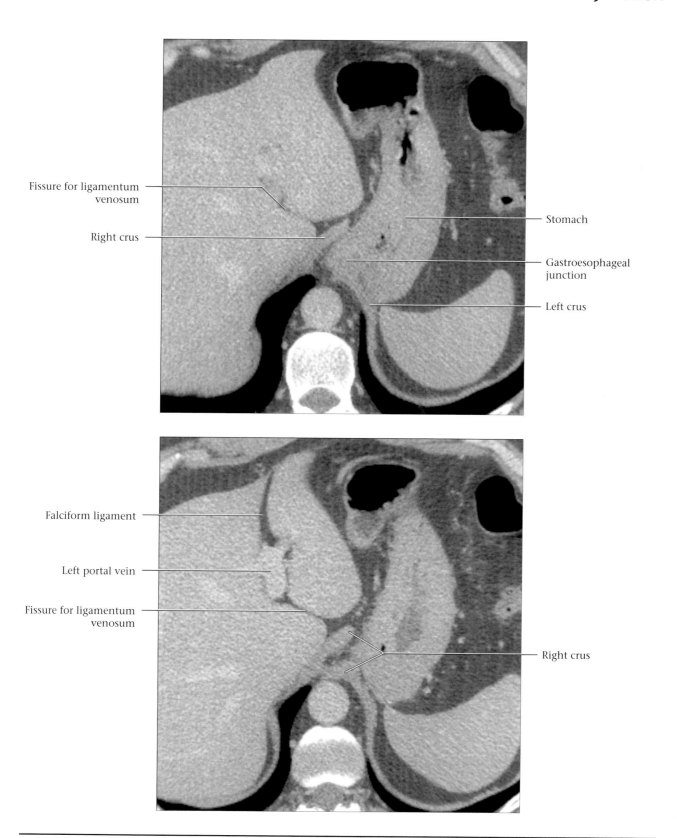

(Top) First of two axial CT sections through the upper abdomen. The esophagus enters the abdomen through fibers of the right crus, and the gastroesophageal junction is normally at about the level of the fissure for the ligamentum venosum. **(Bottom)** The decussation (crossing of fibers) of the right crus is well shown on this CT section.

ESOPHAGUS

PATULOUS DIAPHRAGMATIC HIATUS WITH HERNIA

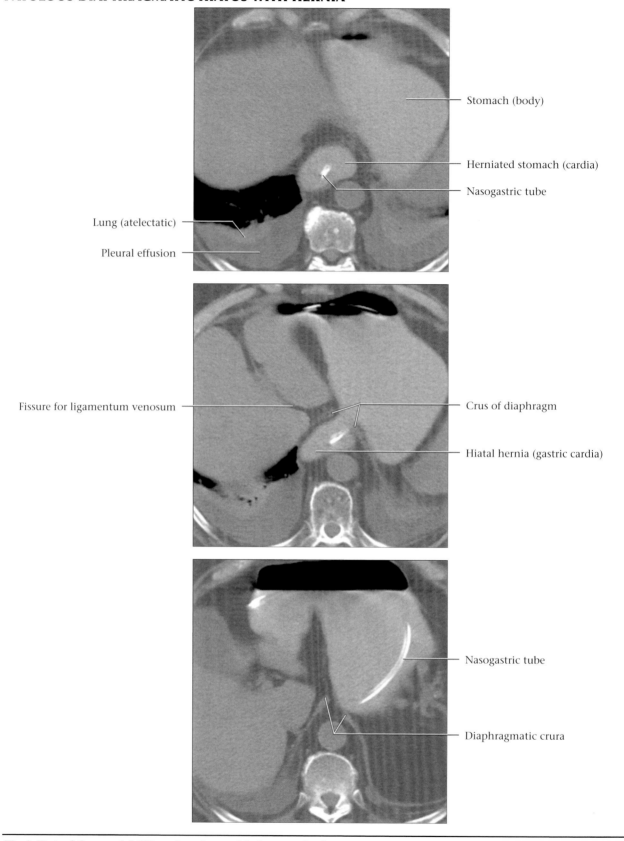

(Top) First of three axial CT sections in an elderly man. In this section through the lower chest, a portion of the stomach is visualized, opacified by oral contrast medium. (Middle) At the level of the fissure for the ligamentum venosum, which should mark the gastroesophageal junction, note the wide opening between the crura of the diaphragm, which has allowed the stomach (gastric cardia) to herniate. This is a sliding hiatal hernia. (Bottom) Most caudal CT section shows a persistent gap between the crura, which should have joined together in the midline at this level.

ESOPHAGUS

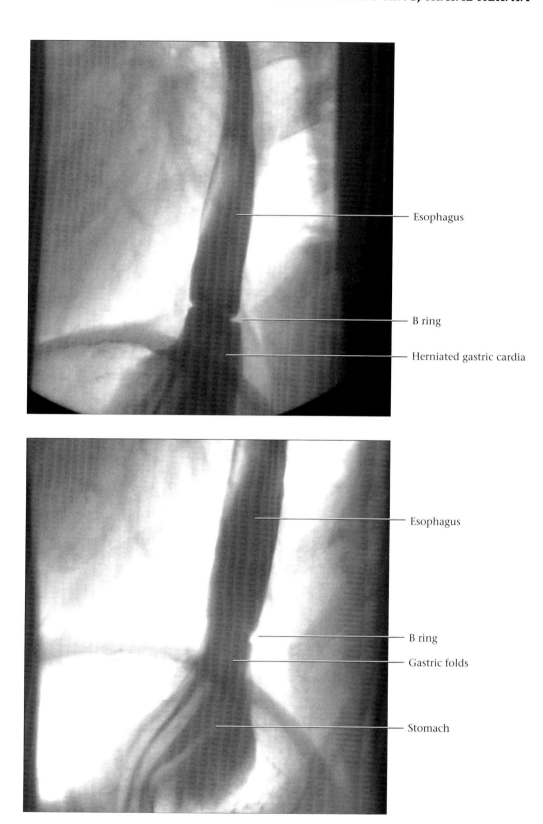

Esophagus

B ring

Herniated gastric cardia

Esophagus

B ring

Gastric folds

Stomach

(Top) First of two films from a barium esophagram shows a web-like narrowing at the gastroesophageal junction, a typical feature of the esophageal B ring, which marks the squamo-columnar junction. The B ring is well seen due to the hiatal hernia and good fluoroscopic technique which has distended the distal esophagus and proximal stomach. (Bottom) Gastric folds extend above the diaphragm to the B ring, another sign of a hiatal hernia.

ESOPHAGUS

STRICTURE AT B RING (SCHATZKI RING)

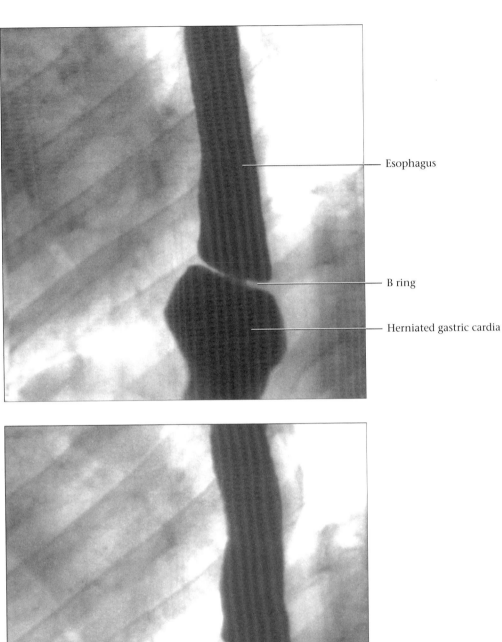

- Esophagus
- B ring
- Herniated gastric cardia

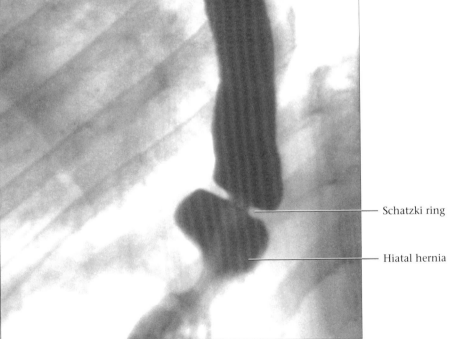

- Schatzki ring
- Hiatal hernia

(Top) First of two films from a barium esophagram shows a narrowed lumen through the B ring, at the gastroesophageal junction. The lower esophageal ring is thickened and the lumen narrowed due to inflammation and scarring, almost always due to gastro-esophageal reflux. (Bottom) When the lumen is narrowed through the B ring, this is sometimes referred to as a "Schatzki" ring after the radiologist who noted that patients with this finding frequently had complaints of reflux and food "sticking" in their esophagus, sometimes requiring endoscopic treatment.

ESOPHAGUS

CRICOPHARYNGEAL ACHALASIA & HIATAL HERNIA

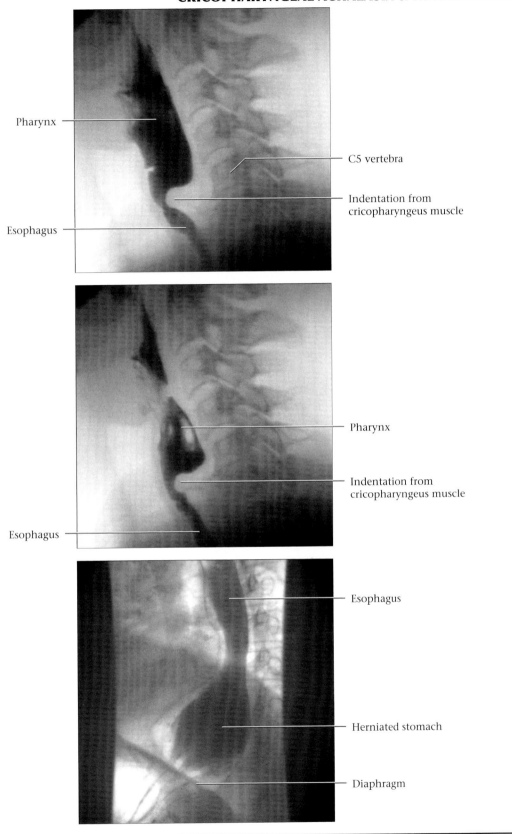

Pharynx

C5 vertebra

Indentation from cricopharyngeus muscle

Esophagus

Pharynx

Indentation from cricopharyngeus muscle

Esophagus

Esophagus

Herniated stomach

Diaphragm

(Top) First of three films from a barium esophagram. This lateral view shows a rounded indentation of the posterior wall of the pharyngo-esophageal junction, at the level of the disk space between the 5th and 6th cervical vertebrae. The pharynx is distended, indicating impaired passage of the barium. These are typical features of spasm or "achalasia" (failure to relax) of the cricopharyngeus muscle, which is part of the upper esophageal sphincter. **(Middle)** The cricopharyngeus normally relaxes in anticipation of the arrival of a bolus of food. This lateral film shows persistent filling of the pharynx and contraction of the cricopharyngeus muscle after the bolus of barium has passed. **(Bottom)** A film of the lower chest shows a hiatal hernia. Cricopharyngeal achalasia is often the indirect result of disordered esophageal motility and acid reflux.

ESOPHAGUS

"FELINE" ESOPHAGUS

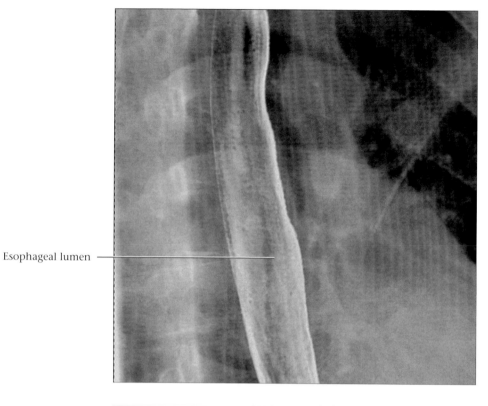

Esophageal lumen ——————

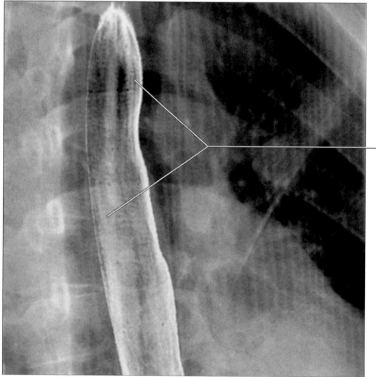

—— "Herringbone" mucosal pattern

(Top) Two films from an air-contrast barium esophagram. Both show a peculiar herringbone surface coating pattern, rather than the normal featureless surface pattern of the esophagus. This is a transient finding and represents the result of contraction of the muscularis mucosa, and usually results from an episode of reflux which "irritates" the esophagus. **(Bottom)** This herringbone-like pattern of barium coating is an uncommon feature in the human esophagus, but is, apparently, a typical feature of the cat esophagus; hence, the descriptive term "feline esophagus".

ESOPHAGUS

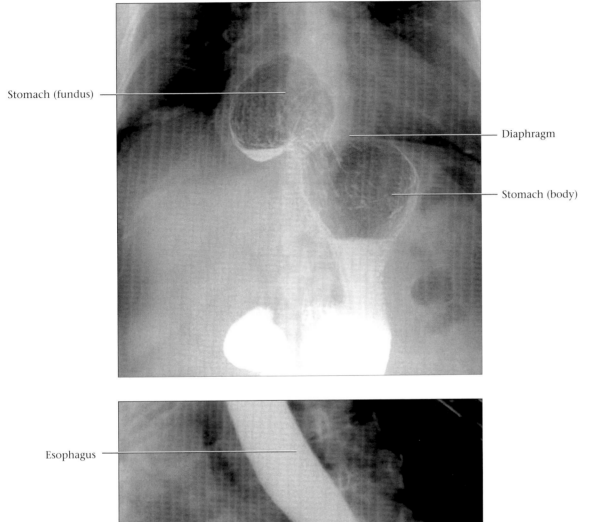

Stomach (fundus)

Diaphragm

Stomach (body)

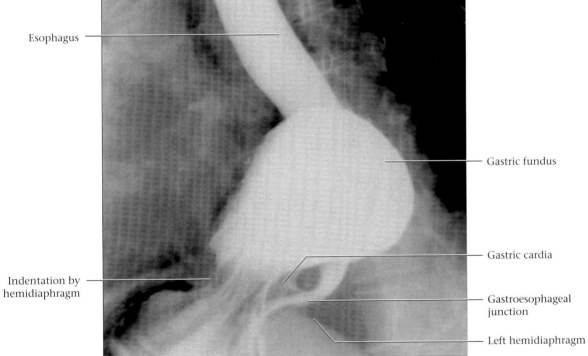

Esophagus

Gastric fundus

Gastric cardia

Indentation by
hemidiaphragm

Gastroesophageal
junction

Left hemidiaphragm

(Top) First of two films from a barium upper GI series, showing herniation of the gastric fundus, as well as the gastric cardia. This constitutes a paraesophageal hernia and is considered a more compelling indication for surgical repair than a simple "sliding" hiatal hernia, which involves only the cardia. **(Bottom)** In most paraesophageal hernias (PEH), the gastroesophageal junction lies above the diaphragm; these are classified as type III PEH. Those in which the GE junction is below the diaphragm are classified as a type II PEH. The term "paraesophageal" refers to the position of the intrathoracic stomach alongside ("para") the esophagus.

ESOPHAGUS

PARAESOPHAGEAL HERNIA

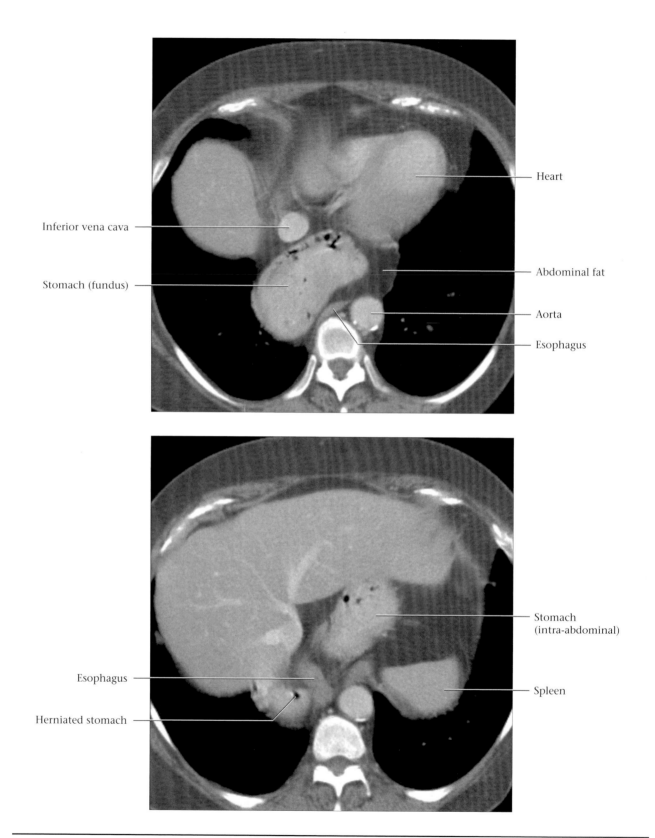

(Top) First of two axial CT sections showing a large paraesophageal hernia. Note the position of the herniated stomach alongside the distal esophagus. Both lie in the mediastinum behind the heart. **(Bottom)** A more caudal section shows the distal esophagus just above the GE junction with stomach herniated beside it, constituting a paraesophageal hernia.

ESOPHAGUS

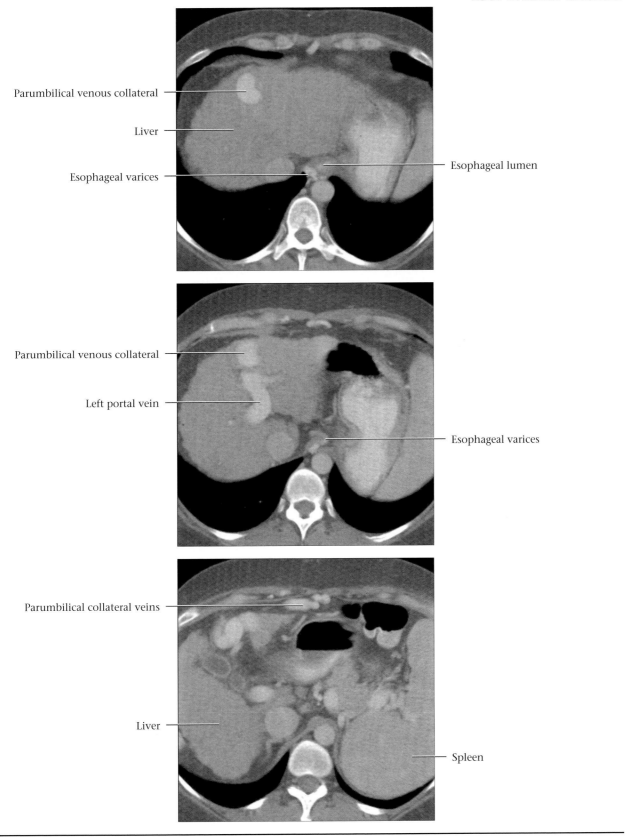

Parumbilical venous collateral

Liver

Esophageal varices

Esophageal lumen

Parumbilical venous collateral

Left portal vein

Esophageal varices

Parumbilical collateral veins

Liver

Spleen

(Top) First of three axial CT sections in a 43 year old woman with alcoholic cirrhosis. The liver appears nodular and heterogeneous, findings typical of cirrhosis. Note the contrast-enhancing venous collaterals in the wall of the esophagus (esophageal varices). **(Middle)** A very large parumbilical collateral vein communicates with the left portal vein and fills due to hepatofugal ("away from the liver") flow as a result of cirrhosis and portal hypertension. **(Bottom)** Most caudal CT section shows the shrunken, scarred, cirrhotic liver, and the spleen which is enlarged due to portal hypertension. The parumbilical collaterals will continue caudally to surround the umbilicus like a group of snakes; hence, the mythologic reference to the head of Medusa ("caput Medusae"), a descriptive term for this physical finding.

GASTRODUODENAL

Terminology

Abbreviations
- Combined positron emission and computed tomography (PET-CT)
- Superior mesenteric artery (SMA)

Gross Anatomy

Overview
- **Stomach**: The alimentary reservoir for mixing and enzymatic digestion of food
  - **Cardia**: Surrounds the esophageal orifice into stomach; lesser and greater curvature meet here
  - **Fundus**: Most cephalic part of stomach; touches left hemidiaphragm
  - **Body**: Main portion; principal site of acid production
  - **Antrum**: Vestibule; pre-pyloric part of stomach
  - **Pylorus**: Sphincter opening into duodenum; formed by thickened middle layer of smooth muscle and a thin fibrous septum
  - **Mural anatomy**
    - Wall consists of 3 layers of smooth muscle (outermost = longitudinal; middle = circular; inner = oblique); circular is thickest
    - **Gastric folds (rugae)**: Redundant folds of the gastric mucosal surface
    - Most evident when the stomach is empty, along greater curve
    - Mucosa is columnar epithelium
    - Gastric glands: Vary in prevalence in different parts of the stomach; produce mucous (which lines and protects gastric surface), pepsinogen (precursor to pepsin), and hydrochloric acid (activates digestive enzymes, assists with breakdown of food)
  - **Vessels, nerves and lymphatics**
    - Lesser curvature: Branches of **left and right gastric arteries** (lie in lesser omentum)
    - Greater curvature: Left and right **gastro-omental (gastroepiploic)** arteries (in greater omentum)
    - Venous drainage into portal vein directly through **left and right gastric veins** and via **splenic and superior mesenteric veins**
    - Lymphatic drainage along course of arteries, then to **celiac nodes** via efferent lymphatic ducts
    - Innervation: Vagus nerve: Parasympathetic, stimulates peristalsis and acid production; sympathetic nerves; celiac and splanchnic ganglia and plexus (also carry pain receptor nerves)
  - Greater curvature attached to transverse colon by **gastrocolic ligament**
    - Carcinoma can cross from stomach to colon and vice versa
- **Duodenum**
  - **Bulb**: Triangular first part
    - Suspended by hepatoduodenal ligament (also contains bile duct, portal vein and hepatic artery)
  - **Descending** (2nd part)
    - Site of major **pancreaticobiliary papilla (of Vater)**; entry of common duct and main pancreatic duct
  - **Transverse** (3rd part)
  - **Ascending** (4th part)
  - **Mural anatomy**
    - Mucosa, submucosa, circular and longitudinal smooth muscle
    - Duodenal bulb is intraperitoneal; remainder retroperitoneal
    - **Brunner glands**: Most prominent in proximal duodenum, secrete fluid with mucous and proteolytic enzymes
  - Anatomic relations
    - 2nd and 3rd portions of duodenum are closely attached to pancreatic head [surgical resection of pancreatic head (**Whipple procedure**) requires resection of duodenum, as well]
    - 2nd part of duodenum lies just anterior to hilum of right kidney (inflammation from duodenal perforation may extend into perirenal space)
    - Duodenojejunal junction usually at about L2 level (about same level as pylorus), suspended by **ligament of Treitz** (extension of right crus of diaphragm)
  - **Vessels and nerves**
    - Arterial supply primarily from celiac artery → gastroduodenal to pancreaticoduodenal arteries
    - **Pancreaticoduodenal artery** receives branches from celiac and SMA; frequent collateral pathway in event of occlusion or narrowing of celiac or SMA

Clinical Implications

Clinical Importance
- Gastric and duodenal ulcers are common
  - Etiology is often multifactorial, often (90%) related to **Helicobacter pylori** infection which erodes the mucosa, making it vulnerable to the caustic effects of acid and digestive enzymes (pepsin) produced by stomach
  - Rich vascular supply makes "upper GI" bleeding a common result
- **Gastric malignancies** are common, though more prevalent in Asia
  - Rich lymphatic & venous drainage makes nodal & liver metastases common at the time of diagnosis
- 3rd part of duodenum is adjacent to aorta
  - Following repair of an abdominal aortic aneurysm, a fistula may form to the duodenum, often with fatal consequences (**aorto-enteric fistula**)
- **Gastric and duodenal diverticula** are common and usually asymptomatic
  - May be mistaken for upper abdominal cystic mass
  - Gastric diverticulum can simulate adrenal mass on CT or MR
  - Duodenal diverticulum can simulate a pancreatic head cystic mass
  - Periampullary duodenal diverticulum may be associated with biliary dysfunction

GASTRODUODENAL

FRONTAL VIEW OF STOMACH & GASTRIC MUCOSA

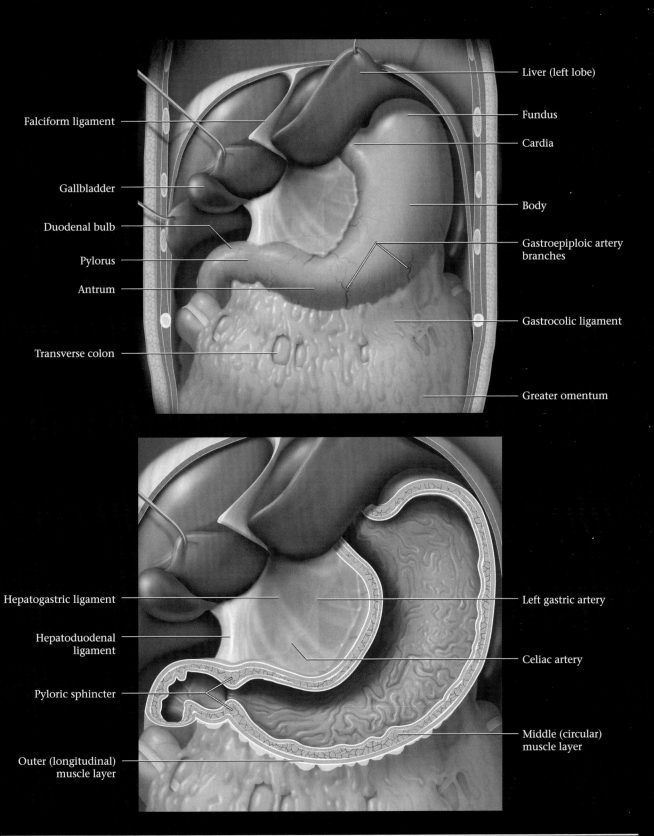

Falciform ligament

Gallbladder

Duodenal bulb

Pylorus

Antrum

Transverse colon

Liver (left lobe)

Fundus

Cardia

Body

Gastroepiploic artery branches

Gastrocolic ligament

Greater omentum

Hepatogastric ligament

Hepatoduodenal ligament

Pyloric sphincter

Outer (longitudinal) muscle layer

Left gastric artery

Celiac artery

Middle (circular) muscle layer

(Top) The liver and gallbladder have been retracted upward. Note that the lesser curvature and anterior wall of the stomach touch the underside of the liver, and the gallbladder abuts the duodenal bulb. The greater curvature is attached to the transverse colon by the gastrocolic ligament, which continues inferiorly as the greater omentum, covering most of the colon and small bowel. **(Bottom)** Lesser omentum extends from the stomach to the porta hepatis, and can be divided into the broader and thinner hepatogastric ligament and the thicker hepatoduodenal ligament. Lesser omentum carries the portal vein, hepatic artery, common bile duct and lymph nodes. Free edge of the lesser omentum forms the ventral margin of the epiploic foramen. Celiac artery can be seen through the surface of the lesser sac. Note the layers of gastric muscle; middle circular layer is thickest.

GASTRODUODENAL

DUODENUM, FRONTAL & INTERNAL FOLD PATTERN

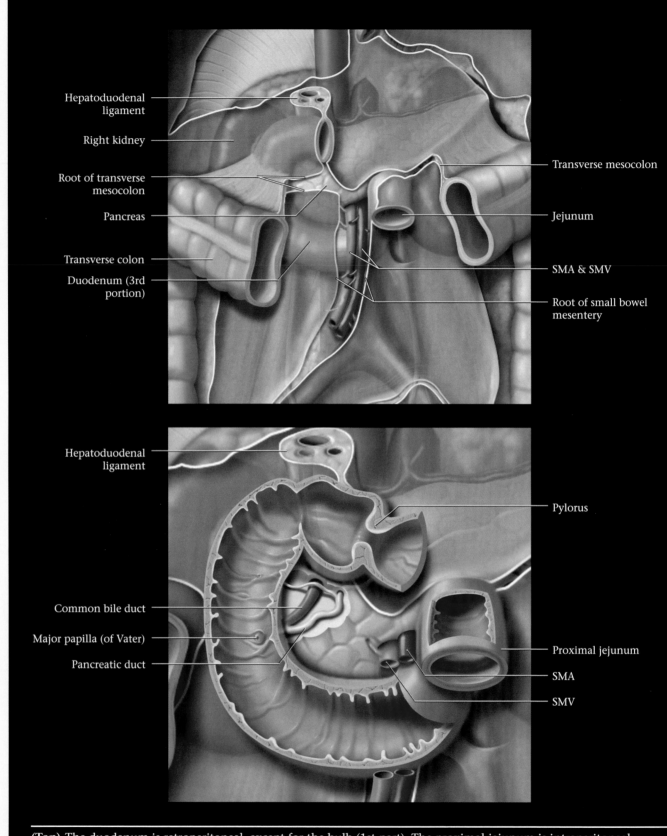

Hepatoduodenal ligament

Right kidney

Root of transverse mesocolon

Pancreas

Transverse colon

Duodenum (3rd portion)

Transverse mesocolon

Jejunum

SMA & SMV

Root of small bowel mesentery

Hepatoduodenal ligament

Common bile duct

Major papilla (of Vater)

Pancreatic duct

Pylorus

Proximal jejunum

SMA

SMV

(Top) The duodenum is retroperitoneal, except for the bulb (1st part). The proximal jejunum is intraperitoneal. Hepatoduodenal ligament attaches the duodenum to the porta hepatis and contains the portal triad (bile duct, hepatic artery, portal vein). The root of the transverse mesocolon and mesentery both cross the duodenum. The third portion of the duodenum crosses in front of the aorta and IVC, and behind the superior mesenteric vessels (SMA and SMV). Second portion of duodenum is attached to pancreatic head and lies close to the hilum of the right kidney. **(Bottom)** Duodenal bulb is suspended by the hepatoduodenal ligament. Duodenal-jejunal flexure is suspended by the ligament of Treitz, an extension of the right crus. The major pancreaticobiliary papilla enters the medial wall of the second portion of the duodenum. Duodenal wall consists of mucosa, submucosa, 2 muscle layers.

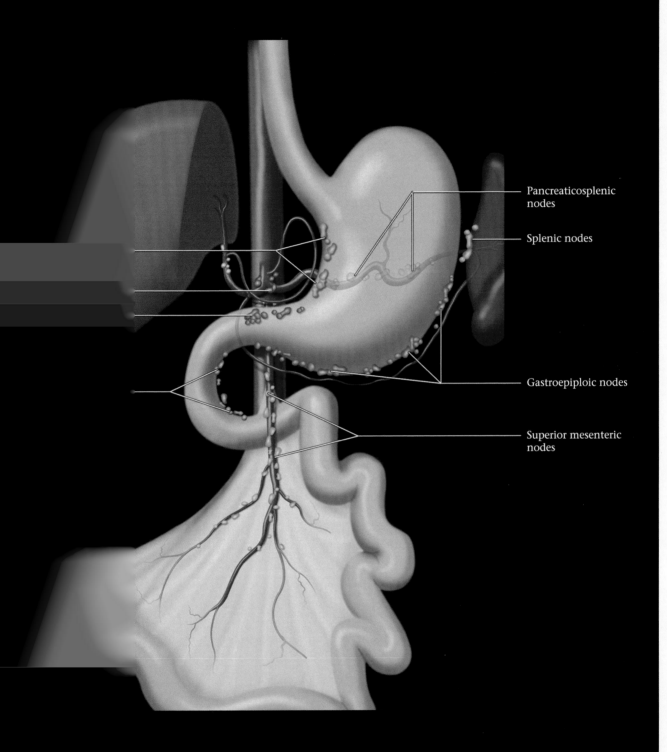

Pancreaticosplenic nodes

Splenic nodes

Gastroepiploic nodes

Superior mesenteric nodes

accompany the arteries of similar names along the greater and lesser curvatures. Lymph
sterior surfaces of the stomach drains to the left gastric and gastroepiploic nodes, along with
odes. The pyloric nodes drain the inferior third of the stomach, primarily from the lesser
l part of the greater curvature and the duodenum drain to the pancreaticoduodenal nodes.
ubsequently drain to the celiac nodes, which are grouped at the base of the celiac artery

GASTRODUODENAL

ARTERIES OF STOMACH AND DUODENUM

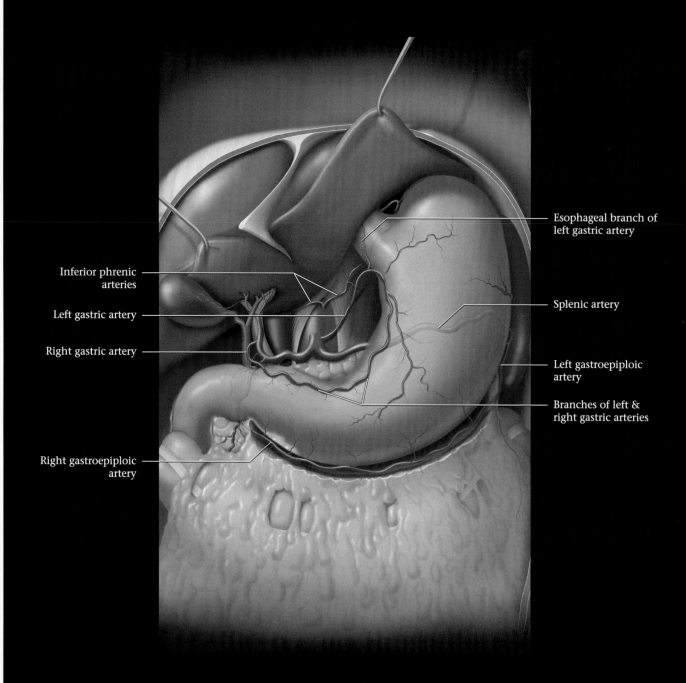

Esophageal branch of left gastric artery

Inferior phrenic arteries

Left gastric artery

Right gastric artery

Splenic artery

Left gastroepiploic artery

Branches of left & right gastric arteries

Right gastroepiploic artery

"Conventional" arterial anatomy of the stomach and duodenum (present in only 50% of population) has the left gastric artery arising from the celiac trunk, supplying the lesser curvature, and anastomosing with right gastric artery, a branch of the proper hepatic artery. The gastroduodenal artery is the first major branch of the common hepatic artery and branches into the superior pancreaticoduodenal and right gastroepiploic arteries. The greater curvature of the stomach is supplied by anastomosing branches of the gastroepiploic arteries, with the left arising from the splenic artery. The duodenum and pancreas are supplied by a rich pancreaticoduodenal "arcade" comprised of multiple, anastomosing branches from the gastroduodenal and superior mesenteric arteries.

PORTAL VENOUS SYSTEM

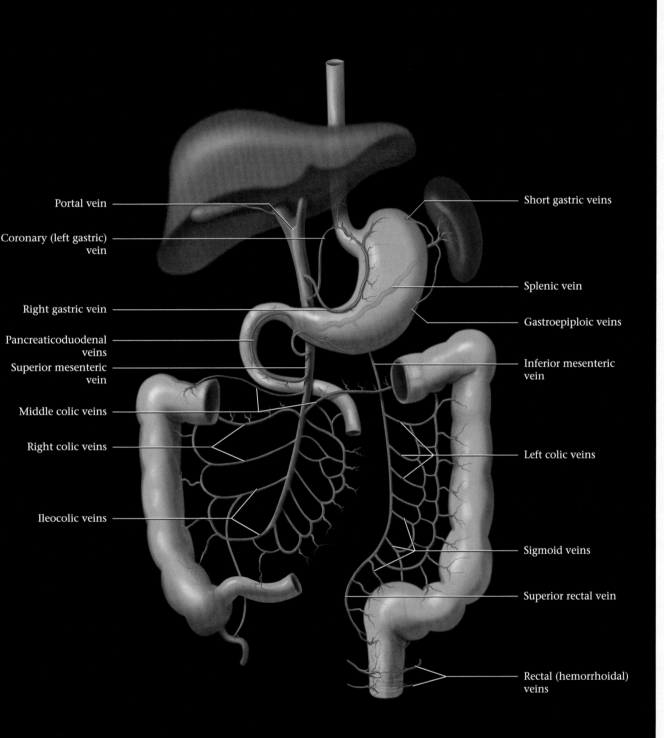

Portal vein

Coronary (left gastric) vein

Right gastric vein

Pancreaticoduodenal veins

Superior mesenteric vein

Middle colic veins

Right colic veins

Ileocolic veins

Short gastric veins

Splenic vein

Gastroepiploic veins

Inferior mesenteric vein

Left colic veins

Sigmoid veins

Superior rectal vein

Rectal (hemorrhoidal) veins

Venous drainage from the stomach, duodenum, small bowel and colon (up to the splenic flexure) is to the superior mesenteric vein. Pancreatic venous drainage is to the splenic and superior mesenteric veins (SMV). The descending and sigmoid colon drain through the inferior mesenteric vein (IMV). The splenic vein, SMV and IMV are the main tributaries of the portal vein. These veins are valveless and freely communicate through numerous collateral pathways, which become important and evident in cases of thrombosis or compression of veins (e.g., splenic vein occlusion by pancreatic cancer, leading to collateral flow through the coronary and short gastric veins ("gastric varices"). There are also extensive potential collaterals to the systemic venous circulation that become important in portal hypertension, especially gastroesophageal, parumbilical, and hemorrhoidal varices.

GASTRODUODENAL

NORMAL STOMACH

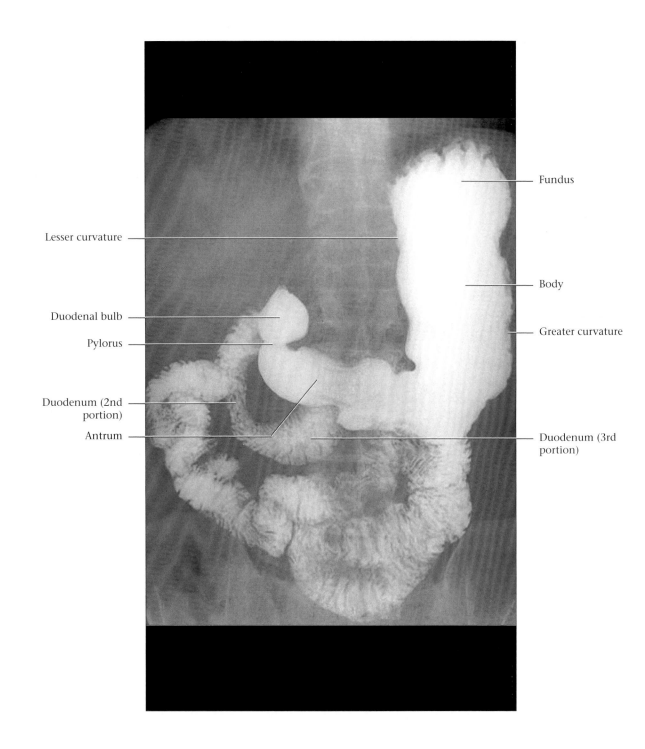

Fundus

Lesser curvature

Body

Duodenal bulb

Greater curvature

Pylorus

Duodenum (2nd portion)

Antrum

Duodenum (3rd portion)

Frontal film from a barium upper GI series. The lesser curvature is the concave border and the greater curvature is the convex border of the stomach. The fundus is the uppermost hood-like portion of the stomach, which intersects with the cardia, where the esophagus enters the stomach, at an acute angle. The body is the main portion and the antrum is the distal part of the stomach which empties into the duodenum through the pylorus.

GASTRODUODENAL

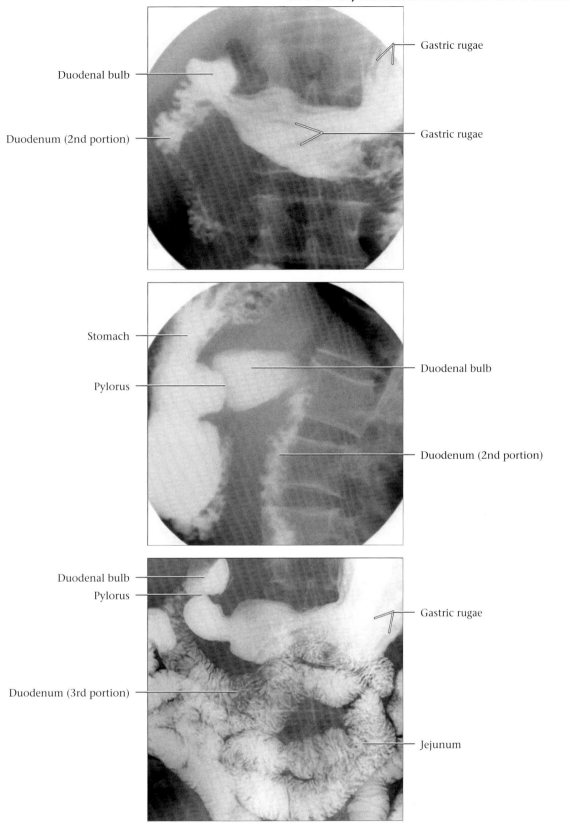

Duodenal bulb

Duodenum (2nd portion)

Gastric rugae

Gastric rugae

Stomach

Pylorus

Duodenal bulb

Duodenum (2nd portion)

Duodenal bulb

Pylorus

Gastric rugae

Duodenum (3rd portion)

Jejunum

(Top) First of three films from a barium upper GI series shows the distal stomach and duodenum. Note the gastric folds, or rugae, as smooth, linear filling defects in the barium pool. **(Middle)** Lateral view from upper GI series shows the anterior and posterior walls of the stomach, as well as the pylorus in profile. The duodenal bulb is well distended, with its normal triangular shape. **(Bottom)** Note the smooth mucosal surface of the duodenal bulb and the feathery fold pattern of the remaining duodenum and jejunum.

GASTRODUODENAL

AXIAL CECT, NORMAL GASTRODUODENAL ANATOMY

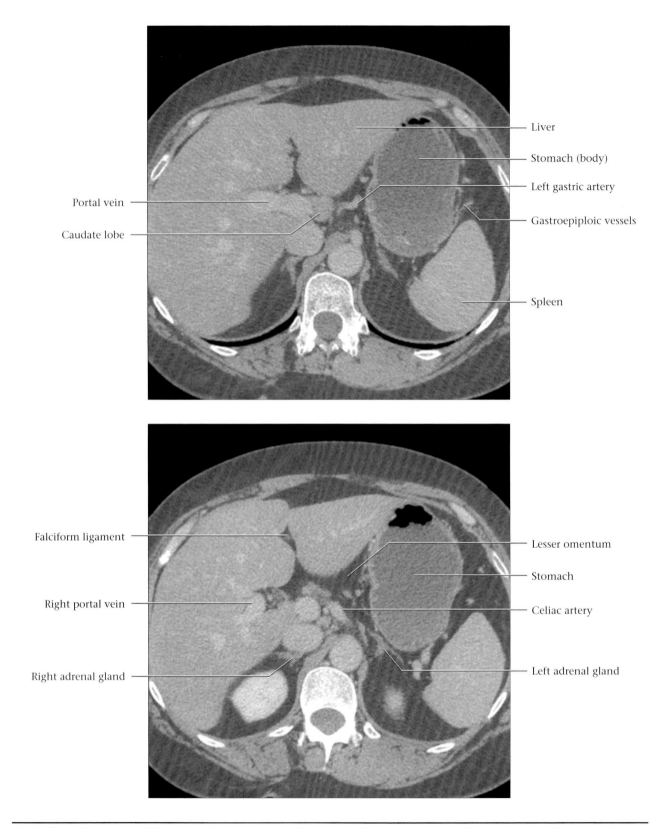

Liver

Stomach (body)

Left gastric artery

Gastroepiploic vessels

Portal vein

Caudate lobe

Spleen

Falciform ligament

Lesser omentum

Stomach

Right portal vein

Celiac artery

Right adrenal gland

Left adrenal gland

(Top) First of four axial CT sections shows the normal relations of the stomach to adjacent organs. Note that the stomach may be compressed by an enlarged liver or spleen. **(Bottom)** Note the fat-containing lesser omentum that carries vessels and lymphatics to the stomach and liver.

GASTRODUODENAL

AXIAL CECT, NORMAL GASTRODUODENAL ANATOMY

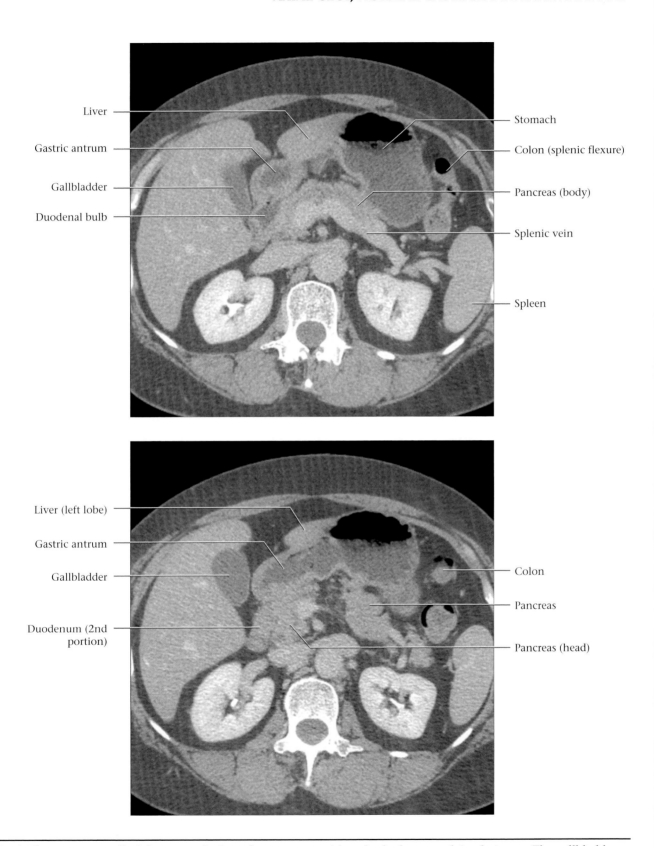

(Top) The posterior wall of the stomach abuts the pancreas, with only the lesser sac lying between. The gallbladder abuts the gastric antrum and duodenal bulb. The greater curvature touches the splenic flexure of colon. **(Bottom)** The gastric antrum abuts the pancreatic head posteriorly and the gallbladder laterally.

GASTRODUODENAL

GASTRIC & DUODENAL ARTERIES

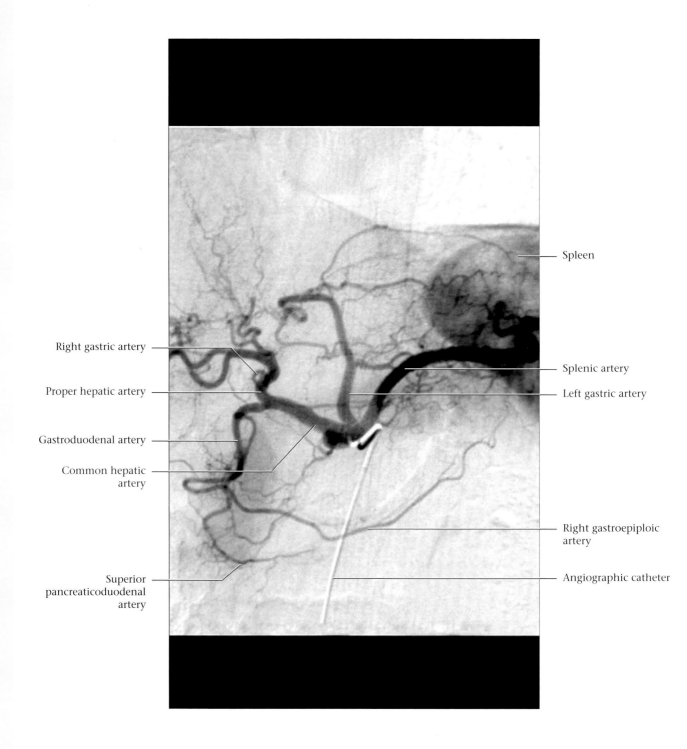

Right gastric artery

Proper hepatic artery

Gastroduodenal artery

Common hepatic artery

Superior pancreaticoduodenal artery

Spleen

Splenic artery

Left gastric artery

Right gastroepiploic artery

Angiographic catheter

Catheter arteriogram, celiac artery. The main branches of the celiac trunk are the left gastric, splenic and common hepatic arteries. The lesser curvature of the stomach is supplied by the left and right gastric arteries, with the latter being a branch of the proper hepatic artery. The greater curvature is supplied by the right and left gastroepiploic arteries, branches of the gastroduodenal and splenic arteries, respectively. The splenic artery also supplies short gastric arteries to the fundus. The gastroduodenal artery gives rise to the superior pancreaticoduodenal arteries which anastomose with branches from the superior mesenteric artery to supply rich flow to the pancreas and duodenum. There are numerous congenital variations in the blood supply to the upper abdominal organs, and many interconnecting pathways of the celiac and superior mesenteric arteries and their branches.

GASTRODUODENAL

CATHETER & CT ANGIOGRAPHY, ARTERIAL VARIATIONS

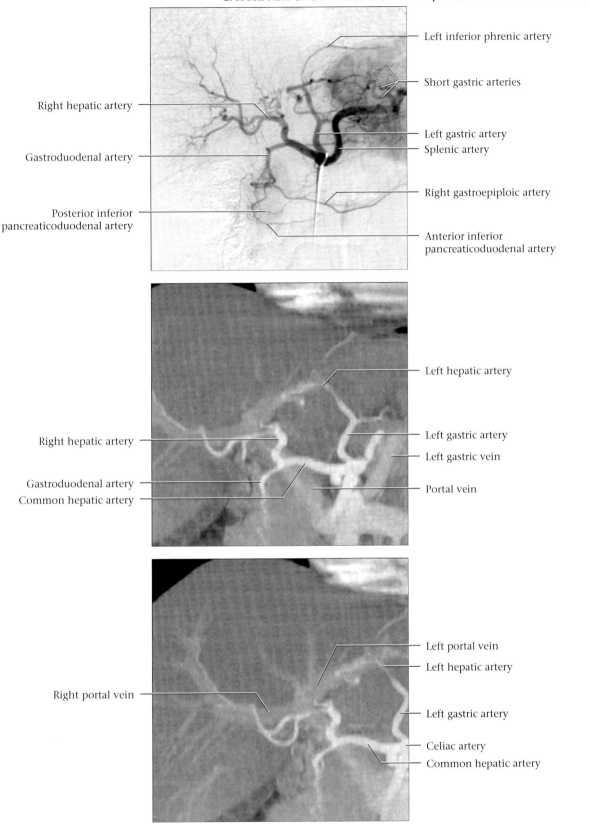

(Top) Catheter angiogram shows the common hepatic artery arising from the celiac axis, its most common arrangement, and giving rise to the gastroduodenal and right hepatic arteries in this individual. **(Middle)** Coronal reformation of a CT scan, displayed as a CT angiogram following IV administration of contrast material. The origin of the left hepatic artery from the left gastric, a common variant, is better shown on the CTA than the catheter angiogram. Branches of the portal venous system are less well opacified due to the deliberate timing of the CT scan to show the arteries preferentially. **(Bottom)** The CT angiogram is a digital creation generated by the initial axial CT data set and it can be rotated into various planes to more optimally display vessels and their origins.

GASTRODUODENAL

ARTERIAL VARIATIONS, SEPARATE ORIGIN OF LEFT GASTRIC ARTERY

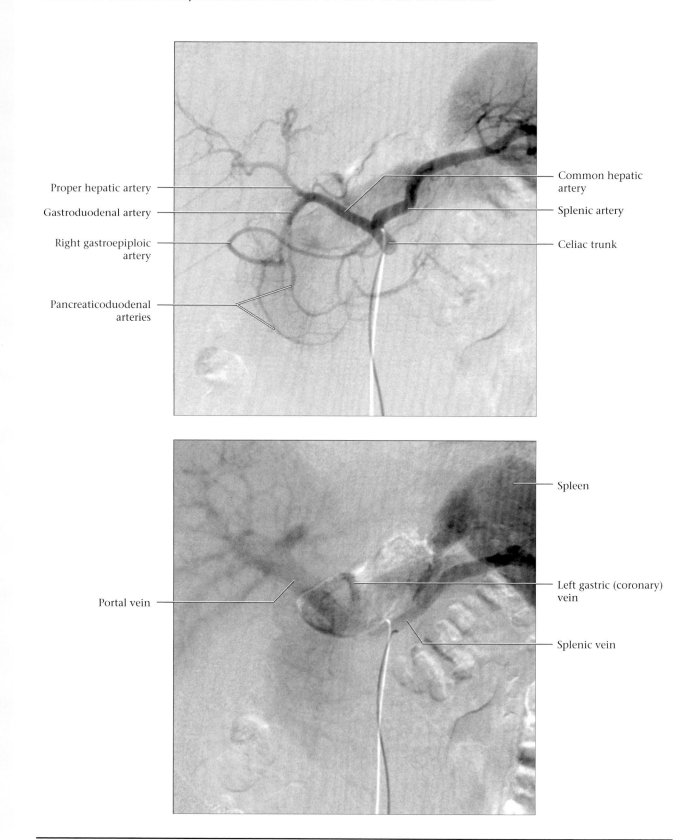

(Top) First of six images of the same patient. Arterial phase of celiac angiogram shows only the common hepatic and splenic arteries arising from the celiac trunk. The left gastric artery has a separate origin from the aorta in this individual, as shown on the subsequent CT scan. **(Bottom)** Venous phase image from celiac angiogram shows the left gastric vein entering the portal vein near its confluence with the splenic vein.

GASTRODUODENAL

ARTERIAL VARIATIONS, SEPARATE ORIGIN OF LEFT GASTRIC ARTERY

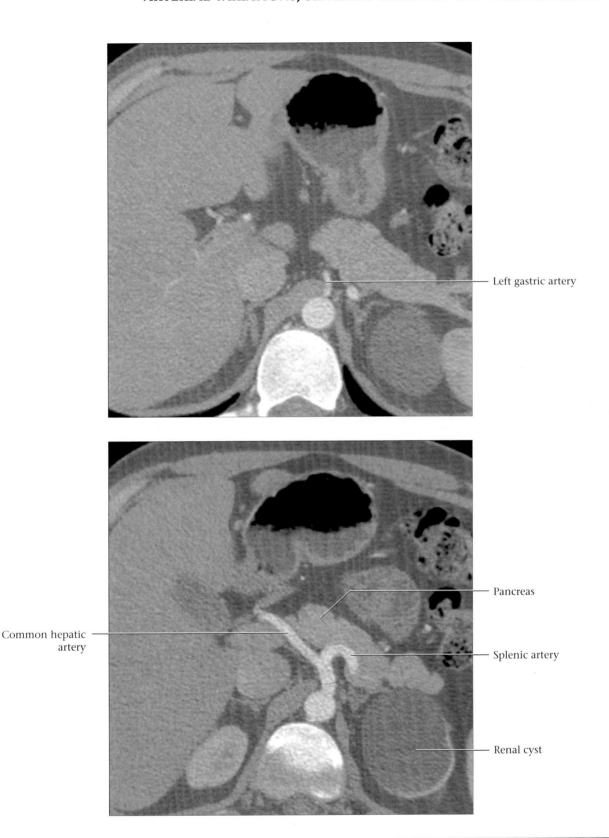

Left gastric artery

Common hepatic artery

Pancreas

Splenic artery

Renal cyst

(Top) Axial CT section through the upper abdomen shows the left gastric artery arising separately from the aorta, rather than having its usual origin from the celiac trunk. **(Bottom)** More caudal CT section through the celiac trunk shows the common hepatic and splenic arteries at their origin. The splenic artery runs a circuitous route, frequently indenting the dorsal surface of the pancreas. (Incidentally noted is a left renal cyst).

GASTRODUODENAL

ARTERIAL VARIATIONS, SEPARATE ORIGIN OF LEFT GASTRIC ARTERY

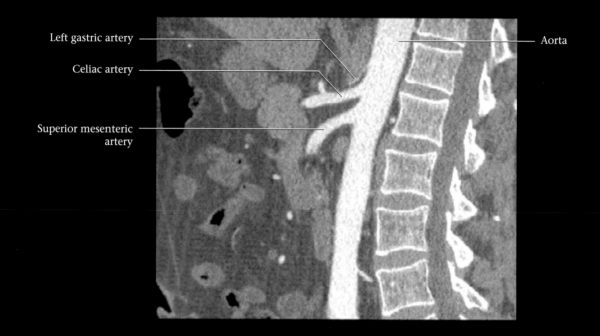

Left gastric artery — Aorta

Celiac artery —

Superior mesenteric artery —

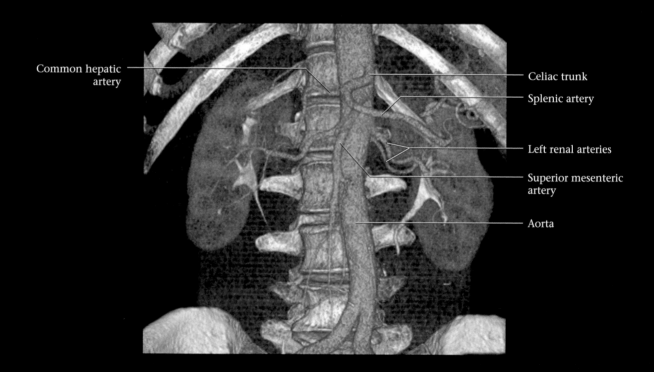

Common hepatic artery — Celiac trunk

Splenic artery

Left renal arteries

Superior mesenteric artery

Aorta

(Top) Sagittal reformation of CT data set shows the origins of the celiac and superior mesenteric arteries from the proximal abdominal aorta. Barely seen is the small left gastric artery, which has a separate origin from the aorta in this man. **(Bottom)** Frontal volume rendered CT angiogram from the same original CT data set demonstrates the major visceral branches of the abdominal aorta. From cephalad to caudal these are the celiac, superior mesenteric, renal and inferior mesenteric arteries.

GASTRODUODENAL

BRUNNER GLAND HYPERPLASIA

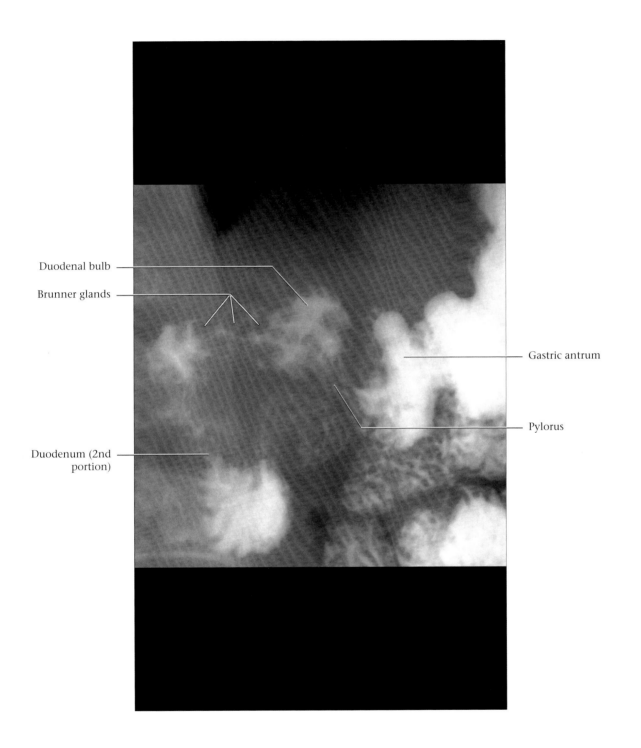

Duodenal bulb

Brunner glands

Gastric antrum

Pylorus

Duodenum (2nd portion)

Film from an upper GI series shows numerous polypoid filling defects in the duodenal bulb characteristic of hyperplastic Brunner glands. These glands are normal constituents of the duodenal wall, more numerous in the bulb and second portion. They are normally only 1 or 2 mm in diameter and are usually not evident on radiographic studies. The Brunner glands secrete a clear fluid that contains mucus and a weak proteolytic enzyme acting in an acid milieu.

PERFORATED DUODENAL ULCER

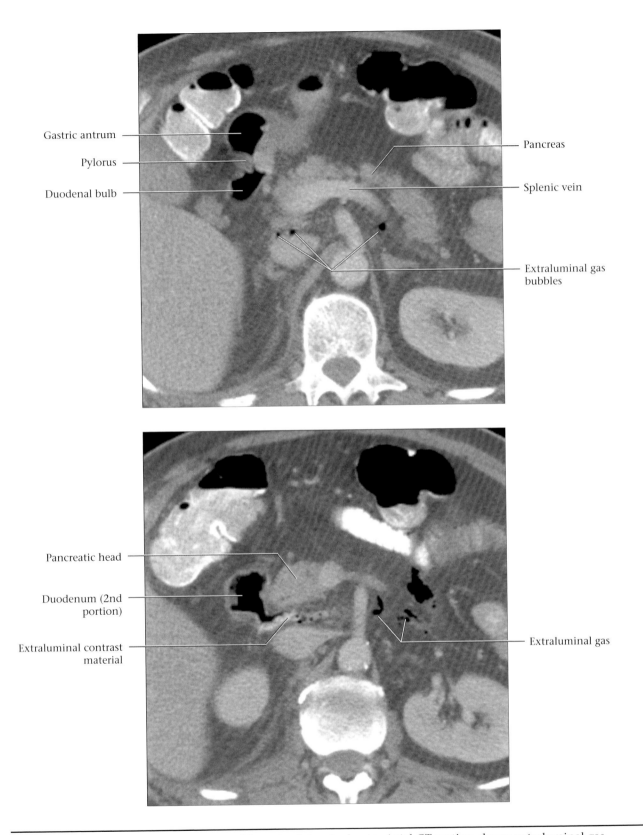

(Top) First of six images in a young man with acute abdominal pain. Axial CT section shows extraluminal gas bubbles dorsal to the pancreas, in the retroperitoneum. **(Bottom)** More caudal CT section shows high density contrast material that has "leaked" out of the lumen of the second portion of the duodenum. The lumen of the duodenum is distorted.

GASTRODUODENAL

PERFORATED DUODENAL ULCER

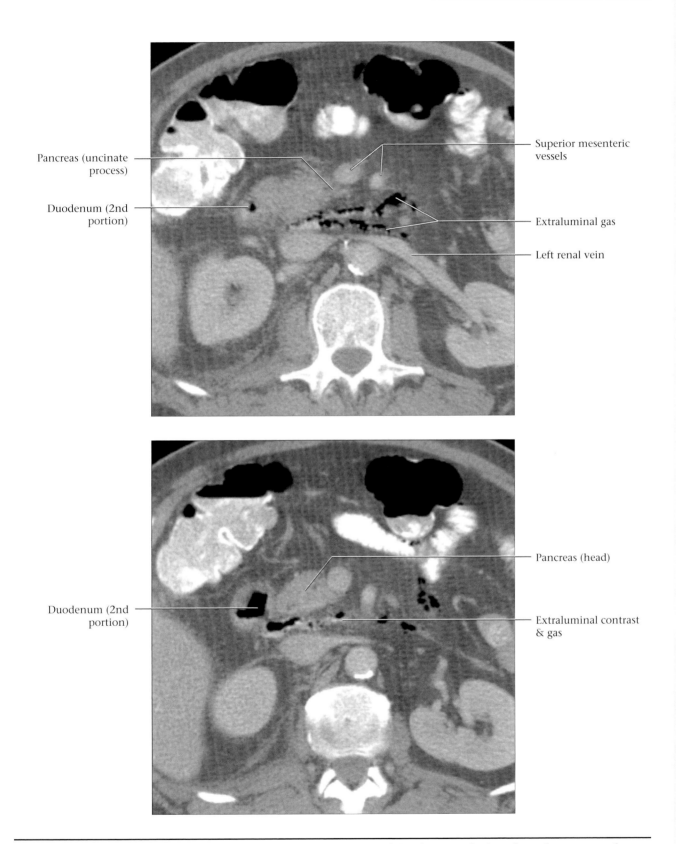

(Top) Extraluminal gas tracks along the course of the third portion of duodenum, which is the only segment of bowel to cross between the aorta and the superior mesenteric vessels. The only other structures that lie in this space are the uncinate process of the pancreas and the left renal vein, both of which appear normal in this patient. **(Bottom)** The lumen of the second portion of duodenum is distorted as usually occurs as a result of ulceration and spasm. The extraluminal gas and contrast material appear to be leaking from the second or third part of the duodenum.

GASTRODUODENAL

PERFORATED DUODENAL ULCER

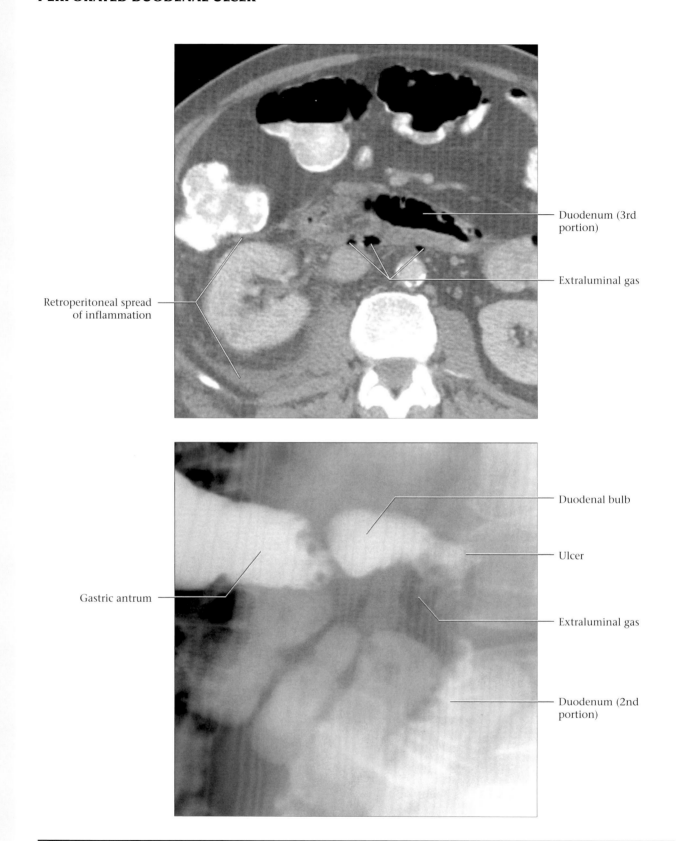

Duodenum (3rd portion)

Extraluminal gas

Retroperitoneal spread of inflammation

Duodenal bulb

Ulcer

Extraluminal gas

Gastric antrum

Duodenum (2nd portion)

(Top) The lumen of the third portion of duodenum appears to be normal, but extraluminal gas is evident behind the duodenum. Also note the inflammatory changes in the retroperitoneal space around the right kidney. **(Bottom)** Oblique film from an upper GI series performed with water-soluble contrast medium shows an ulcer at the apex of the duodenum, which is the post bulbar segment that begins the second portion of the duodenum. The lumen of the adjacent segment of duodenum is narrowed due to spasm. Extraluminal gas is present. A perforated ulcer of the second portion of duodenum was confirmed at surgery. While the duodenal bulb is intraperitoneal, the rest of the duodenum is retroperitoneal, which explains the presence of retroperitoneal inflammation and gas in this case.

GASTRODUODENAL

PERFORATED DUODENAL ULCER; TISSUE PLANES

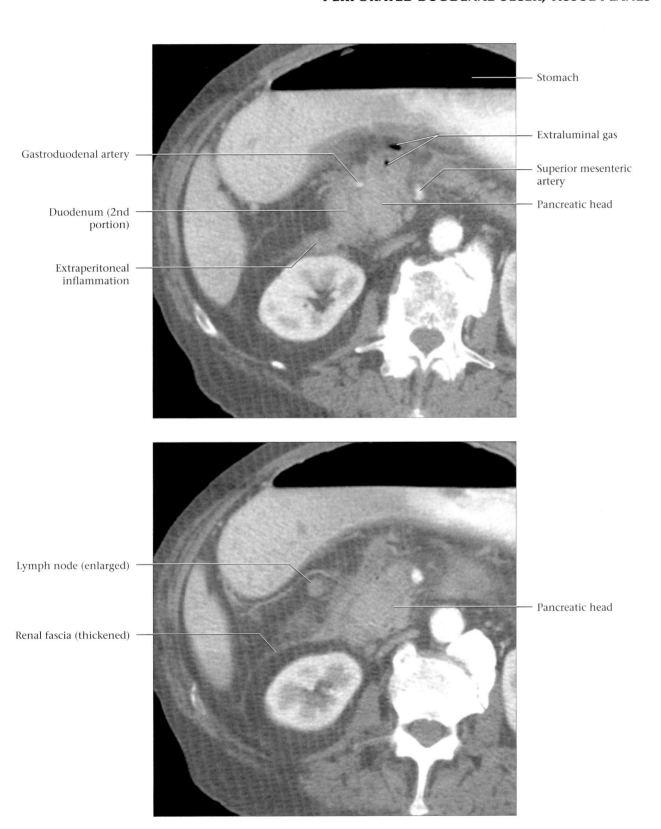

(Top) First of two axial CT sections in an elderly man with acute abdominal pain shows extraluminal gas near the second portion of the duodenum and infiltration of the retroperitoneal (anterior pararenal) space on the right. The gastroduodenal artery lies in a plane between the pancreatic head and the second portion of duodenum. **(Bottom)** The second portion of the duodenum always lies immediately lateral to the pancreatic head. The lumen of the duodenum is collapsed, and the adjacent retroperitoneal fascial planes and spaces are infiltrated. An adjacent lymph node is enlarged due to inflammation (reactive hyperplasia). A perforated ulcer was subsequently confirmed. Inflammation of the pancreas or duodenum will result in infiltration of the anterior pararenal space and thickening of the renal fascia, which forms the dorsal boundary to this space.

GASTRODUODENAL

GASTRIC ULCER, PERFORATED INTO LESSER SAC

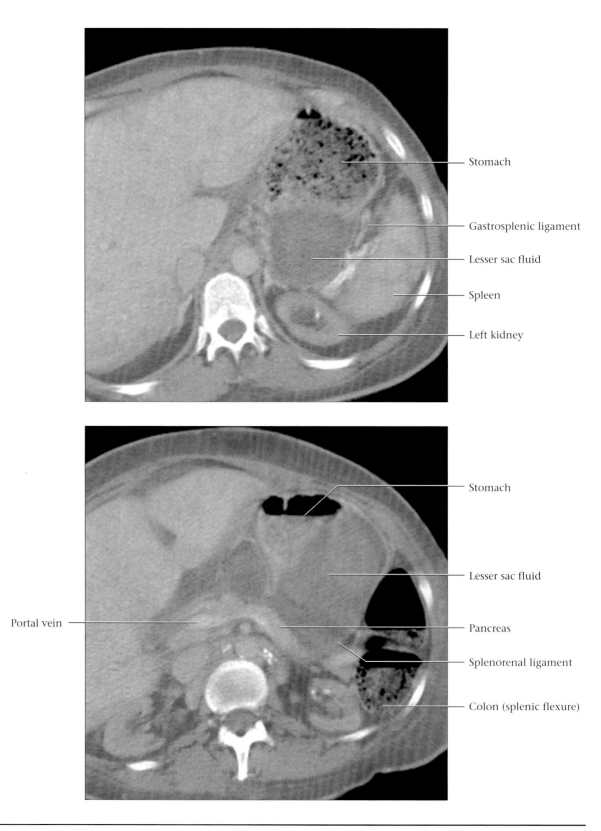

(Top) First of four images in an elderly man with chronic renal failure and acute abdominal pain. Axial CT section shows a heterogeneous retrogastric fluid collection within the lesser sac, bounded laterally by the gastrosplenic ligament. (Bottom) Note the heterogeneity and loculation of the fluid within the lesser sac, representing mostly blood and gastric juice. The kidneys are atrophic due to chronic renal failure.

GASTRODUODENAL

GASTRIC ULCER PERFORATED INTO LESSER SAC

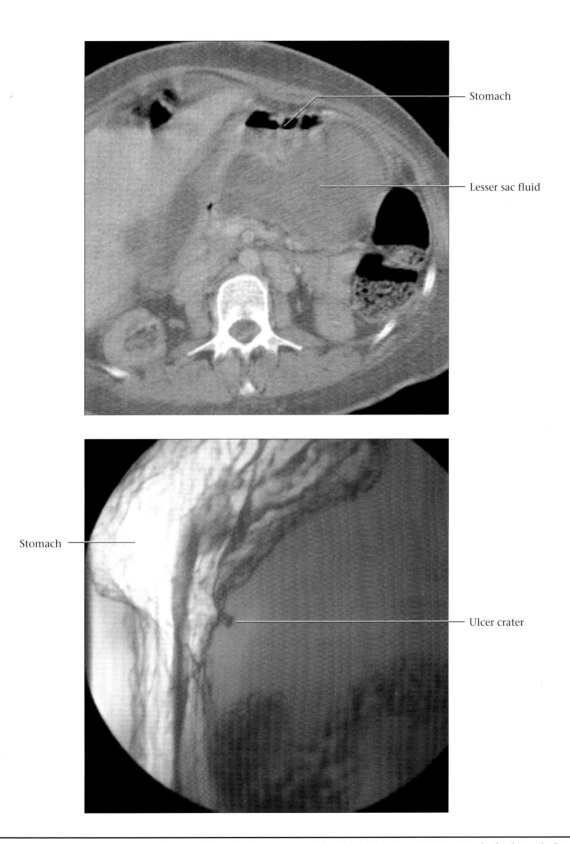

Stomach

Lesser sac fluid

Stomach

Ulcer crater

(Top) The stomach is compressed and displaced by the lesser sac fluid, which is heterogeneous and of relatively high density. Loculated lesser sac fluid collections are usually the result of pancreatitis or a perforated ulcer of the posterior wall of the stomach, since these organs abut the lesser sac. (Bottom) Lateral view from an air contrast upper GI series shows a focal outpouching of barium from the posterior wall of the stomach, diagnostic of a benign gastric ulcer. The ulcer was confirmed by endoscopy and resolved with medical therapy. Recall that the lesser sac lies immediately adjacent to the posterior wall of the stomach.

GASTRODUODENAL

GASTRIC CARCINOMA WITH NODAL METASTASES

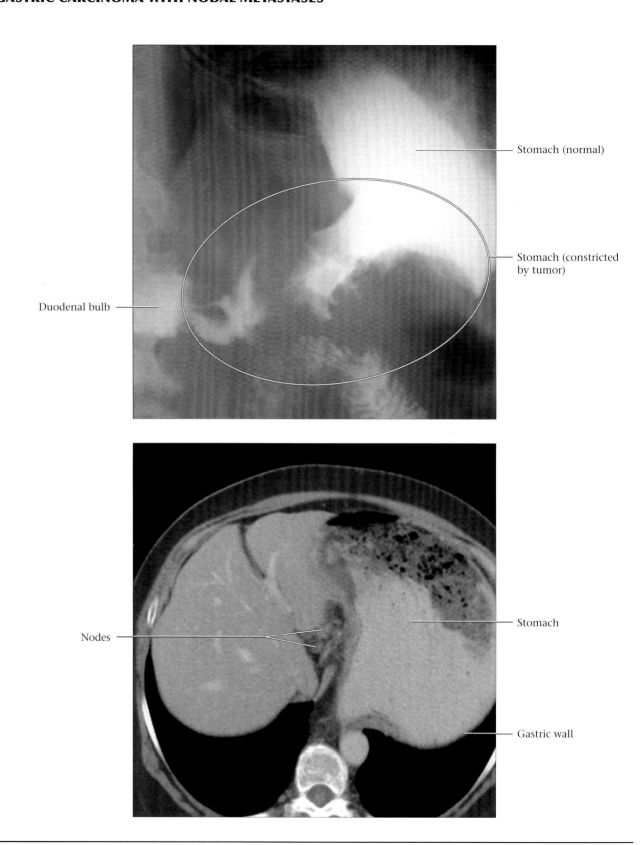

Stomach (normal)

Stomach (constricted by tumor)

Duodenal bulb

Nodes

Stomach

Gastric wall

(**Top**) Frontal film from an upper GI series in an elderly man with early satiety and weight loss shows marked irregular thickening of the wall of the stomach throughout the distal body and antrum. There is an abrupt transition between the normally distensible fundus and proximal body and the fixed, nondistensible distal stomach. The duodenal bulb is normal. (**Bottom**) First of five axial CT sections in the same patient as previous image shows distension of the proximal stomach and a thin, normal gastric wall. Enlarged lymph nodes are present in the gastrohepatic ligament (upper left gastric group) due to metastatic spread of tumor.

GASTRODUODENAL

GASTRIC CARCINOMA WITH NODAL METASTASES

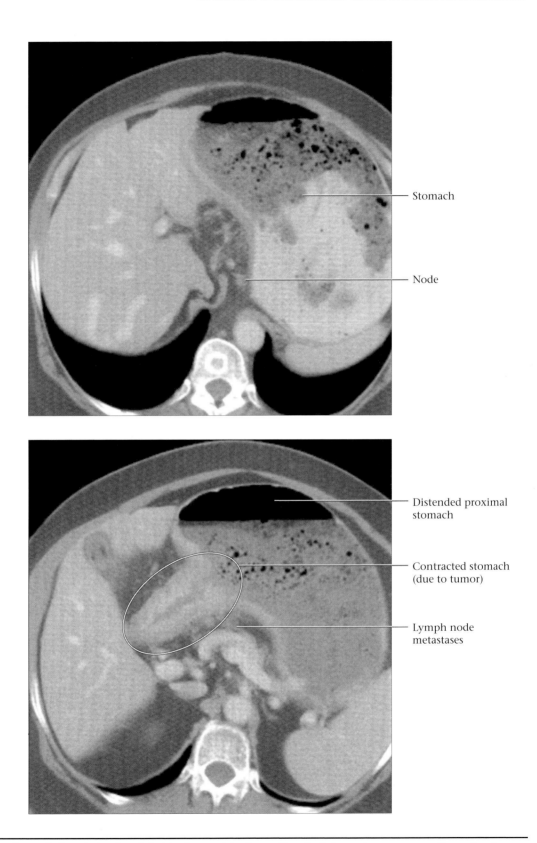

Stomach

Node

Distended proximal stomach

Contracted stomach (due to tumor)

Lymph node metastases

(Top) The stomach is distended with food and fluid, along with the orally administered contrast medium, due to gastric outlet obstruction. (Bottom) Note the abrupt transition from the dilated proximal stomach with its thin wall to the narrowed lumen and thick wall of the distal stomach. When carcinoma affects the distal stomach, it often results in a rigid, nondistensible condition that obstructs gastric emptying. Spread to upper nodal chains is also typical.

GASTRODUODENAL

GASTRIC CARCINOMA WITH NODAL METASTASES

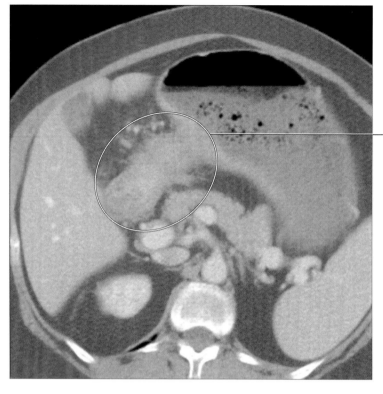

Contracted stomach
(due to tumor)

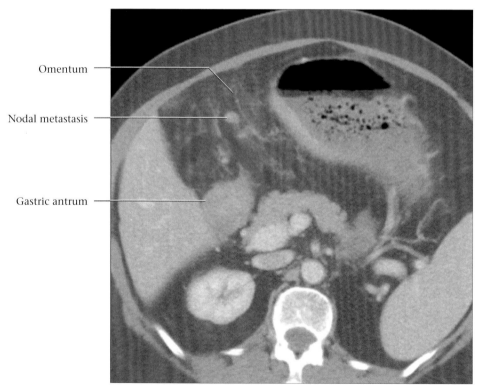

Omentum

Nodal metastasis

Gastric antrum

(Top) More caudal CT section. Note the collapsed, constricted lumen of the distal stomach and the thickened wall due to tumor infiltration. The fat planes next to the stomach are infiltrated due to direct tumor spread through the wall. (Bottom) A nodal metastasis and generalized infiltration are present in the greater omentum. The thickened wall of the gastric antrum is seen in cross section.

GASTRODUODENAL

GASTROCOLIC LIGAMENT TUMOR EXTENSION

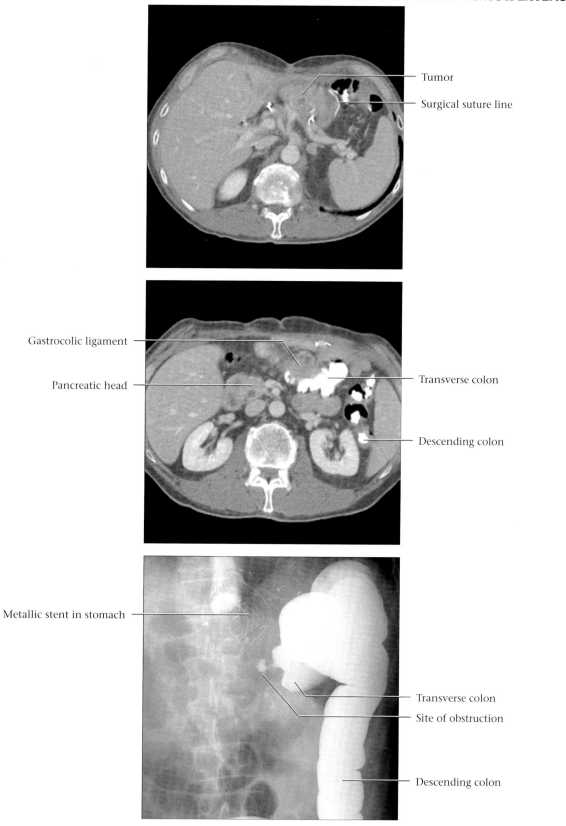

(Top image labels) Tumor / Surgical suture line

(Middle image labels) Gastrocolic ligament / Pancreatic head / Transverse colon / Descending colon

(Bottom image labels) Metallic stent in stomach / Transverse colon / Site of obstruction / Descending colon

(Top) First of three images shows recurrence of gastric carcinoma after prior resection. Axial CT section shows a tumor mass adjacent to a line of sutures that mark the resection margin following partial gastrectomy. **(Middle)** More caudal section shows tumor in the gastrocolic ligament, the portion of the greater omentum that connects the greater curvature of the stomach with the transverse colon. The tumor distorts and narrows the lumen of the transverse colon. **(Bottom)** Frontal film from a barium enema shows complete obstruction to retrograde flow of barium in the transverse colon. Note the metallic stent that had been inserted into the stomach in an attempt to prevent complete gastric outlet obstruction. This serves as a radiologic marker for the gastric tumor, and shows how close the gastric tumor is to the colon, which led to the tumor invasion and obstruction of the colon.

GASTRODUODENAL

DUODENAL COMPRESSION, "SMA SYNDROME"

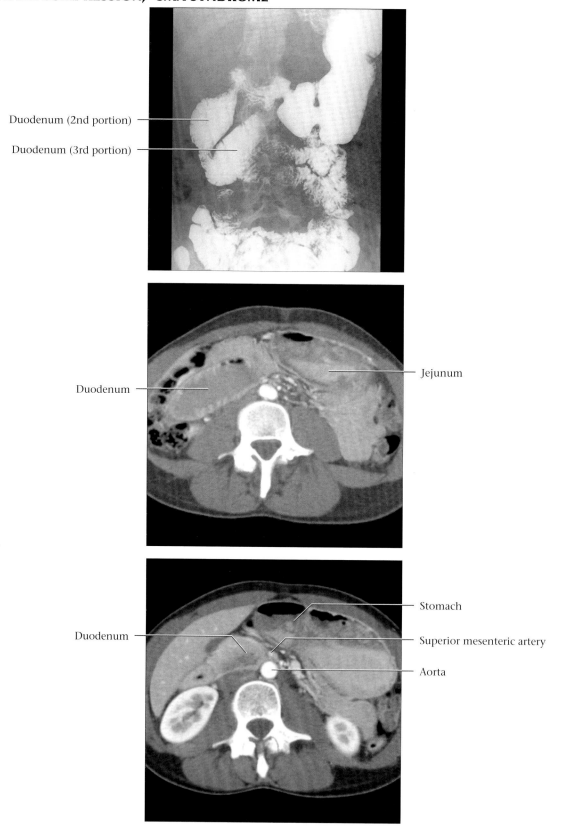

Duodenum (2nd portion)

Duodenum (3rd portion)

Duodenum — Jejunum

Duodenum — Stomach

— Superior mesenteric artery

— Aorta

(Top) First of three images in a young woman with post-prandial pain, nausea and weight loss. A barium upper GI series shows dilation of the second and third portions of duodenum, with an abrupt vertical, band-like narrowing as the duodenum crosses the midline. The remainder of the bowel is normal. **(Middle)** Axial CT section shows marked dilation of the third portion of the duodenum up to the midline. The jejunum and other bowel are normal. **(Bottom)** As the duodenum crosses between the aorta and the superior mesenteric vessels, it is compressed, and the lumen is markedly comarrowed. This is sometimes referred to as the "SMA syndrome" and is felt to cause functional partial obstruction of the duodenum.

GASTRODUODENAL

AORTO-ENTERIC FISTULA

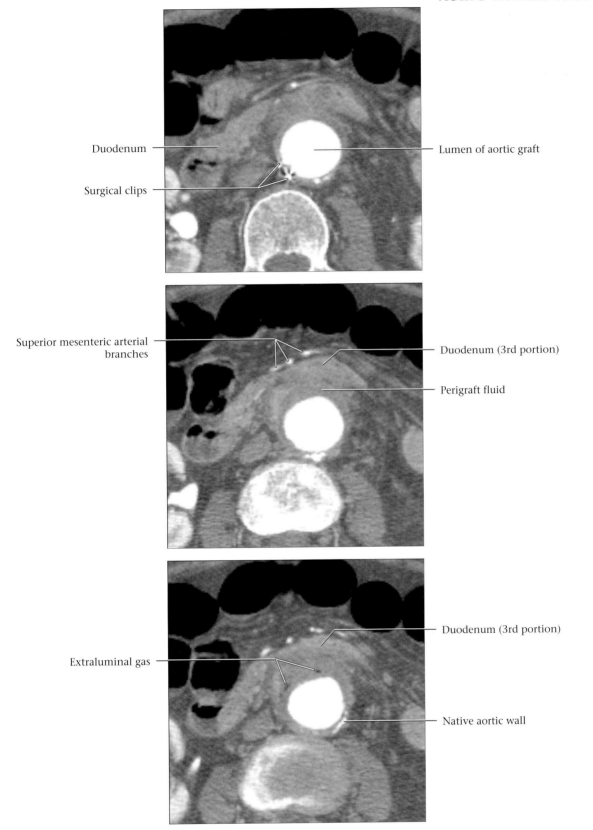

Duodenum — Lumen of aortic graft

Surgical clips

Superior mesenteric arterial branches — Duodenum (3rd portion)

Perigraft fluid

Duodenum (3rd portion)

Extraluminal gas

Native aortic wall

(Top) First of three axial CT sections in a elderly man who had open surgical repair of an abdominal aortic aneurysm. Now has upper GI bleeding. CT shows the cephalic end of the graft which has been placed within the aortic lumen and sutured to the native aortic wall. Note the surgical clips. **(Middle)** Note that the third portion of the duodenum is "draped" over the aorta as it passes behind the superior mesenteric vessels. **(Bottom)** The partially calcified native aortic wall should be closely applied to the synthetic graft. Instead, there are fluid and gas bubbles in the perigraft space between the third portion of duodenum and the aortic lumen. Graft infection and a fistula from the aorta to the duodenum account for the extraluminal gas and fluid. This was repaired at surgery.

GASTRODUODENAL

GASTRIC DIVERTICULUM

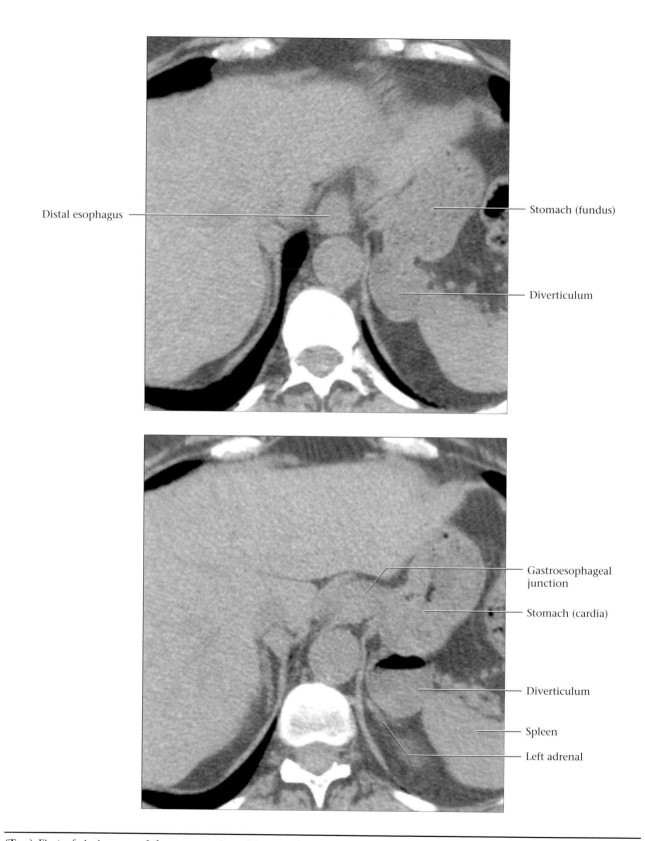

Distal esophagus

Stomach (fundus)

Diverticulum

Gastroesophageal junction

Stomach (cardia)

Diverticulum

Spleen

Left adrenal

(Top) First of six images of the same patient. Most cephalad CT section shows a focal outpouching from the posterior wall of the gastric fundus, near the gastroesophageal junction. **(Bottom)** The air-fluid level within the diverticulum helps to identify its communication with the gastric lumen. Note other adjacent structures, such as adrenal and spleen.

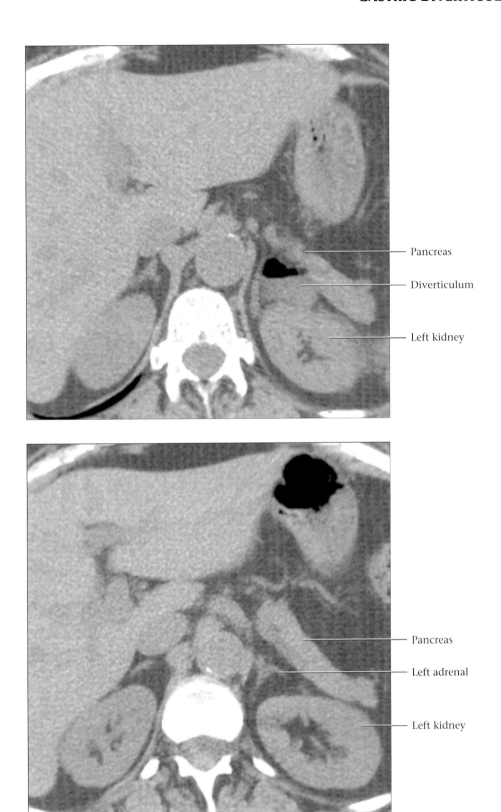

(Top) Even though the diverticulum originates from the intraperitoneal stomach, it appears to be interposed between the pancreas and left kidney, both retroperitoneal organs. **(Bottom)** In cases in which a gastric diverticulum is filled with fluid or food, rather than gas, it can easily be mistaken for a tumor or cyst, such as one arising from the pancreas or adrenal gland.

GASTRODUODENAL

GASTRIC DIVERTICULUM

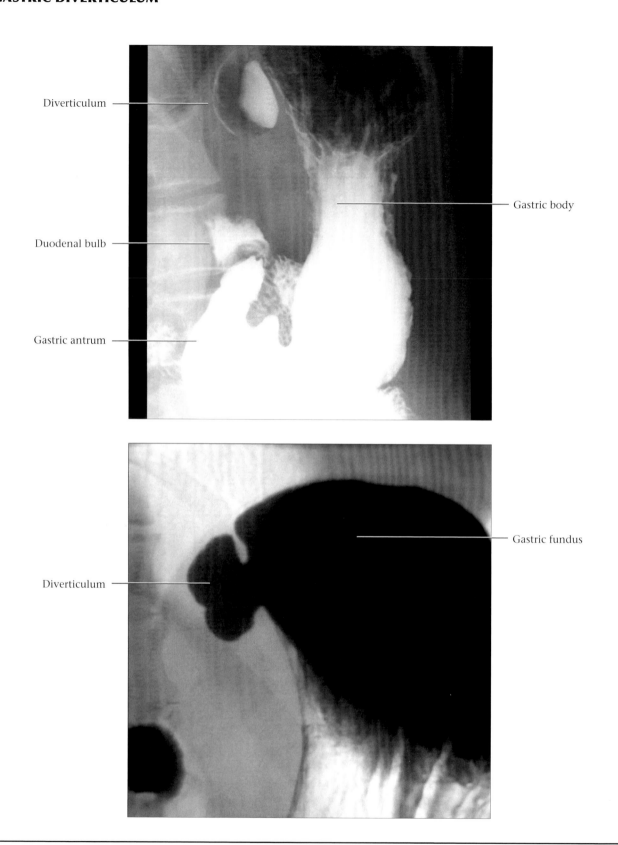

(Top) Lateral film from an upper GI series confirms the gastric diverticulum as an outpouching from the posterior wall of the fundus, just above the gastroesophageal junction. (Bottom) Supine frontal film from upper GI series; spot film with barium displayed as "black". The fundus and diverticulum fill with barium. Note the wide "mouth" of the diverticulum which usually permits free entry and exit of food and fluid.

GASTRODUODENAL

LARGE DUODENAL DIVERTICULUM

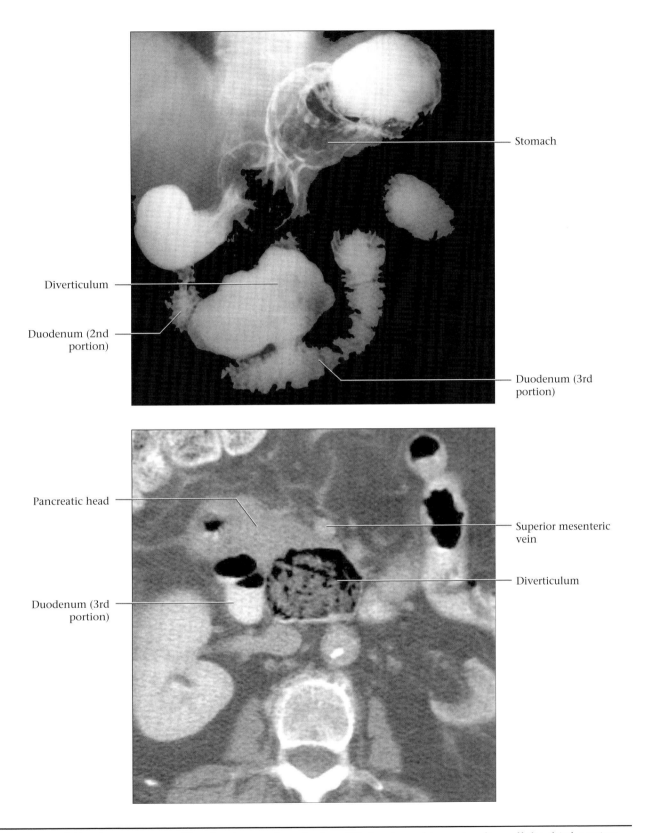

Stomach

Diverticulum

Duodenum (2nd portion)

Duodenum (3rd portion)

Pancreatic head

Superior mesenteric vein

Diverticulum

Duodenum (3rd portion)

(Top) Frontal film from an upper GI series shows a large barium-filled outpouching extending off the third portion of the duodenum. This is a typical location, but an unusually large size, for a duodenal diverticulum. These are usually asymptomatic, but may rupture or bleed, and may be mistaken for ulcers or masses on various imaging tests. **(Bottom)** Axial CT section shows the large diverticulum, filled with food and gas from a recent meal. Orally administered contrast material opacifies the lumen of adjacent bowel loops but fills only the dependent position of the diverticulum.

SMALL INTESTINE

Gross Anatomy

Overview
- Mesenteric small bowel is suspended from the posterior abdominal wall by a fan-shaped **mesentery**

Divisions
- **Jejunum**
  - Begins at **duodenojejunal flexure**
    - Duodenojejunal flexure often acutely angulated; suspended by the musculotendinous **ligament of Treitz (suspensory ligament of the duodenum)**, extension of right crus of diaphragm
  - Constitutes about 40% of the length of the intestine
    - About 2-3 meters long
  - Usually lies in left upper quadrant
  - Thicker, more vascular wall with tall, closely spaced **circular folds** (4-7 folds per inch), few **lymphoid nodules (Peyer patches)** in submucosa
  - Circular folds also referred to as **valvulae conniventes, plicae circulares, folds of Kerckring**
    - Prominence of folds and wall thickness vary by age (more in younger), degree of bowel distention
- **Ileum**
  - No clear point of distinction from jejunum
  - Constitutes distal 60% of intestine (~ 4 meters long)
  - Usually lies in right lower abdomen and pelvis
  - Has thin wall, less vascular, lower and more widely spaced circular folds, more **lymphoid follicles**
  - Ends at ileocecal valve
- **Vessels and nerves**
  - All lie between the layers of the **small bowel mesentery**
  - **Superior mesenteric artery (SMA)** supplies entire intestine
    - Arises from aorta at L1 level, 1 cm caudal to celiac artery
    - Sends ~ 15-18 branches to intestine
    - Arteries unite to form arches (**arterial arcades**) → straight arteries (**vasa recta**)
  - **Superior mesenteric vein (SMV)** drains entire intestine
    - Lies to the right of the SMA
    - Unites with **splenic vein** to form **portal vein** behind the pancreatic neck
- **Lymphatics**
  - Begin within the **intestinal villi** (tiny projection of mucous membrane) as **lacteals**
    - Specialized lymphatic vessels that absorb fat from gut
    - Empty milky chyle into **lymphatic plexuses** in the intestinal walls → **lymphatic vessels** (in mesentery) → lymph nodes
  - **Juxta-intestinal nodes** near wall of intestine
  - **Mesenteric lymph nodes** follow arterial arcades
- **Nerves** are autonomic
  - Sympathetic: Follow SMA and its branches, called the **splanchnic nerves**
    - Effect: Reduce motility, secretion and vascularity
  - Parasympathetic: Follow arterial branches
    - Are branches of **posterior vagal trunks**
    - Increase motility, secretion, vascularity & digestion
  - Includes sensory branches that can detect stretching & distention, but no other pain stimuli; bowel obstruction → distended lumen → spasms of crampy abdominal pain (**colic**); poorly localized

Anatomy-Based Imaging Issues

Imaging Recommendations
- **Bowel ischemia** is a major clinical problem
  - May result from arterial or venous occlusion (SMA or SMV) or hypoperfusion (e.g., from shock, cardiac failure)
  - Demonstrating patency of vessels and perfusion of bowel wall is key
  - Contrast-enhanced CT is best single study; can be combined with CT angiography and 3D imaging
  - MR angiography has similar role as CT
  - Catheter angiography usually reserved for high suspicion of vessel occlusion; allows embolectomy and stent placement
- Bowel wall thickening
  - Almost all acute bowel injuries result in thickening of submucosal layer of wall ("**thickened folds**")
  - Etiology of submucosal thickening may be suggested by the density (attenuation) of the submucosal layer on CT scanning
    - Gas: Pneumatosis, as with infarction
    - High density blood: Acute hemorrhage, as with trauma or spontaneous coagulopathic hemorrhage
    - Fat: Chronic proliferation of fat, as in chronic inflammation from Crohn disease

Clinical Implications

Clinical Importance
- **Bowel obstruction** is a common clinical problem
  - Usual causes are adhesions and hernias (external > internal)
  - Much more commonly affects the intestine than the colon; (intestine is longer, more mobile)

Embryology

Embryologic Events
- Embryological foregut: Esophagus, stomach, duodenum, liver, biliary system
- Midgut: Small intestine and right side colon
- Hindgut: Left side of colon and rectum
- Foregut and midgut are herniated into the early fetal umbilical cord, usually return to abdominal cavity after 270° counterclockwise rotation and then are fixed into position by modification of mesenteries
- Errors in this process are common
  - Malrotation and **midgut volvulus**
    - May present in infants or adults
    - May cause bowel obstruction and ischemia

SMALL INTESTINE

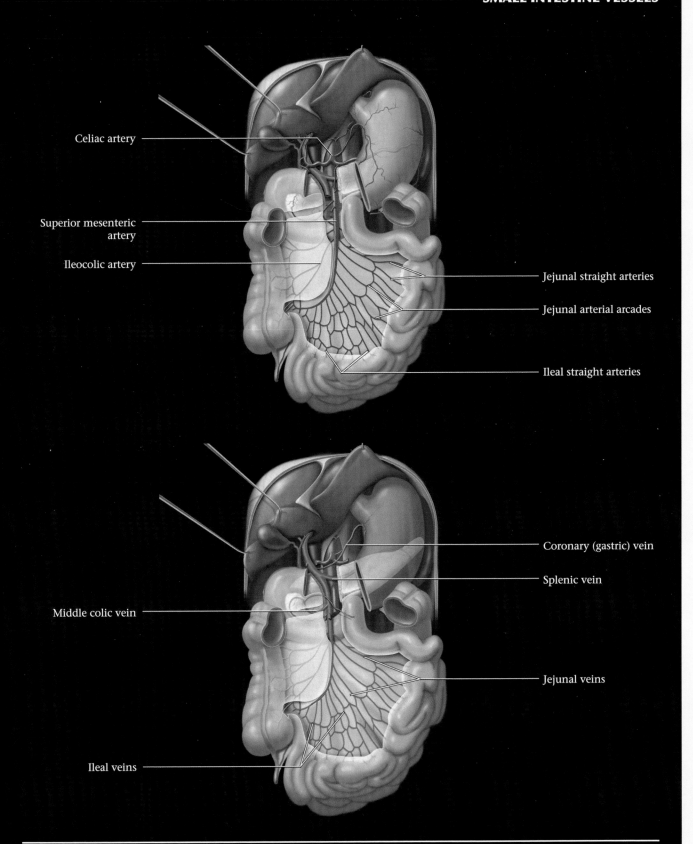

Celiac artery

Superior mesenteric artery

Ileocolic artery

Jejunal straight arteries

Jejunal arterial arcades

Ileal straight arteries

Coronary (gastric) vein

Splenic vein

Middle colic vein

Jejunal veins

Ileal veins

(Top) The superior mesenteric artery supplies the entire small intestine. Arising from the anterior wall of the aorta at about the L1 vertebral level, its first branch is the inferior pancreaticoduodenal artery, which supplies the duodenum & pancreas, and anastomoses freely with branches from the celiac trunk. The next branch is the middle colic, supplying the transverse colon. Arising from the convex or left side of the SMA are numerous branches to the jejunum & ileum. Jejunal arteries are generally larger and longer than those of the ileum. After a straight course the arteries form multiple curvilinear arcades which form lateral communications between the arteries. Finally, straight arteries (arteriae rectae) extend to & penetrate the wall of the intestine. **(Bottom)** In number, point of origin, course & name, the intestinal veins are similar to the arteries.

SMALL INTESTINE

JEJUNUM

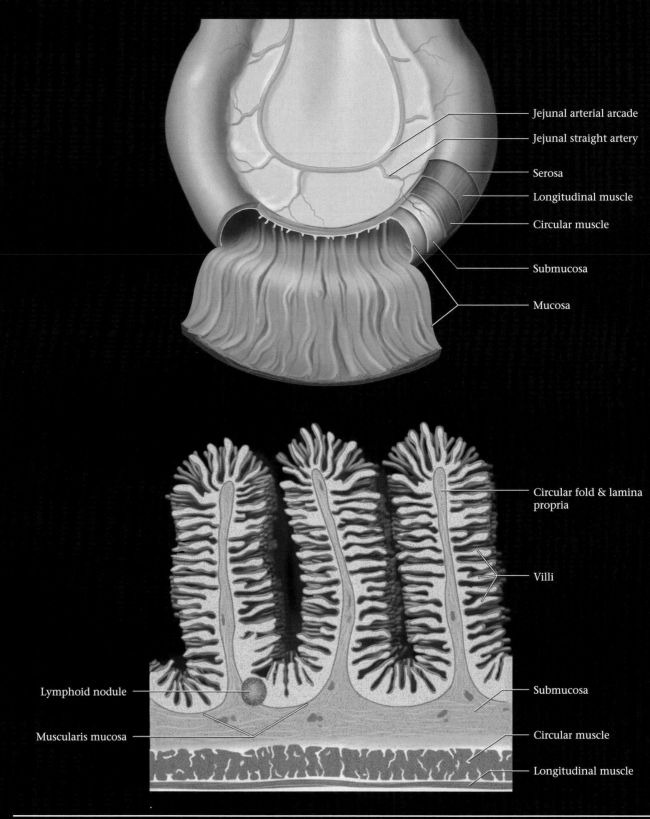

Jejunal arterial arcade

Jejunal straight artery

Serosa

Longitudinal muscle

Circular muscle

Submucosa

Mucosa

Circular fold & lamina propria

Villi

Lymphoid nodule

Submucosa

Muscularis mucosa

Circular muscle

Longitudinal muscle

(Top) There is no sharp point of demarcation between the jejunum & ileum and both have the same basic structure. The jejunum has a richer vascular supply, thicker wall and wider lumen. There are five layers of the bowel wall. The innermost is the mucosa, the absorptive surface of the gut. The jejunal mucosa is extensively plicated (folded) and these transverse ("circular") folds lie perpendicular to the long axis of the bowel. The other layers are the submucosa, circular muscle, longitudinal muscle, and serosa, the peritoneal lining of the bowel. **(Bottom)** The mucosal surface of the jejunum is increased by prominent villi, fingerlike projections of mucosa. The muscularis mucosa separates the mucous membrane from the submucosa. The submucosa has a network of capillaries, lymphatics, and a nerve plexus (of Meissner). The jejunum has few and small, discrete lymphoid nodules.

SMALL INTESTINE

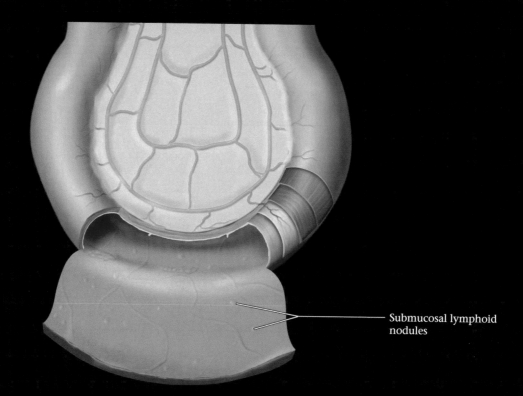

Submucosal lymphoid
nodules

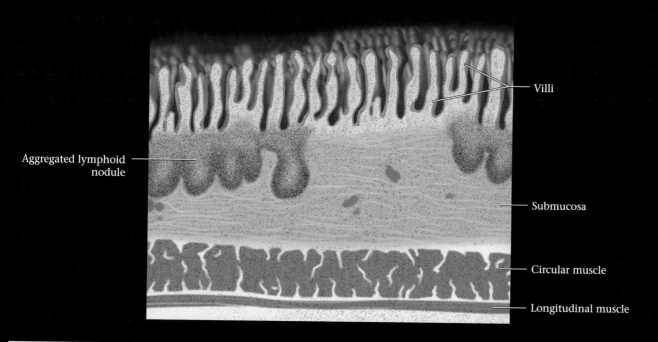

Aggregated lymphoid
nodule

Villi

Submucosa

Circular muscle

Longitudinal muscle

(Top) The ileum is distinguished by a thinner wall, less vascularity, and less prominent transverse folds and villi than the jejunum. It has the same five layers of the bowel wall. **(Bottom)** Low power microscopic view of a section of ileum. The villi in the ileum are shorter and narrower than in the jejunum and the transverse folds are much less prominent. They are often not visible on radiographic studies of the intestine. Conversely, submucosal lymphoid follicles become progressively more prominent along the course of the distal small intestine. In the distal ileum lymphoid follicles may aggregate into macroscopic collections, called Peyer patches, which may be evident as submucosal "masses" of a few millimeters in diameter on barium studies of the small intestine.

SMALL INTESTINE

MESENTERY OUTLINED BY ASCITES

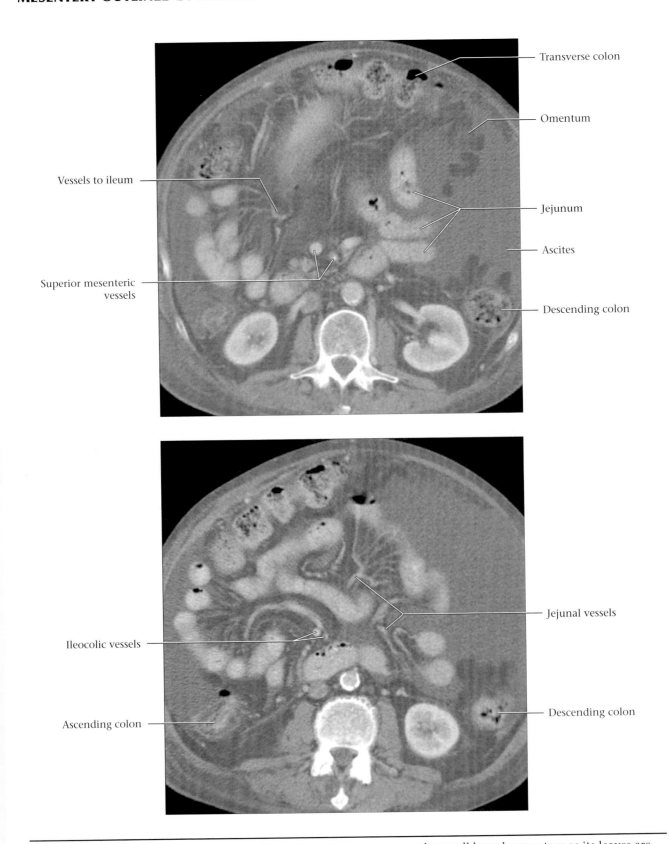

(Top) First of two axial CT sections in a patient with ascites accentuates the small bowel mesentery as its leaves are separated by the fluid. The mesenteric vessels, nerves and lymphatics travel to and from the bowel between the layers of the mesentery, surrounded by a layer of fat and loose connective tissue. Note the superior mesenteric artery and vein at the base of the mesentery. **(Bottom)** A section through the right lower quadrant shows the ileocolic vessels supplying the ileum and ascending colon as well as multiple jejunal vessels to the left of midline. The vessels to the ascending and descending colon travel through the retroperitoneum, rather than through a mesentery.

SMALL INTESTINE

BARIUM STUDY, NORMAL SMALL INTESTINE

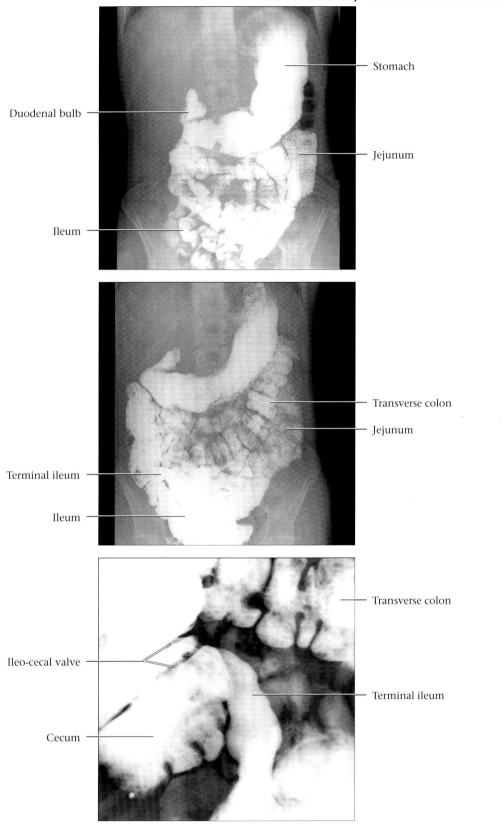

Stomach

Duodenal bulb

Jejunum

Ileum

Transverse colon

Jejunum

Terminal ileum

Ileum

Transverse colon

Ileo-cecal valve

Terminal ileum

Cecum

(Top) First of three images from a barium small bowel follow through shows the normal appearance of the small intestine. Note the position of the jejunum in the left upper quadrant, and its prominent, feathery mucosal fold pattern (in the nondistended state). The ileum lies predominantly in the right lower quadrant and has a less prominent fold pattern. **(Middle)** Later image from the same series shows barium progressively opacifying distal small bowel and colon. Note the difference in spacing between the transverse semilunar folds of the colon and the closely spaced, circular folds of the small bowel. **(Bottom)** Frontal coned down "spot" image from the same series shows the terminal ileum, ileo-cecal valve and cecum.

SMALL INTESTINE

ENTEROCLYSIS, NORMAL SMALL INTESTINE

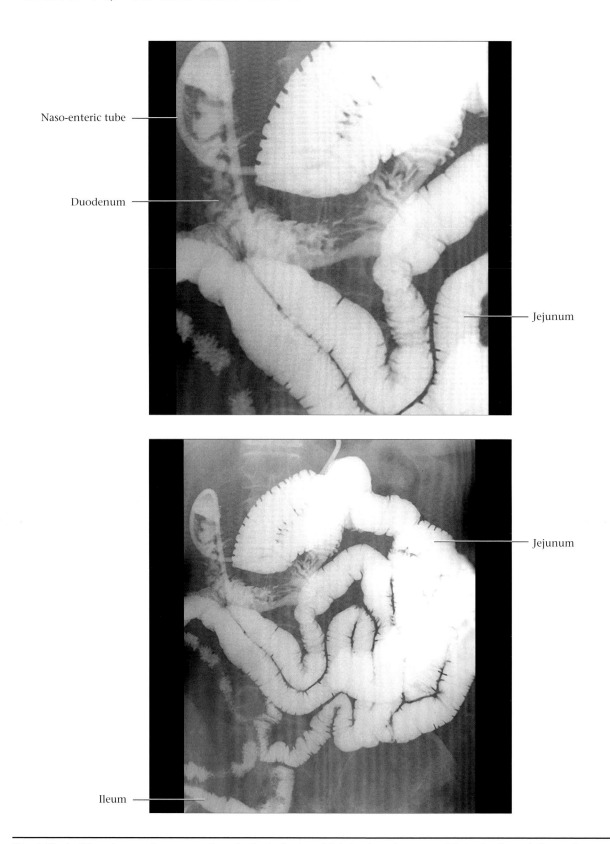

(Top) First of two images from an enteroclysis study, in which barium is pumped into the bowel through a naso-enteric tube, the tip of which has been advanced to the duodenojejunal junction under fluoroscopic control. By bypassing the gastric pylorus and using a pump to infuse barium at about 70 mL per minute, the bowel lumen can be distended optimally, allowing much better visualization of the circular folds. Note how thin and evenly spaced the jejunal folds are, with about 4-7 folds per linear inch in the jejunum, and somewhat fewer and less prominent folds in the ileum, as a general rule. (Bottom) Image from the enteroclysis shows the less prominent fold pattern in the ileum, compared with the jejunum.

SMALL INTESTINE

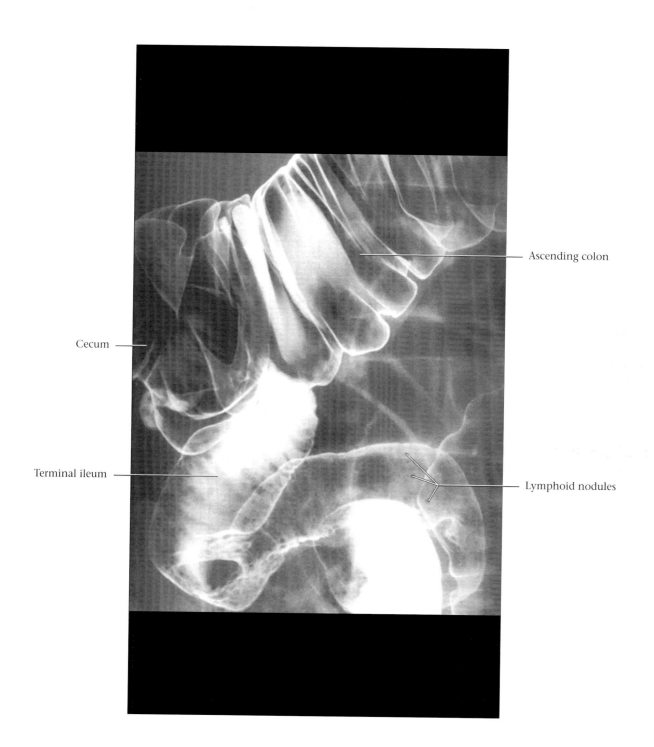

Oblique image from an air-contrast barium enema shows the innumerable small lymphoid nodules (Peyer patches) which are normal aggregates of lymphoid tissue that lie in the submucosa of the bowel wall. These are more prominent in the terminal ileum and in younger patients, in general.

SMALL INTESTINE

CATHETER ANGIOGRAM, SUPERIOR MESENTERIC ARTERY AND VEIN

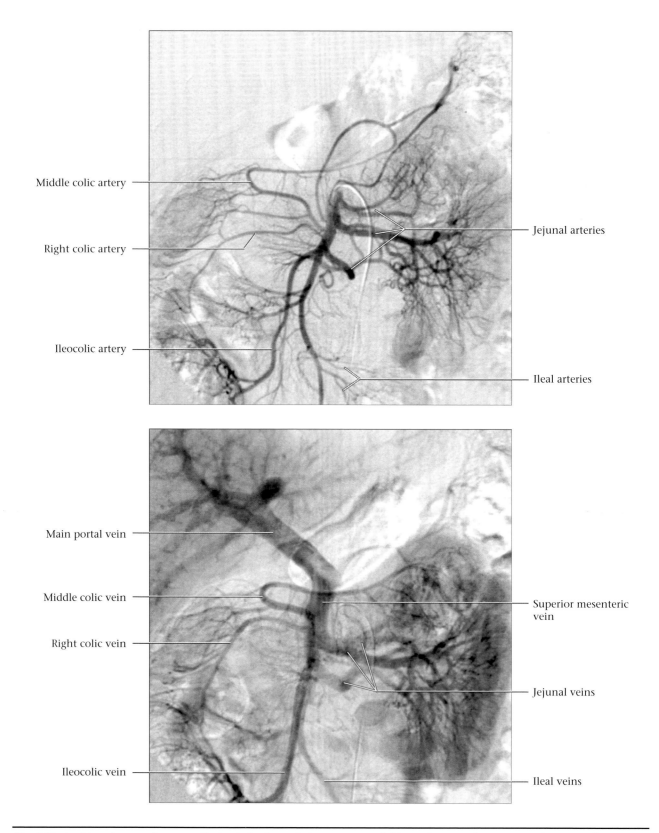

(Top) First of two images from a catheter injection of contrast material into the superior mesenteric artery shows multiple (15-18) arterial branches to the small bowel, as well as 3 major branches to the ascending and transverse colon (ileocolic, right & middle colic arteries). (Bottom) Venous phase image from the same study shows the superior mesenteric vein (SMV) and some of its major tributaries, as well as the portal vein. The veins parallel the arteries and have similar names.

CT ANGIOGRAM, SUPERIOR MESENTERIC ARTERY & VEIN

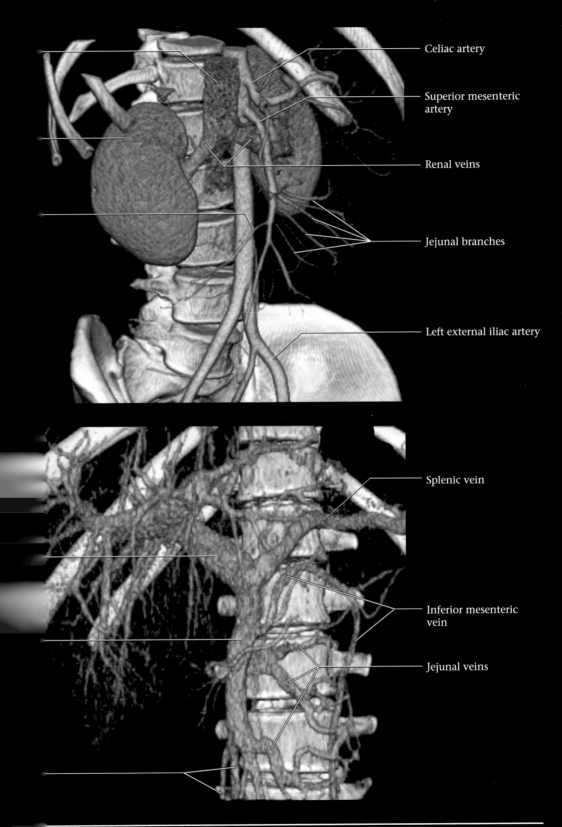

Celiac artery

Superior mesenteric artery

Renal veins

Jejunal branches

Left external iliac artery

Splenic vein

Inferior mesenteric vein

Jejunal veins

from an abdominal CT angiogram, late arterial phase, shows the SMA as the second major
ominal aorta, arising just distal to the celiac artery. The SMA courses over the left renal
branches of the SMA are well shown, with their peripheral portions excluded (deliberately)
The image is rotated to the left. **(Bottom)** Image from the venous phase of the CTA
major venous tributaries of the portal vein, including the superior mesenteric and splenic
inferior mesenteric vein (which drains the left side of the colon) empties into the superior
f into the splenic vein, a common variant (30% of population)

SMALL INTESTINE

MESENTERIC NODES

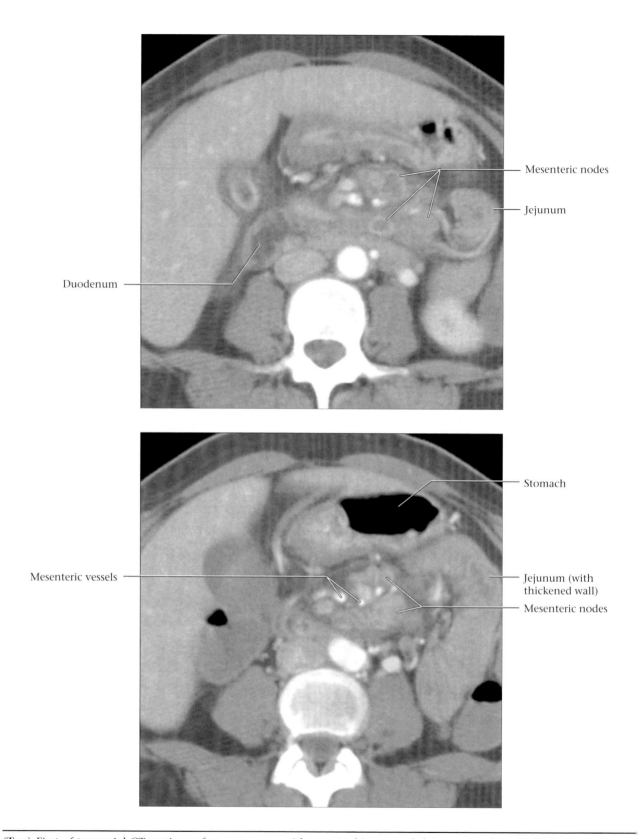

Mesenteric nodes

Jejunum

Duodenum

Stomach

Mesenteric vessels

Jejunum (with thickened wall)

Mesenteric nodes

(Top) First of two axial CT sections of a young man with acquired immunodeficiency syndrome (AIDS) shows multiple enlarged mesenteric nodes, especially prominent near the jejunum. The nodes have a peculiar low density center with contrast-enhancing periphery, findings characteristic of "caseation" and strongly suggestive of mycobacterial disease. In immunosuppressed patients, such as transplant recipients and those with AIDS, infectious agents, such as mycobacteria, may enter through the bowel, causing the jejunal wall thickening seen here, with subsequent involvement of the mesenteric nodes draining these segments of bowel. **(Bottom)** Note the position of the mesenteric nodes, "sandwiching" the mesenteric blood vessels. The jejunal wall is also thickened due to infection and inflammation.

MESENTERIC NODAL & SPLENIC DISEASE

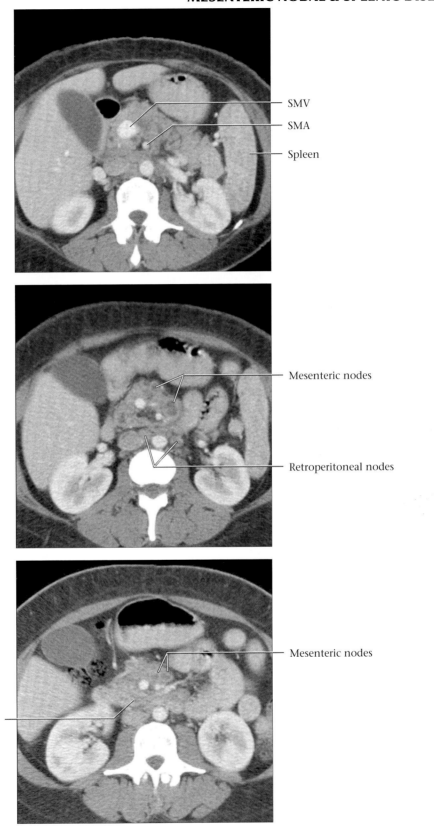

SMV

SMA

Spleen

Mesenteric nodes

Retroperitoneal nodes

Mesenteric nodes

Duodenum

(Top) First of three axial CT sections in another young man with AIDS and disseminated mycobacterium avium-complex shows splenomegaly with innumerable tiny low density lesions, due to infectious granulomas. The duodenal and jejunal walls and the mesenteric nodes have a similar appearance, also due to mycobacterial infection. The nodes almost surround the superior mesenteric vessels. **(Middle)** Mesenteric and retroperitoneal nodes are enlarged with central necrosis or caseation, indicated by the low density centers and contrast-enhancing rims, characteristic of mycobacterial infection. **(Bottom)** Additional mesenteric nodes are seen ventral to the duodenum and the superior mesenteric trunks.

SMALL INTESTINE

CROHN DISEASE

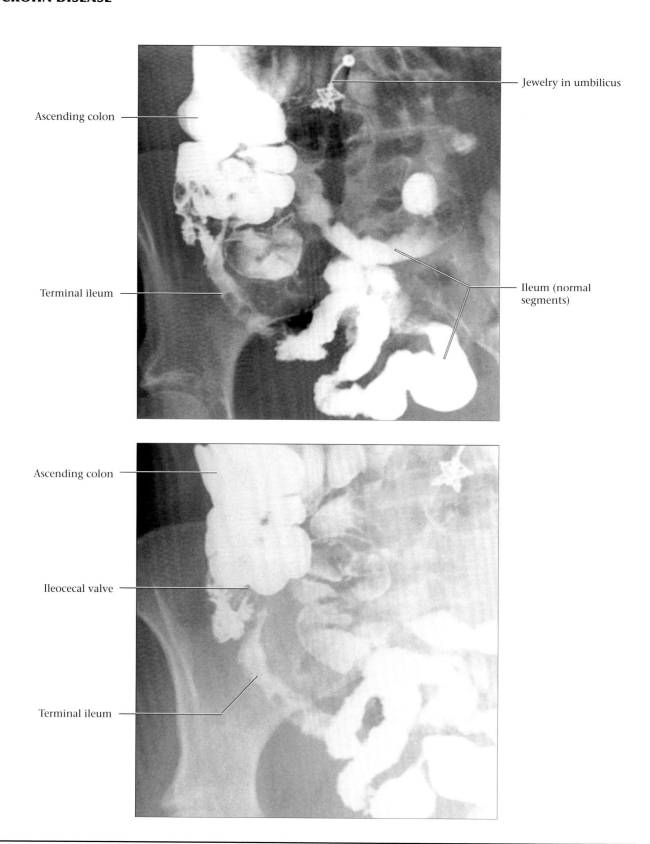

Jewelry in umbilicus

Ascending colon

Ileum (normal segments)

Terminal ileum

Ascending colon

Ileocecal valve

Terminal ileum

(Top) First of five images of a young woman with Crohn disease. First image from a barium small bowel follow through shows irregular nodular thickening of the wall of the terminal ileum. **(Bottom)** The lumen of the terminal ileum is narrowed and the wall is irregularly thickened. This abnormal segment of bowel appears straightened and stands away from other segments of bowel, reflecting bowel wall thickening and infiltration of the mesenteric fat to this segment of bowel. The terminal ileum is usually the first portion of bowel to be inflamed in patients with Crohn disease, a common inflammatory bowel condition of uncertain etiology. The clinical and radiographic features in this case are typical of this disease.

SMALL INTESTINE

CROHN DISEASE

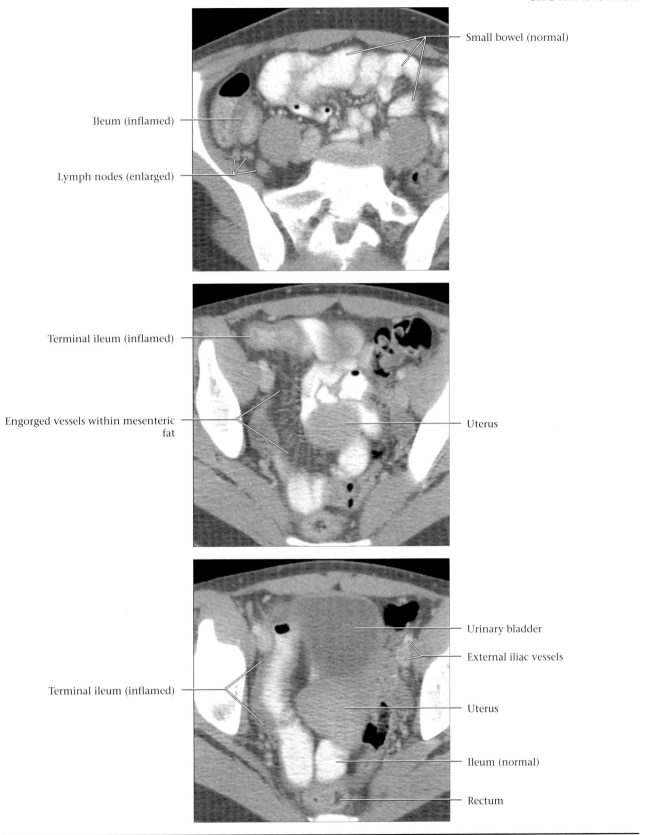

Small bowel (normal)

Ileum (inflamed)

Lymph nodes (enlarged)

Terminal ileum (inflamed)

Engorged vessels within mesenteric fat

Uterus

Terminal ileum (inflamed)

Urinary bladder

External iliac vessels

Uterus

Ileum (normal)

Rectum

(Top) Axial CT section of the same young woman as previous 2 images shows enlarged lymph nodes near the terminal ileum, which has a thickened wall. Compare with the normal, and almost imperceptible wall of other, uninvolved segments of bowel. **(Middle)** Note the thickened wall of the terminal ileum and the thickened segment of mesenteric fat with engorged blood vessels, indicating hyperemia (increased blood flow) of the inflamed segment of bowel. **(Bottom)** The inflamed terminal ileum that is supplied by the engorged blood vessels is best seen on this more caudal section. Note the thickened wall of the inflamed segment as opposed to that of the adjacent, uninvolved ileum.

SMALL INTESTINE

CROHN DISEASE WITH MESENTERIC SCARRING

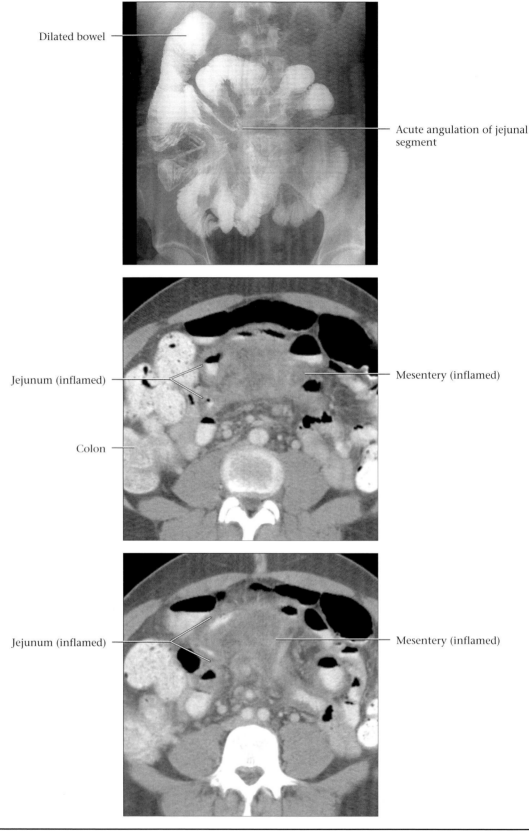

Dilated bowel

Acute angulation of jejunal segment

Jejunum (inflamed)

Mesentery (inflamed)

Colon

Jejunum (inflamed)

Mesentery (inflamed)

(Top) First of six images of a patient with Crohn disease. First image from a barium small bowel follow through shows a peculiar "stellate" arrangement of small bowel segments, with acute angulation of loops. Some portions of the bowel lumen are narrowed while others are dilated, indicating some degree of bowel obstruction. (Middle) Axial CT section shows extensive infiltration of the mesenteric fat, replacing its normal homogeneous fat density. (Bottom) The small bowel mesentery is markedly thickened and inflamed as are the adjacent segments of small bowel, including much of the jejunum.

SMALL INTESTINE

CROHN DISEASE WITH MESENTERIC SCARRING

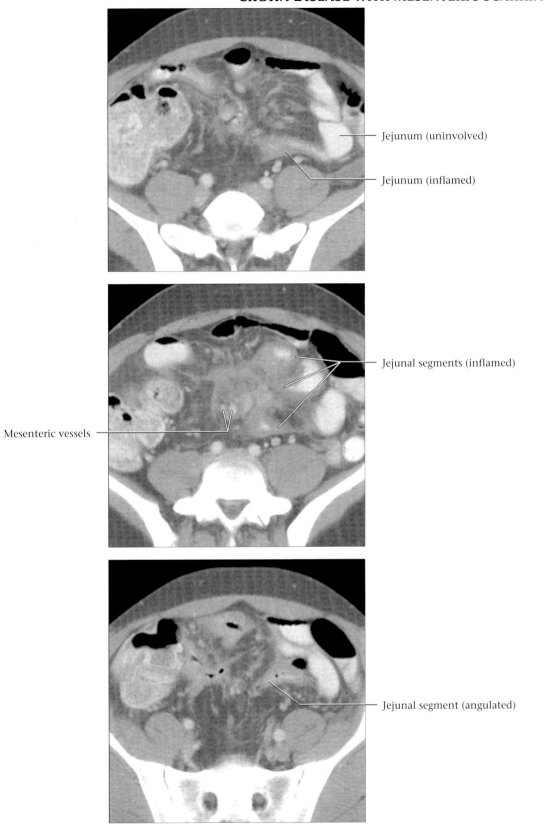

(Top) The mesenteric fat is thickened ("proliferated"), a characteristic feature of chronic inflammatory conditions, such as Crohn disease. (Middle) Note the thick walls and distorted lumen of the involved jejunal segments and the thickened, inflamed mesentery. (Bottom) A more caudal section shows an acutely angulated segment of jejunum, corresponding with similar findings on the small bowel follow through exam.

SMALL INTESTINE

BOWEL ISCHEMIA, SMA STENOSIS

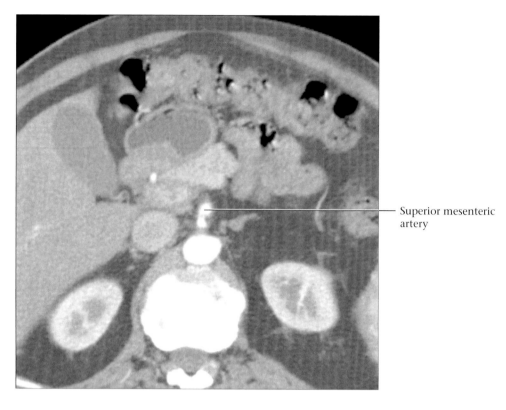

Superior mesenteric
artery

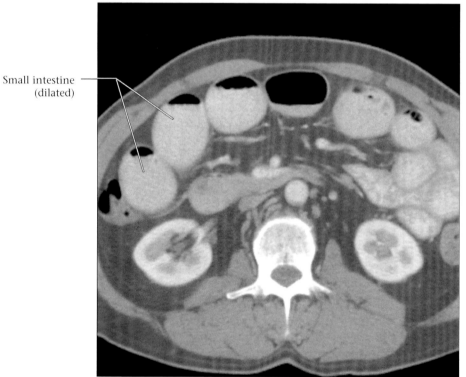

Small intestine
(dilated)

(Top) First of seven images of an elderly patient with chronic abdominal pain, worse after eating. This axial CT section shows marked narrowing at the origin of the superior mesenteric artery due to atherosclerosis. **(Bottom)** A more caudal section shows multiple dilated segments of small bowel, especially ileum.

SMALL INTESTINE

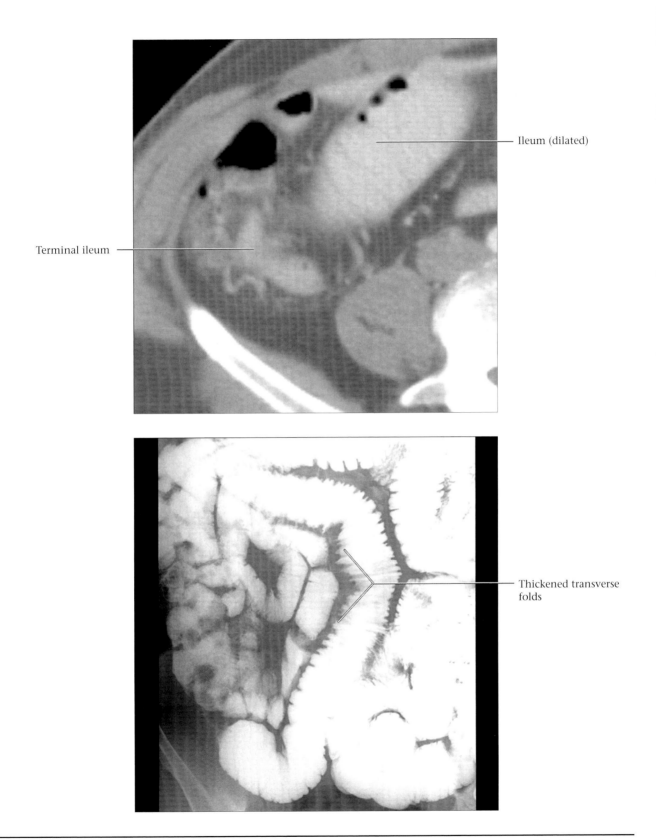

Ileum (dilated)

Terminal ileum

Thickened transverse folds

(Top) The lumen of the terminal ileum is normal or slightly narrowed, while that of more proximal ileal loops is dilated. Findings suggested a functional obstruction of the distal small intestine, but the etiology was unclear at this point. **(Bottom)** Image from a barium small bowel follow through confirms dilation of proximal and mid small bowel, with a transition to collapsed distal bowel. Also evident is thickening of the transverse folds of some of the dilated segments of ileum, indicating some form of injury to the bowel wall causing submucosal swelling.

SMALL INTESTINE

BOWEL ISCHEMIA, SMA STENOSIS

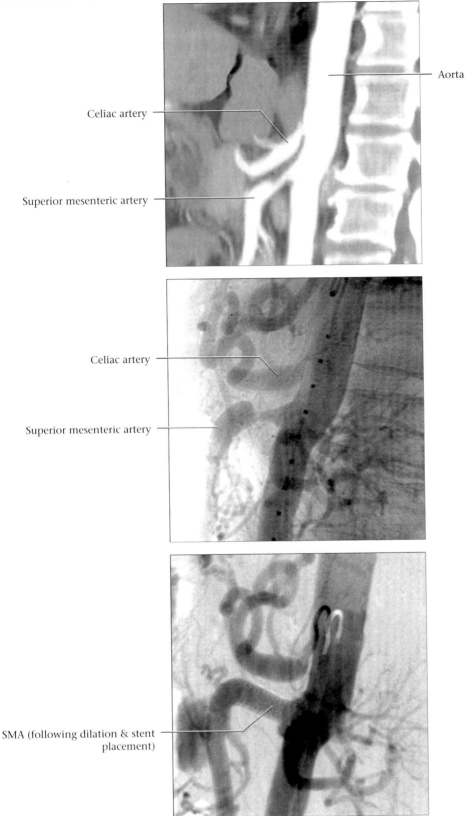

Aorta

Celiac artery

Superior mesenteric artery

Celiac artery

Superior mesenteric artery

SMA (following dilation & stent placement)

(Top) A sagittal reformation of the CT scan shows marked narrowing of the base of the superior mesenteric artery, and moderate narrowing of the celiac artery. (Middle) A lateral view of a catheter angiogram confirms significant atherosclerotic narrowing of the origins of the celiac and superior mesenteric arteries. Balloon dilation of the SMA was performed, followed by placement of a metallic stent to maintain vessel patency. (Bottom) A repeat angiogram in the lateral projection shows the markedly increased diameter of the SMA following dilation and stent placement. The patient's symptoms were attributed to "intestinal angina" and resolved following angioplasty of the SMA.

SMALL INTESTINE

INFARCTION, WITH PNEUMATOSIS

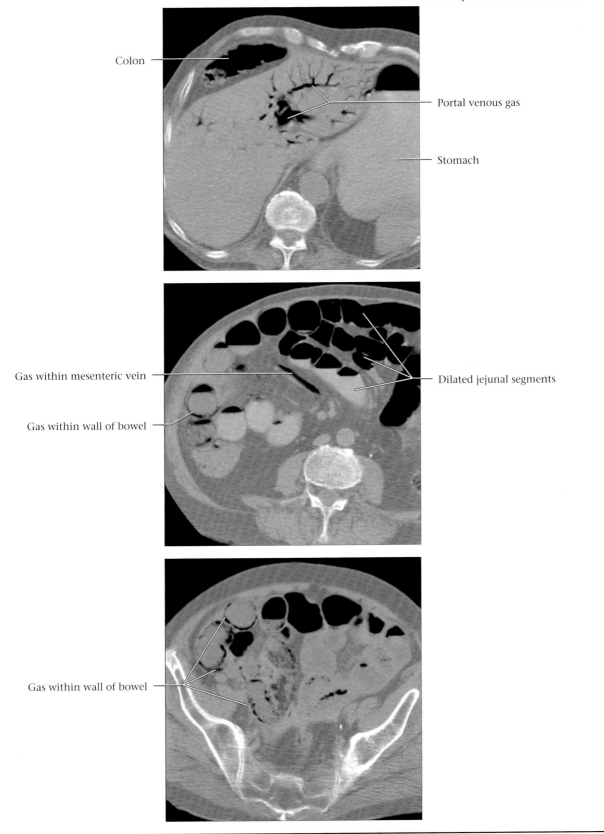

Colon — Portal venous gas — Stomach

Gas within mesenteric vein — Dilated jejunal segments

Gas within wall of bowel

Gas within wall of bowel

(Top) First of three axial CT sections in an elderly patient with severe abdominal pain and hypotension shows extensive gas within the intrahepatic portal vein branches. Portal venous gas is distinguished from biliary gas, as the former flows to the periphery of the liver, while biliary gas collects more centrally as it flows toward the duodenal papilla. (Middle) More caudal section shows gas within the wall of dilated segments of ileum in the right lower quadrant. The jejunum is dilated, but its wall is normal. Gas is present in the mesenteric vein draining the ileal segment with the pneumatosis (intramural gas). (Bottom) More caudal section shows ileal segments with pneumatosis, due to bowel infarction. The ischemic mucosa has broken down, allowing gas from the bowel lumen to enter the submucosal layer. This gas, in turn, enters the mesenteric & portal veins.

SMALL INTESTINE

SMALL INTESTINE INFARCTION, VENOUS THROMBOSIS

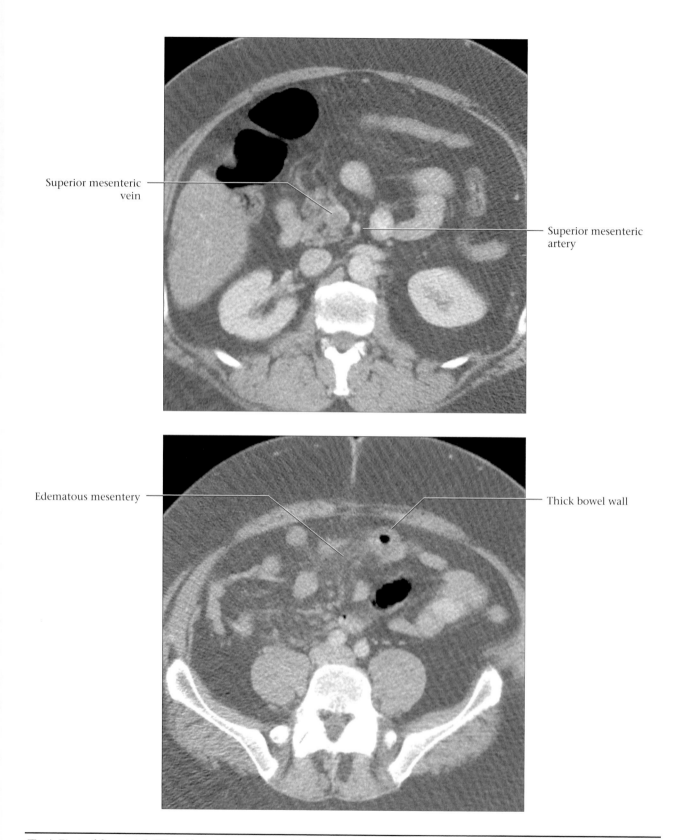

Superior mesenteric vein

Superior mesenteric artery

Edematous mesentery

Thick bowel wall

(Top) First of five axial CT sections in a patient with severe abdominal pain shows a normal caliber and uniformly enhancing lumen of the superior mesenteric artery, while the lumen of the SMV is distended and partly occluded by (non-enhancing) clot. (Bottom) More caudal section shows diffuse edema of the mesentery and a thick-walled segment of small bowel, indicative of some sort of acute injury (in this case, acute ischemia).

SMALL INTESTINE

SMALL INTESTINE INFARCTION, VENOUS THROMBOSIS

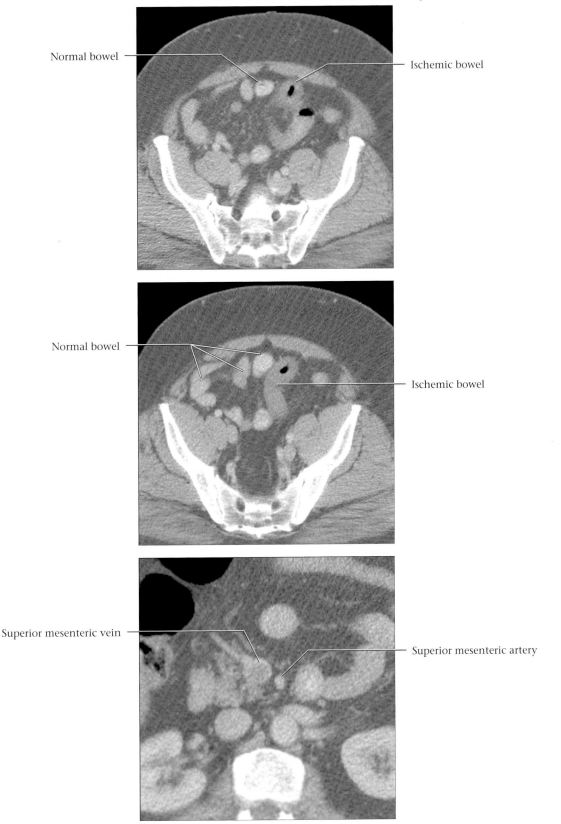

(Top) More caudal CT section shows focal bowel wall thickening. Compare with the almost imperceptible wall thickness of normal bowel. **(Middle)** Note the thickening of the wall of the jejunal segment that was ischemic due to thrombosis of its superior mesenteric venous tributary. **(Bottom)** Magnified view of axial CT section shows thrombosis (nonenhancement) of this portion of the superior mesenteric vein, near the site of entry of the jejunal tributaries. At surgery, a segment of infarcted jejunum was resected and thrombus was removed from the lumen of the SMV. The patient was subsequently confirmed to have a hypercoagulable condition that predisposed him to spontaneous venous thromboses.

SMALL INTESTINE

SMALL INTESTINE OBSTRUCTION

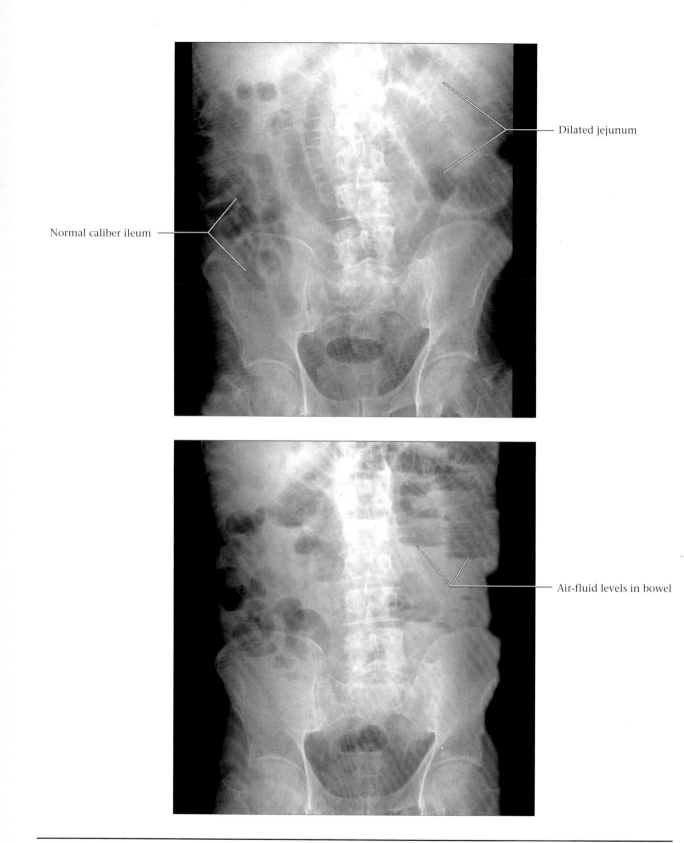

Dilated jejunum

Normal caliber ileum

Air-fluid levels in bowel

(Top) First of four images of a patient with abdominal distention and crampy pain. A supine image of the abdomen shows dilated segments of proximal small bowel (jejunum) in the left upper quadrant. Distal small bowel and colon are of normal caliber. (Bottom) An upright image demonstrates multiple air-fluid levels within the dilated segments of bowel, a characteristic feature of small bowel obstruction.

SMALL INTESTINE

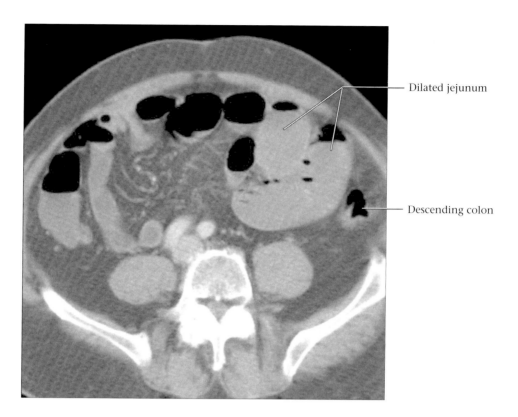

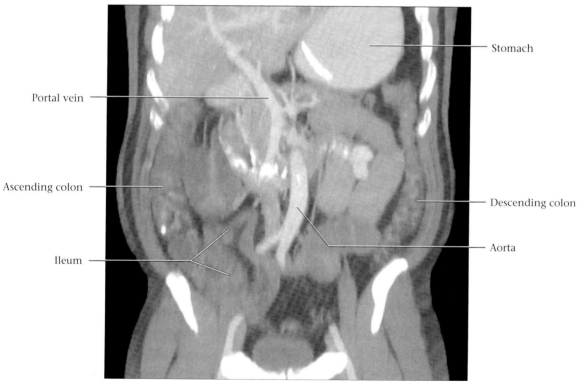

(Top) Axial CT section (same patient as previous 2 images) shows dilated jejunum, with air-fluid levels, and "collapsed", normal caliber ileum and colon. **(Bottom)** Coronal reformation of the CT scan shows the dilated jejunum and the collapsed ileum and colon, which are beyond the point of obstruction. An adhesive band was found at surgery to be the cause of the bowel obstruction.

SMALL INTESTINE

PLAIN IMAGE, MALROTATION

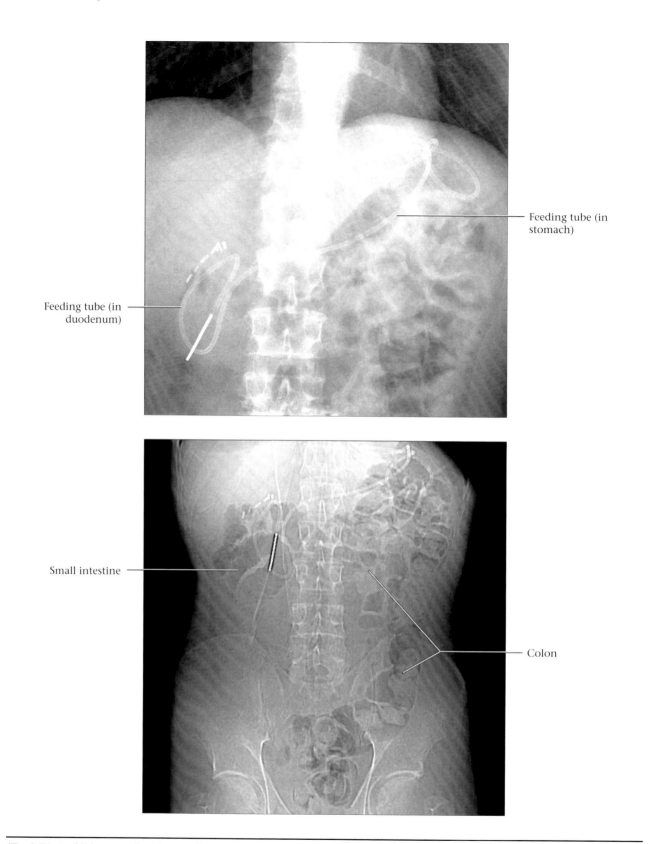

Feeding tube (in stomach)

Feeding tube (in duodenum)

Small intestine

Colon

(Top) First of 5 images showing malrotation. Frontal radiograph shows a feeding tube which has been advanced through the nose and stomach. The course of the tube within the duodenum shows that the duodenum is "looped" upon itself to the right of midline, instead of crossing the midline, as the third portion of the duodenum does normally. **(Bottom)** Frontal radiograph shows the duodenum and small bowel (marked by the feeding tube and gas) in the right upper quadrant. Gas and stool within the colon suggests that all of the colon lies to the left of midline.

SMALL INTESTINE

CT, MALROTATION

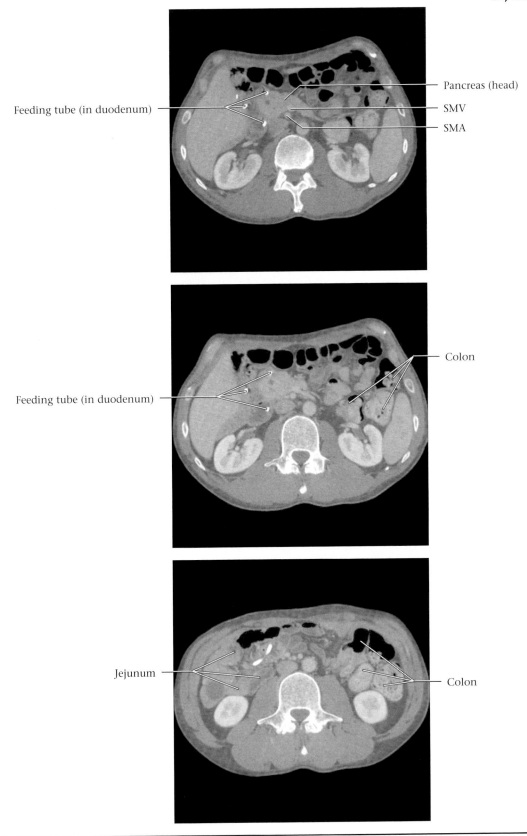

Pancreas (head)

Feeding tube (in duodenum)

SMV

SMA

Feeding tube (in duodenum)

Colon

Jejunum

Colon

(Top) Axial CT section (same patient as previous 3 images) shows the radiopaque feeding tube coiled within the duodenum, all of which lies to the right of midline. The SMV lies ventral and to the left of the SMA, which is opposite to its usual relation. **(Middle)** All four portions of the duodenum lie to the right of midline, as marked by the feeding tube. The colon lies to the left of midline. **(Bottom)** All of the jejunum lies to the right of midline, and all of the colon lies to the left, characteristic of midgut malrotation (nonrotation). At this axial level, the third portion of the duodenum would normally cross the midline between the aorta and the superior mesenteric vessels.

SMALL INTESTINE

BARIUM STUDY, MALROTATION

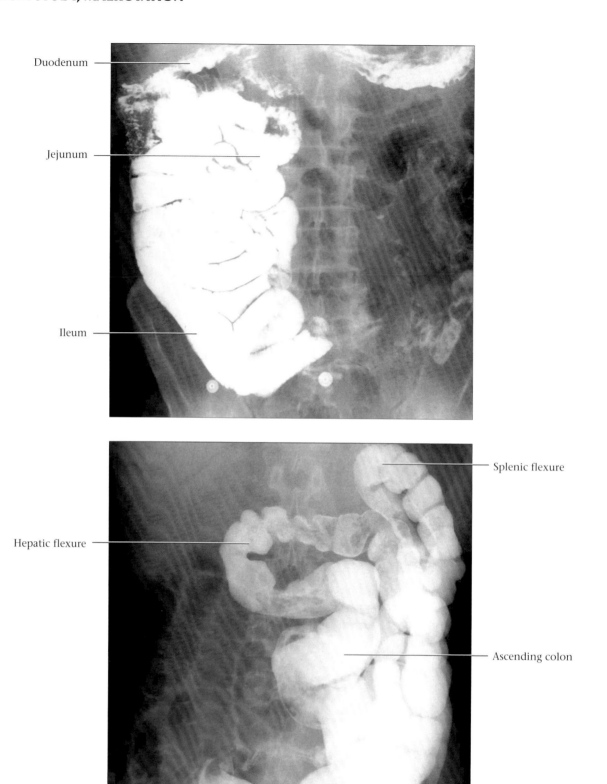

(Top) First of two images from a barium small bowel follow through exam shows essentially all of the small intestine lying to the right of midline. The duodenum never crosses the midline, and the jejunum is not in its usual left upper quadrant location. (Bottom) Delayed frontal image from small bowel study shows all of the colon lying in the left side of the abdomen. The descending and sigmoid colon and rectum, all parts of the embryological hindgut, are in normal position. It is the embryological midgut which has failed to rotate properly on its return from the umbilical cord to the peritoneal cavity, resulting in the abnormal position of the small bowel and right side of colon. This situation can predispose to twisting (volvulus) of the bowel & its blood vessels around an abnormally short mesenteric root with obstruction of the bowel lumen or its vessels.

SMALL INTESTINE

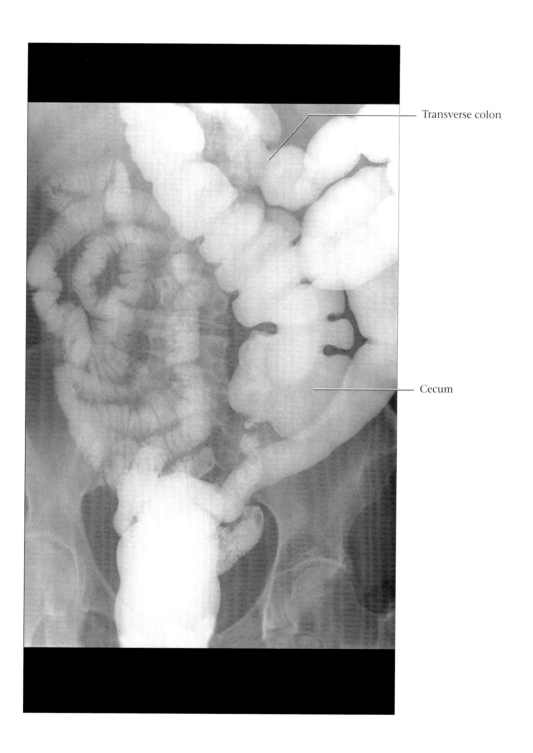

Transverse colon

Cecum

Delayed image from a barium small bowel follow through shows all of the small intestine lying to the right of midline, while all of the colon lies to the left. The embryologic midgut has failed to rotate properly on its return to the abdominal cavity in fetal life, resulting in malrotation of the small intestine and the colon up to the splenic flexure. This subject shows no signs of bowel obstruction or volvulus at the time of this exam.

SMALL INTESTINE

MIDGUT VOLVULUS WITH INFARCTION

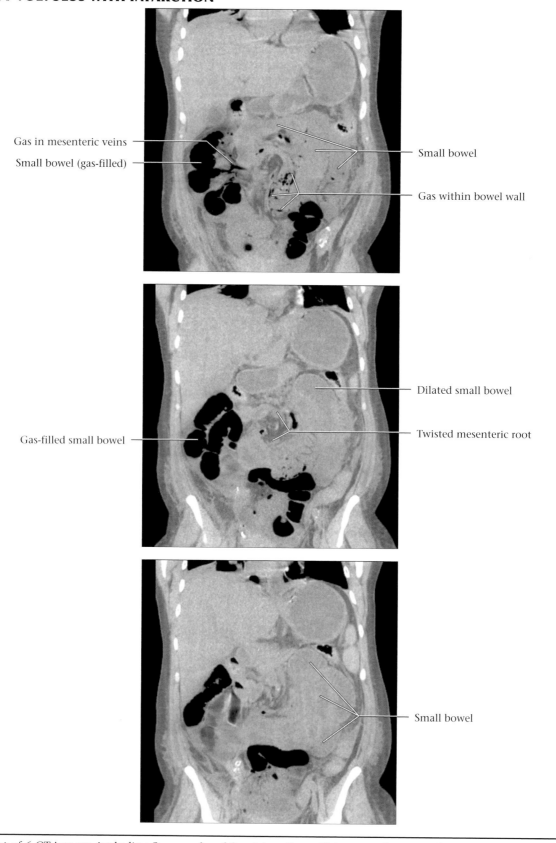

Gas in mesenteric veins

Small bowel (gas-filled)

Small bowel

Gas within bowel wall

Gas-filled small bowel

Dilated small bowel

Twisted mesenteric root

Small bowel

(Top) First of 6 CT images, including 3 coronal and 3 axial sections. This coronal section shows dilated small bowel that is distended with fluid in the left side of the abdomen, while bowel loops in the right side are distended with gas. Branching air density also indicates gas within the intestinal wall and in the mesenteric veins draining the small intestine. Note the "swirled" or twisted appearance of the mesenteric vessels as they converge near the midline; these findings are indicative of midgut volvulus and infarction. (Middle) Coronal section shows the dilated small bowel segments and the twisting of the mesenteric root. (Bottom) Coronal section shows the twisted and distended small bowel segments.

SMALL INTESTINE

MIDGUT VOLVULUS WITH INFARCTION

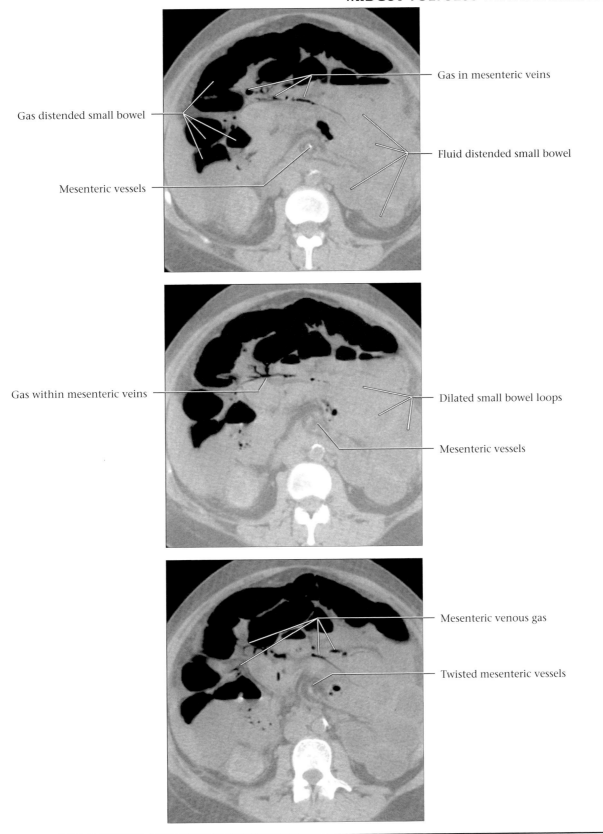

Gas in mesenteric veins

Gas distended small bowel

Fluid distended small bowel

Mesenteric vessels

Gas within mesenteric veins

Dilated small bowel loops

Mesenteric vessels

Mesenteric venous gas

Twisted mesenteric vessels

(Top) Axial CT section shows twisting of the mesenteric vessels, mesenteric venous gas, and small bowel distended with gas or fluid. **(Middle)** Axial section shows distended, thick-walled bowel and mesenteric venous gas, indicative of bowel infarction. The "whirled" (twisted) mesenteric vessels indicate volvulus as the reason for the bowel infarction. **(Bottom)** Axial section shows more of the infarcted bowel and the spiral appearance of the mesenteric root, indicative of volvulus.

SMALL INTESTINE

CONGENITAL DUPLICATION CYST

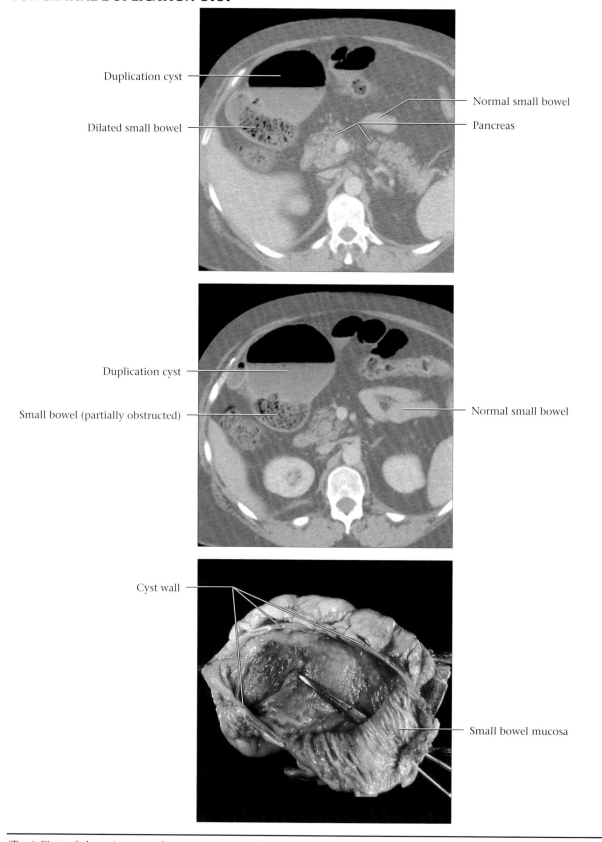

Top image labels: Duplication cyst, Dilated small bowel, Normal small bowel, Pancreas

Middle image labels: Duplication cyst, Small bowel (partially obstructed), Normal small bowel

Bottom image labels: Cyst wall, Small bowel mucosa

(Top) First of three images of a young man with crampy abdominal pain. Axial CT shows a spherical mass with an air-fluid level adjacent to a dilated segment of small bowel that has particulate matter and gas within it, simulating stool, a common feature of small bowel obstruction. (Middle) The cystic mass communicates with the bowel lumen, as shown by its air-fluid level. (Bottom) Surgical specimen photograph shows a probe passing from the small bowel lumen into the cyst, which was lined by intestinal mucosa. Congenital duplications or cysts may occur along the entire length of the alimentary tube. In rare cases, long segments of bowel or colon may be duplicated. These lesions may remain asymptomatic or may become infected or cause bowel obstruction. They may or may not communicate with the lumen of the gut.

MECKEL DIVERTICULUM

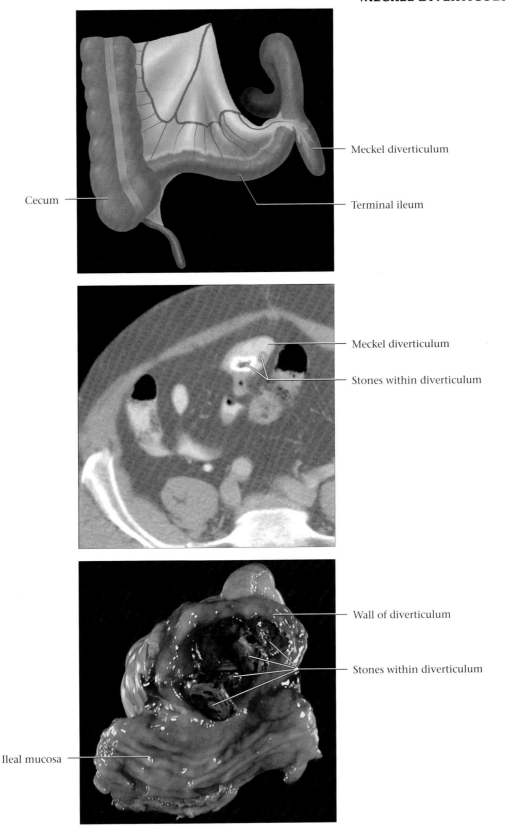

(Top) Graphic labels: Meckel diverticulum, Cecum, Terminal ileum

(Middle) CT labels: Meckel diverticulum, Stones within diverticulum

(Bottom) Photograph labels: Wall of diverticulum, Stones within diverticulum, Ileal mucosa

(Top) First of three images demonstrating a Meckel diverticulum. Graphic shows a blind-ending diverticulum arising from the antimesenteric border of the distal ileum, a characteristic appearance of a Meckel diverticulum. This is a remnant of the embryologic omphalomesenteric or vitelline duct, also known as the yolk stalk, which normally connects the fetal gut to the yolk sac. This connection atrophies and disappears soon after birth in most individuals. **(Middle)** Axial CT section shows a blind-ending sac, or diverticulum, arising from the distal ileum which contains rounded stones or enteroliths. All the remaining bowel was normal in appearance. **(Bottom)** Photograph of the resected specimen shows the opened diverticulum and some of the dark brown stones or enteroliths that had formed within it.

COLON

Gross Anatomy

Overview

- Colon (**large intestine**): Organ responsible for absorption of water from bowel contents (**chyme**) that was not digested and absorbed by small intestine
  - Converts contents into semisolid stool or feces that is stored until defecation occurs

Segments

- **Cecum**: First part of colon, about 7 cm in length
  - Loosely attached to posterior and lateral abdominal wall by **peritoneal (cecal) folds**
  - Receives terminal ileum through **ileocecal valve**
    - Valve lips have variable submucosal fat content usually evident on CT
    - Valve usually prevents reflux of colonic contents into intestine
  - **Appendix** ("vermiform" appendix)
    - Blind intestinal diverticulum 6-15 cm in length
    - Has mesentery (**mesoappendix**)
    - Always arises from tip of cecum but may point and lie in many locations (²/₃ retrocecal)
  - Cecum and appendix supplied by **ileocolic artery** and vein
- **Ascending colon**
  - From cecum (1st semilunar fold at ileocecal valve) to transverse colon
  - Supplied by right colic branch of superior mesenteric artery (SMA) and superior mesenteric vein (SMV) in retroperitoneum
- **Transverse colon**
  - Supplied by middle colic branch of SMA and SMV
  - Vessels, nerves, lymphatics through **transverse mesocolon**
- **Descending colon**
  - Supplied by inferior mesenteric artery (IMA) and inferior mesenteric vein (IMV)
  - Retroperitoneal location
- **Sigmoid colon**
  - Mobile, on long sigmoid mesocolon
  - Supplied by IMA and IMV
  - Quite variable in length, redundancy, location
- **Rectum**
  - Final 15-20 cm of colon; **rectosigmoid junction** at lumbo-sacral level (variable)
  - Lies in extraperitoneal pelvis
  - Has several **rectal folds** (**valves**) analogous to semilunar folds of colon
  - Has continuous layer of longitudinal muscle, rather than taeniae (separate bands of muscle) in colon
  - Has **mesenteric** (superior rectal branches of IMA and IMV) and **systemic vessels** (middle and inferior rectal branches of internal iliac vessels)

Mural (Wall) Anatomy

- Same basic components: Mucosa, submucosa, double layer muscularis, serosa (for intraperitoneal parts) and submucosa (adventitia for extraperitoneal parts)
- Longitudinal muscle layer not continuous (unlike intestine) but separated into taeniae
- Unlike intestine, mucosa of colon not covered with villous projections

- Submucosa contains numerous, discrete **lymphoid follicles** that may be apparent as subtle 3-4 mm nodules on double-contrast barium enema exam
- **Taeniae coli**: Three thickened, flat bands of smooth muscle constituting outer longitudinal layer of smooth muscle
- **Haustra**: Sacculations of colon wall caused by contractions of taeniae, separated by semilunar folds
- **Semilunar folds (plicae semilunares)**
  - Furrows between haustra
  - Consist of mucosa, submucosa and circular muscle; (small bowel folds lack muscle layer)
- **Epiploic (omental) appendages** (or **appendices**)
  - Subserosal pockets of fat extending off colonic surface

Clinical Implications

Clinical Importance

- **Appendicitis**
  - Occlusion of lumen common, leading to appendicitis
  - Initial symptoms are vague periumbilical discomfort due to distention and stretching of wall
    - Localized pain and tenderness in lower quadrant due to inflammation of parietal peritoneum
- **Diverticulosis**
  - All parts of colon except rectum may develop diverticula
    - Most prevalent in sigmoid colon
  - Protrude through weak points in colonic wall where nutrient arteries penetrate muscle coat
  - May perforate (= diverticulitis)
  - Common in Western society with high fat, low fiber diet
- **Epiploic appendagitis**
  - Appendages may twist and infarct
  - Leads to symptoms similar to diverticulitis
- **Colonic volvulus**
  - Sigmoid mesocolon may be long with a narrow base of attachment to posterior abdominal wall
    - Predisposes to volvulus (twisting) of colon that often obstructs lumen and compresses vessels; may lead to ischemia and perforation
  - Cecum and ascending colon may also be on mesentery, also predisposing to volvulus, obstruction and ischemia ("**cecal volvulus**")
- **Rectal carcinoma**
  - Because of systemic and portal venous drainage, may metastasize to systemic sites (lungs, bones, etc.) as well as liver (colon carcinoma almost always metastasizes to liver first)
- **Colonic ischemia** is common, despite frequent anastomoses between branches of SMA and IMA
  - "Watershed" sites (splenic flexure and sigmoid colon) most common sites of ischemia, maybe due to congenital deficiency of vascular anastomoses

COLON

COLON & ITS MESENTERY

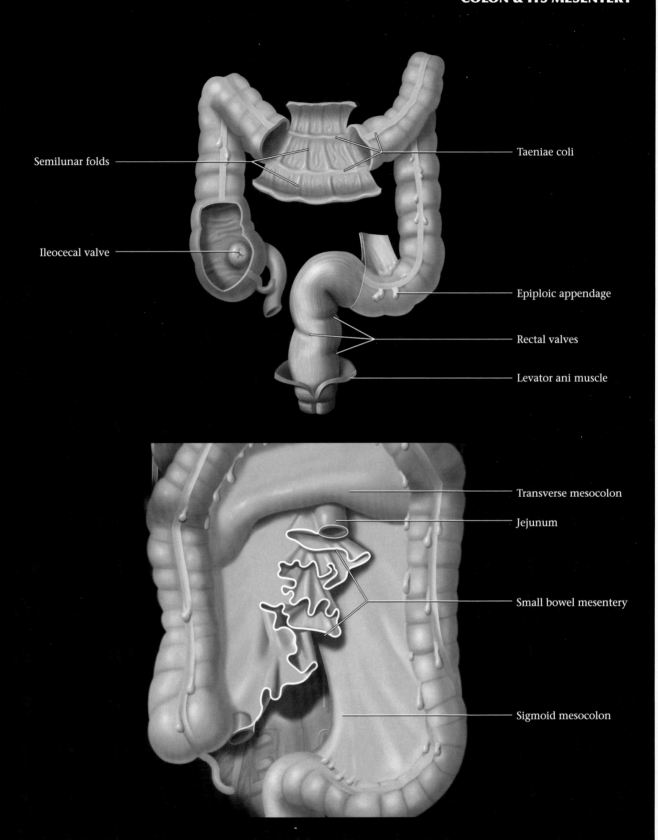

Semilunar folds

Ileocecal valve

Taeniae coli

Epiploic appendage

Rectal valves

Levator ani muscle

Transverse mesocolon

Jejunum

Small bowel mesentery

Sigmoid mesocolon

(Top) Graphic shows surface and mucosal view of the colon. The appendix & ileocecal valve enter the cecum, the first part of the colon, with the ileocecal valve acting as a sphincter to prevent reflux. The semilunar folds lie at right angles to the long axis of the colon and are analogous to the rectal folds (valves). The outpouchings between the folds are the haustra, and the spaces between the transverse folds are wider than in the small intestine. The longitudinal muscle layer of the rectum is continuous, as it is in the small intestine. In the colon, this layer is separated into three thickened flat bands of muscle, called the taeniae coli. (Bottom) The ascending and descending colon are largely retroperitoneal, while the transverse and sigmoid colon have a mesentery (mesocolon). Graphic shows the transverse mesocolon and colon are reflected upward.

COLON

ARTERIES

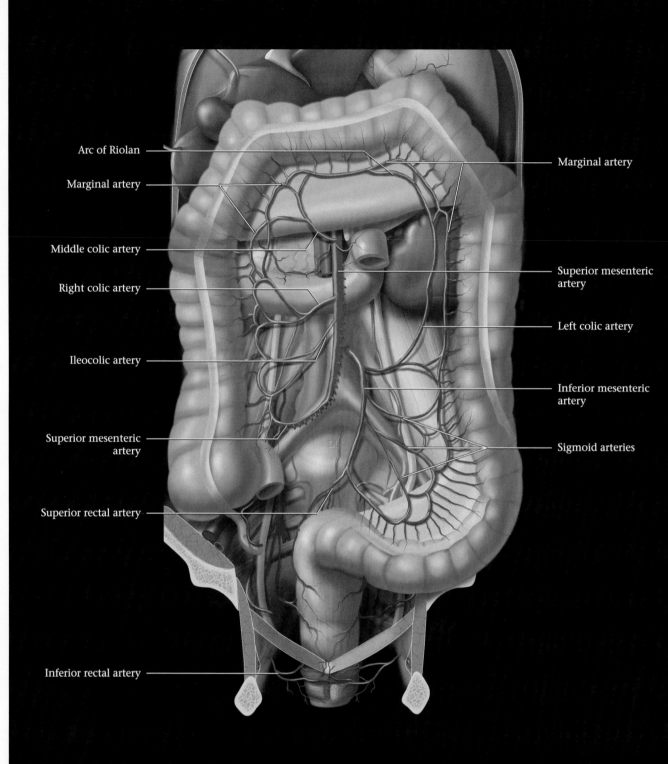

Arc of Riolan

Marginal artery

Middle colic artery

Right colic artery

Ileocolic artery

Superior mesenteric artery

Superior rectal artery

Inferior rectal artery

Marginal artery

Superior mesenteric artery

Left colic artery

Inferior mesenteric artery

Sigmoid arteries

Graphic shows the small intestine has been removed and the transverse colon has been reflected upward. This shows the conventional depiction of the superior mesenteric artery supplying the colon from the appendix through the splenic flexure, and the inferior mesenteric artery supplying the descending colon through the rectum. The cecum is supplied by the ileocolic branch, the ascending colon by the right colic, and the transverse colon by the middle colic artery. These arterial branches are highly variable and all are connected by anastomotic arterial arcades and by the marginal artery (of Drummond) and arc of Riolan which also anastomose with branches of the inferior mesenteric artery that feed the descending & sigmoid colon. The arcades give off the straight arteries (arteriae rectae) to the colonic wall.

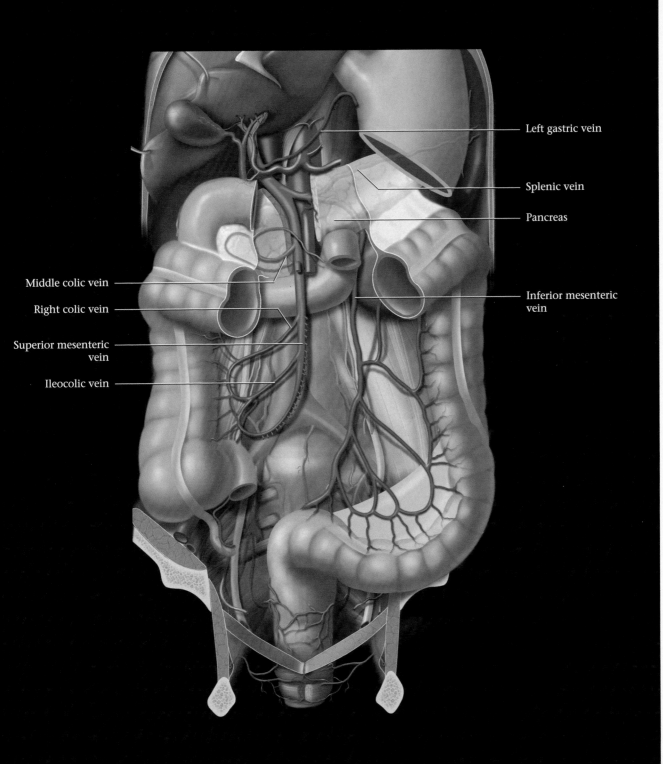

Left gastric vein

Splenic vein

Pancreas

Inferior mesenteric vein

Middle colic vein

Right colic vein

Superior mesenteric vein

Ileocolic vein

The veins that drain the colon generally follow a similar course and have similar names as the arteries that they accompany. The inferior mesenteric vein drains the left colon and empties into the splenic vein, or less commonly, the superior mesenteric or portal vein. The superior and inferior mesenteric veins lie just deep to the neck of the pancreas.

ILEOCECAL REGION

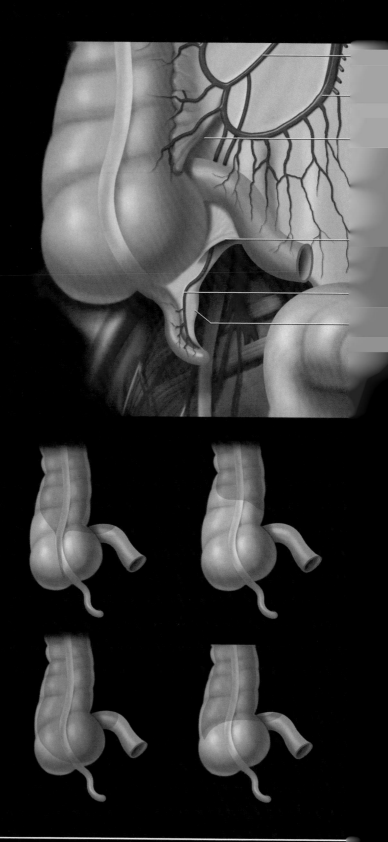

(Top) The cecum is the blind-ending pouch that lies caudal to the ileocecal valve. It is usual[ly]
colon and is easily distended with intestinal gas and the fluid contents that empty into it fro[m]
The cecum usually rests in the right iliac fossa near the external iliac vessels & iliacus muscle[s]
into the pelvis. (Bottom) Graphics show variations of the posterior peritoneal attachments [of]
dark area representing the retroperitoneal attached segment. Note that the cecum is usually [...]
the appendix and terminal ileum, while the ascending colon is usually fixed retroperitoneal[ly]
and often does, lie in a retrocecal space. An especially "free" (unattached) cecum & ascendin[g]

COLON

LATERAL VIEW, RECTOSIGMOID

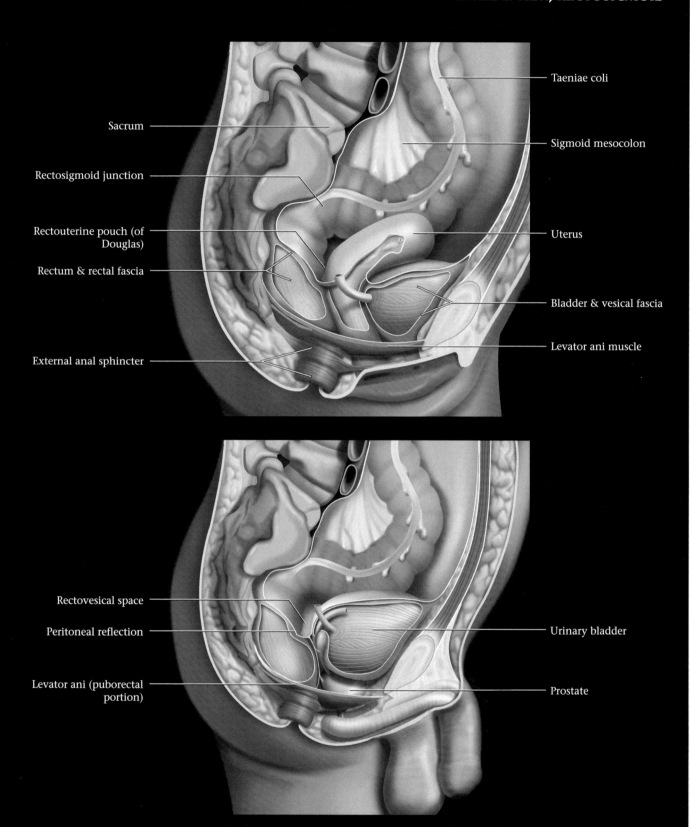

Taeniae coli

Sacrum

Sigmoid mesocolon

Rectosigmoid junction

Rectouterine pouch (of Douglas)

Uterus

Rectum & rectal fascia

Bladder & vesical fascia

Levator ani muscle

External anal sphincter

Rectovesical space

Peritoneal reflection

Urinary bladder

Levator ani (puborectal portion)

Prostate

(Top) The sigmoid colon is on a mesentery while the rectum is retroperitoneal. The anterior surface of the rectum has a peritoneal covering, which extends deep in the pelvis in women, forming the rectouterine pouch (of Douglas) as it is reflected along the posterior surface of the uterus. The rectum is narrowed as it passes through the pelvic diaphragm and then enters the anal canal with three levels of the anal sphincter (deep, superficial & subcutaneous). The rectum has a continuous external longitudinal coat of muscle, unlike the colon with its discontinuous rows of taeniae. **(Bottom)** The rectovesical space (recess) is the most dependent portion of the peritoneal cavity in men. The anterior wall of the rectum has more contiguity with the peritoneal cavity than its lateral or posterior walls.

COLON

RECTAL VEINS & VALVES

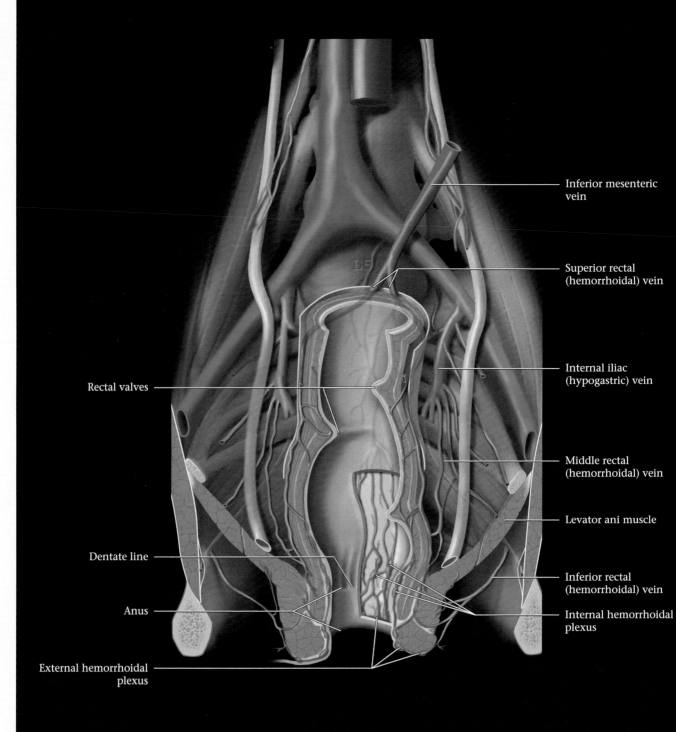

Inferior mesenteric vein

Superior rectal (hemorrhoidal) vein

Internal iliac (hypogastric) vein

Rectal valves

Middle rectal (hemorrhoidal) vein

Levator ani muscle

Dentate line

Inferior rectal (hemorrhoidal) vein

Anus

Internal hemorrhoidal plexus

External hemorrhoidal plexus

The rectal valves (folds) are crescentic infoldings of the wall that include the mucosa, submucosa, & circular muscle layers. The dentate line marks the squamo-columnar boundary. The veins of the rectum return blood to two different systems; the superior rectal to the portal system and the middle & inferior rectal to the inferior vena cava. These anastomose with each other & have important clinical implications (patterns of hematologic spread of rectal cancer; perirectal varices in portal hypertension). The external hemorrhoidal plexus lies in the subcutaneous tissue surrounding the anus, while the internal plexus is in the submucosal tissue of the rectum. These veins have no valves & are easily distended due to portal hypertension or chronic straining at stool, resulting in "hemorrhoids" which are common, painful swellings that may bleed &/or thrombose.

COLON

BARIUM ENEMA, NORMAL COLON

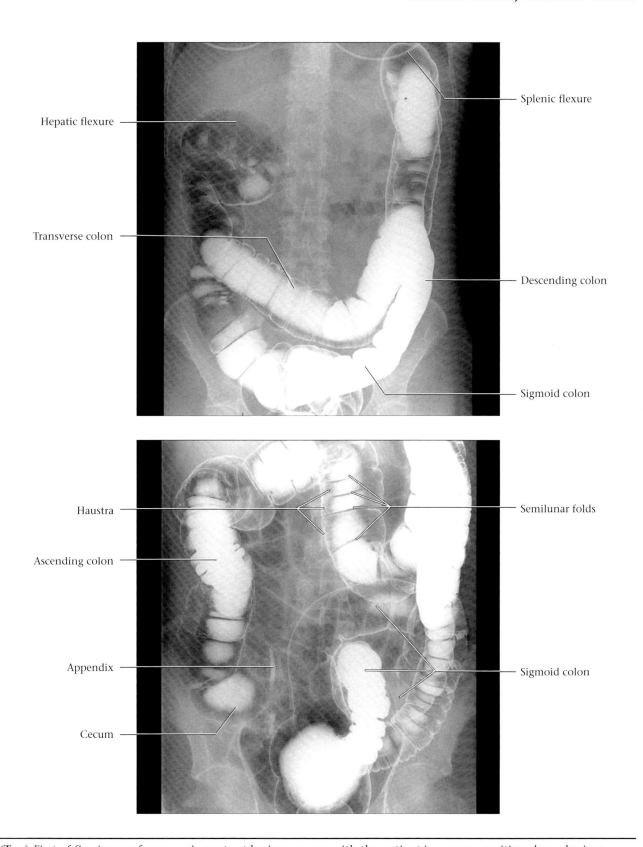

Hepatic flexure

Transverse colon

Splenic flexure

Descending colon

Sigmoid colon

Haustra

Ascending colon

Appendix

Cecum

Semilunar folds

Sigmoid colon

(Top) First of five images from an air-contrast barium enema with the patient in a prone position shows barium pooling in the dependent portions of the transverse and sigmoid colon. Note the "radiologic" hepatic & splenic flexures of the colon, which are the most cephalic portions of the transverse colon. The "anatomic" flexures are the transitions from the retroperitoneal ascending (and descending) colon to the intraperitoneal transverse colon.
(Bottom) In this supine position image, barium pools in the ascending & descending colon, as well as the rectum. Note the transverse semilunar colonic folds, and the haustra, the saccular outpouchings of the lumen between the folds. Colonic transverse folds are spaced farther apart than those in the small intestine, a useful marker in distinguishing among bowel segments on plain radiographs.

COLON

BARIUM ENEMA, NORMAL COLON

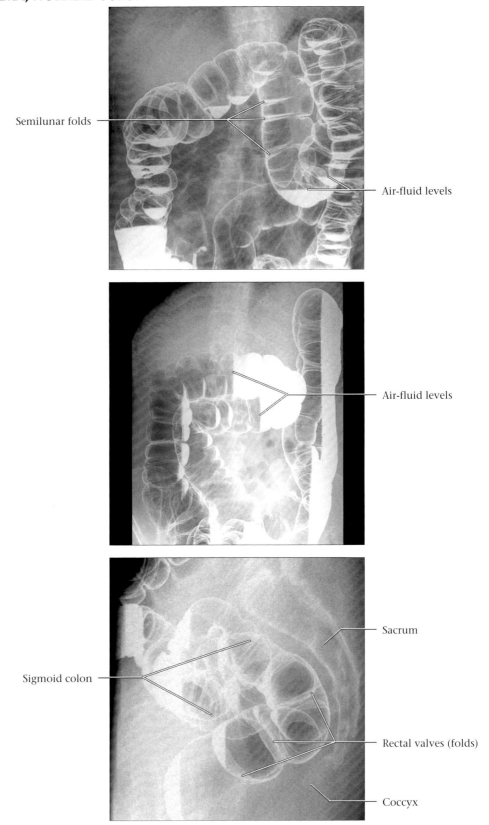

Semilunar folds

Air-fluid levels

Air-fluid levels

Sacrum

Sigmoid colon

Rectal valves (folds)

Coccyx

(Top) Upright position image from an air-contrast barium enema shows barium pooling in dependent haustra and curvatures of the colon. (Middle) A left lateral decubitus image shows barium pooling in the dependent left (descending) colon and within dependent haustra. This patient has a relatively long and curving ("redundant") colon, a common variant of no clinical concern, although this condition makes colonoscopic inspection of the entire colon difficult. (Bottom) A "cross table lateral" image, with the patient in the prone position shows barium pooling along the anterior surface of the rectum & colon. Note the rectal valves (folds), which are analogous to the semilunar folds of the colon.

COLON

NORMAL ILEOCECAL VALVE

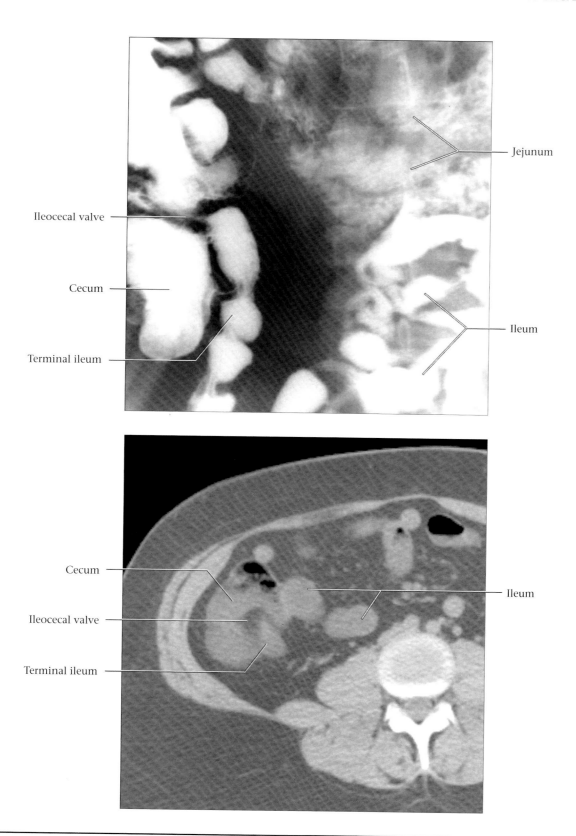

(Top) Barium small bowel follow through image shows a normal ileocecal valve. The "lips" of the ileocecal valve compress the terminal ileum as it enters the cecum. In most patients, this prevents reflux of colonic contents into the small intestine. (Bottom) Axial CT scan from the same patient as the previous image shows normal low attenuation (density) within the "lips" of the ileocecal valve, due to fibro-fatty tissue. This constitutes a useful anatomic marker for identification of the ileocecal valve on CT sections.

COLON

NORMAL APPENDIX

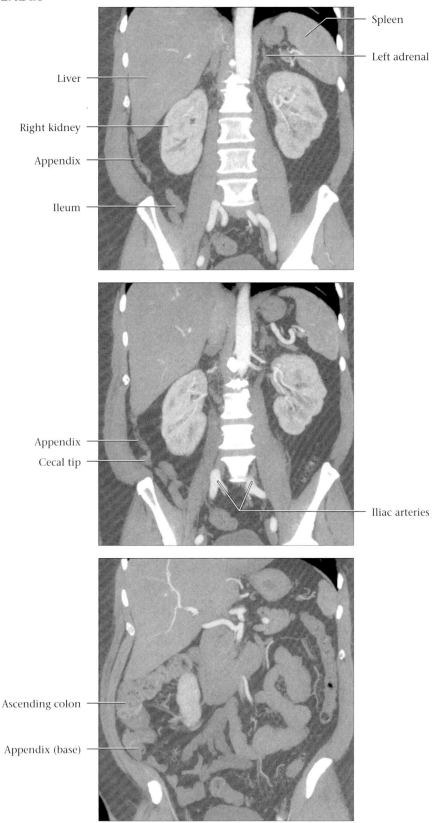

(**Top**) First of six CT sections of a patient with a normal appendix shows the appendix lying in a vertical position with its tip in the right upper quadrant, next to the liver on this coronal section. If this patient were to develop appendicitis, the point of maximum tenderness would not be in the "expected" right lower quadrant site. While the appendix always arises from the tip of the cecum, it may extend on its mesoappendix in any direction, much like the hand of a clock. In this patient, the appendix is pointing to "12 o'clock". (**Middle**) The normal appendix has a small amount of fecal content and gas, with a luminal diameter less than 6 mm and a thin wall. The base of the appendix is seen at the tip of the cecum. (**Bottom**) A more anterior coronal section shows the normal ascending colon and cecum as well as normal small intestine.

COLON

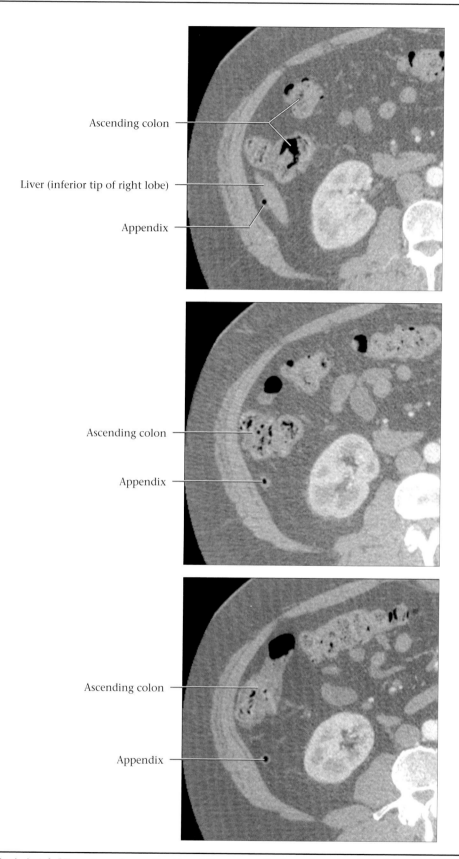

Ascending colon

Liver (inferior tip of right lobe)

Appendix

Ascending colon

Appendix

Ascending colon

Appendix

(Top) Axial CT section shows the tip of the appendix lateral to the right lobe of the liver. (Middle) The appendix commonly lies behind the cecum and ascending colon, as in this subject. The appendix may be intra- or retroperitoneal. (Bottom) Note the thin wall and gas content of the appendix, as well as the homogeneous, noninflamed appearance of the periappendiceal fat planes.

COLON

SUPERIOR MESENTERIC VESSELS

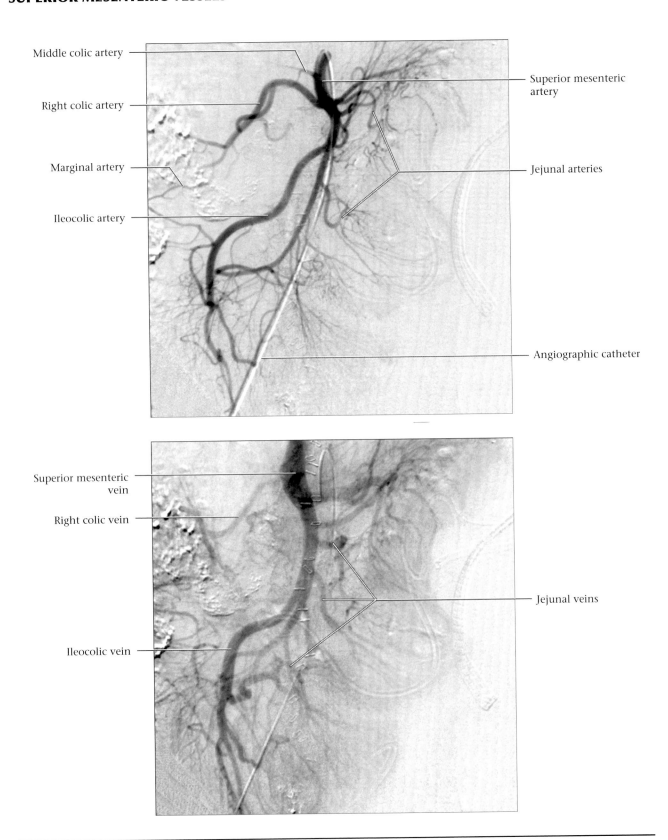

Top image labels:
- Middle colic artery
- Right colic artery
- Marginal artery
- Ileocolic artery
- Superior mesenteric artery
- Jejunal arteries
- Angiographic catheter

Bottom image labels:
- Superior mesenteric vein
- Right colic vein
- Ileocolic vein
- Jejunal veins

(Top) First of two images from a catheter injection of the superior mesenteric artery shows the jejunal arteries arising from the left or convex side of the SMA and the colic branches from the right side. The middle colic is the first colonic branch of the SMA and supplies the transverse colon. The ascending colon is supplied by the right colic, and the cecum, appendix & ileum by the ileocolic artery. There are many variations of this pattern and multiple anastomoses between colonic arteries, most notably through the marginal artery which connects branches of all colonic arteries. **(Bottom)** Venous phase of the angiogram shows opacification of the major branches of the SMV. These follow the same course and have similar names as the major arteries. The SMV usually joins with the splenic vein just behind the neck of the pancreas to form the portal vein.

INFERIOR MESENTERIC VESSELS

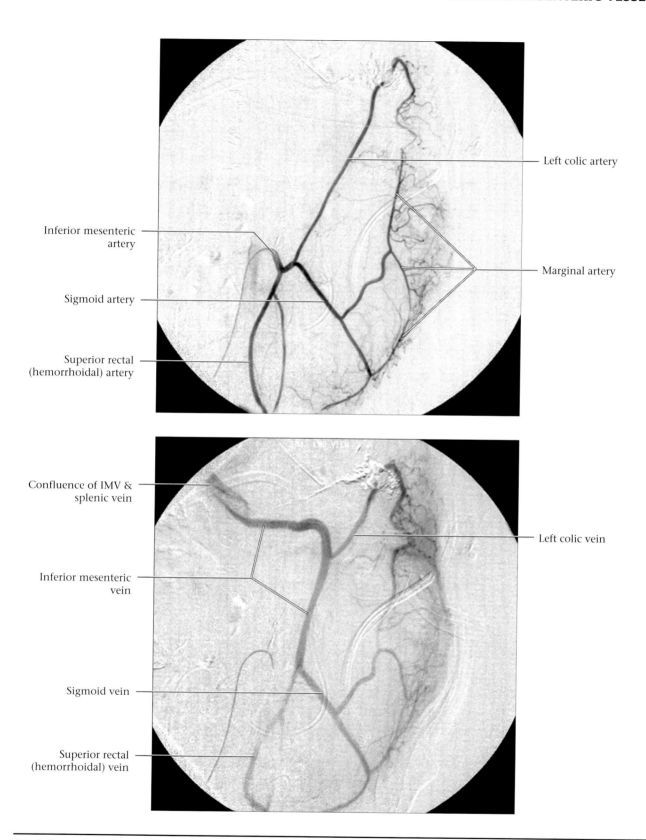

Left colic artery

Inferior mesenteric artery

Marginal artery

Sigmoid artery

Superior rectal (hemorrhoidal) artery

Confluence of IMV & splenic vein

Left colic vein

Inferior mesenteric vein

Sigmoid vein

Superior rectal (hemorrhoidal) vein

(Top) First of two images from a catheter injection of the inferior mesenteric artery shows its major branches, including the left colic (to the descending colon), sigmoid and rectal arteries. The marginal artery parallels the course of the entire colon, gives rise to the terminal straight branches, and forms an important pathway for collateral flow to segments of the colon. The marginal artery connects branches of the SMA and IMA and these collateral vessels may be sufficient to maintain colonic viability even with complete occlusion of the origin of the IMA. The distribution of the SMA and IMA overlap in the "watershed" region of the splenic flexure. In the setting of shock or diminished cardiac output, this region is prone to ischemic injury. **(Bottom)** A venous phase image from the inferior mesenteric angiogram shows the major tributaries of the IMV.

COLON

MESENTERY OUTLINED BY ASCITES

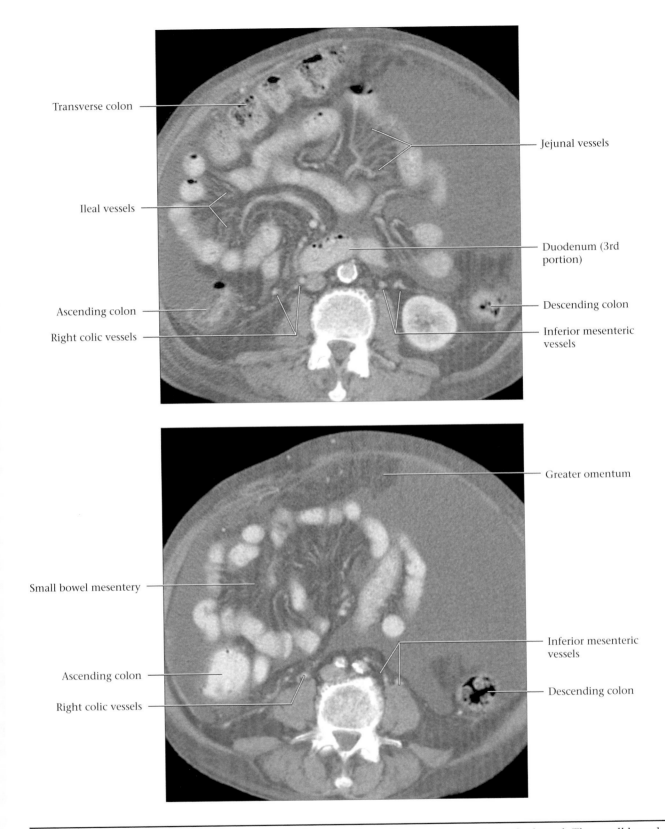

(Top) First of five axial CT sections in a patient with ascites shows the vascular supply to the bowel. The small bowel and transverse colon receive their supply through the mesentery & transverse mesocolon, respectively, and these are highlighted by mesenteric fat and separated by ascites in this subject. The ascending & descending colon are retroperitoneal as are their vessels. The origin of the IMA is seen on this section, arising from the distal aorta just caudal and dorsal to the 3rd portion of the duodenum. **(Bottom)** This section clearly shows the distinction between the intra- and retroperitoneal bowel segments and their blood supplies.

COLON

MESENTERY OUTLINES BY ASCITES

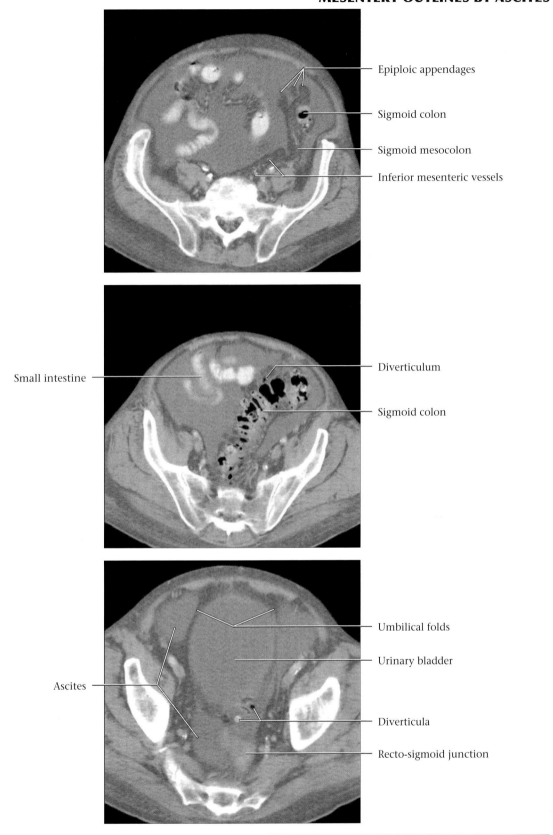

(Top) More caudal section shows the sigmoid colon on its mesocolon which carries the sigmoid branches of the inferior mesenteric vessels. Note the normal epiploic appendages, vestigial fatty tags on the antimesenteric surface of the colon. **(Middle)** The sigmoid colon is mobile on its mesocolon and is surrounded by ascites in this subject. One of many diverticula is identified. **(Bottom)** The recto-sigmoid junction marks the transition from the intraperitoneal sigmoid colon to the extraperitoneal rectum. Diverticula potentially affect all portions of the colon, especially the sigmoid, but spare the rectum.

COLON

INFERIOR MESENTERIC VESSELS, ASCITES

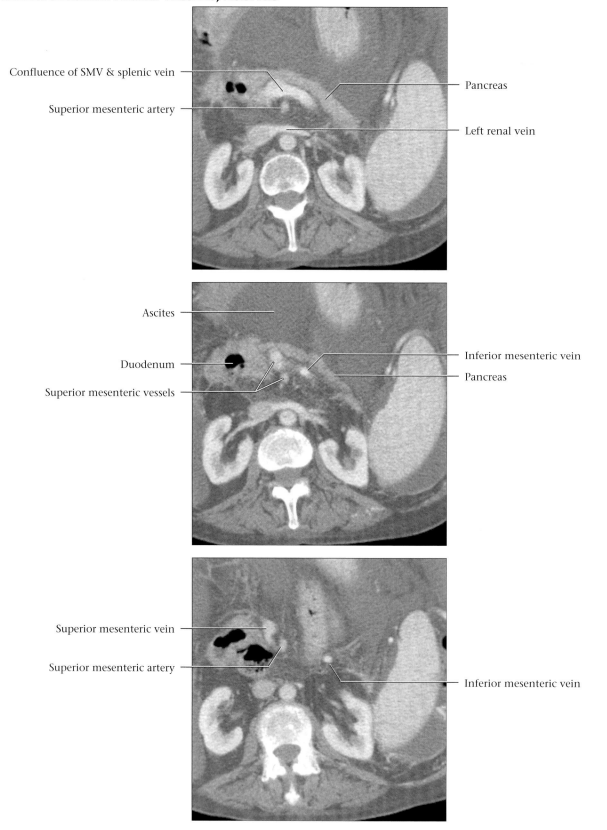

(Top) First of six axial CT sections in a patient with ascites shows the confluence of the splenic and superior mesenteric veins behind the neck of the pancreas, forming the portal vein. (Middle) A more caudal section shows the confluence of the inferior mesenteric and splenic veins behind the body of the pancreas. (Bottom) The inferior mesenteric vein has a cephalo-caudal course and small size, making it difficult to identify on many axial CT studies.

COLON

INFERIOR MESENTERIC VESSELS, ASCITES

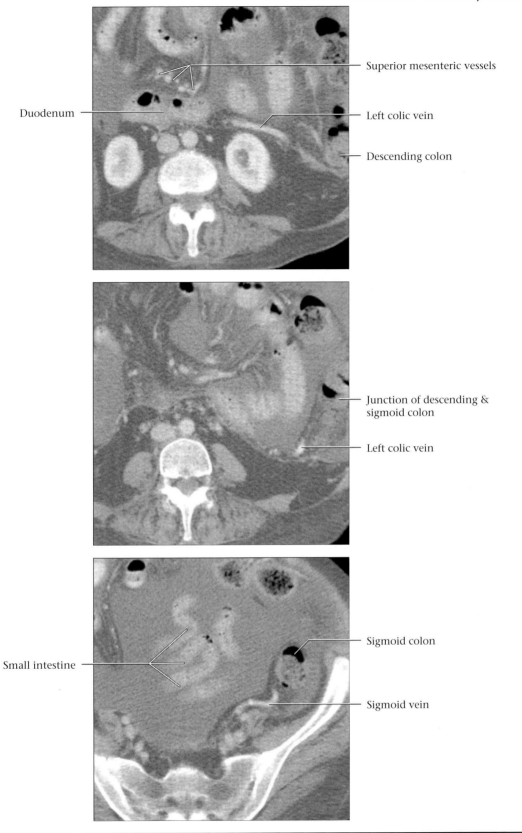

Superior mesenteric vessels

Duodenum

Left colic vein

Descending colon

Junction of descending & sigmoid colon

Left colic vein

Small intestine

Sigmoid colon

Sigmoid vein

(Top) A more caudal section shows the left colic vein draining the descending colon. **(Middle)** The left colic vein joins with tributaries from the sigmoid colon. **(Bottom)** The sigmoid colon and its vessels are seen within the sigmoid mesocolon. Veins are generally larger in caliber and less tortuous than arteries.

COLON

INFERIOR MESENTERIC VESSELS, ASCITES

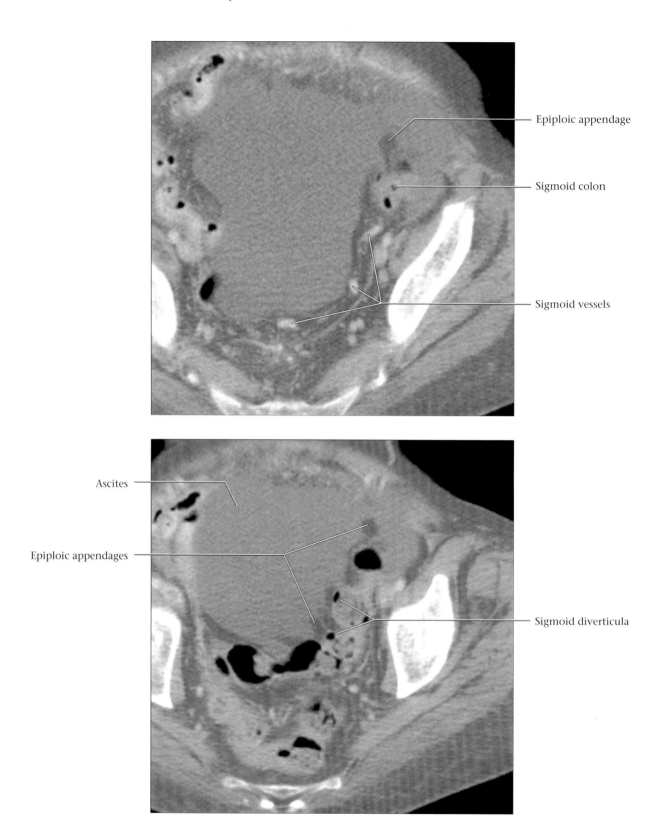

(Top) First of two axial CT sections in a patient with ascites shows the sigmoid colon and its mesocolon which carries the vessels to & from the colon. Note the epiploic appendages, fatty tags on the antimesenteric border that are especially prominent in the sigmoid colon. These are normal anatomic features that are made more evident by the presence of ascites. (Bottom) Another common, though abnormal, feature of the sigmoid colon is the presence of diverticula, which are outpouchings of the mucosa & submucosa through the muscle layers of the colonic wall.

NORMAL EPIPLOIC APPENDAGES

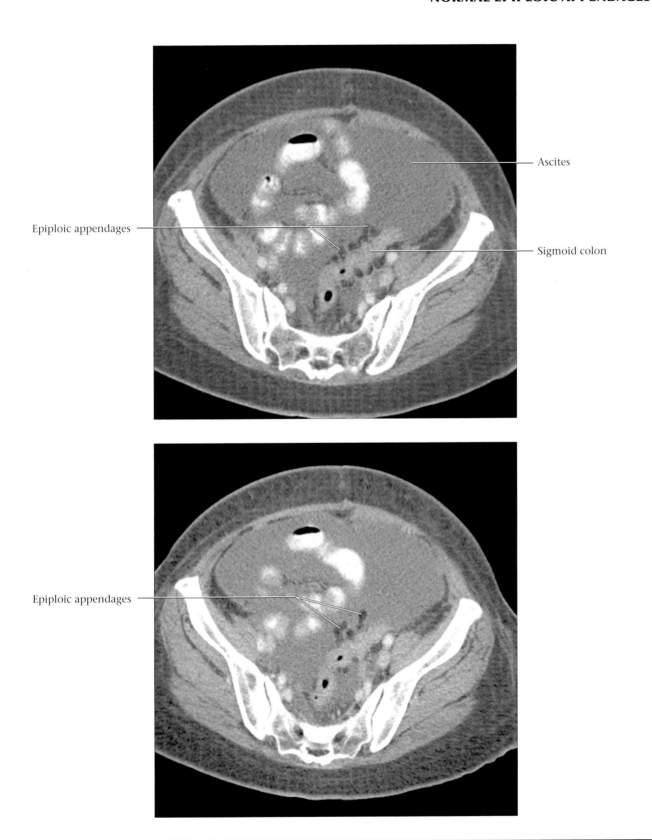

Ascites

Epiploic appendages

Sigmoid colon

Epiploic appendages

(Top) First of two axial CT sections in a patient with ascites shows multiple fat-density epiploic appendages arising from the wall of the sigmoid colon. These are present in nearly all individuals, but are usually not evident on cross-sectional imaging because the fat-density appendages are indistinguishable from the mesenteric & omental fat that normally abut the colon. **(Bottom)** The epiploic appendages can be quite elongated, as in this subject, and may twist and infarct, leading to localized pain and tenderness, symptoms that mimic those of diverticulitis.

COLON

ACUTE APPENDICITIS

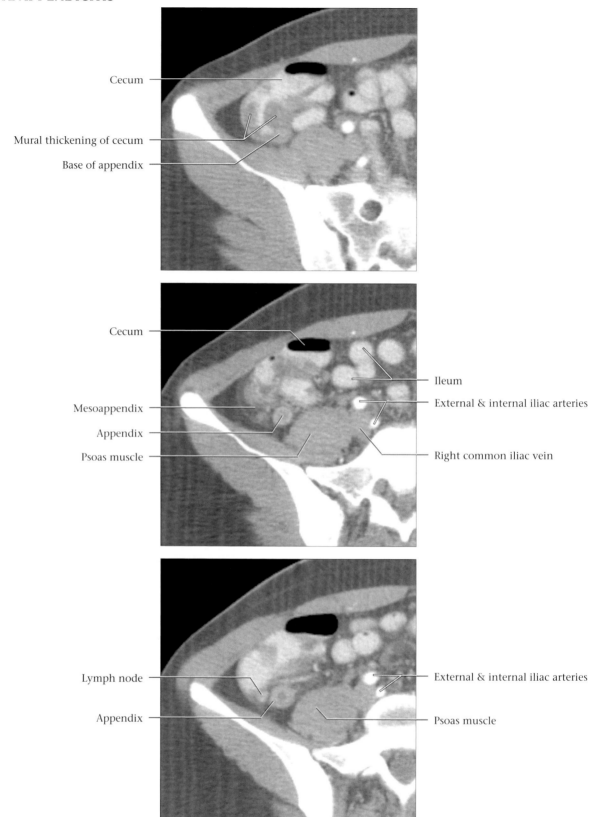

Cecum

Mural thickening of cecum

Base of appendix

Cecum

Mesoappendix

Appendix

Psoas muscle

Ileum

External & internal iliac arteries

Right common iliac vein

Lymph node

Appendix

External & internal iliac arteries

Psoas muscle

(Top) First of five CT sections of a young man with acute appendicitis shows mural thickening of the wall of the cecum at the base of the appendix. (Middle) More caudal section shows normal distal ileum opacified by enteric contrast material. Arteries are densely opacified by IV contrast material, while the veins have not yet become opacified. Vascular and enteric contrast material aid in distinguishing normal structures from the nonopacified lumen of the appendix. Appendicitis occurs when the lumen of the appendix is occluded by inspissated stool (fecalith) with subsequent distention & inflammation of the appendix. Note the enhancing, thickened wall of the appendix and infiltration of the surrounding fat planes. (Bottom) More caudal section shows the inflamed, obstructed appendix and an enlarged reactive lymph node.

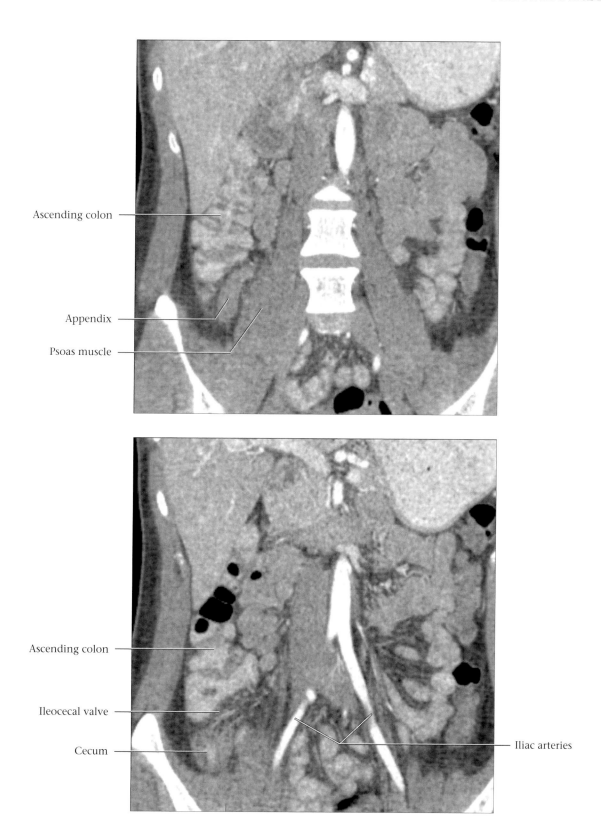

(Top) A coronal CT reformation shows the thick-walled appendix lying medial to the ascending colon and adjacent to the psoas muscle. In patients with acute appendicitis, the psoas muscle is often inflamed, causing pain when the leg is flexed and straightened. **(Bottom)** The wall of the cecum is thickened due to inflammation from the contiguous appendix.

COLON

DIVERTICULITIS

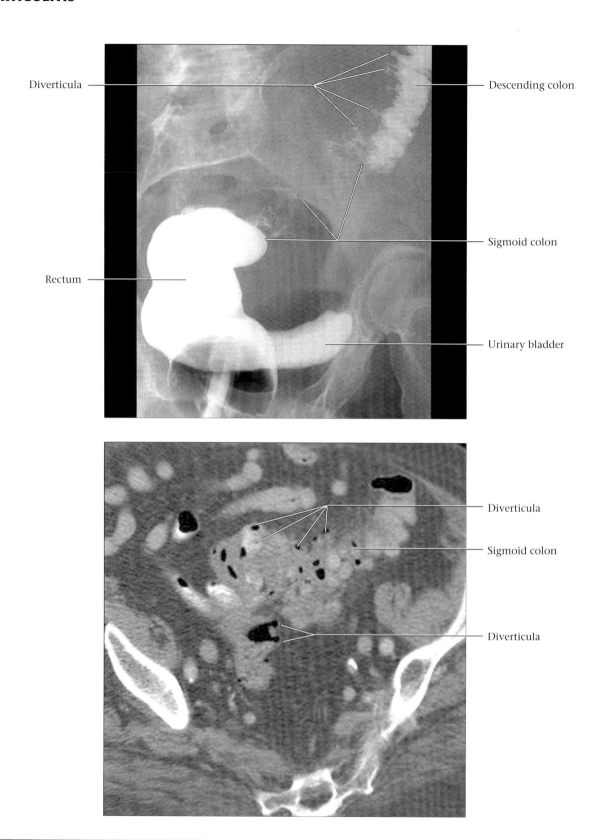

Diverticula — Descending colon

Sigmoid colon

Rectum

Urinary bladder

Diverticula

Sigmoid colon

Diverticula

(Top) First of five images of a patient with diverticulitis and a colo-vesical fistula. An oblique image from a barium enema shows marked spasm and luminal narrowing of the sigmoid colon and opacification of the urinary bladder through a fistula (that is not evident on this image). Numerous diverticula are seen in the descending & sigmoid colon. **(Bottom)** Axial CT section shows multiple gas- and contrast-filled diverticula arising from the sigmoid colon.

DIVERTICULITIS

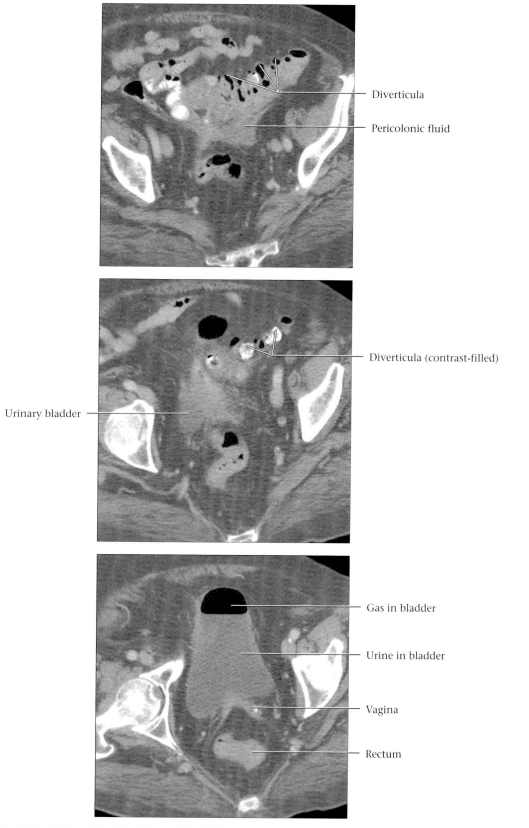

Diverticula

Pericolonic fluid

Diverticula (contrast-filled)

Urinary bladder

Gas in bladder

Urine in bladder

Vagina

Rectum

(Top) More caudal CT section shows extraluminal fluid adjacent to the sigmoid colon, due to perforation of the diverticula and inflammation. **(Middle)** More caudal CT section shows pericolonic fluid & infiltration and several diverticula with high density contents due to retained enteric contrast material. The inflammatory process is contiguous with the top of the urinary bladder. **(Bottom)** More caudal CT section shows a gas-fluid level in the urinary bladder, indicative of a colovesical fistula.

COLON

EPIPLOIC APPENDAGITIS

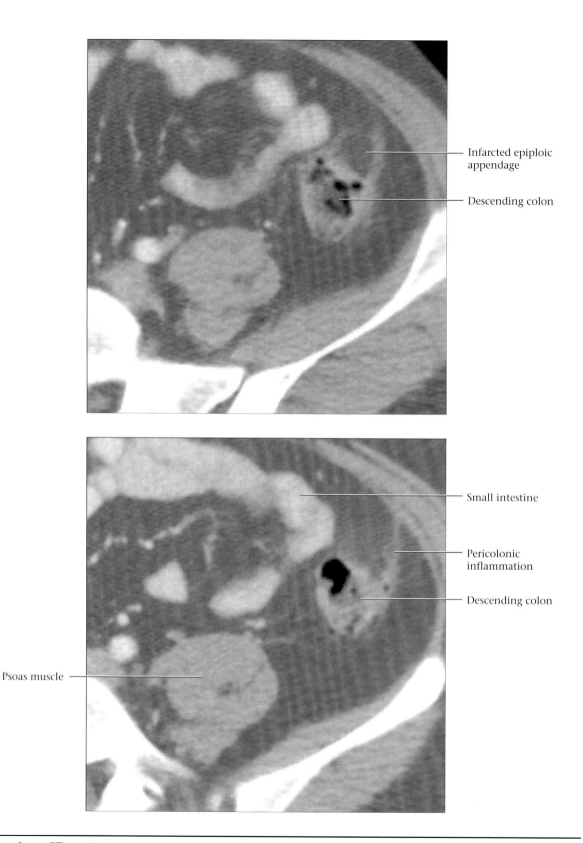

Infarcted epiploic
appendage

Descending colon

Small intestine

Pericolonic
inflammation

Descending colon

Psoas muscle

(Top) First of two CT sections in a patient with acute left lower quadrant pain shows inflammation of the fat planes anterior to the descending colon. In the middle of the inflammation is an oval fat-density lesion that represents an infarcted epiploic appendage. Recall that the normal epiploic appendage is a tag of fat that extends off the antimesenteric border of the colon. (Bottom) The absence of diverticula and the presence of the central fat density in the inflammatory focus help to distinguish epiploic appendagitis from diverticulitis which causes very similar clinical signs & symptoms.

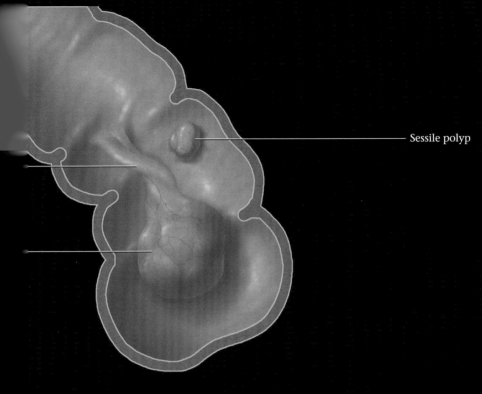

Sessile polyp

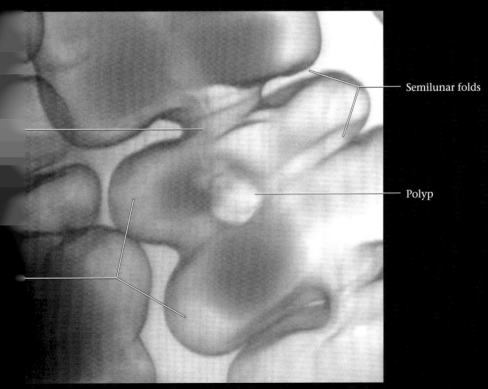

Semilunar folds

Polyp

common shapes of colonic polyps: A pedunculated polyp on an elongated stalk, and a
olyp. In adults, most polyps are adenomatous (gland-forming) and are considered
. For this reason, surveillance techniques, such as colonoscopy and barium enema, are
olyps so that they can be removed before undergoing malignant degeneration. **(Bottom)**
ntrast barium enema reveals a spherical pedunculated polyp on a long thin stalk. A polyp of
ually benign, but should be resected, preferably via colonoscopy.

COLON

SIGMOID VOLVULUS

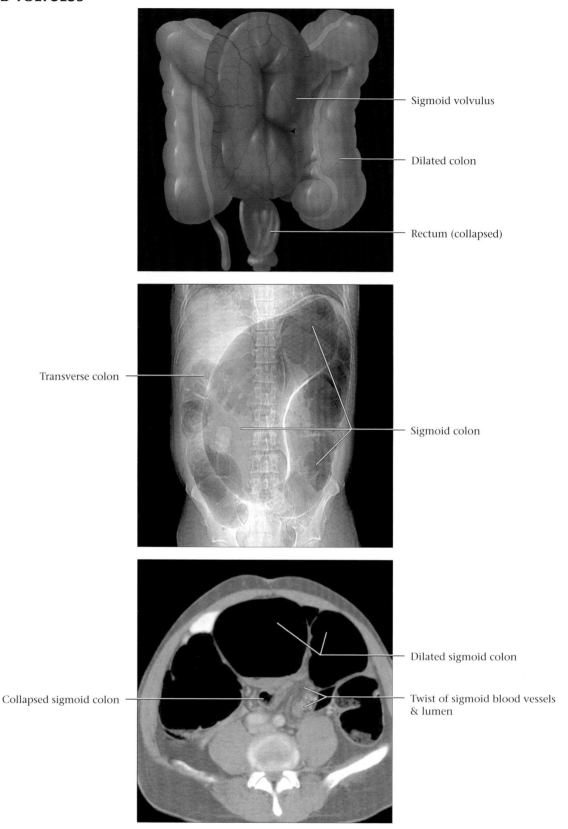

Sigmoid volvulus

Dilated colon

Rectum (collapsed)

Transverse colon

Sigmoid colon

Dilated sigmoid colon

Collapsed sigmoid colon

Twist of sigmoid blood vessels & lumen

(Top) Graphic shows a sigmoid volvulus, in which the sigmoid colon is twisted around the base of its mesocolon. The sigmoid lumen and blood vessels are occluded which may lead to ischemia & perforation. **(Middle)** A frontal abdominal film shows massive distention and elongation of the sigmoid colon, which has a shape likened to a football or coffee bean, with the "seam" representing the apposed walls of the sigmoid. The sigmoid extends above the transverse colon which is only moderately distended with gas. The distal rectosigmoid colon is collapsed. **(Bottom)** Axial CT section through the point of volvulus shows abrupt narrowing & twisting of the sigmoid lumen and its blood vessels. All of the colon upstream from the volvulus is dilated, but especially the sigmoid colon itself.

CECAL VOLVULUS

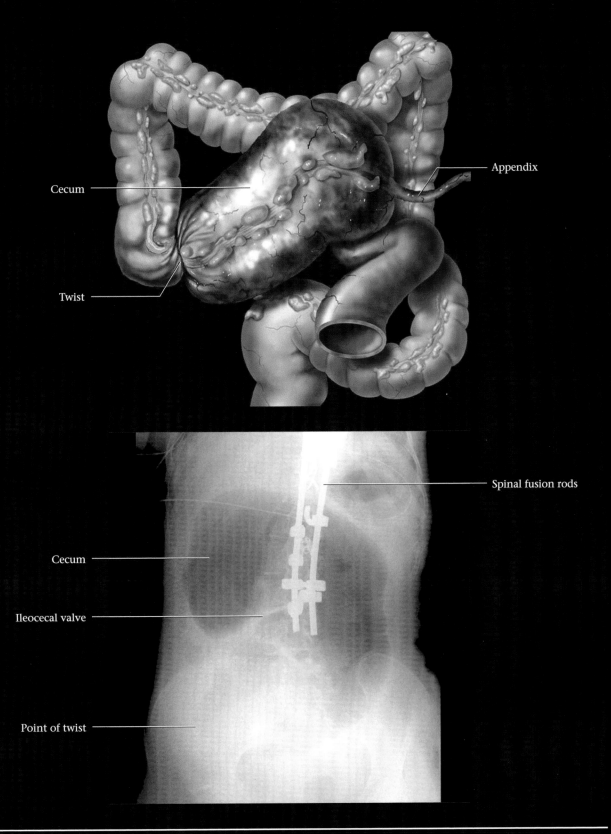

Cecum

Appendix

Twist

Spinal fusion rods

Cecum

Ileocecal valve

Point of twist

(Top) Graphic shows typical cecal volvulus. The ascending colon is usually fixed in a retroperitoneal location. Patients who have an elongated cecum & ascending colon that is on a mesentery are prone to twisting and obstruction of these segments, resulting in obstruction of the bowel lumen and blood vessels of the twisted colonic segment. Note that the cecum is dilated and displaced toward the left upper quadrant. The discoloration represents ischemic injury to the bowel. (Bottom) First of three frontal abdominal radiographs of a patient who had a recent spinal fusion shows massive distention of the right side of the colon, actually, the cecum and a portion of the ascending colon, that are inverted & obstructed.

COLON

CECAL VOLVULUS

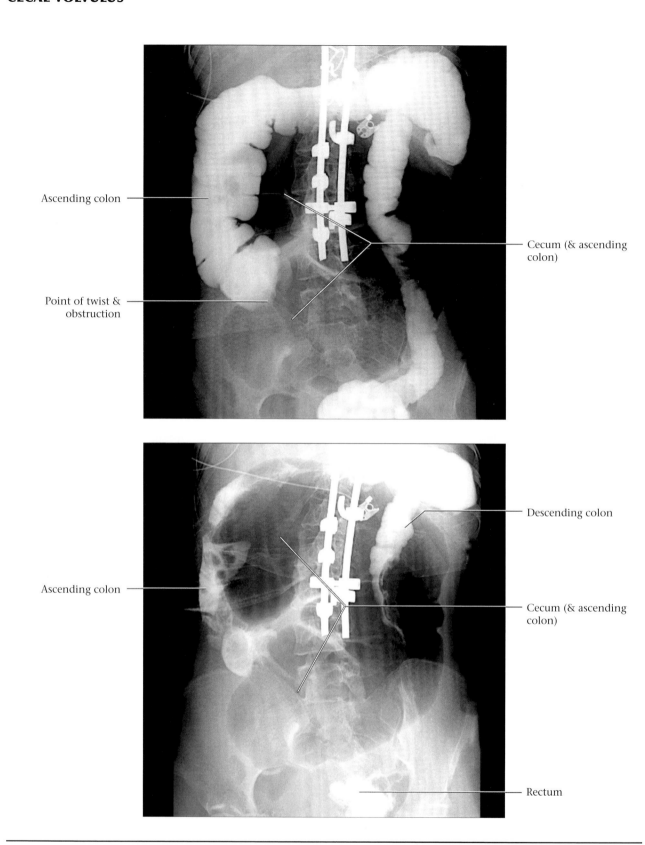

Ascending colon

Cecum (& ascending colon)

Point of twist & obstruction

Descending colon

Ascending colon

Cecum (& ascending colon)

Rectum

(Top) Image from a barium enema shows retrograde opacification of normal colon, with abrupt obstruction in the ascending colon. **(Bottom)** "Post-evacuation" image shows collapsed normal colon and massive distention of the cecum and the twisted portion of the ascending colon, diagnostic of cecal volvulus.

COLON CANCER

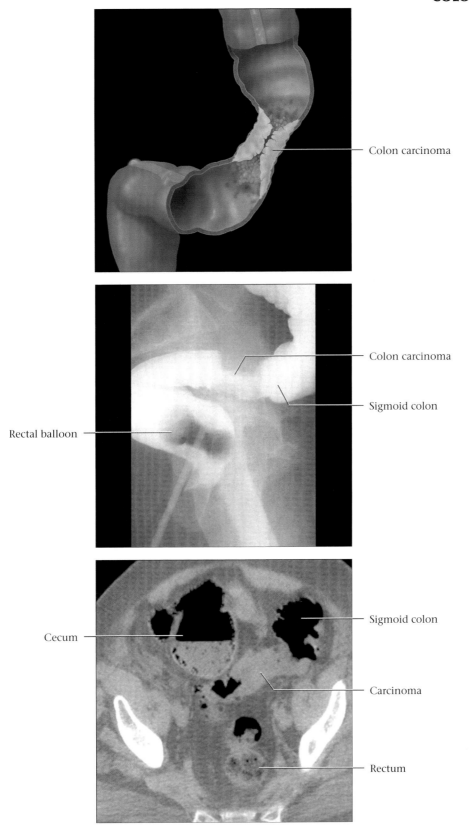

(Top) Graphic shows a typical "apple-core" narrowing of the colonic lumen by a circumferential tumor. Carcinoma is often a scirrhous mass that leads to luminal narrowing and partial obstruction. **(Middle)** A lateral view from a barium enema shows abrupt, irregular narrowing of the sigmoid colon by a carcinoma. **(Bottom)** An axial CT section shows gas and feces within the colon, except for the sigmoid colon where the lumen is markedly narrowed and only a soft tissue mass is seen, representing the primary carcinoma.

COLON

RECTAL CARCINOMA WITH METASTASES

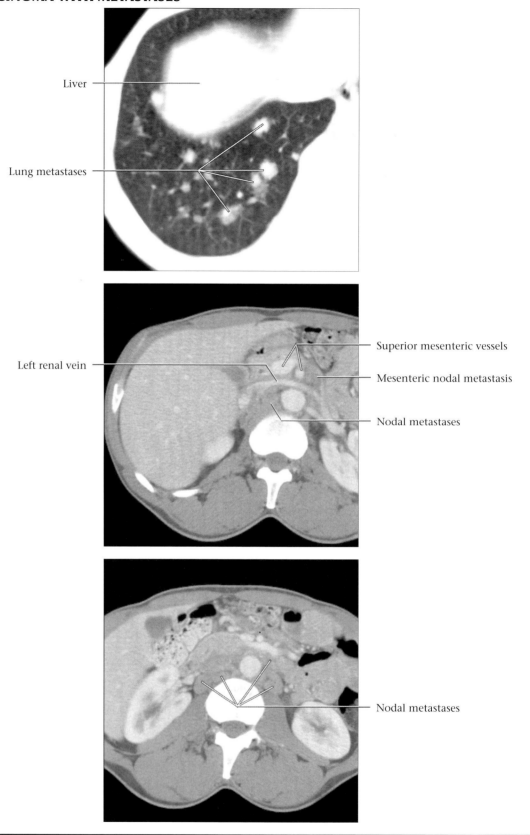

(Top) First of five CT sections of a man with rectal carcinoma shows numerous lung nodules representing pulmonary metastases. **(Middle)** A more caudal section shows lumbar retroperitoneal and mesenteric nodal metastases. Note the absence of liver metastases. Colon carcinoma usually spreads to the liver via the portal venous system, and systemic metastases are encountered less commonly and only late in the disease. Conversely, rectal cancer may spread via systemic venous and lymphatic drainage, bypassing the liver. **(Bottom)** A more caudal section shows extensive retroperitoneal nodal metastases.

RECTAL CARCINOMA WITH METASTASES

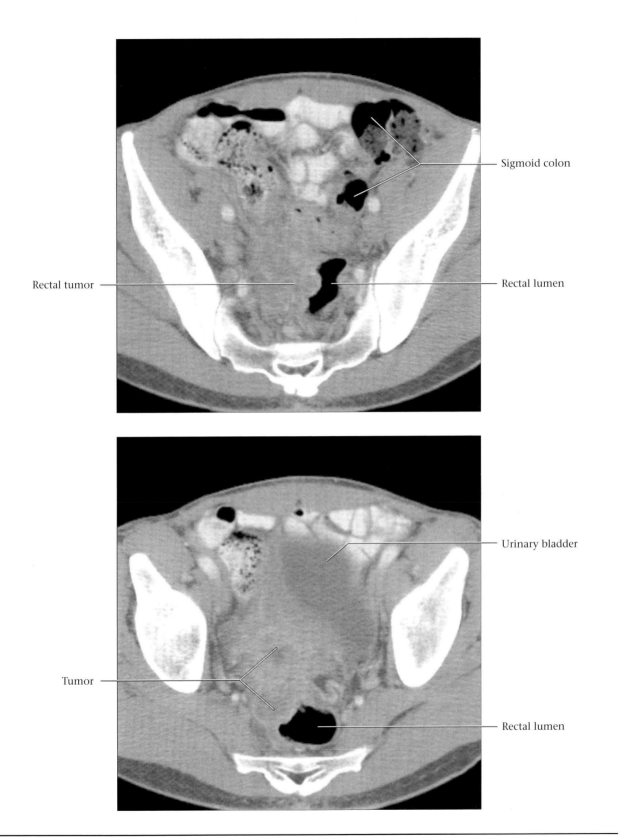

Sigmoid colon

Rectal tumor

Rectal lumen

Urinary bladder

Tumor

Rectal lumen

(Top) Gas in the rectal lumen indicates displacement and narrowing of the rectum by a bulky tumor. **(Bottom)** A more caudal section shows extensive perirectal tumor filling much of the pelvis and displacing the urinary bladder.

ISCHEMIC COLITIS

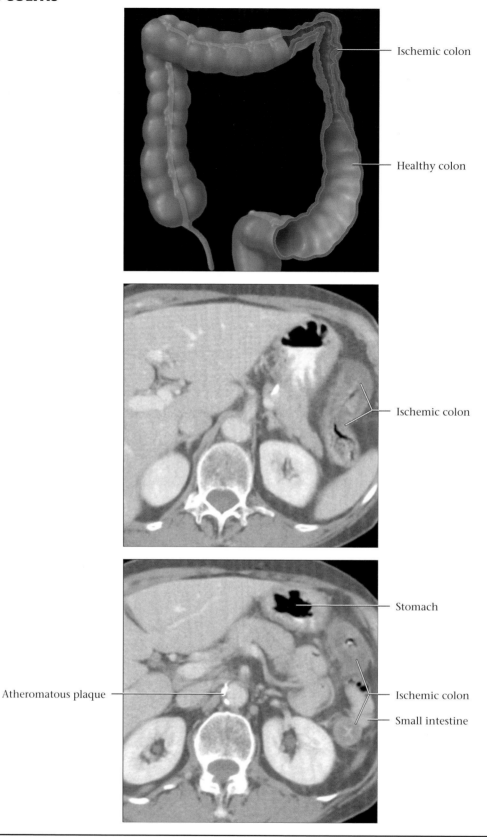

Ischemic colon

Healthy colon

Ischemic colon

Stomach

Atheromatous plaque

Ischemic colon

Small intestine

(Top) Graphic shows the typical effect of hypoperfusion ischemic injury of the colon. The "watershed" region of the splenic flexure, where the distribution of the superior and inferior mesenteric arteries intersect, is the most vulnerable segment. Note the luminal narrowing and wall thickening. **(Middle)** First of five CT sections shows luminal narrowing and submucosal edema within the splenic flexure region of the colon. **(Bottom)** The ischemic injury to the colon extends into the distal transverse and proximal descending colon.

ISCHEMIC COLITIS

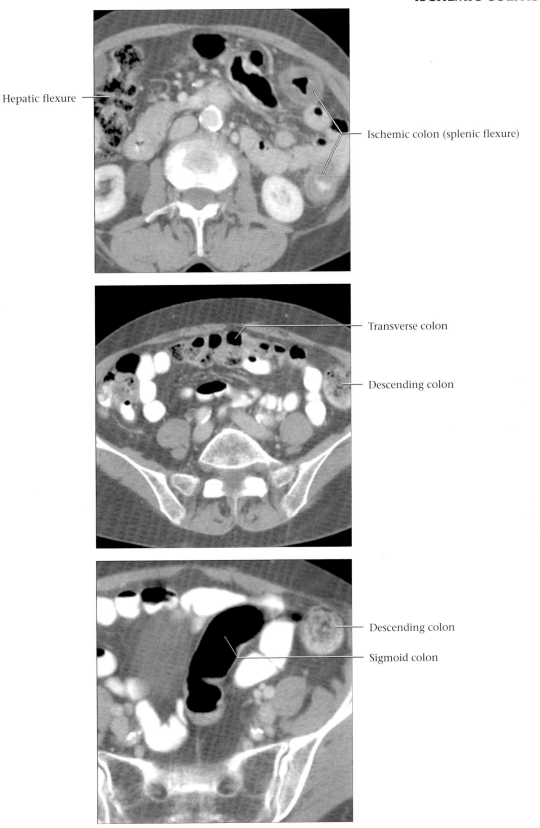

Hepatic flexure

Ischemic colon (splenic flexure)

Transverse colon

Descending colon

Descending colon

Sigmoid colon

(Top) The wall of the hepatic flexure is normal; compare with the thickened wall of the splenic flexure. **(Middle)** The mid transverse and descending colon are normal as is the small intestine. Note the thickness of the normal bowel wall which is almost imperceptible on these sections, measuring only about 2 mm in thickness. **(Bottom)** Most caudal section shows normal distal colon and small intestine.

SPLEEN

Gross Anatomy

Overview

- Spleen is the the largest lymphatic organ
  - Size is variable
    - Usually not more than 12 cm long, 8 cm wide, or 5 cm thick
    - Usual volume range 100-250 cm³, mean 150 cm³ in adults
    - Volume > 470 cm³ = splenomegaly
  - Functions
    - Manufactures lymphocytes, filters blood (removes damaged red blood cells & platelets)
    - Acts as blood reservoir: Can expand or contract in response to changes in blood volume
- **Histology**
  - Soft organ with fibroelastic **capsule** entirely surrounded by peritoneum, except at splenic hilum
  - **Trabeculae**: Extensions of the capsule into the parenchyma; carry arterial & venous branches
  - **Pulp**: Substance of the spleen; **white pulp** = lymphoid nodules; **red pulp** = sinusoidal spaces containing blood
  - Splenic cords (plates of cells) lie between sinusoids; red pulp veins drain sinusoids
- **Relations and vessels**
  - Spleen contacts the posterior surface of the stomach and is connected via the **gastrosplenic ligament** (GSL)
    - GSL is the left anterior margin of the lesser sac
    - GSL carries the **short gastric & left gastroepiploic arteries** and venous branches to spleen
  - Contacts the pancreatic tail and surface of left kidney and is connected to these by the **splenorenal ligament** (SRL)
    - SRL carries **splenic arterial** and venous branches to spleen
    - SRL is the left posterior margin of the **lesser sac** (**omental bursa**)
  - **Splenic vein** runs in groove along dorsal surface of pancreatic body and tail
    - Receives the **inferior mesenteric vein** (IMV)
    - Combined splenic and IMV join **superior mesenteric vein** to form **portal vein**
  - **Splenic artery** (from celiac), often very tortuous

Anatomy-Based Imaging Issues

Key Concepts

- Spleen shows **heterogeneous enhancement** on arterial phase enhanced CT or MR imaging
  - Reflects lack of capillary bed, presence of red and white pulp and sinusoidal architecture
  - Can be mistaken for pathology on abdominal CT or MR exam
- Spleen has highly variable size and shape
  - Imaging accurately detects **splenomegaly** and may suggest its cause (e.g., with cirrhosis = portal hypertension; with lymphadenopathy = lymphoma, mononucleosis, etc.)
- Spleen is **commonly injured** in blunt trauma, especially with fracture of the left lower ribs
  - Parenchymal laceration & capsular tear often result in substantial intraperitoneal bleeding
- Spleen texture
  - Soft & pliable, relatively mobile
  - Easily indented & displaced by masses and even loculated fluid collections
  - Changes position in response to resection of adjacent organs (e.g., post-nephrectomy)

Clinical Implications

Clinical Importance

- Neoplastic involvement
  - Spleen is commonly involved in Hodgkin and non-Hodgkin **lymphoma** and leukemia (often result in massive splenomegaly)
  - Uncommonly involved with other metastatic disease (direct invasion by gastric or pancreatic cancer; metastatic melanoma)
  - Rarely the site of other primary malignancy
- Tail of pancreas contacts splenic hilum
  - Pancreatic tail lies in splenorenal ligament (can be considered intraperitoneal)
  - Pancreatitis can extend into splenic hilum, result in **intrasplenic pseudocyst**
- **Splenic infarction**
  - Relatively common cause of acute left upper quadrant pain
  - Appears as sharply marginated wedge-shaped, poorly enhancing lesion(s) abutting splenic capsule
  - Etiologies
    - Sickle cell and other hemoglobinopathies
    - "Spontaneous" in any cause of splenomegaly
    - Embolic (e.g., I.V. drug abuse, endocarditis, atrial fibrillation)

Embryology

Embryologic Events

- From dorsal mesogastrium during 5th fetal week
- Normally rotates to the left
- Usually fixed into left subphrenic location by peritoneal reflections linking it to diaphragm, abdominal wall, kidney & stomach
- Usually develops as one "fused" mass of tissue

Practical Implications

- **Accessory spleen** found in 10-30% of population
  - Usually small, near splenic hilum
  - Can enlarge & simulate mass, especially after splenectomy
- Spleen may be on a long mesentery
  - "**Wandering spleen**" may be found in any abdominal or pelvic location
- **Asplenia** and **polysplenia**
  - Rare congenital conditions associated with other cardiovascular anomalies, situs inversus, etc.
  - Polysplenia can be simulated by **splenosis** (peritoneal implantation of splenic tissue that may follow traumatic splenic injury)

SPLEEN

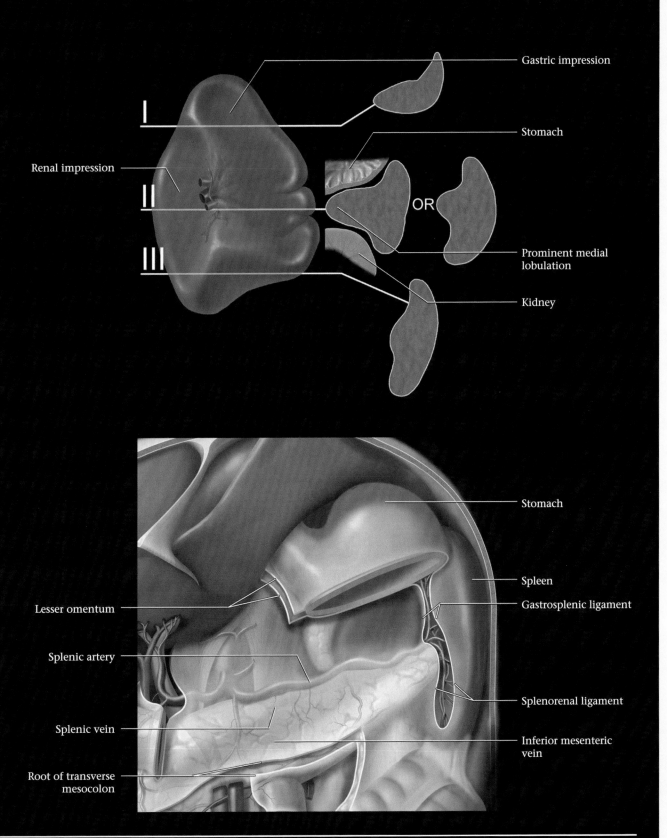

(Top) Graphic shows the medial surface of the spleen & representative axial sections at three levels through the parenchyma. The spleen is of variable shape & size, even within the same individual, varying with states of nutrition and hydration. It is a soft organ that is easily indented by adjacent organs. The medial surface is often quite lobulated as it is interposed between the stomach & the kidney. **(Bottom)** The liver is retracted upward & the stomach transected to reveal the pancreas and spleen. The splenic artery & vein course along the body of the pancreas, & the tail of the pancreas lies within the splenorenal ligament. The gastrosplenic ligament carries the short gastric & left gastroepiploic vessels to the stomach and spleen. The splenic vein receives the inferior mesenteric vein & joins the superior mesenteric vein behind the neck of the pancreas to form the portal vein.

SPLEEN

AXIAL CT, NORMAL SPLEEN

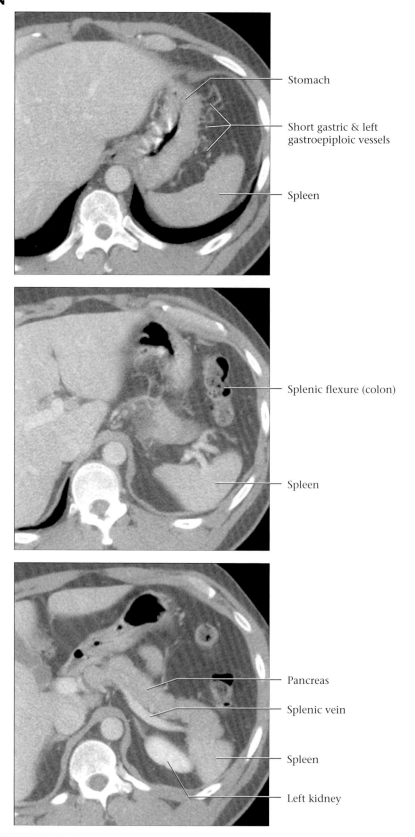

Stomach

Short gastric & left gastroepiploic vessels

Spleen

Splenic flexure (colon)

Spleen

Pancreas

Splenic vein

Spleen

Left kidney

(Top) First of 3 axial CT sections shows a normal spleen abutting the left hemidiaphragm. The short gastric and left gastroepiploic vessels lie in the gastrosplenic ligament and supply both the stomach and spleen. **(Middle)** Note the relation between the spleen and the left ("splenic") flexure of the colon. **(Bottom)** The body of the pancreas courses along the splenic vein and the tail of the pancreas inserts into the splenic hilum. Note the relation of the spleen to the left kidney.

SPLEEN

CORONAL CT, NORMAL SPLEEN

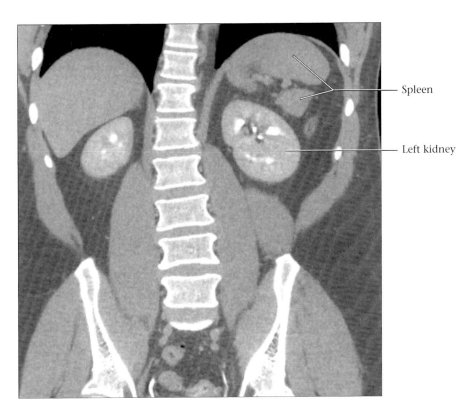

Spleen

Left kidney

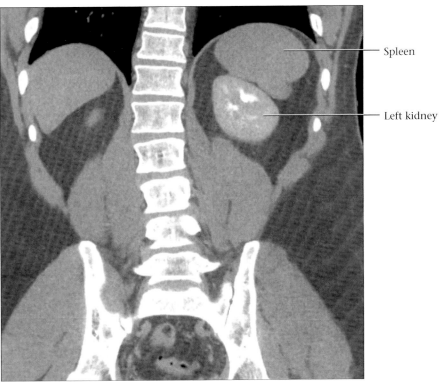

Spleen

Left kidney

(Top) First of two coronal CT images shows a normal spleen in its subdiaphragmatic location. Note the normal fatty clefts in the splenic parenchyma. Infoldings of the splenic capsule into the parenchyma are called trabeculae, and these carry the branches of the splenic vessels. **(Bottom)** Note the close relation between the spleen and the left kidney.

SPLEEN

NORMAL SPLEEN

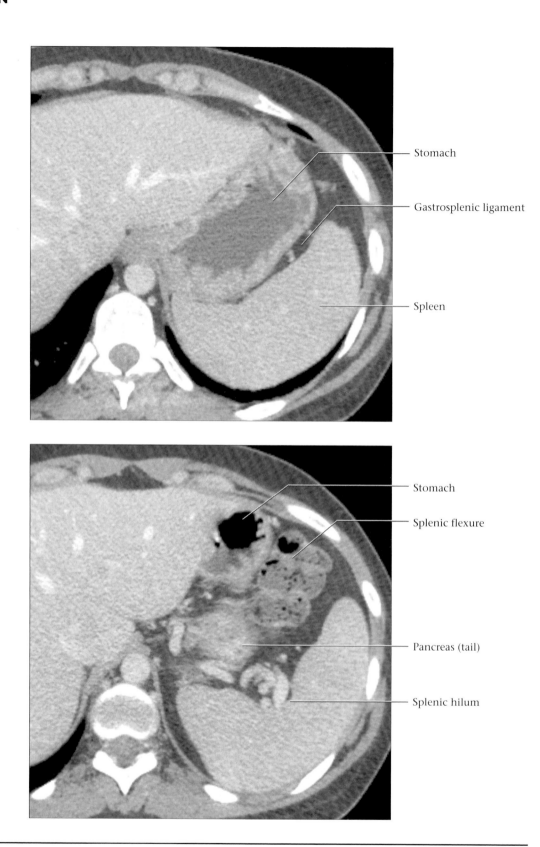

Stomach

Gastrosplenic ligament

Spleen

Stomach

Splenic flexure

Pancreas (tail)

Splenic hilum

(Top) First of five axial CT sections shows a normal spleen and its relations. Note the fat-containing gastrosplenic ligament which carries the short gastric and left gastroepiploic vessels to the stomach and spleen. **(Bottom)** The tail of the pancreas courses with the splenic vessels through the splenorenal ligament and lies in the splenic hilum. The tail of the pancreas is the only intraperitoneal portion of this organ. Processes that affect the pancreatic tail, including pancreatitis and cancer, can easily extend into the splenic hilum and invade the splenic parenchyma.

SPLEEN

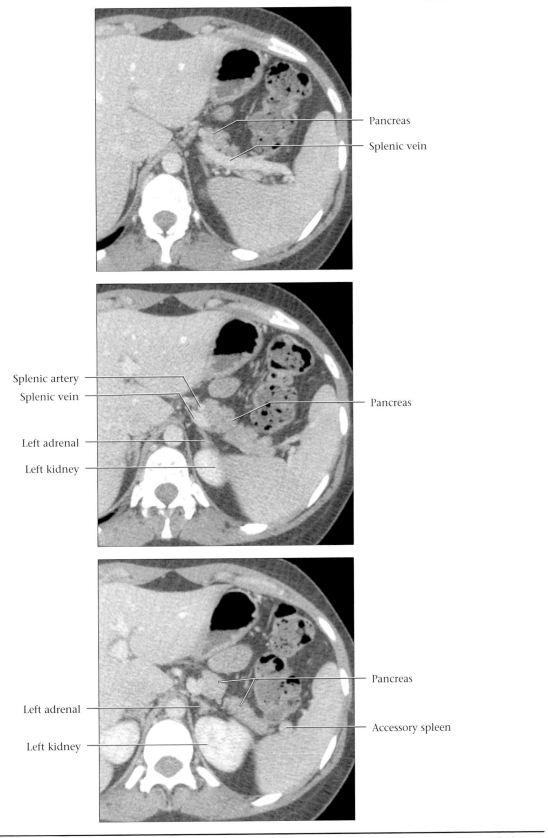

(Top) The splenic vein runs in a transverse plane in a groove in the dorsal surface of the pancreas. This is a reliable anatomic marker to help identify the pancreatic body. (Middle) The splenic artery has a much more circuitous route, especially in older individuals and frequently moves into and out of the axial plane of CT sections. (Bottom) Accessory splenic tissue is found in up to 30% of the population. As in this example, it is usually seen as a small, spherical "mass" in the splenic hilum.

SPLEEN

SPLENIC LIGAMENTS & VESSELS

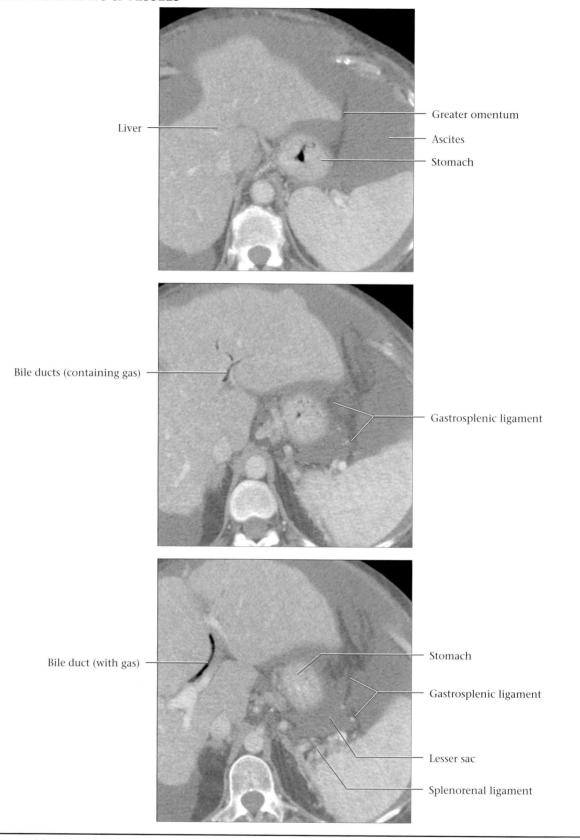

Liver — Greater omentum — Ascites — Stomach

Bile ducts (containing gas) — Gastrosplenic ligament

Bile duct (with gas) — Stomach — Gastrosplenic ligament — Lesser sac — Splenorenal ligament

(Top) First of five axial CT sections in a man with ascites that helps to accentuate the peritoneal ligaments that carry vessels to and from the spleen. Axial image shows ascites surrounding the liver and spleen. **(Middle)** The gastrosplenic ligament is the peritoneal reflection that connects the stomach and spleen; it carries the short gastric and left gastroepiploic vessels to both organs. **(Bottom)** The gastrosplenic and splenorenal ligaments form the left lateral margin of the lesser sac and convey blood vessels, nerves, and lymphatics to the spleen.

SPLEEN

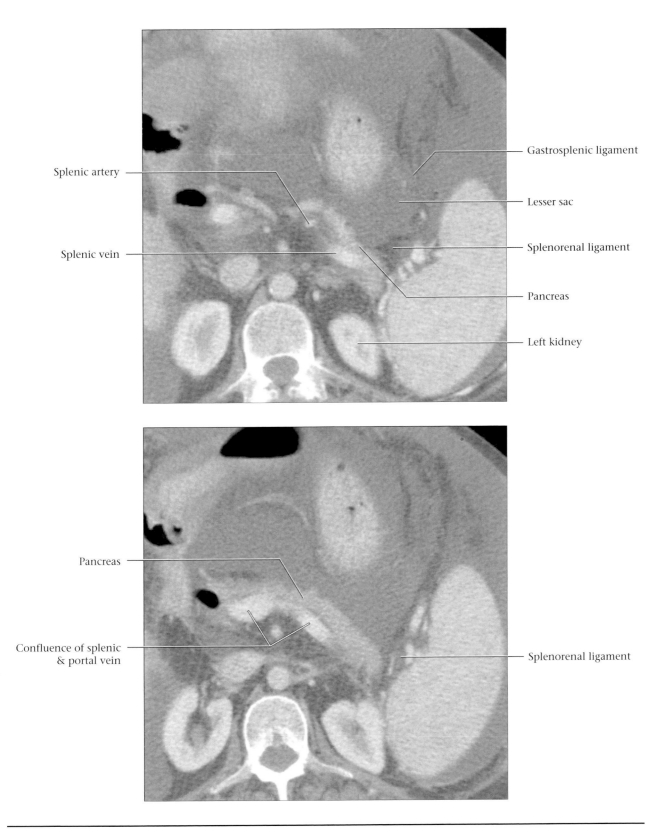

Splenic artery

Splenic vein

Gastrosplenic ligament

Lesser sac

Splenorenal ligament

Pancreas

Left kidney

Pancreas

Confluence of splenic & portal vein

Splenorenal ligament

(Top) The (main) splenic artery and vein course along the pancreas and enter the spleen through the splenorenal ligament. **(Bottom)** The splenic vein runs parallel to the body of the pancreas and lies in a groove along its dorsal margin.

SPLEEN

ANGIOGRAM, SPLENIC VESSELS

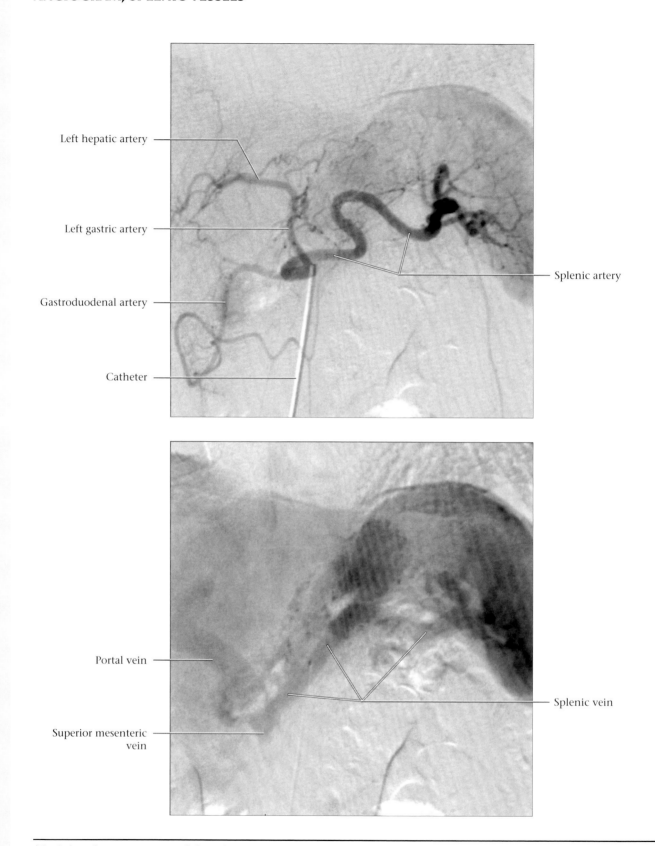

(Top) A catheter injection of the celiac artery shows the typically tortuous course of the splenic artery. This individual exhibits a common variant in which the right hepatic artery arose from the superior mesenteric artery and is, therefore, not opacified on this injection. **(Bottom)** The splenic vein joins the superior mesenteric vein to form the portal vein. The inferior mesenteric vein, draining the left side of the colon, usually joins the splenic vein just prior to its confluence with the superior mesenteric vein.

SPLEEN

HETEROGENEOUS SPLENIC ENHANCEMENT

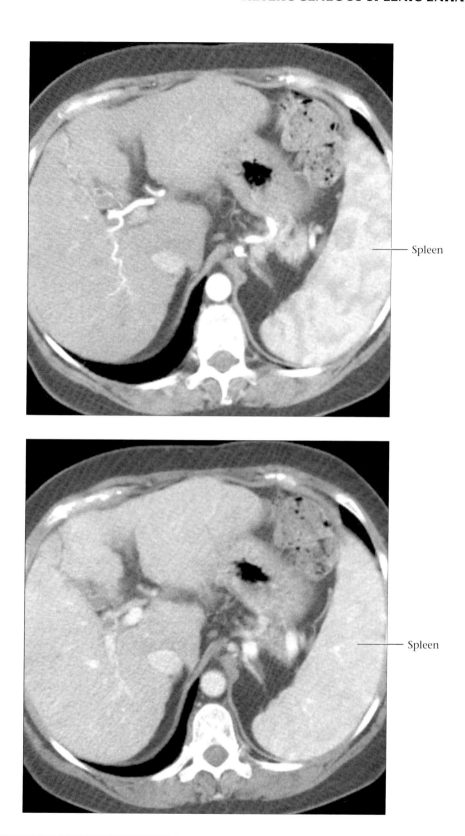

Spleen

Spleen

(Top) First of two axial CT sections through a normal, though prominent, spleen. This image was obtained in the predominantly arterial phase of enhancement (about 45 seconds after the start of the intravenous injection of contrast medium) and shows heterogeneous enhancement of the splenic parenchyma. This reflects the unique histology of the spleen, with cords of tissue and sinusoidal spaces, rather than a capillary bed as is found in most organs. (Bottom) A repeat CT section after about an 80 second delay shows homogeneous enhancement of the splenic parenchyma. The liver is cirrhotic.

SPLEEN

SPLENIC TRAUMA

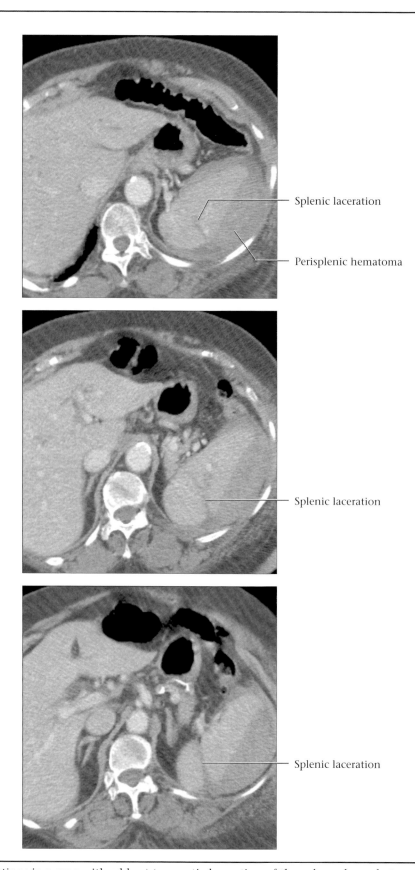

Splenic laceration

Perisplenic hematoma

Splenic laceration

Splenic laceration

(Top) First of three axial CT sections in a man with a blunt traumatic laceration of the spleen shows heterogeneous clotted blood (hematoma) surrounding the spleen. A linear lucency in the lateral side of the spleen represents the splenic laceration. **(Middle)** A more caudal section shows continuation of the irregular parenchymal laceration. **(Bottom)** Note that the lateral surface of the spleen is flattened by the hematoma. The hematoma is lentiform and mostly subcapsular (within the splenic capsule), although the presence of blood lower in the abdomen (not shown) indicates that the capsule was torn, as usually results from significant splenic trauma.

SPLEEN

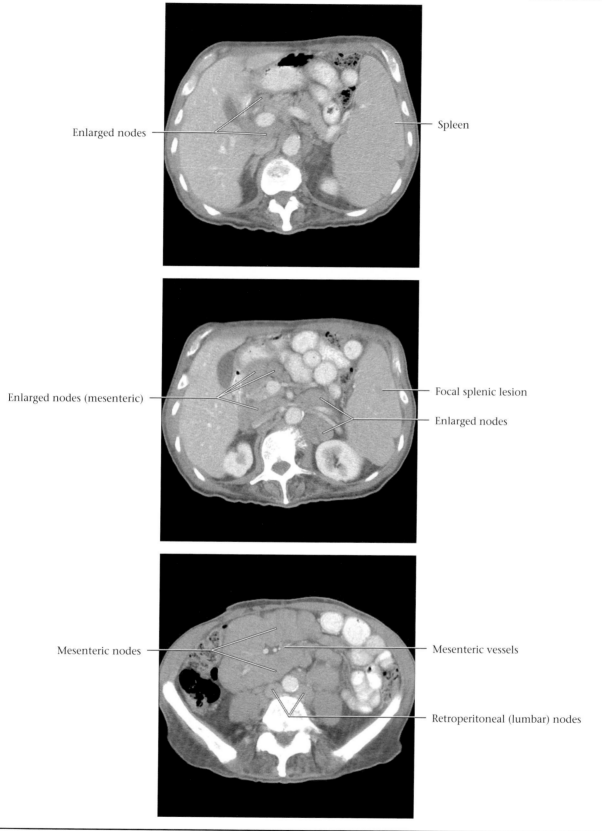

Enlarged nodes — Spleen

Enlarged nodes (mesenteric) — Focal splenic lesion

Enlarged nodes

Mesenteric nodes — Mesenteric vessels

Retroperitoneal (lumbar) nodes

(Top) First of three axial CT sections in a patient with night sweats and fever shows an enlarged spleen and numerous enlarged upper abdominal lymph nodes. **(Middle)** The presence of focal splenic lesions and mesenteric lymphadenopathy is strongly suggestive of non-Hodgkin lymphoma, which was subsequently proven by lymph node biopsy. **(Bottom)** Note how the superior mesenteric vessels are "sandwiched" between massively enlarged nodes, an appearance that is characteristic of widespread non-Hodgkin lymphoma.

SPLEEN

SPLENIC VEIN OCCLUSION, CANCER

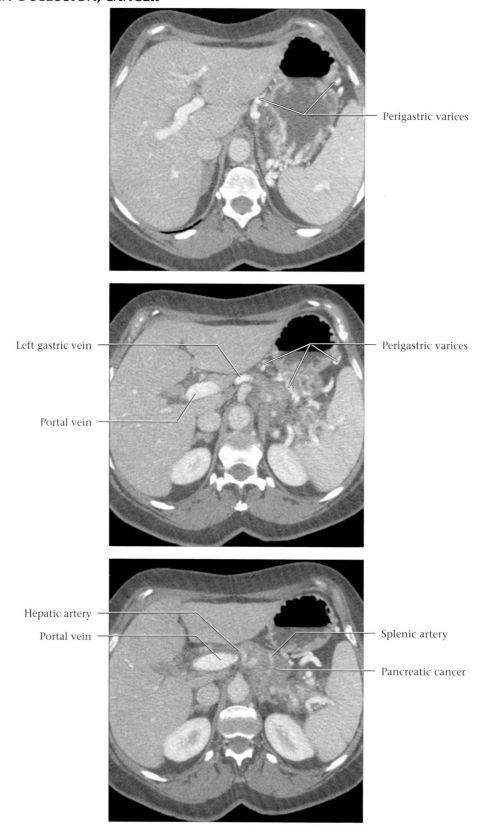

Perigastric varices

Left gastric vein — Perigastric varices

Portal vein

Hepatic artery — Splenic artery
Portal vein — Pancreatic cancer

(Top) First of six CT images from a patient with carcinoma of the pancreas shows enlarged perigastric varices, which are collateral veins connecting with the short gastric veins and splenic vein tributaries. **(Middle)** The splenic vein should be opacified and visible on this section. Instead, collateral perigastric varices return blood to the portal vein via the left gastric (coronary) vein. Note the normal appearance of the liver; perigastric varices in the absence of cirrhosis & portal hypertension are indicative of splenic vein occlusion, usually due to pancreatic carcinoma or chronic pancreatitis. **(Bottom)** A hypodense, poorly enhancing mass is seen in the body of the pancreas, totally encasing the splenic artery & vein, as well as the hepatic artery. This is a typical appearance for pancreatic ductal carcinoma, with vascular invasion precluding surgery.

SPLEEN

SPLENIC VEIN OCCLUSION, CANCER

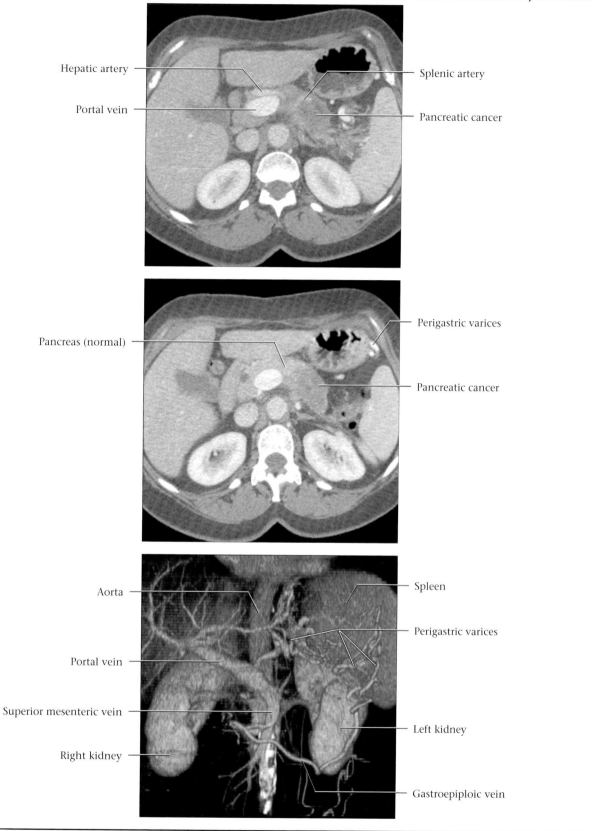

Hepatic artery

Portal vein

Splenic artery

Pancreatic cancer

Pancreas (normal)

Perigastric varices

Pancreatic cancer

Aorta

Spleen

Perigastric varices

Portal vein

Superior mesenteric vein

Left kidney

Right kidney

Gastroepiploic vein

(Top) The pancreatic tumor and its effect on the splenic vessels are well shown on this section. **(Middle)** Note the difference between the normally enhancing neck & head of the pancreas and the hypo-enhancing tumor in the body. **(Bottom)** Coronal reformation of the axial CT sections is displayed to accentuate the vessels in this image obtained during the venous phase of enhancement. Note the absence of filling of the splenic vein, due to encasement by the pancreatic tumor. Blood from the spleen is returned to the liver via collaterals that course along the surface of the stomach, including the short gastric, left gastric and gastroepiploic veins.

SPLEEN

INTRASPLENIC PSEUDOCYST

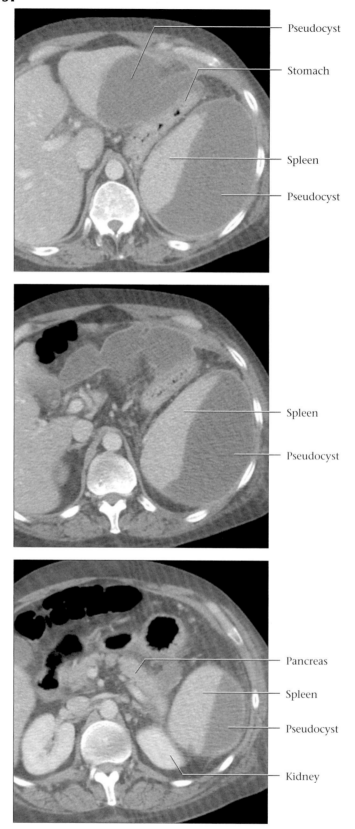

Pseudocyst

Stomach

Spleen

Pseudocyst

Spleen

Pseudocyst

Pancreas

Spleen

Pseudocyst

Kidney

(Top) First of three axial CT sections in a patient with recurrent pancreatitis shows the stomach compressed between two pseudocysts. One of these is within the splenic capsule and causes marked compression of the splenic parenchyma. **(Middle)** More caudal section again shows the encapsulation of the splenic pseudocyst and its effect on the splenic parenchyma. **(Bottom)** There is relatively little infiltration of the peripancreatic fat planes at this time and level. Inflammation from the tail of the pancreas has entered the spleen via the splenic hilum. Recall that the tail of the pancreas lies within the splenorenal ligament, as do the main splenic vessels; spread of inflammation (or tumor) from the pancreatic tail into the spleen is relatively common.

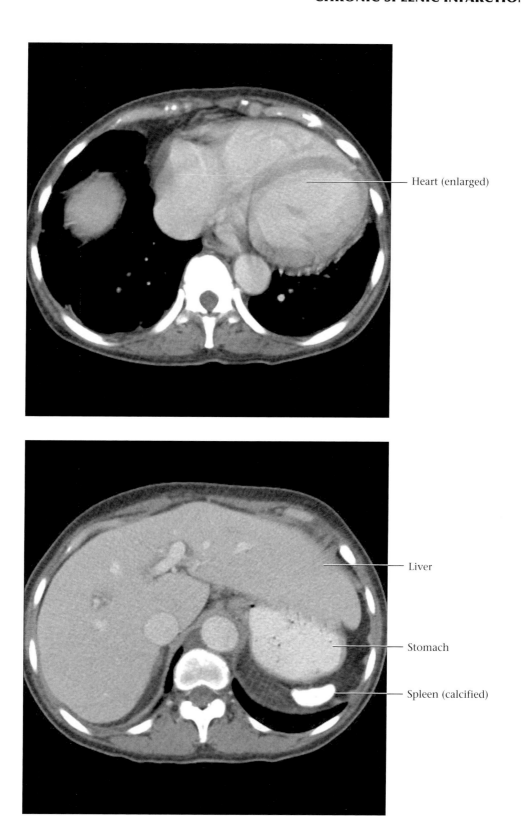

(Top) First of two axial CT sections of a 35 year old man with sickle cell anemia and abdominal pain shows cardiomegaly. (Bottom) More caudal section shows that the spleen is very small and densely calcified, characteristic of chronic splenic infarction that occurs typically in patients with sickle cell disease. The spleen is nonfunctional in this setting and the term "autosplenectomy" is sometimes applied to this condition.

SPLEEN

SPLENIC INFARCTION & CYST

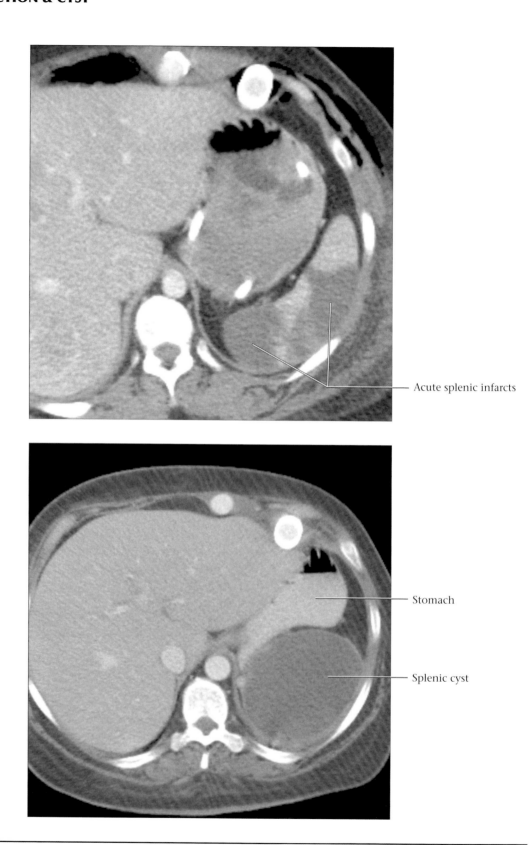

Acute splenic infarcts

Stomach

Splenic cyst

(Top) First of four CT sections of a patient with heart failure, a ventricular assist device, and acute abdominal pain shows wedge-shaped regions of nonenhancing splenic parenchyma that extend to the capsular surface, characteristic of acute splenic infarctions. **(Bottom)** CT image obtained seven days later shows interval development of splenic cysts, near water density lesions that may develop after splenic infarction or other forms of injury.

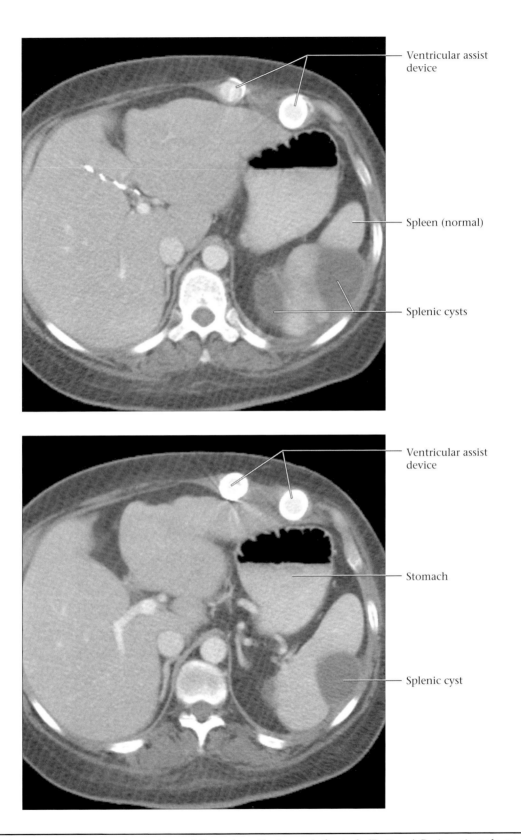

(Top) Additional splenic cysts now occupy the regions of the spleen that were infarcted. **(Bottom)** By imaging alone, it is often impossible to distinguish an acquired splenic cyst (as in this case) from a congenital (epithelial lined) cyst. Patient history and visible evolution of the cyst, as in this subject, are more reliable criteria.

SPLEEN

ACUTE SPLENIC INFARCTION

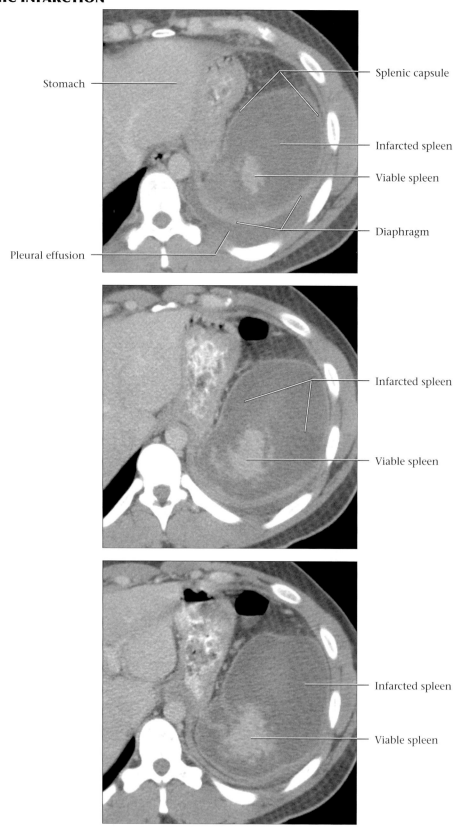

Stomach

Splenic capsule

Infarcted spleen

Viable spleen

Diaphragm

Pleural effusion

Infarcted spleen

Viable spleen

Infarcted spleen

Viable spleen

(Top) First of five axial CT sections in a young man with mononucleosis shows large areas of nonenhancing splenic parenchyma. **(Middle)** The spleen is enlarged due to mononucleosis and the nonenhancing parenchyma is indicative of acute infarction, which may occur in any setting of splenomegaly. **(Bottom)** The infarcted parenchyma is still limited by an intact splenic capsule. Rupture of the capsule might result in intraperitoneal bleeding and would likely require urgent splenectomy for treatment.

SPLEEN

ACUTE SPLENIC INFARCTION

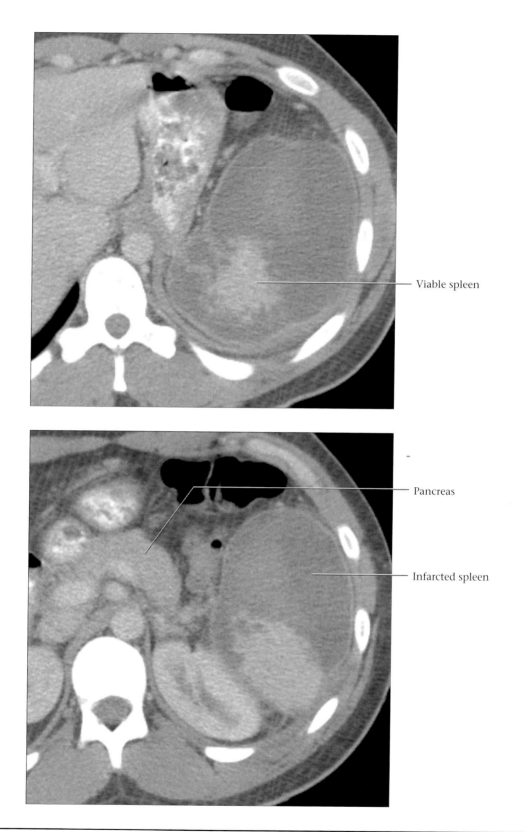

Viable spleen

Pancreas

Infarcted spleen

(Top) A more caudal section shows the infarcted, nonenhancing, portions of the spleen as distinct from the enhancing, viable portions. (Bottom) Some heterogeneity within the infarcted portion of the spleen is due to clotted blood.

SPLEEN

ACCESSORY SPLEENS AFTER SPLENECTOMY

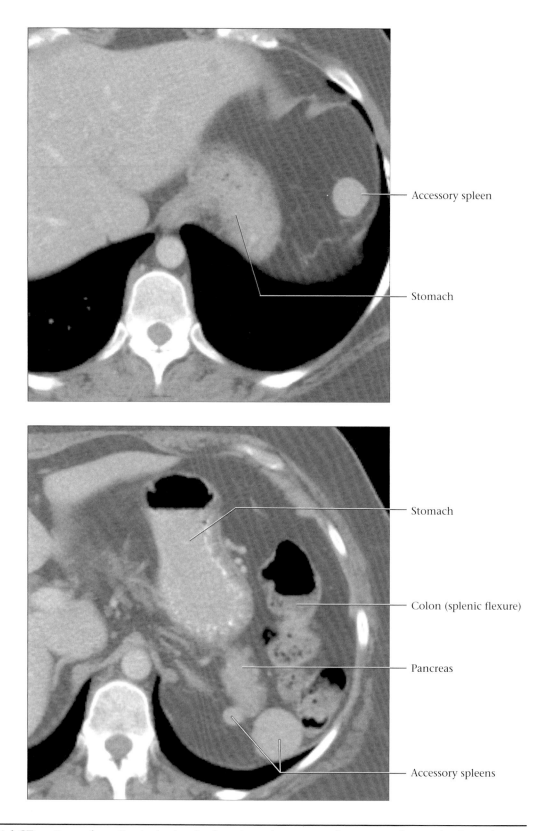

(Top) First of two axial CT sections of a patient who has had a prior splenectomy shows one of several spherical masses in the left upper quadrant. (Bottom) More caudal section shows two more splenic masses that represent enlarged accessory spleens that have hypertrophied to sompensate for the surgical removal of the "main" spleen. A similar situation may occur after trauma, and many small pieces of splenic tissue may implant throughout the peritoneal cavity and acquire a new blood supply, developing into multiple splenic masses. This latter condition is known as "splenosis".

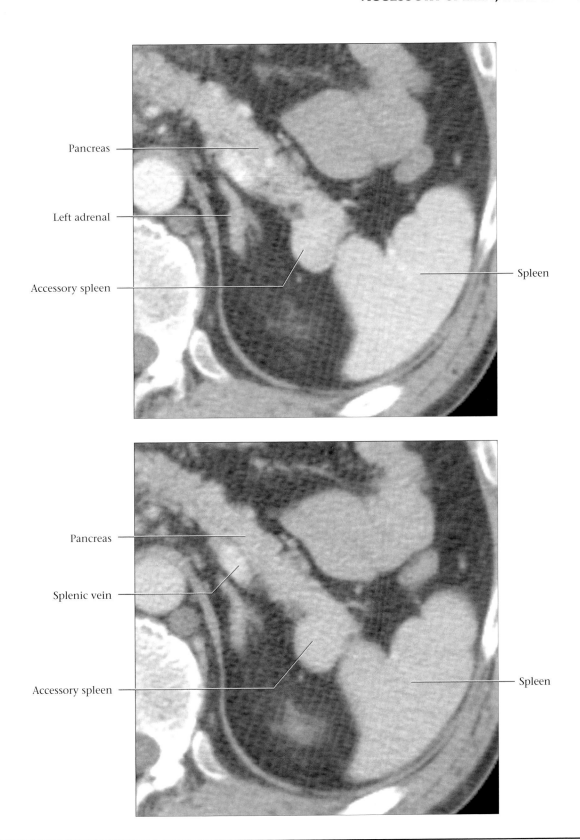

(**Top**) First of two axial CT sections through the same anatomic level. First image obtained during the arterial phase of imaging and shows a spherical, enhancing mass adjacent to the tail of the pancreas and near the splenic hilum. (**Bottom**) A more delayed, venous phase image shows that the "mass" and the spleen enhance to the same degree on both phases, indicating that this is an accessory spleen. Its location in or adjacent to the tail of the pancreas could lead to the erroneous diagnosis of a pancreatic tumor.

SPLEEN

ACCESSORY SPLEEN, ENLARGED IN CIRRHOSIS

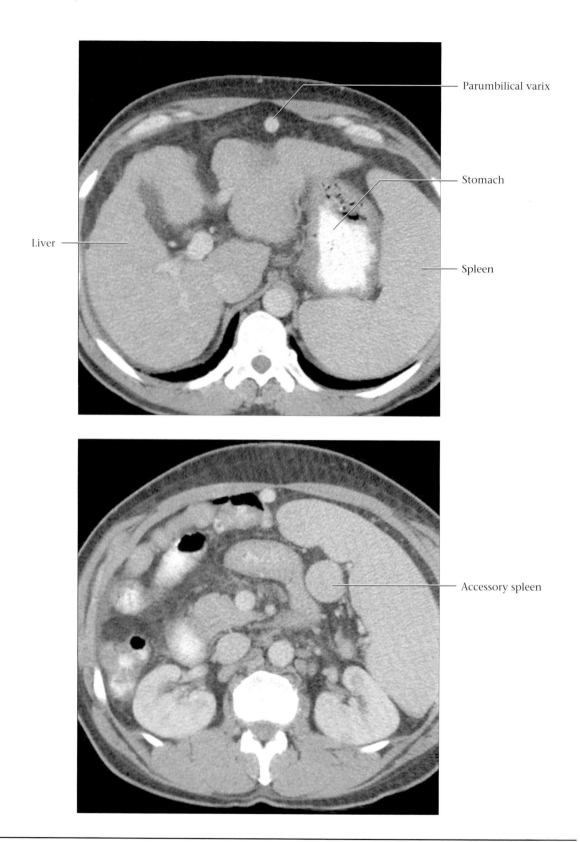

(Top) First of two axial CT sections shows a cirrhotic, nodular liver with evidence of portal hypertension, including varices (enlarged parumbilical vein) and splenomegaly. (Bottom) Near the splenic hilum is a spherical mass representing an enlarged accessory spleen. Processes that result in splenomegaly may also cause increased size of accessory spleens that may be present.

SPLEEN

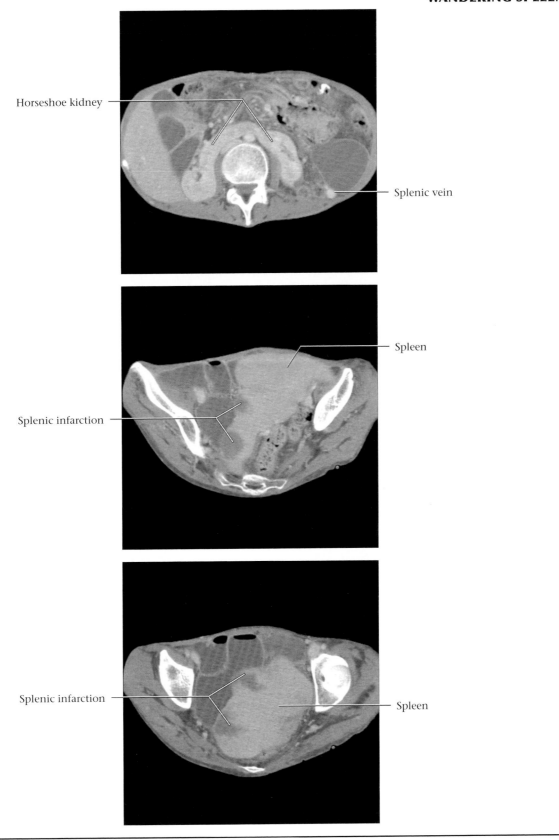

(Top) First of three axial CT sections in a subject with several congenital anomalies shows a horseshoe kidney. Note the splenic vein which could be followed to its junction with the superior mesenteric vein. (Middle) No splenic tissue was evident in the upper abdomen. This pelvic mass was proved to be a "wandering spleen" which was on a long mesentery allowing it to descend into the pelvis. Low density peripheral lesions represent acute splenic infarctions. (Bottom) More caudal section shows more of the enlarged, pelvic spleen and its infarcted portions.

SPLEEN

POLYSPLENIA SYNDROME

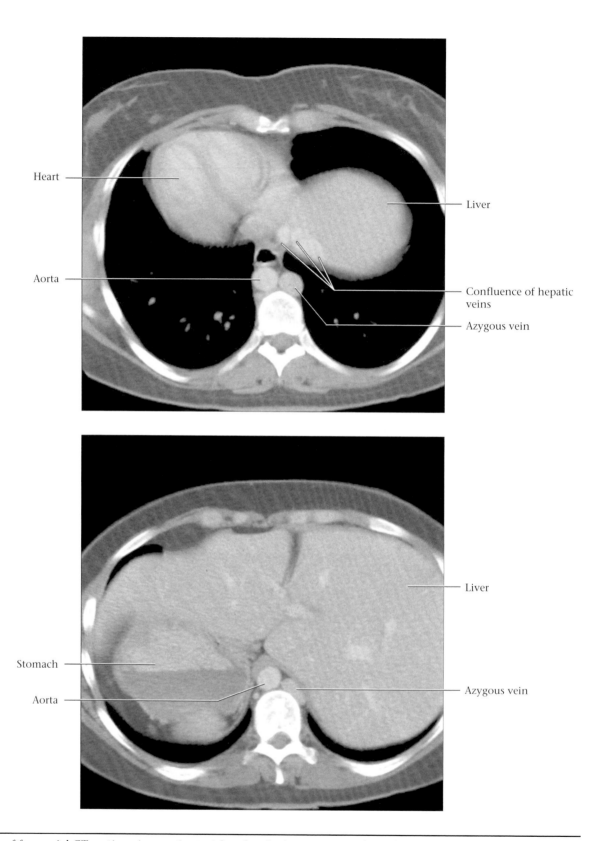

(Top) First of four axial CT sections in a patient with polysplenia, a congenital syndrome associated with multiple anomalies of development, position and rotation of viscera and vessels. This section shows dextrocardia and a left-sided liver, along with an enlarged azygous vein. The hepatic veins empty directly into the right atrium. (Bottom) The stomach and liver are on the "wrong" side, as is the azygous vein which is enlarged due to congenital absence of the suprarenal IVC.

SPLEEN

POLYSPLENIA SYNDROME

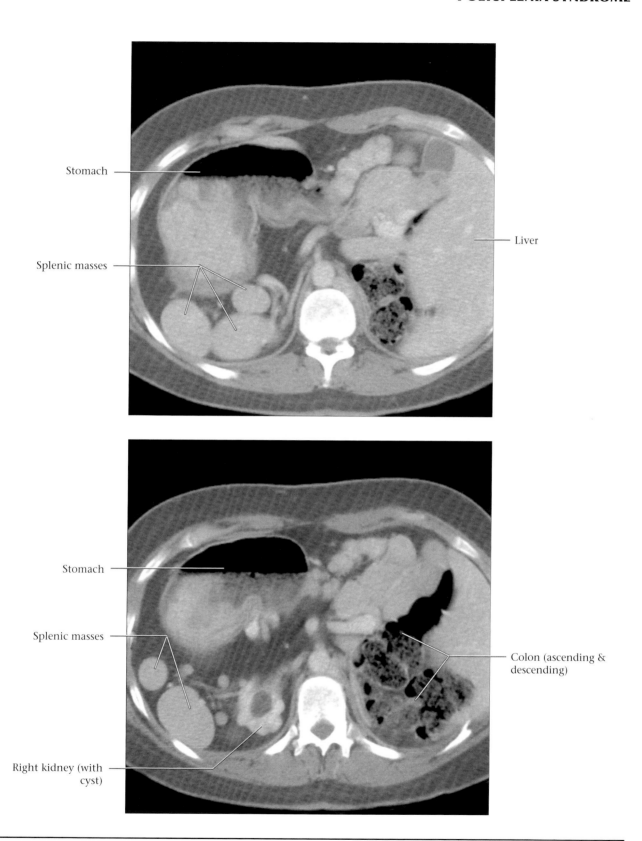

(Top) Multiple splenic "masses" are present on the right side of the abdomen. **(Bottom)** More caudal section shows additional splenic masses. In addition to the inverted position of the spleen, stomach and liver, all of the colon is present on the left side of the abdomen, while the small bowel was predominantly right-sided.

LIVER

Gross Anatomy

Overview

- Liver is largest gland & largest internal organ (average weight = 1500 grams)
  - Functions
    - Processes all nutrients (except fats) absorbed from GI tract; conveyed via **portal vein**
    - Stores glycogen, secretes bile
  - Relations
    - Anterior & superior surfaces are smooth and convex
    - Posterior & inferior surfaces are indented by colon, stomach, right kidney, duodenum, IVC, gallbladder
  - Covered by peritoneum except at **gallbladder fossa**, **porta hepatis** and **bare area**
    - **Bare area**: Nonperitoneal posterior superior surface where liver abuts diaphragm
  - **Porta hepatis**: Site of entry/exit of the portal vein, hepatic artery and bile duct
  - **Falciform ligament**: Extends from liver to anterior abdominal wall
    - Separates right & left **subphrenic peritoneal recesses** (between liver & diaphragm)
    - Marks plane separating medial and lateral segments of left hepatic lobe
    - Carries **round ligament** (lig. **teres**), fibrous remnant of umbilical vein
- Vascular supply (unique dual afferent blood supply)
  - **Portal vein**
    - Carries nutrients from gut and hepatotrophic hormones from pancreas to liver along with oxygen (contains 40% more oxygen than systemic venous blood)
    - 75-80% of blood supply to liver
  - **Hepatic artery**
    - Supplies 20-25% of blood
    - Liver is less dependent than biliary tree on hepatic arterial blood supply
    - Usually arises from celiac artery
    - Variations are common including arteries arising from superior mesenteric artery
  - **Hepatic veins**
    - Usually 3 (right, middle and left)
    - Many variations & accessory veins
    - Collect blood from liver and return it to IVC at the **confluence of hepatic veins** just below diaphragm and entrance of IVC into heart
  - **Portal triad**
    - At all levels of size and subdivision, branches of the hepatic artery, portal vein and bile ducts travel together
    - Blood flows into hepatic sinusoids from interlobular branches of hepatic artery & portal vein → hepatocytes (detoxify blood and produce bile) → bile collects into ducts, blood collects into central veins → hepatic veins
- Segmental anatomy of liver
  - Eight **hepatic segments**
    - Each receives secondary or tertiary branch of hepatic artery and portal vein
    - Each is drained by its own bile duct (intrahepatic) and hepatic vein branch
  - Caudate lobe = segment 1
    - Has independent portal triads and hepatic venous drainage to IVC
  - Left lobe
    - Lateral superior = segment 2
    - Lateral inferior = segment 3
    - Medial superior = segment 4A
    - Medial inferior = segment 4B
  - Right lobe
    - Anterior inferior = segment 5
    - Posterior inferior = segment 6
    - Posterior superior = segment 7
    - Anterior superior = segment 8

Anatomy-Based Imaging Issues

Key Concepts or Questions

- Designating and remembering hepatic segments
  - Portal triads are intra-segmental, hepatic veins are inter-segmental
  - Separating right from left lobe
    - Plane extending vertically through gallbladder fossa & middle hepatic vein
  - Separating right anterior from posterior segments
    - Vertical plane through right hepatic vein
  - Separating left lateral from medial segments
    - Plane of the falciform ligament
  - Separating superior from inferior segments
    - Plane of main right & left portal veins
  - Segments are numbered in **clockwise order** as if looking at anterior surface of liver

Imaging Pitfalls

- Because of variations of vascular & biliary branching within liver (common), it is frequently impossible to designate precisely the boundaries between hepatic segments on imaging studies

Clinical Implications

Clinical Importance

- Advances in hepatic surgery (tumor resection, transplantation) make it essential to depict lobar and segmental anatomy, volume, blood supply, biliary drainage as accurately as possible
  - Combination of axial, coronal, sagittal and 3D imaging by CT, MR and sonography may be needed
  - "Invasive" imaging studies (catheter angiography and percutaneous transhepatic or endoscopic cholangiography) can be avoided in many cases by CT & MR angiography and cholangiography
- **Liver metastases are common**
  - Primary carcinomas of colon, pancreas, & stomach are common
  - Portal venous drainage usually results in liver being initial site of metastatic spread from these tumors
- Primary **hepatocellular carcinoma**
  - Common worldwide, usually result of viral hepatitis B or C, alcoholism

LIVER

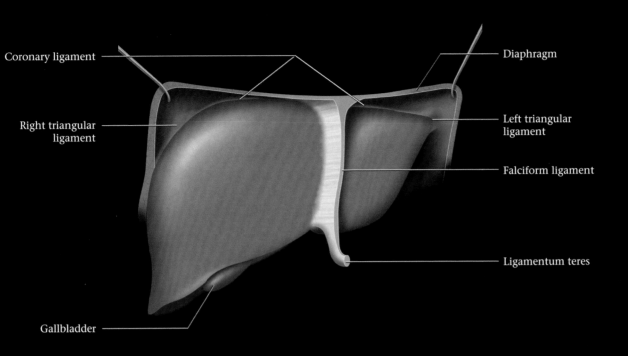

Coronary ligament

Right triangular ligament

Gallbladder

Diaphragm

Left triangular ligament

Falciform ligament

Ligamentum teres

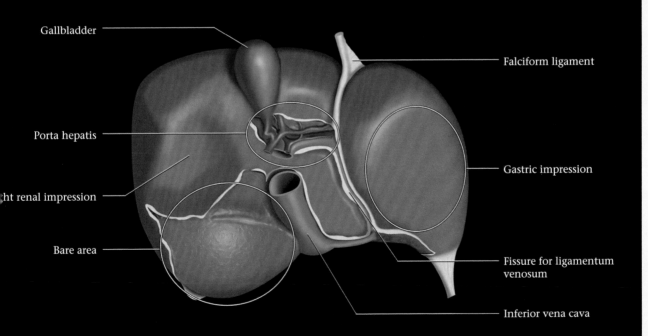

Gallbladder

Porta hepatis

ht renal impression

Bare area

Falciform ligament

Gastric impression

Fissure for ligamentum venosum

Inferior vena cava

b) The anterior surface of the liver is smooth and molds to the diaphragm & anterior abdominal wall. Generally, y the anterior/inferior edge of the liver is palpable on physical exam. The liver is covered with peritoneum, except the gallbladder bed, porta hepatis, and the bare area. Peritoneal reflections form various ligaments that connect liver to the diaphragm & abdominal wall, including the falciform ligament, the inferior edge of which contains ligamentum teres, the obliterated remnant of the umbilical vein. **(Bottom)** Graphic shows the liver inverted, ewhat similar to the surgeon's view of the upwardly retracted liver. The structures in the porta hepatis include portal vein (blue), hepatic artery (red), and the bile ducts (green). The visceral surface of the liver is indented by cent viscera. The bare area is not easily accessible.

LIVER

HEPATIC ATTACHMENTS AND RELATIONS

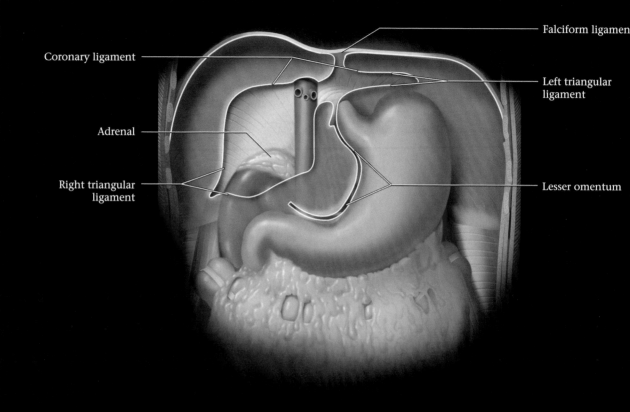

Coronary ligament

Adrenal

Right triangular ligament

Falciform ligament

Left triangular ligament

Lesser omentum

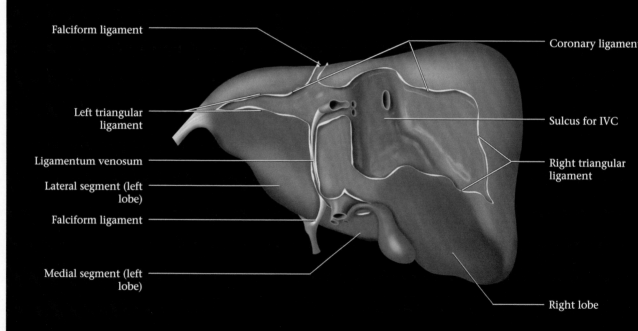

Falciform ligament

Left triangular ligament

Ligamentum venosum

Lateral segment (left lobe)

Falciform ligament

Medial segment (left lobe)

Coronary ligament

Sulcus for IVC

Right triangular ligament

Right lobe

(Top) Liver is attached to the posterior abdominal wall and diaphragm by the left & right triangular and the coronary ligaments. The falciform ligament attaches the liver to the anterior abdominal wall. The bare area is in direct contact with the right adrenal & kidney, and the IVC. **(Bottom)** Posterior view of the liver shows the ligamentous attachments. While these may help to fix the liver in position, abdominal pressure alone is sufficien evidenced by orthotopic liver transplantation, after which the ligamentous attachments are lost without the live shifting position. The diaphragmatic peritoneal reflection is the coronary ligament whose lateral extensions are t right & left triangular ligaments. The falciform ligament separates the medial & lateral segments of the left lobe.

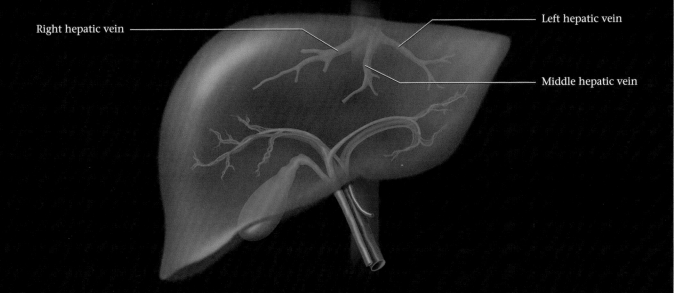

Right hepatic vein

Left hepatic vein

Middle hepatic vein

This graphic emphasizes that, at every level of branching and subdivision, the portal veins, hepatic arteries and bile ducts course together, constituting the "portal triad". Each segment of the liver is supplied by branches of these vessels. Conversely, hepatic venous branches lie between hepatic segments and interdigitate with the portal triads, but never run parallel to them.

LIVER

HEPATIC SEGMENTS

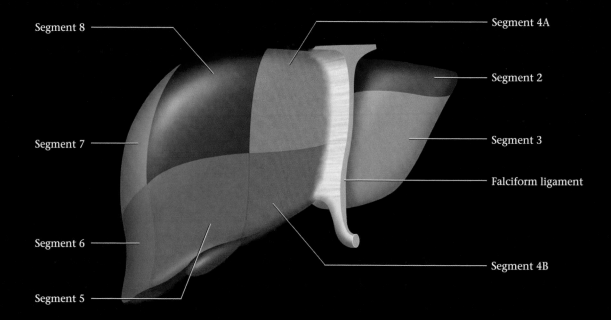

Segment 8 — Segment 4A

Segment 2

Segment 7 — Segment 3

Falciform ligament

Segment 6 — Segment 4B

Segment 5

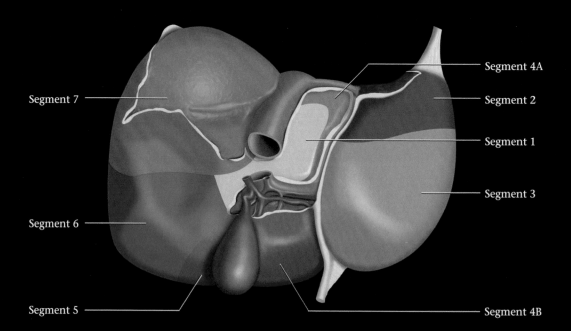

Segment 4A

Segment 7 — Segment 2

Segment 1

Segment 3

Segment 6

Segment 5 — Segment 4B

(Top) First of two graphics demonstrating the segmental anatomy of the liver in a somewhat idealized fashion. Segments are numbered in a clockwise direction, starting with the caudate lobe (segment 1), which can not be seen on this frontal view. The falciform ligament divides the lateral (segments 2 & 3) from the medial (segments 4A & 4B) left lobe. The horizontal planes separating the superior from the inferior segments follow the course of the right and left portal veins. An oblique vertical plane through the middle hepatic vein, gallbladder fossa and IVC divides the right & left lobes. **(Bottom)** Posterior view of the liver shows that the caudate is entirely posterior, abutting the IVC, ligamentum venosum & porta hepatis. A plane through the IVC and gallbladder divides the left & right lobes.

LIVER

Middle hepatic vein — Left hepatic vein

Right hepatic vein — IVC

Middle hepatic vein

Right portal vein (anterior segment)

Right hepatic vein

Medial segment branch — Lateral segment branch

Right portal vein (anterior) — Left portal vein

Right hepatic vein

Right portal vein (posterior)

(Top) First of nine axial CT sections shows the confluence of the hepatic veins with the IVC just below the diaphragm and the entrance of the IVC into the right atrium. **(Middle)** At this level the portal veins run in a predominantly cephalo-caudal direction and bisect the angle made by the hepatic veins. Portal veins generally lie within hepatic segments, while hepatic veins lie between segments. **(Bottom)** The horizontal plane defined by the left portal vein divides the lateral segment into segment 2 (above the vein) and 3 (below).

LIVER

AXIAL CT, NORMAL LIVER

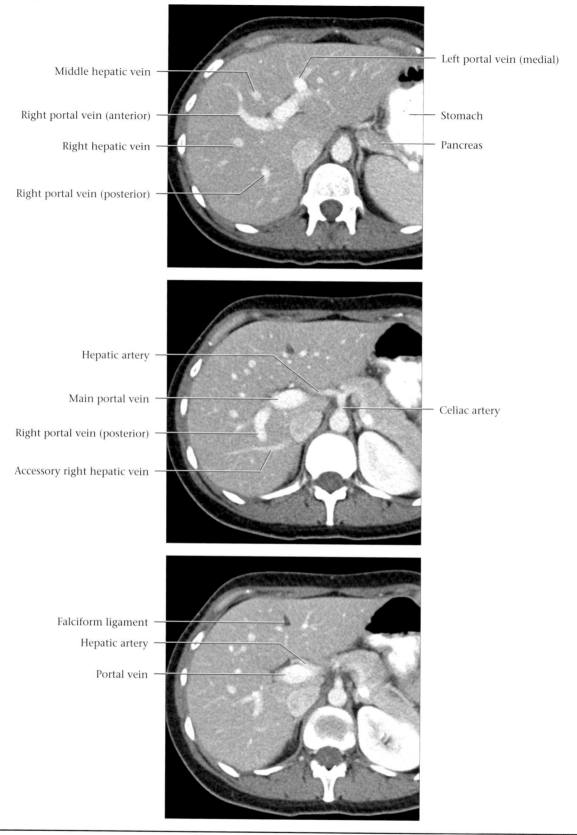

Middle hepatic vein

Right portal vein (anterior)

Right hepatic vein

Right portal vein (posterior)

Left portal vein (medial)

Stomach

Pancreas

Hepatic artery

Main portal vein

Right portal vein (posterior)

Accessory right hepatic vein

Celiac artery

Falciform ligament

Hepatic artery

Portal vein

(Top) The plane of section through the long axis of the right portal vein divides segments 7 & 8 (above) from segments 5 & 6 (below). Note the relations between the liver, stomach, and pancreas. (Middle) The hepatic artery arises conventionally in this subject, from the celiac artery. There is an accessory right hepatic vein that drains directly into the IVC, caudal to the confluence of the other hepatic veins. (Bottom) Note the fissure for the falciform ligament which separates the medial and lateral segments of the liver (segment 4 from segments 2 & 3).

LIVER

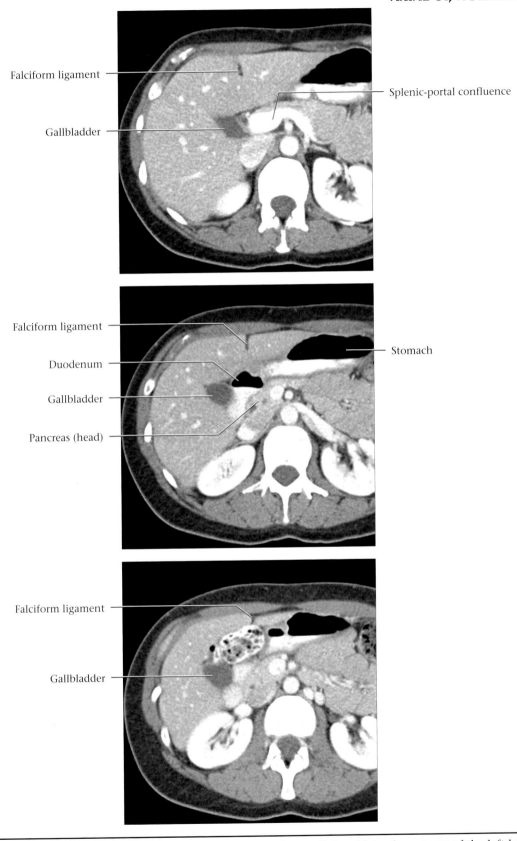

(Top) A vertical plane through the falciform ligament separates the medial and lateral segments of the left lobe, while a vertical plane through the gallbladder fossa and middle hepatic vein separates the right and left lobes. **(Middle)** Note the relations between the liver and adjacent organs. **(Bottom)** The right lobe of the liver extends much more caudally than the left, occasionally, even into the pelvis. The considerable variability of the shape of the liver makes it difficult to identify hepatomegaly by physical examination alone, especially since only the ventral, inferior edge of the liver can be palpated.

LIVER

PORTAL VENOUS SYSTEM

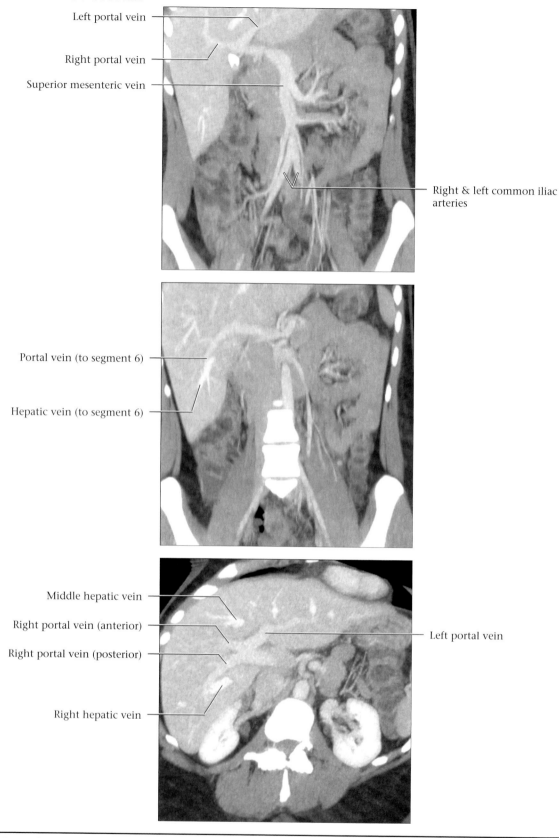

Left portal vein

Right portal vein

Superior mesenteric vein

Right & left common iliac arteries

Portal vein (to segment 6)

Hepatic vein (to segment 6)

Middle hepatic vein

Right portal vein (anterior)

Right portal vein (posterior)

Left portal vein

Right hepatic vein

(Top) First of three CT images emphasizing the portal venous system. This coronal reformation of a CT scan in the venous phase of imaging shows the superior mesenteric vein and its branches as well as the portal vein. The (arbitrary) thickness and plane of the section exclude the splenic vein and include the iliac arteries. **(Middle)** Coronal plane through the posterior segments of the liver shows the hepatic artery and portal vein branches to segment 6. **(Bottom)** Thick reconstructed axial section shows a "trifurcation" pattern of the portal vein, in which the left portal vein and the anterior & posterior branches of the right portal vein all arise directly from the main portal vein.

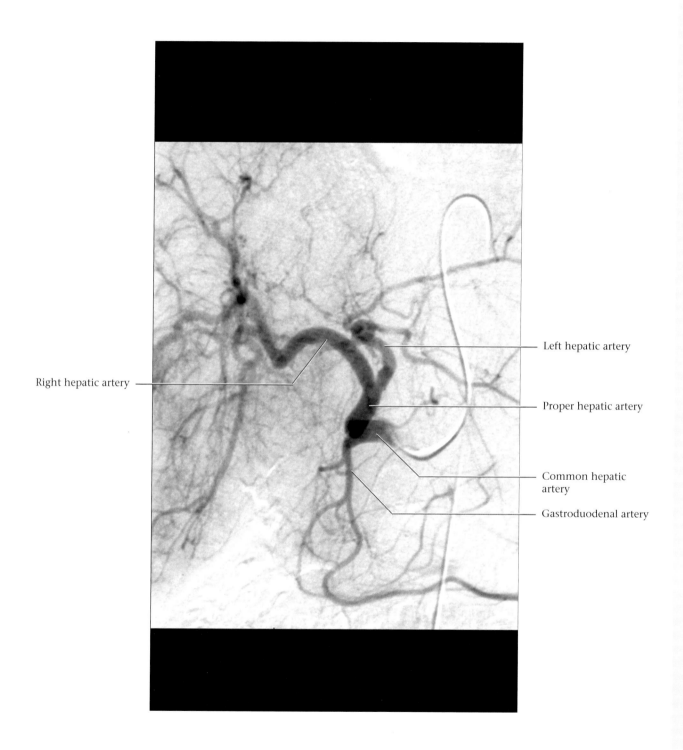

Right hepatic artery

Left hepatic artery

Proper hepatic artery

Common hepatic artery

Gastroduodenal artery

Selective catheterization of the common hepatic artery demonstrates conventional arterial anatomy, in which all the hepatic arteries arise from the celiac axis. Variations in hepatic arterial supply are very common and important to recognize, especially if partial hepatic resection is being considered.

LIVER

CELIAC AND HEPATIC ARTERIES

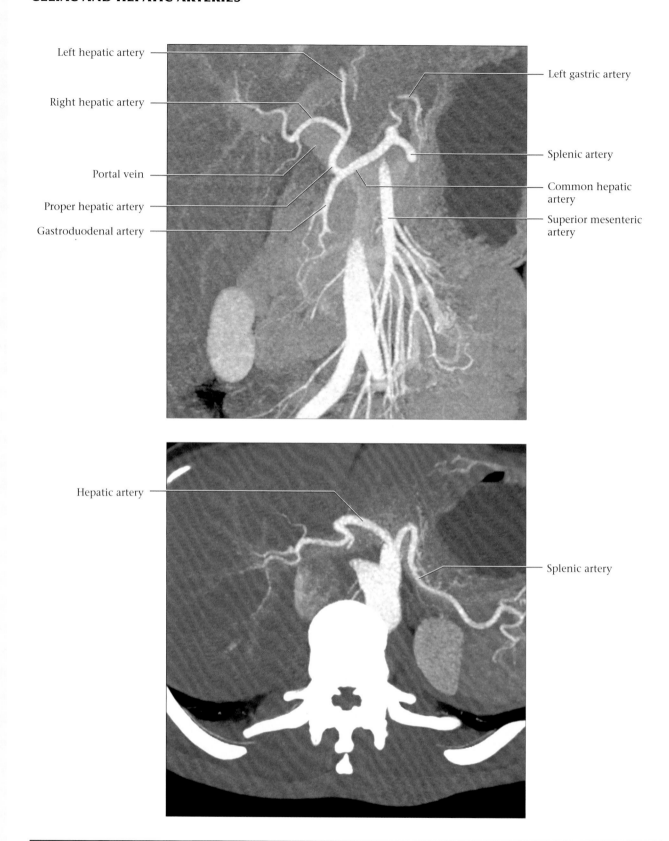

(Top) First of two CT images showing conventional hepatic arterial anatomy. This coronal reformation shows both hepatic arteries arising from the proper hepatic artery which, in turn, arises from the common hepatic artery. Also visible are the portal venous branches, less well opacified as this image was obtained in the predominantly arterial phase of enhancement. (Bottom) A thick axial reconstructed CT image shows the hepatic and splenic arteries arising from the celiac artery.

LIVER

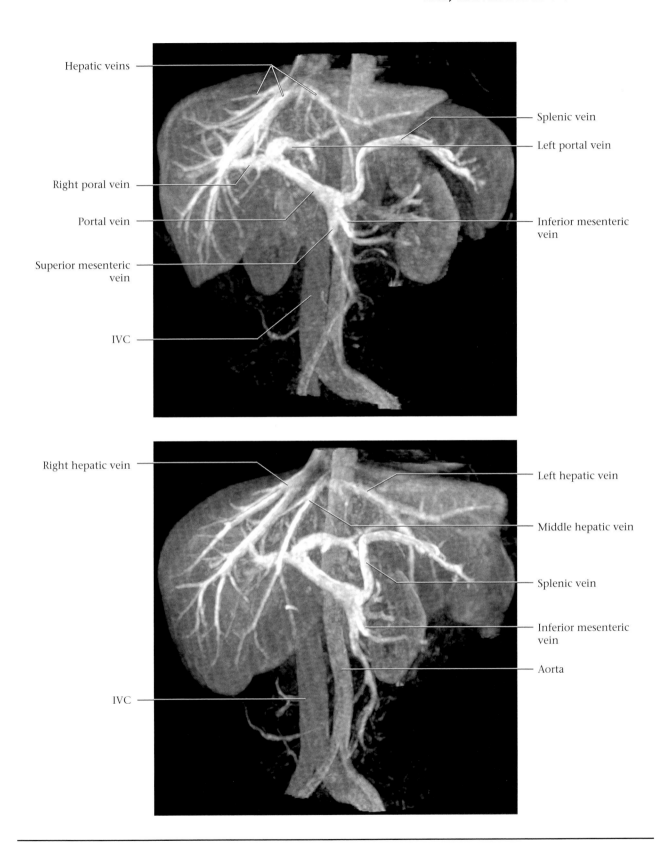

Hepatic veins

Right poral vein

Portal vein

Superior mesenteric vein

IVC

Splenic vein

Left portal vein

Inferior mesenteric vein

Right hepatic vein

IVC

Left hepatic vein

Middle hepatic vein

Splenic vein

Inferior mesenteric vein

Aorta

(**Top**) First of two coronal maximum intensity projection (MIP) images from a contrast-enhanced MR scan shows the major divisions and tributaries of the hepatic and portal veins. Only a few branches of the superior mesenteric vein are included in this plane of section, making it appear artifactually small. (**Bottom**) In this subject the inferior mesenteric vein joins the confluence of the superior mesenteric and splenic veins. Some of the intravenously injected contrast medium is still circulating through the arteries, resulting in opacification of the aorta.

LIVER

SONOGRAPHY, NORMAL ANATOMY

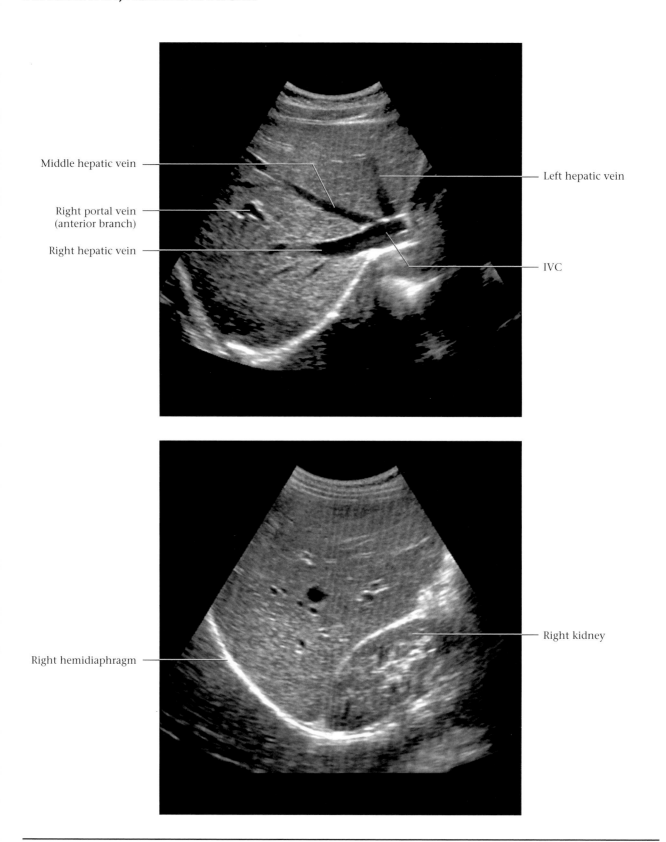

Middle hepatic vein

Right portal vein (anterior branch)

Right hepatic vein

Left hepatic vein

IVC

Right hemidiaphragm

Right kidney

(Top) First of two ultrasound images of the liver. Axial section shows the confluence of the hepatic veins as they enter the IVC. The portal veins generally have a more prominent, echogenic rim. **(Bottom)** Sagittal section through the liver shows its smooth and homogeneous echogenicity with interspersed vessels and small intrahepatic bile ducts.

LIVER

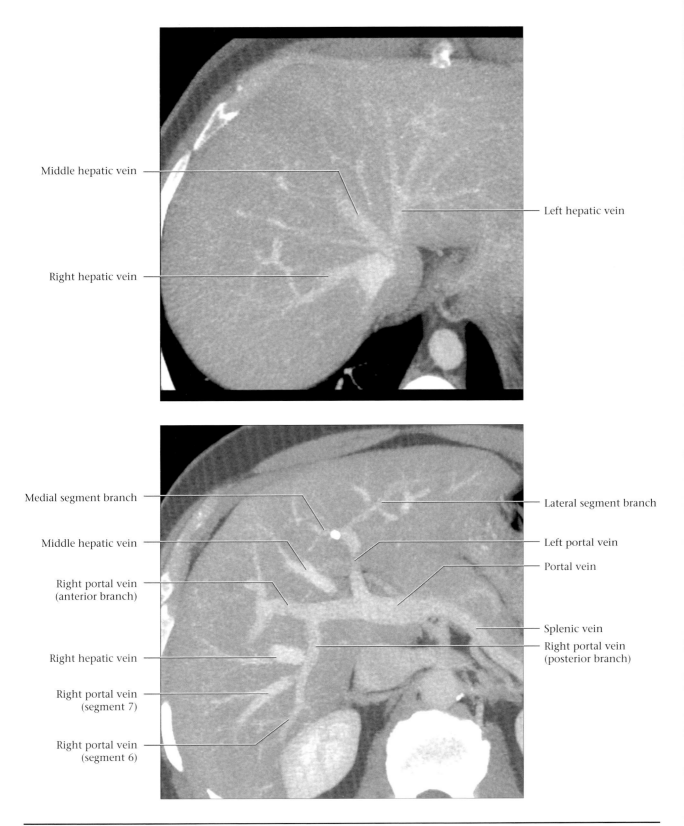

Middle hepatic vein

Right hepatic vein

Left hepatic vein

Medial segment branch

Middle hepatic vein

Right portal vein (anterior branch)

Right hepatic vein

Right portal vein (segment 7)

Right portal vein (segment 6)

Lateral segment branch

Left portal vein

Portal vein

Splenic vein

Right portal vein (posterior branch)

(Top) First of six CT sections through normal liver. This thick axial plane reconstruction shows the confluence of the hepatic veins. **(Bottom)** Another thick axial reconstructed image shows the intrahepatic portal and hepatic veins.

LIVER

MULTIPLANAR CT, NORMAL VESSELS

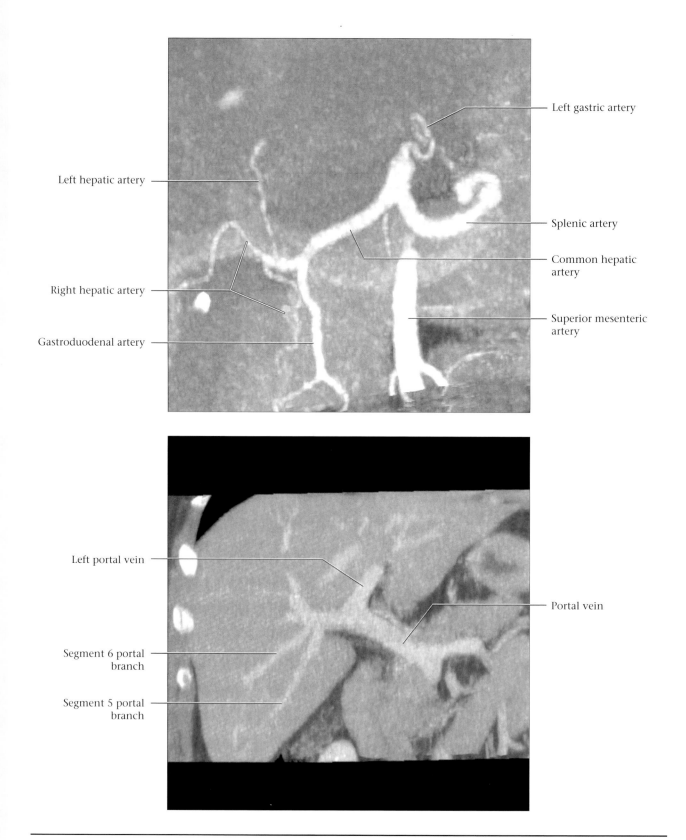

Left gastric artery

Left hepatic artery

Splenic artery

Common hepatic artery

Right hepatic artery

Superior mesenteric artery

Gastroduodenal artery

Left portal vein

Portal vein

Segment 6 portal branch

Segment 5 portal branch

(Top) CT section reformatted into the coronal plane. This image was obtained in the arterial phase of contrast enhancement and shows the origins of the celiac and superior mesenteric arteries. The hepatic arteries arise conventionally from branches of the celiac trunk. (Bottom) A coronal image from the portal venous phase of enhancement shows the major branches of the portal vein.

MULTIPLANAR CT, NORMAL VESSELS

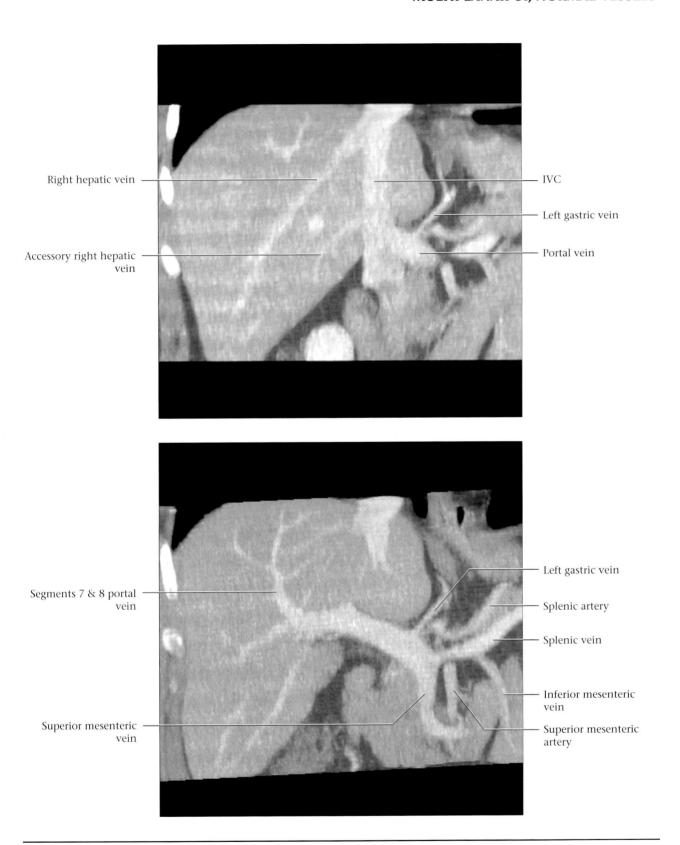

Right hepatic vein

Accessory right hepatic vein

IVC

Left gastric vein

Portal vein

Segments 7 & 8 portal vein

Superior mesenteric vein

Left gastric vein

Splenic artery

Splenic vein

Inferior mesenteric vein

Superior mesenteric artery

(Top) Coronal plane image shows the entry of the right hepatic vein into the IVC. A small accessory right hepatic vein is also present. The thick plane of reconstruction artifactually suggests that the portal vein is entering the IVC. **(Bottom)** Coronal image includes the major tributaries of the portal vein, including the superior & inferior mesenteric veins and the splenic vein. Recirculation of contrast medium results in residual enhancement of some arteries that also lie in this plane of section.

LIVER

AXIAL T2WI FS MR

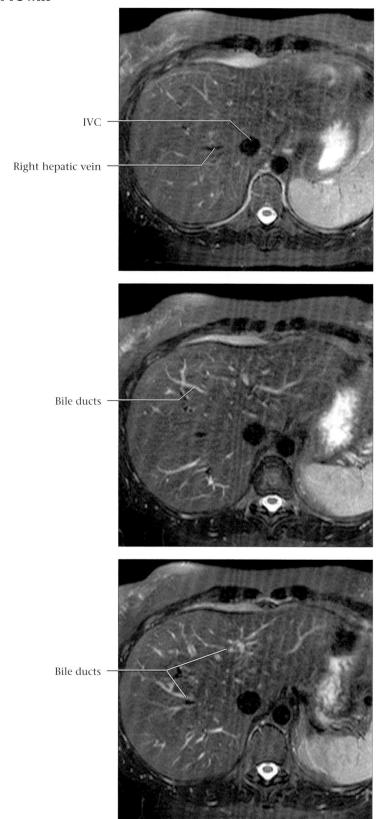

IVC

Right hepatic vein

Bile ducts

Bile ducts

(Top) First of nine axial T2 weighted fat-suppressed MR images shows relatively low signal from the liver parenchyma. Flowing blood appears very dark, while static fluid, such as bile and spinal fluid appears quite bright. **(Middle)** The branching pattern of the intrahepatic bile ducts is evident. **(Bottom)** A more caudal section shows the bile ducts becoming larger as they approach the porta hepatis.

LIVER

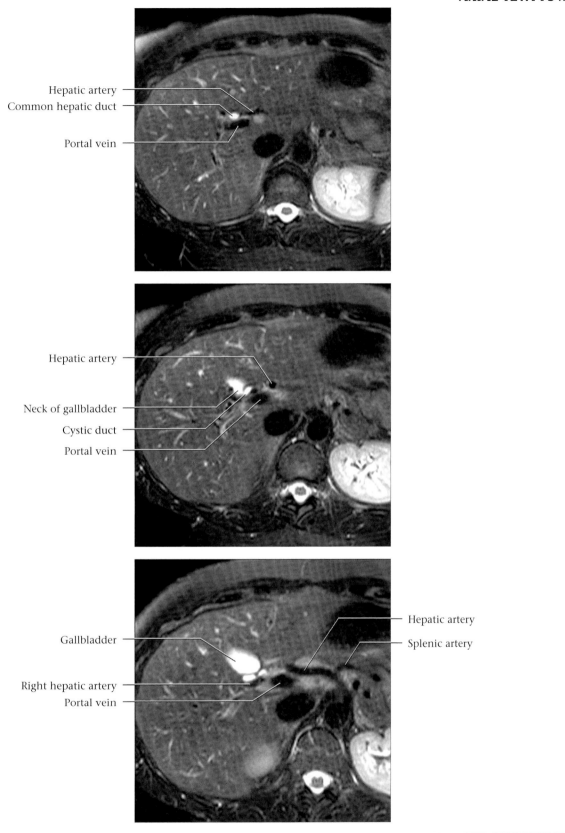

Hepatic artery
Common hepatic duct
Portal vein

Hepatic artery
Neck of gallbladder
Cystic duct
Portal vein

Gallbladder
Right hepatic artery
Portal vein
Hepatic artery
Splenic artery

(Top) More caudal section shows the usual relation between the bile duct, portal vein, and hepatic artery near the porta hepatis. (Middle) The neck of the gallbladder and cystic duct are seen on this section. (Bottom) Section through the porta hepatis shows the hepatic artery and portal vein entering the liver.

LIVER

AXIAL T2WI FS MR

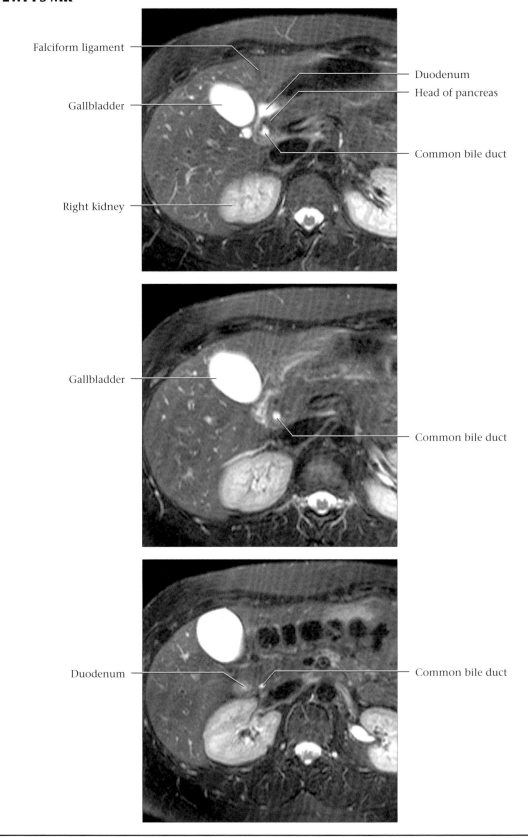

Falciform ligament

Gallbladder

Right kidney

Duodenum

Head of pancreas

Common bile duct

Gallbladder

Common bile duct

Duodenum

Common bile duct

(Top) The common duct leaves the liver, descends medial to the second portion of the duodenum and enters the pancreatic head. **(Middle)** The vertical course of the bile duct within the pancreatic head is seen well on this image. **(Bottom)** The bile duct is seen just proximal to its confluence with the pancreatic duct and their entry into the pancreaticobiliary ampulla in the duodenum.

LIVER

AXIAL T1WI MR, HEPATIC ARTERIAL PHASE

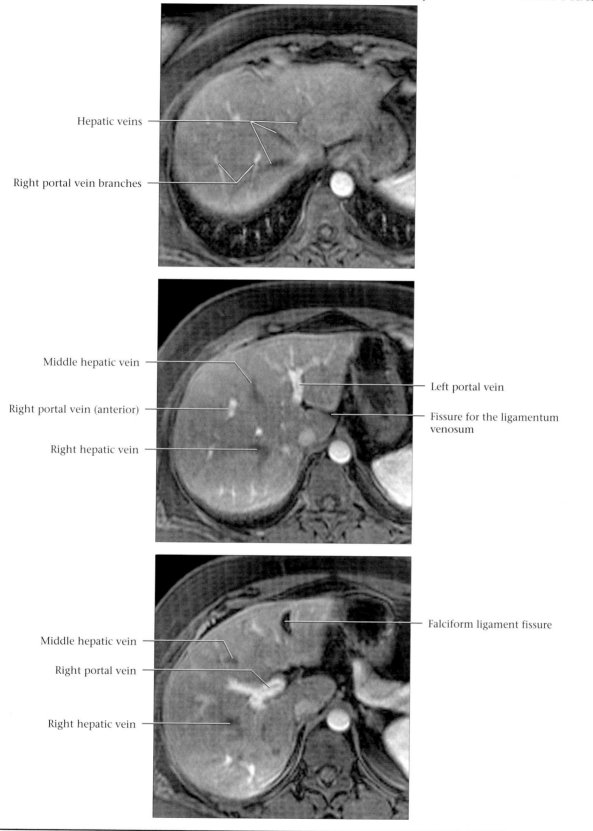

Hepatic veins

Right portal vein branches

Middle hepatic vein

Right portal vein (anterior)

Right hepatic vein

Left portal vein

Fissure for the ligamentum venosum

Middle hepatic vein

Right portal vein

Right hepatic vein

Falciform ligament fissure

(Top) First of six axial T1-weighted MR images obtained during the arterial (portal venous inflow) phase of contrast-enhancement shows the hepatic veins as dark, unenhanced structures, while the aorta, arteries, and portal venous branches are bright due to contrast-enhancement. **(Middle)** The portal and hepatic venous branches are well seen on this section. **(Bottom)** A more caudal section again shows the opacified portal vein branches and the unopacified hepatic veins.

LIVER

AXIAL T1WI MR, HEPATIC ARTERIAL PHASE

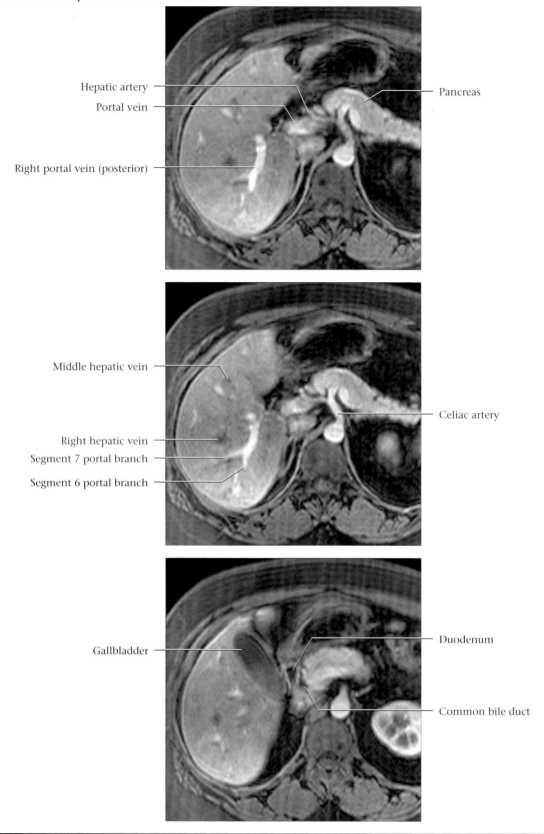

Hepatic artery — Portal vein — Pancreas

Right portal vein (posterior)

Middle hepatic vein — Celiac artery

Right hepatic vein
Segment 7 portal branch
Segment 6 portal branch

Gallbladder — Duodenum — Common bile duct

(Top) The pancreas, arteries, and portal veins are well-opacified on this image. (Middle) Note the intra-segmental position of the portal vein branches, while the hepatic veins lie between segments (in general). (Bottom) On these T1-weighted images, static fluid-containing structures, such as the gallbladder and duodenum, appear dark (low signal).

LIVER

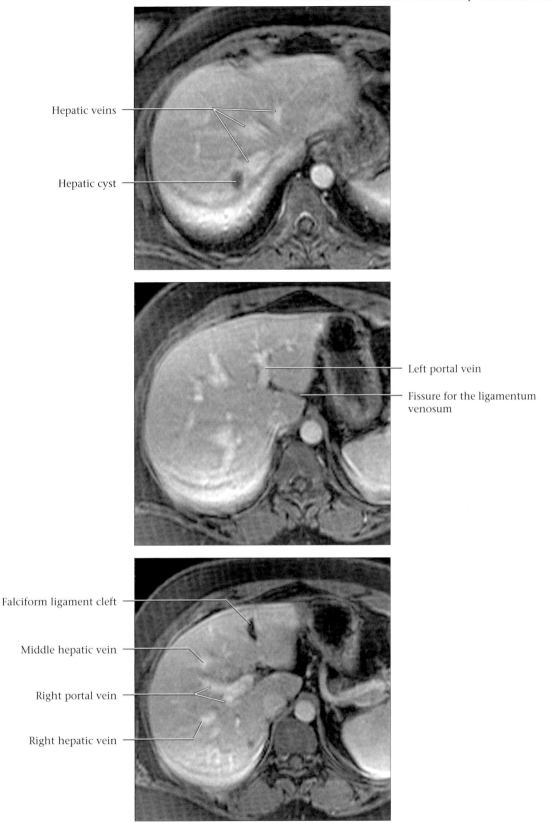

Hepatic veins

Hepatic cyst

Left portal vein

Fissure for the ligamentum venosum

Falciform ligament cleft

Middle hepatic vein

Right portal vein

Right hepatic vein

(Top) First of three axial T1-weighted MR images obtained during the hepatic venous phase of enhancement, when all the vascular structures in the liver are of bright signal due to contrast-enhancement. A small cyst is seen adjacent to the right hepatic vein. (Middle) The portal and hepatic vein branches are all enhanced. (Bottom) The fissures and paths of the major veins are well identified, aiding in the definition of hepatic segmental anatomy.

LIVER

LIVER SEGMENTAL ANATOMY

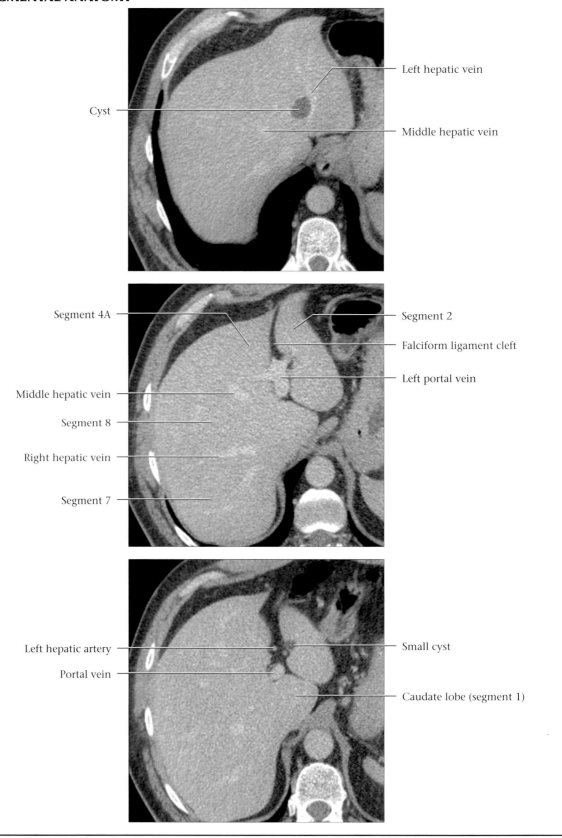

Cyst — Left hepatic vein

Middle hepatic vein

Segment 4A — Segment 2

Falciform ligament cleft

Left portal vein

Middle hepatic vein

Segment 8

Right hepatic vein

Segment 7

Left hepatic artery — Small cyst

Portal vein

Caudate lobe (segment 1)

(**Top**) First of six axial CT sections. Dividing the right and left lobes is a vertical plane connecting the middle hepatic vein and the gallbladder fossa. The plane of the falciform ligament divides the medial (segment 4) from the lateral (segments 2 & 3) left lobe. The cyst is above the plane of the falciform ligament, probably within segment 4A. (**Middle**) A vertical plane passing through the right hepatic vein divides segments 5 & 8 anteriorly from segments 6 & 7 posteriorly. Segments 7 & 8 lie above the plane of the right portal vein, while segments 5 & 6 lie below it. The medial segment is sometimes divided into 4A and 4B, with 4A being the more cephalic. (**Bottom**) A small cyst is seen in segment 3. The caudate lobe (segment 1) lies high along the posterior surface of the liver, bordered by the portal vein and fissure for the ligamentum venosum anteriorly & the IVC posteriorly.

LIVER

LIVER SEGMENTAL ANATOMY

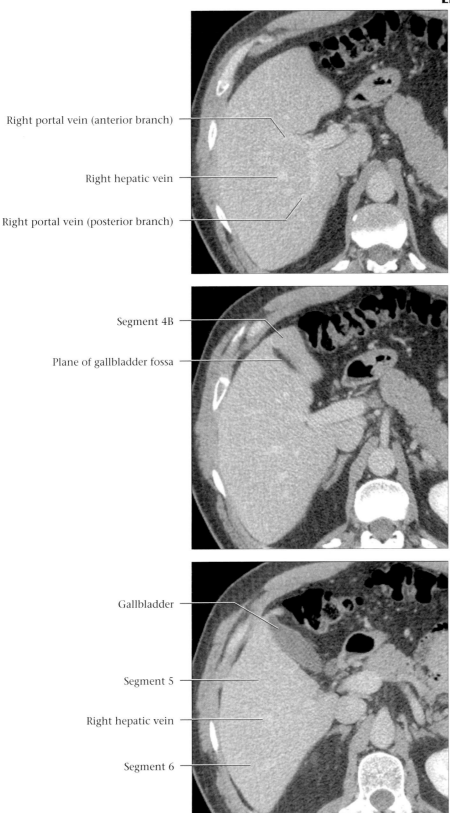

Right portal vein (anterior branch)

Right hepatic vein

Right portal vein (posterior branch)

Segment 4B

Plane of gallbladder fossa

Gallbladder

Segment 5

Right hepatic vein

Segment 6

(Top) The posterior branch of the right portal vein supplies segments 6 & 7, while the anterior branch supplies segments 5 & 8. A vertical plane through the right hepatic vein separates the anterior (segments 5 & 8) from the posterior segments (6 & 7) of the right lobe. Segments 7 & 8 lie above the plane of the right portal vein while 5 & 6 lie below it. **(Middle)** A plane passing vertically through the middle hepatic vein and the gallbladder fossa divides the left and right lobes of the liver. The medial segment (4) lies just medial to this plane. **(Bottom)** The inferior segments of the right lobe are seen on this section, segment 5 anterior to the right hepatic vein, and segment 6 posterior to it.

LIVER

FALCIFORM LIGAMENT

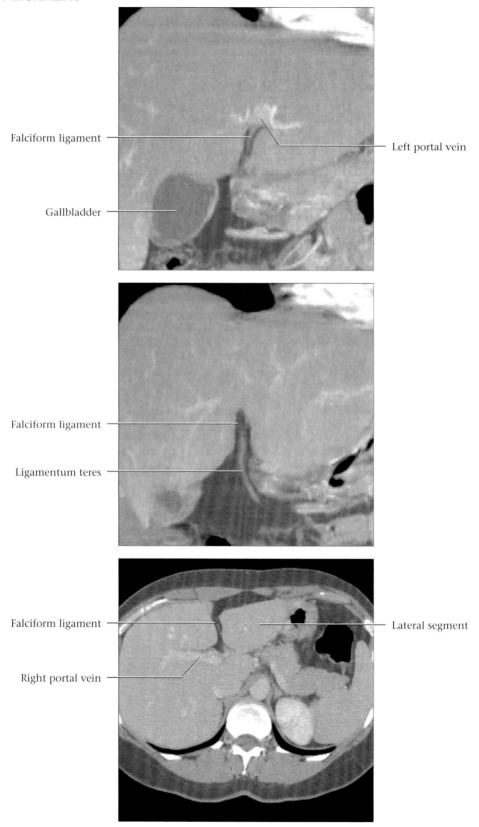

(Top) First of three CT sections showing the falciform ligament in various planes. Coronal reformation through the middle of the liver shows the falciform ligament dividing the medial and lateral segments of the left lobe. The ascending portion of the left portal vein also lies in the falciform ligament. **(Middle)** A more anterior coronal section shows the ligamentum teres, the obliterated remnant of the umbilical vein, which lies in the falciform ligament before leaving the antero-inferior surface of the liver to extend to the umbilicus. **(Bottom)** This axial section shows the ligamentum teres within the falciform ligament.

LIVER

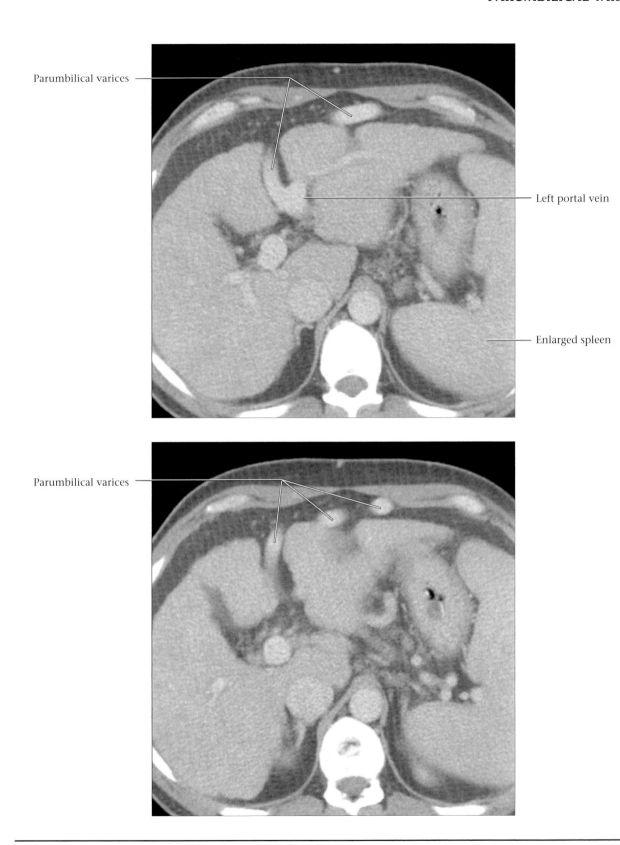

Parumbilical varices

Left portal vein

Enlarged spleen

Parumbilical varices

(Top) First of four axial CT sections in a patient with cirrhosis and portal hypertension shows large parumbilical collateral veins (varices) communicating with the left portal vein. Flow within these vessels is "hepatofugal" (away from the liver), as blood is being diverted away from the liver into the systemic venous system due to the increased resistance to flow into the liver (portal hypertension). **(Bottom)** Note the shrunken, nodular appearance of the liver and the widened fissures, all characteristic of cirrhosis.

LIVER

PARUMBILICAL VARICES

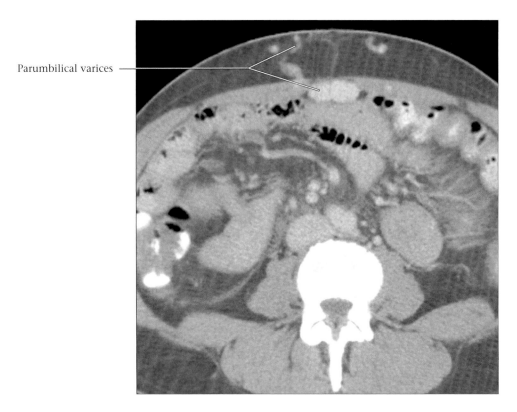

Parumbilical varices

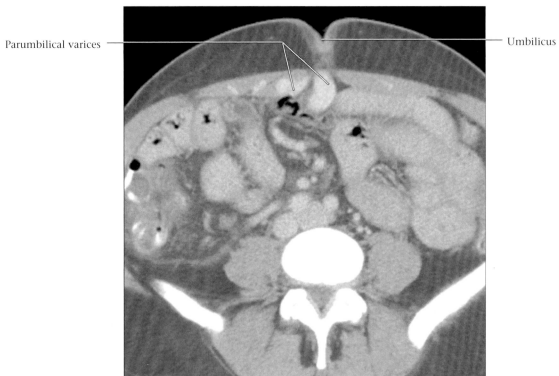

Parumbilical varices — Umbilicus

(**Top**) As the parumbilical varices run caudally, they approach the anterior abdominal wall and surround the umbilicus. These are often visible on physical examination and have been likened to the mythological Medusa, whose hair was a tangle of snakes ("caput Medusae"). (**Bottom**) The parumbilical varices are evident immediately below the umbilicus. In fetal life, there are three common areas in which the systemic and portal venous systems come into contact and form anastomoses, including the parumbilical region, around the distal esophagus, and around the rectum. These, in turn, are the most common sites of portal-systemic shunts (varices) that develop in patients with portal hypertension or other etiologies of increased pressure within the venous system.

LIVER

CONGENITAL HYPOPLASIA OF SEGMENTS

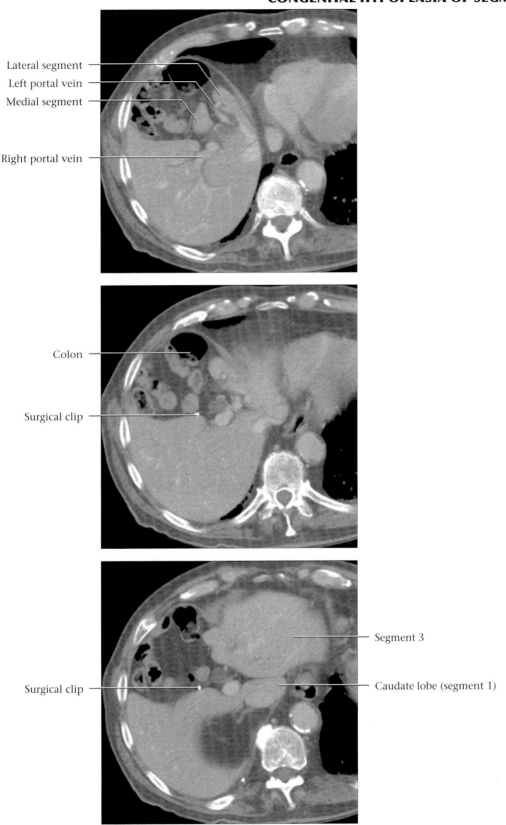

Lateral segment
Left portal vein
Medial segment

Right portal vein

Colon

Surgical clip

Surgical clip

Segment 3

Caudate lobe (segment 1)

(Top) First of three axial CT sections shows colon in the right subphrenic region normally occupied by the anterior and medial segments of the liver. This person is asymptomatic and has not had surgical resection nor a history of liver disease. Note the relative absence of tissue lateral to the left portal vein which lies in the falciform ligament (boundary between the medial & lateral segments). The anterior branch of the right portal vein is absent. **(Middle)** A surgical clip is present from a prior cholecystectomy, during which the congenital hypoplasia of hepatic segments was confirmed. **(Bottom)** Congenital hypoplasia usually affects the anterior and medial segments, though any portion of the liver may fail to develop normally. This is one of the common causes of so-called "interposition" of the colon between the liver and the right hemidiaphragm.

HEPATIC ARTERIAL VARIANTS

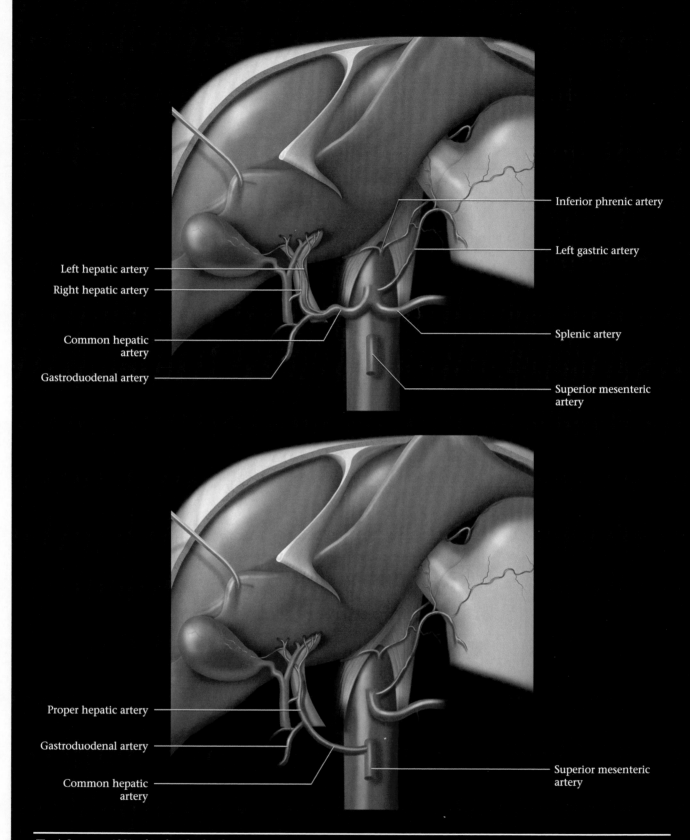

Inferior phrenic artery

Left gastric artery

Left hepatic artery

Right hepatic artery

Common hepatic artery

Gastroduodenal artery

Splenic artery

Superior mesenteric artery

Proper hepatic artery

Gastroduodenal artery

Common hepatic artery

Superior mesenteric artery

(Top) In over 40% of individuals, there are variations in the origin & course of the hepatic arteries that differ from the "conventional" depiction. In this graphic the left hepatic artery arises from the common hepatic artery, proximal to the origin of the gastroduodenal artery. The gallbladder and extrahepatic common bile duct are supplied by the right hepatic artery, as usual. The hepatic artery courses parallel to the portal vein and lies between the vein and the bile duct. **(Bottom)** Graphic shows a completely replaced hepatic artery, arising from the superior mesenteric artery (SMA). In this setting the hepatic artery passes through or behind the head of the pancreas and the portal vein, and may be inadvertently ligated during pancreatic surgery if this variant is not recognized.

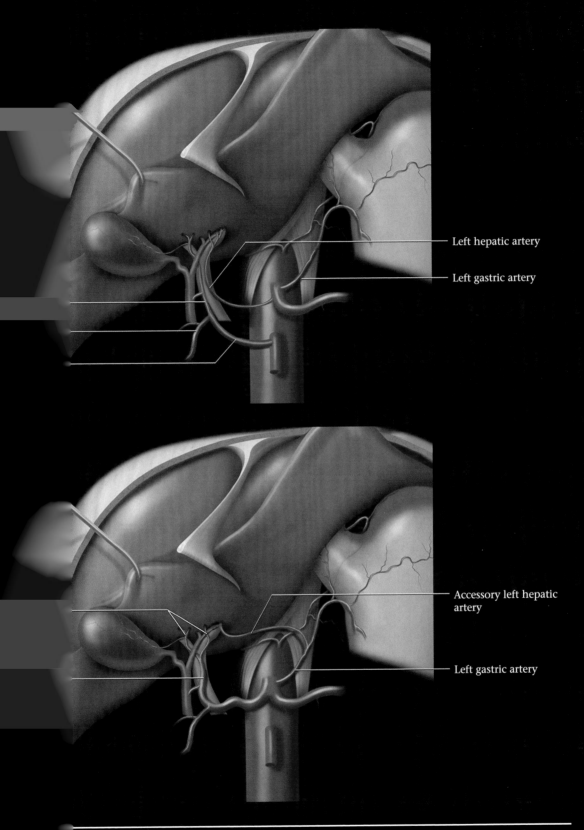

Left hepatic artery

Left gastric artery

Accessory left hepatic artery

Left gastric artery

eparate origin of the left hepatic artery from the celiac trunk. In addition, the right hepatic
g from the SMA. The gastroduodenal & cystic arteries arise from the replaced right hepatic,
riation. **(Bottom)** Graphic depicts an "accessory" left hepatic artery, arising from the left
y artery is a vessel in addition to those originating from the conventional depiction; in this
c artery arising from the proper hepatic artery as well. All of these variations are common
ns for patients undergoing any sort of upper abdominal surgery, especially partial hepatic

LIVER

ACCESSORY RIGHT HEPATIC ARTERY

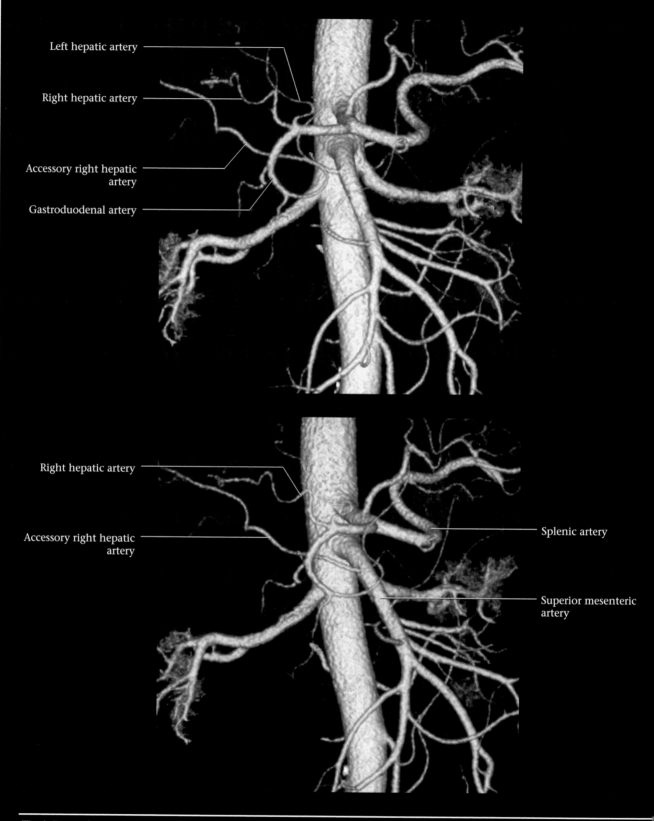

Left hepatic artery

Right hepatic artery

Accessory right hepatic artery

Gastroduodenal artery

Right hepatic artery

Accessory right hepatic artery

Splenic artery

Superior mesenteric artery

(Top) First of two shaded surface display, coronally reformatted CT angiogram images shows only a small right hepatic artery branch from the common hepatic artery. An accessory right hepatic branch arises from the superior mesenteric artery, a common variant. Note the anastomoses between the accessory right hepatic and gastroduodenal arteries. **(Bottom)** Oblique view of the CTA helps to confirm the origin of the accessory hepatic vessel from the SMA.

COMPLETELY REPLACED HEPATIC ARTERY

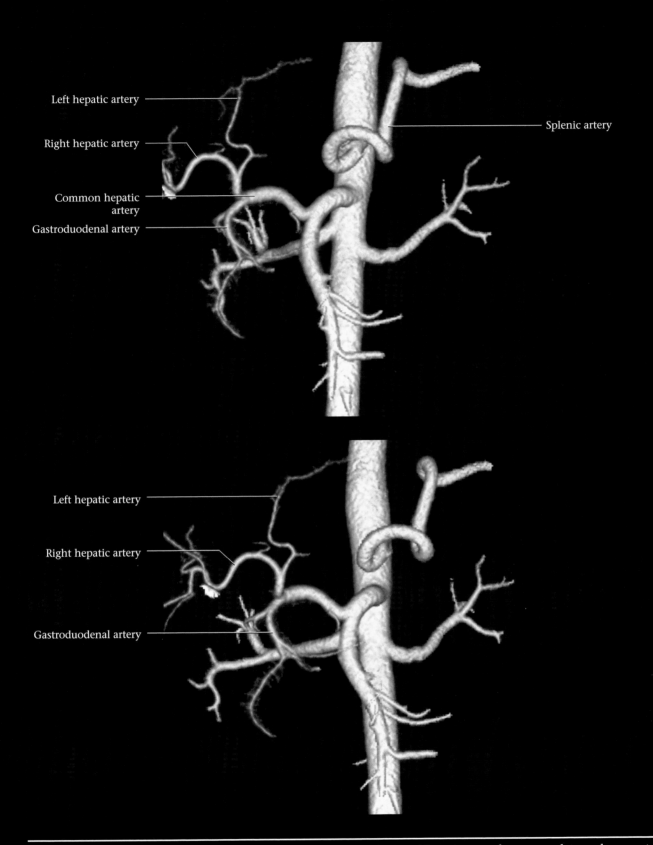

Left hepatic artery

Right hepatic artery

Common hepatic artery

Gastroduodenal artery

Splenic artery

Left hepatic artery

Right hepatic artery

Gastroduodenal artery

(Top) First of two shaded surface, coronally reformatted images from a CT angiogram shows complete replacement of the common hepatic artery from the SMA. Both major hepatic arteries and the gastroduodenal artery arise from the SMA instead of the celiac artery. **(Bottom)** Oblique view helps to confirm the origin of the arteries.

LIVER

REPLACED RIGHT AND LEFT HEPATIC ARTERIES

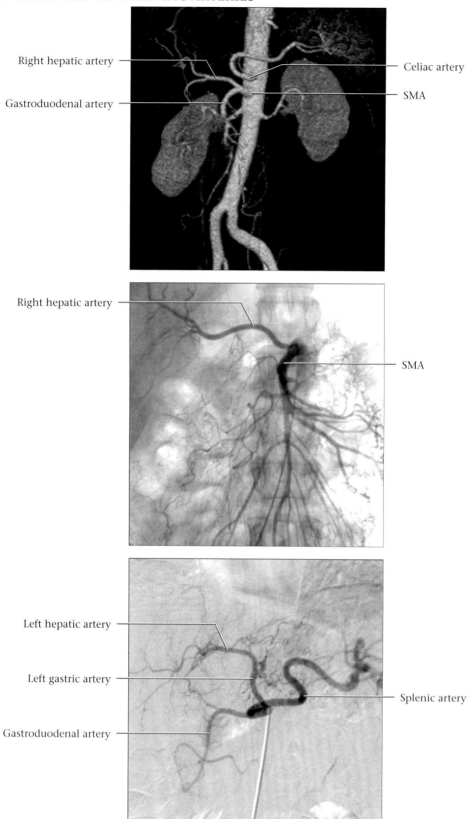

Right hepatic artery — Celiac artery

Gastroduodenal artery — SMA

Right hepatic artery — SMA

Left hepatic artery

Left gastric artery

Gastroduodenal artery — Splenic artery

(Top) First of three images in a person with separately replaced right & left hepatic arteries. Coronal CT angiogram shows the right hepatic artery arising from the SMA. The origin of the left hepatic artery is not shown clearly on this image. (Middle) A frontal film from a conventional catheter angiogram shows the replaced right hepatic artery arising from the SMA. (Bottom) Catheter injection of the celiac axis shows the left hepatic artery arising from the left gastric artery. In this subject the gastroduodenal artery arises directly from the celiac artery. Variations of hepatic arterial anatomy are common and are important to recognize when hepatic transplantation, surgery or other intervention is being considered.

LIVER

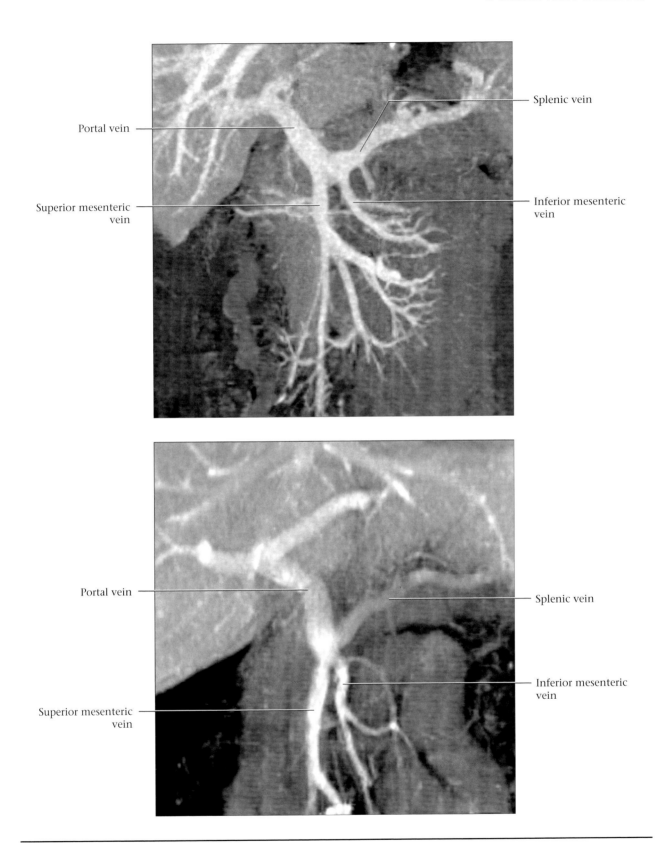

Portal vein

Superior mesenteric vein

Splenic vein

Inferior mesenteric vein

Portal vein

Superior mesenteric vein

Splenic vein

Inferior mesenteric vein

(Top) MR angiogram (venous phase following IV injection of contrast medium) shows the most common arrangement of the major tributaries of the portal vein, in which the inferior mesenteric vein joins the splenic vein just prior to its confluence with the superior mesenteric vein. **(Bottom)** In this person the MRA demonstrates confluence of all three major tributaries at a trifurcated confluence.

LIVER

LIVER VESSELS, UNFAVORABLE FOR TRANSPLANTATION

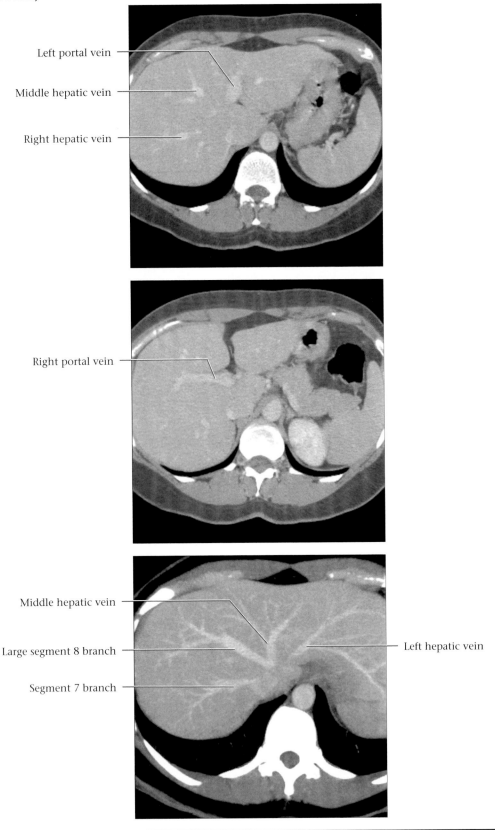

Left portal vein

Middle hepatic vein

Right hepatic vein

Right portal vein

Middle hepatic vein

Large segment 8 branch

Segment 7 branch

Left hepatic vein

(Top) First of five CT images of a person who was being evaluated as a potential partial liver donor, in which the right hepatic lobe would be resected and given to a recipient. This axial section seems normal. (Middle) Axial section also fails to suggest any vascular anomaly. (Bottom) A thick axial reconstructed image shows a large branch from segment 8 (of the right lobe) draining into the middle hepatic vein. In the usual incision used for harvesting the right lobe, the liver is divided just to the right of the middle hepatic vein, which would sever the segment 8 branch and require a separate anastomosis to the recipient IVC.

LIVER

LIVER VESSELS, UNFAVORABLE FOR TRANSPLANTATION

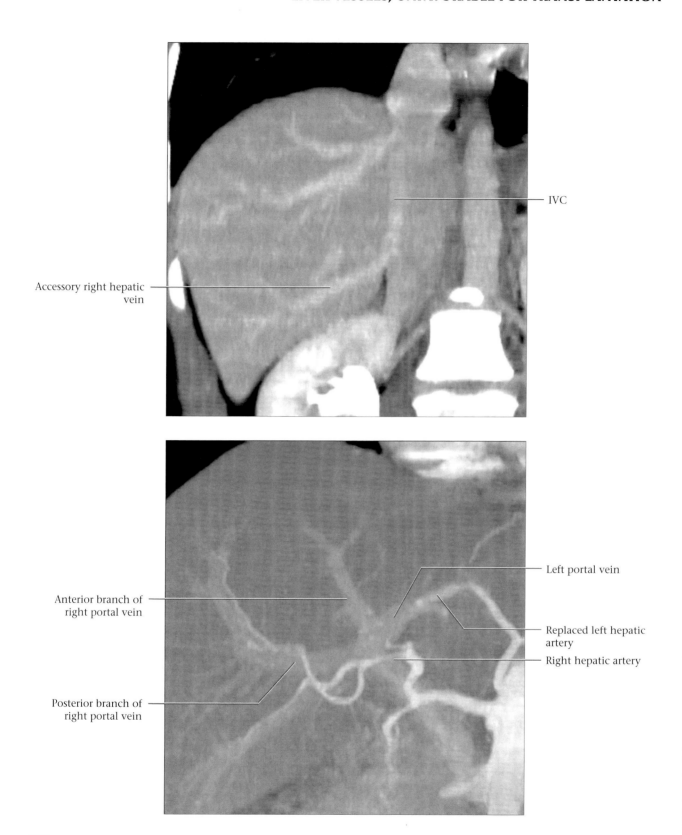

(Top) Coronal reformation shows a large accessory right hepatic vein draining segments 5 & 6 directly into the IVC. If the right lobe were to be used in transplantation, this would require still another separate anastomosis to the recipient IVC. (Bottom) Coronal MIP image in the late arterial, early portal venous phase shows a trifurcation arrangement of the portal vein, in which the anterior & posterior branches of the right portal and the left portal vein all join at the same point. This anatomical variant makes it difficult for the surgeon to transect the right portal vein without jeopardizing the left portal vein which must supply the remaining liver of the donor. Due to the various vascular anatomic variants demonstrated by CT in this person, he was judged to not be a candidate for living donation.

LIVER

COLLATERAL FLOW THROUGH LIVER

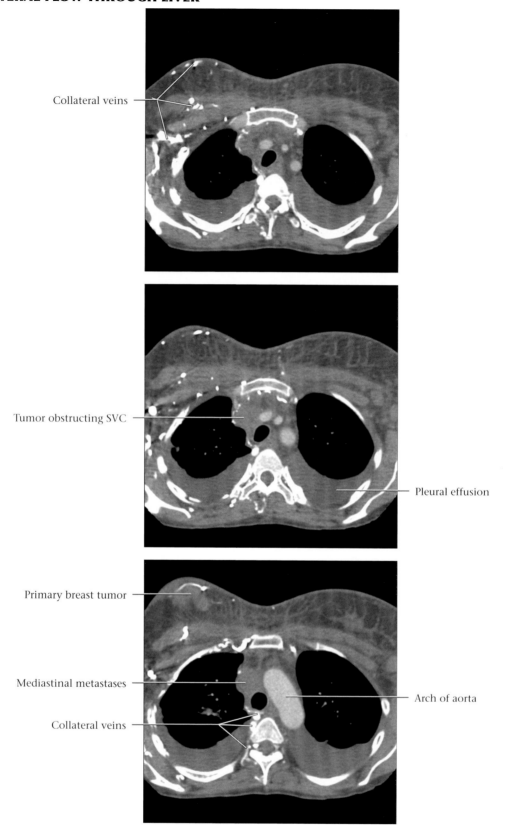

Collateral veins

Tumor obstructing SVC

Pleural effusion

Primary breast tumor

Mediastinal metastases

Arch of aorta

Collateral veins

(Top) First of six CT images in a woman with breast cancer and mediastinal nodal metastases causing obstruction of the superior vena cava. Contrast injection through a right arm vein shows opacification of numerous collateral veins in the chest wall that are bypassing the occluded SVC. (Middle) More caudal section shows continuation of the collateral veins and tumor occluding the SVC. (Bottom) More caudal section shows the primary tumor site in the right breast and additional mediastinal metastases. Numerous collateral veins are noted in the chest wall and paraspinal region.

COLLATERAL FLOW THROUGH LIVER

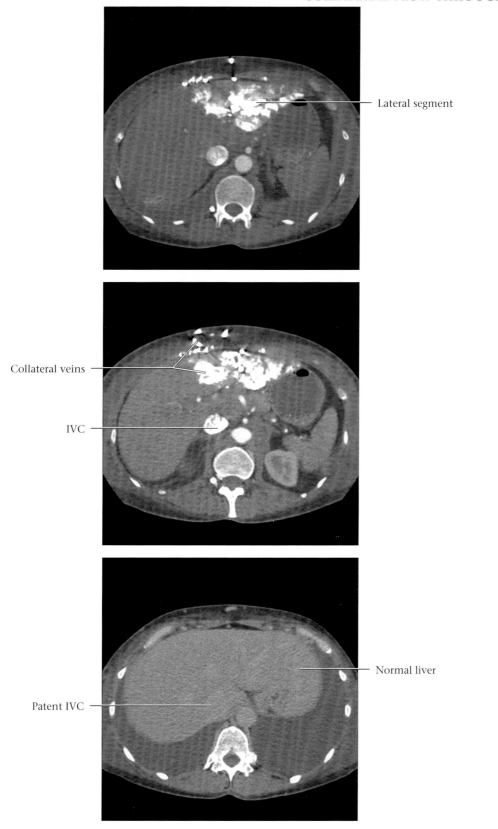

Lateral segment

Collateral veins

IVC

Normal liver

Patent IVC

(**Top**) CT image through the liver in the late arterial phase of imaging shows dense opacification of the left lobe of the liver and opacification of the IVC that is greater than that of the aorta. This is due to collateral blood flow through peridiaphragmatic collateral veins that communicate with hepatic veins and return blood to the IVC. On radionuclide and PET scanning studies this phenomenon may appear as a "hot spot" and be confused for a liver tumor. (**Middle**) More caudal section again emphasizes the collateral flow through the liver to the IVC. (**Bottom**) A delayed phase image through the same segments of the liver shows that the liver is normal and the IVC is patent.

CIRRHOSIS, VARICES

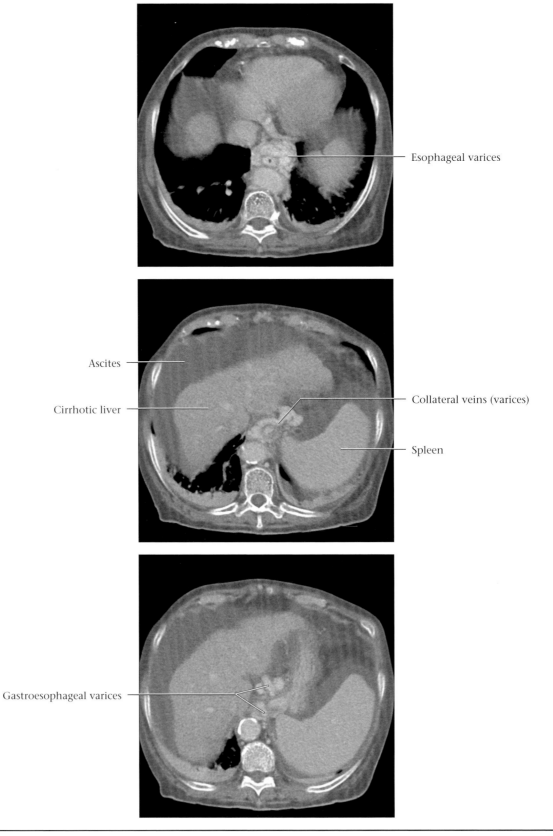

Esophageal varices

Ascites

Cirrhotic liver

Collateral veins (varices)

Spleen

Gastroesophageal varices

(Top) First of three axial CT images in a patient with cirrhosis and portal hypertension shows massive periesophageal varices that carry blood through the mediastinum as collateral veins that are bypassing the cirrhotic liver. **(Middle)** A more caudal section shows the nodular cirrhotic liver and signs of portal hypertension including splenomegaly, ascites and varices. **(Bottom)** A more caudal section shows more of the varices that are present in the wall of the stomach as well as the esophagus.

LIVER

LIVER STEATOSIS

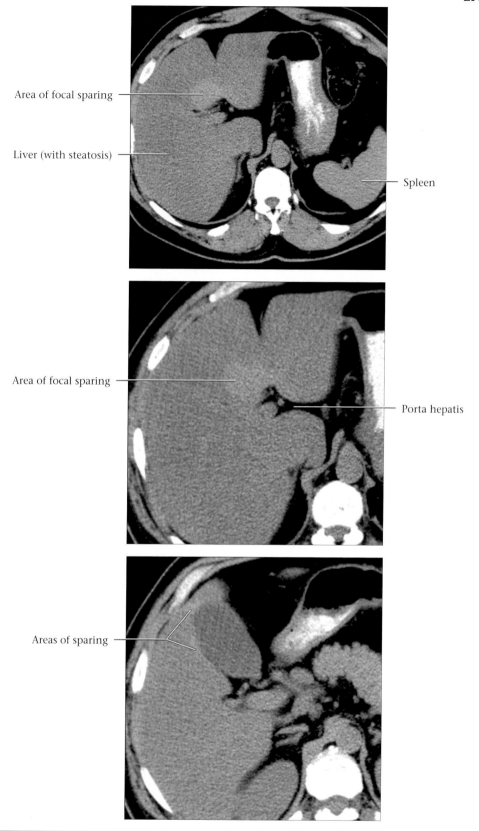

Area of focal sparing

Liver (with steatosis)

Spleen

Area of focal sparing

Porta hepatis

Areas of sparing

(Top) First of three axial nonenhanced CT sections in a patient with hepatic steatosis ("fatty liver") shows that the liver appears darker, or less dense, than the spleen, rather than being slightly more dense (higher in attenuation) as would be normal. Note the rounded area of normal density liver just anterior to the porta hepatis that could be mistaken for a focal liver mass. This area of the liver has been spared from steatosis, generally due to variations in portal venous supply to this part of the liver. **(Middle)** A magnified view of the same axial section shows the area of focal sparing and the diffuse steatosis. Common areas for focal sparing are the those abutting the porta hepatis and gallbladder fossa. **(Bottom)** A thin band of hepatic tissue abutting the gallbladder fossa is also spared and is of greater attenuation than the rest of the liver.

LIVER

MULTIFOCAL STEATOSIS

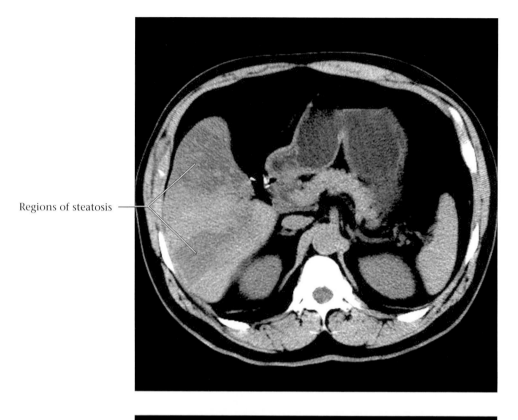

Regions of steatosis —

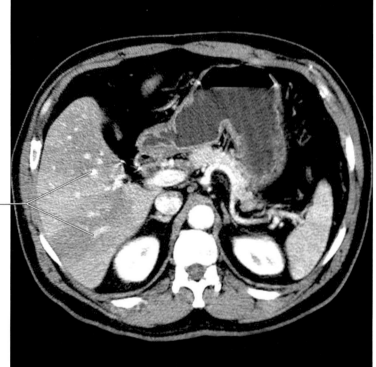

Hepatic vein branches —

(Top) First of two axial CT sections in a patient with multifocal steatosis (fatty infiltration) of the liver. Nonenhanced image shows geographic areas within the right lobe that are lower in density than the spleen. The normal liver is slightly more dense (higher in attenuation) than the spleen on a nonenhanced CT section. **(Bottom)** CT section obtained during the IV injection of contrast material shows a normal distribution of hepatic vessels within the areas of steatosis. The absence of a "mass effect", such as displacement of vessels, helps to distinguish steatosis from a tumor as the etiology of the abnormal low density areas.

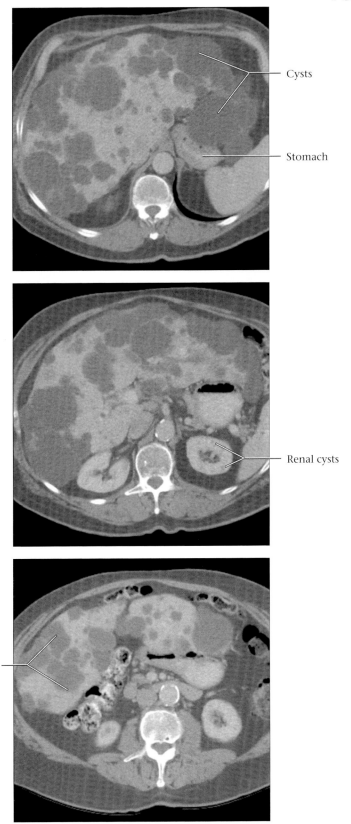

Cysts

Stomach

Renal cysts

Hepatic cysts

(Top) First of three axial CT sections of a patient with autosomal dominant polycystic liver disease shows innumerable water-density masses within the liver. The cysts enlarge and distort the liver and compress the stomach, but rarely cause significant liver dysfunction. **(Middle)** A more caudal section shows relatively few and much smaller renal cysts. Patients with polycystic disease may have severe, mild, or no involvement of either the kidneys and liver. **(Bottom)** Note that the cysts are all of homogeneous low density with no visible wall or mural nodularity, features that help to distinguish these from hepatic tumors or abscesses. Clinical information, such as the presence or absence of fever or a known extrahepatic tumor, are also important diagnostic criteria.

LIVER

LIVER METASTASES

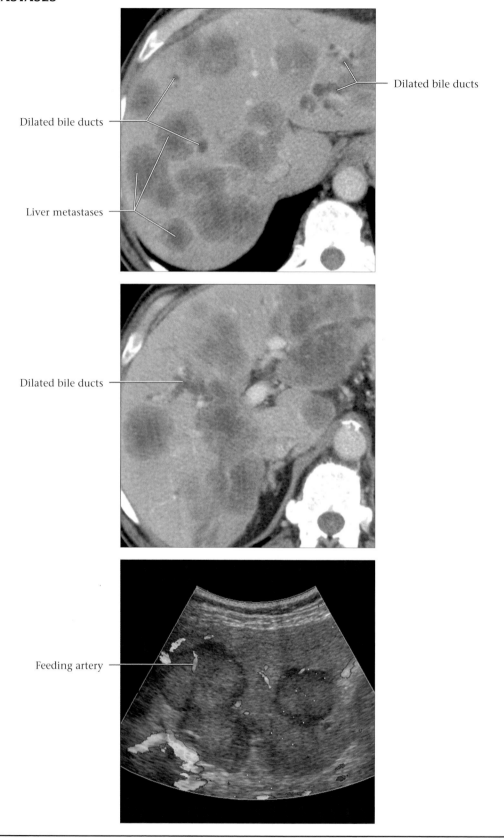

Dilated bile ducts

Dilated bile ducts

Liver metastases

Dilated bile ducts

Feeding artery

(Top) First of three images of a patient with colon carcinoma. Axial CT section shows numerous spherical, heterogeneous masses within all segments of the liver, representing metastatic foci. Some of these have a target appearance, consistent with central necrosis. Dilated bile ducts are seen within both lobes due to mass effect of tumor compressing the bile duct lumen. **(Middle)** Confluent metastases near the porta hepatis cause bile duct obstruction, with dilation of the intrahepatic ducts. **(Bottom)** An axial color Doppler sonographic image also shows the target appearance of the liver metastases. The color Doppler signal is calibrated to show arterial flow as red and venous flow as blue. Both arterial and venous flow are evident within and around the metastases.

LIVER

HEPATOCELLULAR CARCINOMA

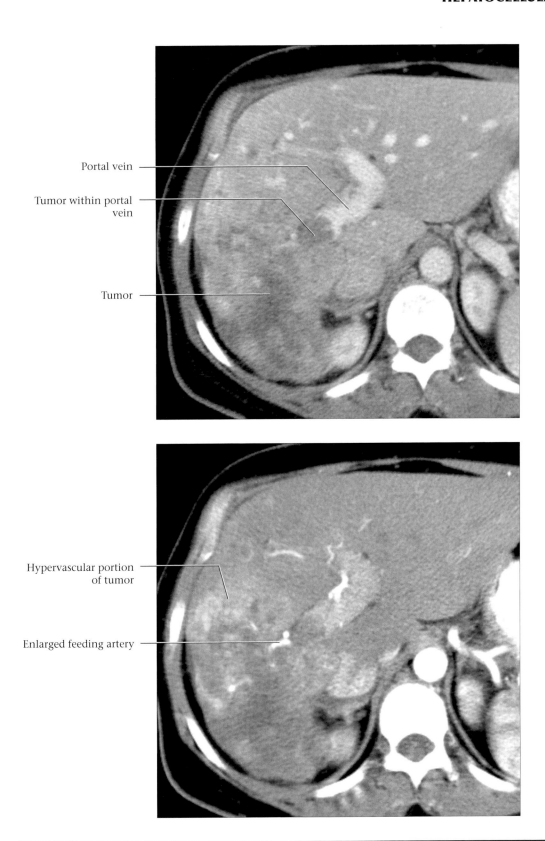

Portal vein

Tumor within portal vein

Tumor

Hypervascular portion of tumor

Enlarged feeding artery

(Top) First of two contrast-enhance axial CT sections of a patient with chronic viral hepatitis shows a heterogeneous tumor filling much of the right lobe of the liver. Tumor invasion of the right portal vein is evident as a filling defect within the contrast-opacified vessel. This is a typical feature of hepatocellular carcinoma and an important staging criterion, precluding liver transplantation or surgical resection as treatment options. (Bottom) A more caudal section shows portions of the tumor that are hypervascular, enhancing to a greater degree than the normal liver. Note the enlarged hepatic arterial branches that have been recruited to feed the tumor.

BILIARY SYSTEM

Imaging Anatomy

Overview

- **Biliary ducts** convey bile from liver to duodenum
  - Bile is produced continuously by liver, stored & concentrated by gallbladder (GB), released intermittently by GB contraction in response to presence of fat in duodenum
  - Hepatocytes form bile → bile canaliculi → interlobular biliary ducts → collecting bile ducts → **right** & **left hepatic ducts** → **common hepatic duct** → **common bile duct**
- Bile duct forms in free edge of lesser omentum by union of cystic duct and common hepatic duct
  - Length of duct: 5-15 cm depending on point of junction of cystic & common hepatic ducts
  - Duct descends posterior & medial to duodenum, lying in a groove on dorsal surface of pancreatic head
  - Bile duct joins with pancreatic duct to form **hepaticopancreatic ampulla (of Vater)** (dilated short segment)
  - Ampulla opens into duodenum through **major duodenal (hepaticopancreatic) papilla**
    - Surrounded by smooth muscle
  - Distal bile duct is thickened into a **sphincter (of Boyden)** and hepaticopancreatic segment is thickened into a **sphincter (of Oddi)**
    - Contraction of these sphincters prevents bile from entering duodenum; forces it to collect in GB
    - Relaxation of sphincters in response to parasympathetic stimulation & cholecystokinin (released by duodenum in response to fatty meal)
- **Vessels, nerves and lymphatics**
  - Arteries
    - Hepatic arteries to intrahepatic ducts
    - **Cystic artery** to proximal common duct
    - **Right hepatic artery** to middle part of common duct
    - **Gastroduodenal** and **pancreaticoduodenal arcade** to distal common duct
    - **Cystic artery** to GB (usually from right hepatic artery; variable)
  - Veins
    - From intrahepatic ducts → hepatic veins
    - From common duct → portal vein (in tributaries)
    - From GB directly into liver sinusoids, bypassing portal vein
  - Nerves
    - Sensory: Right phrenic nerve
    - Parasympathetic & sympathetic from celiac ganglion and plexus; contraction of GB & relaxation at biliary sphincters is caused by parasympathetic stimulation, but more important stimulus is from hormone cholecystokinin
  - Lymphatics
    - Same course and name as arterial branches
    - Collect at celiac lymph nodes and node of omental foramen
    - Nodes draining GB are prominent in the porta hepatis and around pancreatic head
- **Gallbladder**
  - ~ 7-10 cm long, holds up to 50 ml of bile
  - Lies in a shallow fossa on the visceral surface of liver
  - Vertical plane through GB fossa & middle hepatic vein divides left & right hepatic lobes
  - Touches & indents duodenum
  - Fundus is covered with peritoneum & relatively mobile; body & neck are attached to liver & covered by hepatic capsule
  - **Fundus:** Wide tip of GB, projects below liver edge (usually)
  - **Body:** Contacts liver, duodenum & transverse colon
  - **Neck:** Narrowed, tapered and tortuous; joins cystic duct
  - **Cystic duct:** 3-4 cm long, connects GB to common hepatic duct; marked by **spiral folds (of Heister)**; helps to regulate bile flow to & from GB

Anatomy-Based Imaging Issues

Key Concepts

- Direct venous drainage of GB into liver bypasses portal venous system, often results in **sparing of** adjacent liver from generalized **steatosis** (fatty liver)
- **Nodal metastasis from GB carcinoma** to peripancreatic nodes may simulate a primary pancreatic tumor
- **Sonography:** Optimal means of evaluating GB for stones & inflammation (**acute cholecystitis**); best done in fasting state (distends GB)
- Intrahepatic bile ducts follow branching pattern of portal veins
  - Usually lie immediately anterior to portal vein branch; confluence of hepatic ducts just anterior to confluence of right & main portal veins

Clinical Implications

Clinical Importance

- **Common variations of biliary arterial & ductal anatomy** result in challenges to avoid injury at surgery
  - Cystic duct may run in common sheath with bile duct
  - Anomalous right hepatic ducts may be severed at cholecystectomy
- Close apposition of GB to duodenum can result in fistulous connection with chronic cholecystitis and **erosion of gallstone into duodenum**
- **Obstruction of common bile duct** is common
  - **Gallstones** in distal bile duct
  - **Carcinoma** arising in pancreatic head or bile duct
  - Result is **jaundice** due to back up of bile salts into bloodstream

Embryologic Events

- Abnormal embryological development of fetal ductal plate can lead to spectrum of liver & biliary abnormalities including
  - Polycystic liver disease
  - Congenital hepatic fibrosis
  - **Biliary hamartomas**
  - **Caroli disease**
  - **Choledochal cysts**

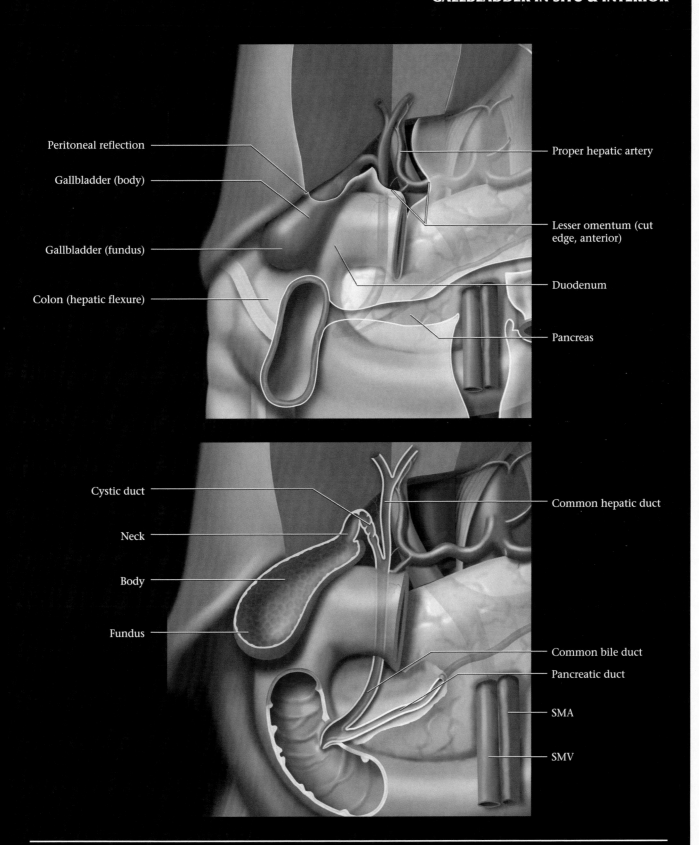

Peritoneal reflection

Gallbladder (body)

Gallbladder (fundus)

Colon (hepatic flexure)

Proper hepatic artery

Lesser omentum (cut edge, anterior)

Duodenum

Pancreas

Cystic duct

Neck

Body

Fundus

Common hepatic duct

Common bile duct

Pancreatic duct

SMA

SMV

(Top) The gallbladder is covered with peritoneum, except where it is attached to the liver. The extrahepatic bile duct, hepatic artery & portal vein run in the lesser omentum. The fundus of the gallbladder extends beyond the anterior-inferior edge of the liver and is in contact with the hepatic flexure of the colon. The body (main portion of the gallbladder) is in contact with the duodenum. **(Bottom)** The neck of the gallbladder narrows before entering the cystic duct, which is distinguished by its tortuous course and irregular lumen. The duct lumen is irregular due to redundant folds of mucosa, called the spiral folds (of Heister), that are believed to regulate the rate of filling and emptying of the gallbladder. The cystic duct joins the hepatic duct to form the common bile duct, which passes behind the duodenum & through the pancreas to enter the duodenum.

BILIARY SYSTEM

VARIANT EXTRAHEPATIC DUCTS

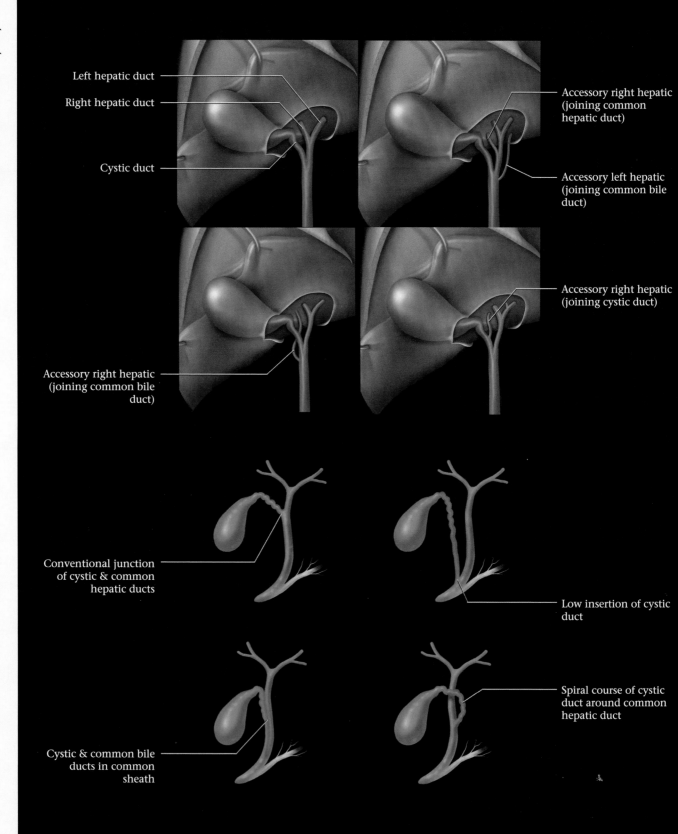

Left hepatic duct

Right hepatic duct

Cystic duct

Accessory right hepatic (joining common hepatic duct)

Accessory left hepatic (joining common bile duct)

Accessory right hepatic (joining cystic duct)

Accessory right hepatic (joining common bile duct)

Conventional junction of cystic & common hepatic ducts

Low insertion of cystic duct

Spiral course of cystic duct around common hepatic duct

Cystic & common bile ducts in common sheath

(Top) Graphic shows the conventional arrangement of the extrahepatic bile ducts, but variations are common (20% of population) and may lead to inadvertent ligation or injury at surgery such as cholecystectomy, where the cystic duct is clamped and transected. Most accessory ducts are on the rsyght side and usually enter the common hepatic duct, but may enter the cystic or common bile duct. Accessory left ducts enter the common bile duct. While referred to as "accessory", these ducts are the sole drainage of bile from at least one hepatic segment. Ligation or laceration can lead to significant hepatic injury or bile peritonitis. **(Bottom)** The course and insertion of the cystic duct are highly variable, leading to difficulty in isolation and ligation at cholecystectomy. The cystic duct may be mistaken for the common hepatic or common bile duct.

BILIARY SYSTEM

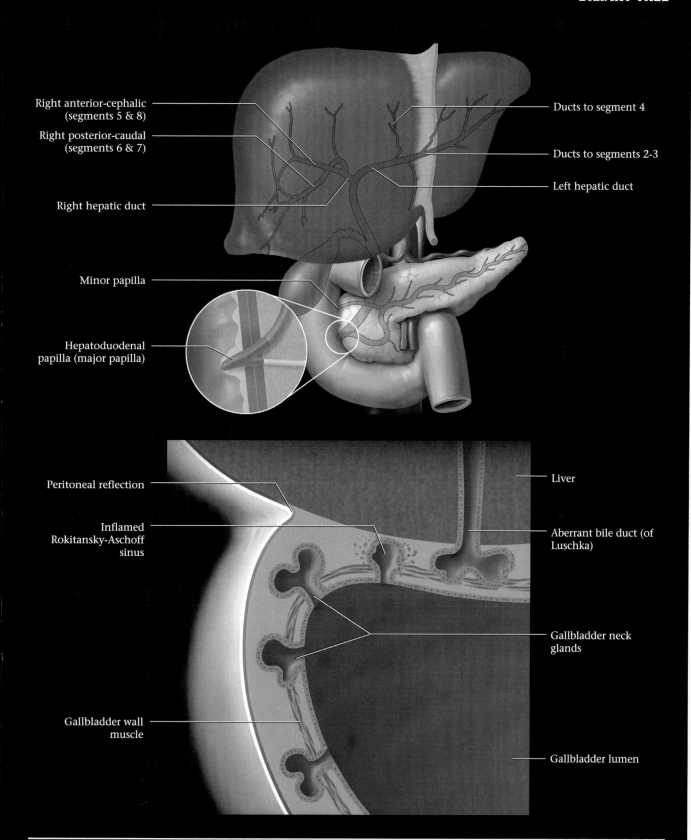

Right anterior-cephalic (segments 5 & 8)

Right posterior-caudal (segments 6 & 7)

Right hepatic duct

Minor papilla

Hepatoduodenal papilla (major papilla)

Ducts to segment 4

Ducts to segments 2-3

Left hepatic duct

Peritoneal reflection

Inflamed Rokitansky-Aschoff sinus

Gallbladder wall muscle

Liver

Aberrant bile duct (of Luschka)

Gallbladder neck glands

Gallbladder lumen

(Top) Note the distribution of the larger intrahepatic bile ducts. The common bile duct usually joins with the pancreatic duct in a common channel or ampulla (of Vater), but may enter the major duodenal papilla separately. The distal bile duct has a sphincteric coat of smooth muscle, the choledochal sphincter (of Boyden), which regulates bile emptying into the duodenum. When contracted, this sphincter causes bile to flow retrograde into the gallbladder for storage. The common hepaticopancreatic ampulla may be surrounded by a smooth muscle sphincter (of Oddi). **(Bottom)** The gallbladder body & neck are adherent to the liver and may be bridged by aberrant bile ducts (of Luschka). Mucus glands are found in the gallbladder neck. Rokitansky-Aschoff sinuses are pseudodiverticula that extend into the wall and may collect debris, becoming inflamed.

BILIARY SYSTEM

CHOLANGIOGRAM

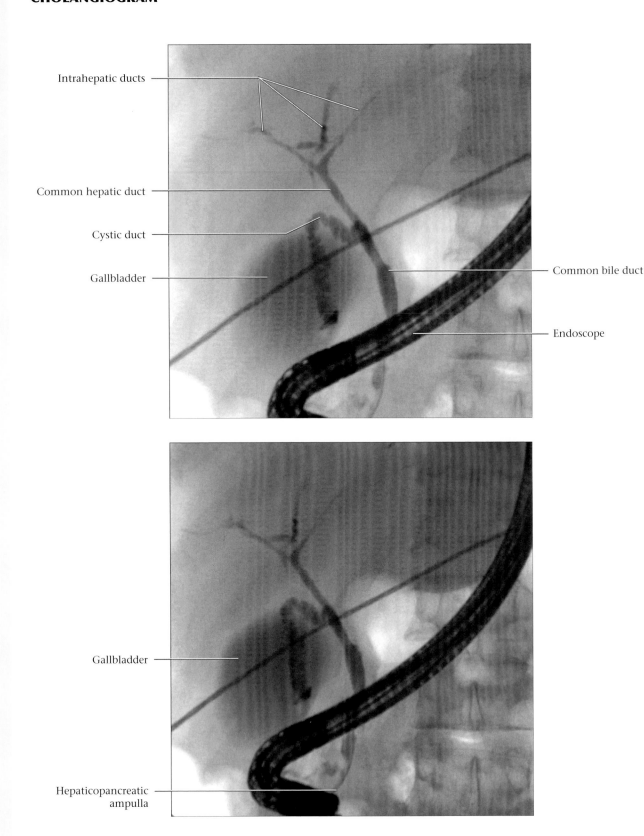

Intrahepatic ducts

Common hepatic duct

Cystic duct

Gallbladder

Common bile duct

Endoscope

Gallbladder

Hepaticopancreatic ampulla

(Top) First of two images from an endoscopic retrograde cholangio-pancreatogram (ERCP) shows normal intra- and extrahepatic bile ducts. Note the irregular contour of the cystic duct caused by the spiral folds of Heister. The gallbladder is opacified by retrograde passage of contrast material, with the tip of the endoscopic cannula inserted into the hepaticopancreatic ampulla (of Vater). **(Bottom)** Portions of the intra- and extrahepatic ducts appear to have an irregular contour, but this is due to incomplete filling. ERCP studies are monitored in real time by X-ray fluoroscopy and multiple films are obtained in different obliquities to distinguish artifacts, such as incomplete filling and air bubbles, from ductal pathology.

BILIARY SYSTEM

MR CHOLANGIO-PANCREATOGRAM

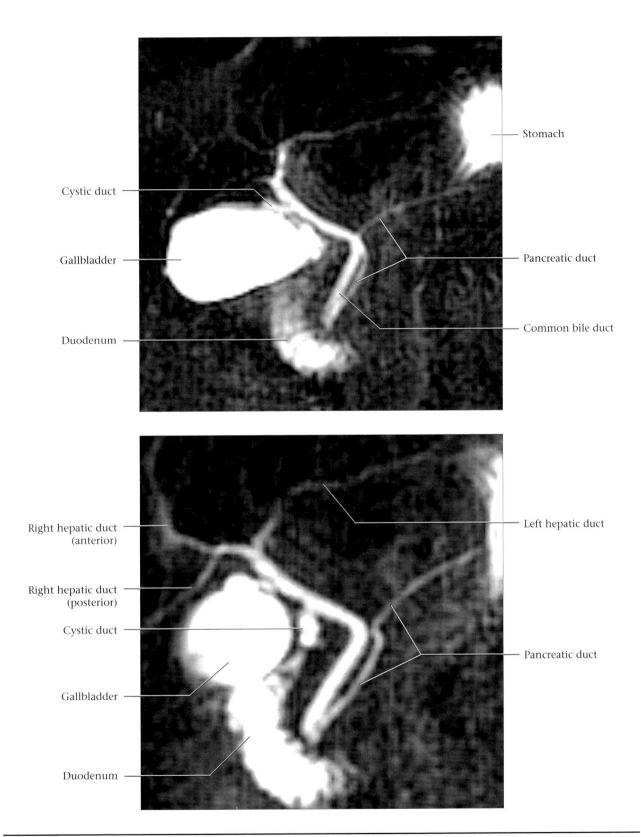

Cystic duct

Gallbladder

Duodenum

Stomach

Pancreatic duct

Common bile duct

Right hepatic duct (anterior)

Right hepatic duct (posterior)

Cystic duct

Gallbladder

Duodenum

Left hepatic duct

Pancreatic duct

(Top) First of two coronal MR cholangio-pancreatogram (MRCP) images, obtained with heavily T2-weighted images that show all static collections of fluid, such as ductal structures and bowel, as very bright. The ducts are all of normal caliber. Note the parallel course of the bile duct and pancreatic duct within the pancreatic head. These ducts usually join just prior to emptying into the duodenum at the papilla of Vater. **(Bottom)** This obliquity shows the main branches of the intrahepatic bile ducts. MRCP and ultrasonography have become the preferred noninvasive methods of determining the presence and cause of biliary ductal obstruction. Direct cholangiography, such as ERCP, is usually reserved for cases of known obstruction when endoscopic intervention, such as placement of a biliary stent, is being considered.

BILIARY SYSTEM

ANGIOGRAM, CYSTIC ARTERY

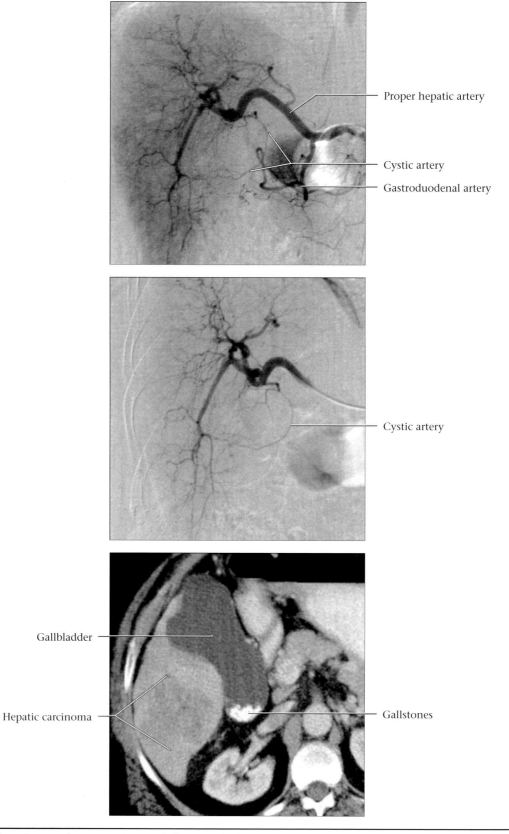

Proper hepatic artery

Cystic artery

Gastroduodenal artery

Cystic artery

Gallbladder

Hepatic carcinoma

Gallstones

(Top) First of three images from a patient with hepatocellular carcinoma. This frontal image from a catheter angiogram shows the cystic artery stretched along the surface of a distended gallbladder. The cystic artery usually arises from the right hepatic artery, though this is quite variable. (Middle) Selective injection of the proper hepatic artery again shows the course of the cystic artery. (Bottom) Axial CT section shows a distended gallbladder with gallstones. The hepatic carcinoma is seen within the right hepatic lobe. The angiogram was obtained in anticipation of treating the tumor with hepatic arterial infusion of chemotherapy.

BILIARY SYSTEM

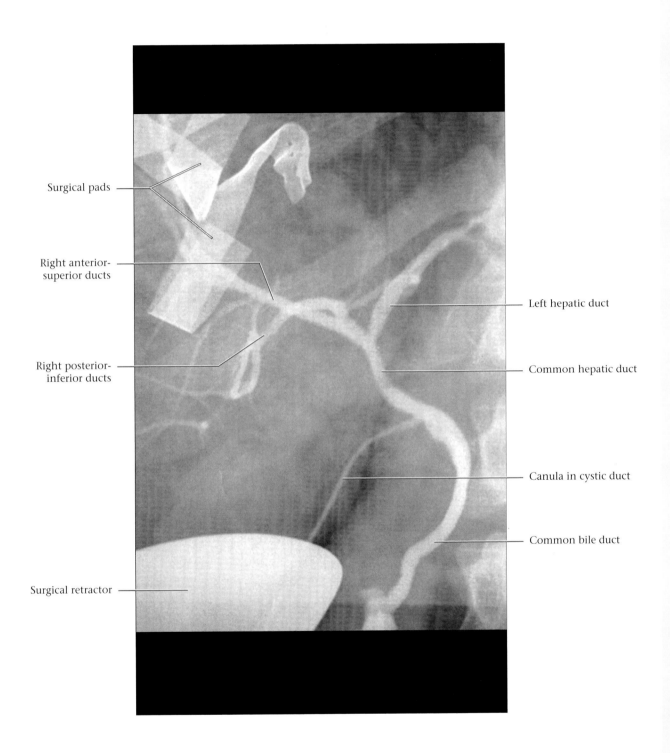

Surgical pads

Right anterior-superior ducts

Right posterior-inferior ducts

Surgical retractor

Left hepatic duct

Common hepatic duct

Canula in cystic duct

Common bile duct

Intra-operative cholangiogram was performed in a subject about to undergo right hepatic lobectomy as a living donor to a relative with liver failure. The cholangiogram shows a trifurcation pattern of the main ducts draining the right and left lobes. This is an unfavorable anatomic variant in this setting because the surgical plane of section will cut across both the anterior and posterior segmental bile ducts, requiring two separate anastomoses to the recipient's biliary (or enteric) system.

BILIARY SYSTEM

GALLSTONE ILEUS

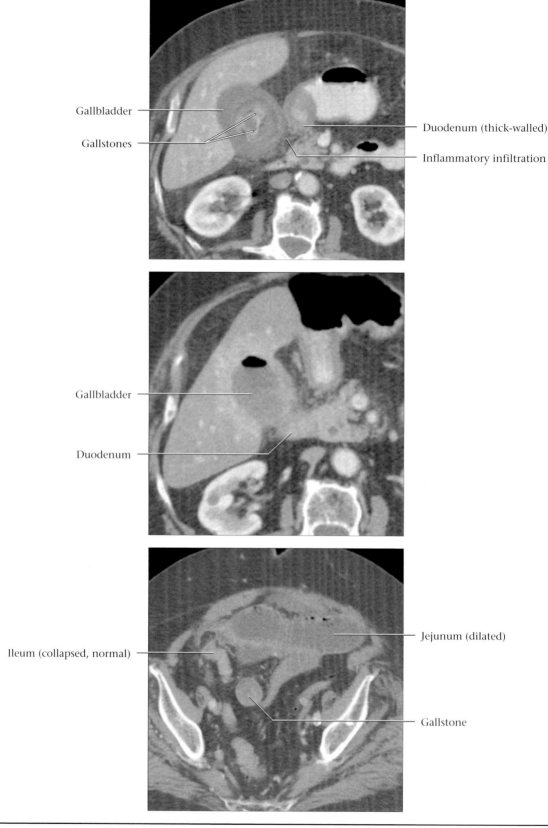

(Top) First of three axial CT sections of an elderly woman. The first image shows large gallstones within a distended gallbladder that is adjacent to a thick-walled duodenum, indicating contiguous inflammation. At this time the patient had symptoms of cholecystitis. (Middle) CT scan was repeated three weeks later when the patient complained of crampy abdominal pain and nausea suggesting bowel obstruction. A section through the gallbladder no longer shows stones, but only gas and fluid. The gallstones had eroded through the wall of the gallbladder directly into the adjacent duodenum. (Bottom) A more caudal section shows small bowel obstruction, with dilated proximal segments and collapsed ileum. At the point of transition there is a spherical "mass" with concentric layers of calcification, representing a large gallstone that is obstructing the lumen.

BILIARY SYSTEM

CT & MR, GALLSTONES

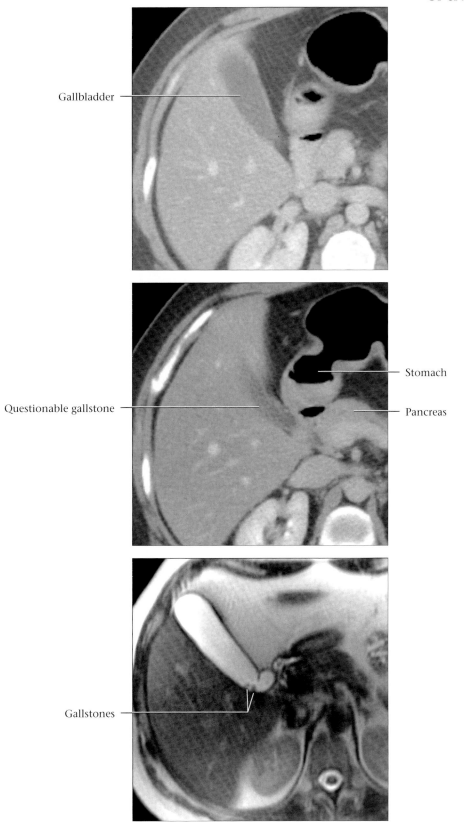

Gallbladder

Questionable gallstone

Stomach

Pancreas

Gallstones

(Top) First of three images of a patient with gallstones in the gallbladder. Axial CT shows a normal appearing gallbladder, with water density bile. **(Middle)** A more caudal CT section shows a subtle focus of heterogeneous density that is suggestive, but not diagnostic of a gallstone. Gallstones can vary in density (attenuation) on CT depending on their chemical composition, from less than water density (pure cholesterol stones), to soft tissue density, to calcific density (calcium bilirubinate stones). CT depicts only about 70-80% of gallstones. **(Bottom)** Axial T2WI MR clearly depicts two calculi in the dependent position of the gallbladder. Gallstones have no mobile protons, and appear as foci of very dark signal, regardless of their chemical composition, and are especially evident on MR sequences that depict fluid as "white" signal.

BILIARY SYSTEM

ACUTE CHOLECYSTITIS

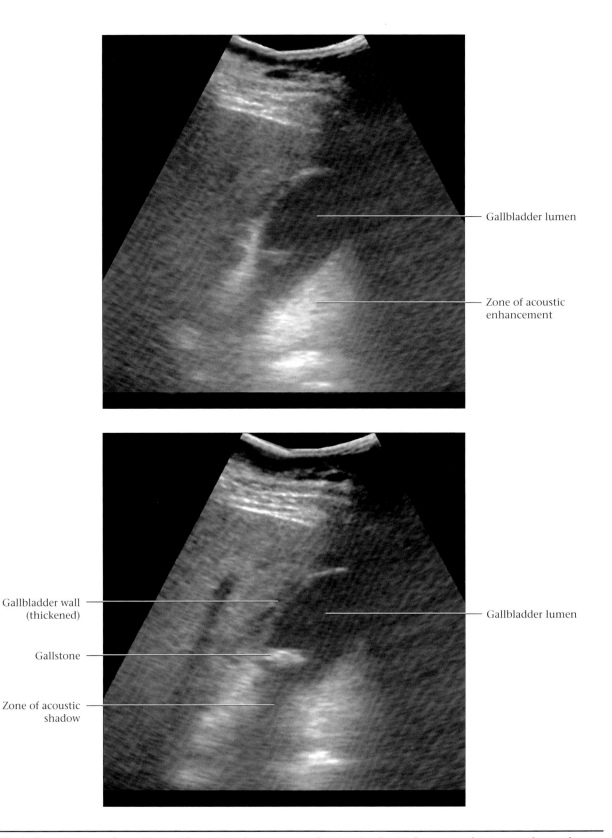

(Top) First of two images of a patient with acute right upper quadrant pain. Sagittal sonographic image shows the sonolucent gallbladder lumen and accentuated through transmission behind the gallbladder, a phenomenon that is due to the sound waves traveling faster through a liquid medium (bile) than the solid tissue of the liver. **(Bottom)** Another sagittal sonogram shows a thickened wall of the gallbladder. A crescentic echogenic gallstone is seen in the dependent gallbladder. All of the ultrasound beam is absorbed or reflected by the stone, resulting in an "acoustic shadow" beyond the stone. Focal tenderness can be elicited by pressing the ultrasound transducer over the gallbladder, inducing the "sonographic Murphy sign". This combination of findings is diagnostic of acute cholecystitis, and sonography is the diagnostic procedure of choice in this setting.

ACUTE CHOLECYSTITIS

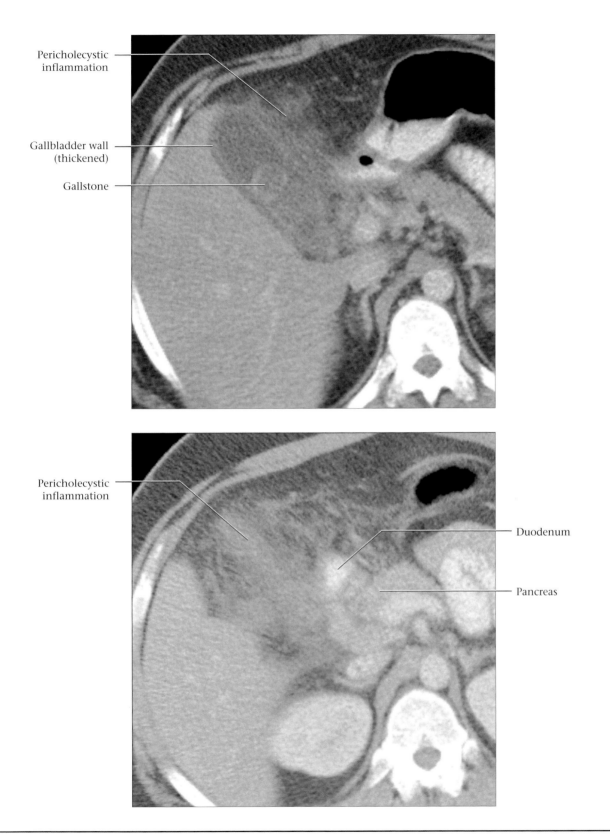

Pericholecystic inflammation

Gallbladder wall (thickened)

Gallstone

Pericholecystic inflammation

Duodenum

Pancreas

(Top) First of two images of a patient who had right upper quadrant pain that resolved, although the patient still appeared ill. CT shows a cholesterol gallstone, essentially isodense (same attenuation) as bile except for a calcified rim. The gallbladder wall is thickened and there is extensive inflammation of the pericholecystic fat planes. **(Bottom)** The pericholecystic inflammation suggests perforation of the gallbladder, which was confirmed at surgery. With severe cholecystitis, the gallbladder wall may become necrotic, effectively causing denervation and perforation of the wall. The nerve damage explains the loss of right upper quadrant pain or tenderness, late in the disease course.

BILIARY SYSTEM

CHOLECYSTITIS & DUCTAL STONES

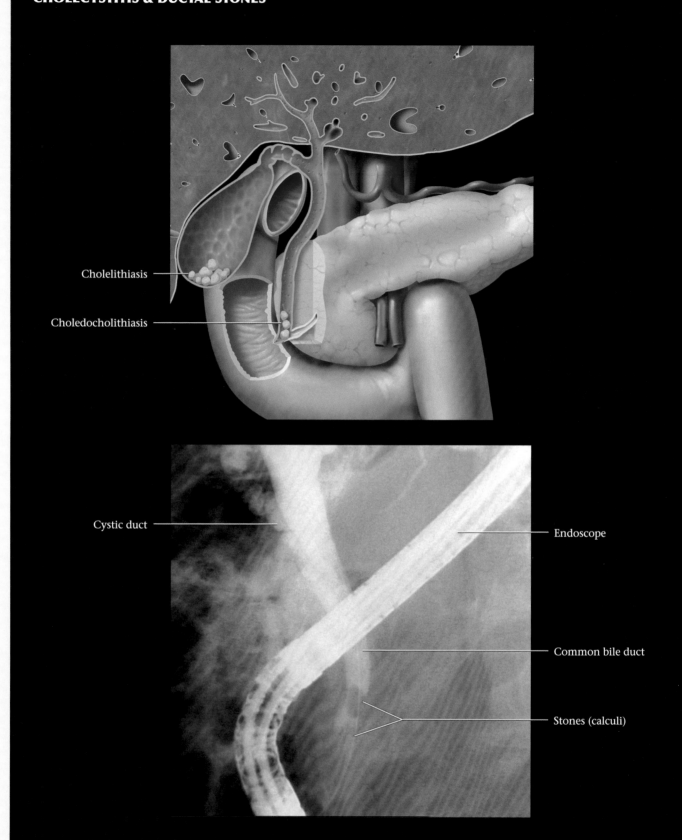

Cholelithiasis

Choledocholithiasis

Cystic duct

Endoscope

Common bile duct

Stones (calculi)

(Top) A graphic and three clinical images demonstrate cholelithiasis (stones in the gallbladder) and choledocholithiasis (stones in the bile ducts). Gallstones are extremely common and may remain asymptomatic. Stones that become impacted, even temporarily, in the gallbladder neck may cause inflammation and distention of the gallbladder, clinically referred to as acute cholecystitis. Stones that pass through the cystic duct often cause biliary colic (spasms of right upper quadrant pain) as they often become trapped within the common bile duct, causing obstruction. **(Bottom)** ERCP shows at least two calculi as filling defects within the contrast opacified distal common bile duct.

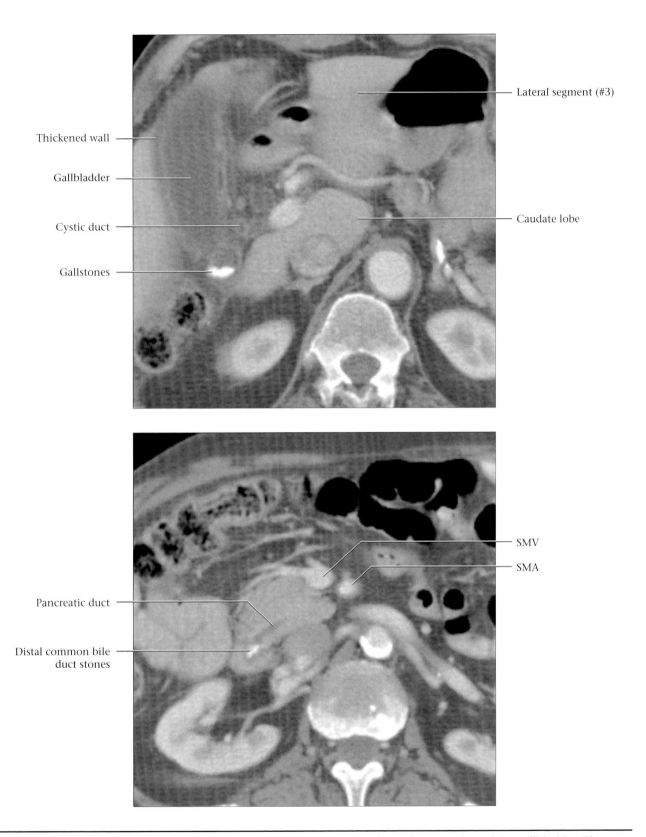

Thickened wall

Gallbladder

Cystic duct

Gallstones

Lateral segment (#3)

Caudate lobe

Pancreatic duct

Distal common bile duct stones

SMV

SMA

(Top) Axial CT shows opaque (calcium bilirubinate) gallstones in the dependent position of the gallbladder. The gallbladder wall is thickened due to acute cholecystitis. **(Bottom)** A more caudal CT section shows small opaque stones within the distal common bile duct as it joins the pancreatic duct at the hepaticopancreatic ampulla (of Vater). Obstruction at this level may cause reflux of bile and pancreatic juice into the pancreatic parenchyma, causing acute pancreatitis.

BILIARY SYSTEM

IATROGENIC BILE DUCT & ARTERIAL OCCLUSION

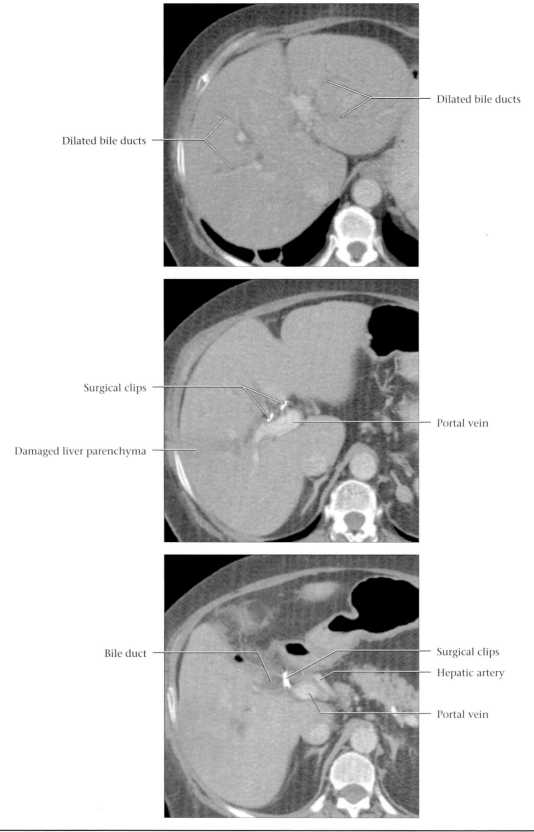

Dilated bile ducts

Dilated bile ducts

Surgical clips

Damaged liver parenchyma

Portal vein

Bile duct

Surgical clips

Hepatic artery

Portal vein

(Top) First of five images of a patient who developed acute hepatic failure following laparoscopic cholecystectomy. An axial CT section shows dilated intrahepatic bile ducts, adjacent to normally enhancing portal veins. **(Middle)** A more caudal section shows surgical clips anterior to the portal vein, at the expected location of the common hepatic bile duct and hepatic artery. **(Bottom)** More caudal CT section shows heterogeneous enhancement of the liver parenchyma, and a dilated bile duct that seems to end abruptly at a surgical clip.

IATROGENIC BILE DUCT & ARTERIAL OCCLUSION

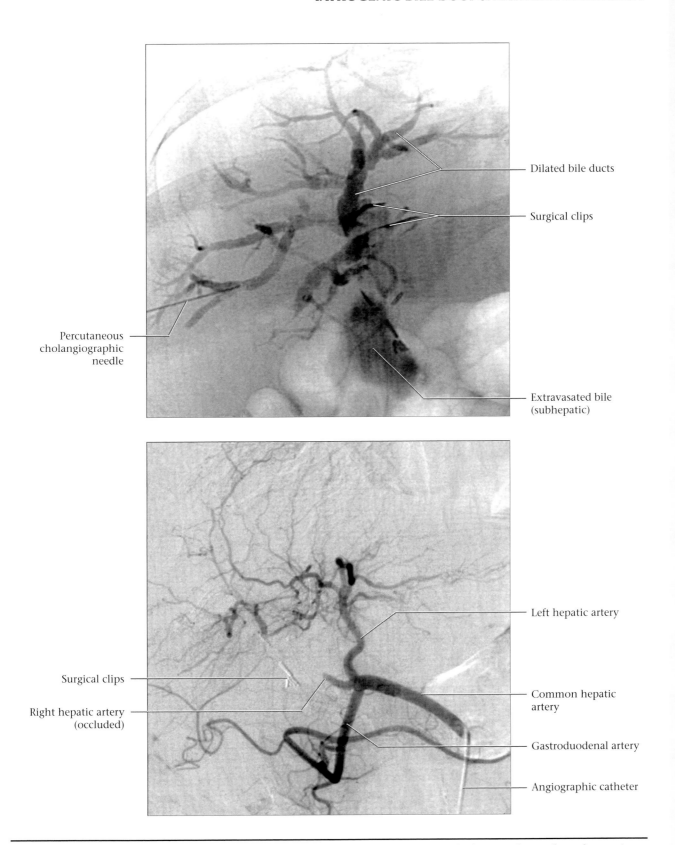

Dilated bile ducts

Surgical clips

Percutaneous cholangiographic needle

Extravasated bile (subhepatic)

Surgical clips

Right hepatic artery (occluded)

Left hepatic artery

Common hepatic artery

Gastroduodenal artery

Angiographic catheter

(Top) A transhepatic cholangiogram shows massive dilation of the intrahepatic bile ducts and complete obstruction near the porta hepatis. A collection of extraluminal bile indicates disruption of the bile duct. **(Bottom)** Hepatic angiography shows complete occlusion of the right hepatic artery adjacent to several surgical clips. At re-exploration, the hepatic artery and bile duct were found to be occluded by surgical clips which required complex reconstructive surgery. Iatrogenic injury to bile ducts and vessels is not rare and is more common with laparoscopic surgical procedures, which may limit visualization of the surgical "field". Due to the complex and highly variable anatomy of the hepatic vessels and biliary system, injuries to these structures have been especially common.

BILIARY SYSTEM

ERCP, COMMON BILE DUCT STONES

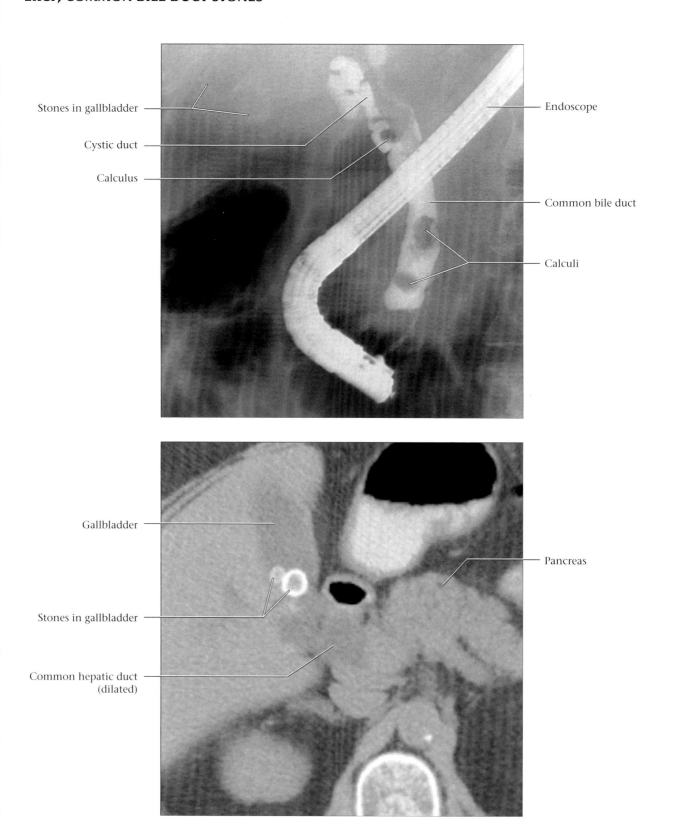

Stones in gallbladder

Cystic duct

Calculus

Endoscope

Common bile duct

Calculi

Gallbladder

Pancreas

Stones in gallbladder

Common hepatic duct
(dilated)

(Top) First of five images of a patient with right upper quadrant pain and abnormal liver function. An ERCP shows multiple filling defects within the common bile duct and cystic duct, representing ductal calculi. The gallbladder has not yet been opacified by retrograde flow of contrast material through the cystic duct. However, gallstones are evident within the gallbladder due to their faint rim of surface calcification. **(Bottom)** Axial CT section shows rim-calcified gallstones within the gallbladder and a dilated common hepatic duct.

BILIARY SYSTEM

ERCP, COMMON BILE DUCT STONES

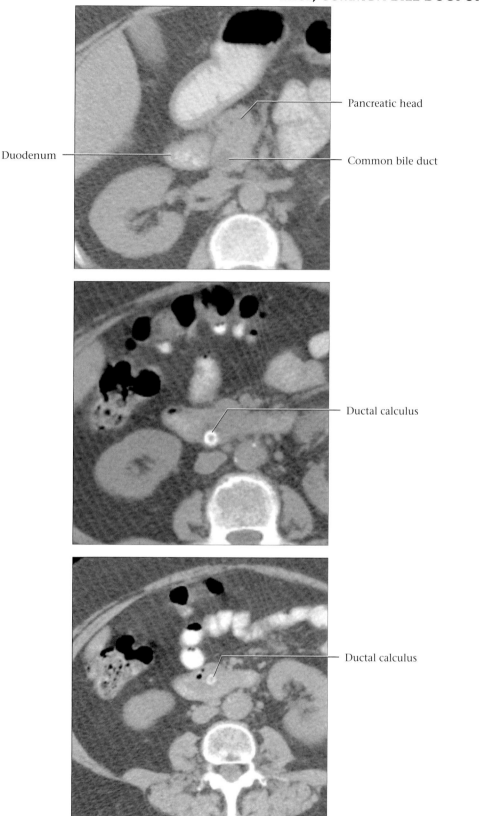

Pancreatic head

Duodenum

Common bile duct

Ductal calculus

Ductal calculus

(Top) A more caudal section shows the dilated common bile duct within the pancreatic head. (Middle) A more caudal section shows a rim-calcified stone within the distal common bile duct, accounting for the dilation of the more proximal duct and the elevated "liver enzymes". (Bottom) Axial section through the hepaticopancreatic ampulla (of Vater) shows an "impacted" stone.

BILIARY SYSTEM

DUCTAL CALCULI

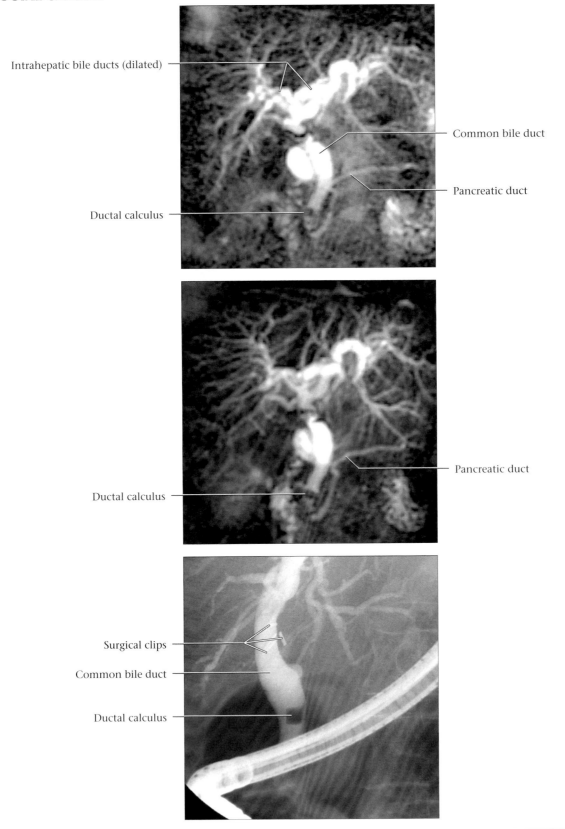

Intrahepatic bile ducts (dilated)

Common bile duct

Pancreatic duct

Ductal calculus

Pancreatic duct

Ductal calculus

Surgical clips

Common bile duct

Ductal calculus

(Top) First of three images of a patient with recurrent right upper quadrant pain one year after cholecystectomy. Coronal MRCP image shows dilated intra- and extrahepatic bile ducts. A discreet focus of low (dark) signal is seen within the distal common bile duct, representing an impacted stone. The pancreatic duct is normal. **(Middle)** Another image helps confirm the ductal stone. MRCP is the preferred noninvasive test for diagnosing biliary obstruction and its specific cause. ERCP is reserved for patients who would benefit from endoscopic intervention, such as extraction of a ductal stone, or placement of a biliary stent to overcome obstruction. **(Bottom)** ERCP demonstrates the ductal stone, having dislodged it from its more distal location near the ampulla. An endoscopic papillotomy was performed and the stone was extracted by basket retrieval.

BILIARY SYSTEM

AMPULLARY CARCINOMA

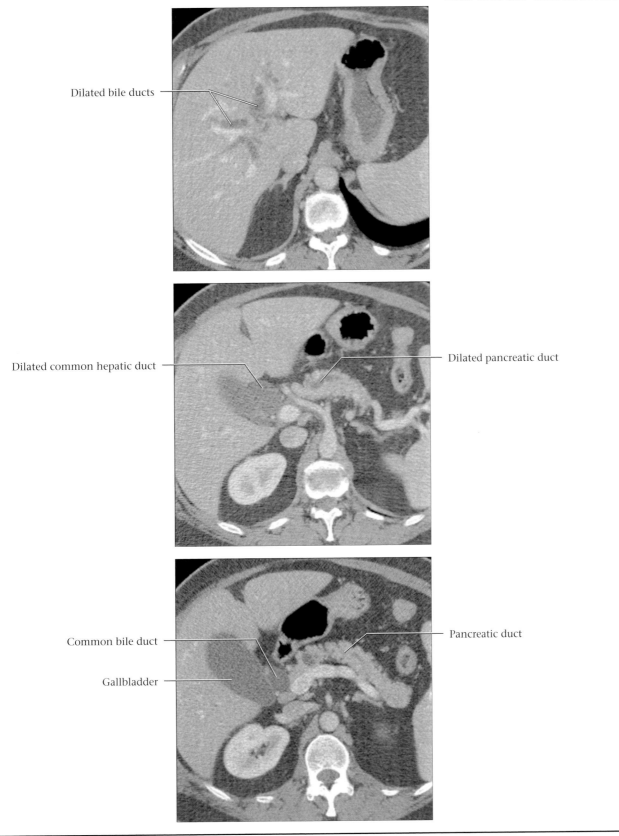

(Top) First of eight images of a patient with painless jaundice. An axial CT section shows dilation of the intrahepatic bile ducts. (Middle) A more caudal section shows dilation of the extrahepatic bile duct and the pancreatic duct. (Bottom) A more caudal section shows dilation of the gallbladder as well as the biliary and pancreatic ducts.

BILIARY SYSTEM

AMPULLARY CARCINOMA

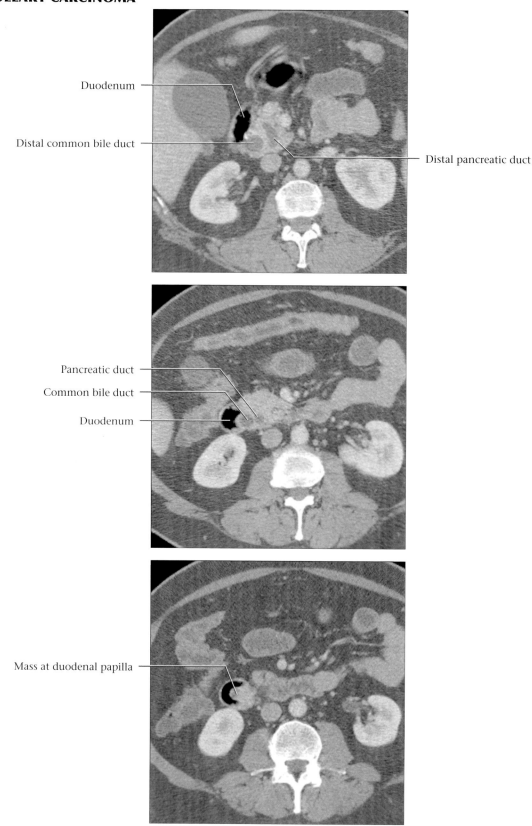

Duodenum

Distal common bile duct

Distal pancreatic duct

Pancreatic duct

Common bile duct

Duodenum

Mass at duodenal papilla

(Top) Axial section through the pancreatic head shows no pancreatic mass, but the bile and pancreatic ducts remain markedly dilated, indicating that the level of obstruction is "downstream" from this point. (Middle) At a level just proximal to the junction of the common bile and pancreatic ducts, both ducts are dilated. The pancreas is normal in appearance. (Bottom) At the level of the hepaticopancreatic (major) papilla, there is a soft tissue density mass that distorts the medial wall of the duodenum, representing an "ampullary" carcinoma. Periampullary tumors of the distal bile duct or pancreatic duct are adenocarcinomas that have a better clinical prognosis than the more common forms of pancreatic or bile duct carcinomas.

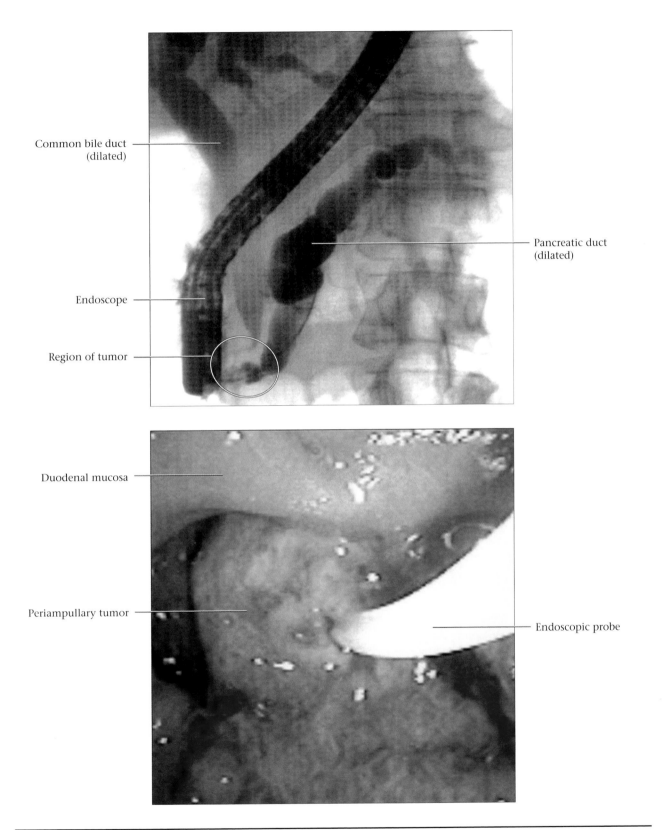

Common bile duct (dilated)

Pancreatic duct (dilated)

Endoscope

Region of tumor

Duodenal mucosa

Periampullary tumor

Endoscopic probe

(Top) An endoscopic probe has been placed through the periampullary mass with contrast opacification of the dilated common bile and pancreatic ducts. **(Bottom)** An endoscopic view of the interior of the duodenum shows the periampullary mass projecting into the lumen. The endoscopic syrobe or canula has been inserted through the tumor to opacify the bile duct and pancreatic duct. The mass was resected and proved to be an ampullary carcinoma.

BILIARY SYSTEM

PANCREATIC HEAD CARCINOMA

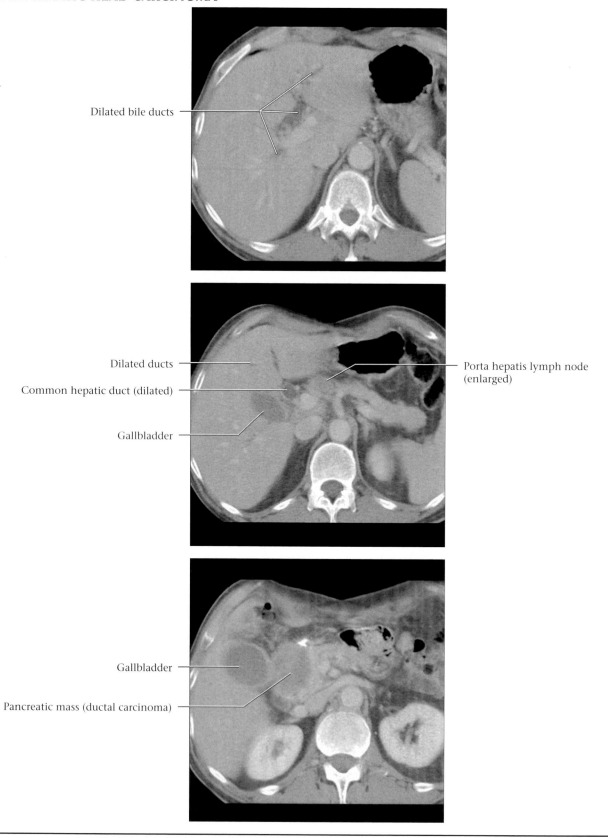

Dilated bile ducts

Dilated ducts

Common hepatic duct (dilated)

Gallbladder

Porta hepatis lymph node (enlarged)

Gallbladder

Pancreatic mass (ductal carcinoma)

(**Top**) First of six images from a patient with painless jaundice. An axial CT section shows a dilated intrahepatic biliary tree. (**Middle**) A more caudal CT section shows dilation of the intrahepatic and common hepatic bile ducts. An enlarged porta hepatis node represents lymphatic metastasis. (**Bottom**) A more caudal section shows a dilated gallbladder and a large heterogeneous mass arising from the head of the pancreas. The pancreatic duct is only mildly dilated, suggesting that the tumor arose from one of the pancreatic ductal side branches, with exophytic growth causing obstruction of the bile duct preferentially.

PANCREATIC HEAD CARCINOMA

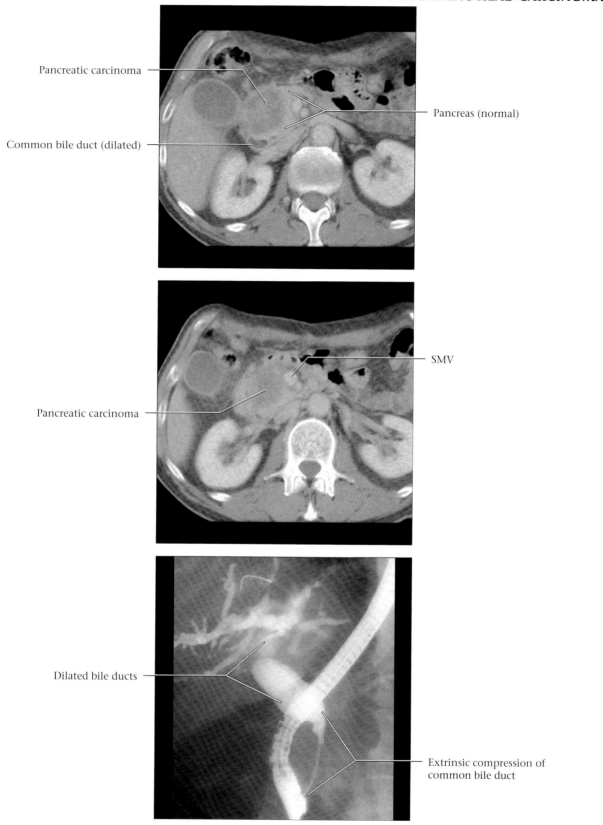

Pancreatic carcinoma

Common bile duct (dilated)

Pancreas (normal)

Pancreatic carcinoma

SMV

Dilated bile ducts

Extrinsic compression of common bile duct

(Top) A more caudal section shows the large, heterogeneous mass arising from the pancreatic head. **(Middle)** Note the irregular contour of the superior mesenteric vein (SMV). At the time of initial symptoms and diagnosis, most patients with pancreatic carcinoma have unresectable tumors due to invasion of critical blood vessels, or metastases. Note this patient's "scaphoid" abdomen, indicative of recent weight loss. **(Bottom)** ERCP film demonstrates the narrowed lumen of the common bile duct as it passes through the head of the pancreas. Pancreatic carcinoma is a scirrhous (hard, fibrotic) tumor that encases and obstructs blood vessels and bile ducts as it surrounds them.

BILIARY SYSTEM

BILIARY HAMARTOMAS

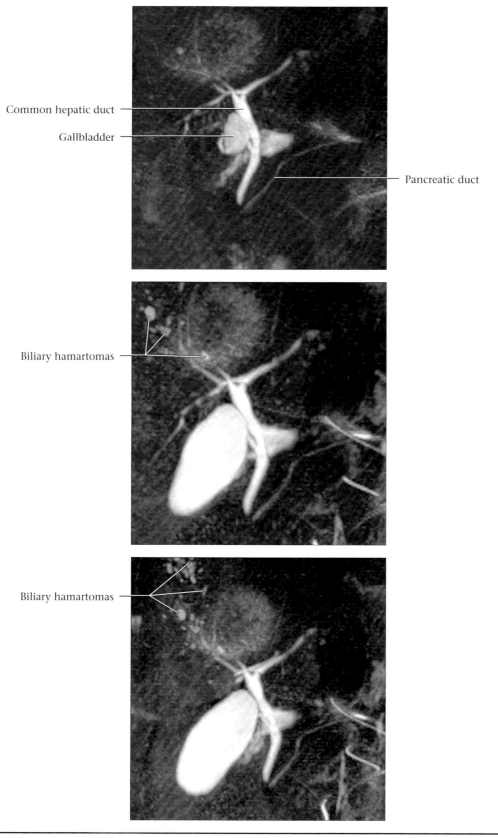

Common hepatic duct

Gallbladder

Pancreatic duct

Biliary hamartomas

Biliary hamartomas

(Top) First of three coronal MRCP images of the liver and biliary tree demonstrates a normal appearance of the gallbladder, biliary tree, and pancreatic duct. **(Middle)** Coronal section shows normal ducts, but there are numerous small "cystic" structures within the liver that are not in continuity with the bile ducts. **(Bottom)** Coronal section shows even more of the dozens of small (< 2 cm) cysts scattered throughout the liver. The large number and small size of the cystic lesions indicate that these represent biliary hamartomas, which are developmental anomalies due to failure of involution of embryonic bile ducts that fail to connect with the normal biliary tree. This is an asymptomatic condition but may be mistaken for more serious conditions such as polycystic disease or liver metastases.

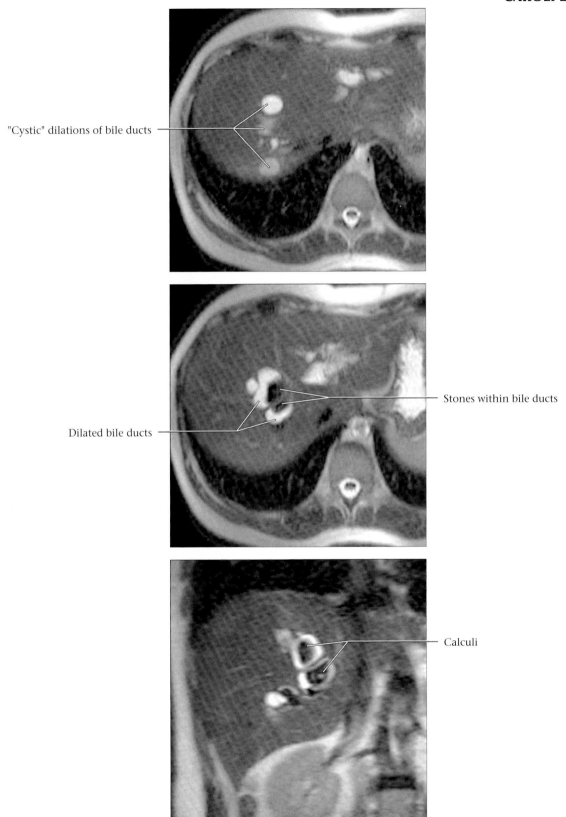

"Cystic" dilations of bile ducts

Stones within bile ducts

Dilated bile ducts

Calculi

(Top) First of three MR images from a patient with Caroli disease (communicating cavernous biliary ectasia), a congenital anomaly that results in multifocal, saccular dilation of the intrahepatic bile ducts. Axial T2WI shows multiple high intensity spherical lesions within the liver, representing dilated bile ducts. **(Middle)** A more caudal section shows large calculi as low intensity lesions within the massively dilated bile ducts. The bile ducts do not "arborize", or branch, in a uniform pattern; they are irregularly dilated in a cystic or fusiform pattern. **(Bottom)** A coronal section shows the extent of the ductal abnormalities and the large calculi within the dilated ducts.

BILIARY SYSTEM

CHOLEDOCHAL CYST

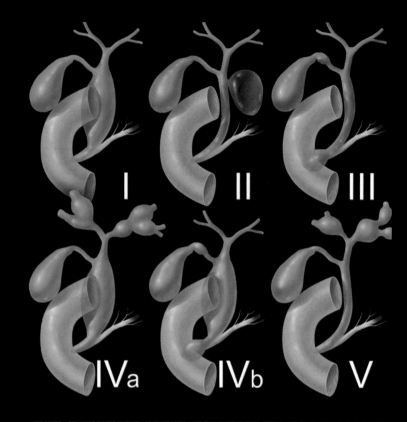

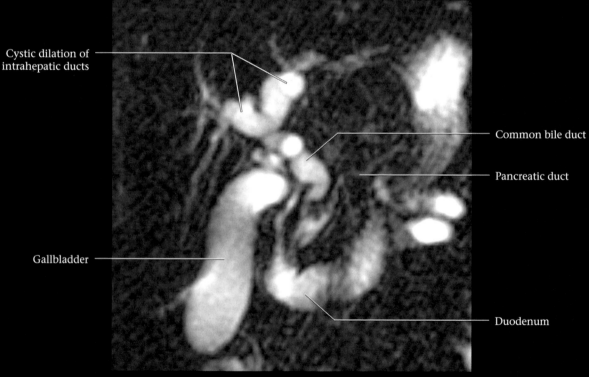

Cystic dilation of intrahepatic ducts

Common bile duct

Pancreatic duct

Gallbladder

Duodenum

(Top) Graphic illustrates the Todani classification of choledochal cysts. Type I is the most common and represents fusiform dilation of the extrahepatic bile duct. Type II is a diverticulum of the extrahepatic bile duct (rare). Type III is also rare, and is a choledochocele, a diverticular expansion of the distal bile duct within the duodenal wall. Type IV is the second most common type and is cystic dilation of the intrahepatic and extrahepatic bile ducts. Type V is cystic dilation of the intrahepatic bile ducts and is synonymous with Caroli disease. **(Bottom)** MRCP of a 2 year old girl with type IV choledochal cyst. There is cystic and fusiform dilation of both the intrahepatic and common bile ducts.

BILIARY SYSTEM

CHOLEDOCHAL CYST

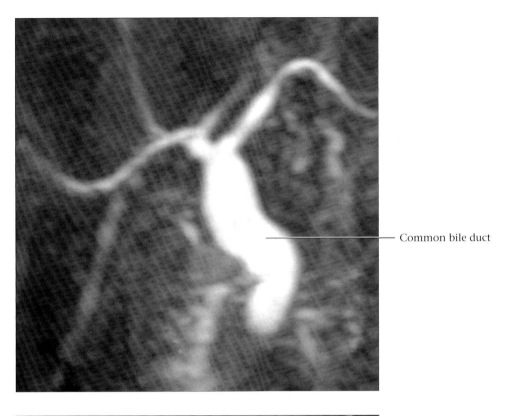

Common bile duct

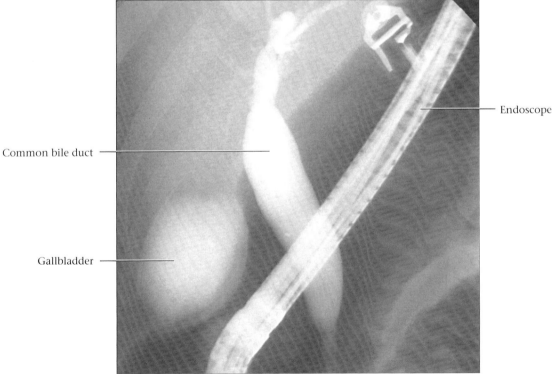

Common bile duct

Endoscope

Gallbladder

(Top) First of two images of a 44 year old woman with recurrent bouts of cholangitis. A coronal MRCP image shows fusiform dilation of the entire extrahepatic bile duct, a type I choledochal cyst. The intrahepatic bile ducts are normal. (Bottom) An ERCP in the same patient as previous image shows fusiform dilation of the entire extrahepatic bile duct.

PANCREAS

Gross Anatomy

Overview

- Pancreas: Accessory digestive gland lying in the retroperitoneum behind stomach
  - Exocrine function: Pancreatic **acinar cells** secrete **pancreatic juice** → **pancreatic duct** → **duodenum**
  - Endocrine: Pancreatic **islet cells** (of **Langerhans**) secrete insulin, glucagon & other polypeptides → portal venous system

Divisions

- **Head:** Thickest part; lies to the right of superior mesenteric vessels (SMA, SMV)
  - Attached to "C" loop of duodenum (2nd & 3rd parts)
  - **Uncinate** process: Head extension, posterior to SMV
  - **Bile duct** lies along posterior surface of head, joins with **pancreatic duct (of Wirsung)** to form **hepatopancreatic ampulla (of Vater)**
  - Main pancreatic & bile ducts empty into **major papilla** in 2nd portion of duodenum
- **Neck:** Thinnest part; lies anterior to SMA, SMV
  - SMV joins splenic vein behind pancreatic neck to form **portal vein**
- **Body:** Main part; lies to left of SMA, SMV
  - **Splenic vein** lies in groove on posterior surface of body
  - Anterior surface is covered with peritoneum forming the back surface of the **omental bursa (lesser sac)**
- **Tail:** Lies between layers of the **splenorenal ligament** in the splenic hilum

Internal Structures

- **Pancreatic duct (of Wirsung)** runs the length of the pancreas, turning inferiorly through the head to join the bile duct
- **Accessory pancreatic duct (of Santorini)** opens into the duodenum at **minor duodenal papilla**
  - Usually communicates with main pancreatic duct
  - Variations are common, including a dominant accessory duct draining most pancreatic juice
- **Vessels, nerves and lymphatics**
  - Arteries to head mainly from **gastroduodenal artery**
    - **Pancreaticoduodenal arcade** of vessels around head also supplied by SMA branches
  - Arteries to body & tail from **splenic artery**
  - Veins are tributaries of the SMV and splenic vein → portal vein
  - Autonomic nerves from **celiac** and **superior mesenteric plexus**
    - Parasympathetic stimulation of pancreatic secretion, but pancreatic juice secretion is mostly under hormonal control (**secretin**, from duodenum)
  - Lymphatics follow the blood vessels
    - Collect in **splenic, celiac, superior mesenteric** and **hepatic nodes**

Anatomy-Based Imaging Issues

Key Concepts

- Shape, size & texture of pancreas are quite variable
  - Largest in young adults
  - Atrophy and fatty infiltration with age (> 70), obesity, diabetes
  - Pancreatic duct also becomes more prominent with age (< 3 mm diameter)
  - Focal bulge or mass effect is abnormal
- Location behind lesser sac
  - Acute pancreatitis often results in lesser sac fluid (not = pseudocyst)
- Pancreas lies in anterior pararenal space (APS)
  - Inflammation (from pancreatitis) easily spreads to duodenum & descending colon (also lie in APS)
  - Inflammation easily spreads into mesentery & mesocolon (roots of these lie just ventral to pancreas)
- **Obstruction of pancreatic duct**
  - Relatively common result of **chronic pancreatitis** (fibrosis &/or stone occluding pancreatic duct), or **pancreatic ductal carcinoma**
- **Acute pancreatitis**
  - Relatively common result of gallstone (lodged in hepatopancreatic ampulla causing bile to reflux into pancreas)
  - May also result from direct damage from alcohol and other toxins
- **Obstruction of splenic vein**
  - Common result of pancreatic ductal carcinoma (> chronic pancreatitis)
  - Causes dilated venous collaterals including **short gastric** and **left gastric veins (gastric varices)**
    - Gastric varices without portal hypertension = splenic vein occlusion

Clinical Implications

Clinical Importance

- **Pancreatic ductal carcinoma** is the 5th leading cause of cancer death
  - Patients are usually unresectable for cure at time of diagnosis due to early spread of cancer to vital structures (liver through portal vein drainage; celiac and superior mesenteric plexus; inaccessible lymph node groups, superior mesenteric or celiac vessels)
  - Role of imaging is to detect tumor & signs of non-resectability to avoid nontherapeutic surgery
- **Pancreatic islet cell tumors**
  - May be benign or malignant
  - "Functional" tumors that secrete excess insulin or glucagon are usually diagnosed early due to characteristic symptoms and laboratory findings
  - "Nonfunctional" malignant tumors often diagnosed late, with extensive liver metastases
  - Are usually very vascular on imaging (unlike pancreatic ductal carcinoma)
- Pancreatic anomalies are relatively common
  - **Pancreas divisum**
    - Failure of fusion of ventral and dorsal pancreas
    - Predisposes to acute/recurrent pancreatitis
  - **Annular pancreas**
    - Error in rotation of ventral pancreas
    - Results in a ring of pancreatic tissue that encircles and narrows duodenum

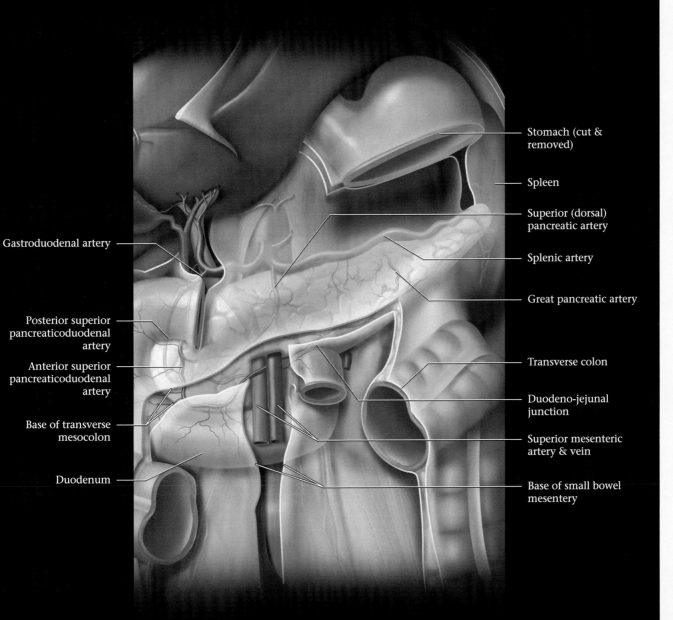

Gastroduodenal artery

Posterior superior
pancreaticoduodenal
artery

Anterior superior
pancreaticoduodenal
artery

Base of transverse
mesocolon

Duodenum

Stomach (cut &
removed)

Spleen

Superior (dorsal)
pancreatic artery

Splenic artery

Great pancreatic artery

Transverse colon

Duodeno-jejunal
junction

Superior mesenteric
artery & vein

Base of small bowel
mesentery

The arterial supply to the body & tail of the pancreas is through terminal branches of the splenic artery, which are variable in number & size. The two largest are usually the dorsal (superior) and great pancreatic arteries, which arise from the proximal & distal splenic artery, respectively. The arteries to the pancreatic head and duodenum come from the pancreaticoduodenal arcades that receive flow from the celiac and superior mesenteric arteries. The superior mesenteric vessels pass behind the neck of the pancreas and in front of the third portion of the duodenum. The root of the transverse mesocolon and small bowel mesentery arise from the surface of the pancreas and transmit the blood vessels to the small bowel & transverse colon. The splenic vein runs along the dorsal surface of the pancreas. The splenic vessels and pancreatic tail insert into the splenic hilum.

PANCREAS

AXIAL CT

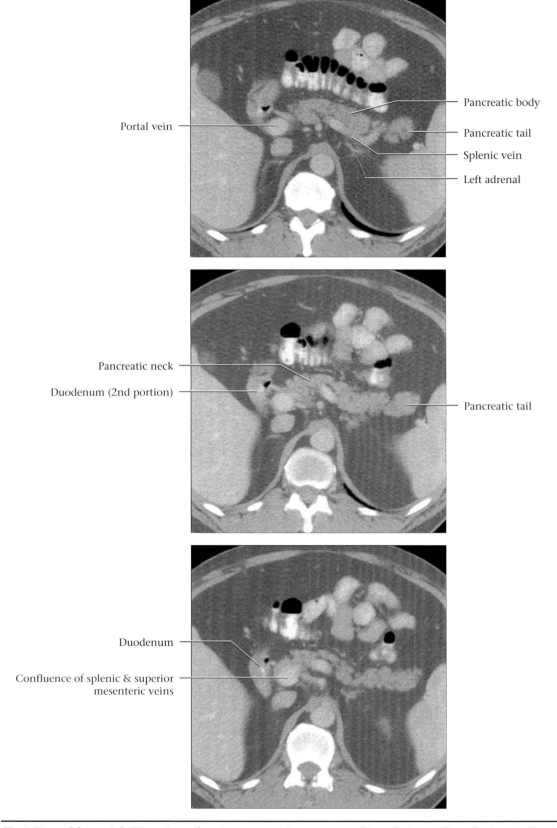

Portal vein

Pancreatic body

Pancreatic tail

Splenic vein

Left adrenal

Pancreatic neck

Duodenum (2nd portion)

Pancreatic tail

Duodenum

Confluence of splenic & superior
mesenteric veins

(Top) First of five axial CT sections showing a normal pancreas and its relations. The splenic vein lies in a groove along the length of the body of the pancreas. The tail of the pancreas lies in the splenic hilum within the splenorenal ligament. **(Middle)** The neck of the pancreas lies just ventral to the superior mesenteric artery and vein. Note the normal degree of fatty lobulation of the pancreas, typical of a young to middle-aged person. **(Bottom)** The head of the pancreas lies between the confluence of the splenic and superior mesenteric veins and the medial wall of the second portion of the duodenum.

PANCREAS

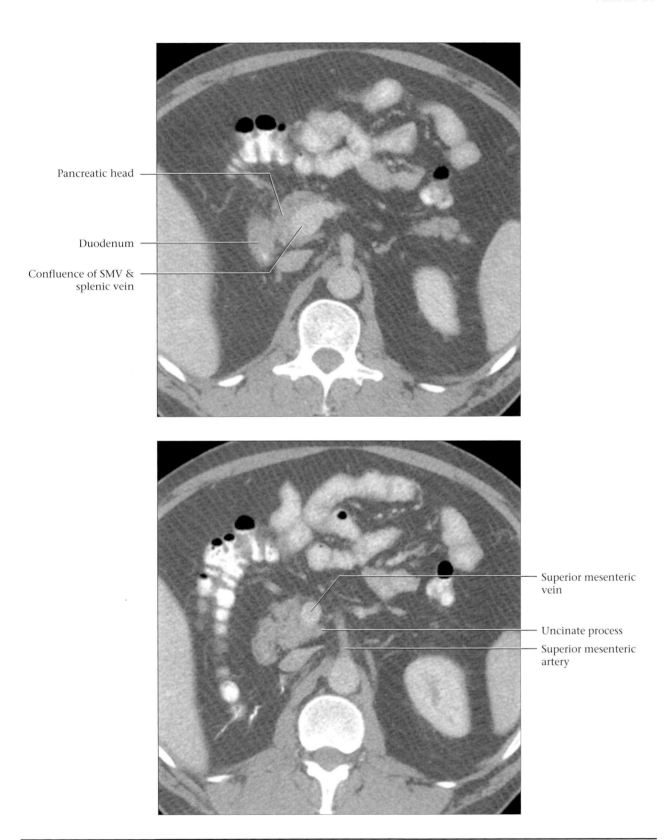

Pancreatic head

Duodenum

Confluence of SMV & splenic vein

Superior mesenteric vein

Uncinate process

Superior mesenteric artery

(Top) The head of the pancreas lies lateral to the superior mesenteric vein (SMV) or SMV-portal vein confluence, while the uncinate process lies dorsal to the SMV. (Bottom) The uncinate process is that portion of the pancreas that extends dorsal to the superior mesenteric vein (SMV).

PANCREAS

CATHETER ANGIOGRAPHY, VESSELS

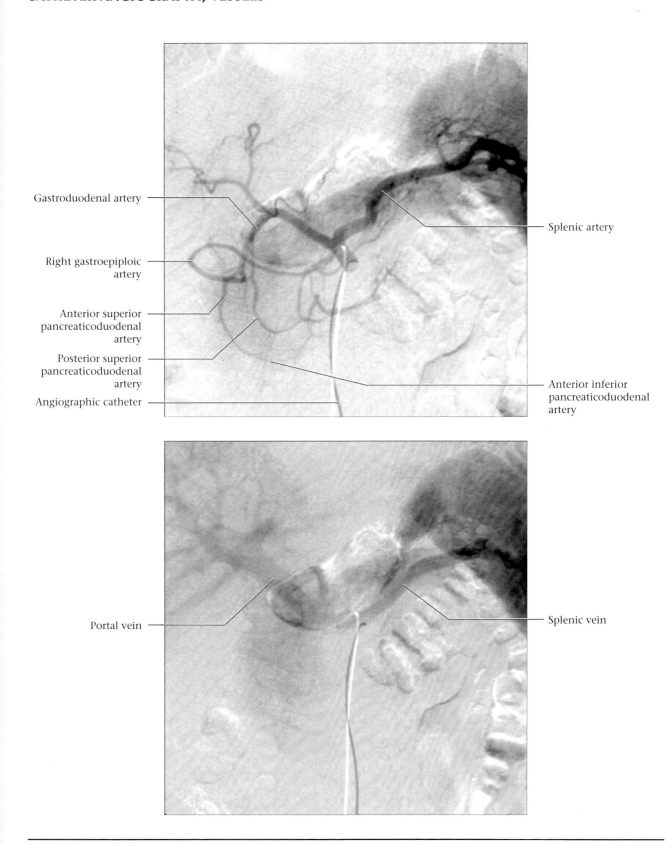

Gastroduodenal artery

Right gastroepiploic artery

Anterior superior pancreaticoduodenal artery

Posterior superior pancreaticoduodenal artery

Angiographic catheter

Splenic artery

Anterior inferior pancreaticoduodenal artery

Portal vein

Splenic vein

(Top) First of two images from a celiac angiogram shows the arterial supply of the pancreas and adjacent organs. Arteries to the pancreatic head and duodenum come from two arcades, the anterior & posterior pancreaticoduodenal arteries, which anastomose with branches from the superior mesenteric artery. The body and tail portions of the pancreas are supplied by branches of the splenic artery which are quite variable in size and distribution. Some are short twigs without specific names, while two are generally larger, the dorsal (superior) and great pancreatic arteries, which originate from the splenic artery proximally and distally, respectively. The gastroduodenal artery courses downward behind the first portion of the duodenum and antero-lateral to the head of the pancreas. (Bottom) The venous drainage of the pancreas is to the splenic, superior mesenteric & portal veins.

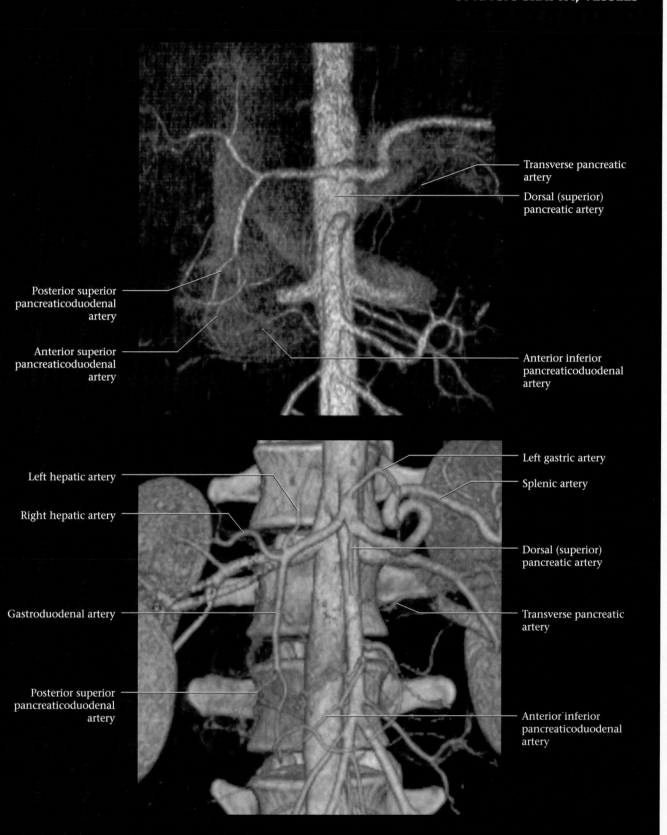

Transverse pancreatic artery

Dorsal (superior) pancreatic artery

Posterior superior pancreaticoduodenal artery

Anterior superior pancreaticoduodenal artery

Anterior inferior pancreaticoduodenal artery

Left gastric artery

Left hepatic artery

Splenic artery

Right hepatic artery

Dorsal (superior) pancreatic artery

Gastroduodenal artery

Transverse pancreatic artery

Posterior superior pancreaticoduodenal artery

Anterior inferior pancreaticoduodenal artery

(Top) Coronal reformation, CT arteriogram demonstrates conventional upper abdominal arteries. The anterior and posterior pancreaticoduodenal arteries arise from the gastroduodenal artery, and their inferior extensions anastomose with the superior mesenteric artery. The dorsal (superior) pancreatic artery arises from the proximal splenic artery. The arterial supply to the pancreas is highly variable and all of the branches anastomose to a considerable degree. The transverse pancreatic artery runs parallel to the splenic artery along the long axis of the pancreas, also sending numerous small, anastomotic branches to the pancreas. (Bottom) A coronal 3D volume rendered CTA in a different patient from previous image shows conventional pancreatic arterial anatomy, but variant hepatic, with the left hepatic artery arising from the common hepatic and the right hepatic from the gastroduodenal artery.

PANCREAS

AXIAL CT, PANCREATIC ARTERIES

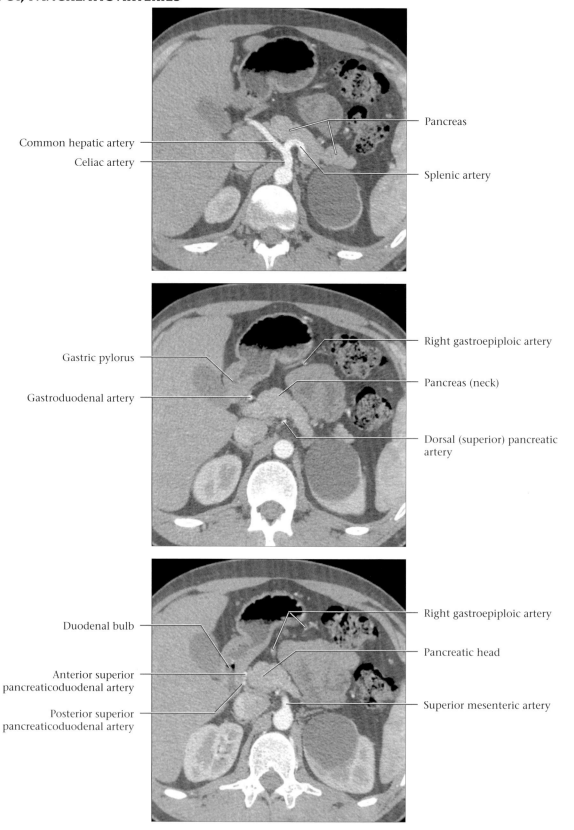

Common hepatic artery

Celiac artery

Pancreas

Splenic artery

Gastric pylorus

Gastroduodenal artery

Right gastroepiploic artery

Pancreas (neck)

Dorsal (superior) pancreatic artery

Duodenal bulb

Anterior superior pancreaticoduodenal artery

Posterior superior pancreaticoduodenal artery

Right gastroepiploic artery

Pancreatic head

Superior mesenteric artery

(Top) First of five axial CT sections in the arterial phase of imaging show normal pancreas and conventional arterial anatomy. The splenic and common hepatic arteries arise from the celiac trunk and supply most of the blood supply to the pancreas through many branches, with a highly variable pattern. **(Middle)** The dorsal (superior) pancreatic artery courses along the posterior surface of the pancreas in a vertical orientation, and is usually the first branch of the splenic artery. The gastroduodenal artery is the first branch of the common hepatic artery and passes behind the gastric pylorus and duodenal bulb and antero-lateral to the pancreatic head. **(Bottom)** The three major branches of the gastroduodenal artery are the right gastroepiploic artery and the anterior and posterior superior pancreaticoduodenal arteries.

PANCREAS

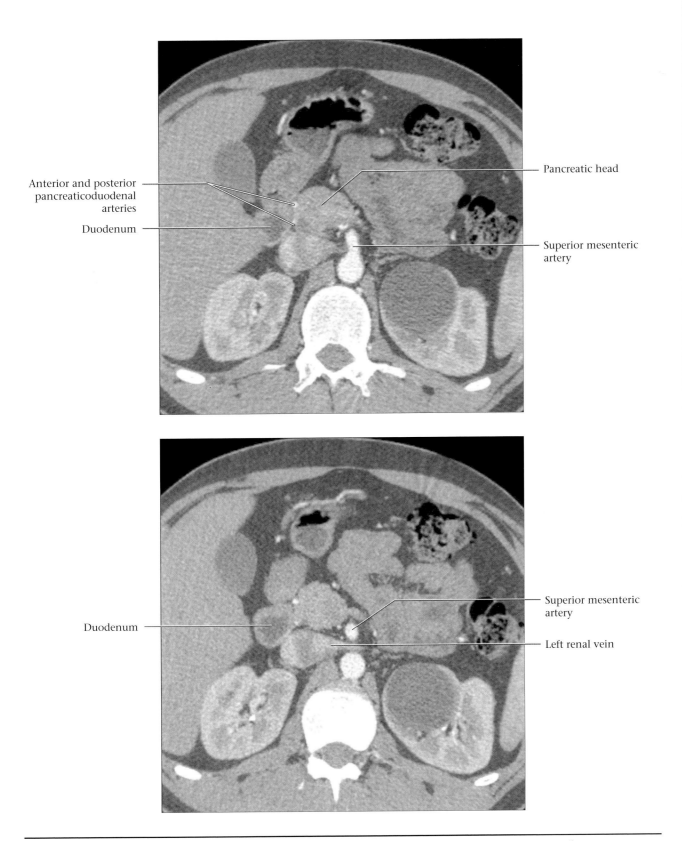

(Top) The anterior and posterior pancreaticoduodenal arcades surround the head of the pancreas and anastomose with the superior mesenteric artery through the inferior branches of these vessels. **(Bottom)** The pancreaticoduodenal arcades send branches laterally to the duodenum and medially to the pancreas.

PANCREAS

AXIAL CT, PARENCHYMA AND VEINS

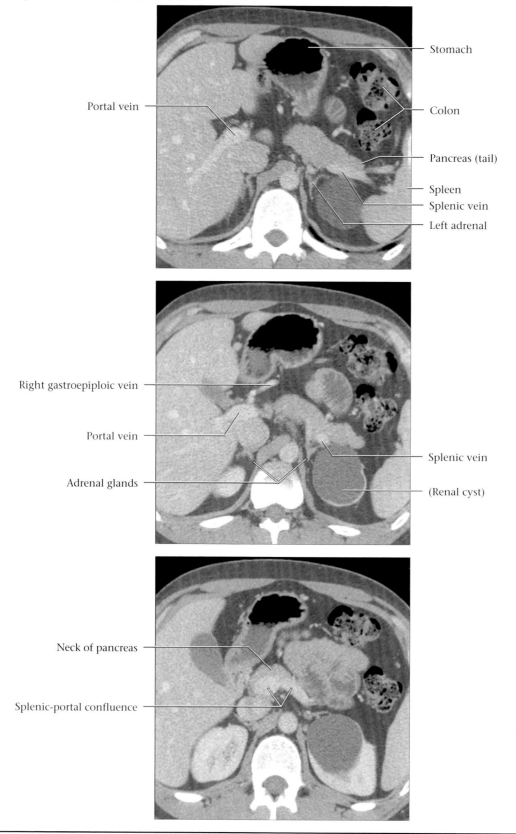

(Top) First of five axial CT sections shows the body and tail of the pancreas lying in a nearly transverse plane, with the splenic vein running in a groove along its dorsal surface. The body of the pancreas lies just ventral to the splenic vein, and the adrenal just dorsal to it. (Middle) There are no reliable measures of "normal" pancreatic dimensions. The normal gland tapers smoothly from the head to the tail, with some thinning through the neck region. Focal areas of enlargement are suggestive of tumor or focal inflammation. (Bottom) The neck of the pancreas lies just ventral to the confluence of the splenic and portal veins.

PANCREAS

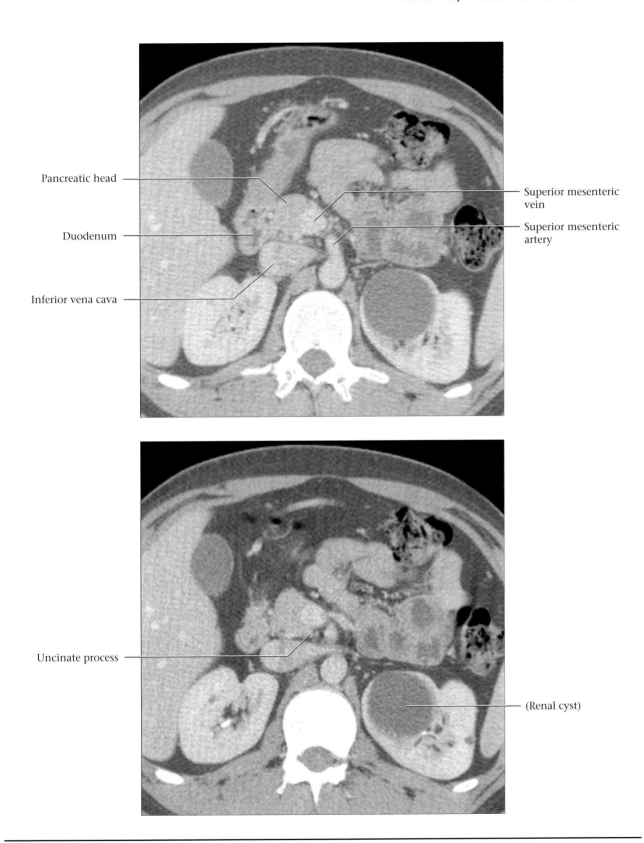

Pancreatic head

Superior mesenteric vein

Duodenum

Superior mesenteric artery

Inferior vena cava

Uncinate process

(Renal cyst)

(Top) The head of the pancreas lies between the second portion of duodenum and the superior mesenteric vessels. The inferior vena cava lies just behind the head of the pancreas. **(Bottom)** The uncinate process lies just behind the superior mesenteric vein.

PANCREAS

CORONAL CT

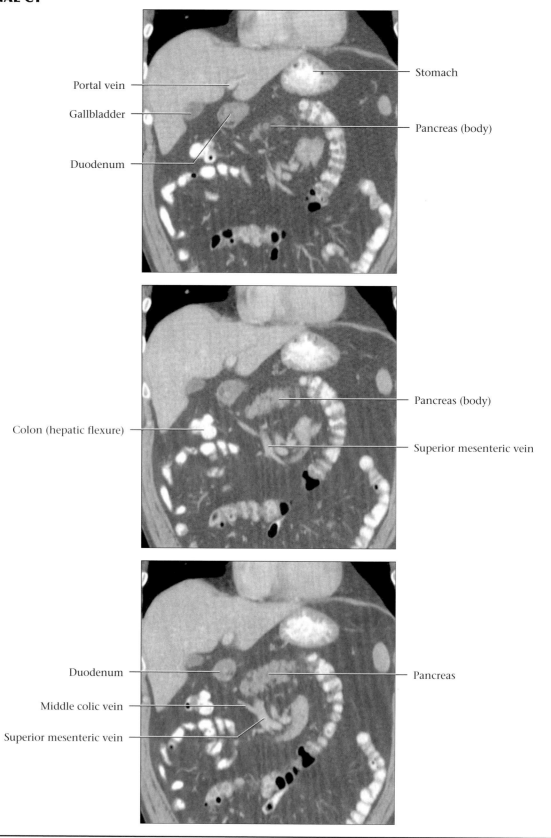

Portal vein

Gallbladder

Duodenum

Stomach

Pancreas (body)

Colon (hepatic flexure)

Pancreas (body)

Superior mesenteric vein

Duodenum

Middle colic vein

Superior mesenteric vein

Pancreas

(Top) First of six coronal CT sections showing normal pancreas and its relations. This most ventral section shows only the anterior surface of the pancreas. **(Middle)** The superior mesenteric vein is seen caudal to the pancreas. **(Bottom)** As the superior mesenteric vein courses toward the liver, it begins to move dorsally, eventually passing behind the neck of the pancreas.

PANCREAS

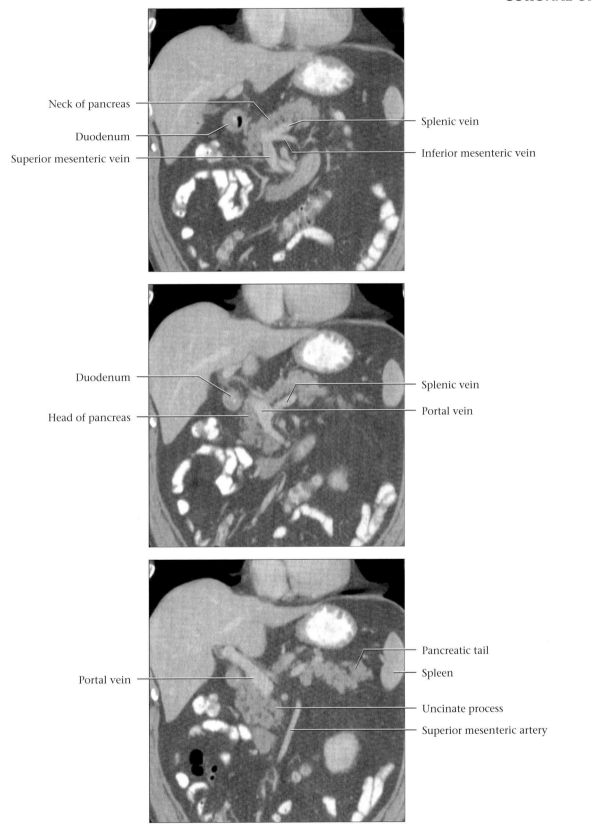

Neck of pancreas

Duodenum

Superior mesenteric vein

Splenic vein

Inferior mesenteric vein

Duodenum

Head of pancreas

Splenic vein

Portal vein

Portal vein

Pancreatic tail

Spleen

Uncinate process

Superior mesenteric artery

(Top) The confluence of the superior & inferior mesenteric veins with the splenic vein is seen, just dorsal and caudal to the neck of the pancreas. The head of the pancreas lies between the mesenteric vessels and the second portion of the duodenum. (Middle) Note the relation between the duodenum and the head of the pancreas. The splenic vein runs in a groove along the posterior surface of the pancreas. Note the thin fat plane between the pancreas and the splenic vein; this plane is often obliterated in cases of pancreatitis or carcinoma. (Bottom) The tail of the pancreas usually lies in the splenic hilum, within the splenorenal ligament.

PANCREAS

AXIAL MR, ARTERIAL PHASE

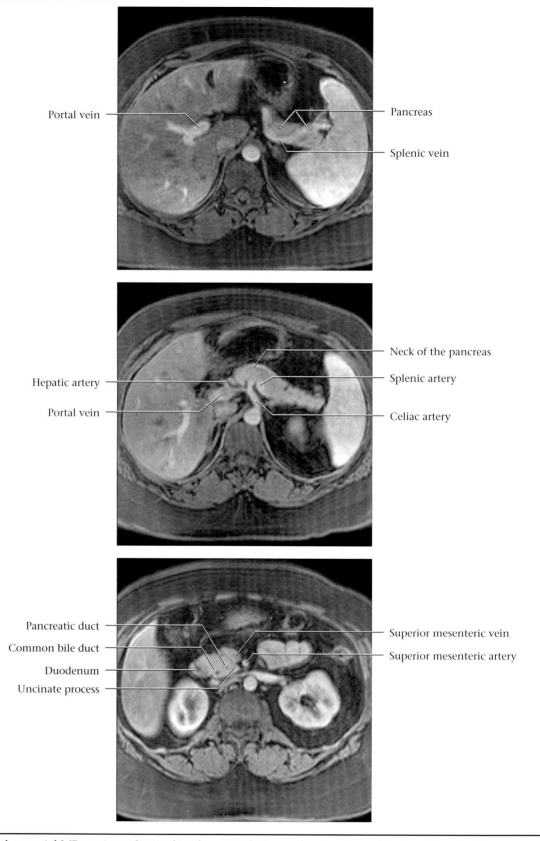

Portal vein

Pancreas

Splenic vein

Neck of the pancreas

Hepatic artery

Splenic artery

Portal vein

Celiac artery

Pancreatic duct

Superior mesenteric vein

Common bile duct

Superior mesenteric artery

Duodenum

Uncinate process

(Top) First of three axial MR sections obtained in the arterial phase of contrast opacification showing the relationship of the body and tail of the pancreas to the splenic vein and the spleen. **(Middle)** The neck of the pancreas is its thinnest portion and lies just ventral to the celiac and superior mesenteric vessels. **(Bottom)** The uncinate process lies behind the superior mesenteric vein (which is not yet well opacified on this arterial phase image). Note the common bile duct and pancreatic duct as low signal "dots", passing vertically through the head of the pancreas.

PANCREAS

Neck of pancreas
Body of pancreas
Celiac artery
Portal vein

Stomach
Neck of pancreas
Portal vein
Splenic vein

Superior mesenteric vein
Duodenum
Left renal vein
Uncinate process

(Top) First of three axial MR sections obtained during the portal venous phase of contrast enhancement shows the neck and body of the pancreas in relation to the celiac and portal vessels. **(Middle)** The neck of the pancreas lies just anterior to the splenic-portal venous confluence. **(Bottom)** The uncinate process lies posterior to the superior mesenteric vein, but does not usually extend behind the artery. The left renal vein often passes between the superior mesenteric vessels and the aorta at this level as well. The third structure that lies in this space is the third portion of the duodenum, which lies about 2 cm more caudal than the uncinate and renal vein.

PANCREAS

MRCP, PANCREATIC & BILE DUCTS

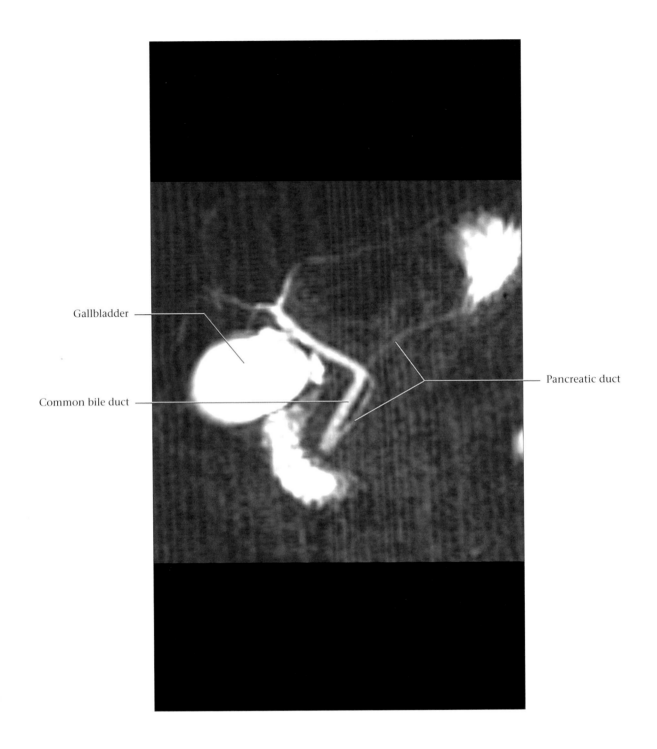

A coronal MR cholangiopancreatogram shows normal caliber pancreatic and bile ducts. The common bile duct & pancreatic duct run a parallel course within the head of the pancreas and join together just prior to emptying into the duodenum at the hepaticopancreatic papilla (of Vater).

PANCREAS

SPLENIC & PANCREATIC ARTERIES

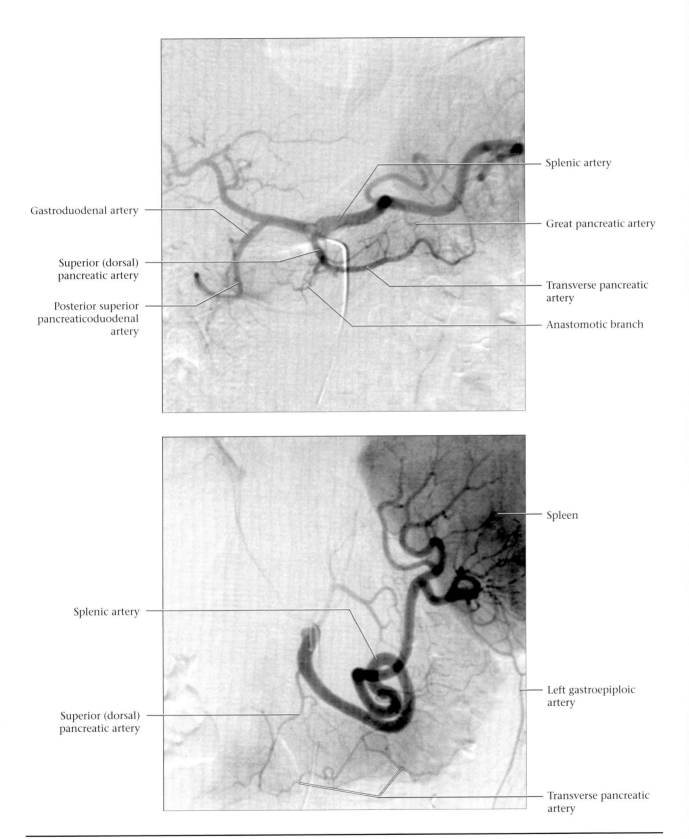

Splenic artery

Gastroduodenal artery

Great pancreatic artery

Superior (dorsal) pancreatic artery

Transverse pancreatic artery

Posterior superior pancreaticoduodenal artery

Anastomotic branch

Splenic artery

Spleen

Superior (dorsal) pancreatic artery

Left gastroepiploic artery

Transverse pancreatic artery

(Top) Selective catheter injection of the celiac artery shows a prominent superior (dorsal) pancreatic artery arising from the celiac artery itself or the proximal splenic artery (its usual source). The transverse pancreatic artery runs along the main axis of the pancreas and receives branches from the superior and great pancreatic arteries and from a separate branch of the SMA, the inferior pancreatic artery. In spite of the name, the "great" pancreatic artery may be relatively small, as in this subject. A branch of the superior pancreatic artery anastomoses with the pancreaticoduodenal arcade. (Bottom) In this subject the splenic artery is very tortuous, a common finding. The pancreatic arterial supply is mostly through unnamed terminal branches of the splenic artery. Neither the superior nor the great pancreatic artery are substantial vessels in this subject.

SENESCENT CHANGE

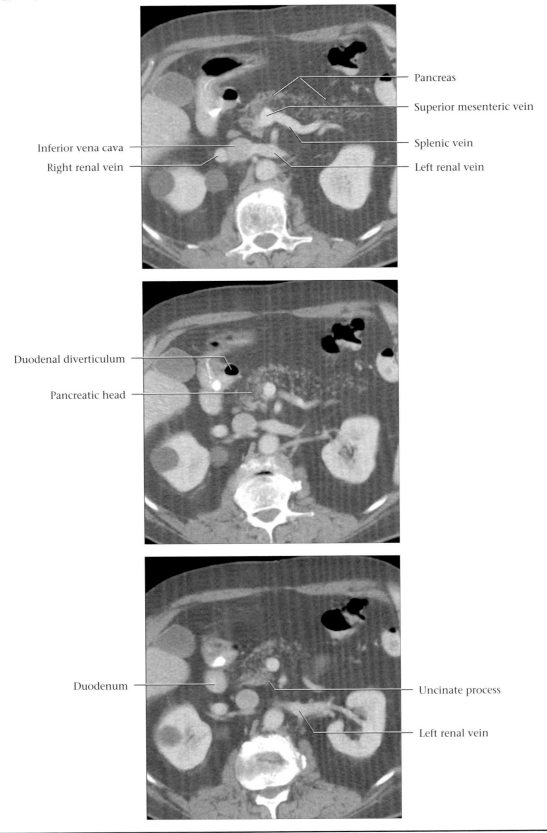

Pancreas

Superior mesenteric vein

Splenic vein

Inferior vena cava

Left renal vein

Right renal vein

Duodenal diverticulum

Pancreatic head

Duodenum

Uncinate process

Left renal vein

(Top) First of three axial CT sections in an elderly patient shows extensive fatty infiltration of the pancreas. While this can be associated with chronic pancreatitis, diabetes and obesity, it is often a normal finding of no clinical significance. The pancreatic parenchyma begins to atrophy and the pancreatic duct may dilate in subjects beyond the age of seventy, without symptoms or signs of pancreatic insufficiency. **(Middle)** In patients with extensive fatty infiltration of the pancreas, as in this subject, the pancreas can be difficult to visualize on ultrasonography, as it is of similar echogenicity as the surrounding retroperitoneal fat. **(Bottom)** In this subject, the degree of fatty infiltration is relatively uniform throughout the gland; as in hepatic steatosis, however, this is not always the case.

PANCREAS

VARIANT, ASYMMETRIC FATTY INFILTRATION

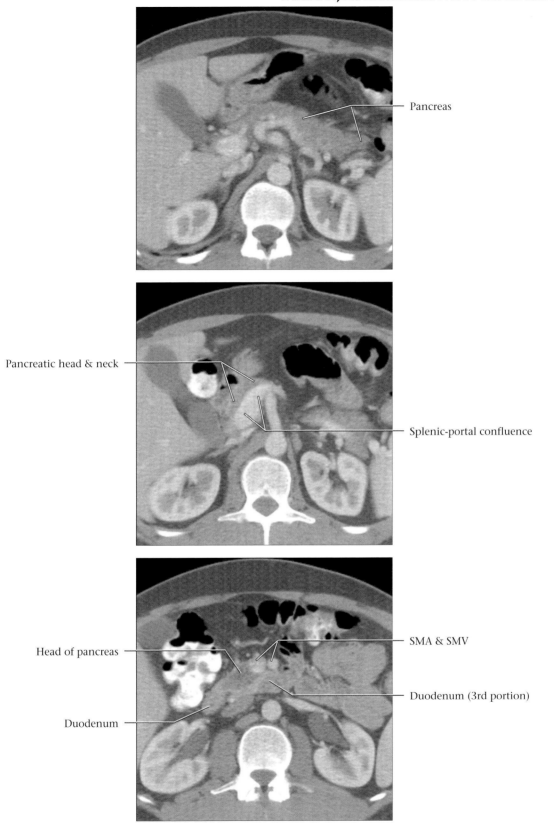

Pancreas

Pancreatic head & neck

Splenic-portal confluence

Head of pancreas

SMA & SMV

Duodenum (3rd portion)

Duodenum

(Top) First of three axial CT sections of a patient with no symptoms or signs of pancreatic disease shows a normal appearing, "soft tissue density" body and tail of pancreas. (Middle) A more caudal section shows that the neck and head of the pancreas are of substantially lower attenuation (density), and might be mistaken for a hypodense, hypovascular mass, such as pancreatic ductal carcinoma. The absence of dilation of the pancreatic or common bile duct correctly suggests the absence of a neoplastic mass in the pancreas. (Bottom) The density of the head of the pancreas is substantially lower than that of the remaining pancreas, but there are no radiographic or clinical signs of tumor or inflammation. The morphology of the pancreatic head may vary from that of the body due to their separate embryologic development, from the ventral and dorsal pancreatic buds.

PANCREAS

ACUTE PANCREATITIS

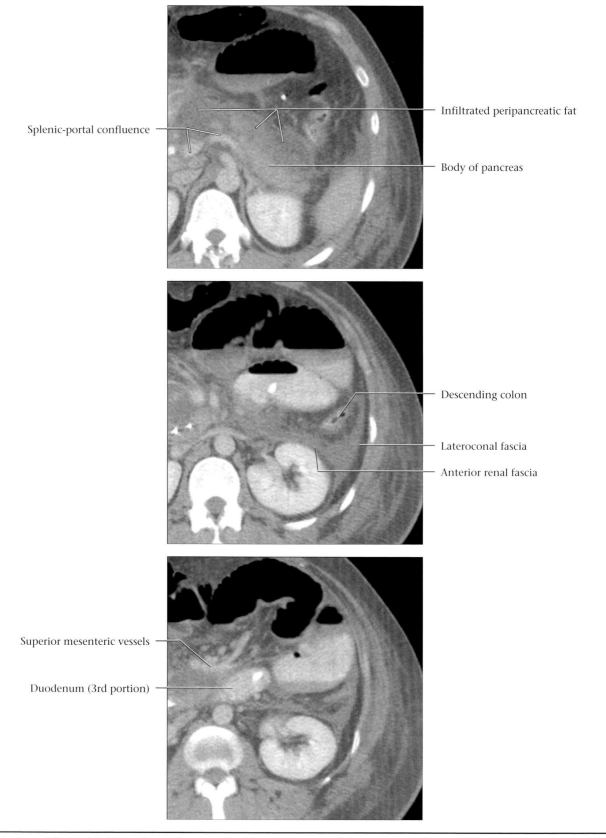

Splenic-portal confluence —

— Infiltrated peripancreatic fat

— Body of pancreas

— Descending colon

— Lateroconal fascia

— Anterior renal fascia

Superior mesenteric vessels —

Duodenum (3rd portion) —

(Top) First of five axial CT sections of a patient with severe upper abdominal pain following heavy alcohol consumption shows diffuse infiltration (blurring) of the fat planes surrounding the pancreas, due to acute pancreatitis. (Middle) The inflammatory process spreads out in all directions. Laterally, it is restrained by the lateroconal fascia, which marks the lateral margin of the anterior pararenal space. Posteriorly, it is restrained by the anterior layer of the renal fascia. The pancreas lies within the anterior pararenal space, along with the duodenum and the ascending & descending colon. (Bottom) The inflammation spreads ventrally and caudally to enter the small bowel mesentery; note the infiltration of the fat planes around the mesenteric vessels. The roots of the small bowel mesentery (& transverse mesocolon) arise from just ventral to the pancreas.

PANCREAS

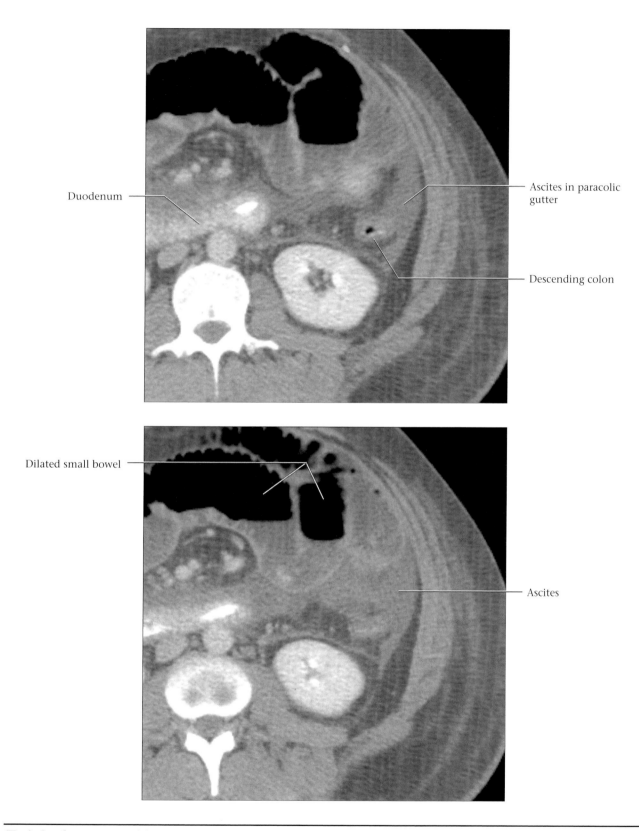

Duodenum

Ascites in paracolic gutter

Descending colon

Dilated small bowel

Ascites

(Top) On this more caudal section, the lateroconal fascia and the parietal peritoneum are adherent to each other. The fluid lateral to the descending colon is in the peritoneal cavity (the paracolic gutter), and represents "pancreatic ascites". (Bottom) Dilated small bowel segments are noted, representing an ileus due to severe abdominal pain and abnormal fluid and electrolyte balances, another result of acute pancreatitis.

PANCREAS

PANCREATITIS WITH PSEUDOCYST

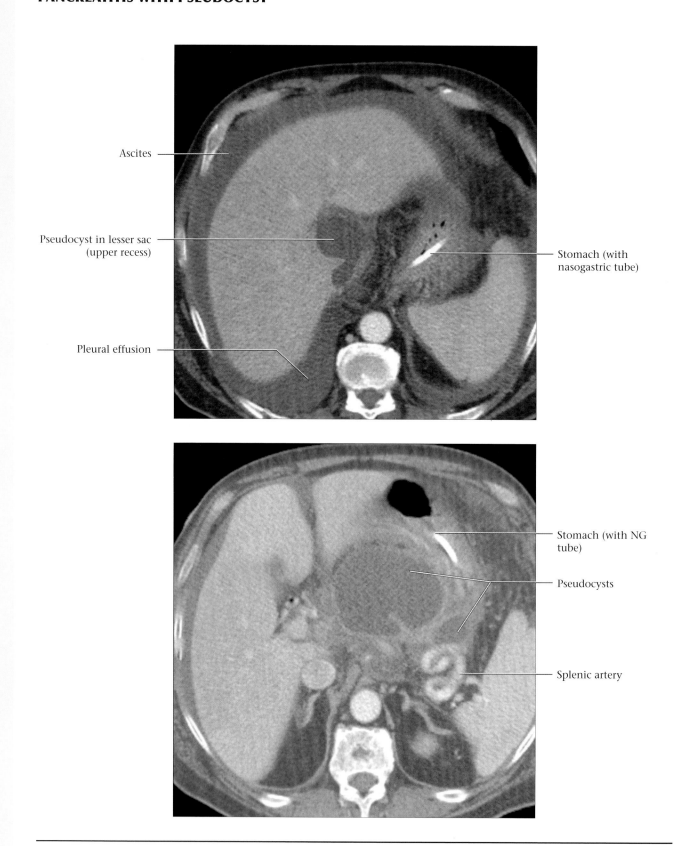

Ascites

Pseudocyst in lesser sac (upper recess)

Stomach (with nasogastric tube)

Pleural effusion

Stomach (with NG tube)

Pseudocysts

Splenic artery

(Top) First of four axial CT sections of a patient with recurrent pancreatitis shows ascites and pleural effusions. In addition, there is a loculated fluid collection in the upper recess of the lesser sac, representing a pseudocyst. (Bottom) Large loculated pseudocysts in the lesser sac displace the stomach forward. Note the contrast-enhancing wall of the pseudocyst. Pseudocysts do not have an epithelial lining but represent loculated collections of pancreatic juice, necrotic debris and inflammatory exudate with an inflammatory and fibrotic wall.

PANCREAS

PANCREATITIS WITH PSEUDOCYST

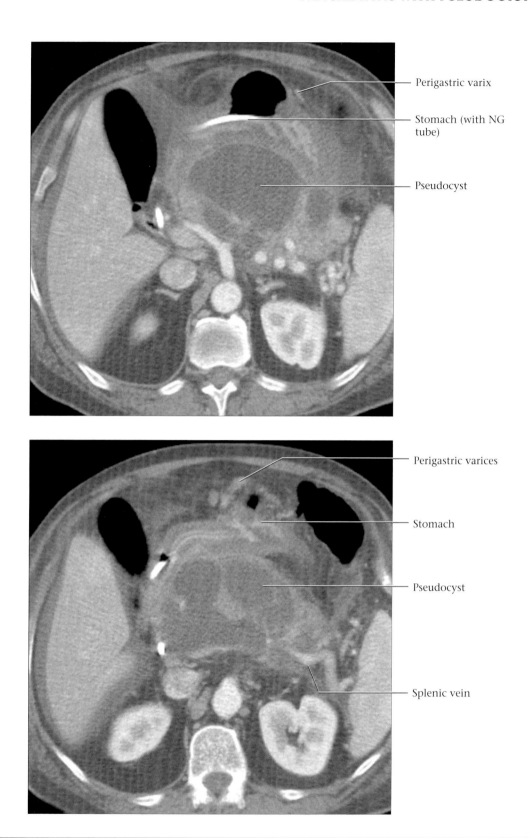

Perigastric varix

Stomach (with NG tube)

Pseudocyst

Perigastric varices

Stomach

Pseudocyst

Splenic vein

(Top) The stomach is displaced and its wall is thickened due to the adjacent pseudocyst. Pseudocysts often resolve spontaneously, but may require drainage due to complications such as infection, hemorrhage, or obstruction of bowel or bile ducts. **(Bottom)** The largest pseudocyst is quite septated, as is common. Note the mass effect on the splenic vein, resulting in narrowing or occlusion of this vessel. Perigastric varices have developed to return blood from the spleen and pancreas to the portal vein, bypassing the obstructed splenic vein. Gastric varices in the absence of portal hypertension implies splenic vein occlusion, usually due to pancreatitis or pancreatic carcinoma.

PANCREAS

CARCINOMA, DUCTAL OBSTRUCTION

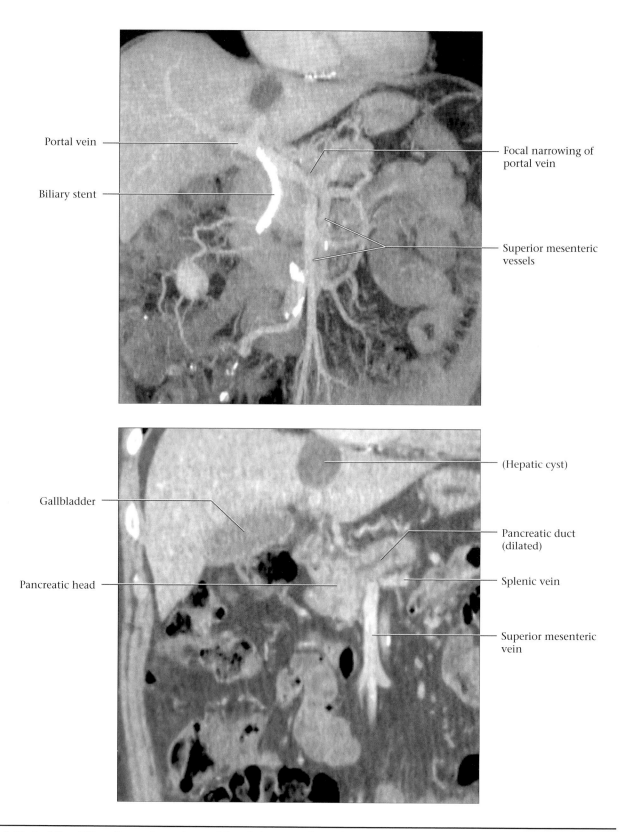

Portal vein

Biliary stent

Focal narrowing of portal vein

Superior mesenteric vessels

(Hepatic cyst)

Gallbladder

Pancreatic duct (dilated)

Splenic vein

Pancreatic head

Superior mesenteric vein

(Top) First of five CT sections of a patient with painless jaundice. This coronal reformation shows a plastic stent in the extrahepatic bile duct, placed endoscopically to bypass an obstruction of the common bile duct. There is a subtle narrowing of the portal vein at its confluence with the superior mesenteric vein. **(Bottom)** A more anterior plane of reformation shows abrupt narrowing of the pancreatic duct as it enters the head of the pancreas. The abrupt transition suggests the presence of a pancreatic tumor, though a discreet mass is not evident.

PANCREAS

CARCINOMA, DUCTAL OBSTRUCTION

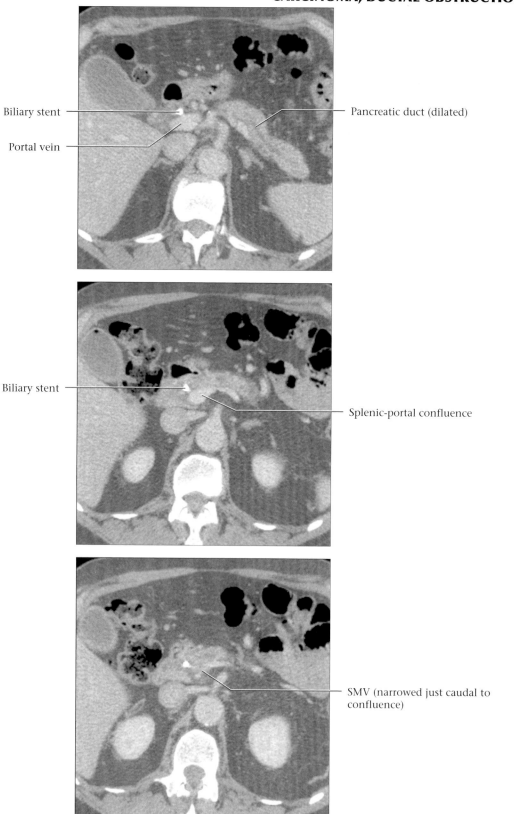

Biliary stent — Pancreatic duct (dilated)

Portal vein

Biliary stent — Splenic-portal confluence

SMV (narrowed just caudal to confluence)

(Top) Axial CT section shows dilation of the pancreatic duct throughout the body and tail segments. (Middle) Axial CT section through the pancreatic neck shows no obvious mass. (Bottom) A section just caudal to the confluence of the superior mesenteric and splenic veins shows abrupt narrowing of the lumen of the SMV. In this patient, the indirect signs of a pancreatic carcinoma, such as biliary and vascular encasement, are more evident than the tumor itself.

PANCREAS

CARCINOMA, VASCULAR OCCLUSION

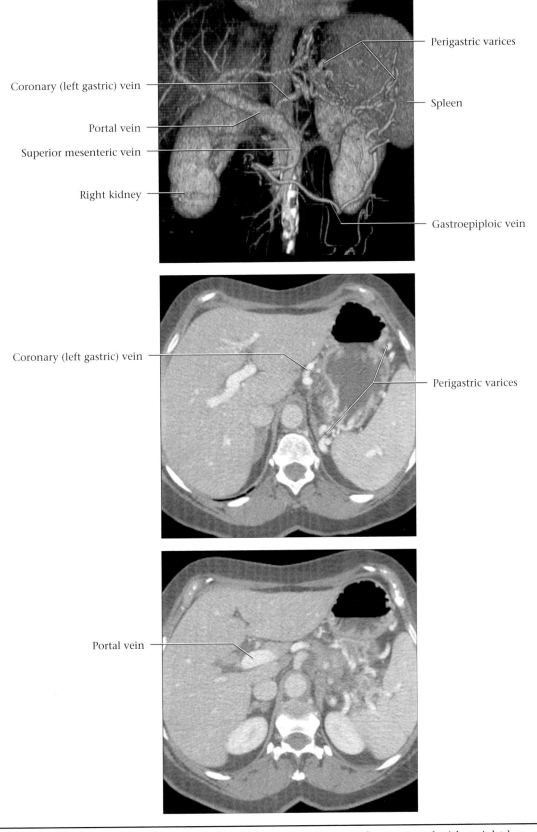

(Top) First of six CT images from a patient with pancreatic carcinoma, who presented with weight loss and upper gastrointestinal bleeding. This coronal reformation highlights the portal venous system and shows complete occlusion of the splenic vein with extensive collateral flow through perigastric varices and the gastroepiploic vein. (Middle) Axial CT shows multiple perigastric varices and an enlarged coronary (left gastric) vein. (Bottom) A more caudal section shows a normal appearing liver and portal vein but no splenic vein. Numerous collateral veins are noted in the splenic hilum near the tail of the pancreas.

PANCREAS

CARCINOMA, VASCULAR OCCLUSION

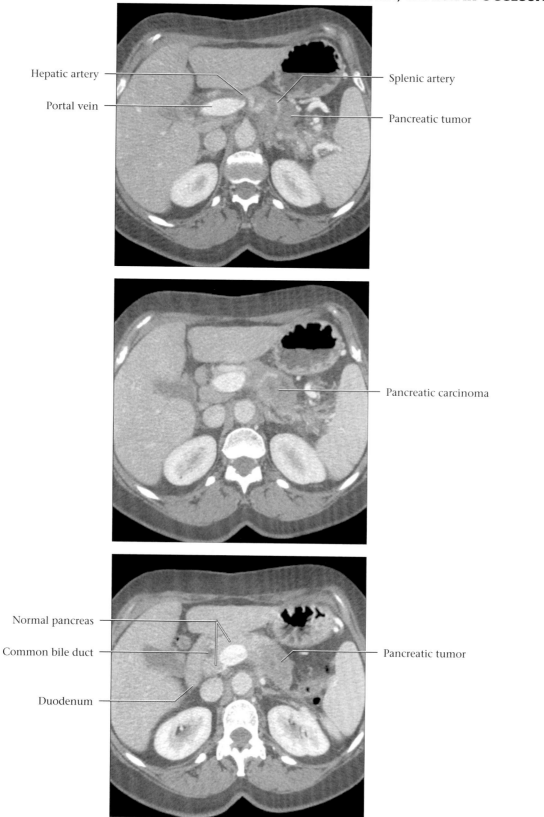

(Top) The hepatic and splenic arteries are encased and narrowed by a large hypodense mass that occupies the body of the pancreas. The splenic vein should be seen coursing from the splenic hilum, along the body of the pancreas, to the portal vein. Instead, it has been occluded along much of its length by the pancreatic carcinoma. (Middle) A more caudal section shows the heterogeneous, hypodense tumor that replaces much of the body of the pancreas. The tumor encases and narrows the hepatic and splenic arteries, indicating that the tumor cannot be resected for cure. (Bottom) Note the difference between the hypodense (dark) appearance of the pancreatic carcinoma and the normal pancreatic head and neck sections. The common bile duct courses normally through the head of the pancreas.

PANCREAS

ISLET CELL TUMOR

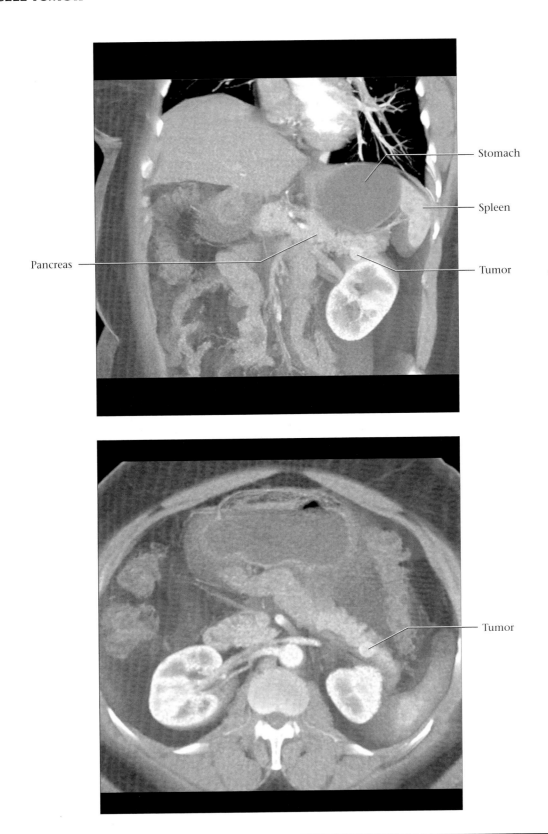

Stomach

Spleen

Pancreas

Tumor

Tumor

(Top) First of two CT sections of a patient with symptoms of palpitations and fainting, found to be due to hypoglycemia. This coronal reformation of a CT scan shows a hypervascular mass in the pancreatic body. This is the typical appearance of an islet cell (neuroendocrine) tumor; a benign insulin-secreting tumor ("insulinoma") was removed at surgery. **(Bottom)** A thick axial reformation also shows the hypervascular islet cell tumor arising from the body of the pancreas. The hypervascularity of the mass and the absence of ductal obstruction are among the imaging features that distinguish islet cell tumors from the more common pancreatic ductal carcinoma.

PANCREAS

PANCREATIC DUCT VARIATIONS

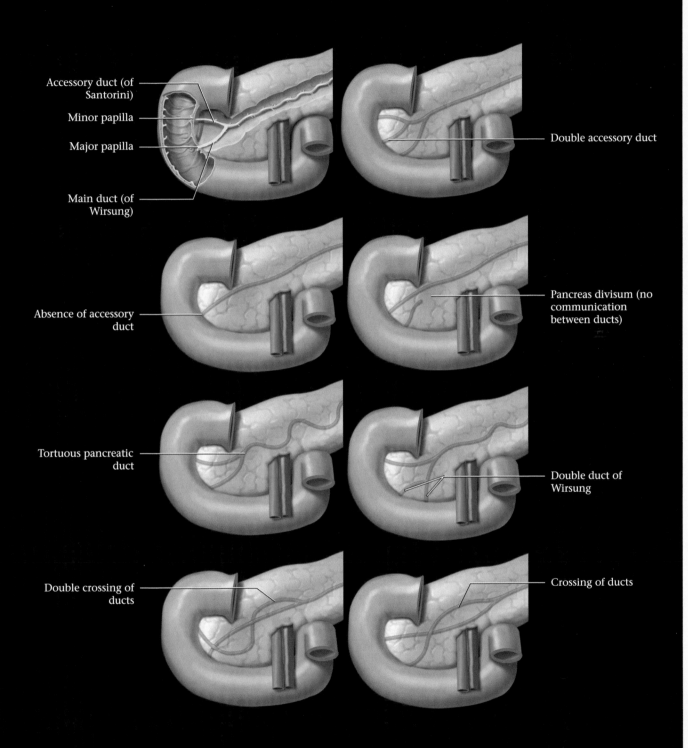

Accessory duct (of Santorini)

Minor papilla

Major papilla

Main duct (of Wirsung)

Double accessory duct

Absence of accessory duct

Pancreas divisum (no communication between ducts)

Tortuous pancreatic duct

Double duct of Wirsung

Double crossing of ducts

Crossing of ducts

The accessory duct (of Santorini) originates with the dorsal pancreatic anlage, which is the larger bud from the embryologic foregut, comprising the pancreatic body & tail. The main duct (of Wirsung) originates with the ventral, smaller, anlage that develops into the pancreatic head and uncinate process. Usually, the main & accessory pancreatic ducts fuse and the main duct becomes the primary conduit for drainage of secretions into the duodenum. The pancreatic duct courses through the center of the gland, and is joined by tributaries that enter it at right angles. In the head, the duct turns caudally & dorsally, and runs parallel to the common bile duct before joining it at the ampulla of Vater and entering the major papilla. The accessory duct usually enters the duodenum more proximally through the minor papilla.

PANCREATIC DIVISUM

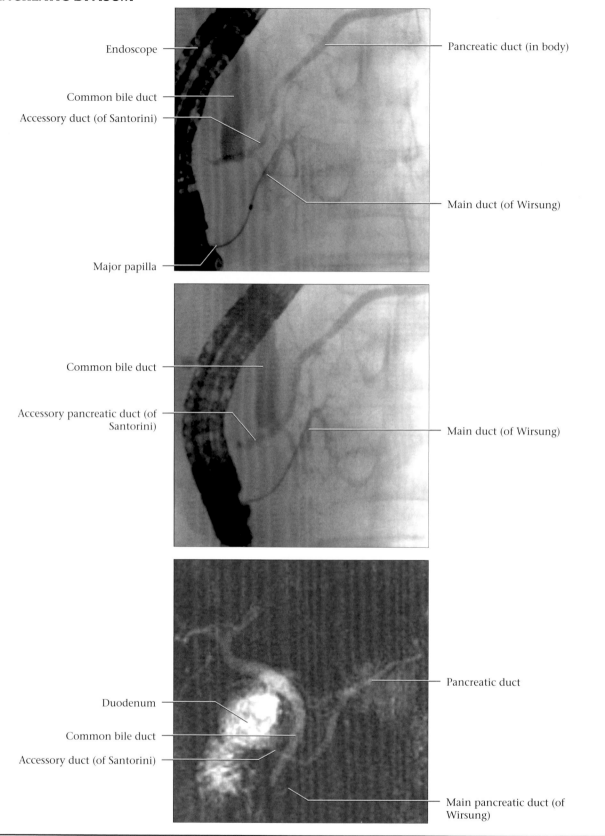

Endoscope

Common bile duct

Accessory duct (of Santorini)

Major papilla

Pancreatic duct (in body)

Main duct (of Wirsung)

Common bile duct

Accessory pancreatic duct (of Santorini)

Main duct (of Wirsung)

Pancreatic duct

Duodenum

Common bile duct

Accessory duct (of Santorini)

Main pancreatic duct (of Wirsung)

(Top) First in series of three images show pancreas divisum, in which the main and accessory ducts fail to fuse. ERCP shows the endoscopic canula in the major papilla with opacification of only the main duct in the pancreatic head and the common bile duct. (Spasm of the choledochal sphincter prevents distention of the distal CBD, which communicated with the main pancreatic duct at the major papilla.) Separate cannulation of the minor papilla had filled the accessory duct of Santorini and the duct throughout the pancreas. **(Middle)** An oblique image from the ERCP shows that the main and accessory pancreatic ducts do not communicate. The accessory duct crosses the common bile duct. **(Bottom)** MRCP shows crossing of the common bile duct and the accessory pancreatic duct, which drains the body of the pancreas in this subject. The main pancreatic duct is small and not in communication.

PANCREAS

ANNULAR PANCREAS

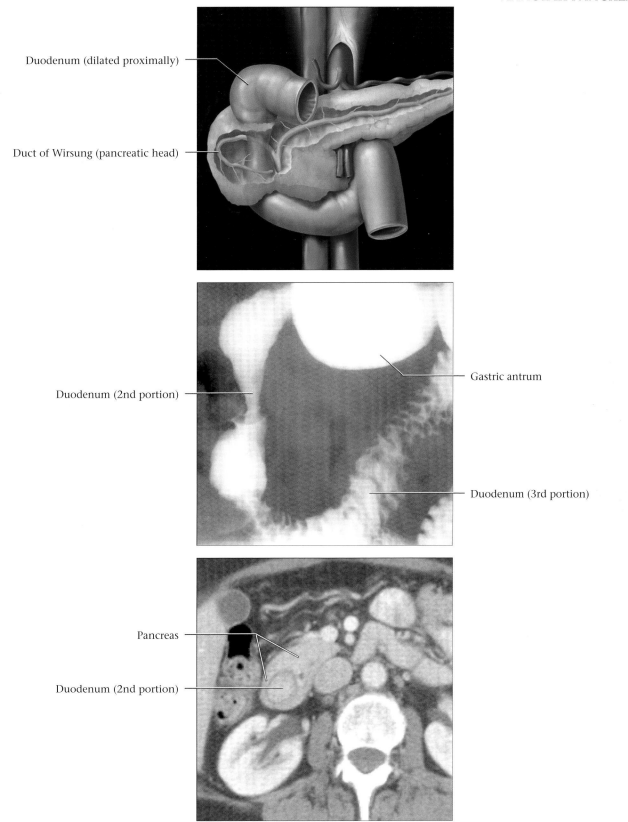

Duodenum (dilated proximally)

Duct of Wirsung (pancreatic head)

Gastric antrum

Duodenum (2nd portion)

Duodenum (3rd portion)

Pancreas

Duodenum (2nd portion)

(Top) First of three images illustrates annular pancreas, in which there is abnormal rotation and fusion of the ventral & dorsal pancreatic anlage, resulting in a circumferential mass of pancreatic tissue that encircles and narrows the duodenum. The duct draining the pancreatic head encircles the second portion of the duodenum. This condition may remain asymptomatic or may result in obstruction of the duodenum, often in neonates. **(Middle)** A spot film from a barium upper GI series shows circumferential narrowing of the second portion of the duodenum in an adult patient with long-standing symptoms of early satiety from an annular pancreas. **(Bottom)** An axial CT section shows pancreatic tissue completely encircling the second portion of the duodenum.

RETROPERITONEUM

Terminology

Abbreviations
- Perirenal space (PS)
- Anterior pararenal space (APS)
- Posterior pararenal space (PPS)

Imaging Anatomy

Overview
- All abdominal contents between **parietal peritoneum** and **transversalis fascia**
- 2 well-defined fascial planes, **(renal & lateroconal fasciae)**, separate the retroperitoneum into 3 compartments
  - **Perirenal space** contains kidney, adrenal, proximal ureter, abundant fat
    - Enclosed by renal fascia
    - Does not extend across abdominal midline
  - **Anterior pararenal space** contains pancreas, duodenum, colon (ascending & descending) and little fat
  - **Posterior pararenal space** contains no organs, some fat; continuous with properitoneal fat
- Renal fascia join and close the perirenal space so that it resembles an inverted cone with tip in iliac fossa
  - Caudal to the perirenal space, the APS and PPS merge to form a single **infrarenal retroperitoneal space**
  - Infrarenal retroperitoneal space communicates directly with the pelvic **prevesical space (of Retzius)**

Anatomic Relationships
- **Parietal peritoneum** separates peritoneal cavity from APS
- **Anterior renal fascia** separates perirenal from APS
- **Posterior renal fascia** separates perirenal from PPS
- **Lateroconal fascia** separates APS from PPS and marks the lateral extent of the APS
- Renal and lateroconal fasciae are laminated planes and can form spaces as pathways of spread for rapidly expanding fluid collections or inflammatory processes (e.g., hemorrhage or pancreatitis)
  - Disease originating in anterior pararenal space (e.g., pancreatitis) can extend posterior to kidney via interfascial plane
- Anterior renal fascia can "split" into a **retromesenteric plane** which is continuous across the midline abdomen
- Posterior renal fascia splits into **retrorenal plane**
- Lateroconal fascia splits into **lateroconal plane**
- All 3 of these planes can be called **interfascial planes** and all communicate at the junction of the lateroconal & renal fasciae
- Interfascial planes communicate across the abdominal midline and extend into pelvis caudal to the perirenal space
- **Great vessels (aorta & IVC)**
  - Occupy poorly defined pre-vertebral portion of retroperitoneum caudal to mediastinum
  - Shared by paraspinal nerve chains (sympathetic), major lymphatic trunks (including chyle cistern & thoracic duct), and ureters

Clinical Implications

Clinical Importance
- **Disease within APS** is common
  - Pancreatic disease > duodenal > colon
  - **Pancreatitis** often spreads inflammation and fluid throughout APS to affect duodenum & descending colon
  - Perforated duodenal ulcer is most common cause of inflammation, fluid, gas in right APS, (may also cause intraperitoneal gas since duodenal bulb is intraperitoneal)
- **Disease in perirenal space** is common
  - Any traumatic, inflammatory or neoplastic process involving kidney or adrenal
  - Renal fascia is strong & effective at containing most primary renal pathology within PS and excluding most other processes from PS
    - Perirenal space is closed and does not communicate across the midline or into the pelvis, but can decompress into interfascial planes which do communicate
    - Perirenal space is divided irregularly by **perirenal bridging septa**; can result in loculated perirenal fluid collections that simulate subcapsular collection; septa may act as conduits for fluid or infiltrative disease (including tumor) to enter or leave perirenal space
- Traumatic or spontaneous **retroperitoneal hemorrhage** is common
  - Causes include anticoagulation therapy, ruptured abdominal aortic aneurysm, bleeding from a renal neoplasm (usually renal carcinoma or angiomyolipoma)
  - Bleeding commonly spreads along fascial planes to involve multiple retroperitoneal and pelvic extraperitoneal compartments, plus rectus and iliopsoas muscle groups (in coagulopathic patients)
- Neoplastic involvement of retroperitoneum
  - Primary carcinoma of kidney, pancreas, colon (ascending or descending) adrenal, duodenum
  - Primary sarcoma, usually **liposarcoma**, often attains huge size displacing abdominal viscera before being diagnosed
  - **Nerve sheath tumors** and **paragangliomas**
  - **Metastases to** retroperitoneal nodes very common (e.g., **lymphoma**, **primary pelvic tumors**, including testes, prostate, uterus, ovary)
- **Retroperitoneal fibrosis**
  - Chronic inflammatory process in lumbar retroperitoneum
  - Encases aorta, IVC, & ureters in fibrotic mantle of tissue
  - Medial deviation and obstruction of ureters

RETROPERITONEUM

RETROPERITONEAL PLANES

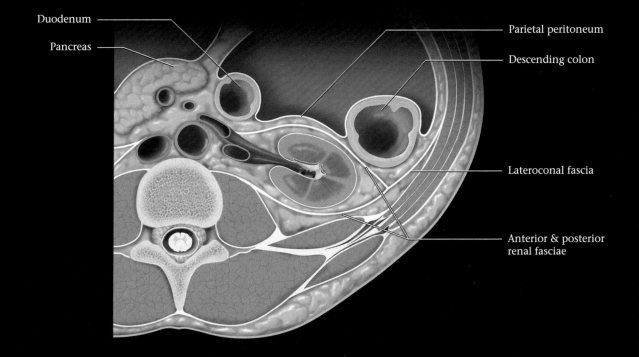

Duodenum

Pancreas

Parietal peritoneum

Descending colon

Lateroconal fascia

Anterior & posterior renal fasciae

The renal and lateroconal fasciae divide the retroperitoneum into three compartments: Anterior pararenal, perirenal (perinephric), and posterior pararenal spaces. The anterior pararenal space (APS) contains the duodenum, pancreas, and the ascending/descending colon. The APS compartment is limited anteriorly by the peritoneum which reflects over the colon to form the paracolic gutter, an intraperitoneal recess. Lateral to the peritoneum covering the lateral abdominal wall is retroperitoneal fat, sometimes called the properitoneal fat stripe. The renal fasciae enclose the perirenal space, and the anterior renal fascia forms the posterior boundary of the APS. The lateroconal fascia forms the lateral margin of the APS and the medial margin of the posterior pararenal space. The posterior renal fascia usually joins with the fasciae of the psoas or quadratus lumborum muscle.

RETROPERITONEUM

RETROPERITONEAL DIVISIONS

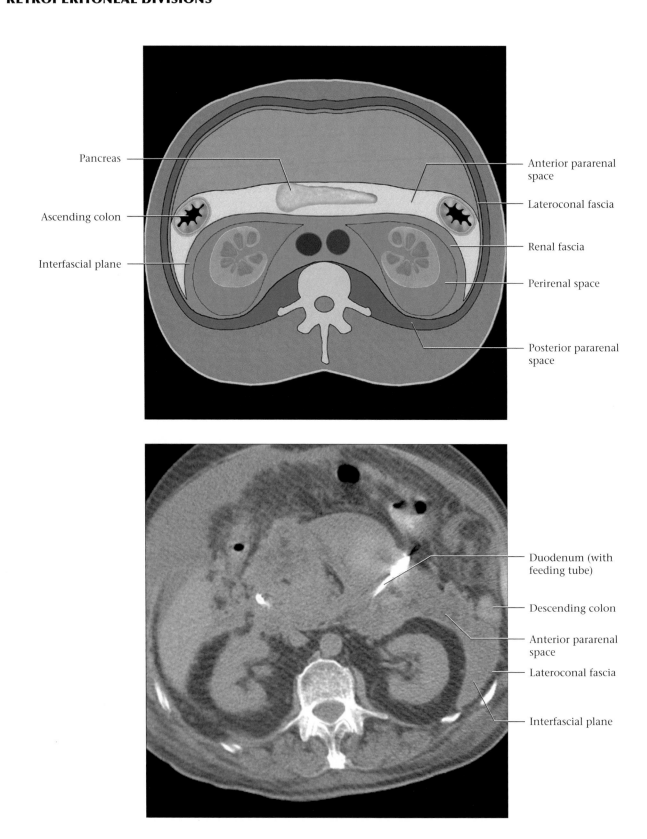

Pancreas
Ascending colon
Interfascial plane

Anterior pararenal space
Lateroconal fascia
Renal fascia
Perirenal space
Posterior pararenal space

Duodenum (with feeding tube)
Descending colon
Anterior pararenal space
Lateroconal fascia
Interfascial plane

(Top) The main divisions of the retroperitoneum are the anterior pararenal space (in yellow), perirenal space (purple) and posterior pararenal space (blue). In addition, the interfascial planes are shown (green). These are the potential spaces created by inflammatory processes that separate the double laminated layers of the renal and lateroconal fasciae. The posterior pararenal space contains no organs, and is synonymous with the properitoneal fat that extends along the lateral and anterior abdominal wall. The perirenal spaces do not communicate across the midline, but the anterior pararenal space and the interfascial planes do so. **(Bottom)** First of 3 CT images of a patient with acute pancreatitis shows fluid distending the anterior pararenal space and interfascial planes. The pancreas, duodenum and vertical colon segments all lie within the anterior pararenal space.

CORONAL & SAGITTAL REFORMATIONS

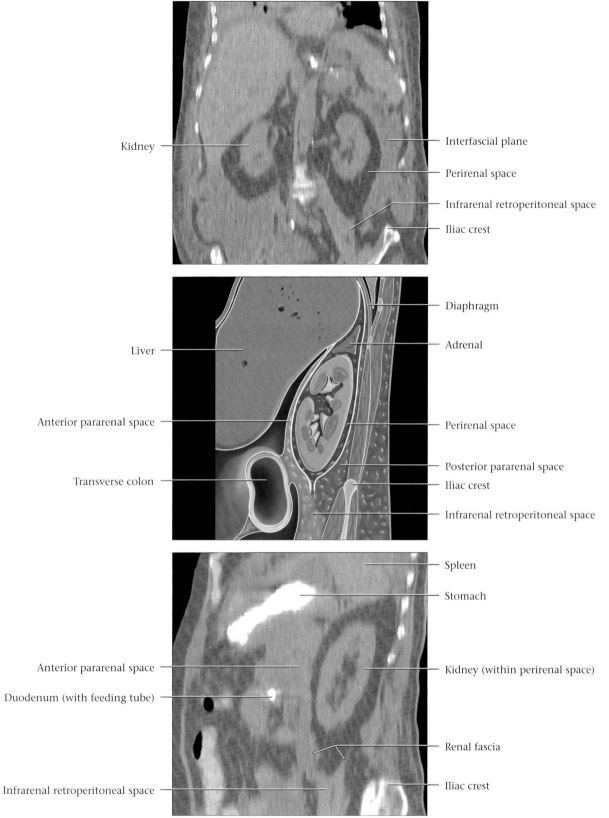

Kidney — Interfascial plane

Perirenal space

Infrarenal retroperitoneal space

Iliac crest

Diaphragm

Liver — Adrenal

Anterior pararenal space — Perirenal space

Transverse colon — Posterior pararenal space

Iliac crest

Infrarenal retroperitoneal space

Spleen

Stomach

Anterior pararenal space — Kidney (within perirenal space)

Duodenum (with feeding tube)

Renal fascia

Infrarenal retroperitoneal space — Iliac crest

(Top) A coronal reformation of the CT scan shows sparing of the perirenal space, which is protected by the renal fascia from the extensive inflammation that fills the anterior pararenal space, interfascial planes and infrarenal retroperitoneal space (caudal to the termination of the renal fascia). **(Middle)** Sagittal graphic through the right kidney shows the three retroperitoneal compartments. Note the confluence of the anterior and posterior renal fasciae at about the level of the iliac crest. Caudal to this, there is only a single infrarenal retroperitoneal space. **(Bottom)** This sagittal reformation through the left kidney shows the shape of the perirenal space which is "protected" in this patient by the renal fascia.

RETROPERITONEUM

AXIAL CT, NORMAL FASCIAL PLANES

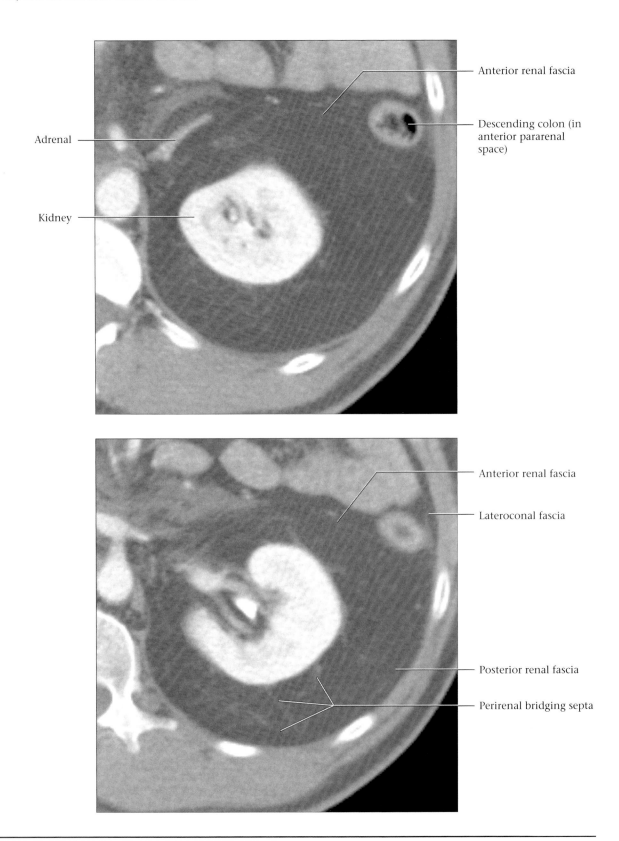

Adrenal

Kidney

Anterior renal fascia

Descending colon (in anterior pararenal space)

Anterior renal fascia

Lateroconal fascia

Posterior renal fascia

Perirenal bridging septa

(Top) First of five axial CT sections that show the renal and lateroconal fasciae that define the retroperitoneal spaces. The renal fascia encloses the perirenal space, which includes the kidney and adrenal, and abundant fat. **(Bottom)** The posterior parietal peritoneum cannot be visualized when normal, but it forms the anterior margin of the anterior pararenal space, whose posterior margin is the anterior layer of the renal fascia. The descending colon can be seen within the anterior pararenal space on this image. Note the perirenal bridging septa that potentially divide the perirenal space into multiple smaller compartments.

RETROPERITONEUM

AXIAL CT, NORMAL FASCIAL PLANES

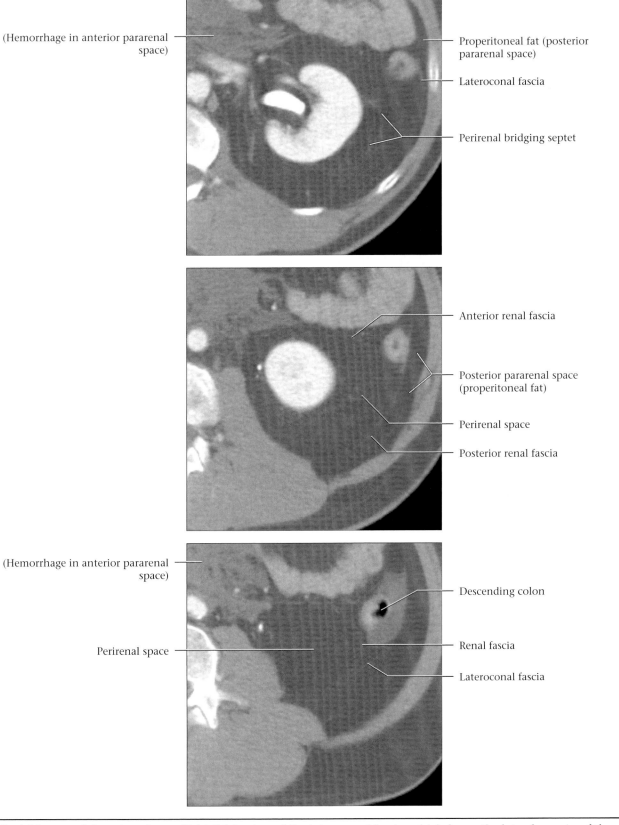

(Hemorrhage in anterior pararenal space)

Properitoneal fat (posterior pararenal space)

Lateroconal fascia

Perirenal bridging septet

Anterior renal fascia

Posterior pararenal space (properitoneal fat)

Perirenal space

Posterior renal fascia

(Hemorrhage in anterior pararenal space)

Descending colon

Perirenal space

Renal fascia

Lateroconal fascia

(Top) More caudal section shows slight thickening of the lateroconal fascia, which forms the lateral margin of the anterior pararenal space. The fat plane between the lateroconal fascia and the transversalis fascia (which is not evident on this image) is known as the properitoneal fat, but also as the posterior pararenal space. No organs or major structures lie within this space, but it is often involved secondarily by inflammation or bleeding that originate elsewhere in the retroperitoneum or abdominal wall. **(Middle)** The posterior pararenal space is broader and more evident on this section. **(Bottom)** Most caudal section below the kidney shows the layers of renal fascia coming together as the perirenal space narrows like an inverted cone.

RETROPERITONEUM

PANCREATITIS DEFINING PLANES & SPACES

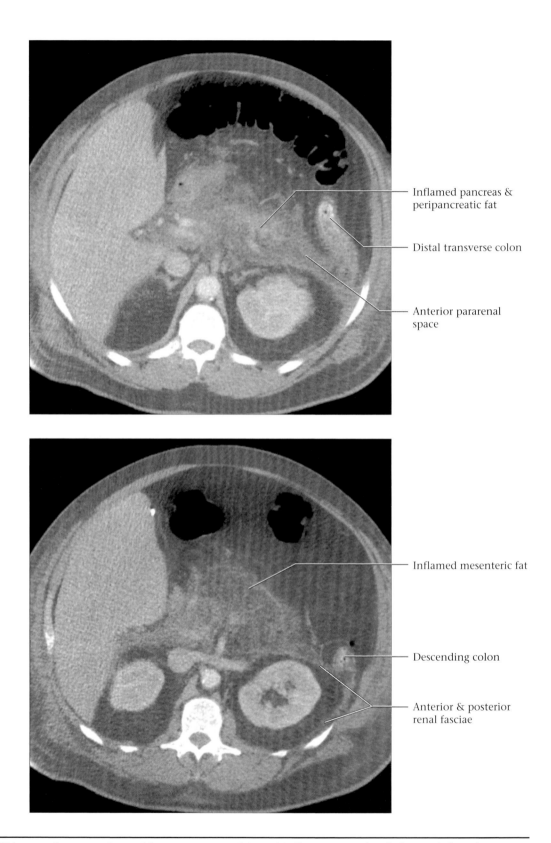

Inflamed pancreas & peripancreatic fat

Distal transverse colon

Anterior pararenal space

Inflamed mesenteric fat

Descending colon

Anterior & posterior renal fasciae

(Top) First of four CT images from a patient with acute pancreatitis and inflammation that helps to define the retroperitoneal spaces. This section shows infiltration of the fat planes surrounding the pancreas, primarily within the anterior pararenal space. The inflammation spreads laterally to the anatomic splenic flexure, where the colon leaves its mesocolon to enter the retroperitoneum as the descending colon. **(Bottom)** The inflammation also spreads caudally and ventrally to enter the mesentery. Recall that the roots of the mesentery and transverse mesocolon arise from just in front of the pancreas, and inflammation easily enters the fatty space between the peritoneal reflections.

RETROPERITONEUM

PANCREATITIS DEFINING PLANES & SPACES

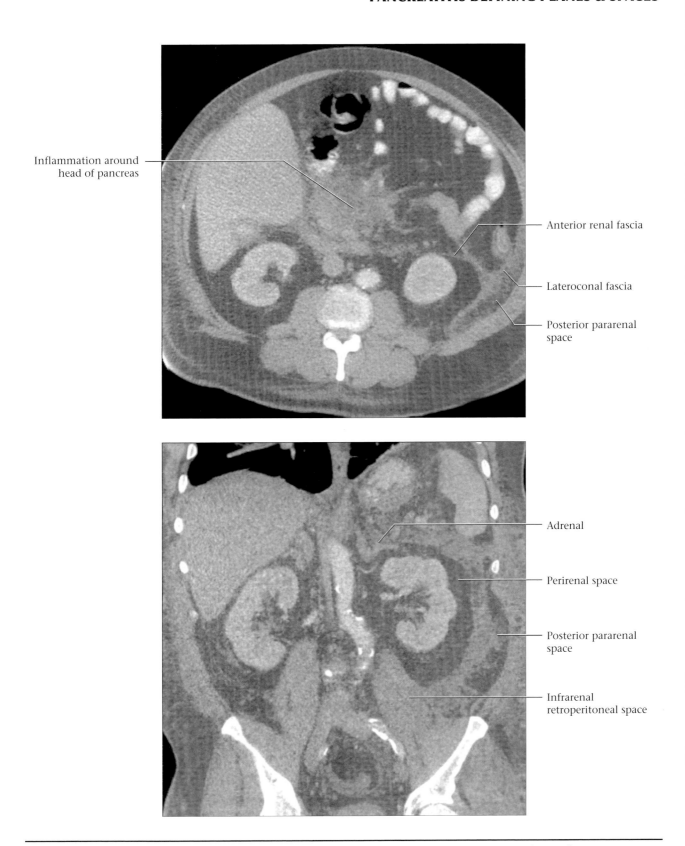

Inflammation around head of pancreas

Anterior renal fascia

Lateroconal fascia

Posterior pararenal space

Adrenal

Perirenal space

Posterior pararenal space

Infrarenal retroperitoneal space

(**Top**) The renal and lateroconal fasciae are thickened by inflammation, which has also spread into the posterior pararenal space lateral to the lateroconal fascia. (**Bottom**) A coronal reformation of the same CT scan shows normal ("spared") fat in the perirenal space, while the fat in the anterior and posterior pararenal spaces is inflamed. Note how the layers of renal fascia close off the perirenal space at about the level of the iliac crest. Caudal to the perirenal space, there is only a single retroperitoneal space, since the anterior and posterior pararenal spaces come together. This helps to explain how the posterior pararenal space becomes involved in inflammatory or hemorrhagic processes that originate in the anterior pararenal space.

RETROPERITONEUM

PANCREATITIS INVOLVING OTHER ORGANS

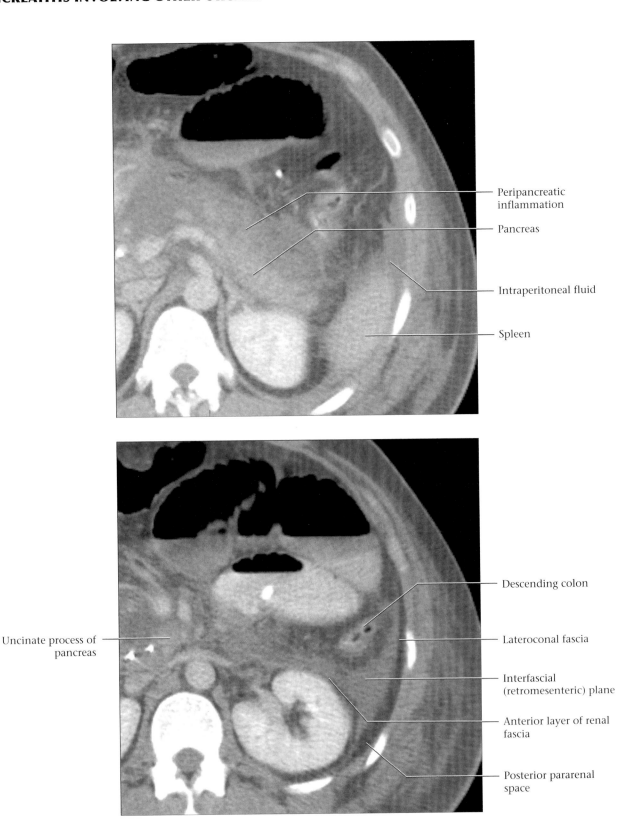

(Top) Peripancreatic inflammation
Pancreas
Intraperitoneal fluid
Spleen

Uncinate process of pancreas

Descending colon
Lateroconal fascia
Interfascial (retromesenteric) plane
Anterior layer of renal fascia
Posterior pararenal space

(Top) First of five axial CT sections of another patient with acute pancreatitis shows extensive infiltration of the fat planes surrounding the pancreas. Fluid around the spleen is ascites, indicating that the inflammatory process has extended through the posterior parietal peritoneum to enter the peritoneal cavity. **(Bottom)** The inflammatory process has spread laterally through the anterior pararenal space but is prevented from entering the posterior pararenal space by the lateroconal fascia. The layers of the renal and lateroconal fasciae are expanded by the inflammation at the point that they join, resulting in fluid tracking through interfascial planes. The descending colon, also residing in the anterior pararenal space, is contacted by the inflammation.

PANCREATITIS INVOLVING OTHER ORGANS

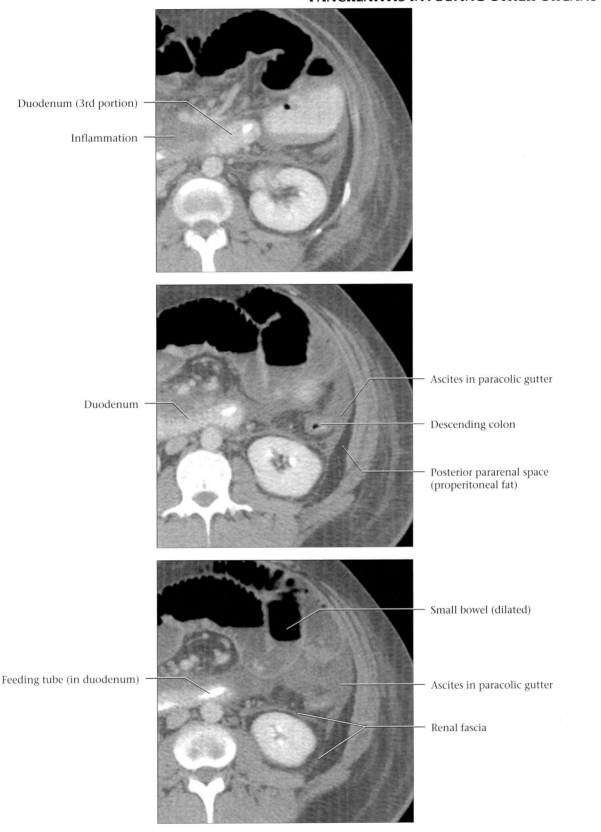

(Top) A more caudal section shows the duodenum surrounded by inflammation as it too lies in the anterior pararenal space. **(Middle)** The parietal peritoneum reflects over the descending colon to form the paracolic gutter, an intraperitoneal recess. The peritoneum is a thin structure, not normally visualized on imaging, and is easily breached by inflammatory and hemorrhagic processes. No clear demarcation can be seen between the retroperitoneal inflammation and the ascites on this section. **(Bottom)** The contiguous involvement of the retroperitoneal and intraperitoneal spaces is evident on this section. The retroperitoneal duodenum is encased by inflammation as are the intraperitoneal small bowel segments, resulting in an ileus (dilated bowel with diminished peristalsis).

PERIRENAL BRIDGING SEPTA

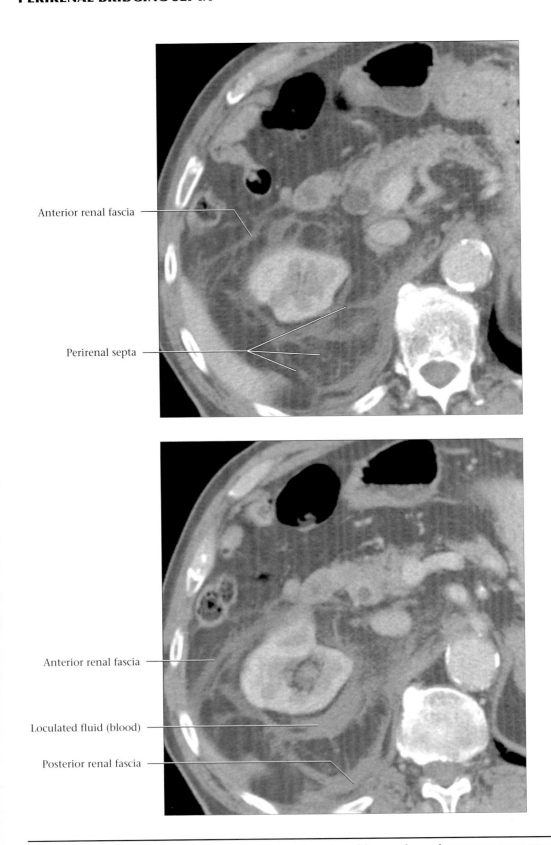

Anterior renal fascia

Perirenal septa

Anterior renal fascia

Loculated fluid (blood)

Posterior renal fascia

(Top) First of two axial CT sections of a patient with perirenal hemorrhage shows numerous curvilinear septations within the perirenal space caused by hemorrhage tracking along the septa that divide the perirenal space into multiple compartments. Blood and inflammatory infiltrate can "decompress" along these planes and spread into other retroperitoneal spaces. (Bottom) Loculated fluid within the perirenal space can mimic subcapsular fluid; note the intact fat plane between the loculated fluid and the surface of the kidney, indicating that the fluid is confined within the perirenal space, but it does not spread diffusely to fill the space because of the perirenal septa.

PERIRENAL SPACE WITH BLOOD

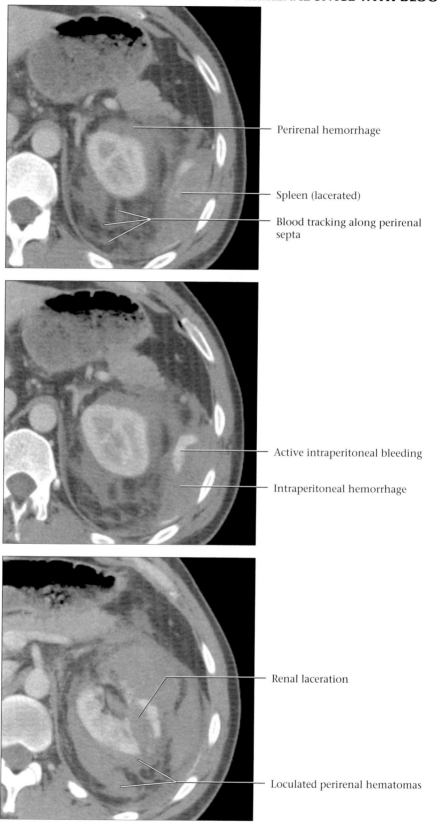

Perirenal hemorrhage

Spleen (lacerated)

Blood tracking along perirenal septa

Active intraperitoneal bleeding

Intraperitoneal hemorrhage

Renal laceration

Loculated perirenal hematomas

(Top) First of three CT images from a patient injured in a motor vehicle crash shows heterogeneous enhancement of the spleen due to parenchymal laceration. Coexisting renal injury has resulted in perirenal hemorrhage that is loculated by perirenal septa. The collection ventral to the kidney simulates a subcapsular hematoma, but spreads along the surface of the kidney without causing compression of the parenchyma. (Middle) A more caudal section just below the spleen shows intraperitoneal hemorrhage, with a collection that is isodense to the contrast-opacified aorta, indicating active arterial bleeding from the splenic injury. Active hemorrhage of this sort requires urgent intervention with surgery or angiographic embolization to occlude the bleeding vessel. (Bottom) A deep renal laceration is seen along with loculated perirenal hematomas.

RETROPERITONEUM

HEMORRHAGE INTO EXTRAPERITONEAL SPACES

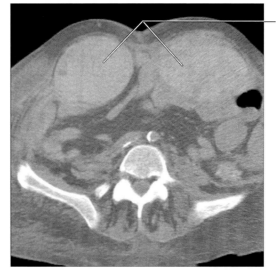

Rectus sheath hematomas

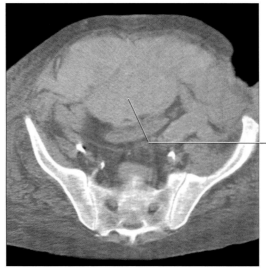

Hemorrhage in prevesical space

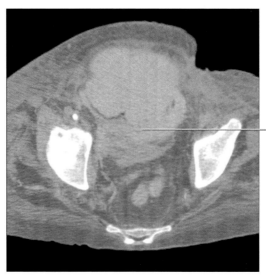

Hemorrhage in prevesical space

(Top) First of five axial CT sections from a patient with spontaneous bleeding from over-anticoagulation. This section shows high density, heterogeneous masses (hematomas) within the rectus sheath bilaterally, a common site for spontaneous bleeding in patients with coagulopathy. (Middle) Because the rectus sheath is incomplete posteriorly along the lower third of the muscle, the bleeding is no longer confined within the rectus sheath, but extends into the adjacent extraperitoneal spaces, including the prevesical space (of Retzius). The prevesical & perivesical spaces communicate superiorly with the infrarenal retroperitoneal space and fluid or inflammation may extend cephalad to involve all three retroperitoneal compartments. (Bottom) A more caudal section shows hemorrhage in the anterior abdominal wall (rectus sheath) and extraperitoneal pelvis (prevesical space).

RETROPERITONEUM

HEMORRHAGE INTO EXTRAPERITONEAL SPACES

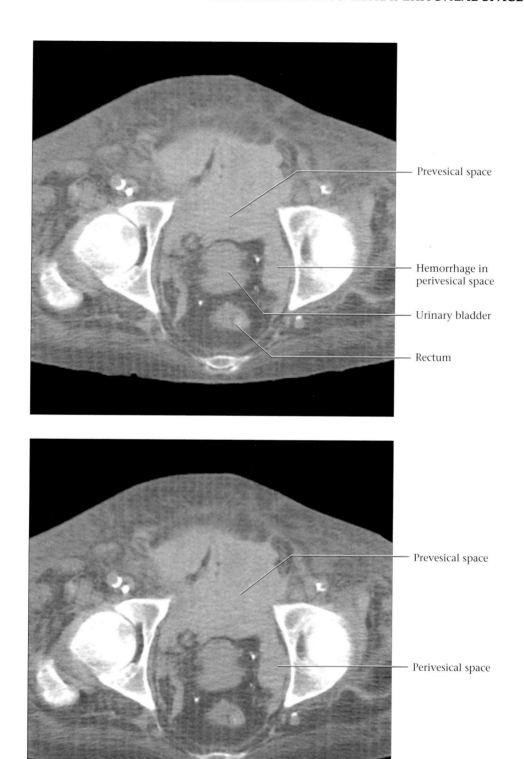

Prevesical space

Hemorrhage in perivesical space

Urinary bladder

Rectum

Prevesical space

Perivesical space

(Top) The prevesical space continues caudally and laterally to involve the perivesical space lower in the pelvis. (Bottom) Hemorrhage spreads extensively through the pelvic extraperitoneal spaces. Involvement of the extraperitoneal pelvic spaces tends to assume a "molar tooth" appearance on axial CT sections, as in this image. The "roots of the tooth" are the extensions into the perivesical space. Extraperitoneal pelvic fluid also commonly extends posteriorly to the presacral space, which is minimally involved in this patient.

RETROPERITONEUM

HEMORRHAGE ACROSS MIDLINE

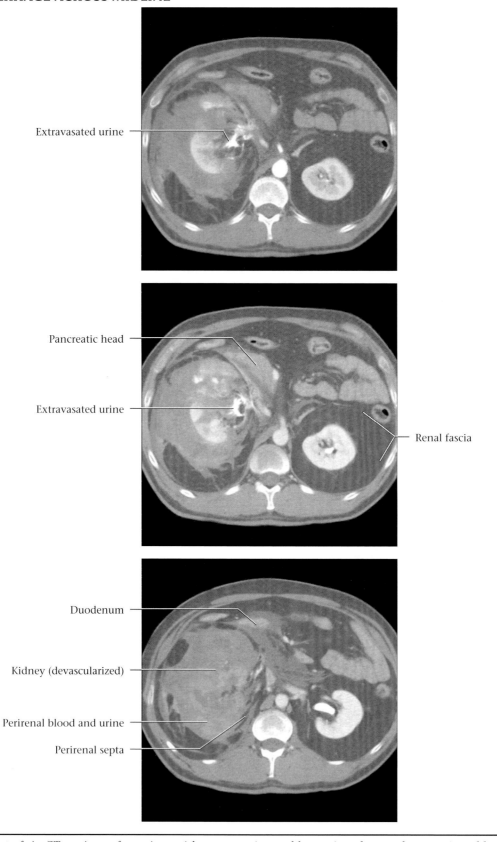

(Top) First of six CT sections of a patient with a traumatic renal laceration shows a large perirenal hemorrhage that fills the perirenal space. The renal parenchyma appears to be fragmented. (Middle) The deep renal lacerations have extended into the collecting system, evident as extravasation of contrast-opacified urine. The pancreatic head and duodenum are displaced by the large perirenal hematoma/urinoma. (Bottom) The lower pole of the right kidney shows no contrast-enhancement, indicating that the renal artery to this segment has been occluded or avulsed. The large perirenal collection of blood and urine is spreading along the perirenal septa to decompress into the interfascial planes. The perirenal space does not extend across the midline; however, the interfascial plane and the anterior pararenal space do cross the midline.

HEMORRHAGE ACROSS MIDLINE

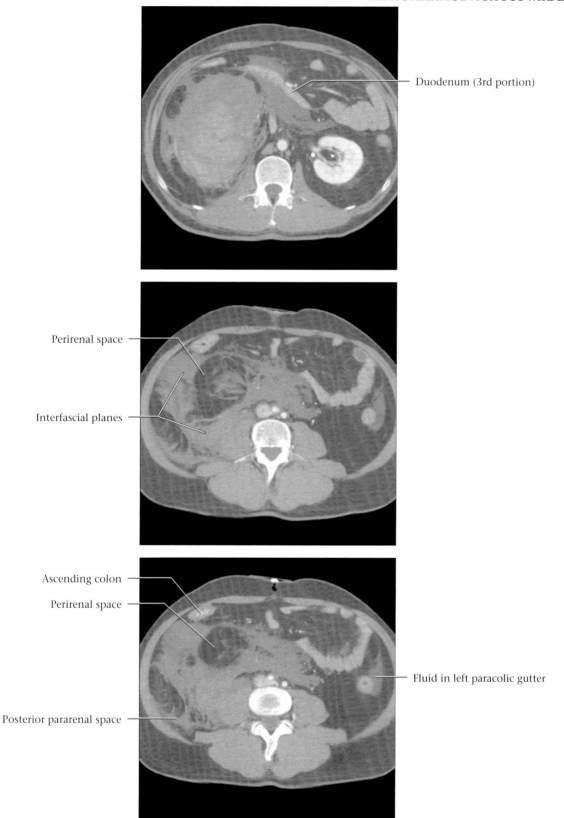

Duodenum (3rd portion)

Perirenal space

Interfascial planes

Ascending colon

Perirenal space

Fluid in left paracolic gutter

Posterior pararenal space

(Top) The fluid crossing the abdominal midline with the duodenum is in the anterior pararenal space and the interfascial plane. These spaces have become involved secondarily after the renal injury resulted in extensive perirenal fluid collections that spread along the perirenal septa and separated the two layers of the renal fascia to form an interfascial plane. **(Middle)** On this more caudal section there is little fluid within the perirenal space, but extensive fluid distention of the interfascial planes. Note the spread of fluid into the contiguous psoas compartment and posterior pararenal space, and the spread across the abdominal midline in front of the aorta and IVC. **(Bottom)** The right anterior pararenal space is relatively spared, as indicated by intact fat planes around the ascending colon. Blood has leaked through the peritoneum into the paracolic gutter.

RETROPERITONEUM

COMMUNICATION AMONG EXTRAPERITONEAL SPACES

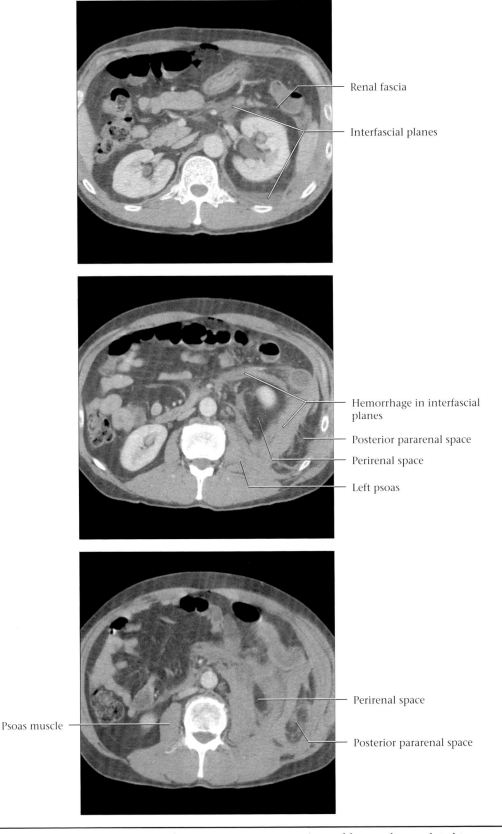

Renal fascia

Interfascial planes

Hemorrhage in interfascial planes

Posterior pararenal space

Perirenal space

Left psoas

Psoas muscle

Perirenal space

Posterior pararenal space

(Top) First of eight axial CT sections in a patient with a spontaneous retroperitoneal hemorrhage related to anticoagulation medication. This section shows only subtle thickening of the left renal fascia and interfascial planes. **(Middle)** Extensive hemorrhage distends the interfascial planes on the left, with contiguous bleeding into the psoas compartment and pararenal spaces. The perirenal space is spared. **(Bottom)** The hemorrhage is spreading along curvilinear planes, corresponding to the interfascial planes and the fasciae covering the left psoas, quadratus lumborum, and transverse abdominal muscles. Coagulopathic hemorrhage often originates in the abdominal wall muscles, especially the rectus and iliopsoas, with subsequent dissection into the retroperitoneal spaces.

COMMUNICATION AMONG EXTRAPERITONEAL SPACES

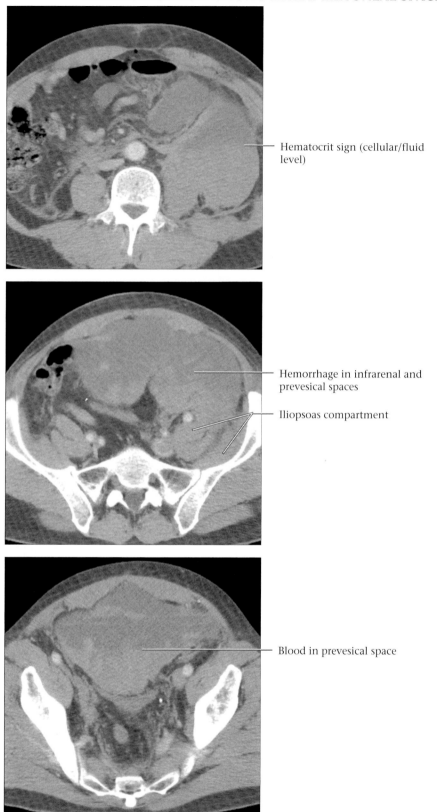

Hematocrit sign (cellular/fluid level)

Hemorrhage in infrarenal and prevesical spaces

Iliopsoas compartment

Blood in prevesical space

(Top) A more caudal section shows massive hemorrhage into the psoas compartment and adjacent retroperitoneum. Note the cellular/fluid level, referred to as the "hematocrit sign", that is almost pathognomonic of a coagulopathic hemorrhage. It indicates gravitational settling of blood cells below a serum level, without clot development. (Middle) Hemorrhage has spread into the infrarenal retroperitoneal space and continues caudally to involve the pelvic extraperitoneal spaces, including the prevesical space. The blood remains contiguous and in communication with the left iliopsoas compartment. (Bottom) Hemorrhage distends the prevesical space.

RETROPERITONEUM

COMMUNICATION AMONG EXTRAPERITONEAL SPACES

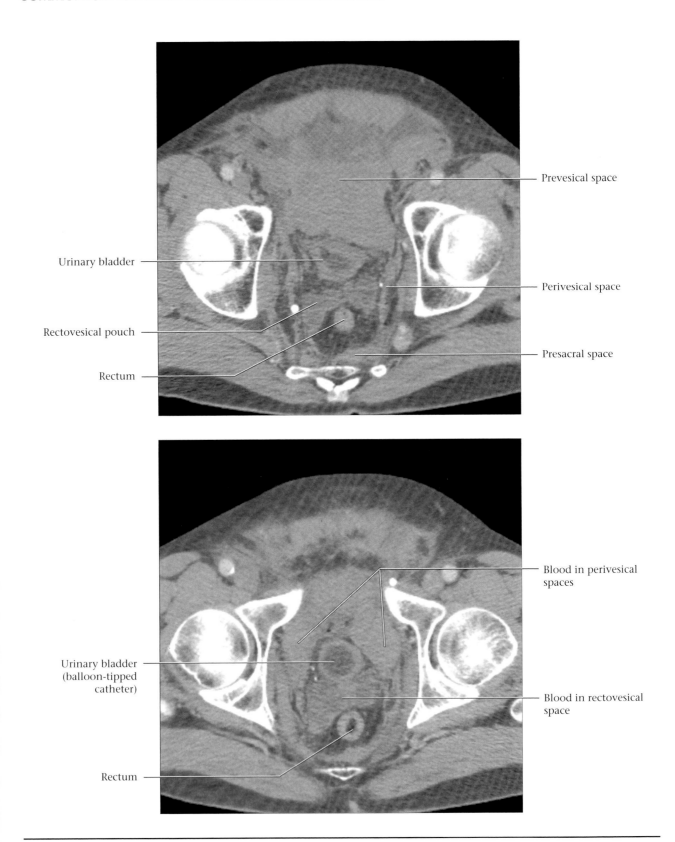

(Top) Blood tracks from the prevesical space into the perivesical and presacral spaces. A small amount of blood has entered the peritoneal cavity and has settled into the rectovesical space or, pouch of Douglas. In this patient, blood has "descended" from its primary site of origin in the abdominal wall and retroperitoneum to the pelvic extraperitoneal spaces. The opposite can also happen, as with a pelvic fracture leading to extensive pelvic extraperitoneal bleeding that extends up into the abdominal retroperitoneum. (Bottom) Note the distinction between the rectovesical space (pouch of Douglas), an intraperitoneal recess, and the perivesical and presacral spaces, divisions of the pelvic extraperitoneal spaces.

RETROPERITONEUM

RETROPERITONEAL LIPOSARCOMA

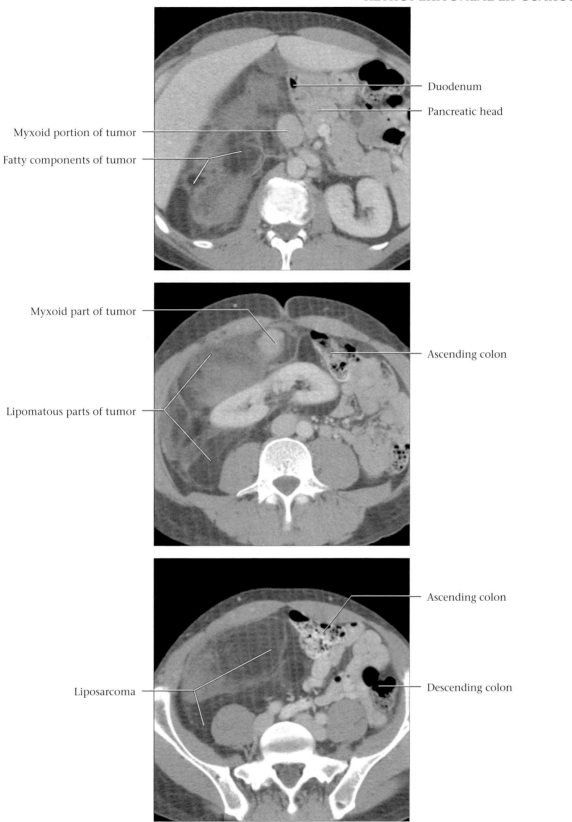

Duodenum

Pancreatic head

Myxoid portion of tumor

Fatty components of tumor

Myxoid part of tumor

Ascending colon

Lipomatous parts of tumor

Ascending colon

Liposarcoma

Descending colon

(Top) First of three axial CT sections of a patient with vague abdominal discomfort, discovered to have a large retroperitoneal liposarcoma. This section shows a large heterogeneous mass in the right side of the abdomen. Its retroperitoneal location is indicated by displacement of other retroperitoneal organs, such as the pancreas, to the left. The mass has large lipomatous (fatty) elements, similar in density to normal fat around the left kidney. A rounded part of the mass, however, is of "soft tissue density", probably due to a myxoid component. (Middle) The tumor compresses and displaces the right kidney, indicating its origin in the perirenal space. The ascending colon is displaced to the left side of the abdomen. (Bottom) All of the bowel is displaced to the left side of the abdomen by the tumor. The tumor was resected, along with the right kidney.

RETROPERITONEUM

RETROPERITONEAL FIBROSIS

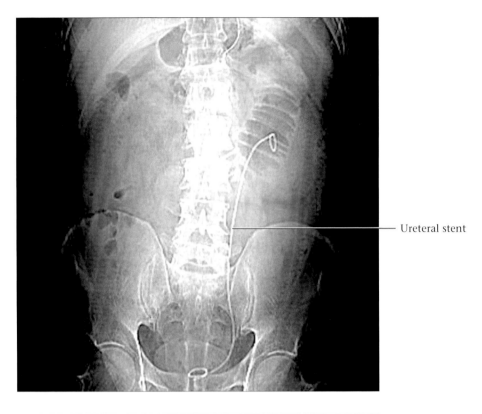

Ureteral stent

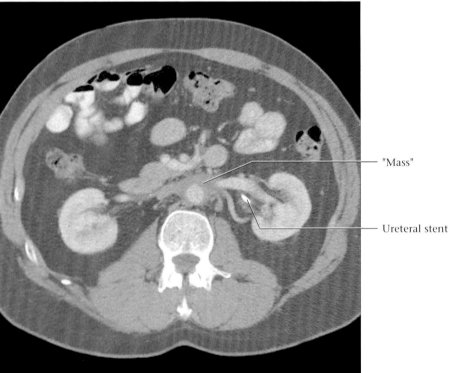

"Mass"

Ureteral stent

(Top) First of four images of a patient with retroperitoneal fibrosis. Frontal radiograph shows a left ureteral stent that was placed to relieve obstruction of the left ureter. The position of the stent indicates medial deviation of the middle part of the ureter. (Bottom) First of three axial CT sections shows a "mass" encasing the aorta and IVC at the level of the 3rd lumbar vertebra.

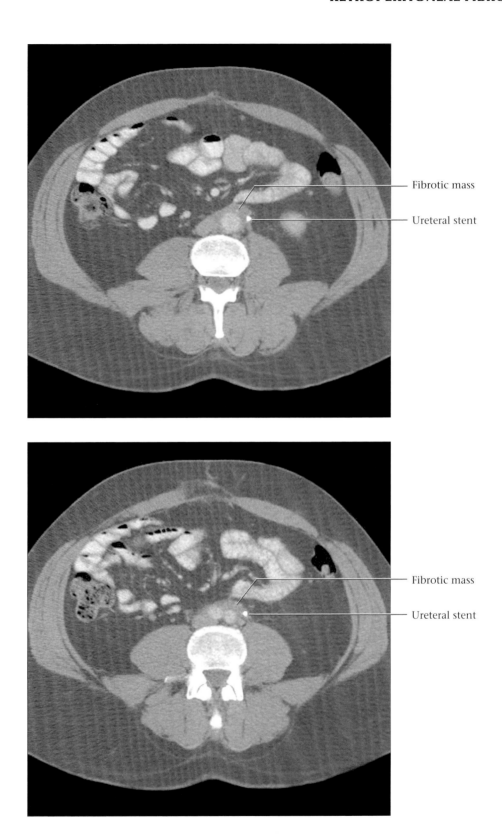

(Top) A more caudal section shows that the periaortic fibrotic mass has encased the left ureter as well as the great vessels. The mass appears as a mantle of tissue around the aorta. **(Bottom)** A more caudal section shows that the periaortic fibrotic mass has encased the left ureter as well as the great vessels. The mass appears as a mantle of tissue around the aorta.

RETROPERITONEUM

NERVE SHEATH TUMOR

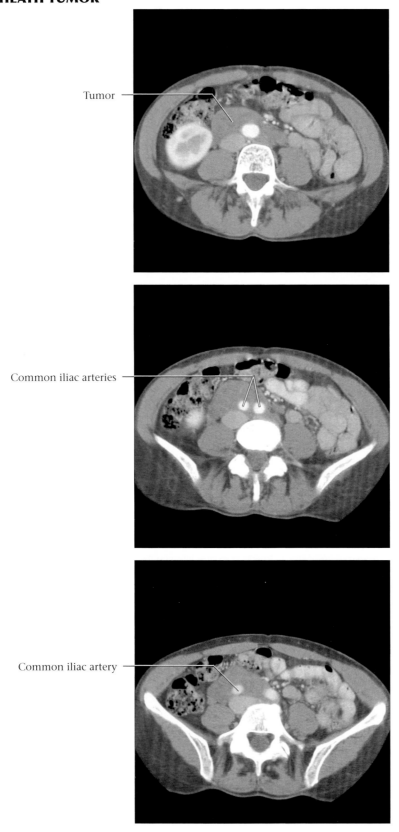

(Top) First of three axial CT sections shows a mass that encases the abdominal aorta with more of a bulky tumor appearance than would be typical for retroperitoneal fibrosis. The mass is eccentric, and appears to arise in the right para-aortic region of the retroperitoneum. (Middle) The mass, a nerve sheath tumor, envelops the common iliac arteries bilaterally. (Bottom) The nerve sheath tumor follows the course of the right common iliac artery. The major autonomic nerve trunks that innervate the abdominal and pelvic viscera run parallel to the spine, and their major branches course parallel to major blood vessels.

LYMPHOMA WITH RETROPERITONEAL LYMPHADENOPATHY

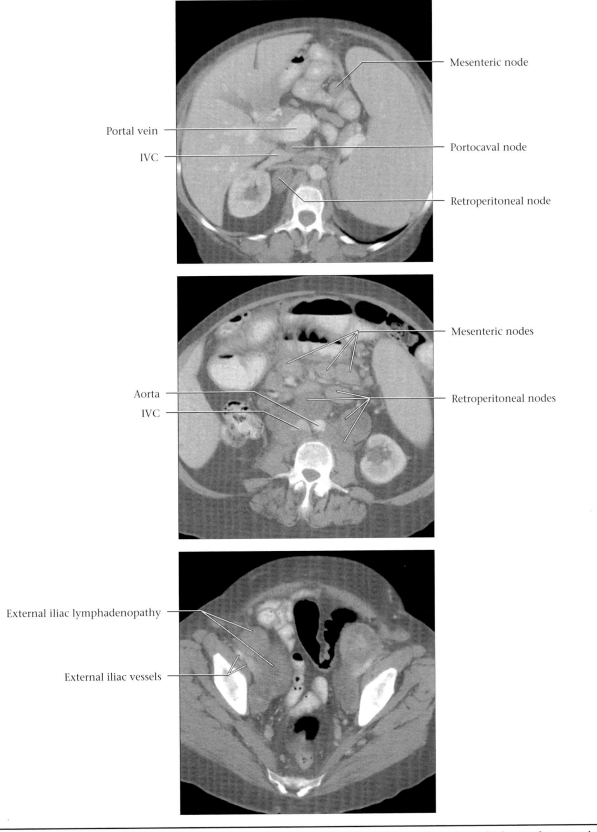

Mesenteric node

Portal vein

Portocaval node

IVC

Retroperitoneal node

Mesenteric nodes

Aorta

IVC

Retroperitoneal nodes

External iliac lymphadenopathy

External iliac vessels

(Top) First of three axial CT sections of a patient who presented with night sweats and weight loss, subsequently diagnosed with non-Hodgkin lymphoma. This section shows splenomegaly and enlarged lymph nodes in several groups, including retroperitoneal. **(Middle)** While enlargement of retroperitoneal nodes is common in lymphoma, tumor involvement of the mesenteric nodes is especially characteristic of this malignancy. **(Bottom)** Massive enlargement of the external iliac lymph nodes bilaterally is also evident. Lymphoma is the most common malignancy that causes widespread lymphadenopathy, involving multiple abdominal nodal chains. Primary pelvic malignancies may also spread to retroperitoneal nodes.

ADRENAL

Terminology

Abbreviations
- Adrenal corticotrophic hormone (ACTH)

Gross Anatomy

Overview
- Adrenal (**suprarenal**) glands are part of the endocrine and neurological systems
  - Essentially different organs within the same structure
  - Lie within the **perirenal space** bilaterally, bounded by the **renal (perirenal) fascia**
  - Lie above and medial to kidneys

Relations
- Right adrenal is more apical in location
  - Lies anterolateral to right crus of diaphragm, medial to liver, posterior to inferior vena cava (IVC)
  - Often pyramidal in shape, inverted "V" shape on transverse section
- Left adrenal is more caudal, lies medial to upper pole of left kidney, lateral to left crus of diaphragm, posterior to splenic vein & pancreas
  - Often crescentic in shape, "lambda" or triangular on transverse section

Divisions
- **Adrenal cortex**
  - Derived from mesoderm
  - Secretes **corticosteroids** (cortisol, aldosterone) and androgens
- **Adrenal medulla**
  - Derived from neural crest
  - Part of the sympathetic nervous system
  - **Chromaffin cells** secrete **catecholamines** (mostly epinephrine) into bloodstream
- **Vessels, nerves & lymphatics**
  - Arteries
    - **Superior adrenal arteries:** (6-8) from inferior phrenic arteries
    - **Middle adrenal artery:** (1) from abdominal aorta
    - **Inferior adrenal artery:** (1) from renal arteries
  - Veins
    - **Right adrenal vein** drains into IVC
    - **Left adrenal vein** drains into left renal vein (usually after joining left inferior phrenic vein)
  - Nerves
    - Extensive sympathetic connection to adrenal medulla
    - Presynaptic sympathetic fibers from paravertebral ganglia end directly on the secretory cells of medulla
  - Lymphatics
    - Drain to **lumbar (aortic** and **caval) nodes**

Anatomy-Based Imaging Issues

Key Concepts
- **Adrenal (cortical) adenomas**

- Very common (at least 2% of general population), but usually cause no symptoms
  - Most are "nonfunctioning" or "non-hyperfunctioning" adenomas; identical on imaging to functional adenomas that cause Cushing or Conn syndrome
  - Usually contain abundant lipid (precursor to steroid hormones)
  - Lipid is intra & intercellular, not in macroscopic deposits of fat
  - Can be identified by CT and MR sequences that show lipid-rich mass
  - Best CT technique: Nonenhanced CT with nodule measuring < 15 HU; or enhanced CT with nodule < 37 HU or showing "washout" (decreased enhancement on delayed CT)
  - Best MR techniques: In - and opposed-phase MR with signal dropout in nodule on opposed phase
- **Cushing syndrome**
  - Due to excess cortisol
  - Signs: Truncal obesity, hirsutism, hypertension, abdominal striae
  - Causes: Pituitary tumors (→ ACTH), exogenous (medications) > adrenal adenoma > carcinoma
- **Conn syndrome** (excess aldosterone)
  - Signs: Hypertension, hypokalemic alkalosis
  - Causes: Adrenal adenomas > hyperplasia > carcinoma
- **Addison syndrome** (adrenal insufficiency)
  - Signs: Hypotension, weight loss, altered pigmentation
  - Causes: Autoimmune > adrenal metastases > adrenal hemorrhage > adrenal infection
- **Pheochromocytoma** (tumor of adrenal medulla)
  - Signs: Headache, palpitations, excessive perspiration (due to excess catecholamines)
  - 90% arise in adrenal, 90% unilateral, 90% benign
    - Similar tumor arising in other chromaffin cells of sympathetic ganglia is called **paraganglioma**
  - May occur in syndromes, including
    - Multiple endocrine neoplasia (often with thyroid & parathyroid tumors)
    - Neurofibromatosis
    - Von Hippel Lindau (along with renal & pancreatic cysts and tumors, CNS hemangioblastomas)

Clinical Implications

Clinical Importance
- Rich blood supply of adrenals reflects important endocrine function
  - Results in adrenal glands being common site for hematologic **metastases** (lung, breast, melanoma, etc.)
- Adrenal glands are designed to respond to stress (trauma, sepsis, surgery, etc.) by secreting more cortisol & epinephrine
  - Overwhelming stress may result in **adrenal hemorrhage**, acute adrenal insufficiency (Addisonian crisis)

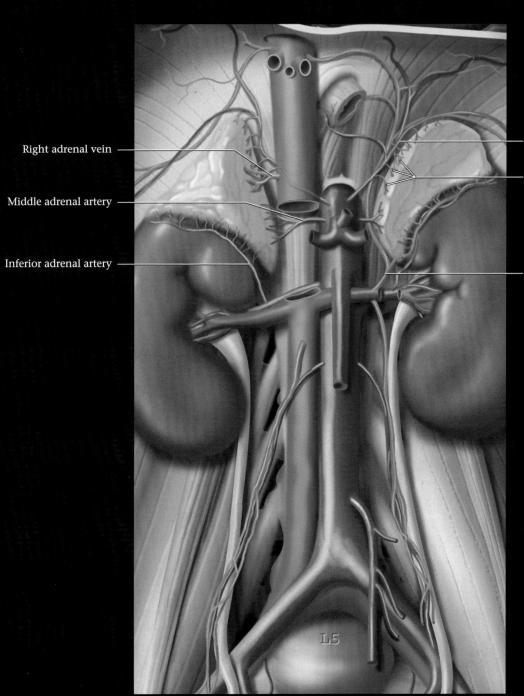

Right adrenal vein

Middle adrenal artery

Inferior adrenal artery

Inferior phrenic artery

Superior adrenal arteries

Left adrenal vein

The adrenal glands rest atop the kidneys, with an interposed layer of fat. Reflecting their critical role in maintaining homeostasis and responding to stress, the adrenal glands have a very rich vascular supply. The superior adrenal arteries are short branches of the inferior phrenic arteries bilaterally. The middle adrenal arteries are short vessels arising from the aorta. The inferior adrenal arteries are branches of the renal arteries. The left adrenal vein drains into the left renal vein, while the right adrenal vein drains directly into the IVC. (The size of the adrenal glands is somewhat exaggerated in this illustration, to facilitate demonstration of the vascular anatomy.)

ADRENAL

ADRENAL AXIAL ANATOMY & RELATIONS

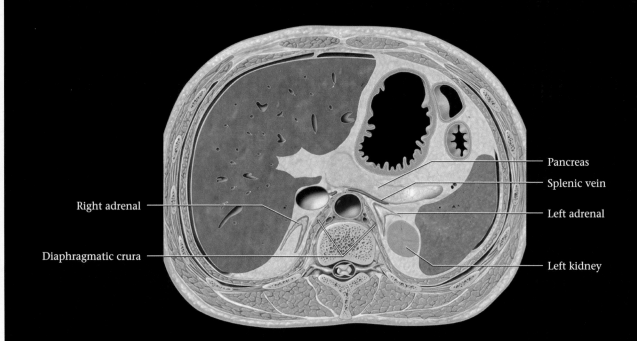

Right adrenal

Diaphragmatic crura

Pancreas

Splenic vein

Left adrenal

Left kidney

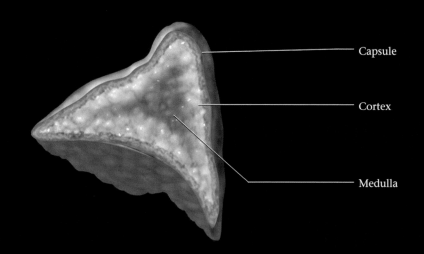

Capsule

Cortex

Medulla

(Top) The right adrenal is often more cephalic in location, and lies above the right kidney, while the left adrenal lies partly in front of the upper pole of the left kidney. The left adrenal lies directly posterior to the splenic vein and body of pancreas, and lateral to the left crus of the diaphragm. The right adrenal lies lateral to the crus, medial to the liver, and directly behind the inferior vena cava. **(Bottom)** The adrenal gland is essentially two organs in a single structure. The cortex is an endocrine gland, secreting primarily cortisol, aldosterone, and androgenic steroids. All of these hormones are derived from cholesterol, which imparts the characteristic lipid-rich appearance and imaging characteristics of the gland. The adrenal medulla is part of the autonomic nervous system and secretes epinephrine and norepinephrine.

ADRENAL

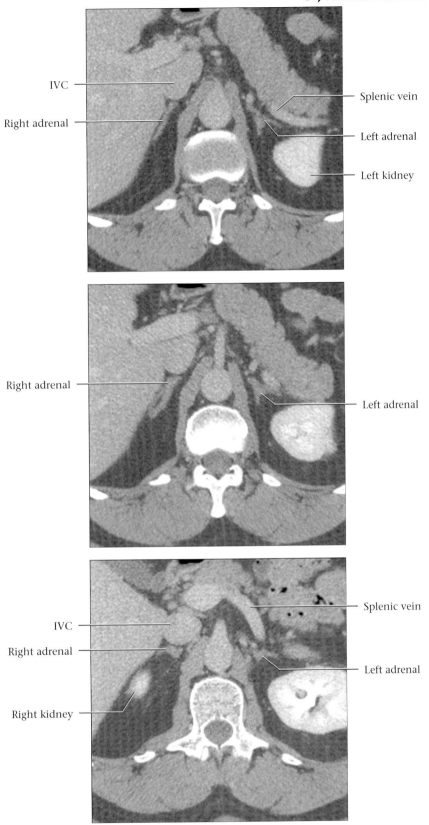

(Top) First of three axial CT sections shows normal adrenal glands bilaterally. The right adrenal is usually suprarenal, touches the back of the IVC and lies lateral to the right crus & medial to the liver. The left adrenal usually lies ventral to the upper pole of the left kidney and behind the splenic vein. The left adrenal often appears as an inverted "Y" shape, while the right is more like an inverted "V". (Middle) Both limbs of the right adrenal are seen on this section. (Bottom) The lowest portions of the adrenals are seen on this section.

ADRENAL

ADRENAL VENOGRAM

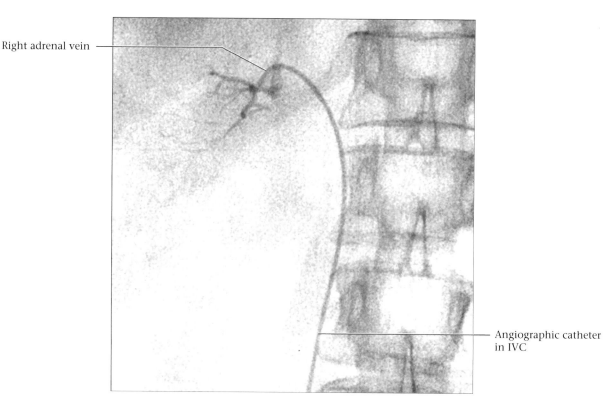

Right adrenal vein —

Angiographic catheter in IVC

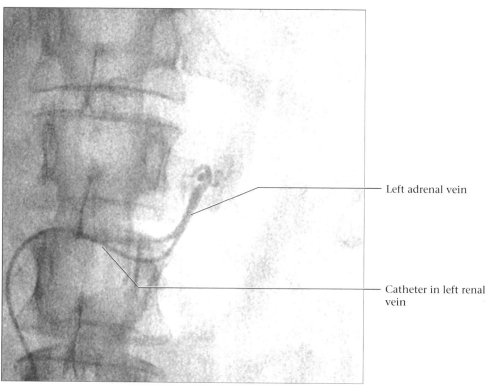

Left adrenal vein

Catheter in left renal vein

(Top) First of two images showing selective catheterization of the adrenal veins in a young woman with hyperaldosteronism, but no definite mass seen on CT. Selective adrenal vein sampling was requested to assess unilateral excess aldosterone secretion. A catheter has been inserted through the right femoral vein and the tip was advanced into the opening of the right adrenal vein. The adrenal veins are very fragile and could be easily ruptured by a forceful injection of contrast medium. The angiographer must know the vascular anatomy and gently probe the venous orifice, confirming the location with a small bolus injection of contrast medium, as shown here. **(Bottom)** A subsequent image shows the catheter repositioned. The tip has been advanced through the left renal vein to enter the left adrenal vein. No attempt is made to opacify the smaller venous tributaries.

ADRENAL

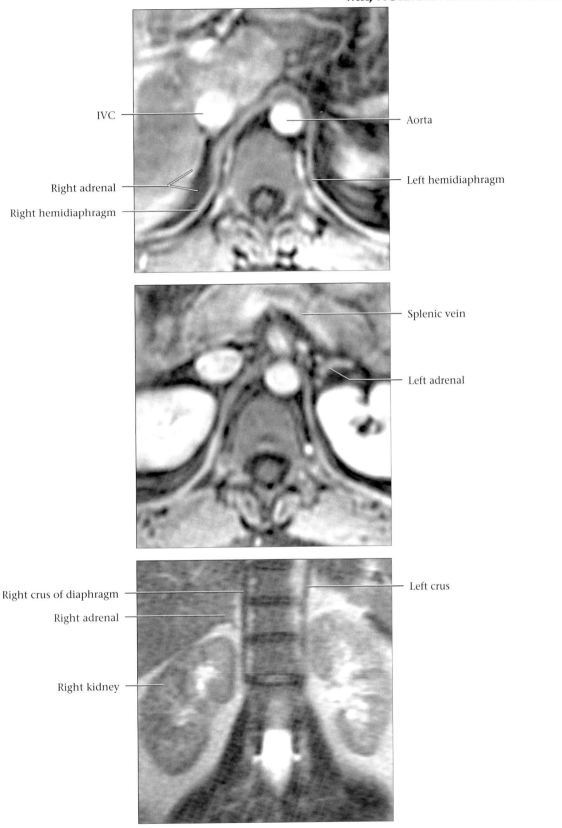

IVC

Right adrenal

Right hemidiaphragm

Aorta

Left hemidiaphragm

Splenic vein

Left adrenal

Right crus of diaphragm

Right adrenal

Right kidney

Left crus

(**Top**) First of three MR images of normal adrenal glands is a contrast-enhanced T1-weighted axial image that shows the thin, parallel limbs of the right adrenal gland. (**Middle**) A more caudal enhanced section shows the left adrenal. (**Bottom**) Coronal T2-weighted image shows the pyramidal shape of the right adrenal gland in its usual suprarenal location. The left adrenal is not included in this plane of section.

ADRENAL

CORONAL, NORMAL ADRENAL ANATOMY

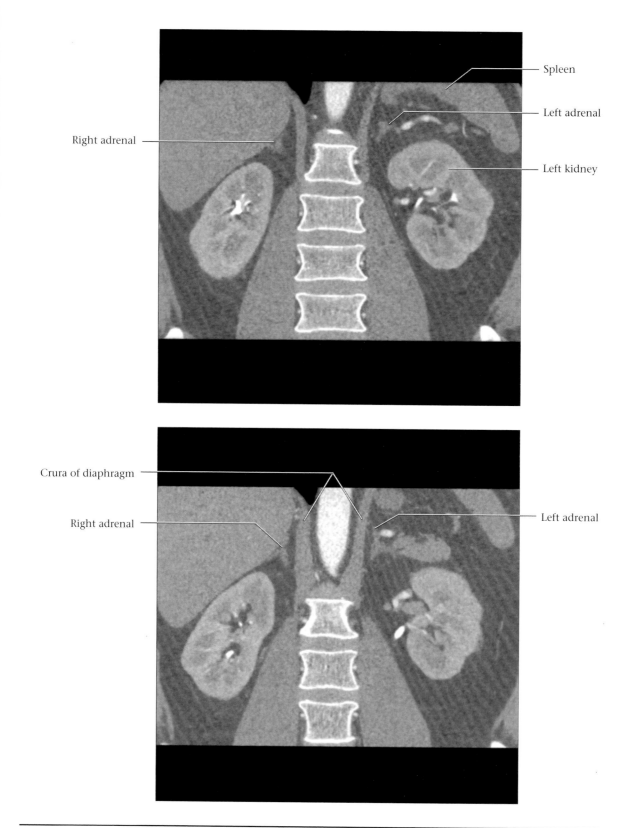

Right adrenal

Spleen

Left adrenal

Left kidney

Crura of diaphragm

Right adrenal

Left adrenal

(Top) First of two coronal CT sections shows the adrenal glands in their suprarenal location, accounting for the alternate name, "suprarenal glands". (Bottom) More anterior coronal CT image shows the adrenal glands and their relations to adjacent structures.

ADRENAL

AXIAL & CORONAL, NORMAL ADRENAL ANATOMY

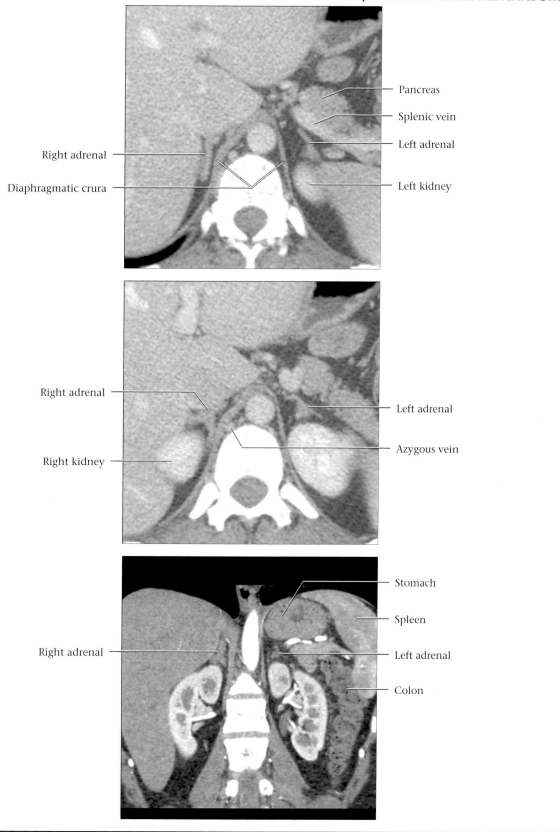

(Top) First of three CT images of a subject with normal adrenal glands shows conventional anatomy. (Middle) More caudal section shows both adrenal glands with an inverted "Y" appearance. There is mild thickening of the left adrenal gland at the confluence of the medial & lateral limbs, a normal finding. (Bottom) This coronal view demonstrates the relation between the adrenals and adjacent organs.

ADRENAL

FETAL ADRENAL & KIDNEY

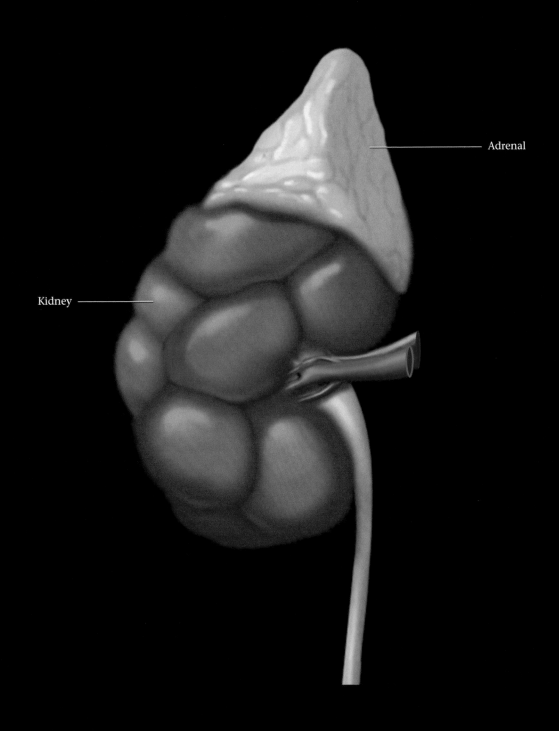

Adrenal

Kidney

Graphic shows the appearance of the adrenal and kidney in the fetus and neonate. The adrenal is much larger relative to the kidney than in the adult. The kidney has a lobulated appearance, reflecting the ongoing fusion of the individual renal lobes, each comprised of one renal pyramid and its associated renal cortex.

ADRENAL

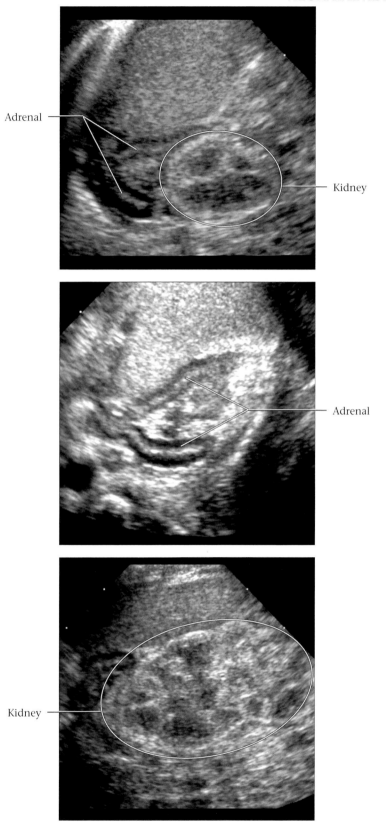

Adrenal

Kidney

Adrenal

Kidney

(**Top**) First of three ultrasound images of a neonate, showing the characteristic prominence of the adrenal gland and the lobation of the renal surface in early infancy. This sagittal image shows the large adrenal gland adjacent to the upper pole of the kidney. (**Middle**) Sagittal ultrasound shows the prominent limbs of the right adrenal gland. (**Bottom**) Sagittal ultrasound of the kidney shows its lobulated contour, a normal finding in the fetus and neonate.

ADRENAL

CT, ADRENAL ADENOMA

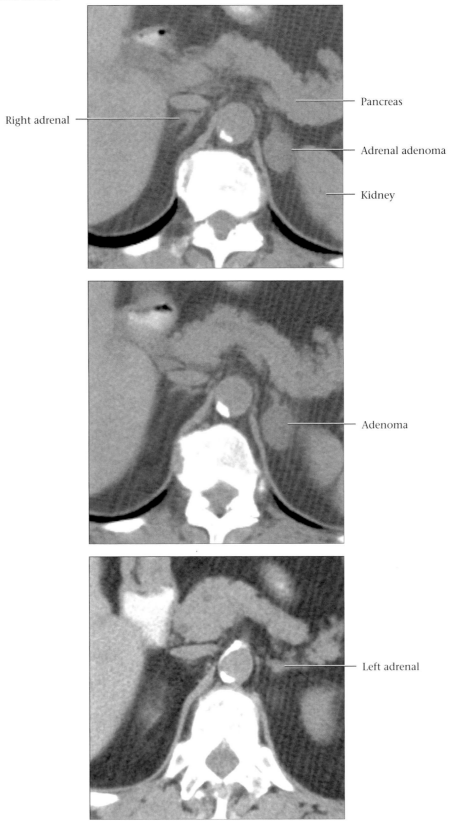

Right adrenal

Pancreas

Adrenal adenoma

Kidney

Adenoma

Left adrenal

(Top) First of three axial CT sections shows a typical adrenal adenoma. Within the left adrenal gland is a homogeneously low density mass (compare with kidney & pancreas). The low density (attenuation) reflects the presence of intra- and extracellular lipid within adenomas, a characteristic feature that allows distinction of adenomas from other types of adrenal masses. **(Middle)** The adenoma is present within an otherwise normal-appearing left adrenal gland. Patients with adenomas may be symptomatic (e.g., signs of excess cortisol or aldosterone) or asymptomatic. Most subjects have the adrenal lesion discovered incidentally on a CT scan performed for some other reason and have no clinical symptoms or signs. In this setting, the adenoma is said to be nonfunctional. **(Bottom)** This section shows a normal appearing lower part of the left adrenal.

ADRENAL

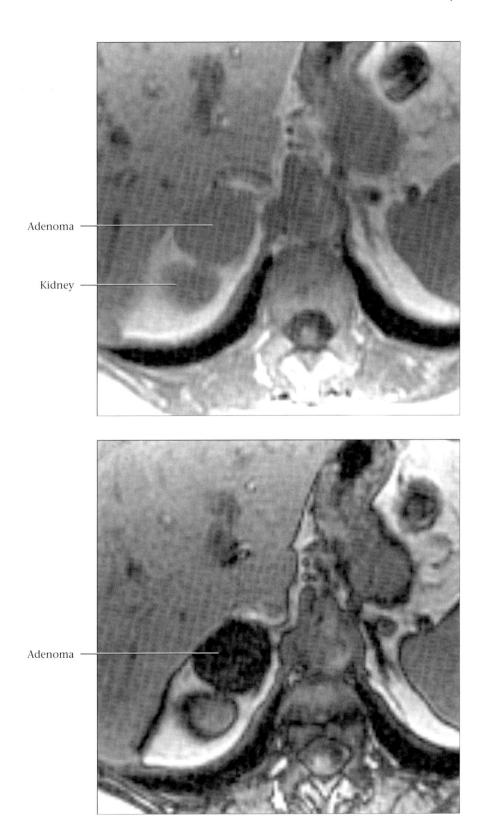

(Top) First of four MR images in a patient with a right adrenal adenoma shows a homogeneous rounded suprarenal mass on a T1-weighted in-phase GRE image. **(Bottom)** An axial T1-weighted opposed-phase GRE image through the same level shows marked loss of signal (lesion darkening) of the adrenal mass, confirming the presence of lipid and water protons evenly distributed throughout the mass. This finding is diagnostic of adrenal adenoma.

ADRENAL

MR, ADRENAL ADENOMA

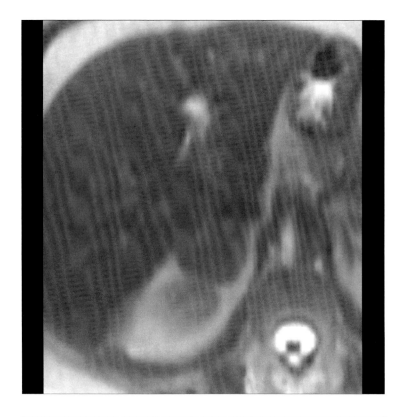

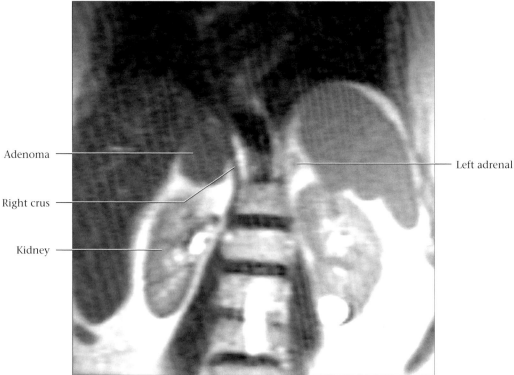

(Top) An axial T2-weighted image through the same level shows that the adenoma is of relatively low signal intensity, unlike the heterogeneous high signal characteristics of most malignant adrenal masses. (Bottom) This coronal image confirms the suprarenal position and homogeneous low signal of the right adrenal adenoma.

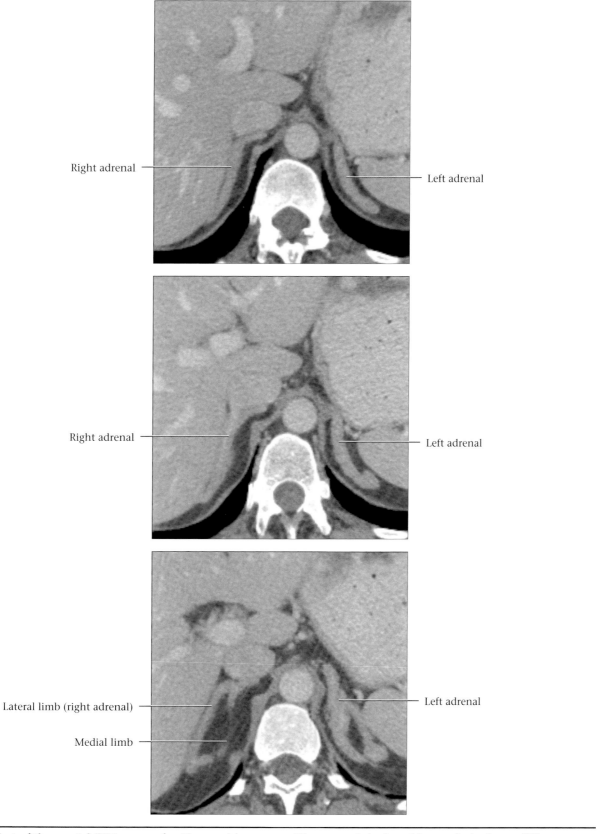

(Top) First of three axial CT images of a 40 year old woman with congenital adrenal hyperplasia shows diffuse enlargement of both adrenal glands, but preservation of their normal shape. **(Middle)** Each limb of the adrenal is in excess of 1 cm in diameter, one criterion used to diagnose or suggest adrenal hyperplasia. Most patients with adrenal hyperplasia have less markedly enlarged glands due to pituitary (or ectopic) production of excess adrenal corticotrophic hormone (ACTH). In many cases the adrenal glands may appear normal by imaging. **(Bottom)** The striking enlargement of the adrenals is evident on this image.

ADRENAL

PHEOCHROMOCYTOMA

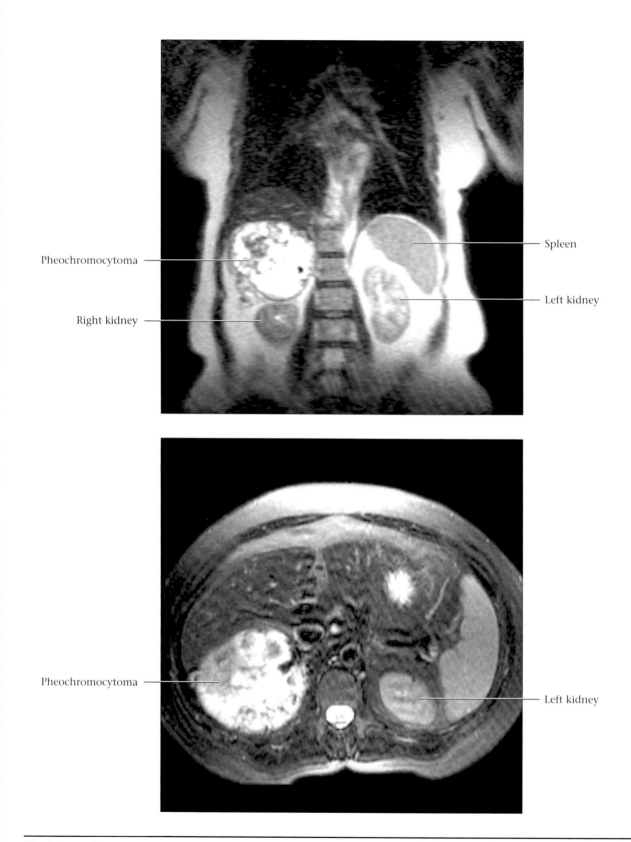

Pheochromocytoma

Right kidney

Spleen

Left kidney

Pheochromocytoma

Left kidney

(Top) First of four MR images of a patient with episodic hypertension, headaches and flushing. This coronal T2WI shows a large heterogeneous, bright mass in the right adrenal region. **(Bottom)** An axial T2WI shows the large heterogeneously bright adrenal mass. This is a typical appearance for an adrenal pheochromocytoma, though diagnosis rests on a combination of clinical, laboratory (excess catecholamines), and imaging criteria.

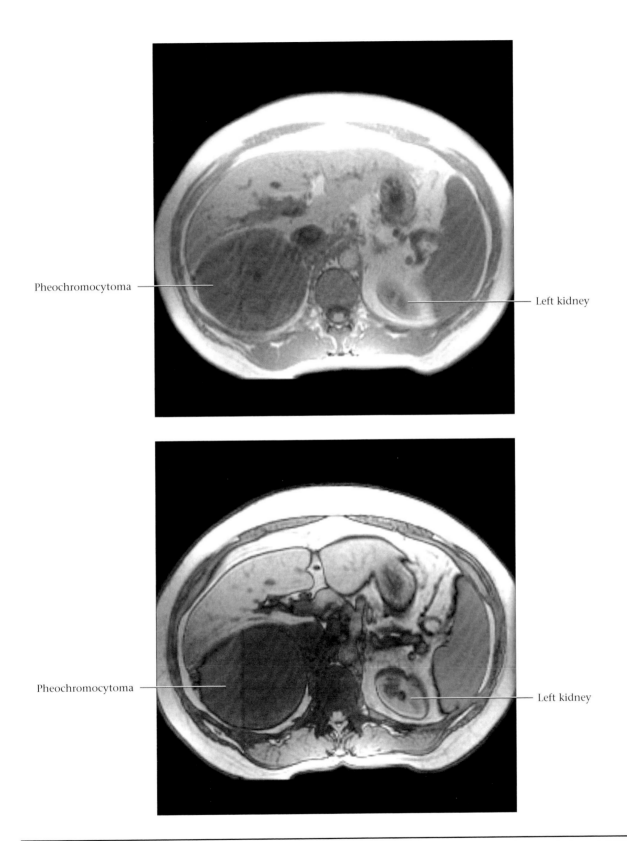

Pheochromocytoma — — Left kidney

Pheochromocytoma — — Left kidney

(Top) An axial T1WI in-phase GRE image shows a heterogeneous, large right adrenal mass. **(Bottom)** An axial T1WI opposed-phase GRE image shows no selective signal dropout from the mass, indicating that it does not contain excess lipid, as would be expected for an adrenal adenoma.

ADRENAL

ADRENAL METASTASES

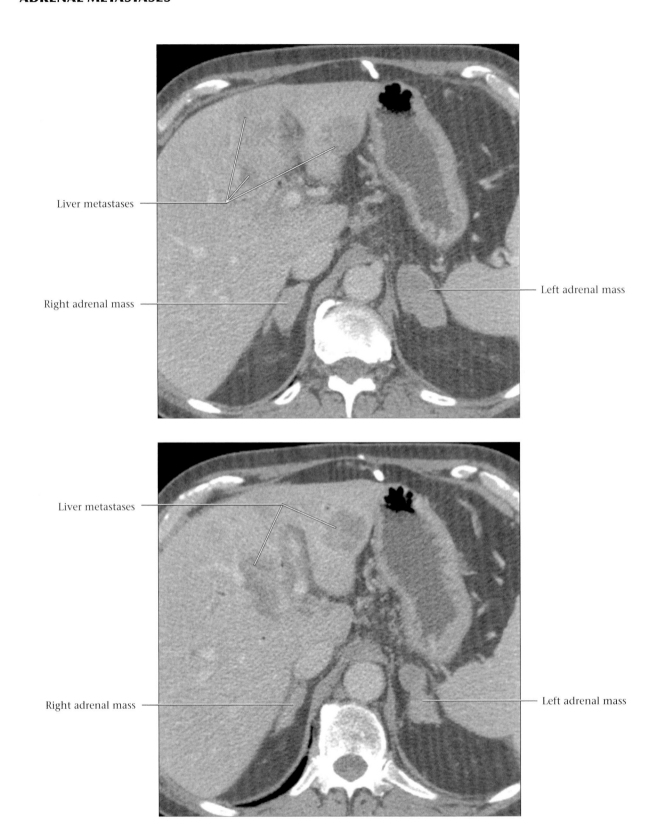

Liver metastases

Right adrenal mass

Left adrenal mass

Liver metastases

Right adrenal mass

Left adrenal mass

(Top) First of two axial CT sections in a patient with pancreatic carcinoma shows bilateral heterogeneous, nodular adrenal masses. Also evident are several heterogeneous, low density liver masses. These all represent metastatic foci. Lung, breast, and renal cancer, along with malignant melanoma frequently metastasize to the adrenal glands due to the rich blood supply of the adrenals. **(Bottom)** A more caudal section shows more of the nodular adrenal metastases.

ADRENAL

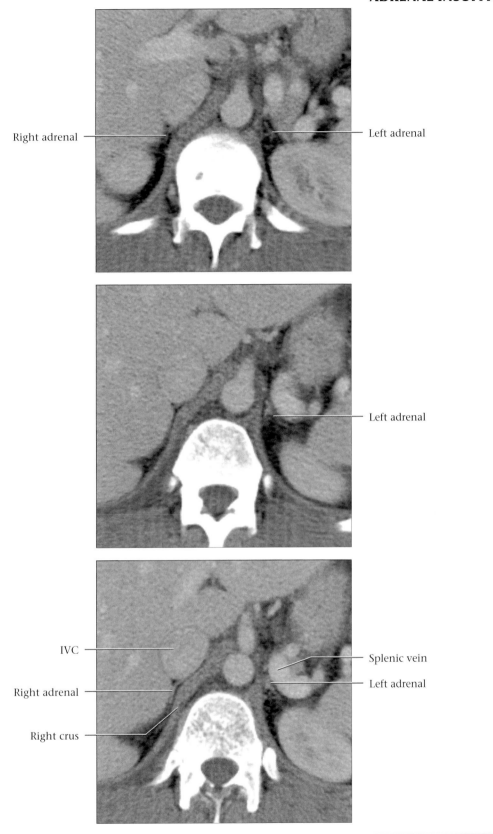

Right adrenal — Left adrenal

Left adrenal

IVC — Splenic vein

Right adrenal — Left adrenal

Right crus

(Top) First of three axial CT sections in a patient with adrenal insufficiency (Addison syndrome) due to autoimmune disease. The adrenal glands are extremely small. (Middle) The small adrenals are again evident. If adrenal insufficiency were due to adrenal tumors, bleeding, or infection, the glands would be enlarged. (Bottom) The adrenal glands have a normal shape but are extremely small.

ADRENAL

ADRENAL HEMORRHAGE

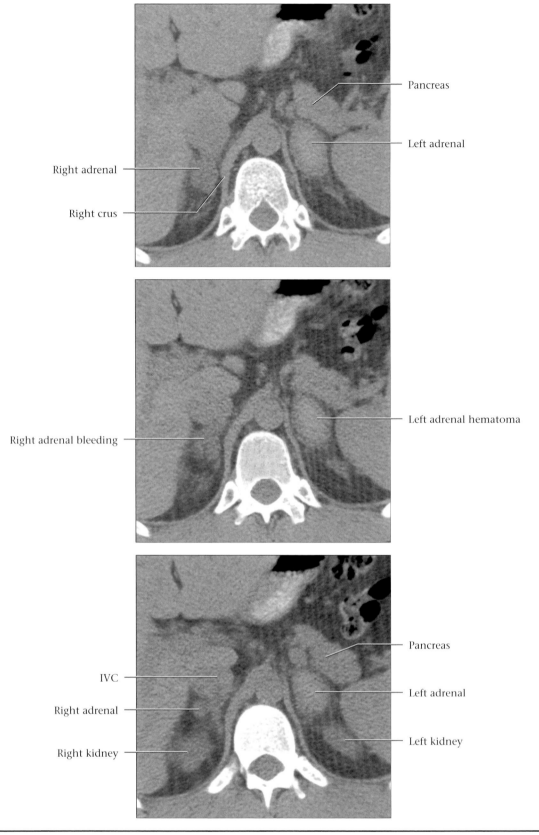

Pancreas

Left adrenal

Right adrenal

Right crus

Left adrenal hematoma

Right adrenal bleeding

Pancreas

IVC

Left adrenal

Right adrenal

Right kidney

Left kidney

(Top) First of five nonenhanced axial CT sections in a patient who was hypotensive from hemorrhage due to blunt abdominal trauma. Both adrenal glands are markedly enlarged and the left adrenal has heterogeneous high density material within it, characteristic of acute hemorrhage. (Middle) Bleeding is evident within and around the adrenal glands. (Bottom) In this, and most patients, the adrenal hemorrhage is in response to the stress of shock, which leads to an outpouring of adrenal cortical and medullary hormones. Excessive stimulation can result in adrenal enlargement or spontaneous adrenal hemorrhage, as in this patient.

ADRENAL

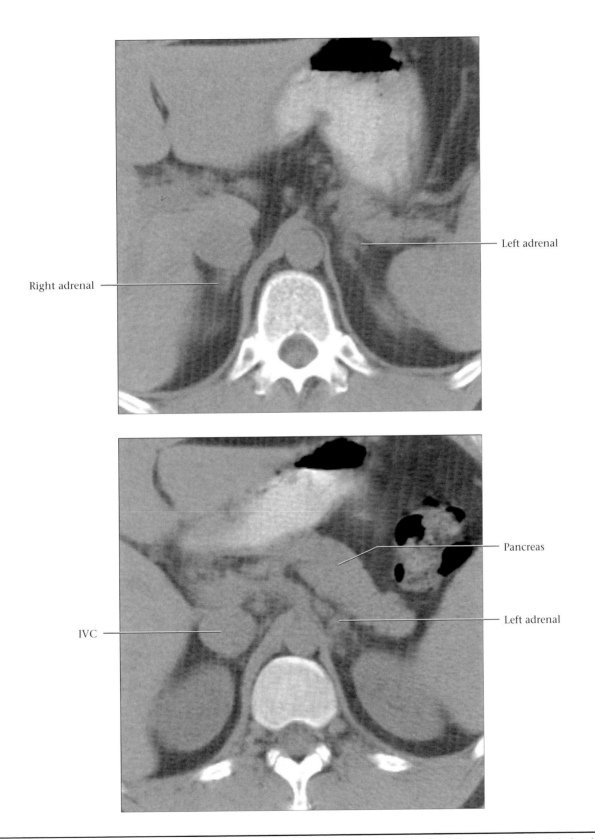

(Top) A repeat CT scan in the same patient three months later shows essentially normal appearing adrenal glands. Adrenal hemorrhage may result in destruction of the glands with adrenal insufficiency, or the adrenal glands may survive without permanent damage. **(Bottom)** The normal left adrenal gland is seen on this section.

ADRENAL

ADRENAL CARCINOMA

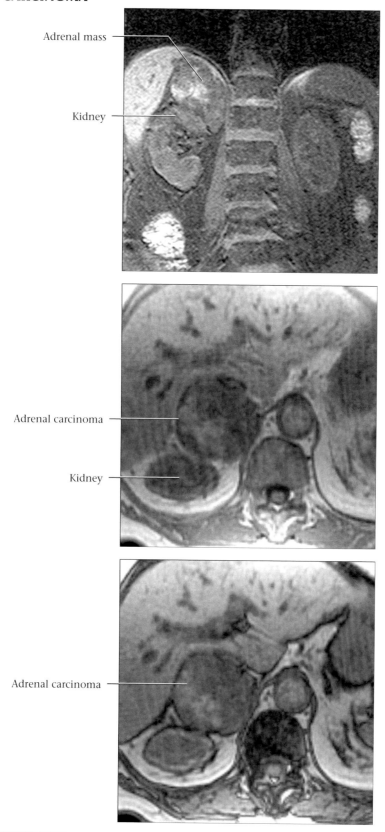

Adrenal mass

Kidney

Adrenal carcinoma

Kidney

Adrenal carcinoma

(Top) First of three MR sections in a patient with Cushing syndrome due to adrenal carcinoma. This coronal T2-weighted MR image shows a heterogeneous, large right adrenal mass. **(Middle)** An axial T1-weighted MR section shows the heterogeneous mass above the right kidney. **(Bottom)** An axial opposed phase GRE image shows no selective dropout of signal from the mass, indicating that it does not contain excess lipid, as would be expected for a benign adrenal adenoma. The size and heterogenicity of the mass are typical for adrenal carcinoma. Tumors arising from the right adrenal gland are especially prone to invasion of the IVC through the short right adrenal vein, leading to lung and systemic metastases.

ADRENAL

GASTRIC DIVERTICULUM SIMULATING ADRENAL MASS

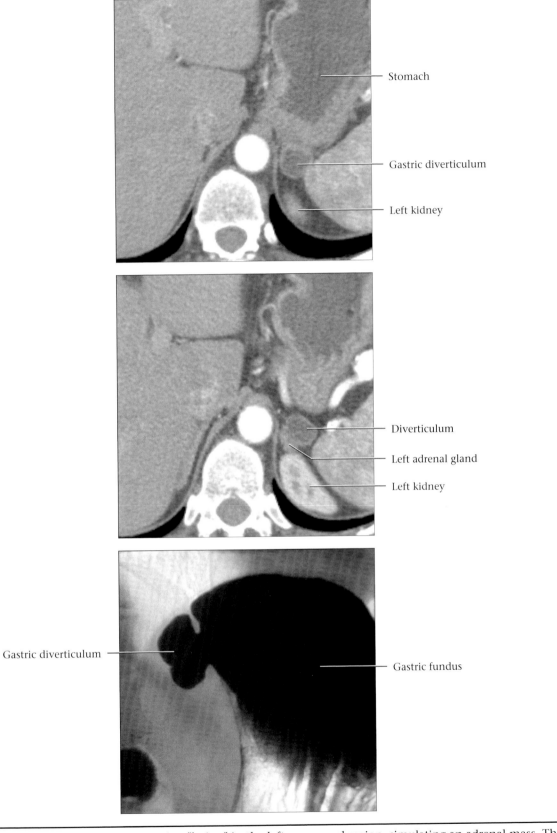

(Top) Axial CT image shows a cystic appearing "lesion" in the left suprarenal region, simulating an adrenal mass. The mass has the same density as the water-filled stomach. (Middle) A more caudal CT section shows part of the normal left adrenal gland, which is displaced medially by the gastric diverticulum. On axial sections, it is difficult to recognize the gastric origin of the diverticulum. Administration of oral contrast medium or gas-producing granules can be helpful in identification. (Bottom) An oblique film from a barium upper GI series shows the barium-filled diverticulum, projecting posteriorly from the gastric cardia.

KIDNEY

Gross Anatomy

Overview
- Kidneys are paired, bean-shaped retroperitoneal organs
  - Function: Remove excess water, salts and wastes of protein metabolism from the blood

Anatomic Relationships
- Lie in retroperitoneum, within **perirenal space**, surrounded by **renal fascia (of Gerota)**
- Each kidney is ~ 10-15 cm in length, 5 cm in width
- Both kidneys lie on **quadratus lumborum muscles**, lateral to **psoas muscles**

Internal Structures
- Kidneys can be considered hollow with renal sinus occupied by fat, renal pelvis, calices, vessels and nerves
- **Renal hilum**: Where artery enters, vein and ureter leave renal sinus
- **Renal pelvis**: Funnel-shaped expansion of the upper end of the ureter
  - Receives **major calices (infundibula)** (2 or 3), each of which receives **minor calices** (2-4)
- **Renal papilla**: Pointed apex of the **renal pyramid** of collecting tubules that excrete urine
  - Each papilla indents a minor calyx
- **Renal cortex**: Outer part, contains renal corpuscles (glomeruli, vessels), proximal portions of collecting tubules & loop of Henle
- **Renal medulla**: Inner part, contains renal pyramids, distal parts of the collecting tubules and loops of Henle
- **Vessels, nerves, and lymphatics**
  - Artery
    - Usually one for each kidney
    - Arise from aorta at about L1-2 vertebral level
  - Vein
    - Usually one for each kidney
    - Lies in front of renal artery and renal pelvis
  - Nerves
    - Autonomic from **renal** and **aorticorenal ganglia** and **plexus**
  - Lymphatics
    - To **lumbar (aortic** and **caval) nodes**

Anatomy-Based Imaging Issues

Key Concepts
- Accessory renal vessels
  - Accessory arteries and veins are common
  - May arise from aorta or common iliac vessels
  - Must be accounted for in planning surgery (e.g., resection, transplantation)

Clinical Implications

Clinical Importance
- Renal colic
  - Calculi ("stones") may form within & obstruct the renal calices or ureter
    - Causes: Dehydration, gout, urinary infection, idiopathic
  - Obstruction plus periodic peristalsis of ureter result in spasms of severe pain, radiating to flank and groin
- Renal carcinoma
  - Tumor invasion of renal vein → lung metastases (common), plus bone & systemic metastases
  - Strong renal fascia usually prevents direct invasion of adjacent organs and body wall
- Renal cysts
  - Extremely common (> 50% of adults have at least one)
  - Etiology unknown, but filled with clear fluid, lined by simple cuboidal epithelium
  - Imaging studies can usually distinguish from neoplasm

Embryology

Embryologic Events
- Congenital anomalies of renal number, position, structure and form are very common
  - Often accompanied by anomalies of other systems
  - **VATER** acronym
    - Vertebral
    - Anorectal (e.g., atresia)
    - Tracheoesophageal (e.g., T-E fistula)
    - Radial (e.g., hand & wrist anomalies or absence)
    - Renal (e.g., agenesis, ectopia)
  - Congenital absence of kidney
    - Commonly associated with ipsilateral anomalies of genital tract (e.g., seminal vesicle absence or cyst; uterovaginal atresia or duplication)
  - Anomalies of position (ectopia) are common
    - Often due to failure to ascend from pelvic location where fetal kidneys lie close together
    - May be accompanied by fusion of kidneys; **crossed fused ectopia** and "**horseshoe kidney**" (1 in 400 adults)
    - Accompanied by anomalies of vessels, ureters
    - More vulnerable to trauma, calculi, hydronephrosis
  - Anomalies of structure
    - Congenitally large **septum of Bertin (lobar dysmorphism)**; asymptomatic, but may simulate mass; in mid-kidney, composed of normal cortex displacing collecting system
    - **Fetal lobulations (lobation)**, single or multiple indentations of the lateral renal contours; represent persistent clefts between renal lobules (must distinguish from cortical scarring from infection or ischemia)
    - **Partial duplication:** Commonly results in enlarged kidney with 2 separate hila, 2 ureters (may join downstream or join bladder separately); duplex kidney = bifid renal pelvis, single ureter
  - **Autosomal dominant polycystic disease:** Common hereditary disorder characterized by multiple renal cysts, progressive renal failure & various systemic manifestations (such as cerebral aneurysms)

KIDNEY

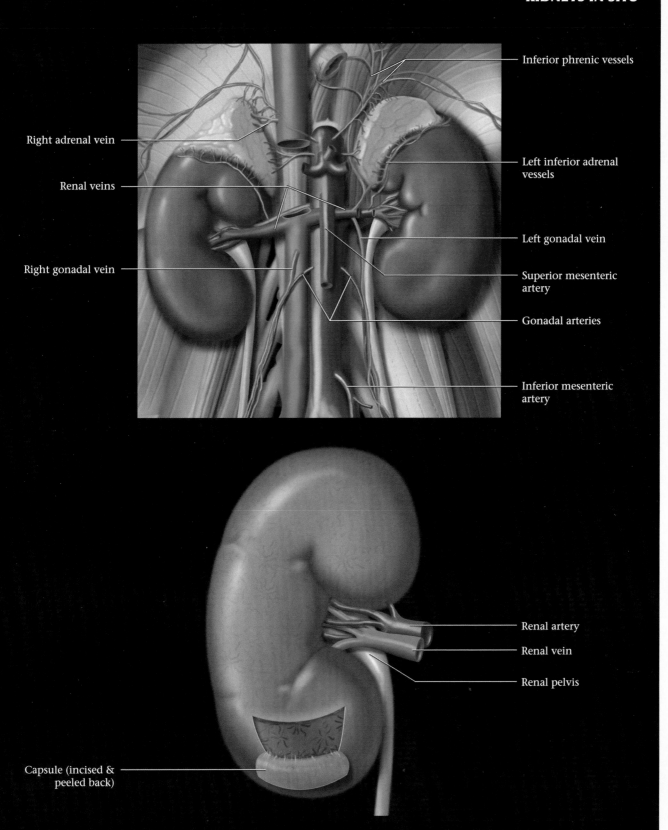

- Inferior phrenic vessels
- Right adrenal vein
- Left inferior adrenal vessels
- Renal veins
- Left gonadal vein
- Right gonadal vein
- Superior mesenteric artery
- Gonadal arteries
- Inferior mesenteric artery

- Renal artery
- Renal vein
- Renal pelvis
- Capsule (incised & peeled back)

(Top) The kidneys are retroperitoneal organs that lie lateral to the psoas and "on" the quadratus lumborum muscles. The oblique course of the psoas muscles results in the lower pole of the kidney lying lateral to the upper pole. The right kidney usually lies 1-2 cm lower than the left, due to inferior displacement by the liver. The adrenal glands lie above and medial to the kidneys, separated by a layer of fat and connective tissue. Peritoneum covers much of the anterior surface of the kidneys. The right kidney abuts the liver, hepatic flexure of colon and duodenum, while the left kidney is in close contact with the pancreas (tail), spleen, and splenic flexure. **(Bottom)** The fibrous capsule is stripped off with difficulty. Subcapsular hematomas do not spread far along the surface of the kidney, but compress the renal parenchyma, unlike most perirenal collections.

KIDNEY

KIDNEY ARTERIES & INTERIOR ANATOMY

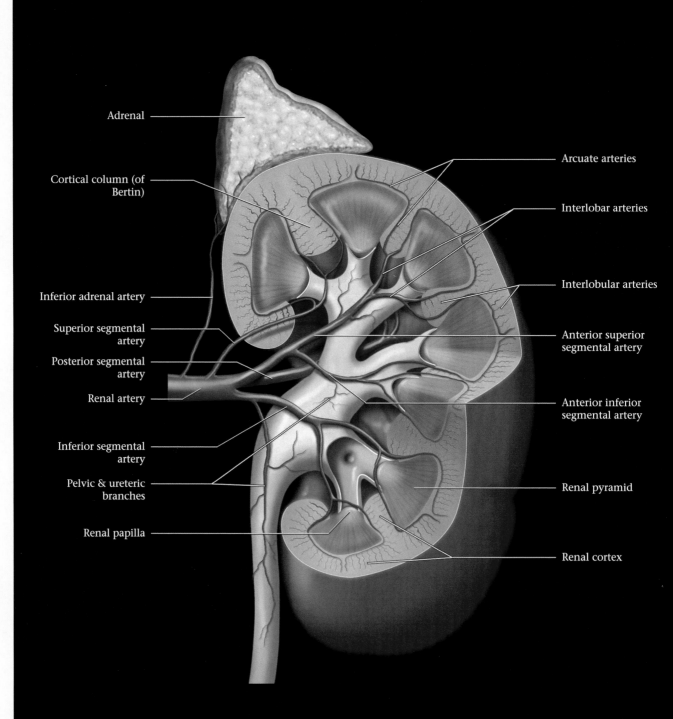

Adrenal

Cortical column (of Bertin)

Inferior adrenal artery

Superior segmental artery

Posterior segmental artery

Renal artery

Inferior segmental artery

Pelvic & ureteric branches

Renal papilla

Arcuate arteries

Interlobar arteries

Interlobular arteries

Anterior superior segmental artery

Anterior inferior segmental artery

Renal pyramid

Renal cortex

The kidney is usually supplied by a single renal artery, the first branch of which is the inferior adrenal artery. It then divides into five segmental arteries, only one of which, the posterior segmental artery, passes dorsal to the renal pelvis. The segmental arteries divide into the interlobar arteries that lie in the renal sinus fat. Each interlobar artery branches into 4 to 6 arcuate arteries that follow the convex outer margin of each renal pyramid. The arcuate arteries give rise to the interlobular arteries that lie within the renal cortex, including the cortical columns (of Bertin) that invaginate between the renal pyramids. The interlobular arteries supply the afferent arterioles to the glomeruli. The arterial supply to the kidney is vulnerable as there are no effective anastomoses between the segmental branches, each of which supplies a wedge-shaped segment of parenchyma.

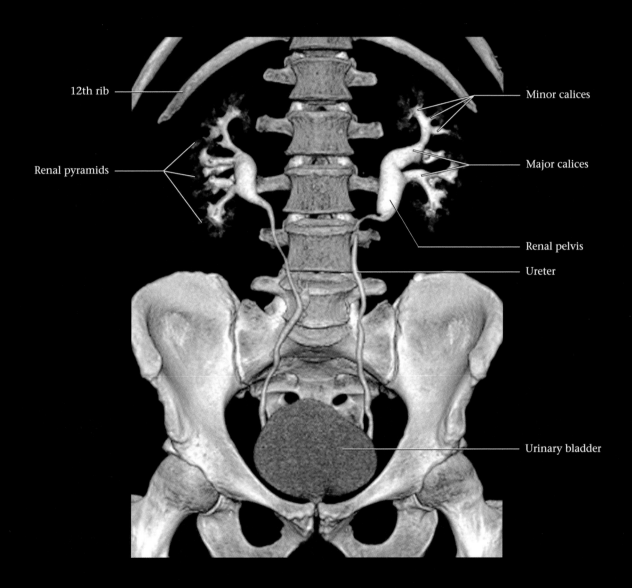

12th rib

Renal pyramids

Minor calices

Major calices

Renal pelvis

Ureter

Urinary bladder

A coronal reconstruction of a series of axial CT sections can be viewed as a surface-rendered 3D image to simulate an excretory urogram. The window levels and workstation controls have been set to display optimally the renal collecting system. The color scale is arbitrary; in this case, opacified urine is displayed as "white". Less dense urine within the renal tubules in the pyramids and the diluted urine within the bladder are displayed as "red". The CT scan was obtained in deep, suspended inspiration, resulting in caudal displacement of the kidneys. In the supine position at quiet breathing, the upper poles of the kidneys usually lie in front of the 12th ribs.

KIDNEY

MULTIPLANAR CT

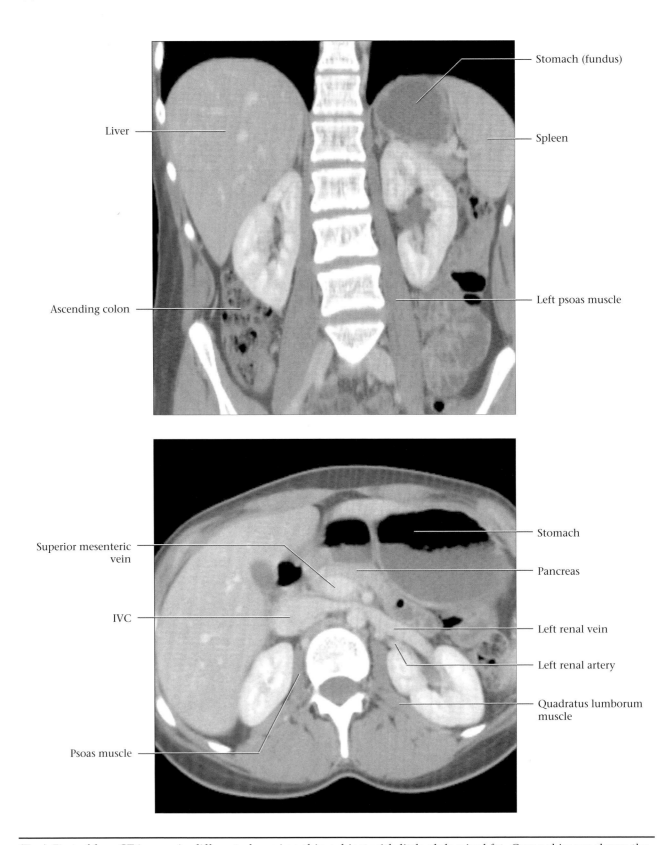

Liver

Ascending colon

Stomach (fundus)

Spleen

Left psoas muscle

Superior mesenteric vein

IVC

Psoas muscle

Stomach

Pancreas

Left renal vein

Left renal artery

Quadratus lumborum muscle

(Top) First of four CT images in different planes in a thin subject with little abdominal fat. Coronal image shows the kidneys and their neighboring organs and structures. The kidneys lie on the quadratus lumborum, and lateral to the psoas muscles. The oblique course of the psoas muscles results in the lower poles of the kidneys lying lateral and ventral to the upper poles. **(Bottom)** This axial image is at the level of the upper pole of the right kidney and the hilum of the left kidney. The left renal vein enters the IVC on this section, after passing behind the superior mesenteric vessels. The renal hila face anteriorly and medially.

KIDNEY

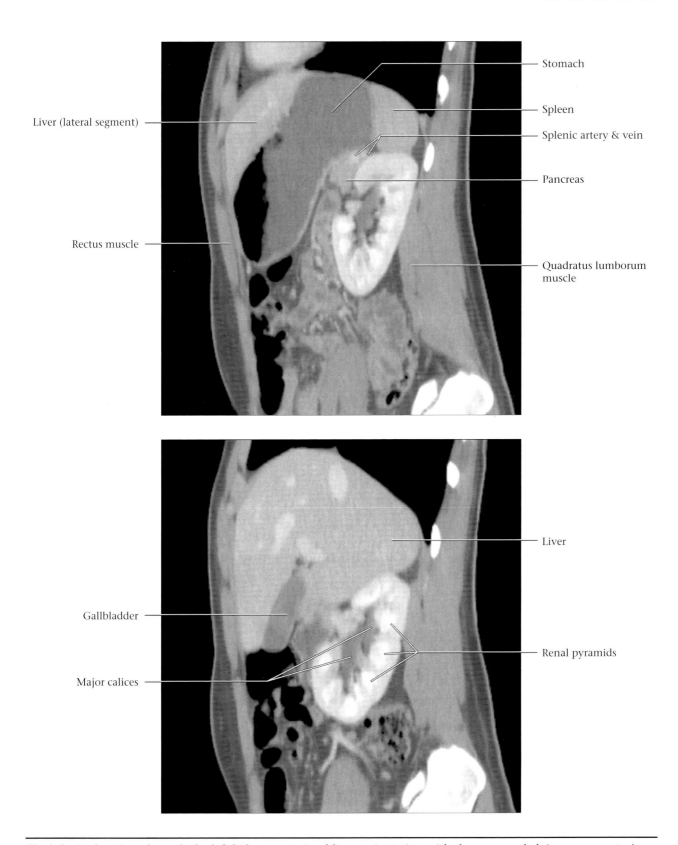

Liver (lateral segment)

Rectus muscle

Stomach

Spleen

Splenic artery & vein

Pancreas

Quadratus lumborum muscle

Gallbladder

Major calices

Liver

Renal pyramids

(Top) Sagittal section through the left kidney; note its oblique orientation with the upper pole lying more posterior than the lower pole. Note the relationship of the left kidney to the spleen and pancreas. **(Bottom)** Sagittal section through the right kidney. The renal pyramids are the groups of renal collecting tubules that appear more dense than the renal cortex on this late parenchymal phase of CT imaging, when the urine is being opacified by contrast material prior to excretion. Urine in the calices is not yet opacified.

KIDNEY

CT, CORTICOMEDULLARY & PYELOGRAPHIC PHASES

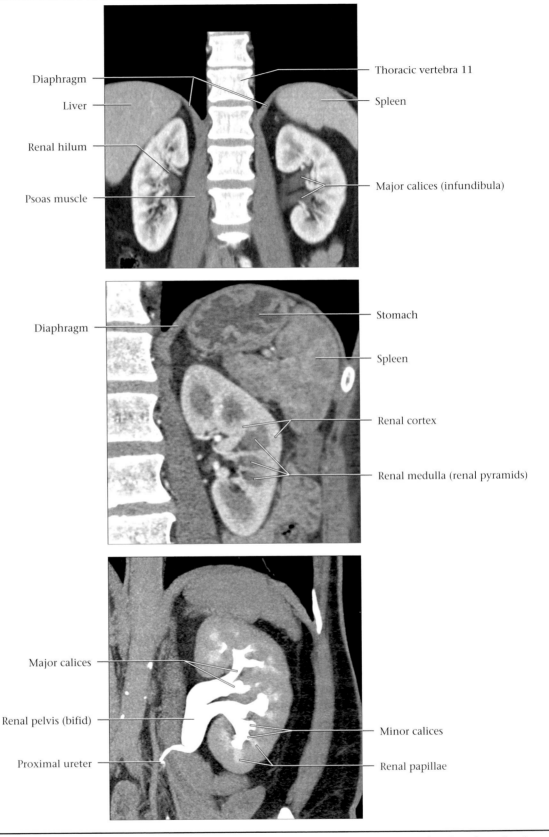

Diaphragm — Thoracic vertebra 11

Liver — Spleen

Renal hilum

Psoas muscle — Major calices (infundibula)

Diaphragm — Stomach

Spleen

Renal cortex

Renal medulla (renal pyramids)

Major calices

Renal pelvis (bifid) — Minor calices

Proximal ureter — Renal papillae

(Top) First of three CT images of the kidneys. In the cortico-medullary phase of contrast opacification the urine in the collecting systems is not yet opacified. The renal pyramids are lucent relative to the cortex. **(Middle)** The cortex contains the renal corpuscles (glomeruli & proximal tubules) while the medulla is comprised of the distal collecting tubules. Note the peripheral renal cortex and the columns of cortex that are interposed between the renal pyramids. The greater enhancement of the cortex reflects its increased blood flow compared with the medulla. **(Bottom)** In this excretory phase image the calices and renal pelvis are filled with densely opacified urine. The renal pelvis is bifid, a normal variant. The renal papillae are the apices of the renal pyramids and these are opacified by urine that is becoming progressively concentrated within the distal collecting tubules.

KIDNEY

EXCRETORY UROGRAM

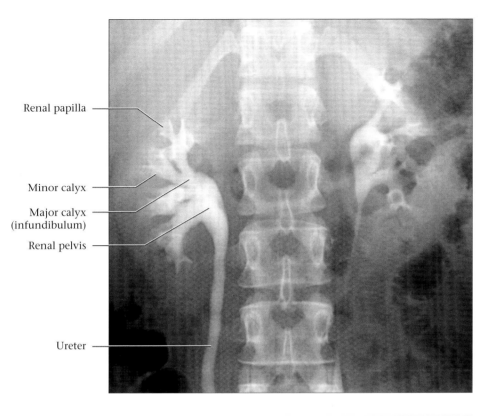

Renal papilla

Minor calyx

Major calyx
(infundibulum)

Renal pelvis

Ureter

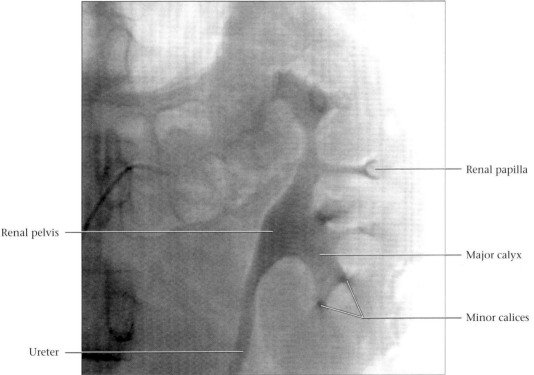

Renal papilla

Renal pelvis

Major calyx

Minor calices

Ureter

(Top) Frontal film from an excretory urogram, also known as an "intravenous pyelogram" (IVP), shows the collecting systems and ureters. The right ureter is dilated due to a distal ureteral stone. The renal pelvis is the funnel-shaped expansion of the upper ureter and it receives two or three major calices (infundibula). Each major calyx receives several minor calices and each minor calyx is indented by a renal papilla, the apex of the renal pyramid from which urine is excreted. Each renal pyramid and its associated cortex form one lobe of the kidney. The renal lobes are readily visible in the human fetus and persist in some adults (and many animals). **(Bottom)** A frontal film following a left renal angiogram shows the collecting system. The number of major and minor calices can be quite variable among individuals without clinical consequence.

KIDNEY

CORONAL OBLIQUE, NORMAL KIDNEY

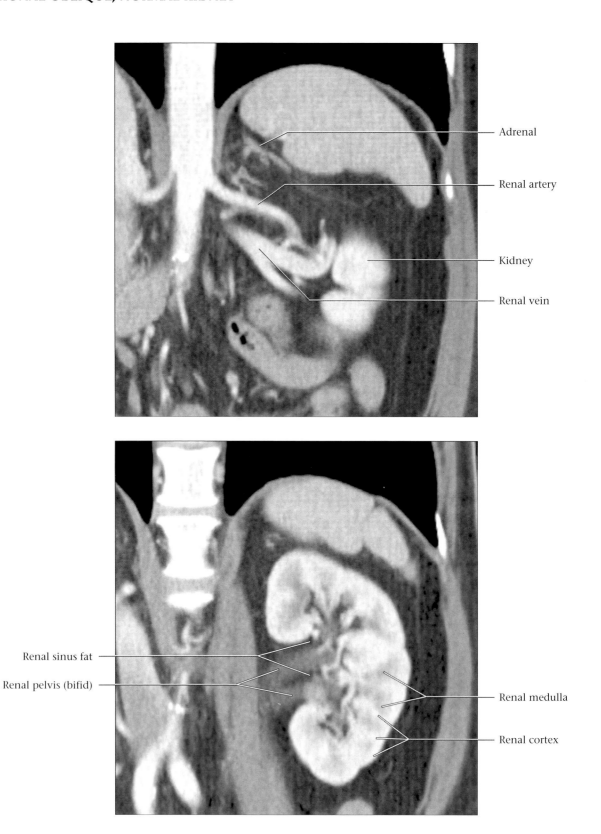

Adrenal

Renal artery

Kidney

Renal vein

Renal sinus fat

Renal pelvis (bifid)

Renal medulla

Renal cortex

(Top) First of four coronal oblique CT images of the left kidney shows the renal artery and vein at the hilum. The vein usually lies ventral to the artery and the renal pelvis. (Bottom) Note the renal sinus fat which accompanies the renal vessels (interlobar) and calices in the central "hollow" core of the kidney. Note the columns of renal cortex (columns or septa of Bertin) that lie between the renal pyramids (medulla).

KIDNEY

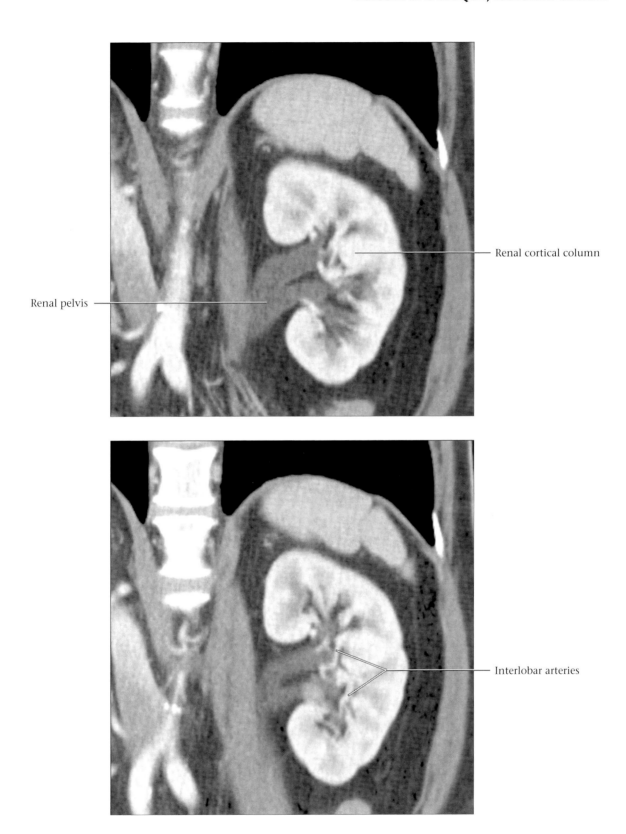

Renal cortical column

Renal pelvis

Interlobar arteries

(Top) Note the prominent, somewhat rounded renal cortical column. These focal collections of cortical tissue may protrude into the renal sinus and separate the pyramids of the renal medulla and may be mistaken for a renal tumor. This is sometimes referred to as a hypertrophied column of Bertin. (Bottom) The renal sinus fat and its accompanying vessels and calices are well depicted on this image.

KIDNEY

NORMAL ULTRASONOGRAPHY

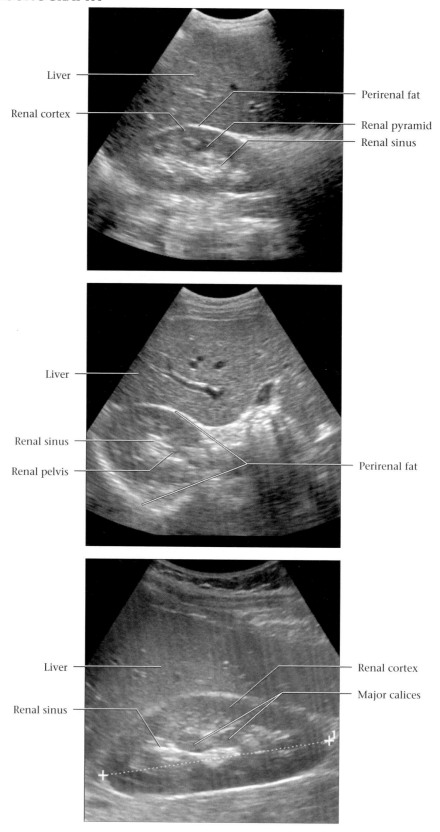

(Top) First of three ultrasonographic images of the right kidney. This sagittal section shows the long axis of the kidney. Renal cortex is usually slightly less echogenic than the liver, while renal sinus fat is quite echogenic. The renal pyramids are relatively sonolucent and the renal pelvis, when distended with urine, is anechoic (no echoes). Fat within the perirenal space creates the echogenic interface between the kidney and the liver. (Middle) This transverse (axial) image of the kidney shows the echogenic fat within the renal sinus and perirenal space in this thin subject. (Bottom) A sagittal sonographic image of the kidney shows an electronic cursor being used to measure the longitudinal axis of the kidney, which is usually 10-15 cm in length.

KIDNEY

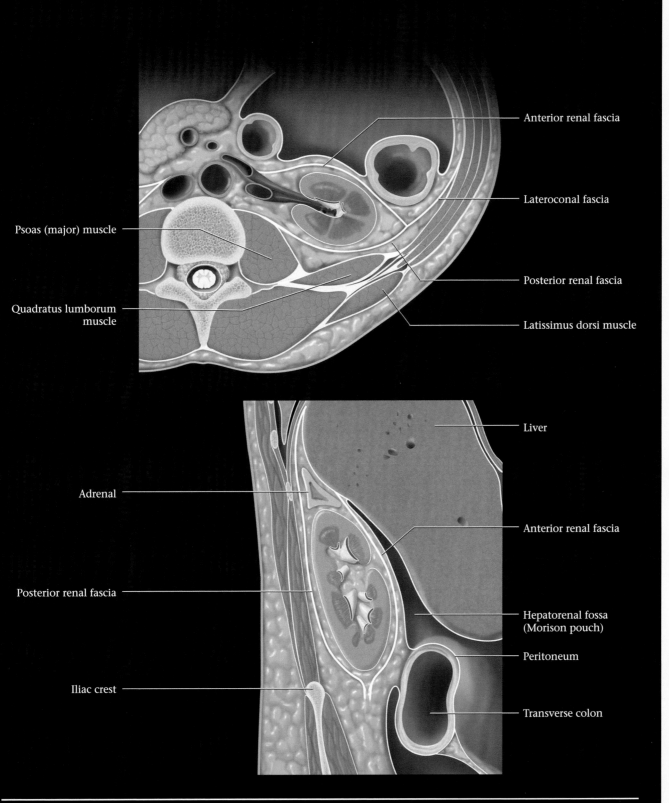

Anterior renal fascia

Lateroconal fascia

Psoas (major) muscle

Posterior renal fascia

Quadratus lumborum muscle

Latissimus dorsi muscle

Liver

Adrenal

Anterior renal fascia

Posterior renal fascia

Hepatorenal fossa (Morison pouch)

Peritoneum

Iliac crest

Transverse colon

(Top) The anterior and posterior layers of the renal fascia envelope the kidneys and adrenals along with the perirenal fat. Medial to the kidneys, the course of the renal fascia is variable (and controversial). The posterior layer usually fuses with the psoas or quadratus lumborum fascia. The perirenal spaces do not communicate across the abdominal midline. However, the renal & lateroconal fasciae are laminated structures that may be distended with fluid collections to form interfascial planes that do communicate across the midline and also inferiorly to the extraperitoneal pelvis. (Bottom) A sagittal section through the right kidney shows the renal fascia enveloping the kidney and adrenal. Inferiorly the anterior and posterior renal fasciae come close together at about the level of the iliac crest. Note the adjacent peritoneal recesses.

KIDNEY

RENAL FASCIA & PERIRENAL SPACE

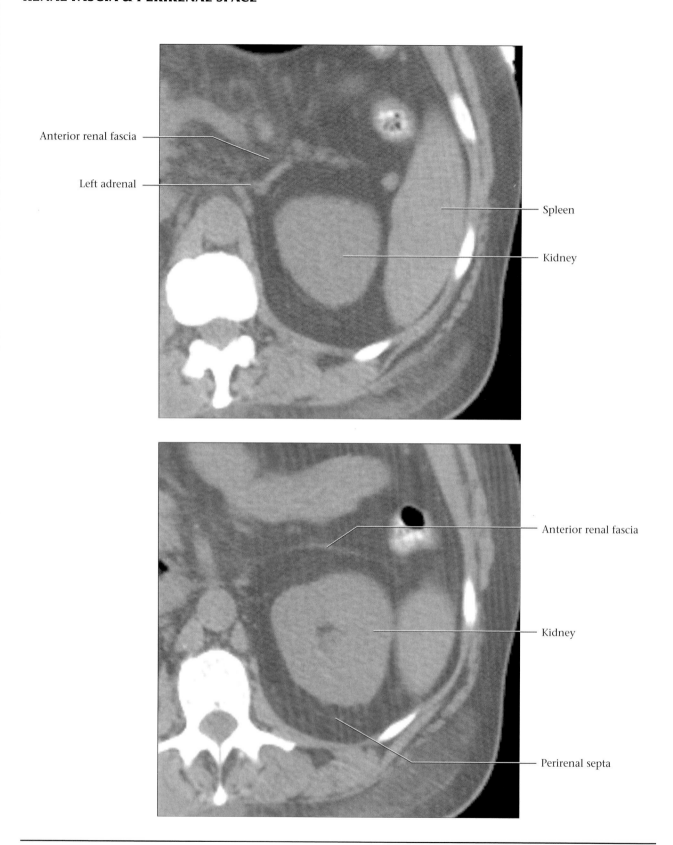

Anterior renal fascia

Left adrenal

Spleen

Kidney

Anterior renal fascia

Kidney

Perirenal septa

(Top) First of five axial CT sections demonstrating the contents and boundaries of the perirenal space. The perirenal space is bounded by the anterior and posterior renal fasciae, and within this space lie the adrenal and kidney, with a variable number of vessels, nerves and lymphatics. **(Bottom)** The anterior renal fascia (also known as Gerota fascia) is well demonstrated on this image. Also note the thin septa within the perirenal fat that may divide this space into multiple, poorly communicating spaces.

KIDNEY

KIDNEY & PERIRENAL SPACE

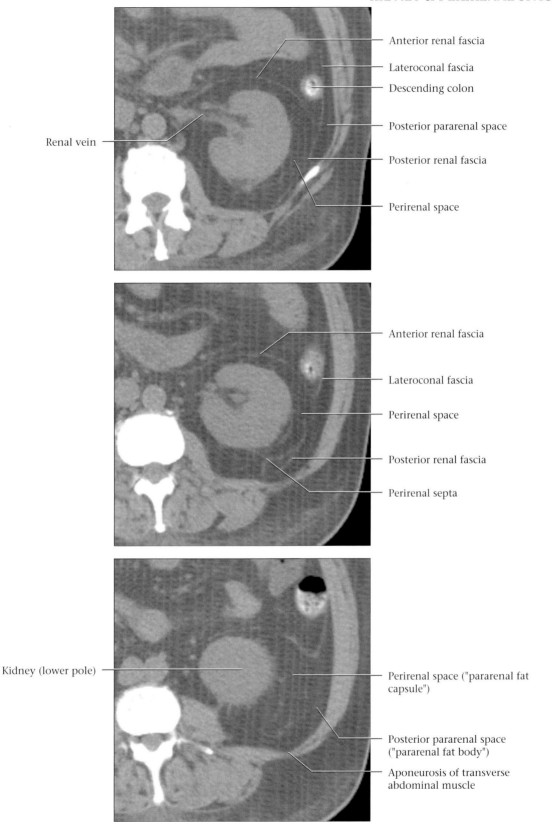

Anterior renal fascia

Lateroconal fascia

Descending colon

Posterior pararenal space

Posterior renal fascia

Perirenal space

Renal vein

Anterior renal fascia

Lateroconal fascia

Perirenal space

Posterior renal fascia

Perirenal septa

Kidney (lower pole)

Perirenal space ("pararenal fat capsule")

Posterior pararenal space ("pararenal fat body")

Aponeurosis of transverse abdominal muscle

(Top) The renal and lateroconal fasciae are the key planes that define the three divisions of the retroperitoneum and they are well demonstrated on this image. The descending colon (plus the duodenum and pancreas) lies in the anterior pararenal space. The lateroconal fascia is the lateral margin of the anterior pararenal space and the medial margin of the posterior pararenal space. (Middle) Note the confluence of the renal and the lateroconal fasciae and the renal with the quadratus lumborum fascia. (Bottom) A flank incision may be used to approach the kidney, and usually involves dividing the aponeurosis of the transverse abdominal muscle to enter the retroperitoneum. First encountered is the fat within the posterior pararenal space, sometimes referred to as the "pararenal fat body". The renal fascia is next seen, within which lies the perirenal space, also known as the "pararenal fat capsule".

KIDNEY

PERIRENAL PLANES

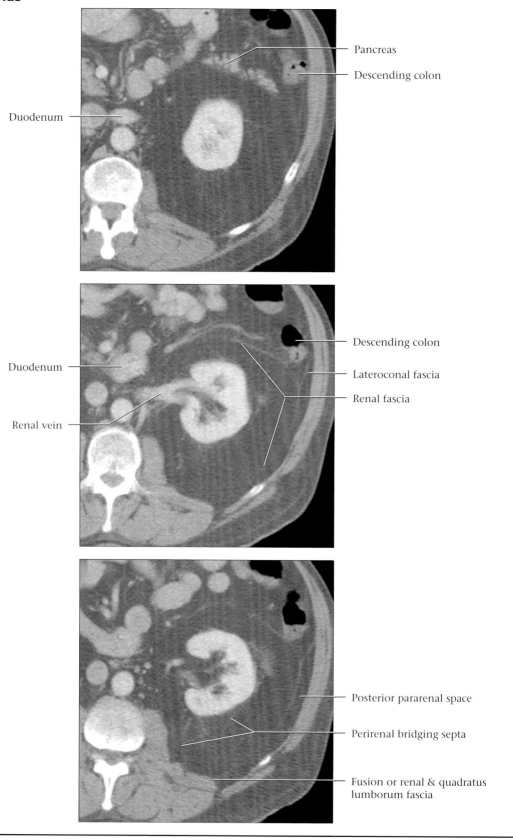

Pancreas

Descending colon

Duodenum

Duodenum

Descending colon

Lateroconal fascia

Renal fascia

Renal vein

Posterior pararenal space

Perirenal bridging septa

Fusion or renal & quadratus lumborum fascia

(Top) First of six axial CT sections shows the upper pole of the left kidney surrounded by extensive fat within the perirenal space. The pancreas, duodenum and ascending/descending colon lie anterior to the renal fascia, within the anterior pararenal space. **(Middle)** The renal and lateroconal fascia are evident on this section. **(Bottom)** The posterior pararenal space lies lateral to the lateroconal fascia and is synonymous with the "properitoneal fat stripe" seen on abdominal radiographs. Note the fusion of the posterior renal fascia with the quadratus lumborum fascia. Several perirenal bridging septa are visible within the perirenal space.

KIDNEY

PERIRENAL PLANES

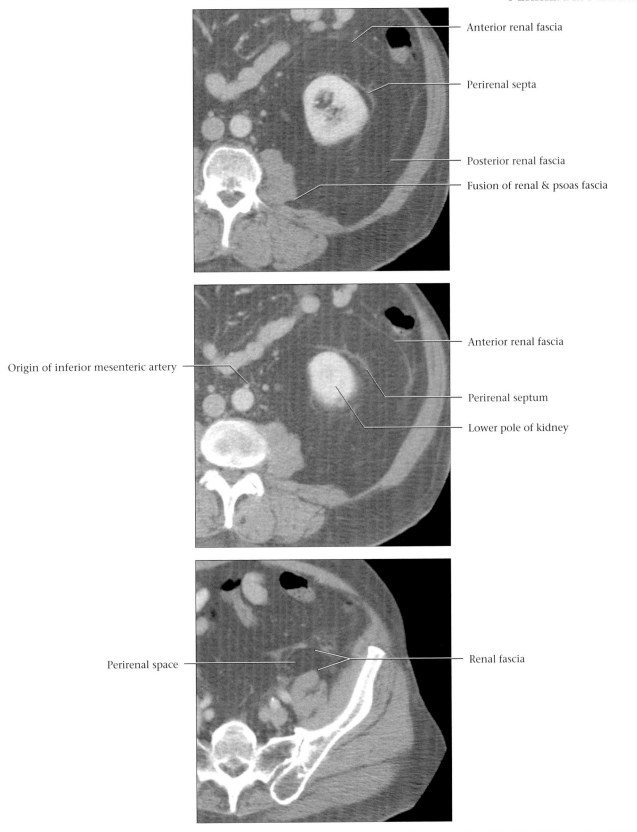

Anterior renal fascia

Perirenal septa

Posterior renal fascia

Fusion of renal & psoas fascia

Origin of inferior mesenteric artery

Anterior renal fascia

Perirenal septum

Lower pole of kidney

Perirenal space

Renal fascia

(Top) On this section the renal fascia courses medially to fuse with the psoas fascia. **(Middle)** Some of the perirenal bridging septa course parallel to the renal capsule and renal fascia and could be mistaken for the renal fascia. **(Bottom)** At a level just caudal to the iliac crest the layers of the renal fascia come close together to almost seal off the lower portion of the perirenal space.

KIDNEY

CATHETER ANGIOGRAM

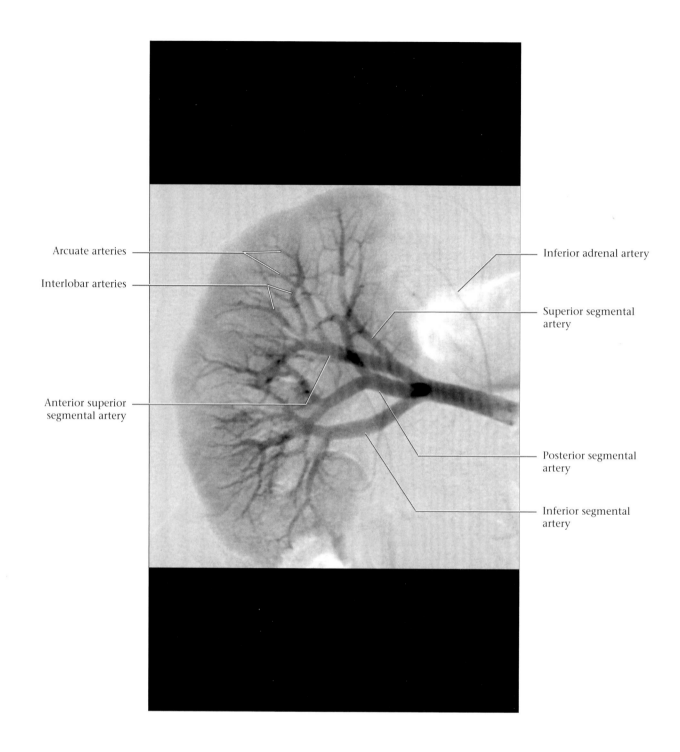

Arcuate arteries

Interlobar arteries

Anterior superior
segmental artery

Inferior adrenal artery

Superior segmental
artery

Posterior segmental
artery

Inferior segmental
artery

A selective catheter injection of the right renal artery depicts the vessels to the level of the arcuate arteries, which course along the convex surface of each renal pyramid.

KIDNEY

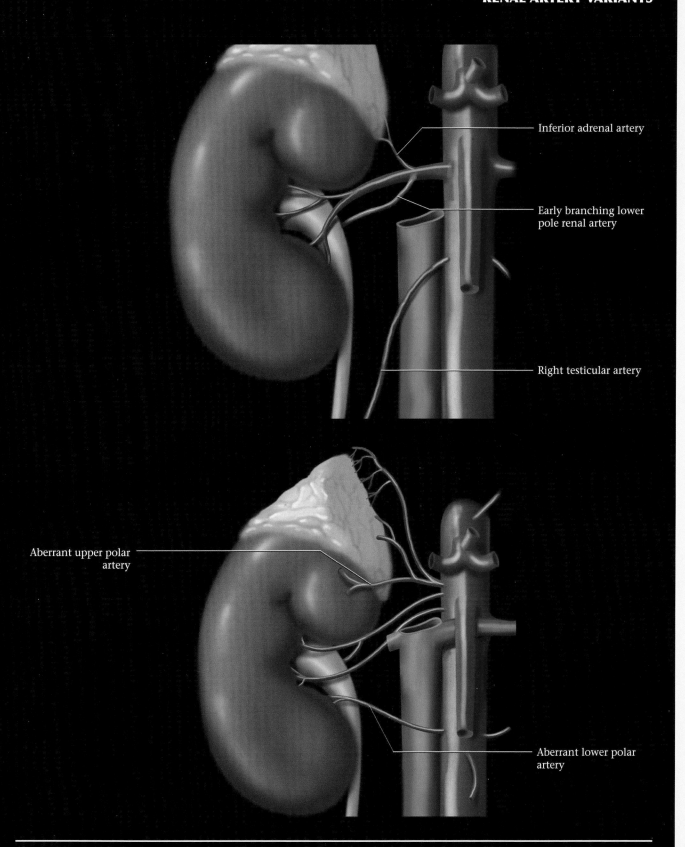

Inferior adrenal artery

Early branching lower pole renal artery

Right testicular artery

Aberrant upper polar artery

Aberrant lower polar artery

(Top) This graphic depicts proximal ramification (early branching) of the renal artery. This may have important implications if renal surgery is being considered. For instance, a person with this vascular anatomy might be considered a poor candidate as a potential living renal kidonr, as "harvesting" this kidney might jeopardize the inferior adrenal and lower pole renal arteries. **(Bottom)** This graphic depicts supernumerary renal arteries arising directly from the aorta. Some of these enter the kidney at locations other than the renal hilum, close to the renal poles. These "polar" or "extrahilar" arteries may be ligated or transected unintentionally during renal, aortic, or other retroperitoneal abdominal surgeries. These are sometimes referred to as "accessory" renal arteries, but each is an end artery and the sole arterial supply to a substantial portion of the renal parenchyma.

KIDNEY

MULTIPLE RENAL ARTERIES

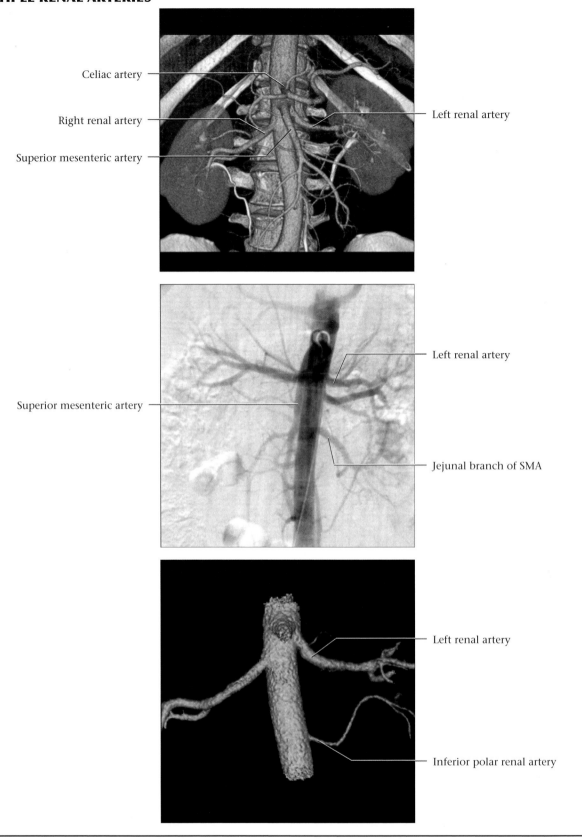

(Top) First of three images of a person being evaluated as a potential living renal donor. This CT angiogram seems to show normal visceral arterial branches of the abdominal aorta. Overlap between the branches of the left renal and superior mesenteric arteries prevents confident interpretation, based on this 3D rendering alone. **(Middle)** A "flush" aortogram in a single frontal projection also leaves questions about renal and superior mesenteric arterial branches. **(Bottom)** A workstation manipulation of the CT angiogram permits subtraction of extraneous overlying vessels to reveal clearly a substantial aberrant left inferior polar artery arising directly from the aorta. The transplant surgeons elected to harvest the right kidney for transplantation.

KIDNEY

RENAL VEIN VARIATIONS

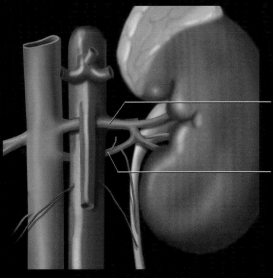

Conventional preaortic renal vein

Retroaortic renal vein

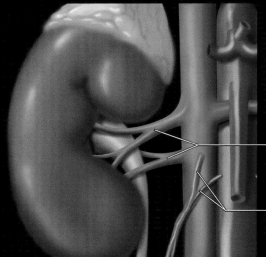

Supernumerary renal veins

Right gonadal vessels

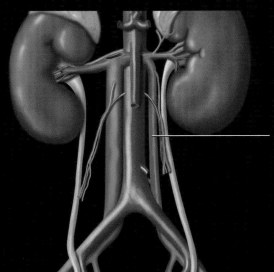

Left sided IVC (empties into left renal vein)

(Top) Anomalies of the renal veins are less common than those of the arteries, but are encountered in clinical practice and may have important implications. All anomalies are variations of the embryologic development and persistence of portions of the paired longitudinal channels, the subcardinal and supracardinal veins, which form a ladderlike collar around the aorta. Normally only the anterior components persist, becoming the renal veins, which course anterior to the aorta. Persistence of the whole collar results in a circumaortic renal vein, which is depicted in this graphic. This anomaly is more common than an isolated retroaortic renal vein. **(Middle)** Persistence variation the collar of veins on the right results in supernumerary right renal veins that encircle the renal pelvis. **(Bottom)** Persistence of the left supracardinal vein below the kidney results in a "duplicated" IVC.

KIDNEY

CIRCUMAORTIC LEFT RENAL VEIN

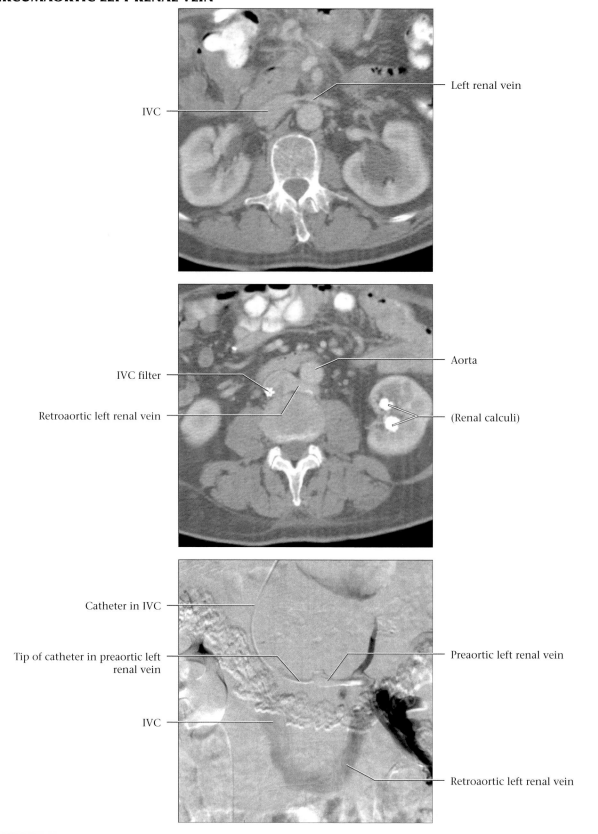

(Top) First of three images demonstrating a circumaortic left renal vein. This CT section shows a small preaortic (conventional) left renal vein as it joins the IVC. **(Middle)** A more caudal section shows a larger retroaortic left renal vein joining the IVC. Also note the tip of an IVC filter, placed to prevent propagation of blood clots into the lungs (pulmonary embolism). Knowledge of renal venous anomalies is important to avoid inadvertent injury to the renal vein during interventional or surgical procedures involving the IVC or aorta. **(Bottom)** Frontal film from inferior vena cavagram preceding the CT scan. A catheter has been inserted through an arm vein and advanced so that its tip is in the left renal vein. Injection of contrast has passed retrograde through the preaortic left renal vein and is flowing antegrade through the larger, more caudal retroaortic renal vein.

KIDNEY

LEFT RENAL VEIN COMPROMISED BY SMA

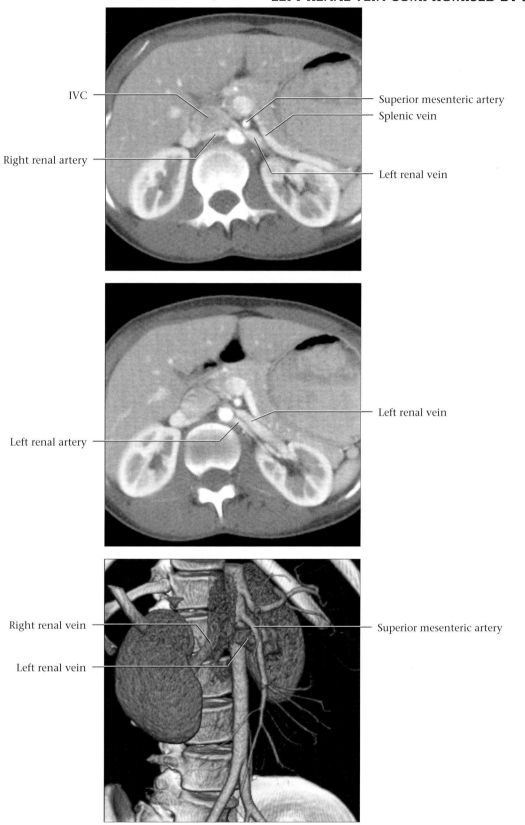

IVC

Superior mesenteric artery

Splenic vein

Right renal artery

Left renal vein

Left renal artery

Left renal vein

Right renal vein

Superior mesenteric artery

Left renal vein

(Top) First of three images showing compression of the left renal vein. This axial CT section shows marked narrowing of the left renal vein as it passes between the aorta and the superior mesenteric artery in this thin woman. (Middle) A more caudal section shows distention of the renal vein "upstream" from the compressed portion. This may result in increased pressure within the renal vein with hematuria and flank pain, as in this patient. (Bottom) This oblique coronal CT angiogram shows the left renal vein as it passes between the aorta and the SMA.

KIDNEY

STAGHORN CALCULI

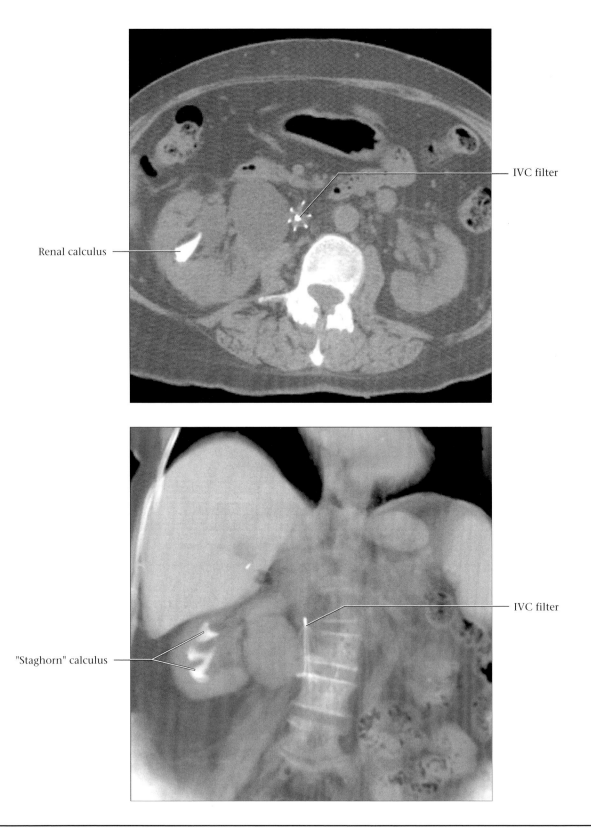

IVC filter

Renal calculus

IVC filter

"Staghorn" calculus

(Top) First of two CT sections showing renal calculi. This non-enhanced axial CT section shows a large hyperdense stone within the right kidney. **(Bottom)** A coronal reformation of the CT scan shows that the renal calculus fills and conforms to the right renal calices, resembling the horns of a deer ("staghorn calculus"). Essentially all renal calculi are dense and easy to recognize on CT scans, while many stones are too small or insufficiently opaque to diagnose on plain abdominal radiographs.

KIDNEY

MR, RENAL CELL CARCINOMA

(Top) First of three MR sections showing a large renal cell carcinoma in the left kidney. This coronal section shows a large mass that replaces most of the left kidney. There is a large filling defect within the IVC, the tip of which extends almost to the level of the hepatic veins. (Middle) A coronal section through the left kidney shows extension of the tumor into the left renal vein and IVC. (Bottom) Renal cell carcinoma often invades the renal vein and extends into the IVC. Shedding of tumor cells within the IVC frequently results in lung and other systemic metastases.

KIDNEY

CT, RENAL CELL CARCINOMA

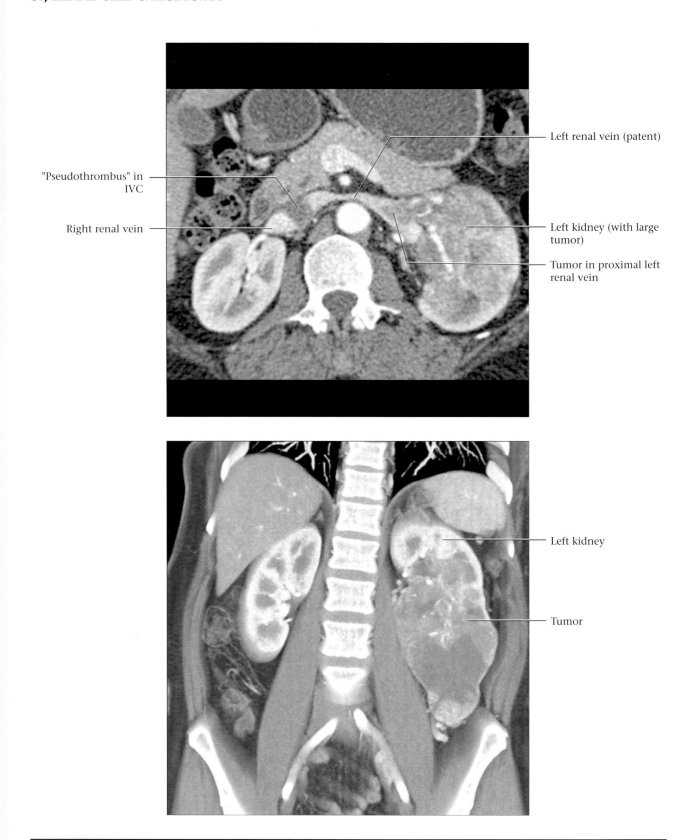

(Top) First of four CT images of a patient with a large renal cell carcinoma in the left kidney. This axial contrast-enhanced section shows tumor filling this portion of the left kidney. The tumor extends into the proximal portion of the left renal vein, but not into the IVC. Note the "pseudothrombus" of the IVC due to mixing of unopacified blood from the legs and opacified blood from the renal veins. **(Bottom)** This coronal section shows the large tumor that replaces most of the left kidney.

KIDNEY

CT, RENAL CELL CARCINOMA

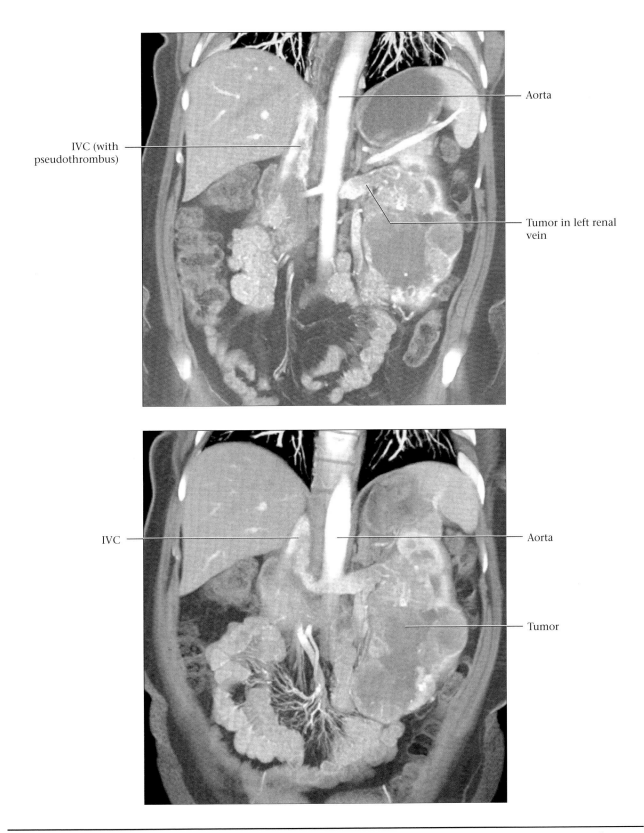

IVC (with pseudothrombus)

Aorta

Tumor in left renal vein

IVC

Aorta

Tumor

(Top) This coronal section shows tumor extending into the left renal vein. Turbulent flow and poor mixing of opacified and unopacified blood within the IVC simulates tumor invasion. **(Bottom)** This coronal section also shows the heterogeneous enhancement of the IVC that could be misinterpreted as invasion by the tumor. Careful analysis of the axial and coronal sections is essential to avoid this clinically important misdiagnosis.

KIDNEY

TRANSITIONAL CELL CARCINOMA

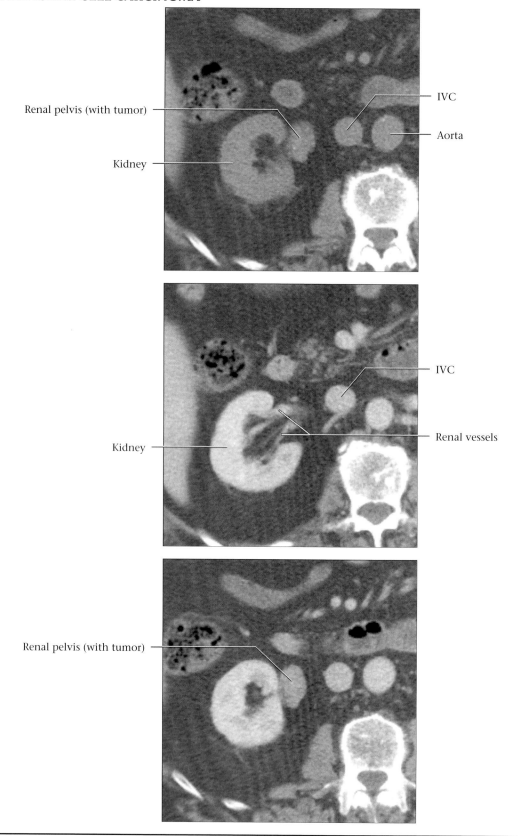

Renal pelvis (with tumor)

Kidney

IVC

Aorta

Kidney

IVC

Renal vessels

Renal pelvis (with tumor)

(**Top**) First of six images of a patient with transitional cell carcinoma of the right renal pelvis. This axial non-enhanced CT section shows a subtle hyperdense mass within the right renal pelvis, but it is much less dense than a renal calculus. (**Middle**) The right kidney appears normal on this section. (**Bottom**) This section shows the renal pelvis filled with tumor that, on cursor measurement, showed slight contrast-enhancement. The urine is not yet contrast-opacified.

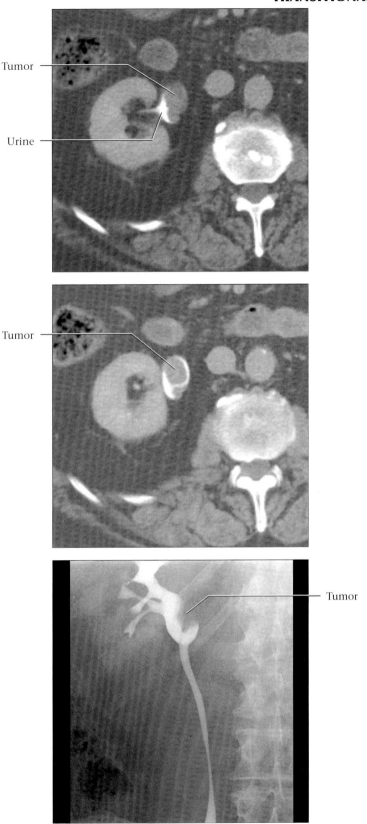

(Top) A repeat axial section after a 10 minute delay shows contrast-opacified urine and tumor within the renal pelvis. (Middle) A more caudal section shows the tumor as a filling defect within the opacified urine in the renal pelvis. (Bottom) A frontal film from a retrograde pyelogram shows the transitional cell carcinoma that arose from the epithelium of the renal pelvis.

KIDNEY

PELVIC KIDNEY

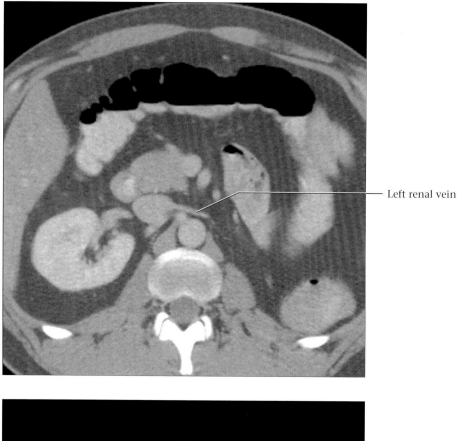

Left renal vein

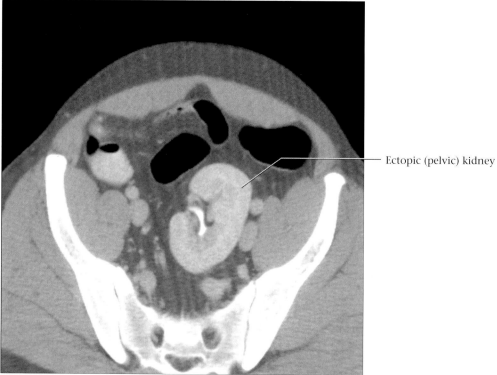

Ectopic (pelvic) kidney

(Top) First of two CT sections shows a normal right kidney in its usual location. The left kidney is not seen, though the left renal vein is present. **(Bottom)** A CT section through the pelvis shows an ectopic, malrotated, pelvic, kidney. In the early embryo, both kidneys lie in the pelvis. As the fetus grows, the kidneys usually "ascend" to their normal abdominal position, successively recruiting more proximal arterial and venous branches from the aorta and IVC. Ectopic kidneys are invariably low in position and usually are malrotated with aberrant blood supply from the distal aorta or iliac arteries.

KIDNEY

TRANSITIONAL CELL CARCINOMA

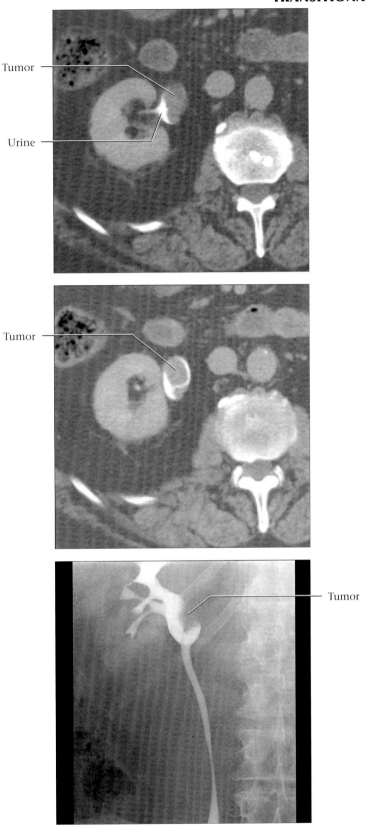

(Top) A repeat axial section after a 10 minute delay shows contrast-opacified urine and tumor within the renal pelvis. (Middle) A more caudal section shows the tumor as a filling defect within the opacified urine in the renal pelvis. (Bottom) A frontal film from a retrograde pyelogram shows the transitional cell carcinoma that arose from the epithelium of the renal pelvis.

KIDNEY

SIMPLE CYST

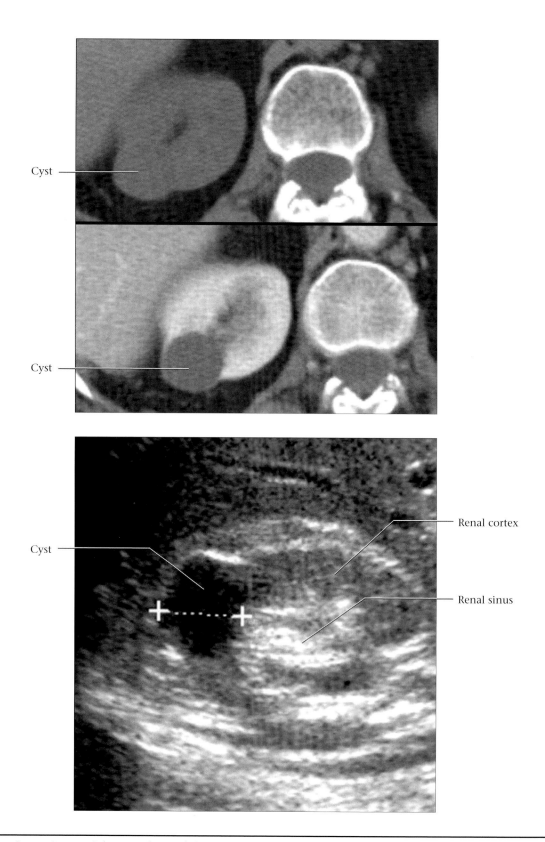

(Top) The top image is an axial non-enhanced CT section that shows a water density spherical mass in the right kidney. The lower image shows that there is no enhancement of the mass or its contents, and there is no visible wall. These findings are diagnostic of a simple renal cyst. Renal cysts are present in almost 50% of individuals over the age of 50, and are usually of no clinical concern. (Bottom) An axial sonogram shows a "sonolucent" mass (no internal echoes), with no visible wall or mural nodularity, findings diagnostic of a simple cyst. The electronic cursor is used to measure its size.

KIDNEY

CONGENITAL ABSENCE OF KIDNEY

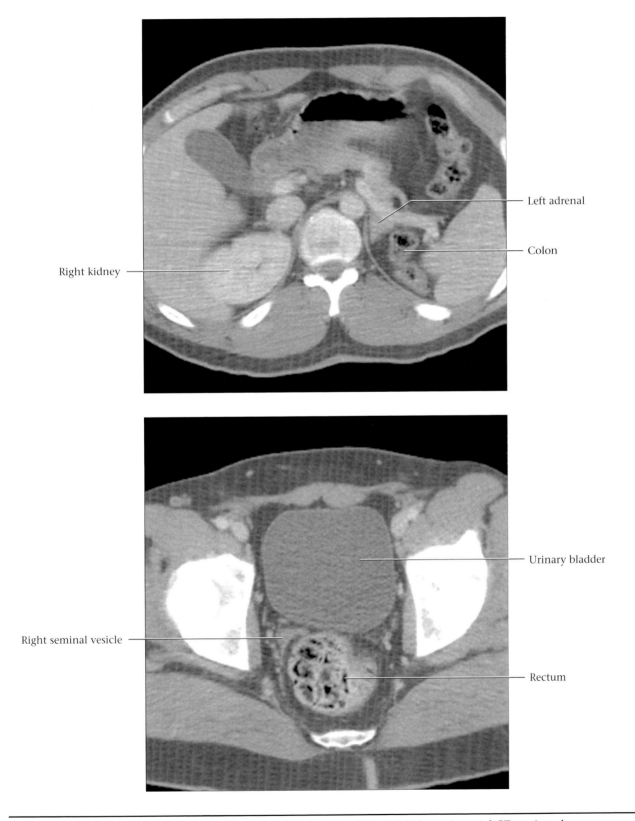

Right kidney

Left adrenal

Colon

Right seminal vesicle

Urinary bladder

Rectum

(Top) First of two images of a patient with congenital absence of the left kidney. An axial CT section shows a normal right kidney and left adrenal gland, but no left kidney. No kidney was found in an ectopic location. **(Bottom)** A more caudal section shows a normal right seminal vesicle, but no left seminal vesicle. Congenital absence of the kidney is often accompanied by anomalies in other organ systems, including musculoskeletal, cardiovascular, and genital. Congenital anomalies of the kidney and genital organs usually occur ipsilaterally (on the same side).

KIDNEY

PELVIC KIDNEY

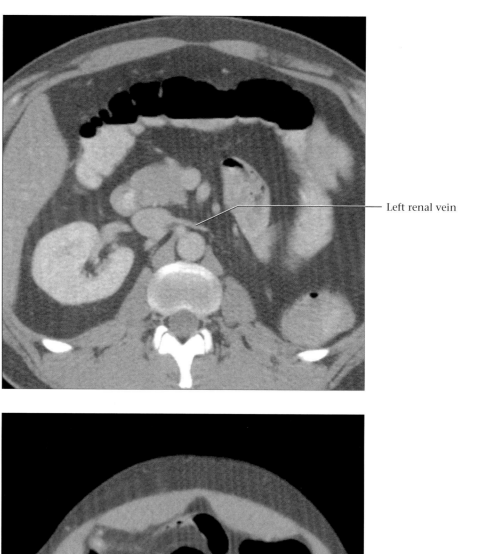

Left renal vein

Ectopic (pelvic) kidney

(Top) First of two CT sections shows a normal right kidney in its usual location. The left kidney is not seen, though the left renal vein is present. **(Bottom)** A CT section through the pelvis shows an ectopic, malrotated, pelvic, kidney. In the early embryo, both kidneys lie in the pelvis. As the fetus grows, the kidneys usually "ascend" to their normal abdominal position, successively recruiting more proximal arterial and venous branches from the aorta and IVC. Ectopic kidneys are invariably low in position and usually are malrotated with aberrant blood supply from the distal aorta or iliac arteries.

KIDNEY

CROSSED FUSED ECTOPIA

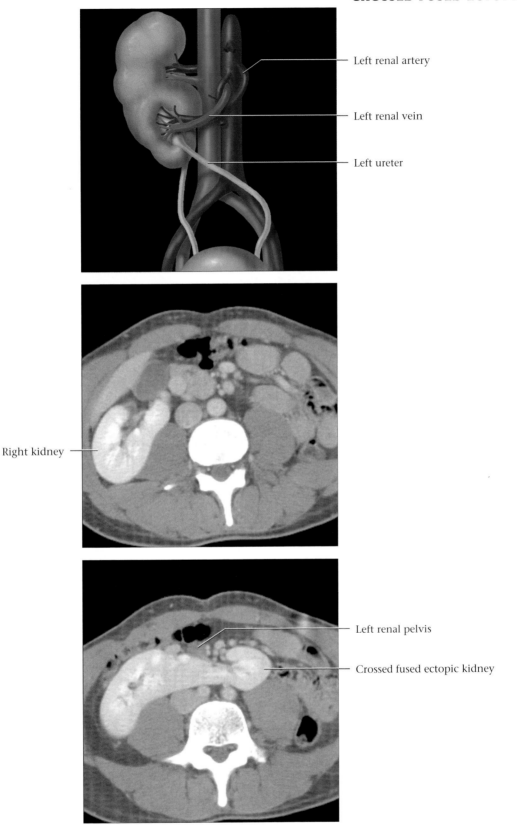

Left renal artery

Left renal vein

Left ureter

Right kidney

Left renal pelvis

Crossed fused ectopic kidney

(Top) This graphic illustrates the typical appearance of a crossed fused ectopic kidney. The right renal unit develops normally with conventional vascular anatomy. The left renal unit is fused to the lower pole of the right unit. The left renal vessels and ureter have their normal origins and insertions, but cross the midline to the left renal unit. Ectopic kidneys are more vulnerable to trauma, calculi, and hydronephrosis. **(Middle)** This axial CT section shows a normal appearing right kidney. **(Bottom)** A more caudal section shows the left renal unit is fused to the lower pole of the right kidney, and its hilum is directed anteriorly.

KIDNEY

HORSESHOE KIDNEY

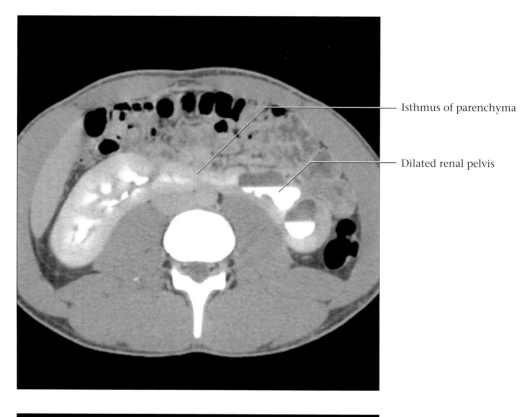

Isthmus of parenchyma

Dilated renal pelvis

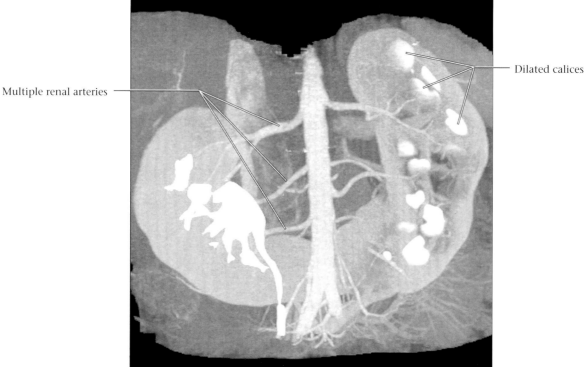

Multiple renal arteries

Dilated calices

(Top) First of four CT images of a horseshoe kidney. This axial section shows the two renal units whose lower poles are joined across the midline by an isthmus of functioning renal parenchyma. The collecting system of the left renal unit is dilated (hydronephrotic), indicating ureteral or pelvic obstruction. **(Bottom)** A coronal MIP image shows the "U" or horseshoe-shaped kidney with the lower poles joined across the midline. Note the multiple renal arteries supplying each half of the kidney. The left-sided hydronephrosis is evident. Hydronephrosis is common in this anomaly and may be caused by aberrant arteries that compress the collecting system, aberrant & multiple ureters, renal calculi or even tumor.

KIDNEY

HORSESHOE KIDNEY

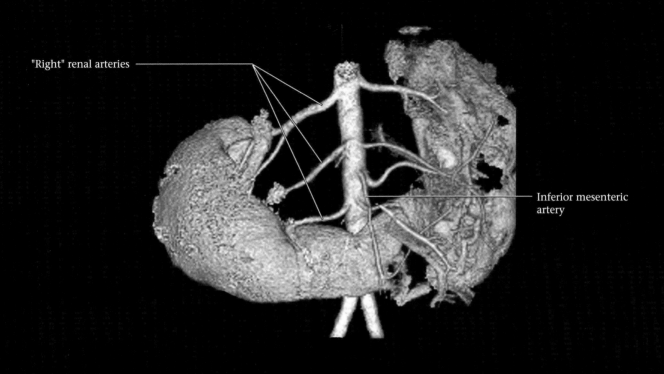

"Right" renal arteries

Inferior mesenteric artery

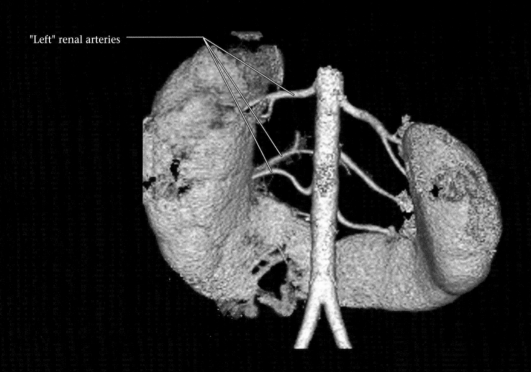

"Left" renal arteries

(Top) Frontal view, shaded surface 3D depiction of the CT scan shows the horseshoe kidney crossing the midline between the aorta and the inferior mesenteric artery. The multiple renal arteries are evident. The left renal unit appears "moth-eaten" as a result of its hydronephrosis kidney decreased parenchymal enhancement, relative to the right side. The window display was set to display normal density renal parenchymal and arterial enhancement. **(Bottom)** A posterior view of the horseshoe kidney is displayed. Note the multiple renal arteries.

KIDNEY

HYPERTROPHIED COLUMN OF BERTIN

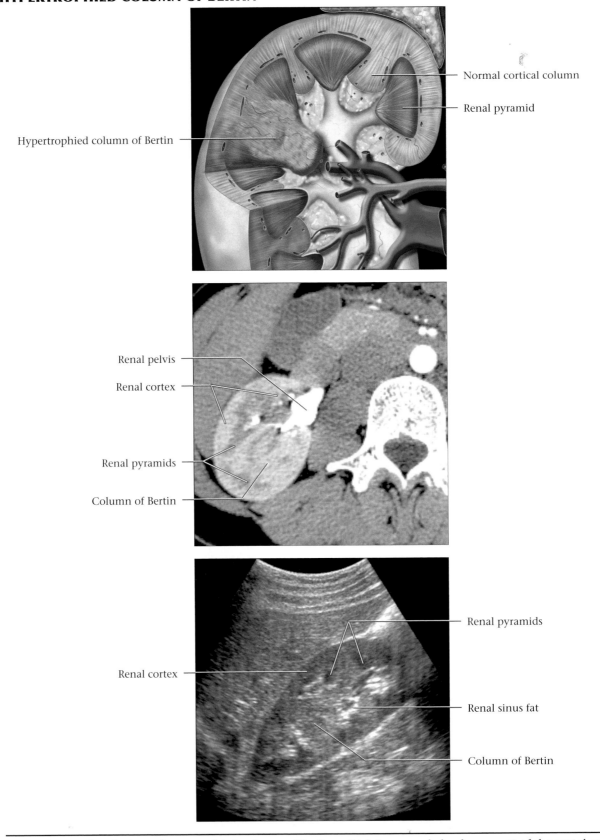

(Top) This graphic depicts a hypertrophied column of Bertin, which is a rounded enlargement of the septal cortical tissue that separates the renal pyramids. This is normal tissue with the same imaging features as other renal cortex, but it may protrude into the renal sinus fat and may be mistaken for a renal mass. (Middle) This corticomedullary phase CT section shows a rounded, prominent "mass" of cortical tissue projecting deep into the renal sinus, seemingly compressing and displacing the renal pyramids in the midpole of the right kidney. The opacified urine is the result of a prior "timing bolus" of contrast material. (Bottom) A sagittal sonogram shows a rounded "mass", a hypertrophied column of Bertin, projecting into and displacing renal sinus fat. This has the same echogenicity as other cortical tissue. The location, between the upper and midpole of the kidney, is typical.

KIDNEY

FETAL LOBATION

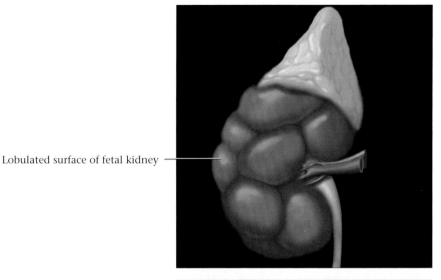

Lobulated surface of fetal kidney

Left kidney

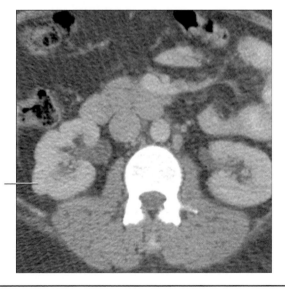

Right kidney

(Top) This graphic depicts the typical lobulated appearance of the kidney in fetal life, reflecting the development of the kidney from numerous lobes, each consisting of a renal pyramid and its associated cortex. This may persist into infancy and occasionally into adult life, though to a lesser degree. Note that the adrenal gland is relatively large compared with the kidney in fetal life and childhood. (Middle) An axial contrast-enhanced CT section of an asymptomatic adult shows a lobulated surface of each kidney, representing persistent fetal lobation (lobulation). This must be distinguished from cortical scarring, in which renal tissue is lost as a result of ischemia or inflammation. (Bottom) A more caudal section shows the lobulated surface of the right kidney.

KIDNEY

DUPLICATION OF COLLECTING SYSTEM

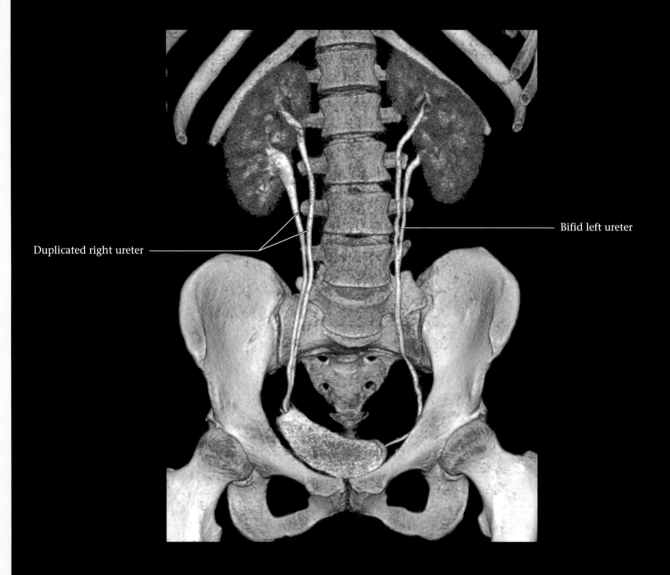

Duplicated right ureter —

Bifid left ureter

Coronal reformatted CT urogram shows a bifid left ureter, with two separate ureters leaving the kidney, but joining distally to form a single ureter. The entire right ureter is duplicated, with separate ureteral orifices into the bladder. Each kidney in this subject had two hila with supernumerary arteries and veins.

KIDNEY

POLYCYSTIC KIDNEY DISEASE

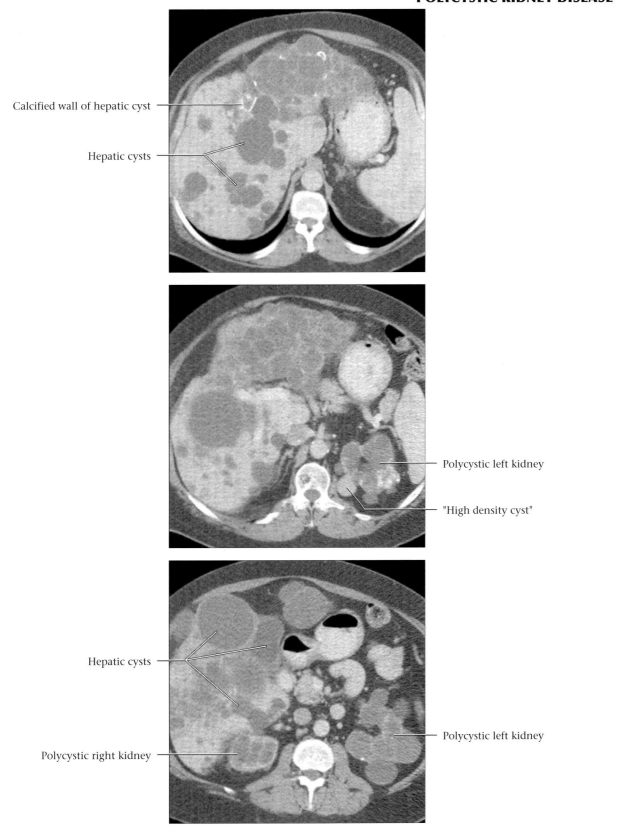

(Top) First of three axial CT sections of a patient with autosomal dominant polycystic disease of the kidneys and liver. This section shows innumerable cysts within the liver, some of which have calcified walls due to prior episodes of spontaneous bleeding within the cyst. (Middle) In spite of the gross enlargement and distortion of the liver, hepatic function is normal in this and most patients with polycystic liver disease. Conversely, the polycystic renal disease is progressive and usually results in renal failure by the sixth decade. This section shows that the left kidney is virtually replaced by cysts, many of which are of increased density due to spontaneous hemorrhage. (Bottom) A more caudal section shows cystic disease of the right kidney as well.

URETER AND BLADDER

Gross Anatomy

Ureter

- Muscular tubes (25-30 cm long) that carry urine from kidneys to bladder
  - Course along posterior abdominal wall in retroperitoneum, just behind parietal peritoneum
    - Proximal ureters lie in **perirenal space**
    - In lower abdomen, lie on psoas muscles
  - In pelvis, lie along lateral walls near internal iliac vessels
    - At the level of ischial spines, ureters curve anteromedially to enter bladder at level of seminal vesicles (men) or cervix (women)
    - **Ureterovesical junction**: Ureters pass obliquely through muscular wall of bladder, creating a valve effect, preventing reflux of urine
  - Three points of physiological narrowing: **Ureteropelvic junction**, pelvic brim and **ureterovesical junction**
- **Vessels, nerves and lymphatics**
  - Arterial branches are numerous and variable, from aorta, and renal, gonadal, internal iliac, vesical, rectal arteries
    - Arterial branches anastomose along length of ureter
  - Venous branches & lymphatics follow the arteries with similar names
  - Innervation
    - Autonomic from adjacent plexuses
    - Cause ureteral peristalsis
    - Also carry pain (stretch) receptors; "stone" in abdominal ureter perceived as back & flank pain; stone in pelvic ureter causes lower abdominal & groin pain
  - Lymphatics to **external & internal iliac nodes** (pelvic ureter), **aorto-caval nodes** (abdomen)

Bladder

- Hollow, distensible viscus with a strong muscular wall
- Lies in **extraperitoneal (retroperitoneal)** pelvis
- Peritoneum covers dome of bladder
  - Reflections of peritoneum form deep recesses in the pelvic peritoneal cavity
  - **Rectovesical pouch** is most dependent recess in men (and in women following hysterectomy)
  - **Vesicouterine pouch** and **rectouterine pouch (of Douglas)** are most dependent in women
- Bladder is surrounded by loose connective tissue and fat
  - **Perivesical space** (contains bladder and urachus)
  - **Prevesical (of Retzius)** between bladder and symphysis pubis; communicates superiorly with **infrarenal retroperitoneal compartment**; communicates posteriorly with presacral space
  - Spaces can expand to contain large amounts of fluid (as in extraperitoneal rupture of the bladder, and hemorrhage from pelvic fractures)
- Wall of bladder composed mostly of detrusor muscle
  - **Trigone of bladder**: Triangular structure at base of bladder with apices marked by 2 **ureteral orifices** and **internal urethral orifice**
- **Vessels, nerves and lymphatics**
  - Arteries from internal iliac
    - **Superior vesical arteries** and other branches of internal iliac arteries in both sexes
  - Venous drainage
    - Men: **Vesical & prostatic venous plexuses** → internal iliac and internal vertebral veins
    - Women: **Vesical and uterovaginal plexuses** → internal iliac vein
  - Autonomic innervation
    - Parasympathetic from pelvic splanchnic & inferior hypogastric nerves (causes contraction of detrusor muscle and relaxation of internal urethral sphincter to permit emptying of the bladder)
    - Sensory fibers follow parasympathetic nerves

Clinical Implications

Clinical Importance

- Ureters are often injured inadvertently during abdominal or gynecological surgery due to traction, causing interruption of their fragile, short arterial supply
- **Ectopic ureter**
  - Usually (80%) associated with complete ureteral duplication
  - Much more common in females (10x)
  - Ureter from upper renal pole often becomes obstructed & inserts ectopically (not at trigone)
  - Causes constant urine dribbling in females (ectopic insertion below urethral sphincter)
  - **Weigert-Meyer** rule: Ureter from upper pole inserts inferior & medial to lower pole ureter
- **Ureterocele:** Cystic dilation of distal ureter
  - Simple (orthotopic) at trigone, with single ureter
  - Ectopic; inserts below trigone
- **Ureteral duplication**
  - **Bifid ureter** drains a duplex kidney; ureters unite before entering bladder
- **Extraperitoneal bladder rupture**
  - Urine and blood distend prevesical space; looks like a "molar tooth" on transverse CT section
  - Urine often tracks posteriorly into presacral space, superiorly into retroperitoneal abdomen
  - Usually caused by pelvic fractures
- **Intraperitoneal bladder rupture**
  - Urine flows up paracolic gutters into peritoneal recesses and surrounds intestine
  - Usually caused by blunt trauma to an overdistended bladder
- Fetal **urachus** forms conduit between umbilicus and bladder
  - Usually becomes obliterated → **median umbilical ligament**
  - May persist as channel "cyst" or diverticulum
  - May become infected or lead to carcinoma
- **Bladder diverticula** are common
  - Congenital: **Hutch diverticulum**
    - Near ureterovesical junction
  - Acquired (usually due to bladder outlet obstruction)
  - Can lead to infection, stones, tumor

URETER AND BLADDER

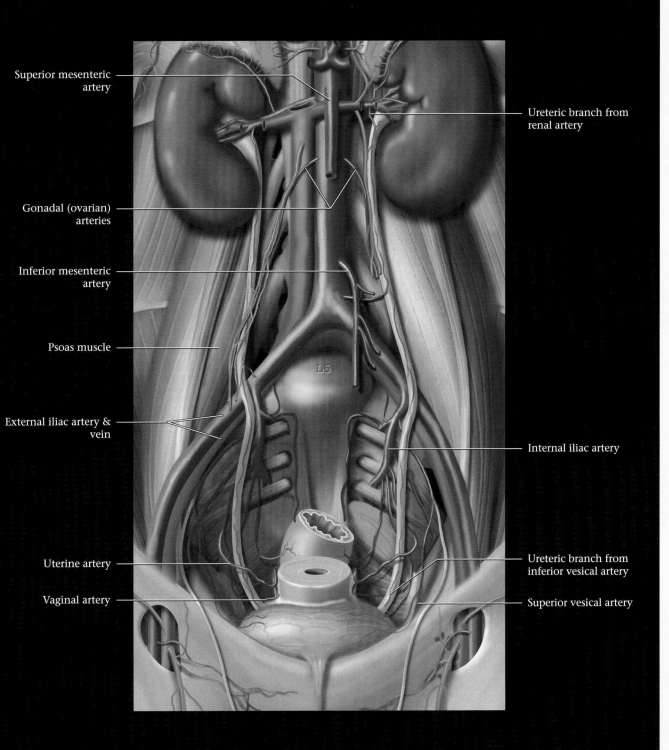

Superior mesenteric artery

Gonadal (ovarian) arteries

Inferior mesenteric artery

Psoas muscle

External iliac artery & vein

Uterine artery

Vaginal artery

Ureteric branch from renal artery

Internal iliac artery

Ureteric branch from inferior vesical artery

Superior vesical artery

L5

The ureters receive numerous and highly variable arterial branches from the aorta, and the renal, gonadal, and internal iliac arteries. These vessels are short and can be easily ruptured by retraction of the ureter during surgical procedures. The arterial supply to the bladder is also quite variable. Both genders receive supply from the superior vesical arteries and from various branches of the internal iliac arteries. Branches to the prostate & seminal vesicles (men) also send branches to the inferior bladder wall. In women, branches to the vagina send arteries to the base of the bladder. Note how the ureters deviate anteriorly as they cross the external (or common) iliac vessels & pelvic brim. This may constitute a point of relative narrowing where the passage of ureteral calculi (stones) may be impeded. In the abdomen the ureters course along the psoas muscles.

URETER AND BLADDER

EXCRETORY UROGRAM, NORMAL IVP

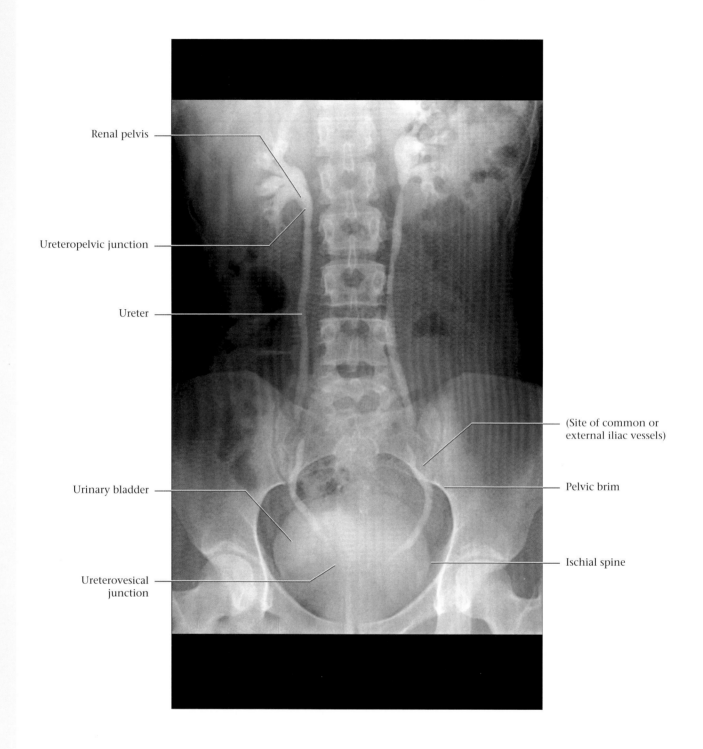

Renal pelvis

Ureteropelvic junction

Ureter

(Site of common or external iliac vessels)

Pelvic brim

Urinary bladder

Ischial spine

Ureterovesical junction

Frontal film of the abdomen obtained ten minutes following the IV administration of iodinated contrast medium. The IV contrast media utilized for excretory urography (also known as intravenous pyelography, or IVP) is identical to that used for a contrast-enhanced CT scan. Because the CT scan can also reveal so much more than the morphology of the renal collecting system, ureters & bladder, it has largely replaced the IVP for most purposes. The ureteropelvic junction (UPJ) lies at about the L2 level (lower on standing), while the ureterovesical junction (UVJ) lies at the level of the ischial spine, or, as shown on axial CT, at the level of the seminal vesicles (men) or the cervix (women). Note the subtle deviation of the ureters as they cross the iliac vessels and pelvic brim.

URETER AND BLADDER

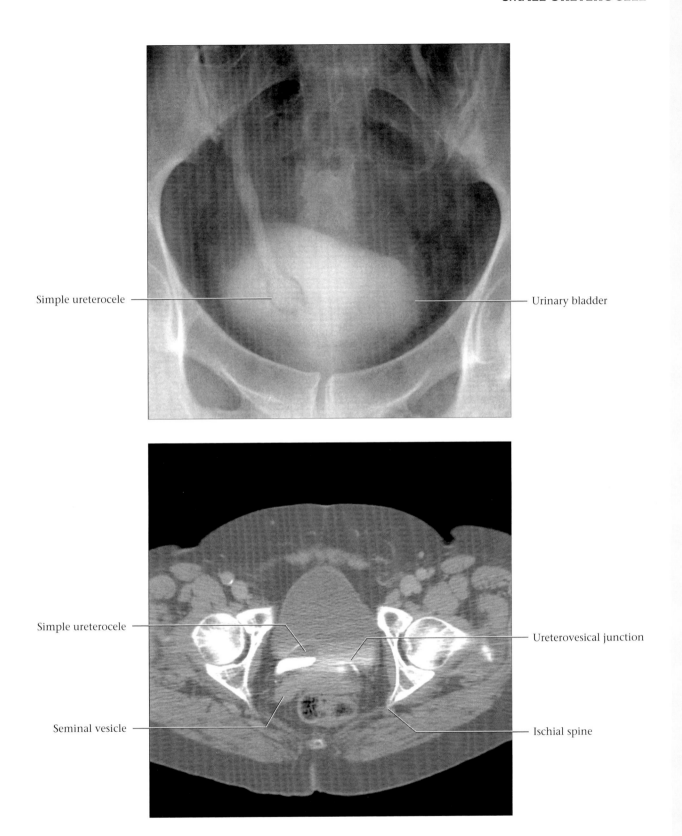

Simple ureterocele — Urinary bladder

Simple ureterocele — Ureterovesical junction

Seminal vesicle — Ischial spine

(Top) A frontal film from an excretory urogram shows a dilated right ureter that terminates in a cystic dilation within the bladder wall. The appearance of this simple ureterocele has been likened to the head of a spring onion or a cobra. **(Bottom)** An axial CT section obtained several minutes after IV contrast administration shows a fluid level within the ureterocele with unopacified urine "floating" on top of the heavier contrast-opacified urine. Note the ureterovesical junctions (UVJ) are at the same level as the seminal vesicles and ischial spines. A ureterocele that occurs at the trigone (the normal site of the UVJ) is called a simple ureterocele, as opposed to an ectopic ureterocele at the tip of a duplicated ureter that inserts in an aberrantly low position.

URETER AND BLADDER

CT UROGRAM, URETERAL DUPLICATION

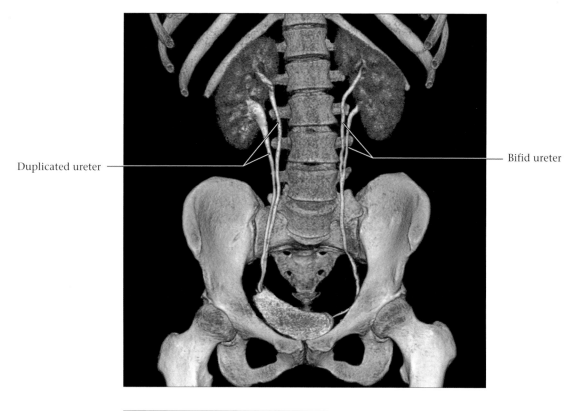

Duplicated ureter —

Bifid ureter

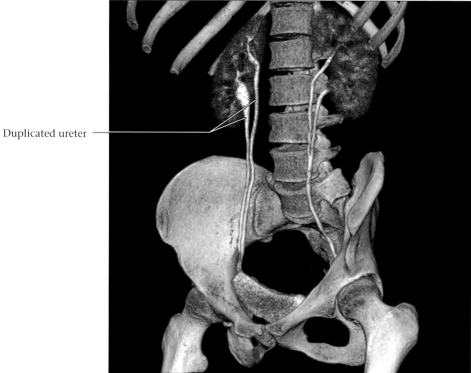

Duplicated ureter —

(Top) First of two CT urographic images, reformatted from a series of axial, contrast-opacified CT sections. This subject has complete duplication of the right ureter and partial duplication of the left (a "bifid ureter"). The ureter draining the upper pole of the right kidney inserted into the bladder just below and medial to the ureteral orifice of the lower pole ureter. In this subject there was no ureteral obstruction. (Bottom) An oblique rotation of the CT urogram confirms the duplicated and bifid ureters. The kidneys in this subject would each have two sets of hilar structures (artery, vein, renal pelvis).

URETER AND BLADDER

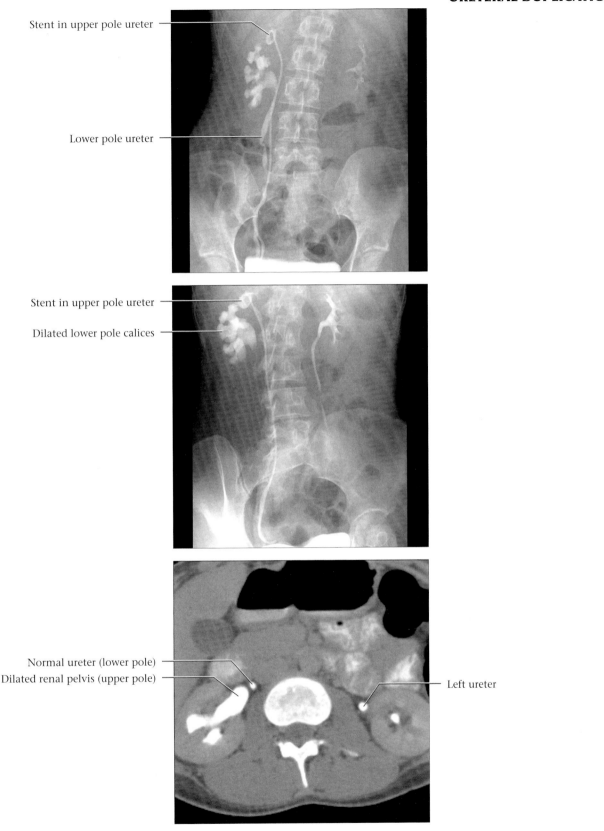

Stent in upper pole ureter

Lower pole ureter

Stent in upper pole ureter

Dilated lower pole calices

Normal ureter (lower pole)
Dilated renal pelvis (upper pole)

Left ureter

(Top) First of three images from a patient with right flank pain. This frontal film from an excretory urogram shows a ureteral stent within the ureter draining the upper pole of the right kidney, which had been noted to be hydronephrotic (dilated) prior to stent placement. The collecting system of the right lower pole is also somewhat dilated due to vesico-ureteral reflux. These are both manifestations of the Weigert-Meyer rule that the ureter draining the upper pole moiety inserts ectopically and is prone to obstruction, while the lower pole ureter is prone to reflux. (Middle) The lower pole collecting system may be displaced and rotated, as in this subject, resembling a "drooping lily". (Bottom) An axial CT section shows the dilated collecting system of the right upper pole and the normal caliber ureter draining the lower pole.

ECTOPIC DUPLICATED URETER

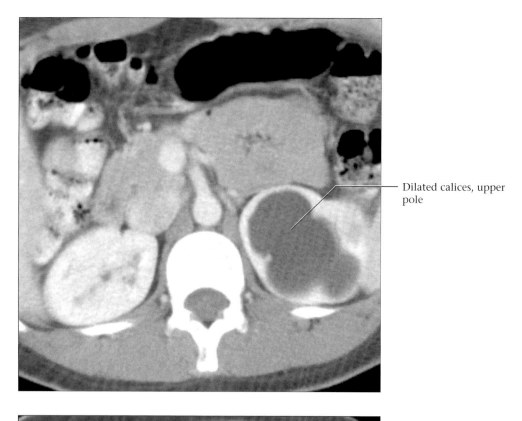

Dilated calices, upper pole

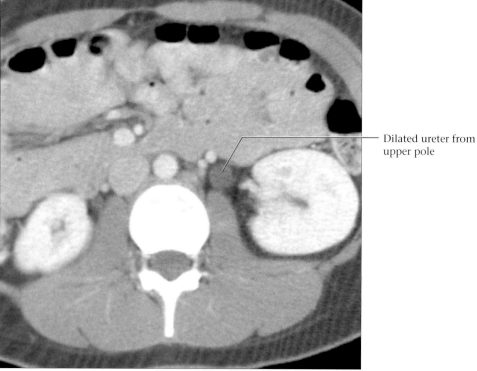

Dilated ureter from upper pole

(Top) First of four images from a patient with an ectopic duplicated ureter. This axial CT section shows a markedly hydronephrotic upper pole of the left kidney. (Bottom) A more caudal section shows the dilated, unopacified ureter from the left upper pole, lying medial to the lower pole, which shows no hydronephrosis.

ECTOPIC DUPLICATED URETER

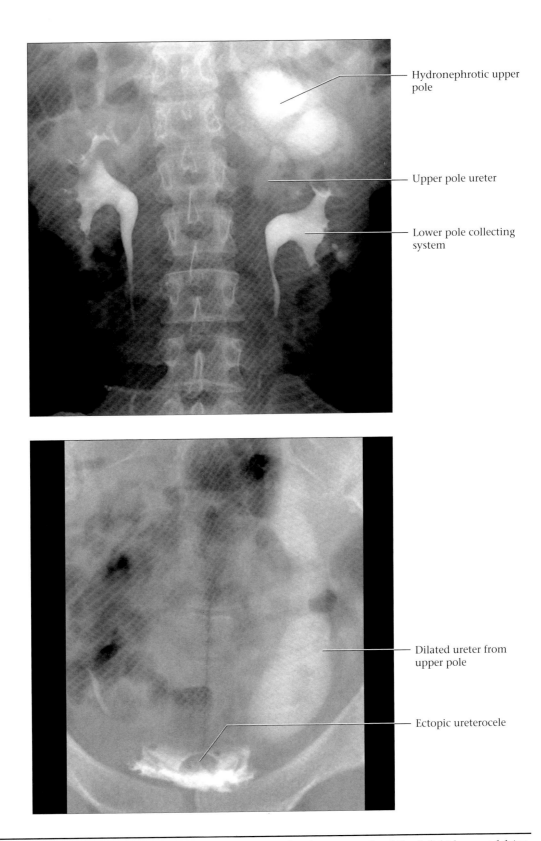

Hydronephrotic upper pole

Upper pole ureter

Lower pole collecting system

Dilated ureter from upper pole

Ectopic ureterocele

(Top) Frontal film from an excretory urogram shows a grossly hydronephrotic upper pole of the left kidney and faint opacification of its ureter. The collecting system of the lower pole is intrinsically normal but is displaced inferiorly, resembling a "drooping lily". **(Bottom)** A delayed "post voiding" film of the pelvis shows the dilated ureter from the upper pole terminating in an ectopic ureterocele near the base of the bladder.

RETROCAVAL URETER

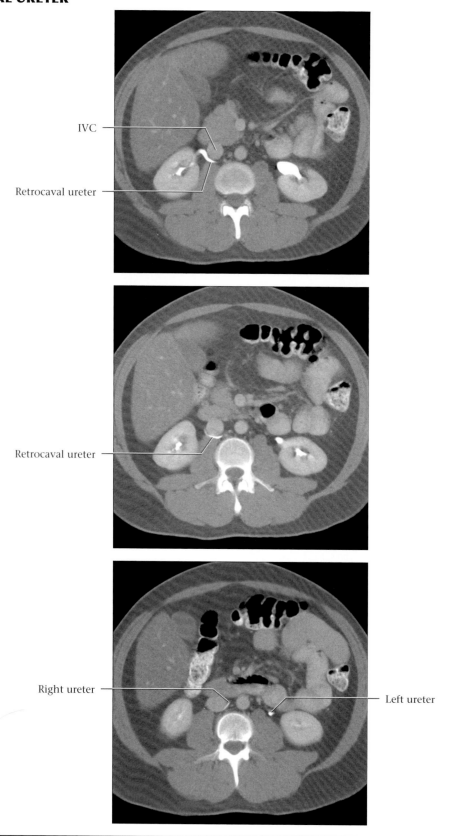

IVC

Retrocaval ureter

Retrocaval ureter

Right ureter

Left ureter

(Top) First of five axial CT sections of a subject with a retrocaval ureter. This section shows the proximal right ureter being compressed as it passes behind the inferior vena cava. The ureter usually runs parallel to the IVC. This is a congenital anomaly of the IVC rather than the ureter, representing a persistent subcardinal vein that traps the right ureter and may result in partial ureteral obstruction. **(Middle)** A more caudal section shows the ureter passing behind the IVC. **(Bottom)** After passing behind the IVC the right ureter is of normal caliber.

URETER AND BLADDER

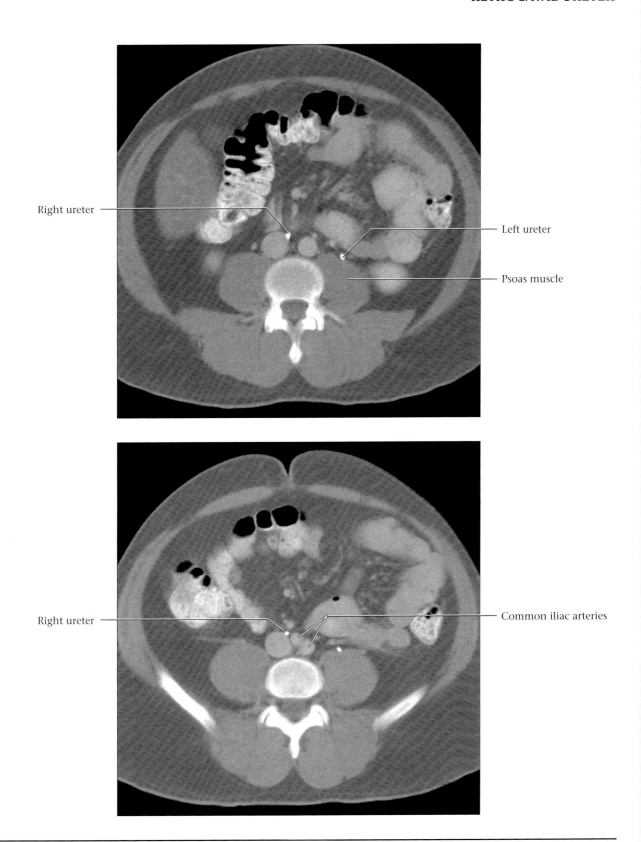

Right ureter

Left ureter

Psoas muscle

Right ureter

Common iliac arteries

(Top) The ureters normally course along the surface of the psoas muscles. Note the anterior and medial course of the right ureter, which follows the course of the IVC after passing behind it. **(Bottom)** The right ureter continues along the anterior surface of the IVC, rather than lying on the psoas muscle as does the normal left ureter.

URETER AND BLADDER

UPJ OBSTRUCTION

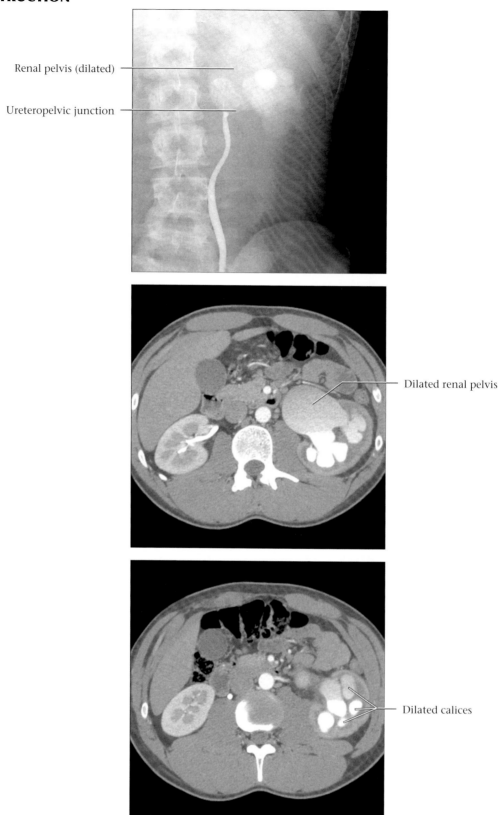

Renal pelvis (dilated)

Ureteropelvic junction

Dilated renal pelvis

Dilated calices

(Top) First of six images of a patient with congenital obstruction of the ureteropelvic junction (UPJ). A frontal film from a retrograde pyelogram shows a sharp transition from the normal ureter to a grossly dilated renal pelvis. UPJ obstruction may be congenital or acquired. (Middle) An axial CT section shows the hydronephrotic left kidney. (Bottom) A more caudal section shows caliectasis (dilated calices).

URETER AND BLADDER

UPJ OBSTRUCTION

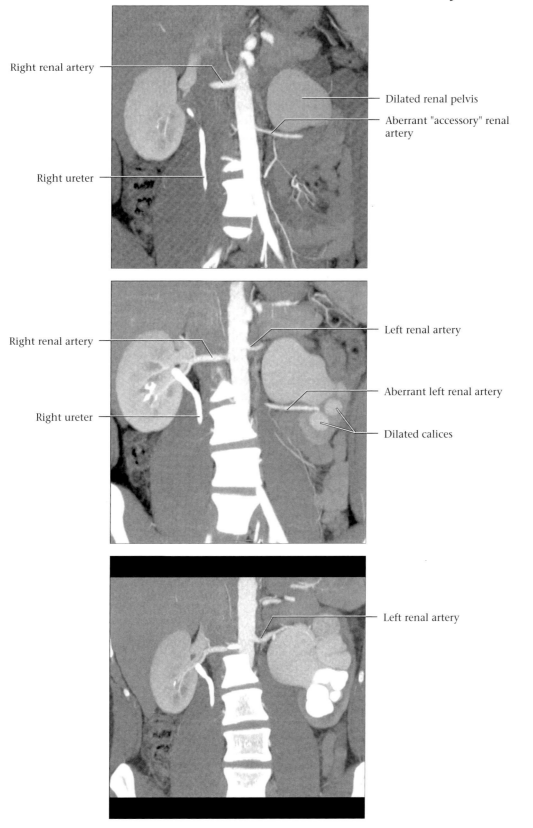

Right renal artery

Right ureter

Dilated renal pelvis

Aberrant "accessory" renal artery

Right renal artery

Right ureter

Left renal artery

Aberrant left renal artery

Dilated calices

Left renal artery

(Top) A coronal reformation MIP CT image from the CT scan shows an accessory (aberrant supernumerary) left renal artery crossing the left UPJ and possibly accounting for the obstruction. Regardless of whether the aberrant vessel is responsible for the UPJ obstruction, it is important to recognize the close relation between the vessel and the UPJ to avoid inadvertent injury to the artery if surgical repair of the UPJ is contemplated. **(Middle)** The normal origins of the right and left renal arteries are shown on this coronal section. **(Bottom)** The left renal artery and its relation to the grossly hydronephrotic left kidney are well shown on this coronal section.

URETER AND BLADDER

CANCER OF URETER

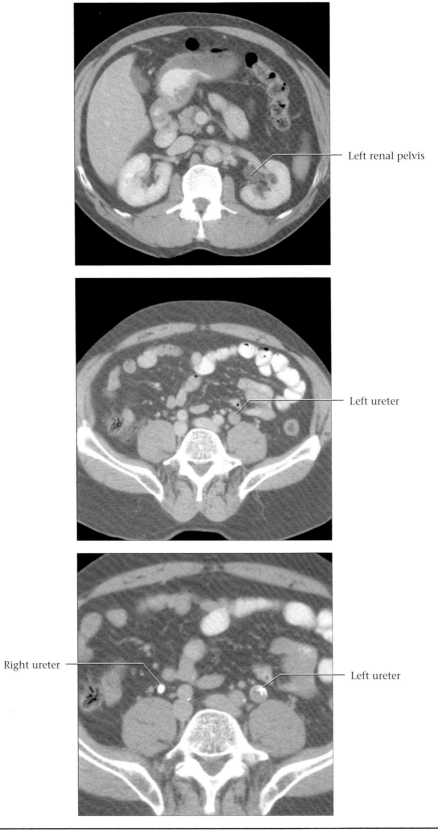

(Top) First of five CT images from a patient with a transitional cell carcinoma of the left ureter. This axial section in the nephrographic phase of enhancement shows a dilated left renal pelvis. **(Middle)** A more caudal section, also in the nephrographic phase, shows a dilated left ureter. No stone or extrinsic mass was seen to explain the ureteral obstruction. **(Bottom)** An axial section from the pyelographic phase of enhancement (10 minute delay) shows a soft tissue mass within the lumen of the left ureter.

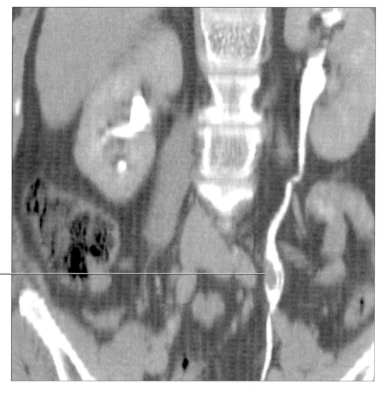

Tumor within ureter

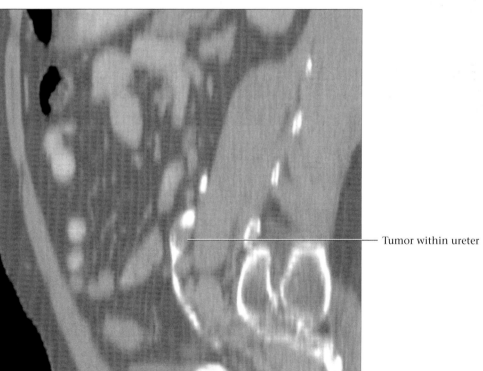

Tumor within ureter

(Top) A coronal reformation, obtained as part of the CT urogram protocol, shows the mass within the left ureter, expanding its lumen and causing partial obstruction. **(Bottom)** This sagittal section through the distal left ureter confirms the presence of the mass, a transitional cell carcinoma, within the ureter. CT allows confident distinction among the various intrinsic and extrinsic causes of ureteral obstruction.

URETER AND BLADDER

FEMALE AND MALE BLADDER

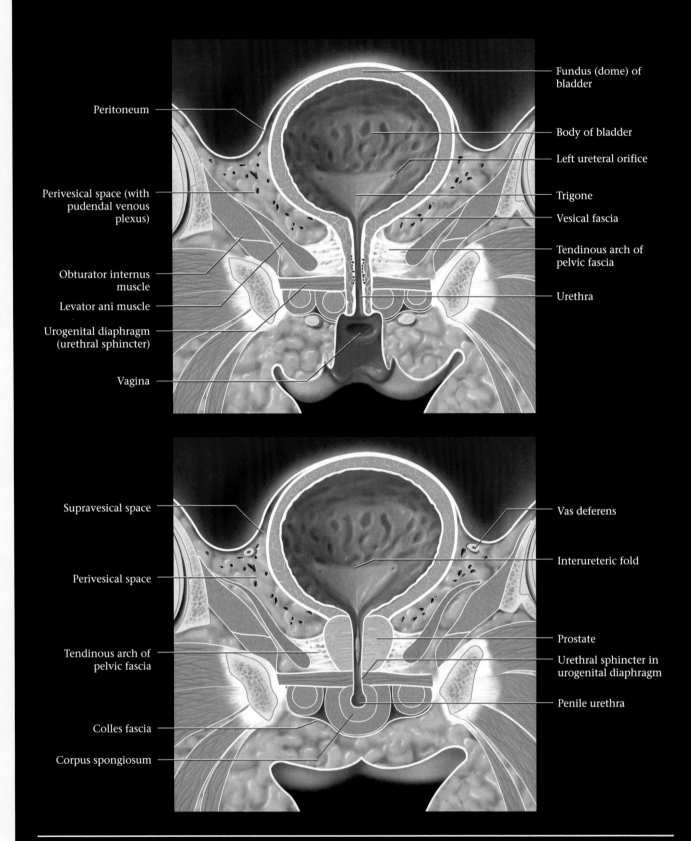

Peritoneum

Perivesical space (with pudendal venous plexus)

Obturator internus muscle

Levator ani muscle

Urogenital diaphragm (urethral sphincter)

Vagina

Fundus (dome) of bladder

Body of bladder

Left ureteral orifice

Trigone

Vesical fascia

Tendinous arch of pelvic fascia

Urethra

Supravesical space

Perivesical space

Tendinous arch of pelvic fascia

Colles fascia

Corpus spongiosum

Vas deferens

Interureteric fold

Prostate

Urethral sphincter in urogenital diaphragm

Penile urethra

(Top) A frontal (coronal) section of the female bladder shows that it rests almost directly on the muscular floor of the pelvis. The dome of the bladder is covered with peritoneum. The trigone is the distinct triangular base of the bladder whose apices are formed by the ureteral and urethral orifices. The bladder is surrounded by a layer of loose fat and connective tissue (the prevesical & perivesical spaces) that communicate superiorly with the retroperitoneum.
(Bottom) A coronal section of the male bladder shows that it rests on the prostate, which separates it from the muscular pelvic floor. The bladder wall is muscular, strong, and very distensible. The ureters enter the bladder through an oblique anteromedial course that helps to prevent urinary reflux into the ureters. The mucosal surface of the ureters is continuous with the bladder and is the same transitional cell type.

URETER AND BLADDER

INTRAPERITONEAL BLADDER RUPTURE

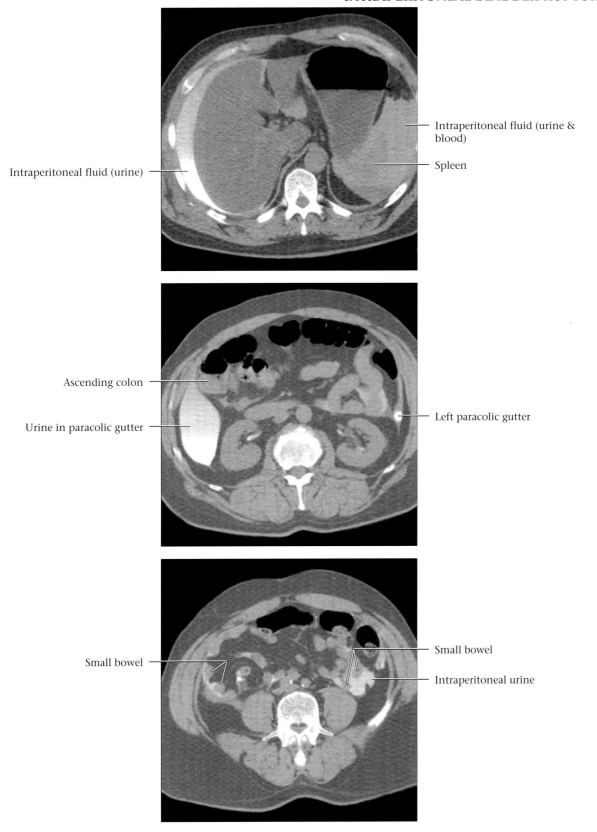

Intraperitoneal fluid (urine)

Intraperitoneal fluid (urine & blood)

Spleen

Ascending colon

Urine in paracolic gutter

Left paracolic gutter

Small bowel

Small bowel

Intraperitoneal urine

(Top) First of nine CT images showing intraperitoneal rupture of the urinary bladder. The CT scan was obtained after installation of contrast medium into the bladder. This section shows dense intraperitoneal fluid (urine) surrounding the liver in the right subphrenic space. The fluid surrounding the spleen is diluted by blood. **(Middle)** The right paracolic gutter is distended with intraperitoneal urine. Note that the right paracolic gutter is more dependent and more voluminous than the left. **(Bottom)** A more caudal section shows dense urine surrounding small intestinal loops, confirming the intraperitoneal location of the fluid.

URETER AND BLADDER

INTRAPERITONEAL BLADDER RUPTURE

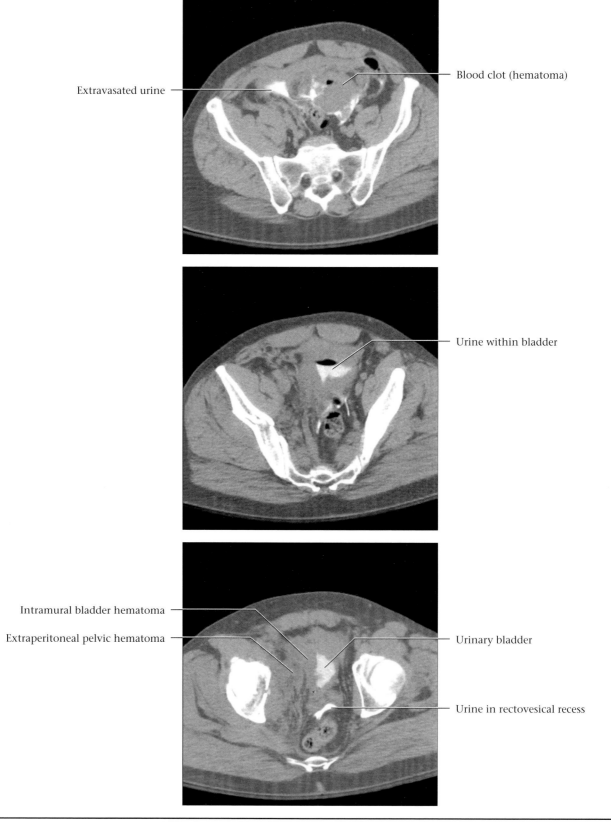

Extravasated urine

Blood clot (hematoma)

Urine within bladder

Intramural bladder hematoma

Extraperitoneal pelvic hematoma

Urinary bladder

Urine in rectovesical recess

(Top) A section near the dome of the bladder shows a hematoma, surrounded by extravasated urine. **(Middle)** This section shows opacified urine within the urinary bladder. The bladder wall is thickened due to mural hematoma and its collapsed state. **(Bottom)** Densely opacified urine settles into the rectovesical recess, the deepest intraperitoneal recess. The bladder is displaced to the left by the pelvic hematoma.

URETER AND BLADDER

INTRAPERITONEAL BLADDER RUPTURE

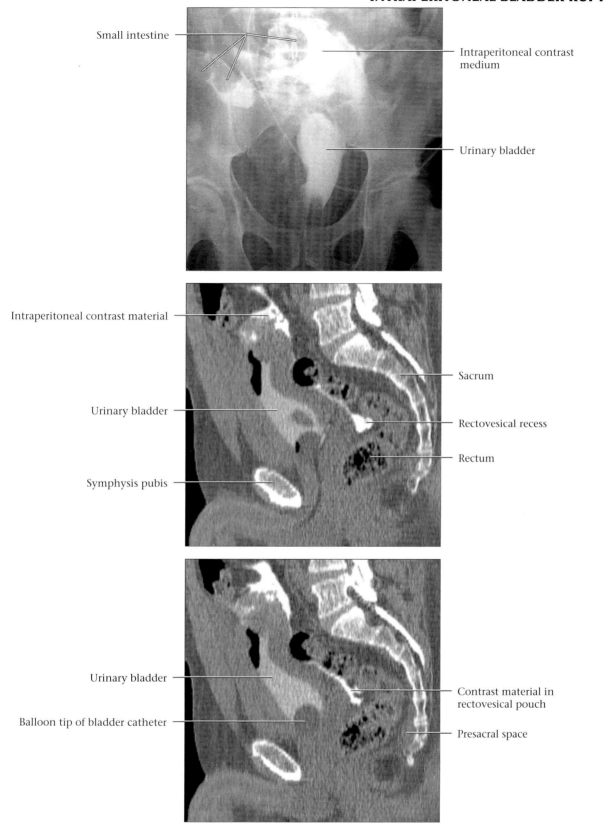

Small intestine — Intraperitoneal contrast medium

Urinary bladder

Intraperitoneal contrast material

Urinary bladder — Sacrum

— Rectovesical recess

Symphysis pubis — Rectum

Urinary bladder — Contrast material in rectovesical pouch

Balloon tip of bladder catheter — Presacral space

(Top) A frontal film from the cystogram that preceded the CT scan shows rupture of the dome of the bladder, with intraperitoneal spill of opacified urine/contrast medium. Note the absence of contrast medium in the perivesical and prevesical (extraperitoneal) spaces, and the contrast medium outlining small intestinal loops, seen as "filling defects" in the pool of contrast medium. The urinary bladder is displaced to the left by a pelvic hematoma. (Middle) A sagittal reformation of the CT scan shows dense contrast material outlining bowel loops and filling the rectovesical recess, both findings indicating an intraperitoneal rupture of the bladder. The bladder is distorted and contains diluted urine and gas, the latter from prior catheterization and contrast instillation. (Bottom) Note the absence of extravasated urine in the extraperitoneal spaces, including the presacral space.

URETER AND BLADDER

EXTRAPERITONEAL BLADDER RUPTURE

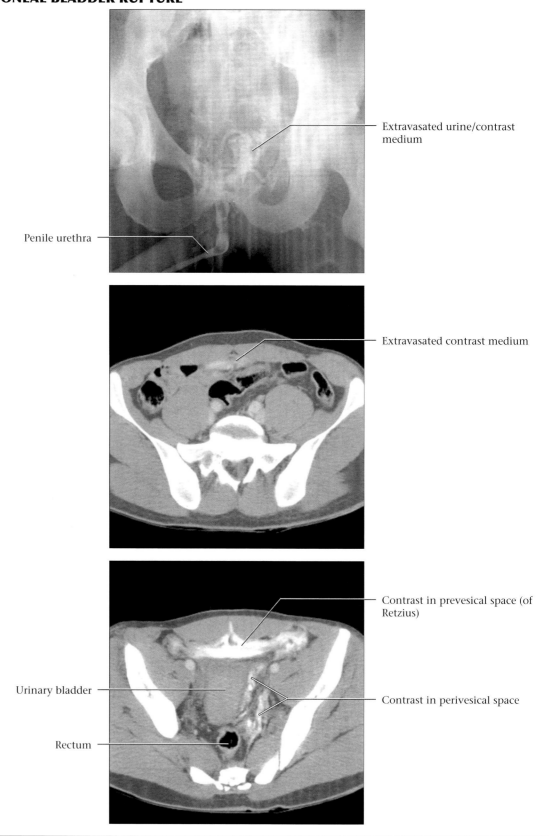

Extravasated urine/contrast medium

Penile urethra

Extravasated contrast medium

Contrast in prevesical space (of Retzius)

Urinary bladder

Contrast in perivesical space

Rectum

(Top) First of six images of a patient with pelvic fractures and an extraperitoneal rupture of the bladder. This frontal film from a cystogram shows contrast medium being instilled through a catheter placed into the penile urethra. There is little or no opacification of the urinary bladder, only an amorphous, streaky collection in the pelvis. **(Middle)** This CT section shows no contrast medium or urine in the paracolic gutters, as would be expected for an intraperitoneal bladder rupture. There is a collection of contrast material just deep to the anterior abdominal wall. **(Bottom)** Dense contrast material is present within the prevesical space (of Retzius), the extraperitoneal compartment that separates the bladder from the anterior abdominal wall and symphysis pubis. Contrast material is also present in the perivesical space, immediately surrounding the bladder.

EXTRAPERITONEAL BLADDER RUPTURE

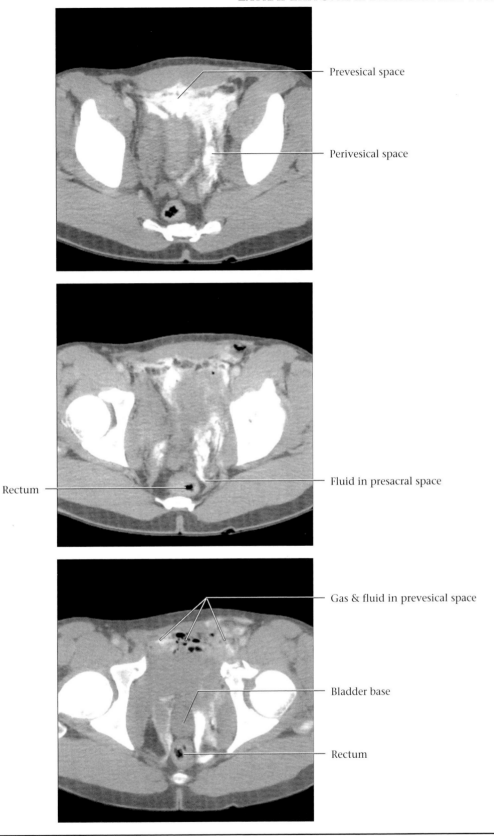

Prevesical space

Perivesical space

Rectum

Fluid in presacral space

Gas & fluid in prevesical space

Bladder base

Rectum

(Top) Contrast material dissects through the extraperitoneal spaces in the pelvis, all of which communicate. **(Middle)** The extravasated fluid extends to the pelvic side walls and to the presacral space, all extraperitoneal. Note the absence of contrast within the rectovesical pouch. **(Bottom)** Again note the absence of intraperitoneal fluid in the rectovesical recess and the large amount of extraperitoneal fluid. The loose areolar tissue (fat and connective tissue) that occupies the prevesical and perivesical spaces is easily displaced and these spaces may expand to collect large amounts of extravasated blood (or other fluids).

URACHAL CYST

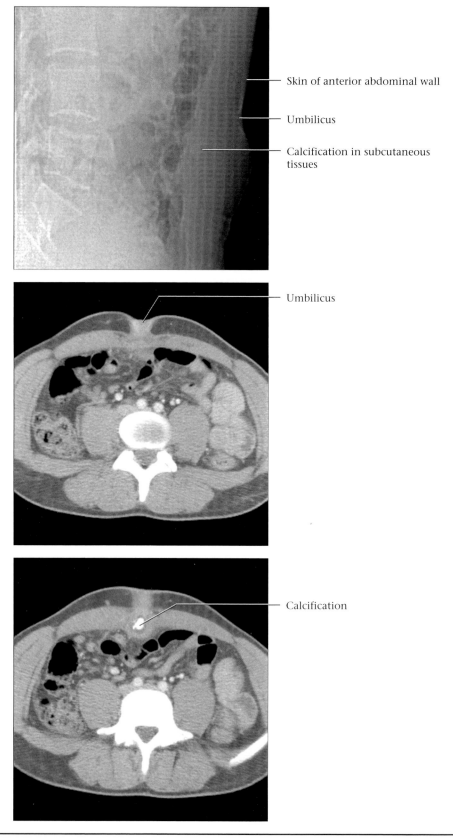

Skin of anterior abdominal wall

Umbilicus

Calcification in subcutaneous tissues

Umbilicus

Calcification

(Top) First of five images of a patient with a urachal cyst who presented with infraumbilical pain and a palpable, tender mass. This lateral film shows a faint calcification in the abdominal wall just inferior to the umbilicus. **(Middle)** An axial CT section shows the umbilicus and subtle infiltration of the abdominal fat just deep to it. **(Bottom)** A more caudal section shows a calcified lesion within a rounded focus of inflammation. This is a typical site for the urachus. Chronic inflammation, which can occur within a urachal cyst, often develops calcification.

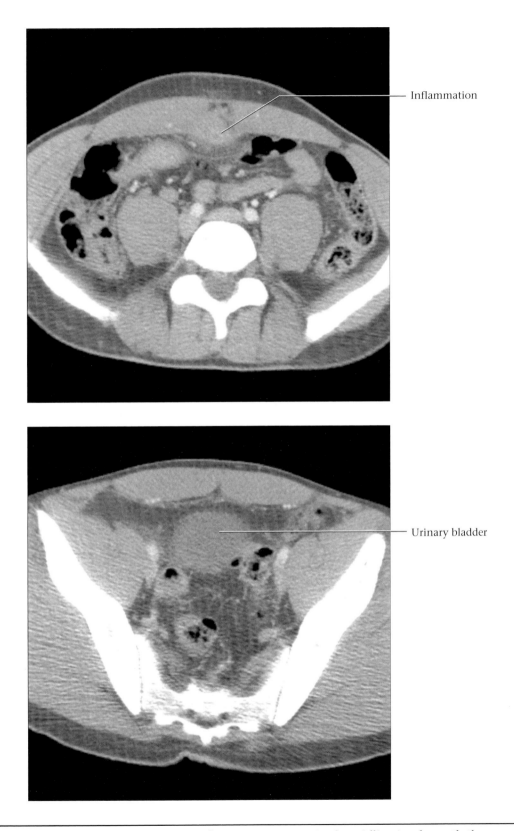

Inflammation

Urinary bladder

(Top) A more caudal section shows continuation of the inflammatory process in the midline just beneath the anterior abdominal wall, again typical for a urachal inflammatory process. **(Bottom)** The dome of the urinary bladder is seen just inferior to the midline inflammatory process. At surgery an infected urachal cyst was excised.

URETER AND BLADDER

URACHAL CANCER

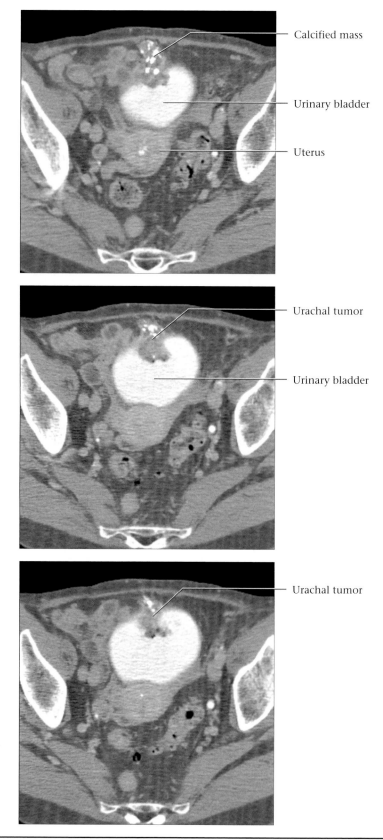

Calcified mass

Urinary bladder

Uterus

Urachal tumor

Urinary bladder

Urachal tumor

(Top) First of three axial CT sections of a woman with a palpable infraumbilical midline abdominal wall mass. The mass is heavily calcified and indents the dome of the urinary bladder while also touching the anterior abdominal wall, a typical location and appearance for a urachal mass. **(Middle)** The mass is quite elongated and extends obliquely between the umbilicus and the urinary bladder. **(Bottom)** A more caudal section suggests that the mass is invading the anterior superior wall of the bladder. A urachal carcinoma was excised at surgery, along with a portion of the bladder.

URETER AND BLADDER

BLADDER DIVERTICULA AND STONES

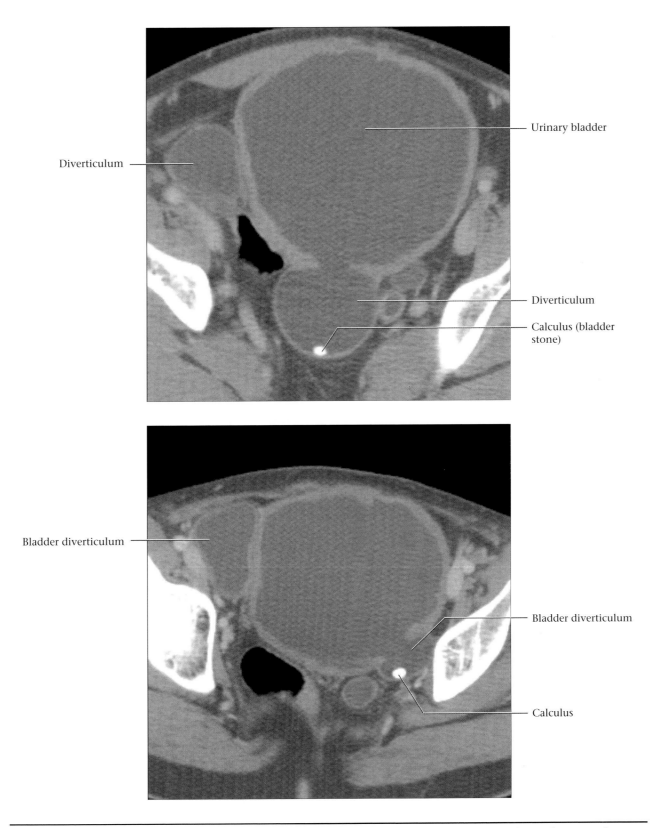

Urinary bladder

Diverticulum

Diverticulum

Calculus (bladder stone)

Bladder diverticulum

Bladder diverticulum

Calculus

(Top) First of two axial CT sections of an elderly man with hematuria and dysuria. This unenhanced section shows multiple outpouchings from the urinary bladder that represent bladder diverticula. A calculus is present in the dependent position within one of the diverticula. **(Bottom)** Additional diverticula and additional stones are seen on other sections.

BLADDER DIVERTICULUM WITH CARCINOMA

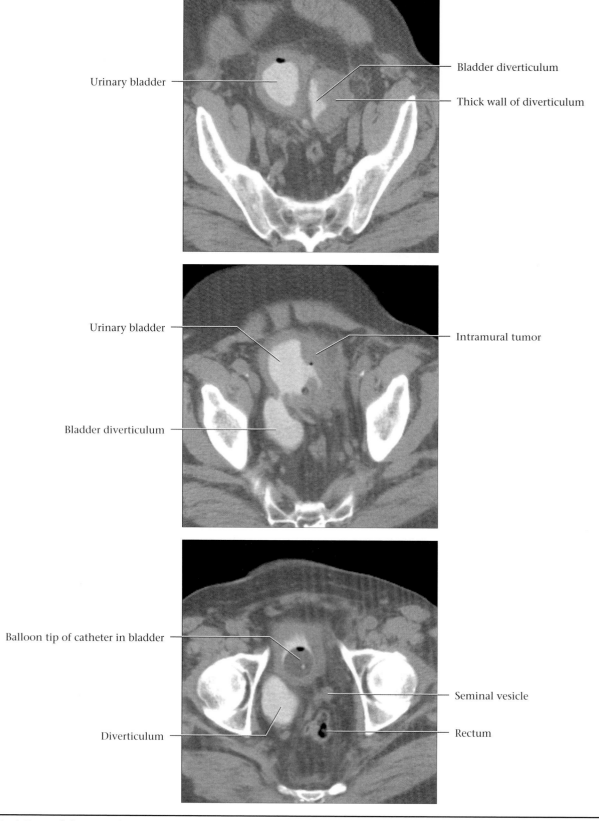

Urinary bladder — Bladder diverticulum

Thick wall of diverticulum

Urinary bladder — Intramural tumor

Bladder diverticulum

Balloon tip of catheter in bladder

Seminal vesicle

Diverticulum — Rectum

(Top) First of three axial CT sections of an elderly man with chronic dysuria and recent gross hematuria. This section shows a thick-walled urinary bladder, often seen in elderly men with bladder outlet obstruction due to prostatic hypertrophy (BPH). BPH also predisposes to the formation of bladder diverticula and urinary stasis within the diverticula. Also seen on this section is an eccentric mass, representing a bladder diverticulum, with a very thick wall. **(Middle)** As seen within the more dependent right-sided diverticulum, the wall is usually thin, since it does not contain all the muscle components of the bladder wall. The wall of the right-sided diverticulum is markedly thickened, and was found to contain invasive carcinoma at surgery. **(Bottom)** Some debris is present within the dependent portion of the right-sided diverticulum, but this was not malignant.

URETER AND BLADDER

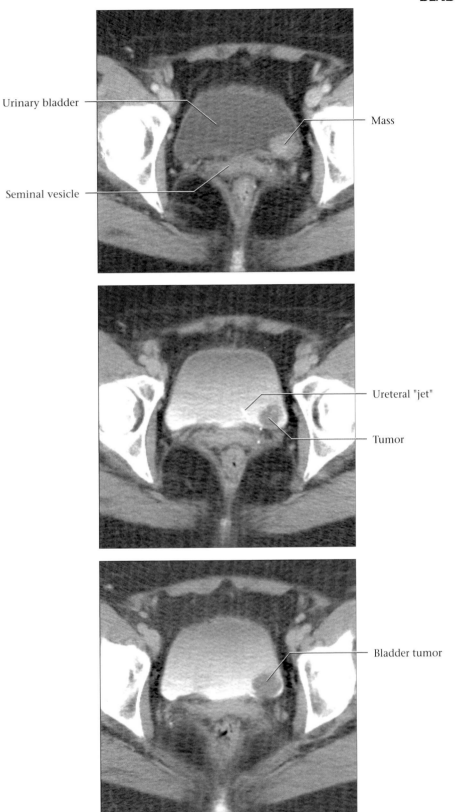

Urinary bladder — Mass

Seminal vesicle —

Ureteral "jet"

Tumor

Bladder tumor

(Top) First of three axial CT sections of a man with gross hematuria. This nonenhanced section shows a soft tissue density mass within the urinary bladder. A calculus would be much higher in density. **(Middle)** A section obtained about 2 minutes after the IV administration of iodinated contrast medium shows the mass as a filling defect within the bladder. Note the "jet" of contrast-opacified urine entering the bladder through the left ureteral orifice, indicating that the tumor is not obstructing the orifice. **(Bottom)** The mass is arising from the base of the bladder. No invasion of the surrounding perivesical fat planes is evident. The mass was resected via an endoscope placed into the bladder via the penis and was a transitional cell carcinoma. The bladder is the most common site of transitional cell tumors, though they may also occur within the kidneys and ureters.

PART III
Pelvis

Pelvic Wall and Floor

Vessels, Lymphatic System and Nerves

Female Pelvic Ligaments and Spaces

Uterus

Ovaries

Testes and Scrotum

Penis and Urethra

Prostate and Seminal Vesicles

PELVIC WALL AND FLOOR

Imaging Anatomy

Anatomic Boundaries

- Iliac crest to perineum
- Divided into **false (major) and true (minor) pelvis**
  - Dividing point from sacral promontory, along arcuate and iliopectineal lines to pubic crest
    - Arcuate line divides flared iliac fossa from inferior, narrowed portion of iliac bone
  - False pelvis wide "bowl" above line
  - True pelvis below arcuate line
    - **Pelvic inlet** upper border of true pelvis (tilts forward approximately 60° from horizontal)
    - **Pelvic outlet** formed by ischiopubic rami, ischial spines, inferior symphysis pubis, sacrotuberous ligaments and coccyx

Skeletal Anatomy

- 4 components
  - Paired innominate bones, each with three parts
    - Ilium, ischium and pubis
  - Sacrum
  - Coccyx
- Key ligamentous attachments and foramina
  - **Sacrospinous ligament**: From sacrum to ischial spine
    - Divides **greater sciatic foramen above** ligament from **lesser sciatic foramen below**
  - **Sacrotuberous ligament**: From sacrum to ischial tuberosity
    - Posterior boundary of lesser sciatic foramen
  - **Inguinal ligament**: From anterior superior iliac spine to pubic tubercle
    - Formed from fibers of external oblique aponeurosis
  - **Obturator foramen**
    - Formed by body and rami of pubic and ischial bones
- **Male vs. female pelvis**
  - Male pelvis
    - Pubic arch (angle formed by inferior pubic rami at symphysis pubis) < 90°
    - Heart-shaped pelvic inlet with narrow outlet
    - Round obturator foramen
    - Narrow sciatic notch
    - Larger, thicker bones
  - Female pelvis
    - Flattened pubic arch (> 90°)
    - Oval pelvic inlet with larger pelvic outlet
    - Oval obturator foramen
    - Wide sciatic notch
    - Thinner, more delicate bones

Anterior Pelvic Wall

- Continuation of upper abdominal muscles
  - **External oblique muscle**: Largest and most superficial of the 3 flat muscles
    - Fibers course inferomedially
  - **Internal oblique muscle**: Middle flat muscle
    - Runs superomedially at right angles to external oblique muscle in abdomen
    - Muscle fibers become more horizontal in pelvis and become inferiorly directed more caudally

- **Transversus abdominis muscle**: Inner most flat muscle with horizontal course
- **Rectus abdominis muscle**
  - Vertically directed strap muscle
- **Linea alba**
  - Midline fibrous raphe formed by aponeuroses of flat muscles
- **Rectus sheath**
  - Strong fibrous sheath, which **invests rectus abdominis muscles** and superior and inferior epigastric vessels
  - Formed by aponeuroses of external oblique, internal oblique and transversus abdominis muscles
  - Internal oblique aponeurosis splits in upper portion of abdominal wall
    - Anterior portion joins external oblique aponeurosis to form **anterior rectus sheath**
    - Posterior portion joins transversus abdominis aponeurosis to form **posterior rectus sheath**
  - Lower third of abdominal wall (below anterior superior iliac spine) all aponeurosis join and course anterior to rectus abdominis muscles
    - Creates **arcuate line** on posterior surface of abdominal wall
    - Wall below arcuate line covered only by **transversalis fascia**, which is separated from parietal peritoneum by extraperitoneal fat

Inguinal Canal

- Passage through anterior abdominal wall
  - Conveys spermatic cord in males and round ligament in females
  - Formed embryologically by evagination of processus vaginalis through anterior abdominal wall
- **Internal or deep ring**
  - Opening through transversalis fascia
  - Located above mid-portion of inguinal ligament
  - Lateral to inferior epigastric artery
- **External or superficial ring**
  - Triangular opening of external oblique aponeurosis
  - Just lateral to pubic tubercle
- **Hesselbach triangle**
  - Area of weakness in pelvic wall
    - Site of direct inguinal hernias
  - Medial border: Lateral edge of rectus sheath
  - Lateral border: Inferior epigastric artery
  - Inferior border: Inguinal ligament

Posterior Pelvic Wall (False Pelvis)

- Psoas and iliacus muscles fuse caudally to form iliopsoas muscle
  - Inserts on lesser trochanter and is powerful hip flexor

Pelvic Floor

- Curved bowl so distinct walls not clearly defined
- Posterior wall: Sacrum, coccyx, and piriformis, coccygeus muscles
- Lateral wall: Ilium, ischium and piriformis, obturator internus, levator ani muscles
- Anterior wall: Symphysis pubis, anterior portion of obturator internus muscle, levator ani muscle
- Floor: **Pelvic diaphragm** (levator ani and fascia)
- Key muscles

PELVIC WALL AND FLOOR

○ **Obturator internus**
  ▪ Runs from inner surface of obturator membrane to greater trochanter
  ▪ Covered by thick fascia (**arcus tendineus**), which is origin of pelvic diaphragm
○ **Coccygeus**
  ▪ Runs from ischial spine to sacrum and coccyx
○ **Levator ani forms pelvic diaphragm**
  ▪ **Formed by 3 muscles: Iliococcygeus, pubococcygeus and puborectalis**
  ▪ All muscles covered by fascial sheath
  ▪ Pierced by urethra, rectum and vagina
  ▪ Primary **support for pelvic organs**
  ▪ Critical for maintaining continence, as well as normal micturition and defecation

Perineum

- **Space inferior to levator ani**
- **Central tendon of perineum (perineal body)** formed in midline
  ○ Behind vagina in females
  ○ Behind urethra in males
- Diamond-shaped area bordered by pubic symphysis, ischial tuberosities and coccyx
  ○ **Subdivided into 2 spaces** (urogenital and anal triangles) by line drawn slightly anterior to ischial tuberosities, along superficial transverse perineus muscle
- **Urogenital triangle** contains urethra and external genitalia
  ○ Muscle development greater in male
    ▪ Paired muscles: Superficial and deep transverse perineus, bulbocavernosus and ischiocavernosus
  ○ **Urogenital diaphragm:** Deep transverse perineus muscle and fascia, urethral sphincter
  ○ Female: **Bartholin glands** (greater vestibular glands) and vestibular bulbs
  ○ Male: **Penile bulb**
- **Anal triangle** contains anus
  ○ Identical in both sexes
  ○ Circular **external anal sphincter** surrounds anus and maintains continence
    ▪ 3 muscle components: Subcutaneous, superficial and deep
    ▪ Fibers extend posteriorly to form **anococcygeal ligament**
  ○ **Ischiorectal fossa** located in posterior and lateral portion of triangle
    ▪ Filled with fat
    ▪ Communicates posteriorly, forming U-shape around levator ani and anus
    ▪ Bounded posteriorly by sacrotuberous ligament and gluteus maximus

Clinical Implications

Clinical Importance

- **Pelvic wall musculature** protects and supports pelvic viscera, stabilizes pelvis for ambulation, increases abdominal pressure for defecation, micturition and parturition
  ○ Laxity or diastasis of musculature results in hernias

  ▪ Incarceration may lead to bowel obstruction
- **Pelvic floor musculature** stabilizes lower pelvis, controls defecation and micturition, and maintains continence
  ○ Laxity results in pelvic floor descent with cystoceles/rectoceles, urinary incontinence, fecal incontinence or constipation

Inguinal Hernia

- May be either indirect or direct
- **Indirect inguinal hernia**
  ○ Passes **through internal inguinal ring**, traverses inguinal canal to external ring
    ▪ May extend into scrotum in males and labia majora in females
  ○ Passes **lateral to inferior epigastric vessels** and has an oblique inferior course
  ○ Considered a congenital defect and associated with a patent processus vaginalis
  ○ 5x more common than direct inguinal hernias
- **Direct inguinal hernia**
  ○ Protrusion through Hesselbach triangle
    ▪ Generally does not extend into scrotum
  ○ Passes **medial to inferior epigastric vessels**
  ○ Considered an acquired defect
- Inguinal hernias 5-10x more common in men

Femoral Hernia

- Begins posterior to medial portion of inguinal ligament
  ○ Traverses **femoral canal to fossa ovalis**
- Herniated contents are **below inguinal ligament**, lateral to pubic tubercle and medial to femoral vessels
- More common in older women

Obturator Hernia

- **Herniation through obturator canal** (superolateral aspect of obturator foramen)
- Herniated contents may lie between obturator muscles or between pectineus and obturator externus
- More common in older women

Sciatic Hernia

- Herniation through greater sciatic foramen laterally into subgluteal region

Perineal Hernia

- Posterior: Through levator ani and coccygeus muscles
- Anterior: Through urogenital diaphragm

Pelvic Floor Relaxation

- Weakness in pelvic floor fascia, muscles and ligaments
  ○ Almost exclusively in women
    ▪ Incidence increases with age (> 50% of women over 50 years old) and number of pregnancies
- May involve 3 different compartments
  ○ Anterior: **Cystocele**
  ○ Middle: **Vaginal prolapse, uterine prolapse, enterocele**
  ○ Posterior: **Rectocele**
- Must examine both relaxed and straining with fast T2WI or fluoroscopy
- Graded on degree of descent relative to pubococcygeal line

PELVIC WALL AND FLOOR

3D CT, MALE PELVIS

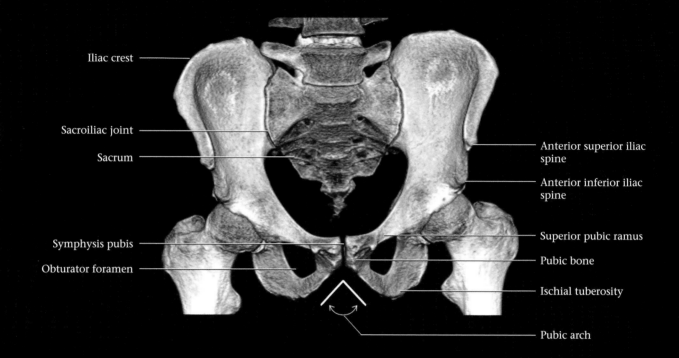

Iliac crest

Sacroiliac joint

Sacrum

Symphysis pubis

Obturator foramen

Anterior superior iliac spine

Anterior inferior iliac spine

Superior pubic ramus

Pubic bone

Ischial tuberosity

Pubic arch

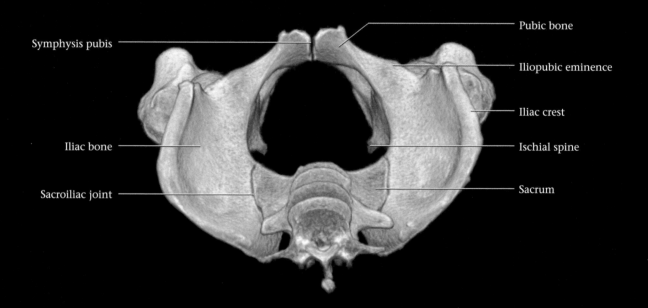

Symphysis pubis

Iliac bone

Sacroiliac joint

Pubic bone

Iliopubic eminence

Iliac crest

Ischial spine

Sacrum

(Top) 3D CT reconstructions of the male pelvis. There are several striking differences between the male and female pelvic bones. The bones are thicker and heavier in the male. The pubic arch is higher, with a more narrow angle. The pelvic inlet is more heart-shaped, and both the inlet and outlet are much narrower compared to the female pelvis. **(Bottom)** Superior view of the pelvic inlet. Note the ischial spines are easily visible, as the pelvis continues to narrow at the outlet.

PELVIC WALL AND FLOOR

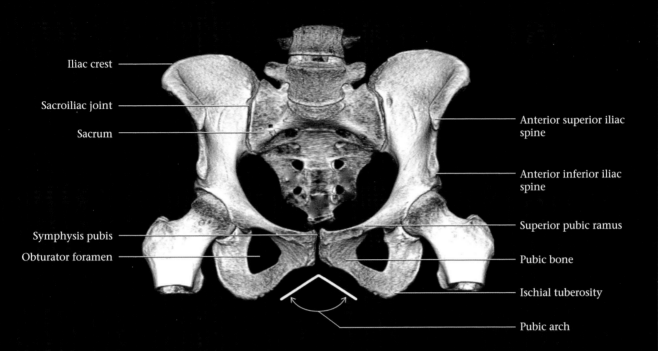

Iliac crest

Sacroiliac joint

Sacrum

Symphysis pubis

Obturator foramen

Anterior superior iliac spine

Anterior inferior iliac spine

Superior pubic ramus

Pubic bone

Ischial tuberosity

Pubic arch

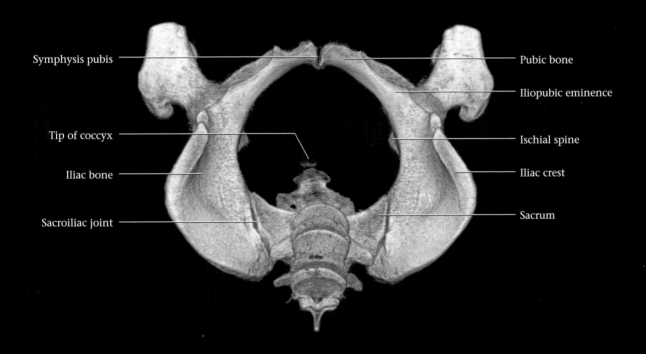

Symphysis pubis

Tip of coccyx

Iliac bone

Sacroiliac joint

Pubic bone

Iliopubic eminence

Ischial spine

Iliac crest

Sacrum

(Top) 3D CT reconstructions of the female pelvis. There are several striking differences between the male and female pelvic bones. The bones are thinner and more delicate in the female. The pubic arch is flatter, creating a wider angle. The pelvic inlet is more oval, and the inlet and outlet are much wider to accommodate childbirth. **(Bottom)** Superior view of the pelvic inlet. Note the more widely spaced ischial spines, compared to the male pelvis.

PELVIC WALL AND FLOOR

3D CT, FEMALE PELVIS

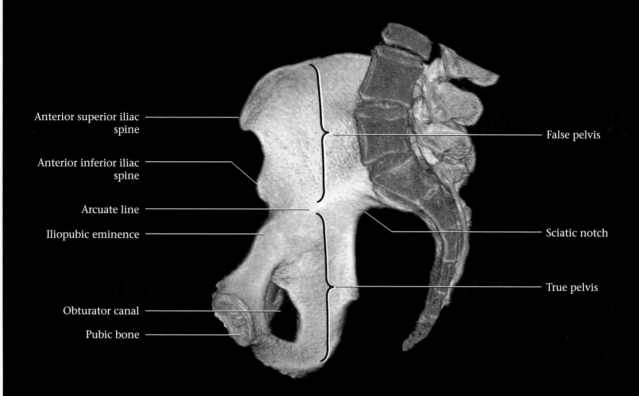

Anterior superior iliac spine

Anterior inferior iliac spine

Arcuate line

Iliopubic eminence

Obturator canal

Pubic bone

False pelvis

Sciatic notch

True pelvis

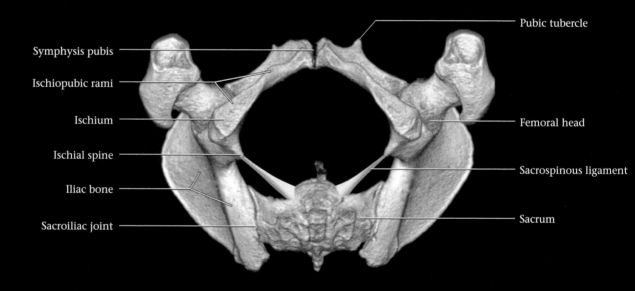

Symphysis pubis

Ischiopubic rami

Ischium

Ischial spine

Iliac bone

Sacroiliac joint

Pubic tubercle

Femoral head

Sacrospinous ligament

Sacrum

(Top) 3D CT reconstruction of the female pelvis viewed from the medial surface. The arcuate line is a bony prominence, which courses from the sacral promontory anteriorly towards the iliopubic eminence. The false pelvis is above the arcuate line, while the true pelvis is below it. **(Bottom)** 3D CT reconstruction of the pelvic outlet, graphically enhanced to show sacrospinous ligament. The pelvic outlet is formed by the ischiopubic rami, ischial spines, inferior symphysis pubis, sacrospinous ligaments and coccyx.

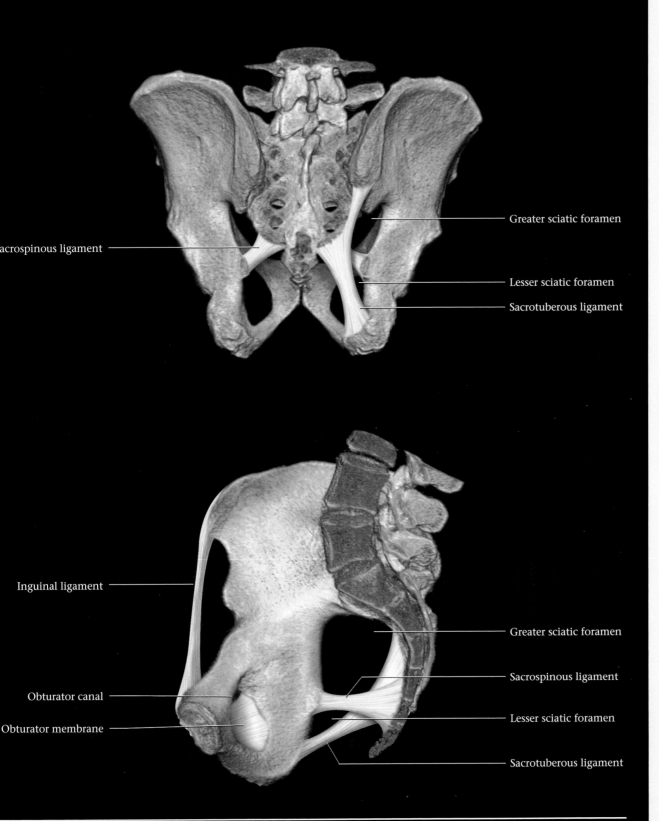

Sacrospinous ligament

Greater sciatic foramen

Lesser sciatic foramen

Sacrotuberous ligament

Inguinal ligament

Obturator canal

Obturator membrane

Greater sciatic foramen

Sacrospinous ligament

Lesser sciatic foramen

Sacrotuberous ligament

(Top) 3D CT reconstruction of the pelvis, graphically enhanced to show the key ligaments. The sacrospinous ligament extends between the sacrum and ischial spine. The greater sciatic foramen is above the sacrospinous ligament and the lesser sciatic foramen is below it. The sacrotuberous ligament has a somewhat broader attachment to the sacrum and extends to the ischial tuberosity. It forms the posterior boundary of the lesser sciatic foramen. (Bottom) The inguinal ligament extends from the anterior superior iliac spine to the pubic tubercle. The obturator foramen is covered by a membrane except for the obturator canal, which is in the superolateral aspect of the foramen. The obturator vessels and nerve pass through this opening.

ANTERIOR PELVIC WALL

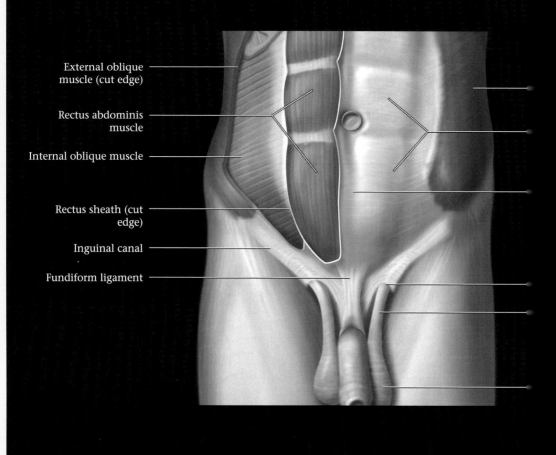

External oblique
muscle (cut edge)

Rectus abdominis
muscle

Internal oblique muscle

Rectus sheath (cut
edge)

Inguinal canal

Fundiform ligament

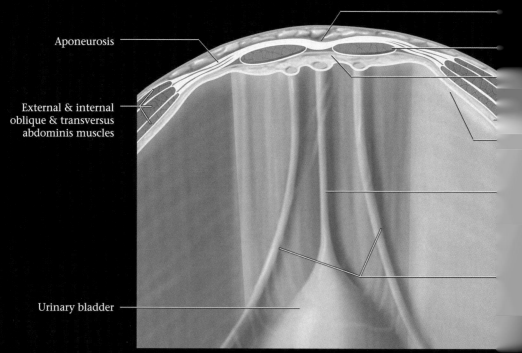

Aponeurosis

External & internal
oblique & transversus
abdominis muscles

Urinary bladder

(Top) Anterior abdominal wall muscles. **(Bottom)** Inner aspect of the anterior abdominal w
arcuate line. The rectus sheath, which is formed by the aponeuroses of the external and inte
transversus abdominis muscles, encloses the rectus muscle both anteriorly and posteriorly ir
the pelvis, at the level of the anterior superior iliac spine, the sheath is present only anterior
this occurs is called the arcuate line. Only the transversalis fascia covers the posterior rectus
as depicted in this graphic. Extraperitoneal fat separates the transversalis fascia from the pai

PELVIC WALL AND FLOOR

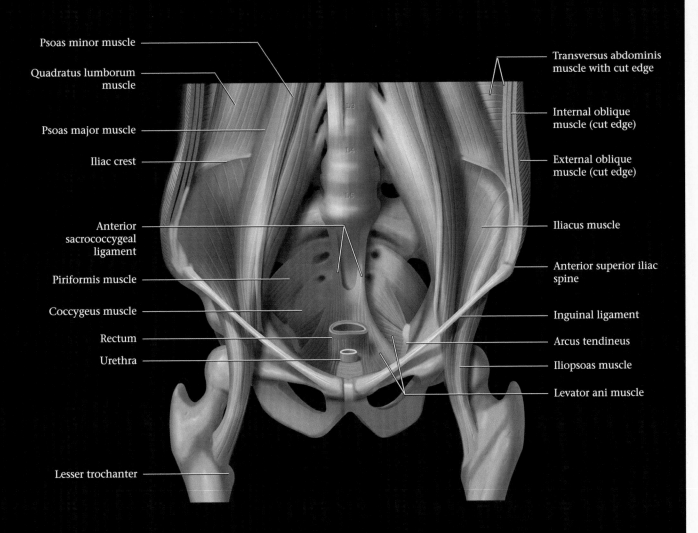

Psoas minor muscle

Quadratus lumborum muscle

Psoas major muscle

Iliac crest

Anterior sacrococcygeal ligament

Piriformis muscle

Coccygeus muscle

Rectum

Urethra

Lesser trochanter

Transversus abdominis muscle with cut edge

Internal oblique muscle (cut edge)

External oblique muscle (cut edge)

Iliacus muscle

Anterior superior iliac spine

Inguinal ligament

Arcus tendineus

Iliopsoas muscle

Levator ani muscle

The posterior wall of the false pelvis is formed by the iliac bones, sacrum, and the iliacus and psoas muscles. These two muscles fuse caudally to form the iliopsoas muscle, which passes anterior to the hip joint to insert onto the lesser trochanter of the femur. The posterior wall of the true pelvis if formed by the sacrum, coccyx, and the piriformis and coccygeus muscles. The inguinal ligament is formed by the external oblique aponeurosis and is continuous with the fascia lata of the thigh.

PELVIC WALL AND FLOOR

AXIAL CT

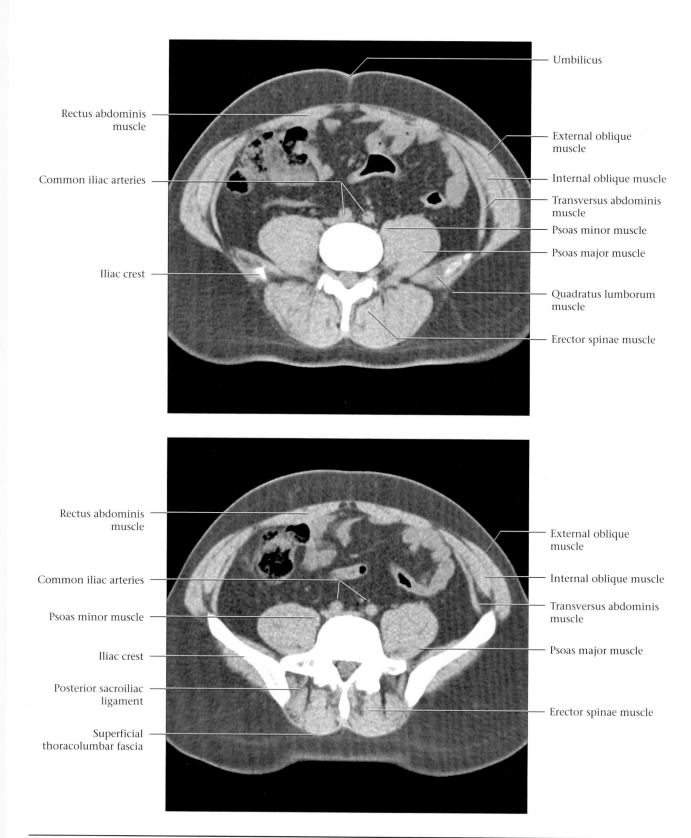

Umbilicus

Rectus abdominis muscle

External oblique muscle

Common iliac arteries

Internal oblique muscle

Transversus abdominis muscle

Psoas minor muscle

Psoas major muscle

Iliac crest

Quadratus lumborum muscle

Erector spinae muscle

Rectus abdominis muscle

External oblique muscle

Common iliac arteries

Internal oblique muscle

Psoas minor muscle

Transversus abdominis muscle

Iliac crest

Psoas major muscle

Posterior sacroiliac ligament

Superficial thoracolumbar fascia

Erector spinae muscle

(**Top**) First of fourteen axial CT images through the pelvis. The pelvis begins at the top of the iliac crest and extends to the perineum. (**Bottom**) The flat muscles that form the lateral anterior abdominal wall include (from external to internal) the external oblique, internal oblique and transversus abdominis muscles. The rectus abdominis muscles are paired, vertically oriented, strap-like muscle running on either side of the midline.

PELVIC WALL AND FLOOR

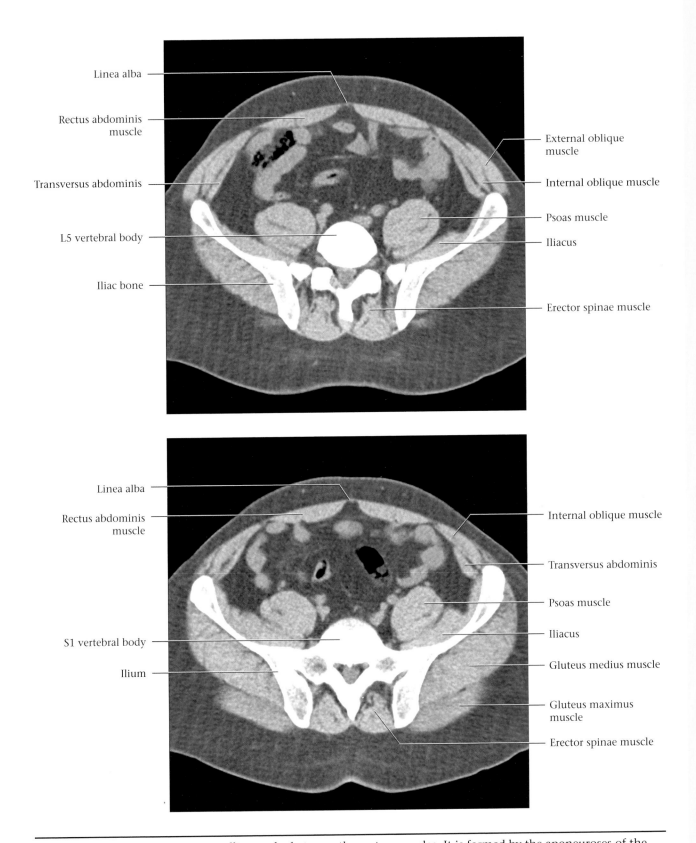

Linea alba — Rectus abdominis muscle — Transversus abdominis — L5 vertebral body — Iliac bone — External oblique muscle — Internal oblique muscle — Psoas muscle — Iliacus — Erector spinae muscle

Linea alba — Rectus abdominis muscle — S1 vertebral body — Ilium — Internal oblique muscle — Transversus abdominis — Psoas muscle — Iliacus — Gluteus medius muscle — Gluteus maximus muscle — Erector spinae muscle

(Top) The linea alba is a fibrous, midline raphe between the rectus muscles. It is formed by the aponeuroses of the flat muscles (external oblique, internal oblique and transversus abdominis muscles). **(Bottom)** The arcuate line (not radiographically visible) occurs at roughly the level of the anterior superior iliac spine. Above this line, the aponeurosis of the internal oblique splits. The anterior portion joins the external oblique aponeurosis to form the anterior rectus sheath. The posterior portion joins the transversus abdominis aponeurosis to form the posterior rectus sheath.

PELVIC WALL AND FLOOR

AXIAL CT

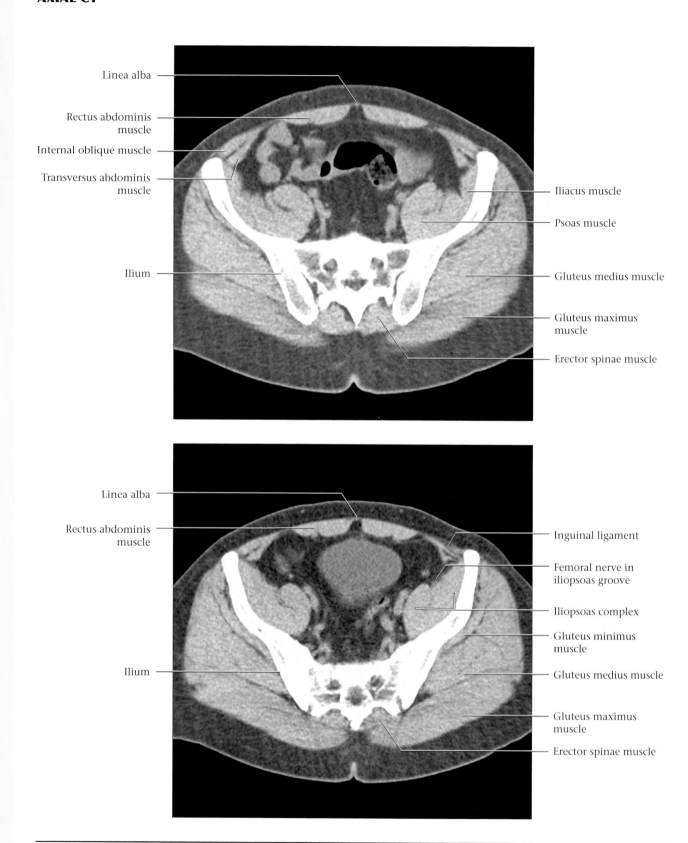

Linea alba

Rectus abdominis muscle

Internal oblique muscle

Transversus abdominis muscle

Ilium

Iliacus muscle

Psoas muscle

Gluteus medius muscle

Gluteus maximus muscle

Erector spinae muscle

Linea alba

Rectus abdominis muscle

Ilium

Inguinal ligament

Femoral nerve in iliopsoas groove

Iliopsoas complex

Gluteus minimus muscle

Gluteus medius muscle

Gluteus maximus muscle

Erector spinae muscle

(Top) Below the arcuate line, all three aponeuroses join and course anterior to the rectus muscle, making the caudal portion of the posterior rectus sheath incomplete. In this region, the posterior rectus abdominis muscle is covered only by the transversalis fascia, which is separated from the parietal peritoneum by a layer of extraperitoneal fat. Because the rectus sheath is incomplete in this area, a rectus hematoma or abscess may extend into the extraperitoneal space. **(Bottom)** The psoas and iliacus muscles merge to form the iliopsoas muscle, which continues inferiorly to insert on the lesser trochanter and serves as a powerful hip flexor. The femoral nerve lies in the iliopsoas groove on its way to the inguinal canal.

PELVIC WALL AND FLOOR

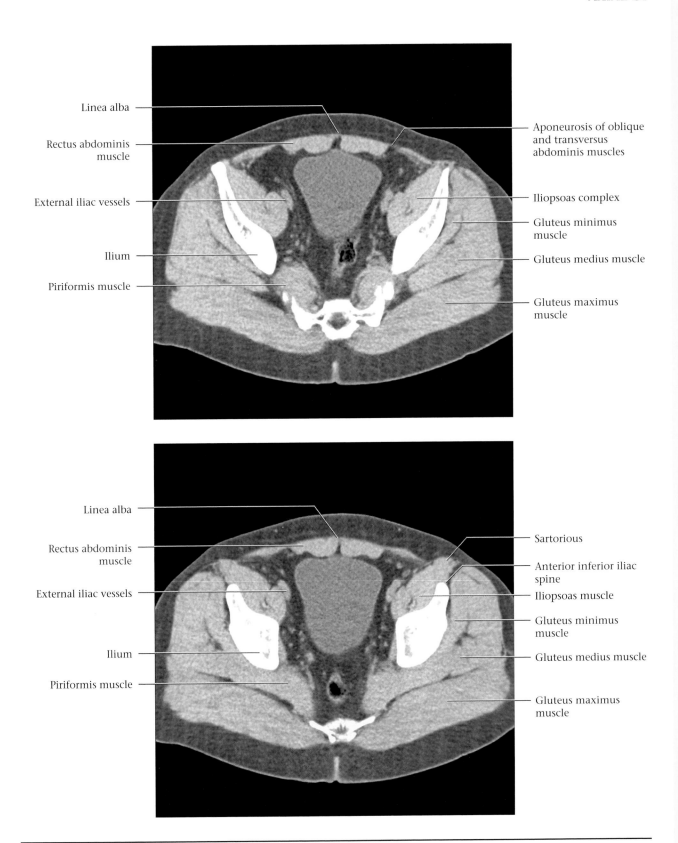

Linea alba

Rectus abdominis muscle

External iliac vessels

Ilium

Piriformis muscle

Aponeurosis of oblique and transversus abdominis muscles

Iliopsoas complex

Gluteus minimus muscle

Gluteus medius muscle

Gluteus maximus muscle

Linea alba

Rectus abdominis muscle

External iliac vessels

Ilium

Piriformis muscle

Sartorious

Anterior inferior iliac spine

Iliopsoas muscle

Gluteus minimus muscle

Gluteus medius muscle

Gluteus maximus muscle

(Top) Note the thinning of the abdominal wall lateral to the rectus muscle. This is the aponeurosis of the internal oblique muscle, external oblique muscle and transversus abdominis muscle. This is a point of inherent weakness and a Spigelian hernia may occur through this area. The piriformis muscle forms an important part of the posterior and lateral wall of the true pelvis. **(Bottom)** Note how the pelvis narrows inferiorly as it transitions from the false pelvis to the true pelvis.

PELVIC WALL AND FLOOR

AXIAL CT

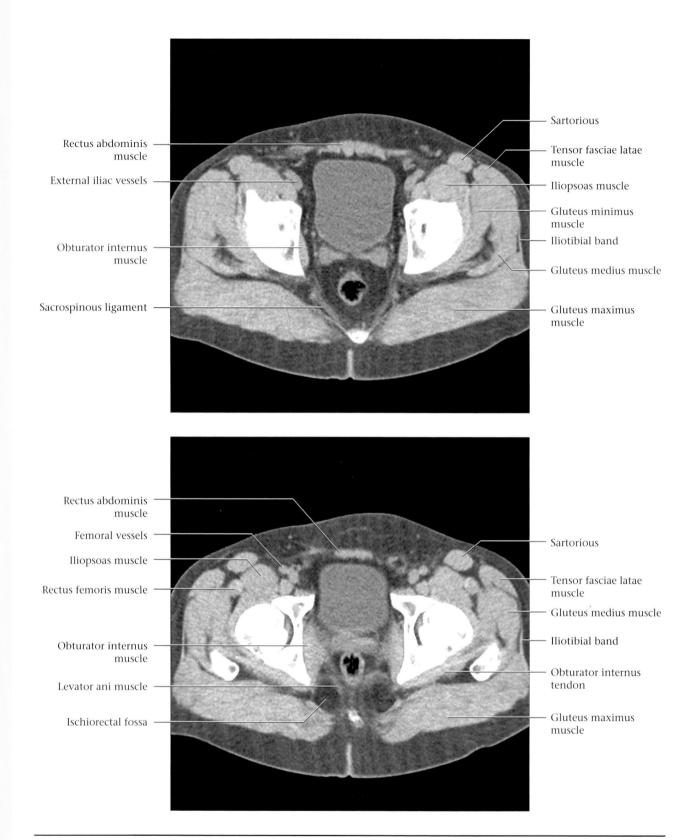

Rectus abdominis muscle

External iliac vessels

Obturator internus muscle

Sacrospinous ligament

Sartorious

Tensor fasciae latae muscle

Iliopsoas muscle

Gluteus minimus muscle

Iliotibial band

Gluteus medius muscle

Gluteus maximus muscle

Rectus abdominis muscle

Femoral vessels

Iliopsoas muscle

Rectus femoris muscle

Obturator internus muscle

Levator ani muscle

Ischiorectal fossa

Sartorious

Tensor fasciae latae muscle

Gluteus medius muscle

Iliotibial band

Obturator internus tendon

Gluteus maximus muscle

(Top) The sacrospinous ligament is an important anatomic landmark, with the greater sciatic foramen being above this ligament and the lesser sciatic foramen below it. (Bottom) The obturator internus muscle, an important part of the lateral pelvic floor, exits the pelvis through the lesser sciatic foramen. The tendon of the obturator internus fuses with the gemellus muscle before inserting on the medial surface of the greater trochanter. Within the pelvis, the fascia of the obturator internus forms the arcus tendineus, which serves as the origin for the levator ani muscles. The obturator internus also forms the lateral wall of the ischiorectal fossa.

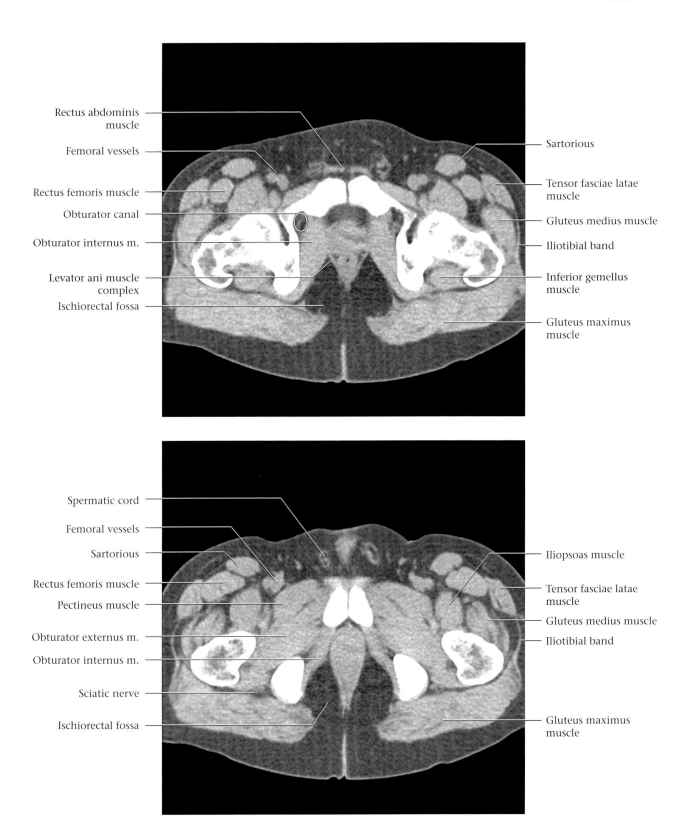

Rectus abdominis muscle

Femoral vessels

Rectus femoris muscle

Obturator canal

Obturator internus m.

Levator ani muscle complex

Ischiorectal fossa

Sartorious

Tensor fasciae latae muscle

Gluteus medius muscle

Iliotibial band

Inferior gemellus muscle

Gluteus maximus muscle

Spermatic cord

Femoral vessels

Sartorious

Rectus femoris muscle

Pectineus muscle

Obturator externus m.

Obturator internus m.

Sciatic nerve

Ischiorectal fossa

Iliopsoas muscle

Tensor fasciae latae muscle

Gluteus medius muscle

Iliotibial band

Gluteus maximus muscle

(Top) Inferiorly, the rectus abdominis muscle thins and inserts on the pubic symphysis. **(Bottom)** The ischiorectal fossa is filled with fat and communicates across the midline, forming a U-shape around the levator ani and anus. A perirectal abscess may extend into this space.

PELVIC WALL AND FLOOR

AXIAL CT

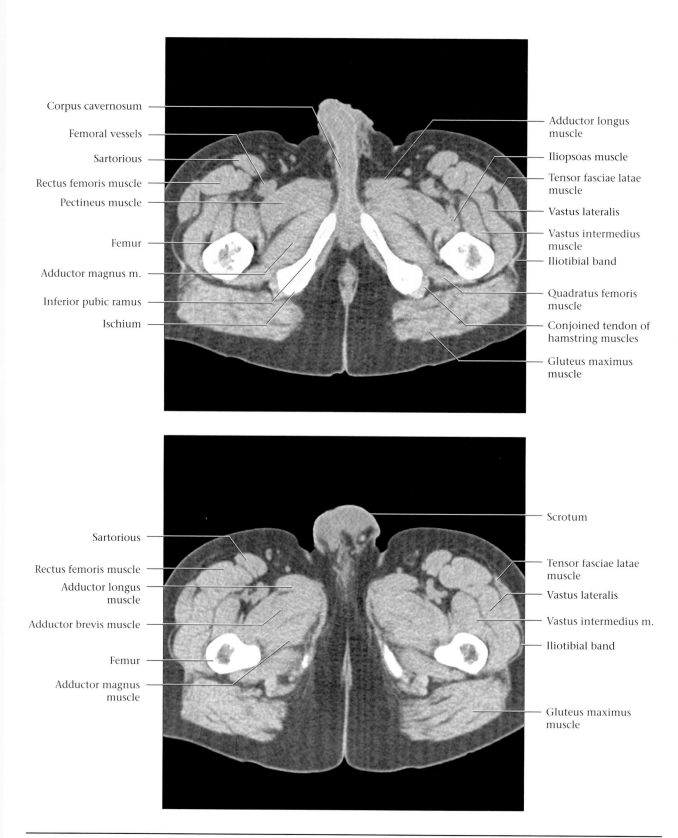

Corpus cavernosum

Femoral vessels

Sartorious

Rectus femoris muscle

Pectineus muscle

Femur

Adductor magnus m.

Inferior pubic ramus

Ischium

Adductor longus muscle

Iliopsoas muscle

Tensor fasciae latae muscle

Vastus lateralis

Vastus intermedius muscle

Iliotibial band

Quadratus femoris muscle

Conjoined tendon of hamstring muscles

Gluteus maximus muscle

Sartorious

Rectus femoris muscle

Adductor longus muscle

Adductor brevis muscle

Femur

Adductor magnus muscle

Scrotum

Tensor fasciae latae muscle

Vastus lateralis

Vastus intermedius m.

Iliotibial band

Gluteus maximus muscle

(**Top**) The perineum is the space below the levator ani and includes external genitalia, urethra and anus. (**Bottom**) More inferiorly, the powerful adductor muscle group is seen.

PELVIC WALL AND FLOOR

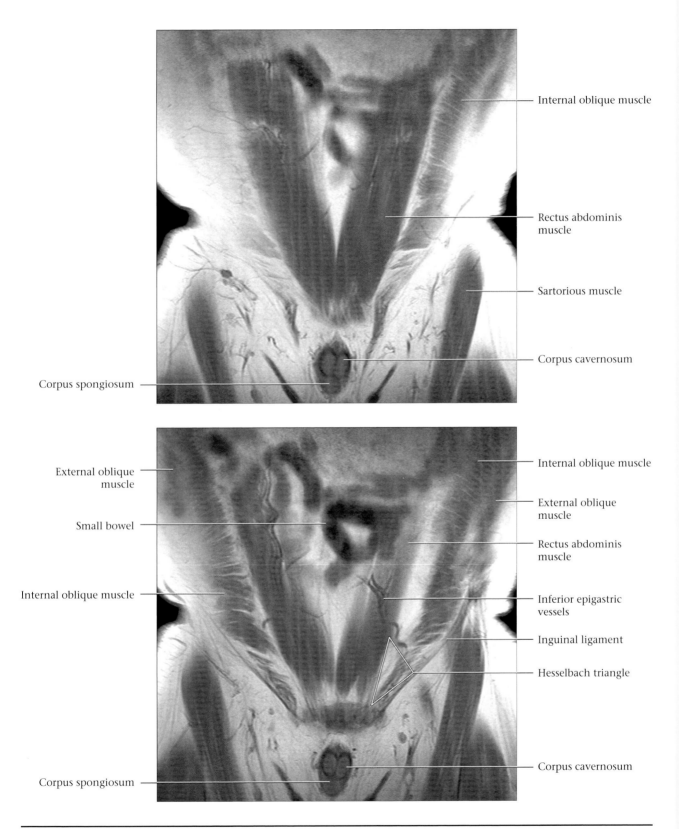

Internal oblique muscle

Rectus abdominis muscle

Sartorious muscle

Corpus cavernosum

Corpus spongiosum

External oblique muscle

Small bowel

Internal oblique muscle

Corpus spongiosum

Internal oblique muscle

External oblique muscle

Rectus abdominis muscle

Inferior epigastric vessels

Inguinal ligament

Hesselbach triangle

Corpus cavernosum

(Top) First of fourteen coronal T1 MR images through the abdominal wall. The rectus abdominis muscle originates from the pubic symphysis and crest, courses superiorly and inserts onto the anterior surface of the xiphoid process and medial portion of the 5th-7th costal cartilages. (Bottom) The fibers of the external oblique muscle (partially seen) are directed inferomedially. The internal oblique muscle runs superomedially in the abdomen but becomes more horizontal, and eventually courses inferiorly, low in the pelvis. The inguinal ligament extends from the anterior superior iliac spine to the pubic tubercle. The triangular area bounded by the lateral aspect of the rectus sheath medially, the inferior epigastric vessels laterally and the inguinal ligament inferiorly is the Hesselbach triangle, an area of weakness of the anterior abdominal wall.

PELVIC WALL AND FLOOR

CORONAL T1 MR

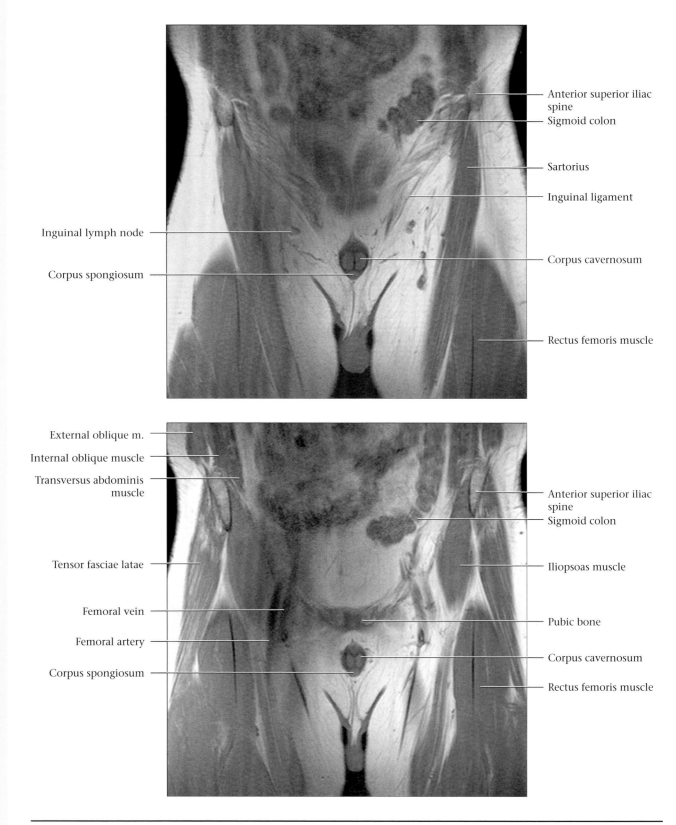

Anterior superior iliac spine

Sigmoid colon

Sartorius

Inguinal ligament

Inguinal lymph node

Corpus spongiosum

Corpus cavernosum

Rectus femoris muscle

External oblique m.

Internal oblique muscle

Transversus abdominis muscle

Anterior superior iliac spine

Sigmoid colon

Tensor fasciae latae

Iliopsoas muscle

Femoral vein

Pubic bone

Femoral artery

Corpus cavernosum

Corpus spongiosum

Rectus femoris muscle

(Top) The inguinal ligament is formed by fibers of the external oblique aponeurosis. The inguinal lymph nodes drain the regional structures including the lower abdominal wall, perineum (including vulva and vagina), anal canal, scrotum, penis and the lower limb. They drain into the external iliac lymph nodes along the external iliac vessels. **(Bottom)** The femoral vessels and nerve pass underneath the inguinal ligament through the femoral canal. Contents of the femoral canal include (from lateral to medial): The femoral nerve, artery and vein. The femoral canal is normally a tight space, but occasionally becomes large enough to allow herniation of abdominal contents into the canal. Femoral hernias are particularly at risk of becoming incarcerated and strangulated.

PELVIC WALL AND FLOOR

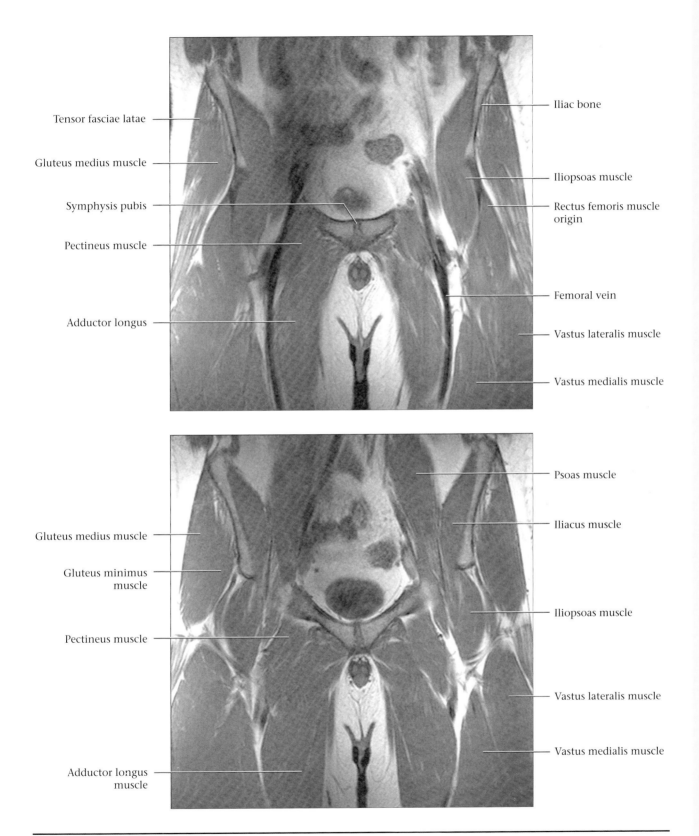

Tensor fasciae latae

Gluteus medius muscle

Symphysis pubis

Pectineus muscle

Adductor longus

Iliac bone

Iliopsoas muscle

Rectus femoris muscle origin

Femoral vein

Vastus lateralis muscle

Vastus medialis muscle

Gluteus medius muscle

Gluteus minimus muscle

Pectineus muscle

Adductor longus muscle

Psoas muscle

Iliacus muscle

Iliopsoas muscle

Vastus lateralis muscle

Vastus medialis muscle

(Top) The pectineus is a flat, quadrangular muscle in the femoral triangle. It arises from the pectineal line of the pubis and passes posterolaterally to insert below the lesser trochanter. **(Bottom)** The iliacus and psoas muscles, the largest muscles within the pelvic cavity, fuse caudally to form the iliopsoas muscle, a powerful hip flexor. After leaving the pelvis, it inserts on the lesser trochanter of the femur. An iliopsoas bursa, which may communicate with the hip joint cavity, separates the tendon from the pubic bone and the hip joint capsule.

CORONAL T1 MR

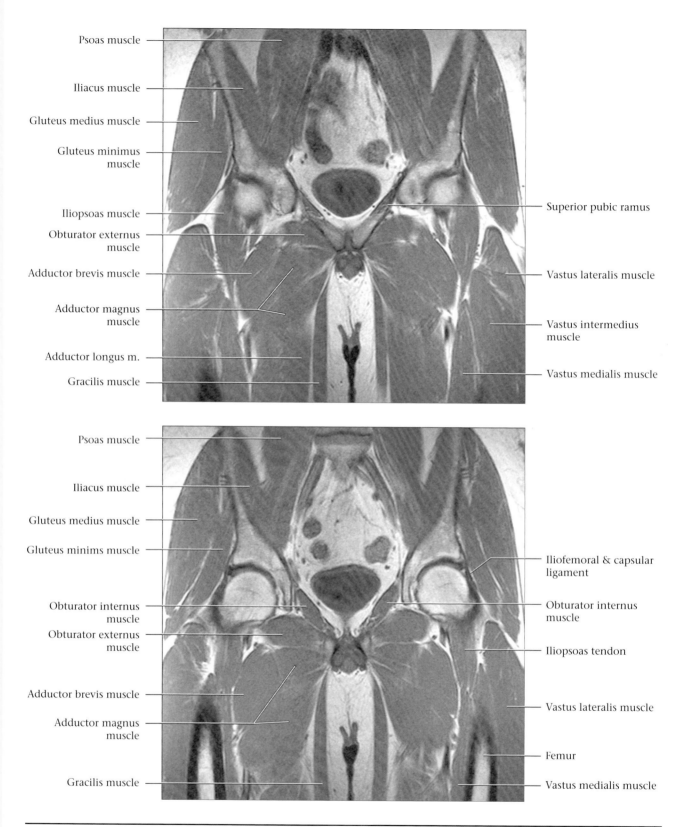

Psoas muscle
Iliacus muscle
Gluteus medius muscle
Gluteus minimus muscle
Iliopsoas muscle
Obturator externus muscle
Adductor brevis muscle
Adductor magnus muscle
Adductor longus m.
Gracilis muscle

Superior pubic ramus
Vastus lateralis muscle
Vastus intermedius muscle
Vastus medialis muscle

Psoas muscle
Iliacus muscle
Gluteus medius muscle
Gluteus minims muscle
Obturator internus muscle
Obturator externus muscle
Adductor brevis muscle
Adductor magnus muscle
Gracilis muscle

Iliofemoral & capsular ligament
Obturator internus muscle
Iliopsoas tendon
Vastus lateralis muscle
Femur
Vastus medialis muscle

(Top) The superior pubic ramus forms the superior border of the obturator foramen, which is covered by a strong membrane. The obturator externus muscle arises from the outer surface of the obturator membrane. **(Bottom)** The obturator internus arises from the inner surface of the obturator membrane and the adjacent inner surfaces of the pubic bone and ischium. It passes posterolaterally along the lateral wall of the pelvis to form a tendon that traverses the lesser sciatic foramen. Inferior to the ischial spine it turns laterally to insert into the medial aspect of the greater trochanter of the femur.

PELVIC WALL AND FLOOR

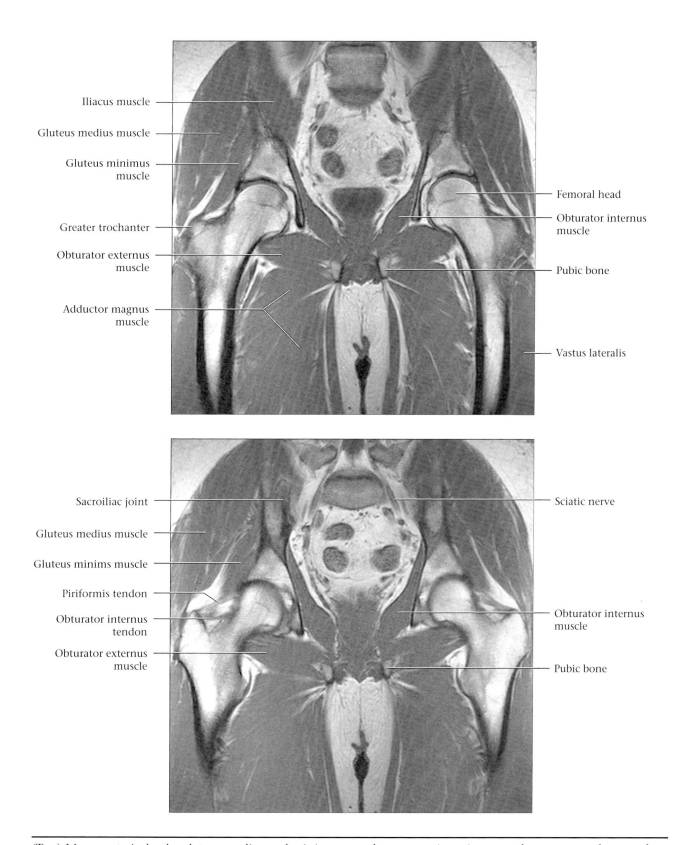

Iliacus muscle

Gluteus medius muscle

Gluteus minimus muscle

Greater trochanter

Obturator externus muscle

Adductor magnus muscle

Femoral head

Obturator internus muscle

Pubic bone

Vastus lateralis

Sacroiliac joint

Gluteus medius muscle

Gluteus minims muscle

Piriformis tendon

Obturator internus tendon

Obturator externus muscle

Sciatic nerve

Obturator internus muscle

Pubic bone

(Top) More posteriorly, the gluteus medius and minimus muscles are seen inserting onto the greater trochanter of the femur. Both muscles are powerful abductors of the thigh. The obturator externus muscle passes behind the neck of femur to insert onto the greater trochanter. **(Bottom)** The piriformis and obturator internus tendon are seen inserting onto the greater trochanter of the femur. Both muscles are lateral rotators of the hip.

PELVIC WALL AND FLOOR

CORONAL T1 MR

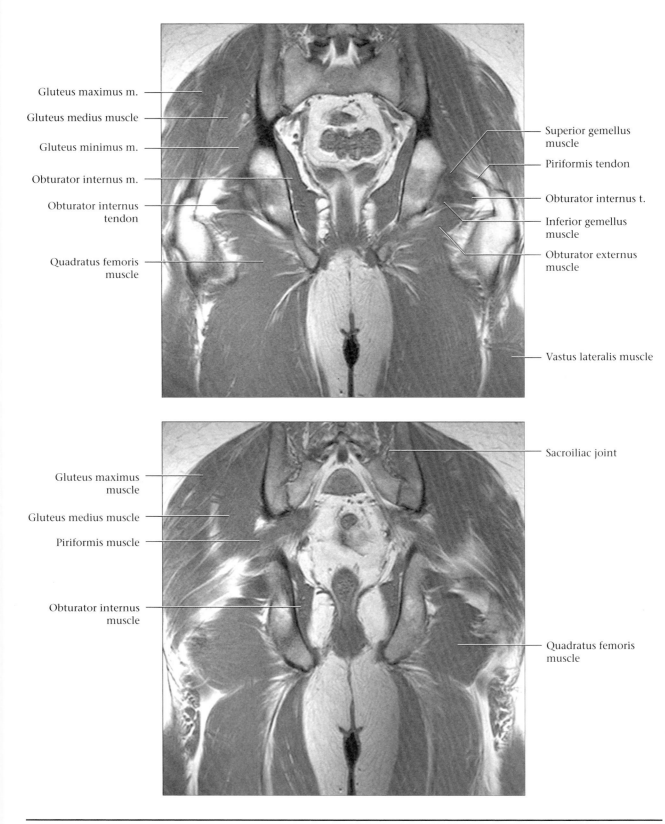

Gluteus maximus m.

Gluteus medius muscle

Gluteus minimus m.

Obturator internus m.

Obturator internus tendon

Quadratus femoris muscle

Superior gemellus muscle

Piriformis tendon

Obturator internus t.

Inferior gemellus muscle

Obturator externus muscle

Vastus lateralis muscle

Sacroiliac joint

Gluteus maximus muscle

Gluteus medius muscle

Piriformis muscle

Obturator internus muscle

Quadratus femoris muscle

(Top) Slightly posteriorly, the obturator externus tendon is shown inserting on the medial aspect of the greater trochanter of the femur. It, too, rotates the hip laterally. **(Bottom)** The piriformis muscle is seen exiting the pelvis through the greater sciatic foramen. Once outside the pelvis, it runs inferior to the gluteus medius and may fuse with it.

PELVIC WALL AND FLOOR

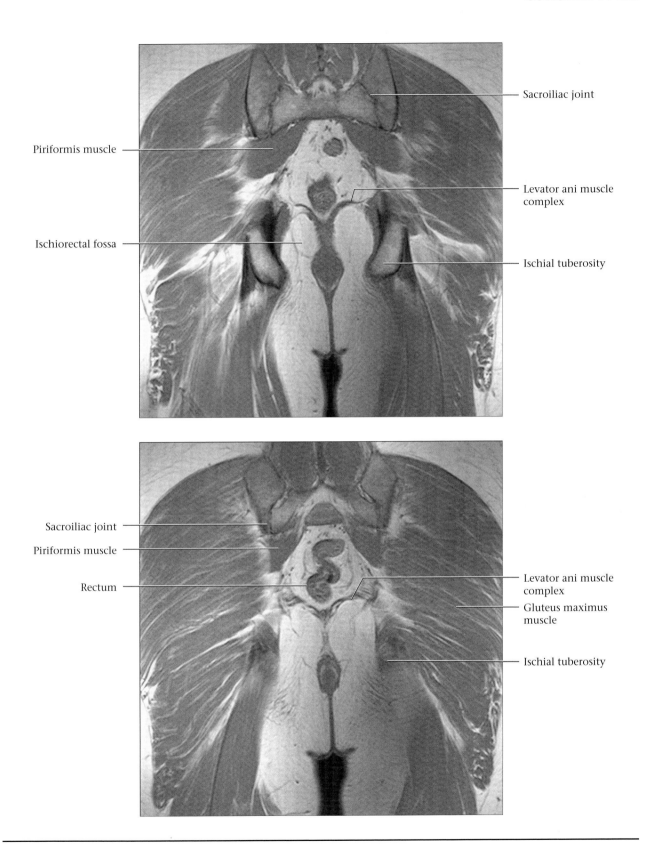

Sacroiliac joint

Piriformis muscle

Levator ani muscle complex

Ischiorectal fossa

Ischial tuberosity

Sacroiliac joint

Piriformis muscle

Rectum

Levator ani muscle complex

Gluteus maximus muscle

Ischial tuberosity

(Top) The ischiorectal fossa is a pyramid-shaped space, with its base towards the perineum and its apex at the origin of the levator ani muscle. The ischiorectal fossa lies between the ischial tuberosity and the obturator internus muscle laterally, and the external anal sphincter and the levator ani muscle medially. The space contains fat, fibrous septa, pudendal and rectal nerves and vessels **(Bottom)** The piriformis muscle arises from the anterior surface of the sacrum and gluteal surface of ilium. Note the close relationship to the rectum, especially on the left.

PELVIC WALL AND FLOOR

SAGITTAL T2 MR

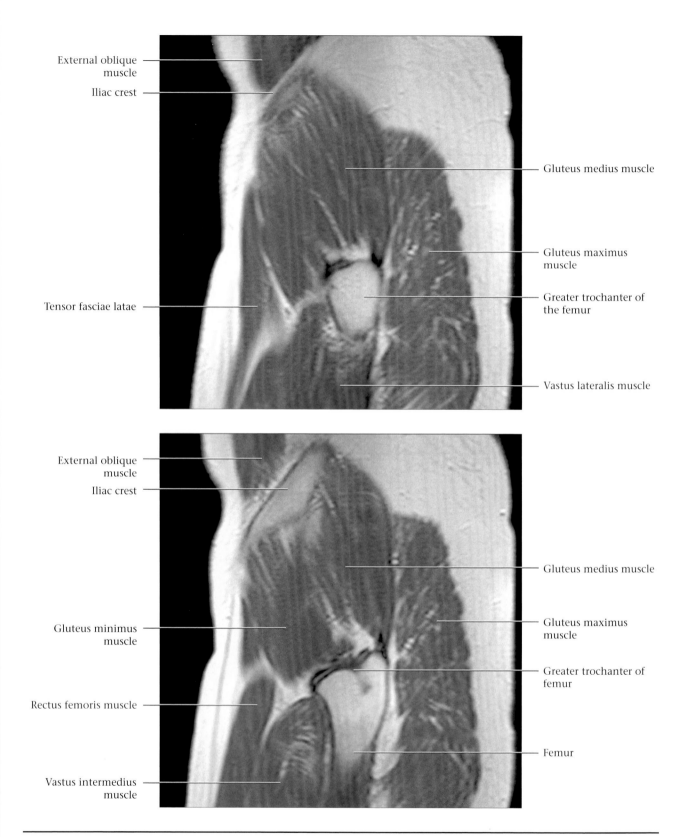

External oblique muscle

Iliac crest

Tensor fasciae latae

Gluteus medius muscle

Gluteus maximus muscle

Greater trochanter of the femur

Vastus lateralis muscle

External oblique muscle

Iliac crest

Gluteus minimus muscle

Rectus femoris muscle

Vastus intermedius muscle

Gluteus medius muscle

Gluteus maximus muscle

Greater trochanter of femur

Femur

(Top) First of twelve sagittal T2 MR images through the pelvic wall presented from lateral to medial. Both the gluteus medius and minimus muscles arise from the dorsal ilium inferior to the iliac crest. The gluteus medius muscle inserts onto the lateral and superior surfaces of greater trochanter, while the gluteus minimus muscle attaches to the anterior surface of the greater trochanter. Both muscles are hip abductors. **(Bottom)** The gluteus maximus is the largest muscle in the body. Its origin includes the posterior gluteal line, portions of medial iliac crest, sacrum, coccyx and sacrotuberous ligament. It inserts on the iliotibial tract of the fascia lata and gluteal tuberosity of the femur. It is the principle extensor of the thigh.

PELVIC WALL AND FLOOR

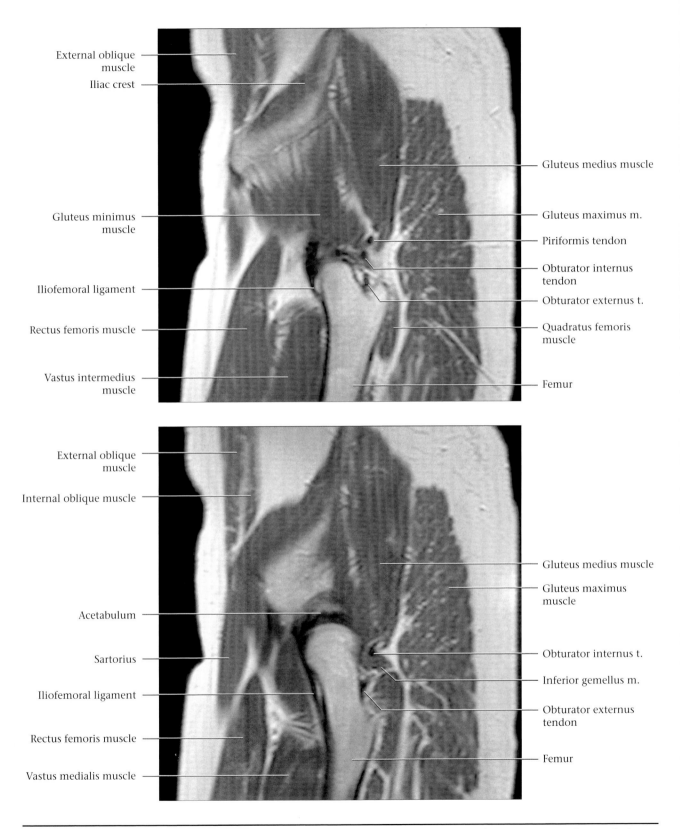

External oblique muscle
Iliac crest
Gluteus minimus muscle
Iliofemoral ligament
Rectus femoris muscle
Vastus intermedius muscle

Gluteus medius muscle
Gluteus maximus m.
Piriformis tendon
Obturator internus tendon
Obturator externus t.
Quadratus femoris muscle
Femur

External oblique muscle
Internal oblique muscle
Acetabulum
Sartorius
Iliofemoral ligament
Rectus femoris muscle
Vastus medialis muscle

Gluteus medius muscle
Gluteus maximus muscle
Obturator internus t.
Inferior gemellus m.
Obturator externus tendon
Femur

(Top) The tendons of the piriformis, obturator internus and obturator externus muscles are seen coursing to their insertions on the greater trochanter. This group of muscles helps to laterally rotate and abduct the thigh. **(Bottom)** The sartorius muscle arises from the anterior, superior iliac spine and courses inferiorly to insert on the medial surface of the tibial shaft, near the tibial tuberosity.

SAGITTAL T2 MR

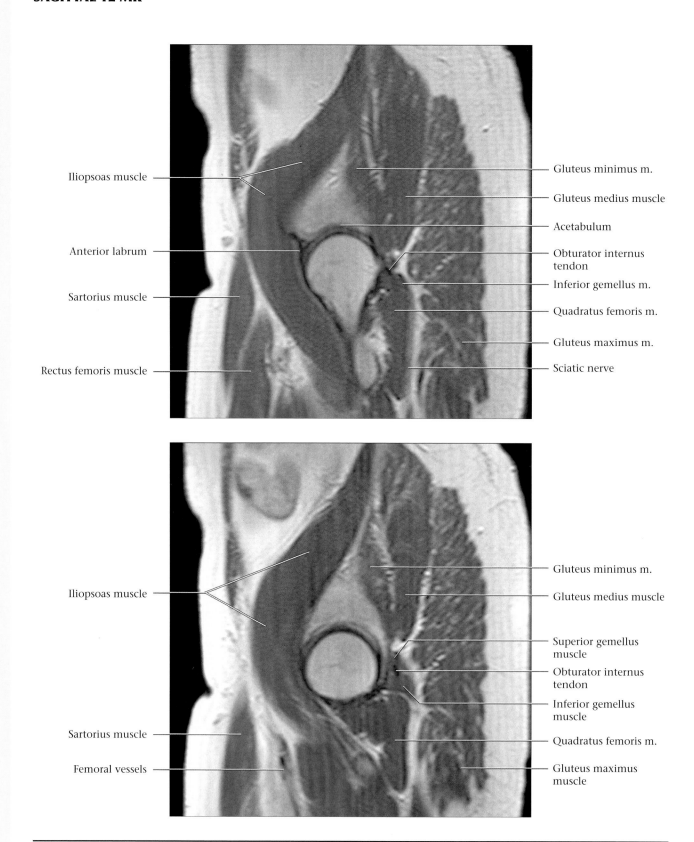

Iliopsoas muscle

Anterior labrum

Sartorius muscle

Rectus femoris muscle

Gluteus minimus m.

Gluteus medius muscle

Acetabulum

Obturator internus tendon

Inferior gemellus m.

Quadratus femoris m.

Gluteus maximus m.

Sciatic nerve

Iliopsoas muscle

Sartorius muscle

Femoral vessels

Gluteus minimus m.

Gluteus medius muscle

Superior gemellus muscle

Obturator internus tendon

Inferior gemellus muscle

Quadratus femoris m.

Gluteus maximus muscle

(Top) The sciatic nerve is seen posterior to the quadratus femoris muscle, where is descends after leaving the pelvis through the greater sciatic foramen, below the piriformis muscle. (Bottom) The superior gemellus muscle arises from the ischial spine, while the inferior gemellus muscle arises from the ischial tuberosity. Both muscles insert on the medial surface of the greater trochanter of the femur, along with the obturator internus tendon. All three muscles rotate the hip laterally.

PELVIC WALL AND FLOOR

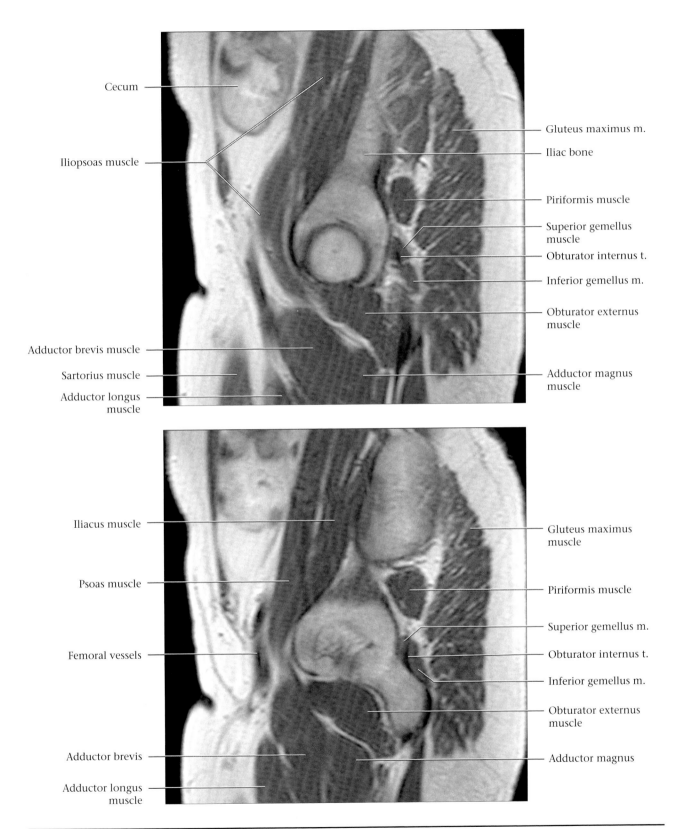

Cecum

Iliopsoas muscle

Gluteus maximus m.

Iliac bone

Piriformis muscle

Superior gemellus muscle

Obturator internus t.

Inferior gemellus m.

Obturator externus muscle

Adductor brevis muscle

Sartorius muscle

Adductor longus muscle

Adductor magnus muscle

Iliacus muscle

Psoas muscle

Femoral vessels

Adductor brevis

Adductor longus muscle

Gluteus maximus muscle

Piriformis muscle

Superior gemellus m.

Obturator internus t.

Inferior gemellus m.

Obturator externus muscle

Adductor magnus

(Top) The close relation between the iliopsoas muscle and the cecum explains the "psoas sign": Pain on extension of right thigh in patients with an inflamed retrocecal appendix. Inflammation in this area may irritate the iliopsoas muscle and cause spasm. (Bottom) The piriformis muscle exits the pelvis through the greater sciatic foramen and is anterior to the gluteus maximus muscle.

PELVIC WALL AND FLOOR

SAGITTAL T2 MR

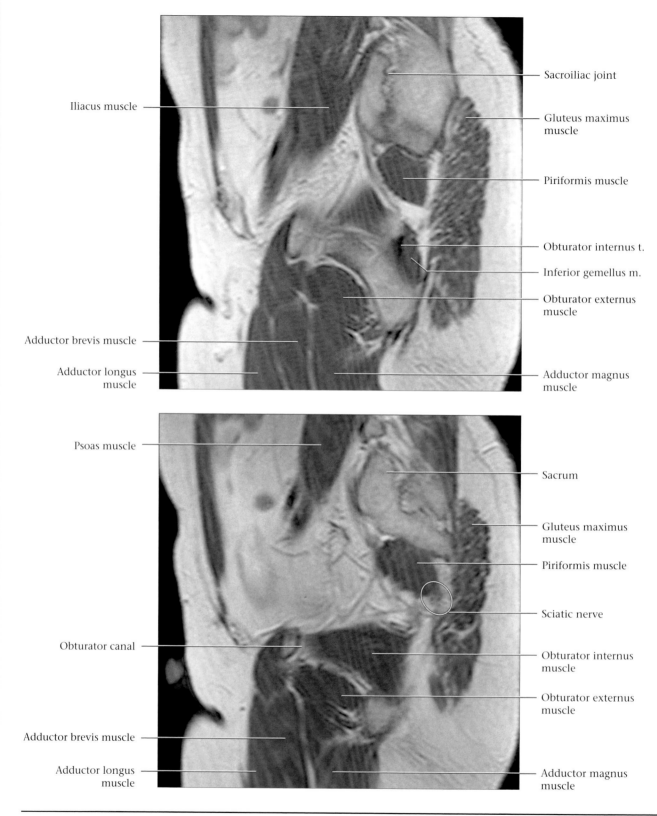

Iliacus muscle

Sacroiliac joint

Gluteus maximus muscle

Piriformis muscle

Obturator internus t.

Inferior gemellus m.

Obturator externus muscle

Adductor brevis muscle

Adductor longus muscle

Adductor magnus muscle

Psoas muscle

Sacrum

Gluteus maximus muscle

Piriformis muscle

Sciatic nerve

Obturator canal

Obturator internus muscle

Obturator externus muscle

Adductor brevis muscle

Adductor longus muscle

Adductor magnus muscle

(Top) More medially, the powerful group of adductor muscles (longus, brevis and magnus) are seen anterior and inferior to the obturator externus muscle. **(Bottom)** The sciatic nerve exits the pelvis through the greater sciatic foramen, inferior to the piriformis muscle. The piriformis syndrome is a condition in which the piriformis muscle irritates the sciatic nerve, causing pain in the buttocks and referred pain along the course of the sciatic nerve.

PELVIC WALL AND FLOOR

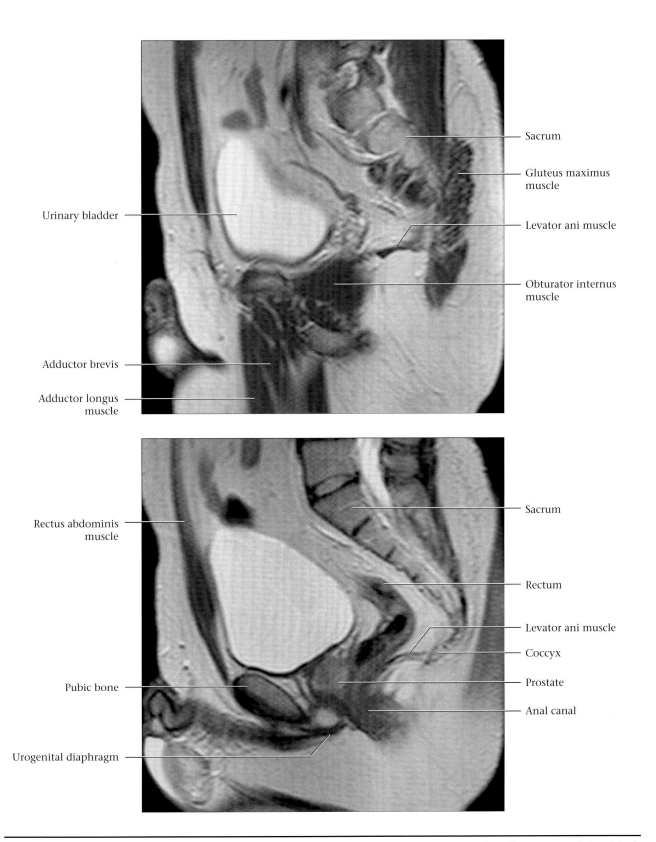

Sacrum

Gluteus maximus muscle

Levator ani muscle

Obturator internus muscle

Urinary bladder

Adductor brevis

Adductor longus muscle

Rectus abdominis muscle

Sacrum

Rectum

Levator ani muscle

Coccyx

Prostate

Anal canal

Pubic bone

Urogenital diaphragm

(Top) The levator ani muscle constitutes the pelvic diaphragm and provides support to the pelvic organs. It is critical for maintaining continence and aiding in normal micturition and defecation. **(Bottom)** The bladder neck, prostate and rectoanal junction are above or at the level of the pubococcygeal line, which extends from the last joint of the coccyx to the lower border of the symphysis pubis.

PELVIC WALL AND FLOOR

INGUINAL CANAL

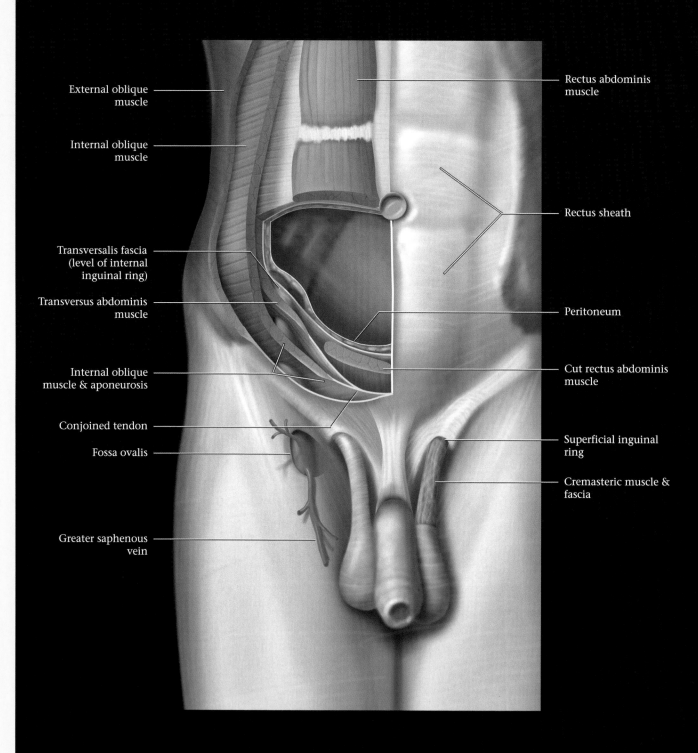

External oblique muscle

Internal oblique muscle

Transversalis fascia (level of internal inguinal ring)

Transversus abdominis muscle

Internal oblique muscle & aponeurosis

Conjoined tendon

Fossa ovalis

Greater saphenous vein

Rectus abdominis muscle

Rectus sheath

Peritoneum

Cut rectus abdominis muscle

Superficial inguinal ring

Cremasteric muscle & fascia

The muscle layers of the anterior pelvic wall have been separated to show the inguinal canal. The inguinal canal extends from the internal (deep) inguinal ring, an opening through transversalis fascia, to the external (superficial) inguinal ring, a triangular opening in the external oblique aponeurosis. The canal courses inferomedially and transmits the spermatic cord in males and the round ligament in females. It is formed embryologically by the processus vaginalis, an evagination of peritoneum through the abdominal wall. Failure of closure of the processus vaginalis (patent processus vaginalis) puts the patient at risk for an indirect inguinal hernia.

PELVIC WALL AND FLOOR

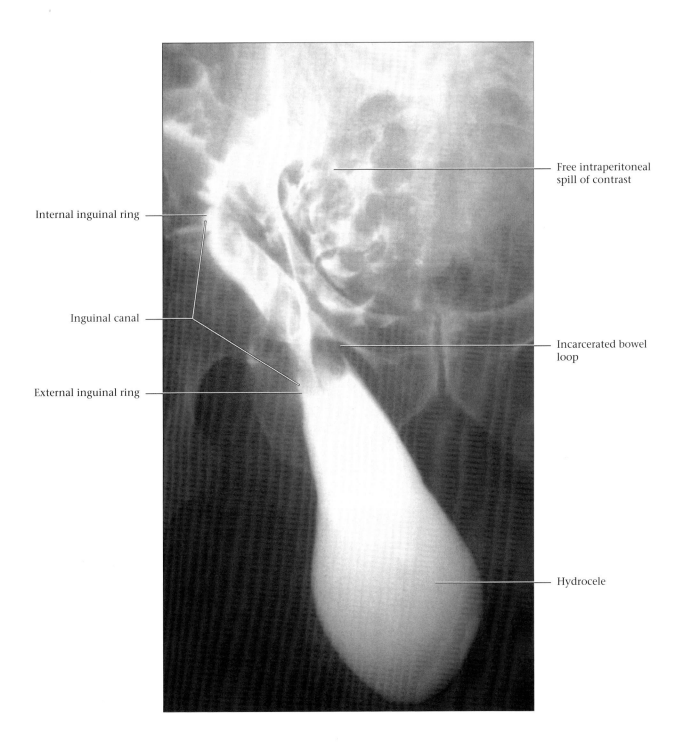

Internal inguinal ring

Inguinal canal

External inguinal ring

Free intraperitoneal spill of contrast

Incarcerated bowel loop

Hydrocele

Herniogram in a man with an indirect inguinal hernia. The right hemiscrotum was injected with contrast material and shows a patent processus vaginalis, with a large associated communicating hydrocele. A loop of bowel is seen as a filling defect within the inguinal canal. Surgery confirmed an indirect inguinal hernia, with an incarcerated small bowel loop at the external inguinal ring. Herniograms are an antiquated examination but it nicely demonstrates the course of the inguinal canal, which roughly parallels the superior pubic ramus.

CT, INDIRECT INGUINAL HERNIA

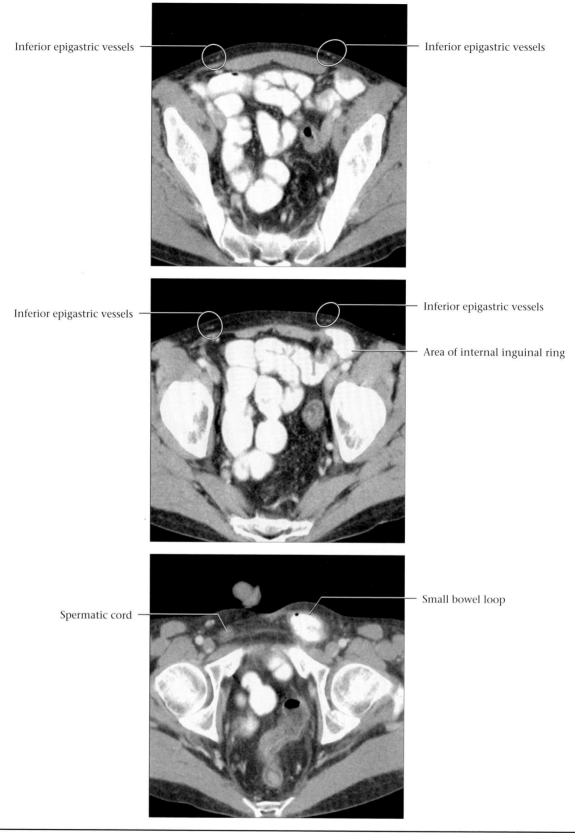

Inferior epigastric vessels — Inferior epigastric vessels

Inferior epigastric vessels — Inferior epigastric vessels

Area of internal inguinal ring

Spermatic cord — Small bowel loop

(Top) First of three CT images of a man with an indirect inguinal hernia. He had a palpable groin mass but no bowel obstruction. **(Middle)** The initial bulge through the abdominal wall is lateral to the inferior epigastric vessels. This represents the area of the internal inguinal ring. **(Bottom)** The course of an indirect inguinal hernia is lateral to medial, following the course of the spermatic cord (round ligament in females). The spermatic cord is being obscured by the hernia but the normal cord is seen on the opposite side. Herniated contents may extend into the scrotum in males or labia majora in females.

PELVIC WALL AND FLOOR

Rectus abdominis muscle

Inferior epigastric vessels

Area of Hesselbach triangle

Infarcted omentum in hernia

Inferior epigastric vessels

Infarcted omentum in hernia

Inferior epigastric vessels

Inferior epigastric vessels

(Top) First of three CT images of a man with a direct inguinal hernia. Direct inguinal hernias occur through Hesselbach triangle, a weakness in the lower pelvic wall. The triangle is formed by the inferior epigastric artery laterally, lateral edge of the rectus sheath medially, and inguinal ligament inferiorly. (Middle) The hernia is medial to the inferior epigastric vessels, which is an important imaging feature used to diagnose a direct inguinal hernia. (Bottom) Direct hernias are broad-based and dome-shaped, and seldom extend into the scrotum. A piece of infarcted omentum was found at surgery.

CT, FEMORAL HERNIA

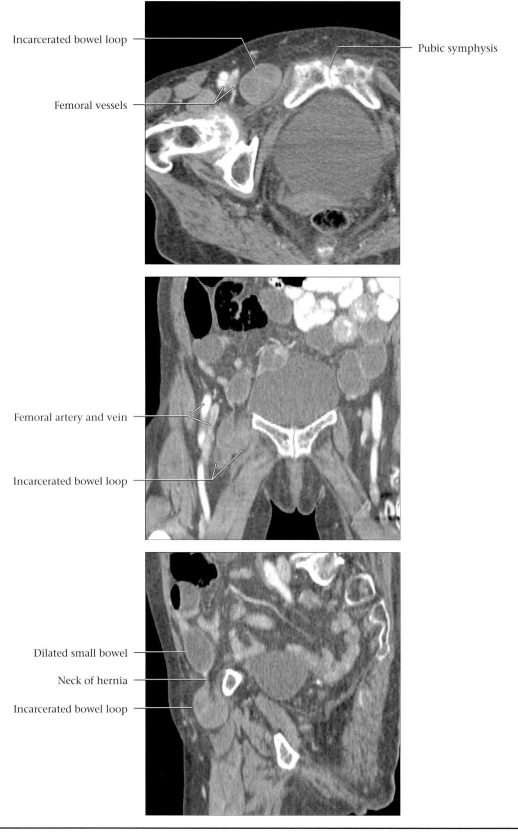

Incarcerated bowel loop

Pubic symphysis

Femoral vessels

Femoral artery and vein

Incarcerated bowel loop

Dilated small bowel

Neck of hernia

Incarcerated bowel loop

(Top) First of three CT images of an elderly woman with a small bowel obstruction secondary to an incarcerated femoral hernia. Femoral hernias traverse the femoral canal, which begins posterior to the medial portion of the inguinal ligament and ends at the fossa ovalis. Herniated contents are below the inguinal ligament, medial to the femoral vessels and lateral to the pubic tubercle. (Middle) Coronal reconstruction shows the proximity of the hernia to the femoral vessels. The neck is narrow, giving it a characteristic pear shape. (Bottom) Sagittal reconstruction shows the narrow neck of the femoral hernia, as the bowel loop passes underneath the inguinal ligament.

PELVIC WALL AND FLOOR

CT, OBTURATOR HERNIA

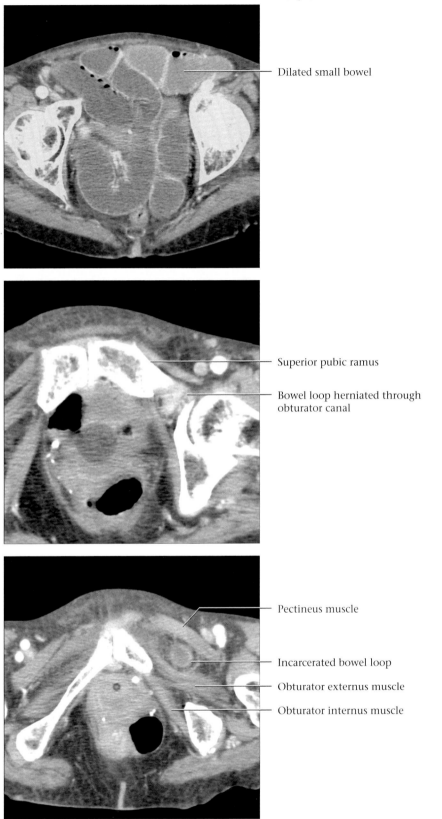

Dilated small bowel

Superior pubic ramus

Bowel loop herniated through obturator canal

Pectineus muscle

Incarcerated bowel loop

Obturator externus muscle

Obturator internus muscle

(Top) First of three CT images of a an elderly woman with a small bowel obstruction from an incarcerated obturator hernia. (Middle) The herniated loop of bowel is seen passing just beneath the superior pubic ramus. This is the obturator canal, which in the superolateral aspect of the obturator foramen. Normally only the obturator vessels and nerve pass through this foramen. (Bottom) The incarcerated bowel loop is between the pectineus and obturator externus muscles.

PELVIC WALL AND FLOOR

CT, SCIATIC HERNIA

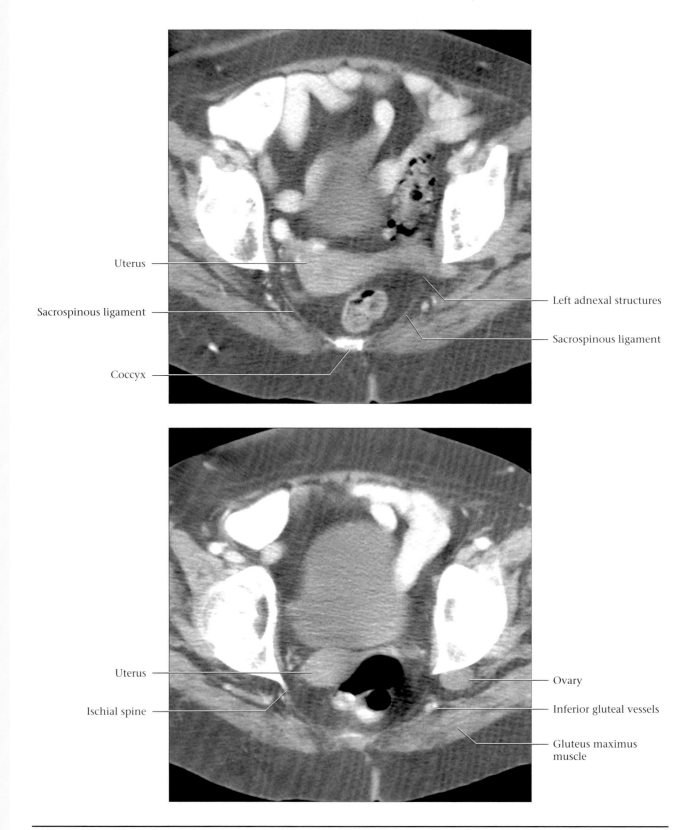

Uterus

Sacrospinous ligament

Coccyx

Left adnexal structures

Sacrospinous ligament

Uterus

Ischial spine

Ovary

Inferior gluteal vessels

Gluteus maximus muscle

(Top) First of two CT scans shows herniation of the left adnexa, including the ovary, fallopian tube and ligamentous supports through the greater sciatic foramen. The greater sciatic foramen is above the sacrospinous ligament, which runs from the ischial spine to the sacrum and coccyx. **(Bottom)** The ovary completely herniated through the greater sciatic foramen and is seen between the posterior acetabulum and gluteus maximus muscle.

PELVIC WALL AND FLOOR

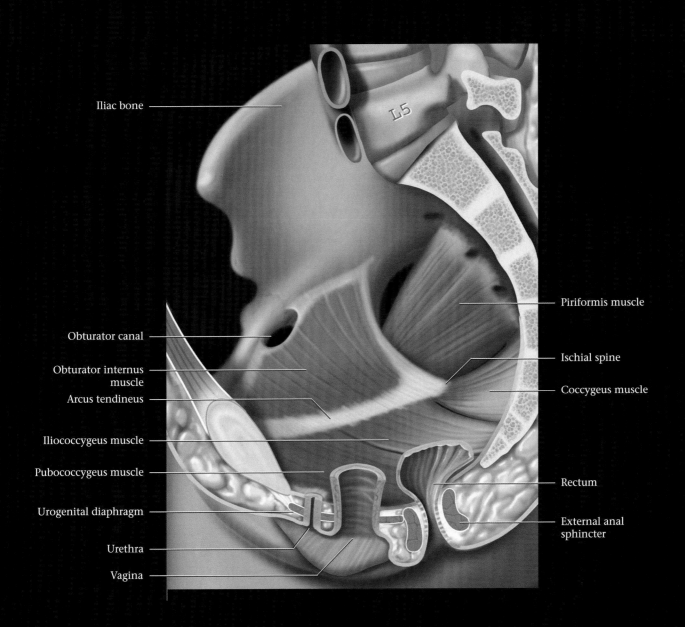

Iliac bone

Obturator canal

Obturator internus
muscle

Arcus tendineus

Iliococcygeus muscle

Pubococcygeus muscle

Urogenital diaphragm

Urethra

Vagina

L5

Piriformis muscle

Ischial spine

Coccygeus muscle

Rectum

External anal
sphincter

The true pelvis is bowl-shaped, so designation of walls is somewhat arbitrary. The pelvic floor is formed by the coccygeus muscles and the pelvic diaphragm (levator ani muscles and fascia). The levator ani is composed of three separate muscles: pubococcygeus, ileococcygeus and puborectalis. The levator ani is attached to the pubic bones anteriorly, the ischial spines laterally and to the arcus tendineus (thickening in the obturator fascia) between the bony attachments. The pelvic diaphragm separates the pelvic cavity from the perineum. The lateral and posterior walls of the true pelvis are formed by the obturator internus and piriformis muscles.

PELVIC WALL AND FLOOR

FEMALE PELVIC FLOOR/PERINEUM, INFERIOR VIEW

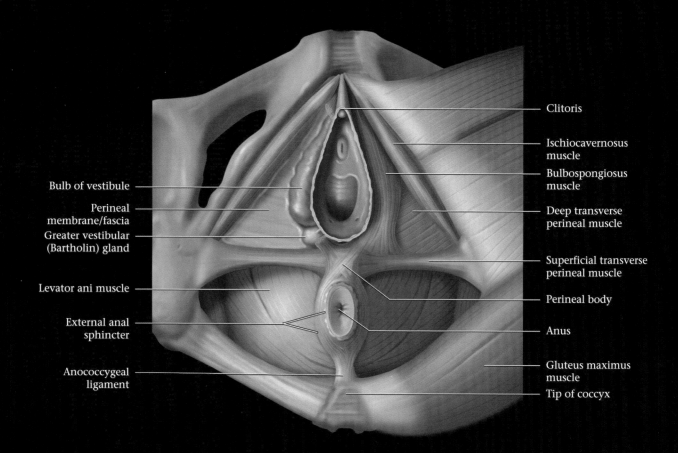

Bulb of vestibule

Perineal membrane/fascia

Greater vestibular (Bartholin) gland

Levator ani muscle

External anal sphincter

Anococcygeal ligament

Clitoris

Ischiocavernosus muscle

Bulbospongiosus muscle

Deep transverse perineal muscle

Superficial transverse perineal muscle

Perineal body

Anus

Gluteus maximus muscle

Tip of coccyx

The perineal body is a thickened, midline condensation of fibrous tissue at the midpoint of a line joining the ischial tuberosities. It is located between vagina and anus in females and between urethra and anus in males. At this point, several important muscles converge and are attached: The external anal sphincter, the paired bulbospongiosus muscles, the paired superficial transverse perineal muscles, and fibers of the levator ani. Stretching and tearing of the attachments of the perineal muscles from the perineal body can occur during childbirth, resulting in loss of support to the pelvic floor. This results in prolapse of pelvic viscera (cystocele, rectocele and/or enterocele).

PELVIC WALL AND FLOOR

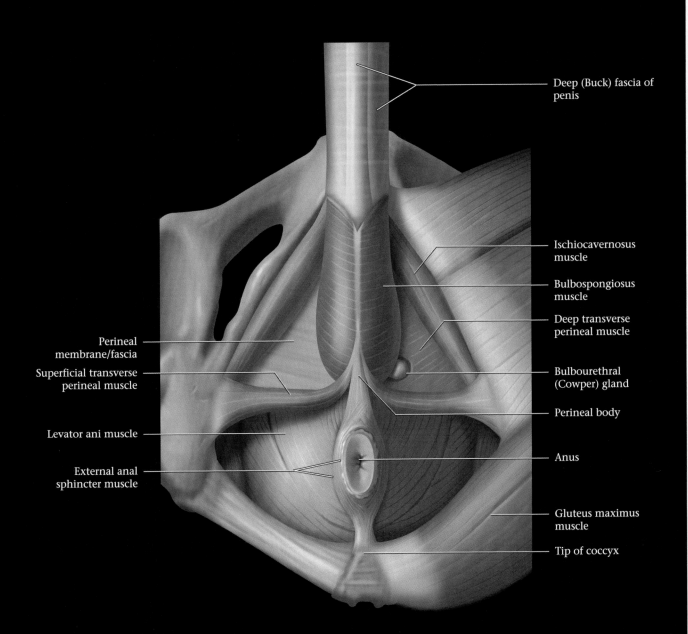

Deep (Buck) fascia of penis

Ischiocavernosus muscle

Bulbospongiosus muscle

Deep transverse perineal muscle

Bulbourethral (Cowper) gland

Perineal body

Anus

Gluteus maximus muscle

Tip of coccyx

Perineal membrane/fascia

Superficial transverse perineal muscle

Levator ani muscle

External anal sphincter muscle

The deep transverse perineal muscle is covered by a thin sheet of tough deep fascia called the perineal membrane. The membrane is pierced by the urethra (also vagina in females) and branches of the pudendal neurovascular bundle. The deep transverse perineal muscle and membrane form the urogenital diaphragm, and provide an attachment for the external genitalia. No such membrane exists posterior to the transverse perineal muscles (anal triangle). Note that in the male, the ischiocavernosus and bulbospongiosus muscles are far more developed than in the female.

PELVIC WALL AND FLOOR

UROGENITAL & ANAL TRIANGLE

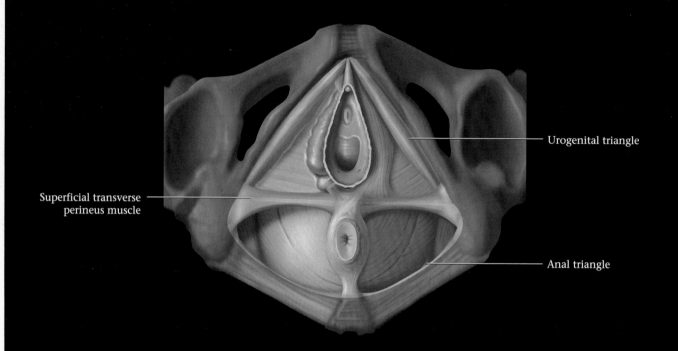

Urogenital triangle

Superficial transverse perineus muscle

Anal triangle

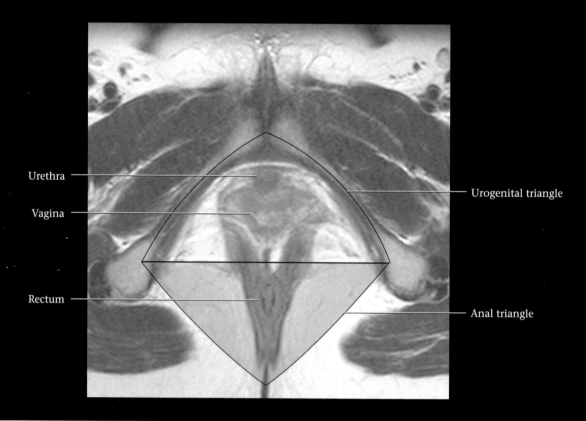

Urethra

Vagina

Rectum

Urogenital triangle

Anal triangle

(Top) The perineum is bordered by the symphysis pubis, ischial tuberosities and coccyx creating a diamond shape. It can be subdivided into two triangular compartments by a line drawn slightly anterior to the ischial tuberosities along the superficial transverse perineus muscle, creating the urogenital triangle anteriorly and the anal triangle posteriorly. **(Bottom)** Axial T2 MR of the perineum in a woman, with the urogenital and anal triangles superimposed. The urogenital triangle contains the urethra and vagina and the anal triangle contains the anus.

PELVIC WALL AND FLOOR

FEMALE PELVIC FLOOR, SUPERIOR & CORONAL VIEW

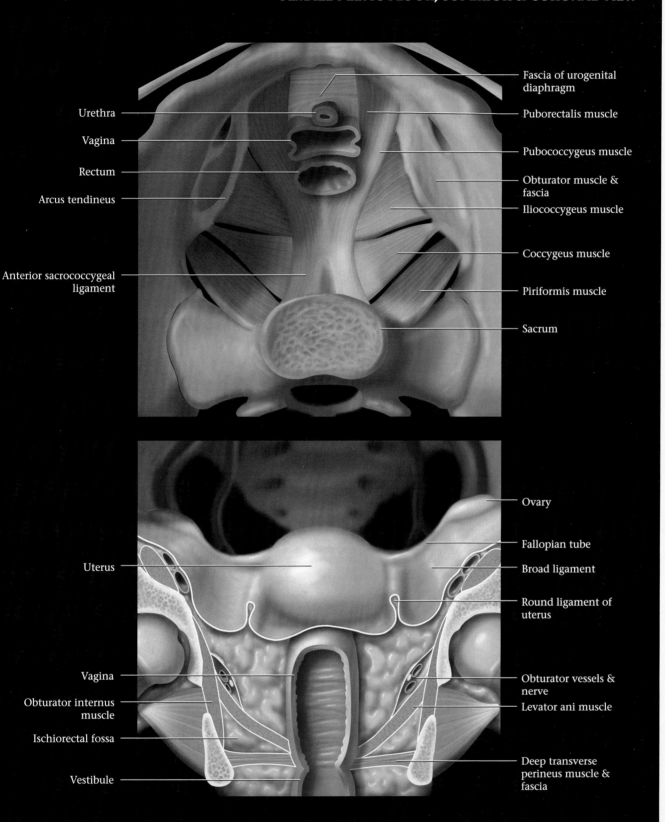

(Top) Superior view of the pelvic floor in a female. The levator ani is formed by the puborectalis, pubococcygeus and iliococcygeus muscles. The obturator internus is covered by a fascia, which forms a thick band, the arcus tendineus or tendinous arch of the levator ani. This is a crucial area of attachment for the levator ani. **(Bottom)** Coronal view of the pelvic floor in a female at the level of the vagina. The levator ani muscles form the pelvic floor through which the urethra, vagina and rectum pass, and is the main support for the pelvic organs. The perineum is space below the levator ani and includes the external genitalia. The deep transverse perineus muscle and fascia, along with the urethral sphincter, form the urogenital diaphragm.

PELVIC WALL AND FLOOR

AXIAL PELVIC FLOOR, FEMALE

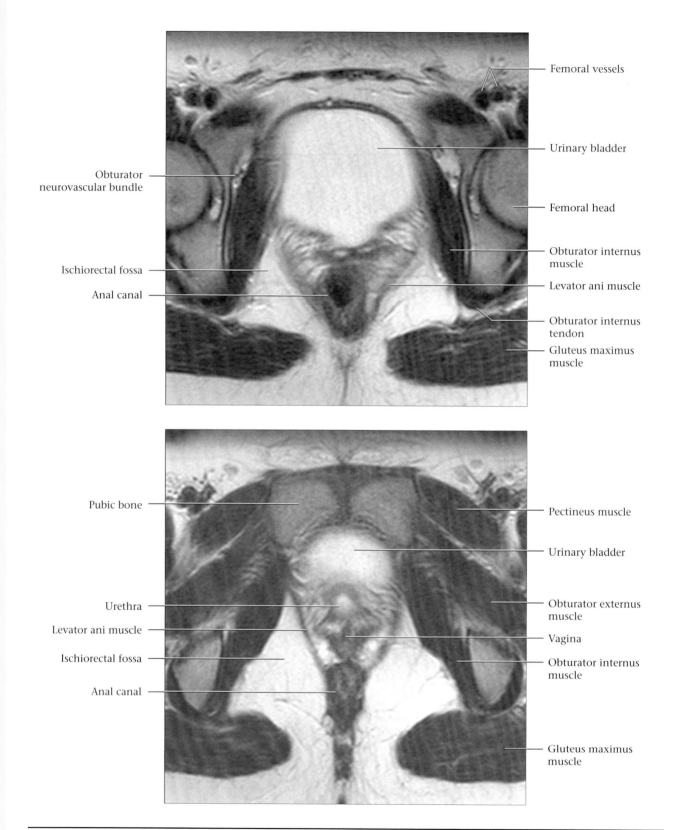

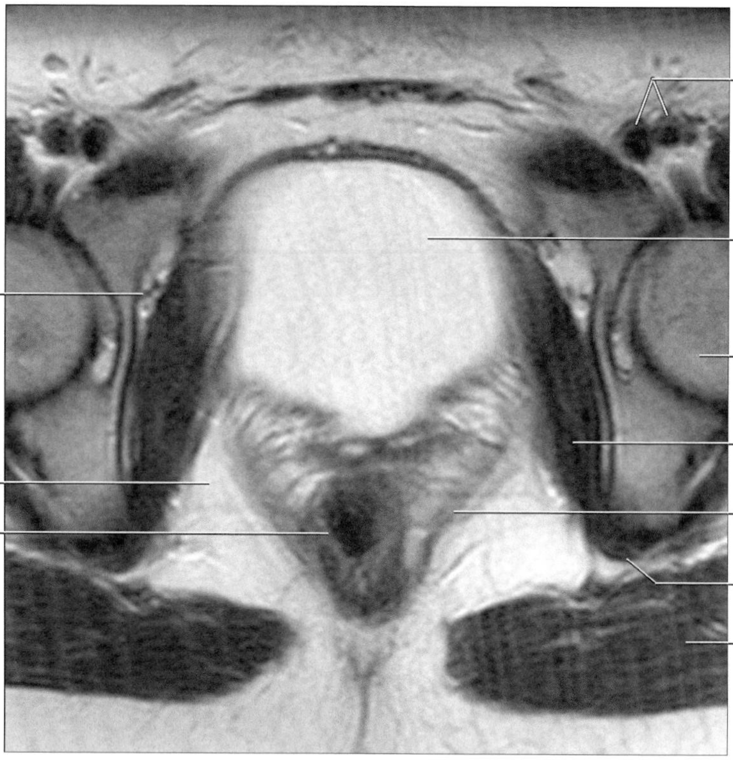
Femoral vessels
Urinary bladder
Obturator neurovascular bundle
Femoral head
Obturator internus muscle
Ischiorectal fossa
Levator ani muscle
Anal canal
Obturator internus tendon
Gluteus maximus muscle

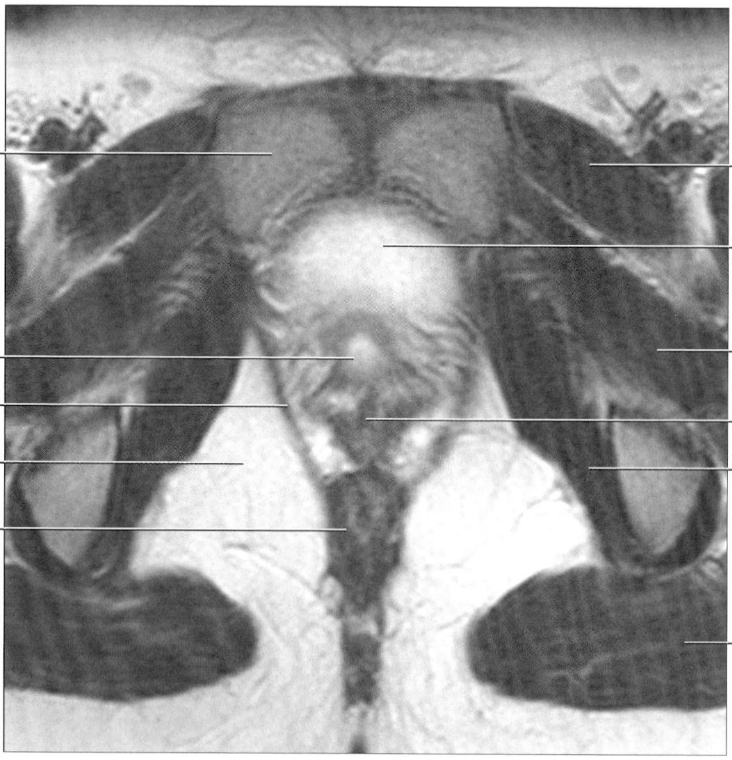
Pubic bone
Pectineus muscle
Urinary bladder
Urethra
Obturator externus muscle
Levator ani muscle
Vagina
Ischiorectal fossa
Obturator internus muscle
Anal canal
Gluteus maximus muscle

(Top) First of four axial T2 MR images of the pelvic floor in a female. **(Bottom)** The levator ani is composed of three muscles: The pubococcygeus, iliococcygeus and puborectalis muscles. The muscle fibers blend and therefore can not be discerned as three separate muscles by imaging. The iliococcygeus arises from the ischial spines and arcus tendineus and is the broadest, most posterior portion of the levator ani. Its most posterior fibers form the anococcygeal ligament. The pubococcygeus is more anterior arising from the posterior surface of the pubis and arcus tendineus.

PELVIC WALL AND FLOOR

AXIAL PELVIC FLOOR, FEMALE

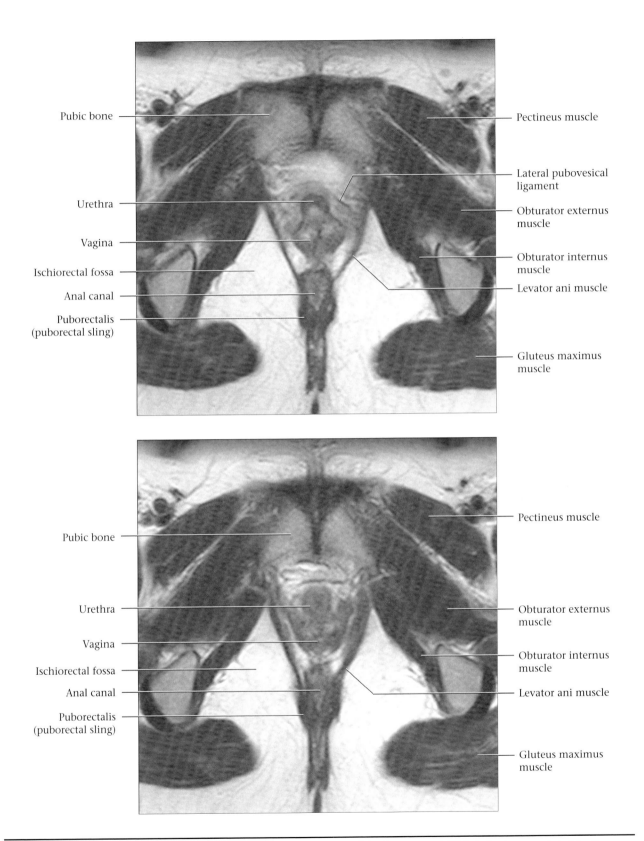

Pubic bone

Urethra

Vagina

Ischiorectal fossa

Anal canal

Puborectalis
(puborectal sling)

Pectineus muscle

Lateral pubovesical
ligament

Obturator externus
muscle

Obturator internus
muscle

Levator ani muscle

Gluteus maximus
muscle

Pubic bone

Urethra

Vagina

Ischiorectal fossa

Anal canal

Puborectalis
(puborectal sling)

Pectineus muscle

Obturator externus
muscle

Obturator internus
muscle

Levator ani muscle

Gluteus maximus
muscle

(Top) The puborectalis is the third and most prominent portion of the levator ani. This is best appreciated in the axial plane. It fuses with fibers from the opposite side to form puborectal sling, which along with the external anal sphincter, maintains fecal continence. Several studies have shown that the left side of the puborectal sling is thicker than the right side. **(Bottom)** The urethra, vagina and rectum are surrounded by the levator ani muscles and ultimately pass through them into the perineum. The vagina often has an H- or U-shaped configuration which is the result of lateral fascial support provided by the levator ani.

PELVIC WALL AND FLOOR

CORONAL PELVIC FLOOR, MALE

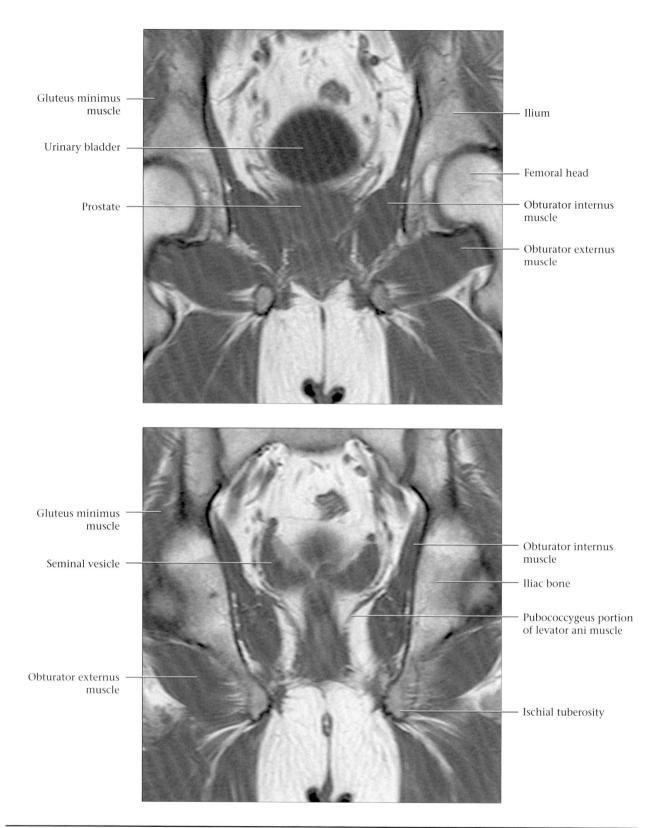

Gluteus minimus muscle

Urinary bladder

Prostate

Ilium

Femoral head

Obturator internus muscle

Obturator externus muscle

Gluteus minimus muscle

Seminal vesicle

Obturator externus muscle

Obturator internus muscle

Iliac bone

Pubococcygeus portion of levator ani muscle

Ischial tuberosity

(Top) First of four coronal T1 MR images of the pelvic floor in a male. The true pelvis in a male is much more narrow than that of the female. **(Bottom)** The bowel-shaped nature of the levator ani is well appreciated on the coronal view. Although it can not be discerned as a separate muscle by imaging, the most anterior portion of the levator ani is the pubococcygeus muscle.

PELVIC WALL AND FLOOR

CORONAL PELVIC FLOOR, MALE

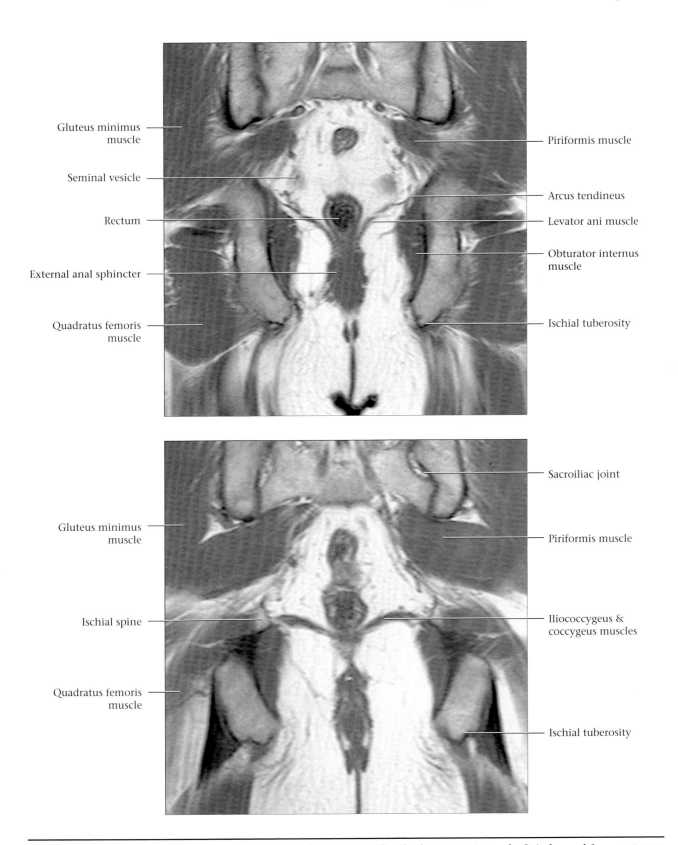

Gluteus minimus muscle

Seminal vesicle

Rectum

External anal sphincter

Quadratus femoris muscle

Piriformis muscle

Arcus tendineus

Levator ani muscle

Obturator internus muscle

Ischial tuberosity

Gluteus minimus muscle

Ischial spine

Quadratus femoris muscle

Sacroiliac joint

Piriformis muscle

Iliococcygeus & coccygeus muscles

Ischial tuberosity

(Top) The arcus tendineus is an important source of attachment for the levator ani muscle. It is formed from a strong fascial membrane covering the obturator internus muscle. **(Bottom)** The iliococcygeus forms the most posterior portion of the levator ani muscle. It arises from the arcus tendineus and ischial spines, and inserts on the sacrum and coccyx. The coccygeus muscle also arises from the ischial spine and likewise inserts on the sacrum and coccyx. The coccygeus forms the most posterior support of the pelvic floor. It may not be seen as a discrete muscle but note the thickening of muscle fibers in this area.

PELVIC WALL AND FLOOR

CORONAL PELVIC FLOOR, FEMALE

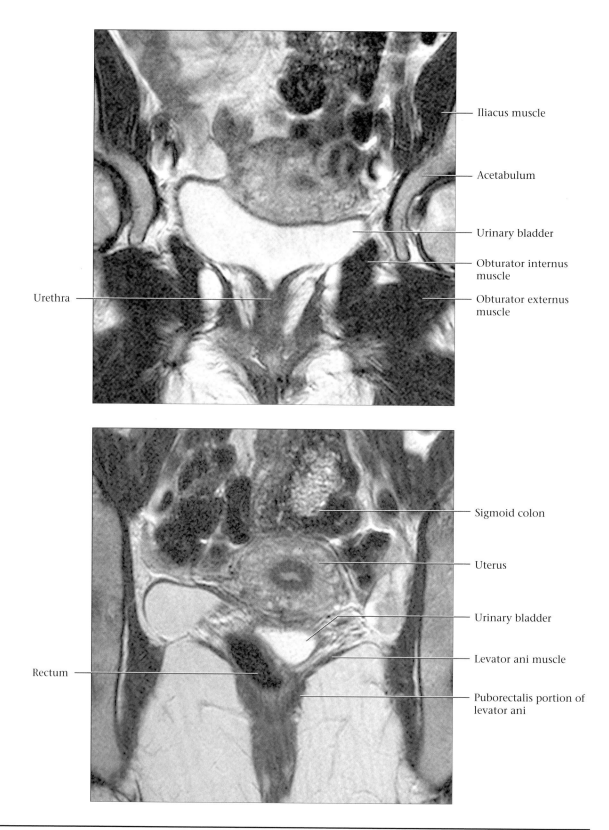

Iliacus muscle

Acetabulum

Urinary bladder

Obturator internus muscle

Obturator externus muscle

Urethra

Sigmoid colon

Uterus

Urinary bladder

Levator ani muscle

Puborectalis portion of levator ani

Rectum

(Top) First of four coronal T2 MR images of the pelvic floor in a female. (Bottom) At the rectum, muscle fibers from the puborectalis portion of the levator ani (puborectal sling) merge with those of the external anal sphincter.

PELVIC WALL AND FLOOR

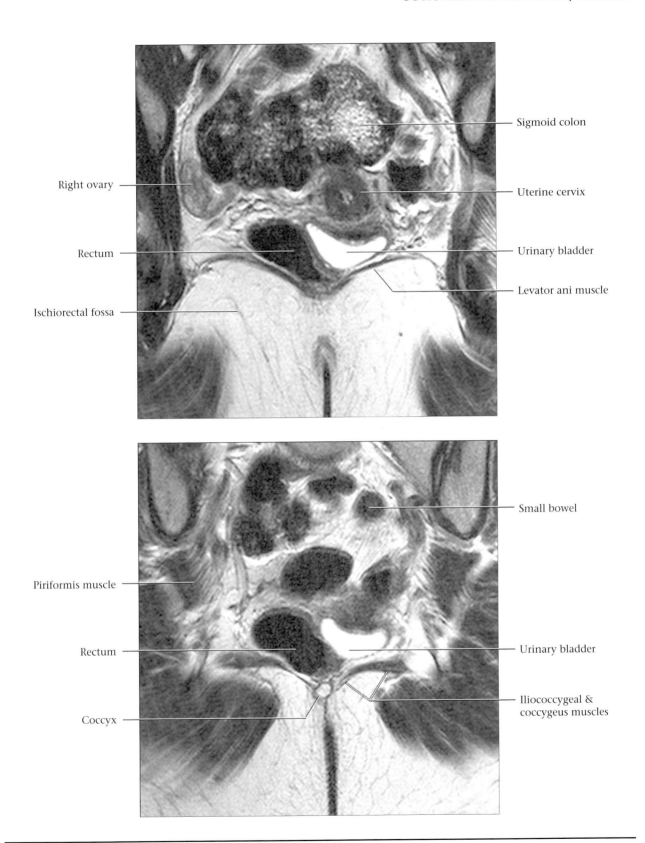

Sigmoid colon

Right ovary

Uterine cervix

Rectum

Urinary bladder

Levator ani muscle

Ischiorectal fossa

Small bowel

Piriformis muscle

Rectum

Urinary bladder

Coccyx

Iliococcygeal & coccygeus muscles

(Top) The levator ani muscles forms the pelvic diaphragm and is the primary support for the pelvic viscera. The coronal plane nicely shows the levator ani separating the pelvic organs above, from the perineum and ischiorectal fossa below. Also note how wide the true pelvis is when compared to the male. **(Bottom)** Both the iliococcygeus (posterior portion of levator ani muscle) and coccygeus muscles insert on the coccyx and sacrum.

PELVIC WALL AND FLOOR

SAGITTAL PELVIC FLOOR, MALE

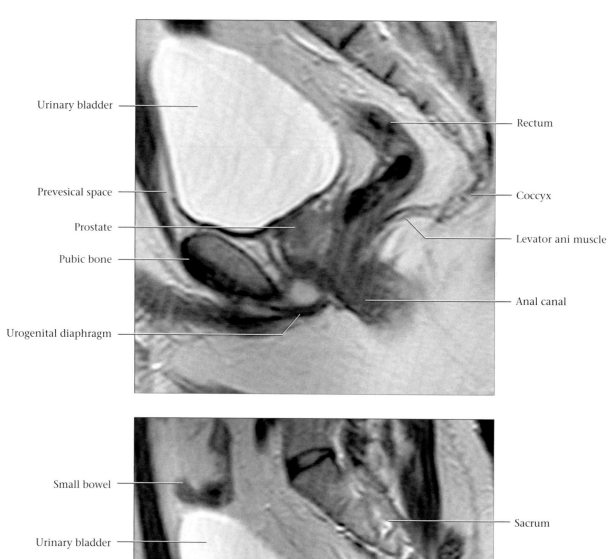

Urinary bladder

Prevesical space

Prostate

Pubic bone

Urogenital diaphragm

Rectum

Coccyx

Levator ani muscle

Anal canal

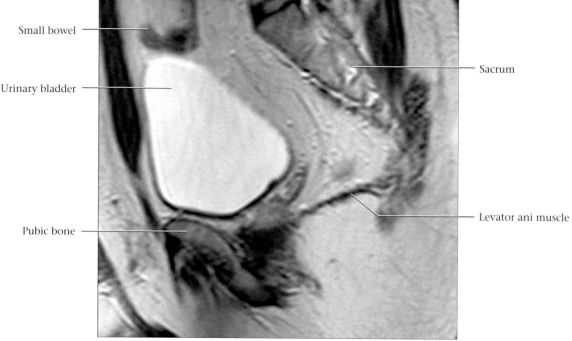

Small bowel

Urinary bladder

Pubic bone

Sacrum

Levator ani muscle

(**Top**) First of two sagittal T2 MR images of the pelvic floor in a male. The urogenital diaphragm is formed by the deep transverse perineus muscle and fascia and the urethral sphincter. Urethral injury following trauma is most common in this area. (**Bottom**) The levator ani extends posteriorly to insert on the coccyx and sacrum.

PELVIC WALL AND FLOOR

SAGITTAL PELVIC FLOOR, FEMALE

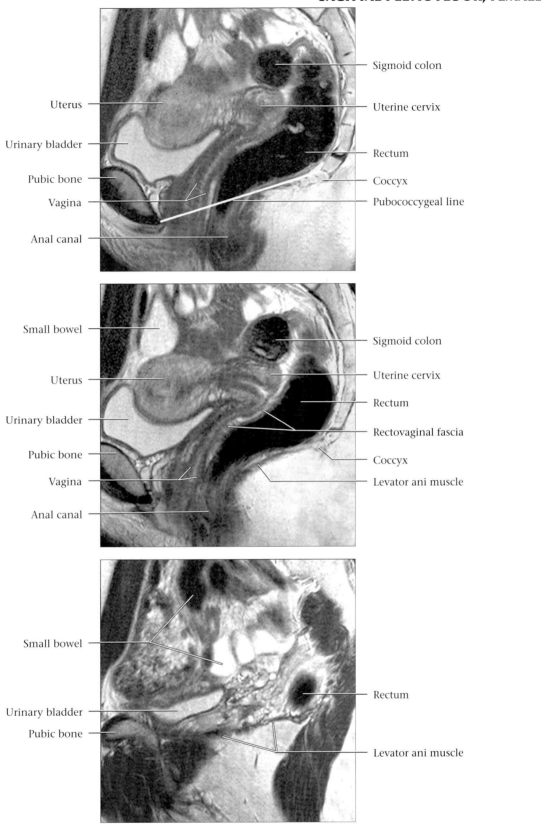

Uterus

Urinary bladder

Pubic bone

Vagina

Anal canal

Sigmoid colon

Uterine cervix

Rectum

Coccyx

Pubococcygeal line

Small bowel

Uterus

Urinary bladder

Pubic bone

Vagina

Anal canal

Sigmoid colon

Uterine cervix

Rectum

Rectovaginal fascia

Coccyx

Levator ani muscle

Small bowel

Urinary bladder

Pubic bone

Rectum

Levator ani muscle

(Top) The first of three sagittal T2 MR images of the pelvis in a female showing the relationship of the pelvic organs to a line extending from the lower border of the pubic symphysis to the last joint of the coccyx (pubococcygeal line). This line represents the plane of pelvic floor. In normal, continent women the bladder neck, vaginal fornices and anorectal junction are at or above the pubococcygeal line. **(Middle)** The posterior vaginal wall and fascial condensation called the rectovaginal fascia support the rectum and prevent formation of an enterocele or rectocele. **(Bottom)** The full length of the pelvic diaphragm is well appreciated on a sagittal view lateral to the midline. The levator ani muscle group has a broad area of attachment including the pubic bones, arcus tendineus, ischial spines, sacrum and coccyx.

PELVIC FLOOR RELAXATION

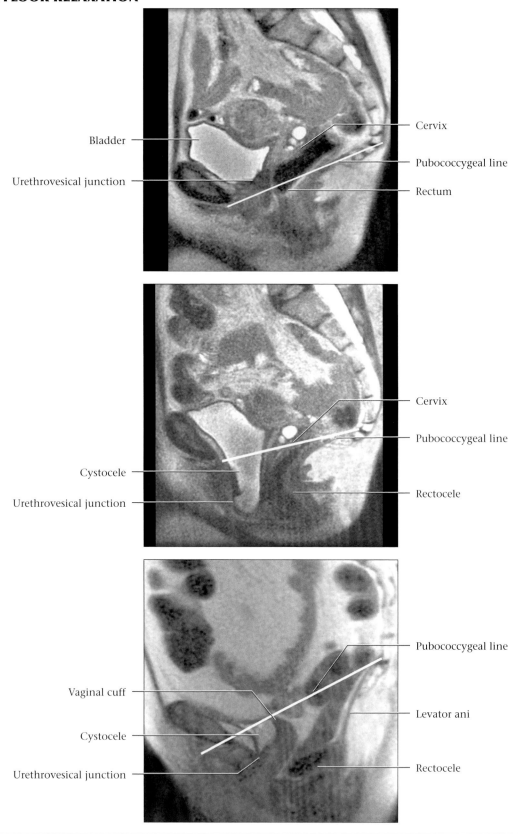

Bladder

Urethrovesical junction

Cervix

Pubococcygeal line

Rectum

Cystocele

Urethrovesical junction

Cervix

Pubococcygeal line

Rectocele

Vaginal cuff

Cystocele

Urethrovesical junction

Pubococcygeal line

Levator ani

Rectocele

(Top) First of two dynamic T2 MR images in a women with pelvic floor descent. On the relaxed view, the urethrovesical junction and cervix lie above the pubococcygeal line. **(Middle)** With straining, there is pelvic floor descent with a cystocele and rectocele. The uterus has also descended, with the external os now at the pubococcygeal line. **(Bottom)** Sagittal T2 MR taken during straining in a different patient shows a cystocele, vaginocele and rectocele. Note the abnormal vertical orientation of the levator ani.

PELVIC WALL AND FLOOR

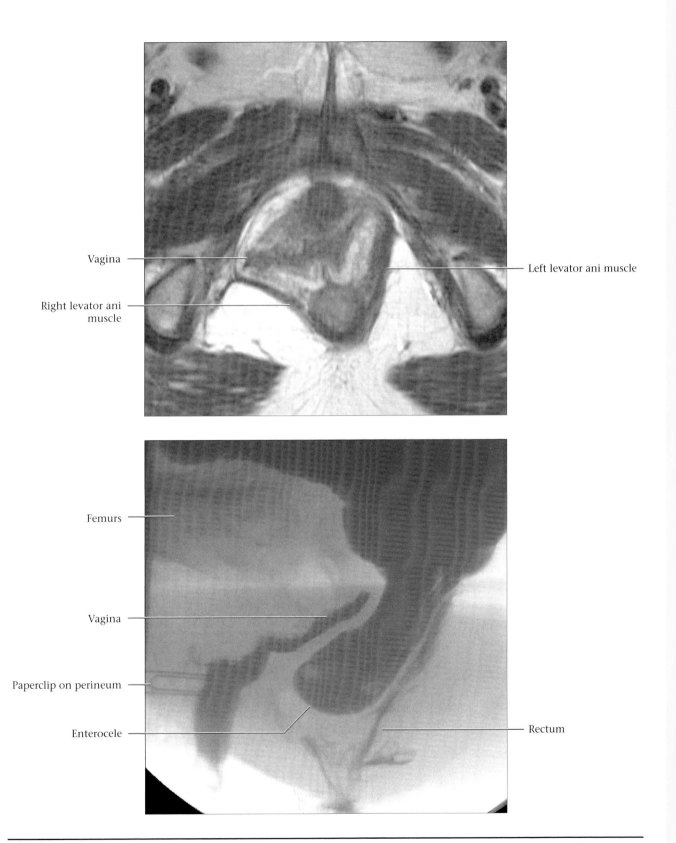

Vagina

Right levator ani muscle

Left levator ani muscle

Femurs

Vagina

Paperclip on perineum

Enterocele

Rectum

(Top) Axial T2 MR shows an abnormal right levator ani muscle in a woman with pelvic floor relaxation. Note the loss of support for the right side of the vagina, which now is directed horizontally rather than maintaining the H-shape configuration as seen on the left. **(Bottom)** Enterocele in an elderly woman. The small bowel is filled with barium, with a small amount in the vagina and rectum to serve as markers (the perineum is marked by a paperclip). The patient is placed in the lateral position and images are obtained at rest and with straining. During straining (image shown), there is pelvic floor descent with small bowel prolapsing between the vagina and rectum. Normally, the rectovaginal fascia forms a supporting barrier, and bowel can not descend into this space.

VESSELS, LYMPHATIC SYSTEM AND NERVES

Imaging Anatomy

Arteries

- **Abdominal aorta**
  - **Testicular and ovarian arteries** originate below renal arteries
  - **Median (middle) sacral artery** is small, unpaired branch from posterior aspect of distal aorta
  - Divides into common iliac arteries at L4-5
- **Common iliac arteries**
  - Run anterior to iliac veins and inferior vena cava (IVC)
  - Usually no major branches
    - Rarely, gives off aberrant iliolumbar or accessory renal arteries
  - Approximately 4 cm long
- **External iliac artery**
  - No major branches
  - Exits pelvis beneath inguinal ligament
  - Larger than internal iliac artery
  - **Inferior epigastric** (medial) and **deep iliac circumflex** (lateral) arteries demarcate junction between external iliac and common femoral arteries
- **Internal iliac (hypogastric) artery**
  - Principal vascular supply of pelvic organs
  - Divides into anterior and posterior trunk
    - Anterior trunk to pelvic viscera
    - Posterior trunk to pelvic musculature
- **Anterior trunk of internal iliac artery**
  - Branching pattern quite variable
  - **Umbilical artery**
    - Only pelvic segment remains patent after birth
    - Remainder becomes the fibrous **medial umbilical ligament**
  - **Obturator artery**
    - Exits pelvis through obturator canal to supply medial thigh muscles
  - **Superior vesicle artery**
    - Supplies bladder and distal ureter
    - Gives off branch to ductus deferens in males
  - **Inferior vesicle artery** (male)
    - May arise from middle rectal artery
    - Supplies prostate, seminal vesicles and lower ureters
  - **Uterine artery** (female)
    - Courses through cardinal ligament, at base of broad ligament
    - Passes over ureter at level of cervix ("water under the bridge")
    - Anastomoses with vaginal and ovarian arteries
  - **Vaginal artery** (women)
  - **Middle rectal artery** runs above pelvic floor and anastomoses with superior and inferior rectal arteries to supply rectum
    - Superior rectal artery continuation of inferior mesenteric artery
    - Inferior rectal artery is branch of internal pudendal artery and runs below pelvic floor
    - Also anastomoses with inferior vesicle artery to help supply prostate and seminal vesicles
  - **Internal pudendal artery**
    - Supplies external genitalia (penis, clitoris) and rectum

- Long complex course
- Exits pelvis through greater sciatic foramen
- Curves around sacrospinous ligament to enter perineum through lesser sciatic foramen
  - **Inferior gluteal (sciatic) artery**
    - Largest and terminal branch of anterior division of hypogastric artery
    - Passes between either 1st and 2nd or 2nd and 3rd sacral nerves
    - Exits pelvis below piriformis muscle
    - Supplies muscles of pelvic floor, thigh, buttocks and sciatic nerve
- **Posterior division of internal iliac artery**
  - **Iliolumbar artery**
    - Ascends laterally to supply iliacus, psoas and quadratus lumborum muscles
  - **Lateral sacral artery**
    - Runs medially toward sacral foramina to anastomose with middle sacral artery
  - **Superior gluteal artery**
    - Largest and terminal branch of posterior division
    - Exits pelvis through greater sciatic foramen, superior to piriformis muscle
    - Supplies piriformis and gluteal muscles

Veins

- **External iliac vein**
  - Upward continuation of femoral vein at level of inguinal ligament
  - Receives inferior epigastric, deep iliac circumflex, and pubic veins
- **Internal iliac vein** begins near upper part of greater sciatic foramen
  - Gluteal, internal pudendal and obturator veins have origins outside pelvis
  - Pelvic viscera drain into multiple, deep pelvic venous plexuses
    - These drain into veins, which roughly parallel pelvic arteries
- **Right gonadal vein** drains into IVC, **left gonadal vein** drains into left renal vein
- **Common iliac vein** is formed by union of external and internal iliac veins
  - Unites with contralateral side to form IVC

Lymphatics

- **Superficial inguinal nodes**
  - In superficial fascia parallel to inguinal ligament, along cephalad portion of greater saphenous vein
  - Receive lymphatic drainage from superficial lower extremity, superficial abdominal wall and perineum
  - Flow into deep inguinal and external iliac nodes
- **Deep inguinal nodes**
  - Along medial side of femoral vein, deep to fascia lata and inguinal ligament
  - Receive lymphatic drainage from superficial inguinal and popliteal nodes
  - Flow into external iliac nodes
  - Deep inguinal node in femoral canal is called gland or node of Cloquet
- **External iliac nodes**
  - Along external iliac vessels
  - Primary drainage from inguinal nodes
  - Flow into common iliac nodes

VESSELS, LYMPHATIC SYSTEM AND NERVES

- **Internal iliac nodes**
  - Along internal iliac vessels
  - Drainage from inferior pelvic viscera, deep perineum and gluteal region
  - Flow into common iliac nodes
- **Common iliac nodes**
  - Along common iliac vessels
  - Drainage from external iliac, internal iliac and sacral nodes
  - Flow into lumbar (lateral aortic) chain of nodes

Nerves

- **Sacral plexus**
  - Coalescence of lumbar and sacral nerves
    - L4 (minor branch), L5
    - S1-3 (ventral rami), S4 (minor branch)
- **Sciatic nerve**
  - Upper band and major branch of sacral plexus
  - Runs on ventral surface of piriformis muscle
  - Broadest nerve in body (2 cm)
  - **Exits pelvis through greater sciatic foramen**, below piriformis
  - Innervates capsule of hip joint, posterior thigh and leg muscles
- **Pudendal nerve**
  - Lower band of sacral plexus
    - Ventral rami of S2-4
  - Follows internal pudendal artery
    - Exits pelvis through greater sciatic foramen
    - Curves around sacrospinous ligament to enter perineum through lesser sciatic foramen
    - **Pudendal canal** on lateral wall of ischiorectal fossa
  - Major nerve supply to perineum and external anal sphincter
- **Obturator nerve**
  - Anterior branches of L2-4 ventral rami
  - Follows obturator vessels, exiting pelvis through obturator foramen
  - Innervates hip adductors
- **Femoral nerve**
  - Posterior branches of L2-4 ventral rami
  - Descends through psoas muscle into iliopsoas groove
  - Exits pelvis beneath inguinal ligament through **femoral canal**
    - Most lateral structure in femoral canal
    - Acronym for **femoral canal** contents from lateral to medial = NAVL (nerve, artery, vein, lymphatic)
  - Branches innervate anteromedial thigh

Anatomy-Based Imaging Issues

Imaging Recommendations

- CT angiography (CTA) and MR angiography (MRA) are imaging modalities of choice to evaluate pelvic vessels
  - 3D reconstructions and maximum intensity projections (MIP) rotated in 360° for complete evaluation
- Delayed imaging (180 seconds) for evaluation of pelvic veins
- Conventional angiography for therapy (embolization)

Clinical Implications

Arterial

- **Collateral circulation**
  - Rich, complex collateral circulation helps ensure delivery of blood to pelvic organs and lower limbs in event of proximal obstruction
  - **Common iliac artery obstruction**
    - Ipsilateral lumbar and contralateral lateral sacral→ internal iliac → retrograde into external iliac artery
  - **Internal iliac artery obstruction**
    - Lumbar → iliolumbar arteries
    - Median sacral → lateral sacral arteries
    - Superior rectal → inferior rectal arteries
    - Deep femoral artery → femoral circumflex branches → inferior gluteal arteries
  - **External iliac artery obstruction**
    - Posterior trunk of internal iliac → deep iliac circumflex artery → common femoral artery
    - Anterior trunk of internal iliac → circumflex femoral branches of deep femoral artery

Venous

- **Rectal plexus** is a major site of porto-systemic collaterals in patients with portal hypertension
  - Hemorrhoids represent engorged collaterals
- **Ovarian vein thrombosis**
  - Postpartum septic thrombosis of ovarian vein
  - 90% occur on right side
- **May-Thurner syndrome**
  - Compression, thrombosis and eventually occlusion of upper left common iliac vein as it passes between the right common iliac artery and spine
- **Rectal carcinoma**
  - Hematogenous spread of metastases depends on location of primary tumor
  - Lower two thirds→ internal iliac veins→ lungs
  - Upper third→ inferior mesenteric vein→ liver

Lymphatic

- **Testicular carcinoma** drains according to site of primary tumor
  - Lymphatics follow venous drainage
  - Right-sided tumors first spread to infrarenal, precaval and aortocaval nodes
  - Left-sided tumors initially spread to left para-aortic nodes near renal hilum
- Ovarian lymphatics follow same course, however, ovarian cancer more often spreads by direct peritoneal seeding

Nerves

- **Piriformis syndrome**
  - Piriformis muscle may irritate sciatic nerve, causing pain in buttocks and referred pain along course of sciatic nerve
- **Pudendal nerve block**
  - Not as frequently utilized secondary to increased use of epidurals
  - Performed either transvaginally or perineally
  - Needle directed toward ischial spine where pudendal nerve curves around into pudendal canal

VESSELS, LYMPHATIC SYSTEM AND NERVES

PELVIC ARTERIES

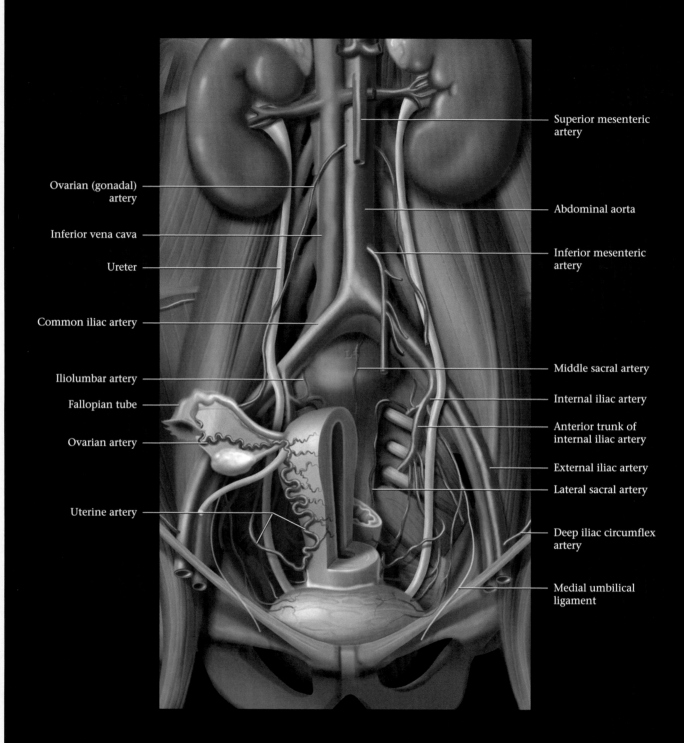

Ovarian (gonadal) artery

Inferior vena cava

Ureter

Common iliac artery

Iliolumbar artery

Fallopian tube

Ovarian artery

Uterine artery

Superior mesenteric artery

Abdominal aorta

Inferior mesenteric artery

Middle sacral artery

Internal iliac artery

Anterior trunk of internal iliac artery

External iliac artery

Lateral sacral artery

Deep iliac circumflex artery

Medial umbilical ligament

Frontal graphic of the abdominal aorta, inferior vena cava, and the iliac vessels in a female. The inferior mesenteric artery is the smallest of the anterior mesenteric branches of the aorta and continues in the pelvis as the superior rectal artery. The paired ovarian arteries arise from the aorta below the renal arteries and pass inferiorly on the posterior abdominal wall to enter the pelvis. The ureters cross anterior to the bifurcation of the common iliac arteries on their way to the urinary bladder. The common iliac artery divides into the external iliac artery, which supplies the lower extremity and the internal iliac (hypogastric) artery, which supplies the pelvis. The internal iliac artery divides into an anterior trunk for the pelvic viscera and a posterior trunk for the muscles of the pelvis.

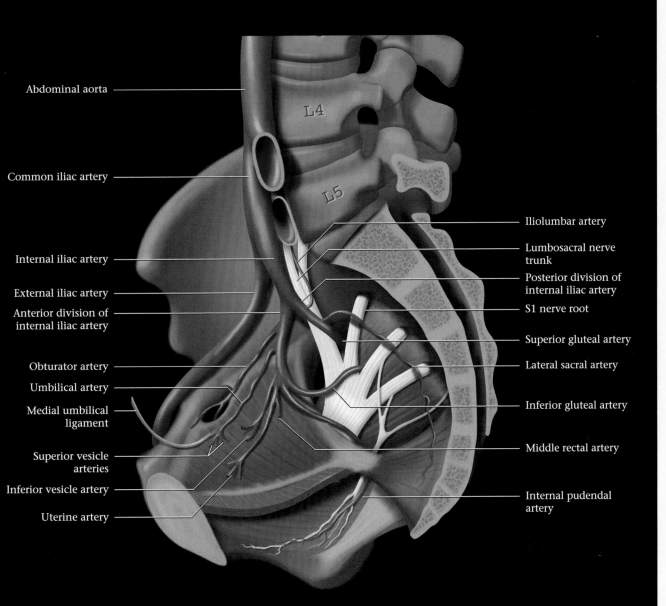

Abdominal aorta

Common iliac artery

Internal iliac artery

External iliac artery

Anterior division of internal iliac artery

Obturator artery

Umbilical artery

Medial umbilical ligament

Superior vesicle arteries

Inferior vesicle artery

Uterine artery

Iliolumbar artery

Lumbosacral nerve trunk

Posterior division of internal iliac artery

S1 nerve root

Superior gluteal artery

Lateral sacral artery

Inferior gluteal artery

Middle rectal artery

Internal pudendal artery

Graphic of the pelvic arteries and their relation to the sacral nerves. The superior gluteal artery passes posteriorly and runs between the lumbosacral trunk and the anterior ramus of the S1 nerve, whereas the inferior gluteal artery usually runs between the S1-2 or S2-3 nerve roots to leave the pelvis through the inferior part of the greater sciatic foramen. Only the proximal portion of the umbilical arteries remains patent after birth, while the distal portion obliterates forming the medial umbilical ligaments. Arteries to the deep pelvic viscera include the superior and inferior vesicle, uterine, middle rectal and internal pudendal. The individual branching pattern is quite variable.

PELVIC VEINS

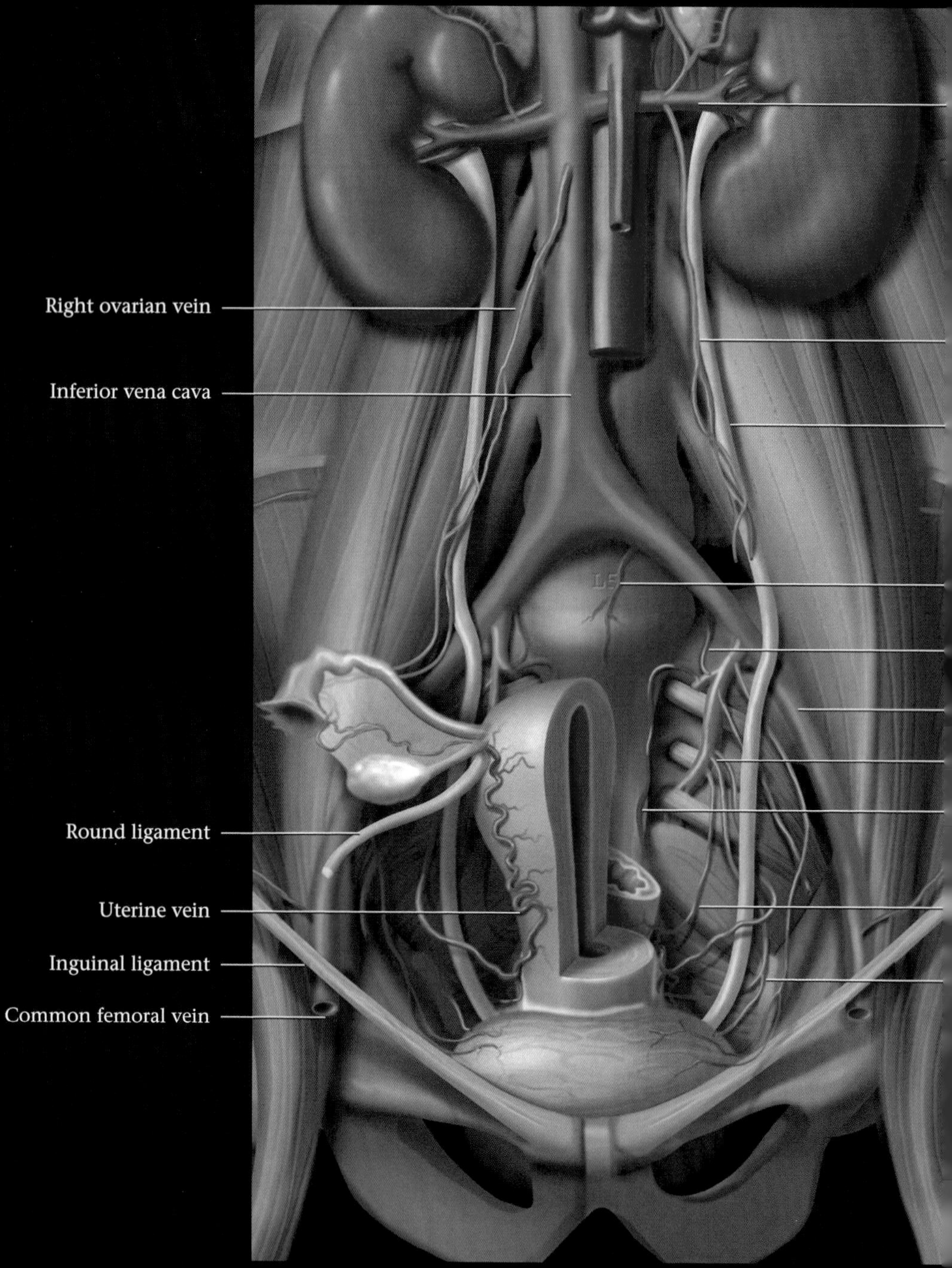

Right ovarian vein

Inferior vena cava

Round ligament

Uterine vein

Inguinal ligament

Common femoral vein

Graphic of the veins of the pelvis. The left ovarian vein drains into the left renal vein, wherea
drains directly into the inferior vena cava. Multiple intercommunicating pelvic venous plexu
prostatic, uterine and vaginal) drain mainly to the internal iliac veins. There is a communica
veins and the intraspinal epidural plexus of veins through the sacral venous plexus.

VESSELS, LYMPHATIC SYSTEM AND NERVES

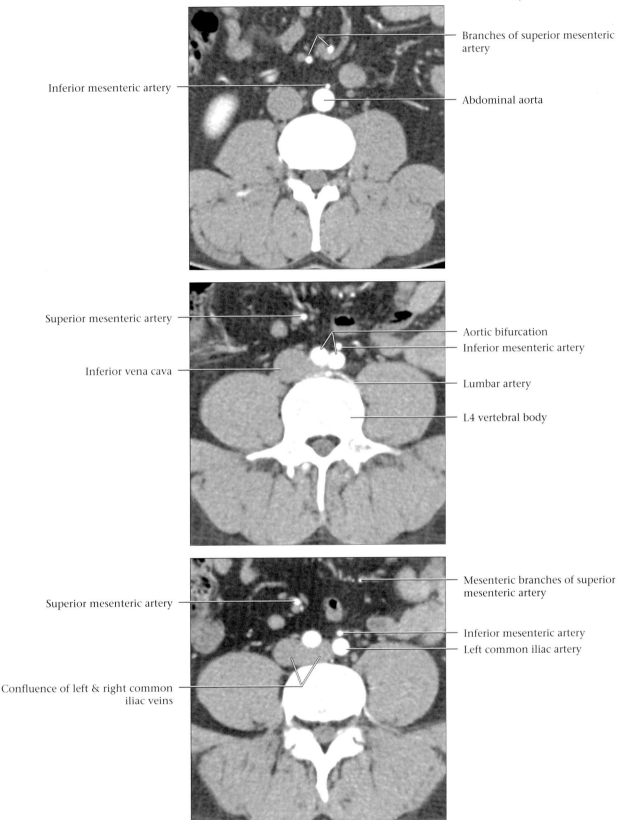

Branches of superior mesenteric artery

Inferior mesenteric artery

Abdominal aorta

Superior mesenteric artery

Aortic bifurcation

Inferior mesenteric artery

Inferior vena cava

Lumbar artery

L4 vertebral body

Superior mesenteric artery

Mesenteric branches of superior mesenteric artery

Inferior mesenteric artery

Left common iliac artery

Confluence of left & right common iliac veins

(Top) First of twelve CECT images of the pelvic vessels. The inferior mesenteric artery, the smallest of the mesenteric arteries, is an anterior branch of the abdominal aorta. It continues in the pelvis as the superior rectal artery. It supplies the distal transverse colon, splenic flexure, descending and sigmoid colon, and the upper part of the rectum. **(Middle)** The aorta bifurcates at the level of L4 into the two common iliac arteries. **(Bottom)** The inferior vena cava is formed below the aortic bifurcation by the joining of the common iliac veins. The left iliac vein passes between the left common iliac artery and the L5 vertebral body. Chronic iliac vein compression syndrome, or May-Thurner syndrome, is deep vein thrombosis resulting from the chronic compression of the left common iliac vein by the overlying right common iliac artery. Patients frequently present with left lower extremity swelling or pain.

VESSELS, LYMPHATIC SYSTEM AND NERVES

AXIAL CECT, PELVIC VESSELS

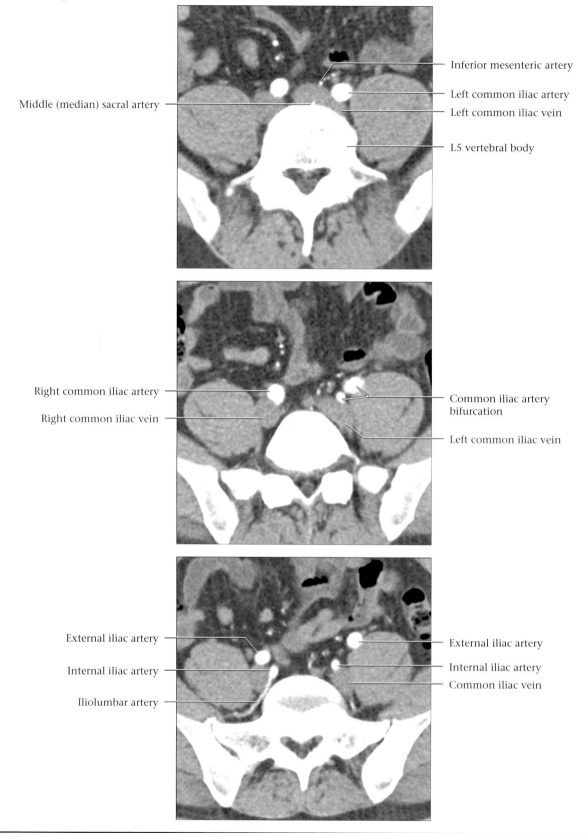

Middle (median) sacral artery

Inferior mesenteric artery

Left common iliac artery

Left common iliac vein

L5 vertebral body

Right common iliac artery

Right common iliac vein

Common iliac artery bifurcation

Left common iliac vein

External iliac artery

Internal iliac artery

Iliolumbar artery

External iliac artery

Internal iliac artery

Common iliac vein

(Top) The middle or median sacral artery is a small unpaired vessel, which comes off the posterior aorta and descends in the midline to the coccyx. The common iliac arteries usually give off no visceral branches. They may, however, give origin to accessory renal arteries. **(Middle)** The common iliac arteries divide, at the level of L5-S1, into two branches, the external and internal iliac (hypogastric) arteries. The external iliac artery supplies the lower extremity, while the hypogastric artery supplies the pelvic viscera and muscles of the pelvis. **(Bottom)** The iliolumbar artery, usually a branch of the posterior trunk of the internal iliac artery, arises in this subject from the main internal iliac artery.

VESSELS, LYMPHATIC SYSTEM AND NERVES

Inferior epigastric artery

External iliac artery

Internal iliac artery

Inferior mesenteric vein

Inferior mesenteric artery

Inferior epigastric artery

External iliac artery

Internal iliac artery

Inferior mesenteric artery

Anterior division, internal iliac artery

Posterior division, internal iliac artery

Inferior epigastric artery

External iliac artery

External iliac vein

Internal iliac vein

Anterior division internal iliac artery

Posterior division internal iliac artery

(**Top**) The inferior mesenteric vein, a continuation of the superior rectal vein, accompanies the inferior mesenteric artery and usually drains into the splenic vein. The rectum is an important site of porto-systemic anastomoses. In patients with portal hypertension, blood is shunted from the high pressure portal venous system through the inferior mesenteric vein to the middle and lnferior rectal veins, which drain into the internal iliac vein. (**Middle**) The internal iliac artery divides into an anterior and posterior trunk. The anterior trunk mainly supplies the pelvic viscera, whereas the posterior trunk supplies the pelvic musculature. (**Bottom**) The internal iliac vein receives blood from multiple pelvic venous plexuses. It unites with the external iliac vein, a continuation of the common femoral vein, to form the common iliac vein.

VESSELS, LYMPHATIC SYSTEM AND NERVES

AXIAL CECT, PELVIC VESSELS

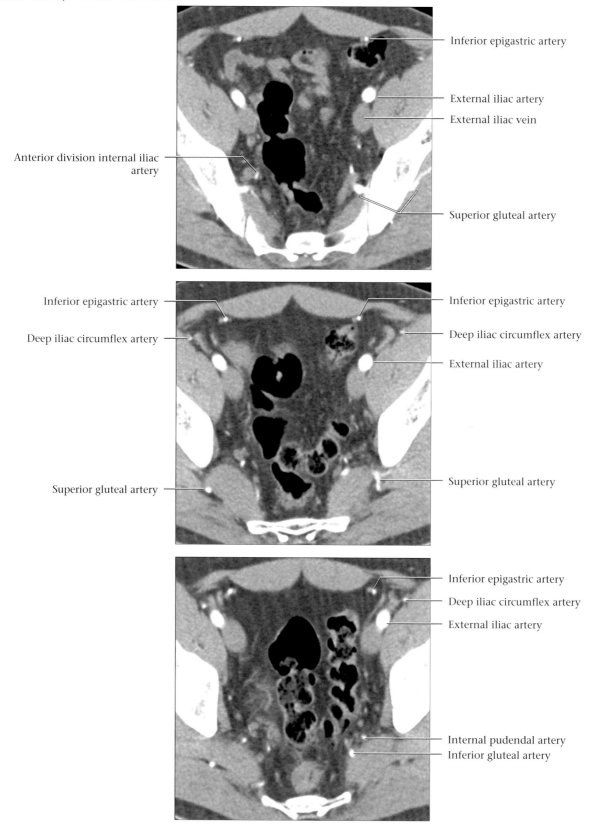

Inferior epigastric artery

External iliac artery

External iliac vein

Anterior division internal iliac artery

Superior gluteal artery

Inferior epigastric artery

Deep iliac circumflex artery

Inferior epigastric artery

Deep iliac circumflex artery

External iliac artery

Superior gluteal artery

Superior gluteal artery

Inferior epigastric artery

Deep iliac circumflex artery

External iliac artery

Internal pudendal artery

Inferior gluteal artery

(Top) The superior gluteal artery runs posteriorly between the lumbosacral trunk and the first sacral nerve. It exits the pelvis through the greater sciatic foramen, above the piriformis muscle. **(Middle)** The inferior epigastric and deep iliac circumflex arteries arise from the external iliac artery just above the inguinal ligament. These are important landmarks on angiography to determine the point where the external iliac artery becomes the common femoral artery. **(Bottom)** The internal pudendal artery and inferior gluteal arteries are the terminal branches of the anterior trunk of the internal iliac artery. They exit the pelvis through the greater sciatic foramen beneath the piriformis muscle. The internal pudendal artery then curves around the sacrospinous ligament to enter the perineum through the lesser sciatic foramen.

VESSELS, LYMPHATIC SYSTEM AND NERVES

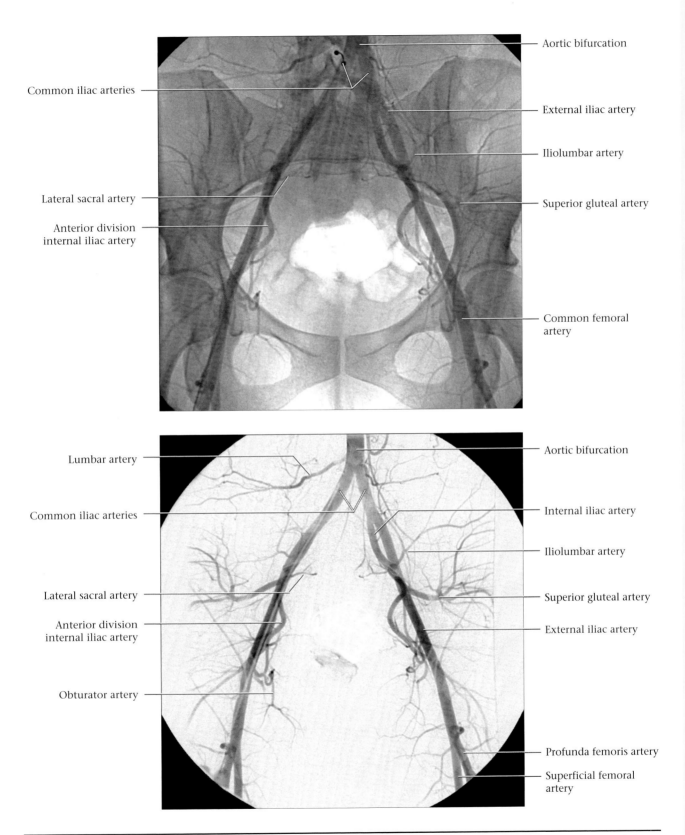

(Top) Conventional angiogram of the pelvic arteries. Note the overlap between the various visceral branches of the internal iliac artery, making it difficult to identify individual arteries. Oblique views are commonly obtained for better visualization of the individual branches. Note that the internal and external iliac arteries are almost in the same sagittal plane. (Bottom) Digital subtraction angiography allows better visualization of the pelvic arteries.

VESSELS, LYMPHATIC SYSTEM AND NERVES

3D CT, ARTERIES

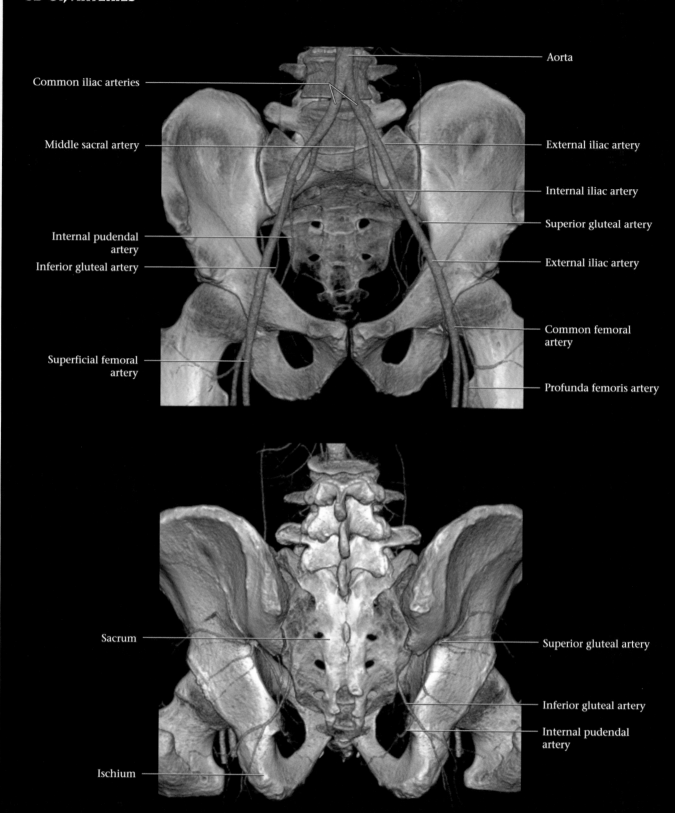

Aorta

Common iliac arteries

Middle sacral artery

External iliac artery

Internal iliac artery

Superior gluteal artery

Internal pudendal artery

External iliac artery

Inferior gluteal artery

Common femoral artery

Superficial femoral artery

Profunda femoris artery

Sacrum

Superior gluteal artery

Inferior gluteal artery

Internal pudendal artery

Ischium

(Top) 3D volume rendering frontal image of the iliac arteries. The aorta bifurcates at the level of L4 into the common iliac arteries and the common iliac arteries bifurcate at the level of L5-S1 into the external and internal iliac arteries. **(Bottom)** 3D volume rendering posterior image of the pelvis showing the superior gluteal artery, the continuation of the posterior trunk of the the internal iliac artery, and the inferior gluteal artery, a branch of the anterior trunk. Note the proximity of the superior gluteal artery to the iliac bone making it vulnerable to injury in cases of pelvic fractures.

VESSELS, LYMPHATIC SYSTEM AND NERVES

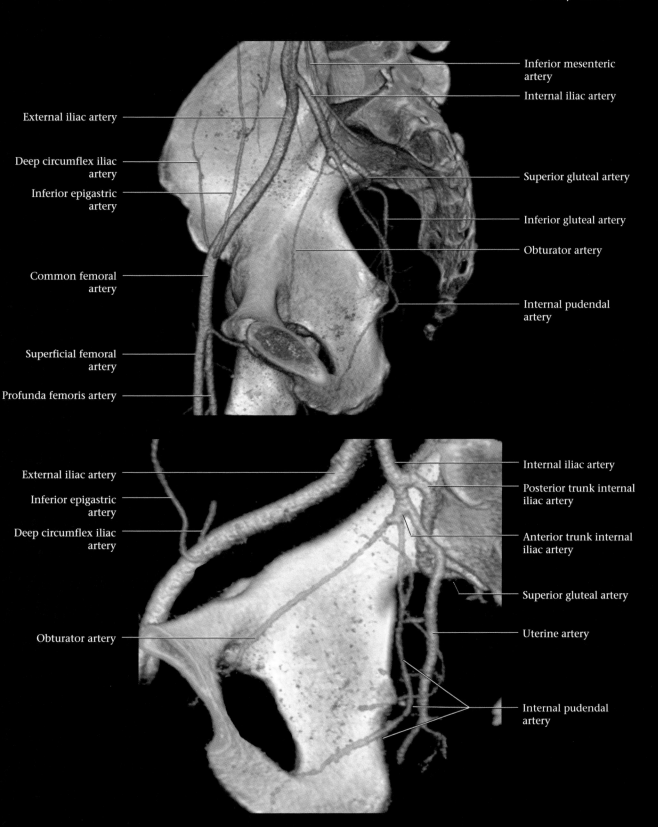

External iliac artery

Deep circumflex iliac artery

Inferior epigastric artery

Common femoral artery

Superficial femoral artery

Profunda femoris artery

Inferior mesenteric artery

Internal iliac artery

Superior gluteal artery

Inferior gluteal artery

Obturator artery

Internal pudendal artery

External iliac artery

Inferior epigastric artery

Deep circumflex iliac artery

Obturator artery

Internal iliac artery

Posterior trunk internal iliac artery

Anterior trunk internal iliac artery

Superior gluteal artery

Uterine artery

Internal pudendal artery

(Top) 3D volume rendered side view of the iliac arteries. The deep iliac circumflex artery arises opposite the inferior epigastric artery just above the level of the inguinal ligament. They demarcate the external iliac artery above, from the common femoral artery below. **(Bottom)** 3D volume rendered oblique side view of the iliac arteries in a female shows a large uterine artery. The obturator artery, a branch of the anterior trunk of the internal iliac artery, runs along the pelvic side wall and leaves the pelvis through the obturator canal. Occasionally, an aberrant obturator artery can come from the inferior epigastric artery. Note the tortuous course of the internal pudendal artery, as it curves around the sacrospinous ligament to enter the perineum through the lesser sciatic foramen.

VESSELS, LYMPHATIC SYSTEM AND NERVES

MRA MIP

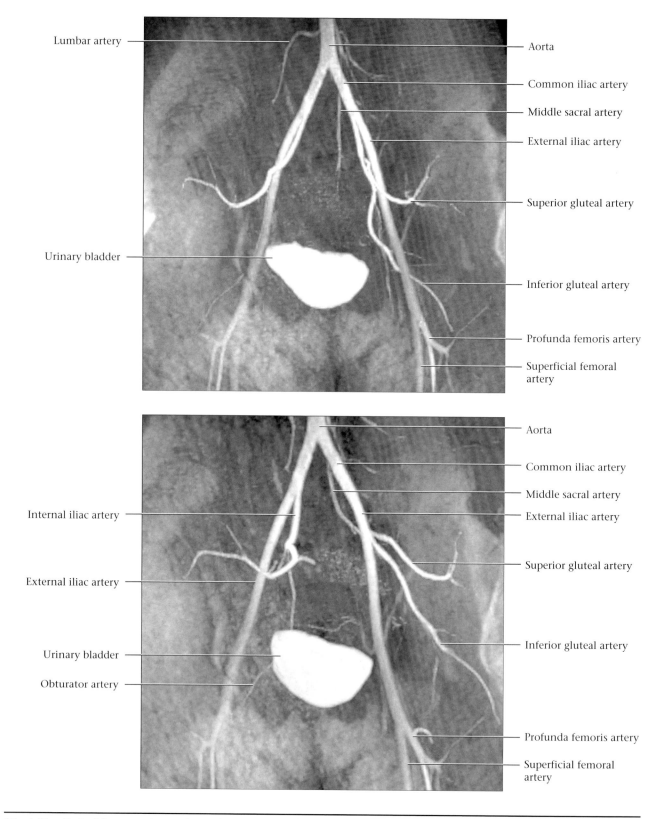

Lumbar artery — Aorta

Common iliac artery

Middle sacral artery

External iliac artery

Superior gluteal artery

Urinary bladder

Inferior gluteal artery

Profunda femoris artery

Superficial femoral artery

Aorta

Common iliac artery

Middle sacral artery

Internal iliac artery — External iliac artery

Superior gluteal artery

External iliac artery

Urinary bladder

Inferior gluteal artery

Obturator artery

Profunda femoris artery

Superficial femoral artery

(Top) The first of four maximum intensity projection (MIP) images obtained from a gadolinium-enhanced MRA of the pelvis. This is a thick MIP image and the small visceral branches are not well seen. **(Bottom)** Oblique thick MIP image of the pelvic arteries again shows the large branches of the iliac arteries. The obturator artery is seen running anterolaterally along the lateral wall of the pelvis. It exits the pelvis through the obturator foramen to supply the medial thigh muscles.

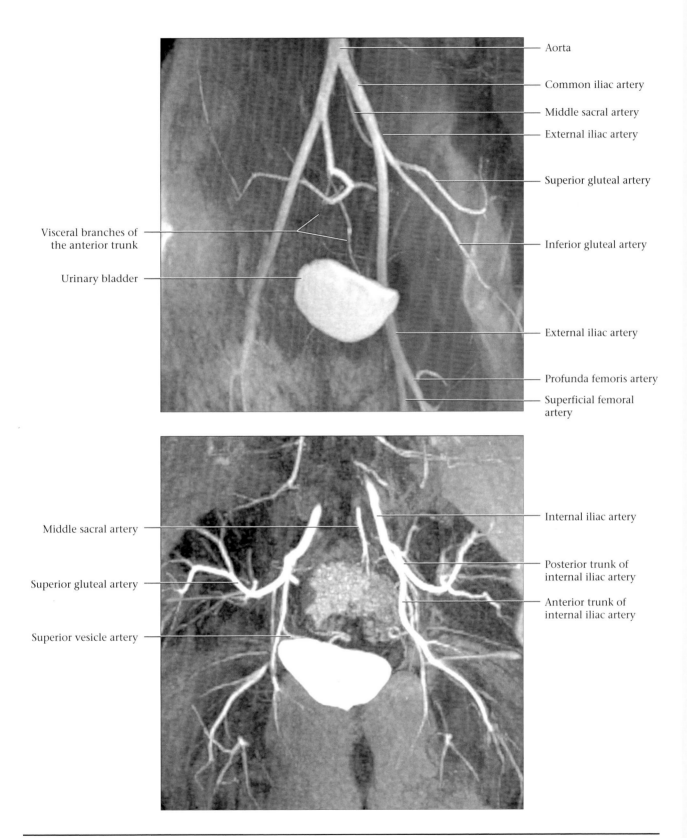

Aorta

Common iliac artery

Middle sacral artery

External iliac artery

Superior gluteal artery

Visceral branches of the anterior trunk

Inferior gluteal artery

Urinary bladder

External iliac artery

Profunda femoris artery

Superficial femoral artery

Middle sacral artery

Internal iliac artery

Superior gluteal artery

Posterior trunk of internal iliac artery

Superior vesicle artery

Anterior trunk of internal iliac artery

(Top) A steeper obliquity shows the superior and inferior gluteal arteries. **(Bottom)** A thin MIP image of the internal iliac arteries shows the branching vessels in much greater detail.

UTERINE ARTERIES

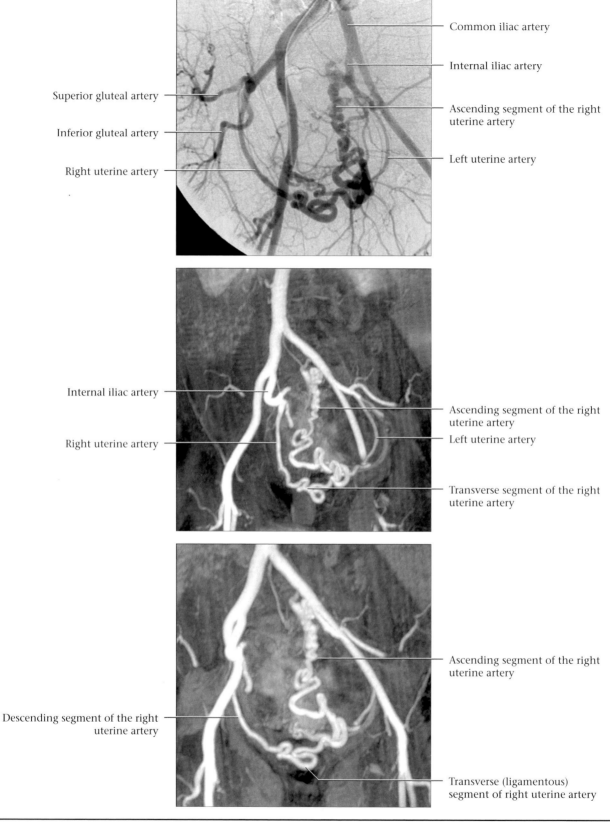

Common iliac artery

Internal iliac artery

Ascending segment of the right uterine artery

Left uterine artery

Superior gluteal artery

Inferior gluteal artery

Right uterine artery

Internal iliac artery

Right uterine artery

Ascending segment of the right uterine artery

Left uterine artery

Transverse segment of the right uterine artery

Descending segment of the right uterine artery

Ascending segment of the right uterine artery

Transverse (ligamentous) segment of right uterine artery

(Top) Oblique view during conventional pelvic angiography shows dilated uterine arteries bilaterally (right > left) in a patient with multiple uterine leiomyomas. **(Middle)** First of two maximum intensity projection images from a gadolinium-enhanced MRA in the same patient as previous image. This closely resembles the appearance on conventional angiography. MRA and CTA have essentially replaced diagnostic conventional angiography for evaluation of pelvic vascular structures and delineation of vascular anatomy, prior to surgical and interventional procedures. **(Bottom)** The uterine artery has a characteristic U-shaped course, which consists of a descending segment running downward and medially, a transverse segment which courses medially through the cardinal ligament, and the marginal or ascending segment running along the side of the uterus.

OVARIAN VEINS

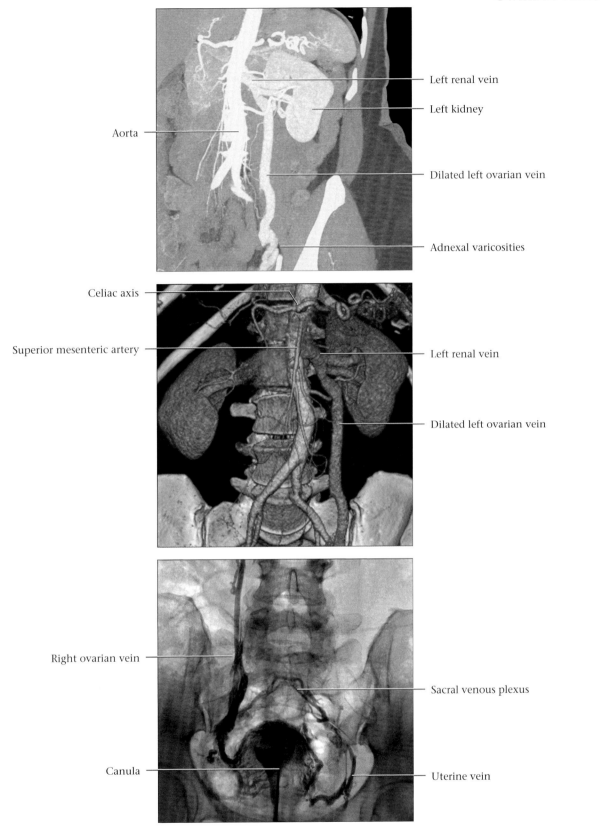

Left renal vein

Left kidney

Aorta

Dilated left ovarian vein

Adnexal varicosities

Celiac axis

Superior mesenteric artery

Left renal vein

Dilated left ovarian vein

Right ovarian vein

Sacral venous plexus

Canula

Uterine vein

(Top) First of two images in a patient with pelvic congestion syndrome. On this oblique MIP CT image the dilated, tortuous, left ovarian vein is seen draining into the left renal vein. The left ovarian vein shows early, dense opacification when compared to the other pelvic venous structures, which are not opacified. This is secondary to reflux of contrast from the left renal vein into the left ovarian vein. **(Middle)** The 3D volume rendered image shows compression of the left renal vein by the superior mesenteric artery. This compression contributes to venous reflux down the ovarian vein and has been called the "nutcracker syndrome". **(Bottom)** Pelvic venogram in a different patient, obtained after insertion of a canula into the myometrium, shows filling of a normal-sized right ovarian vein. The right ovarian vein flows directly into the IVC, and therefore, is at less risk for reflux.

VESSELS, LYMPHATIC SYSTEM AND NERVES

AXIAL CECT, THROMBOSED RIGHT OVARIAN VEIN

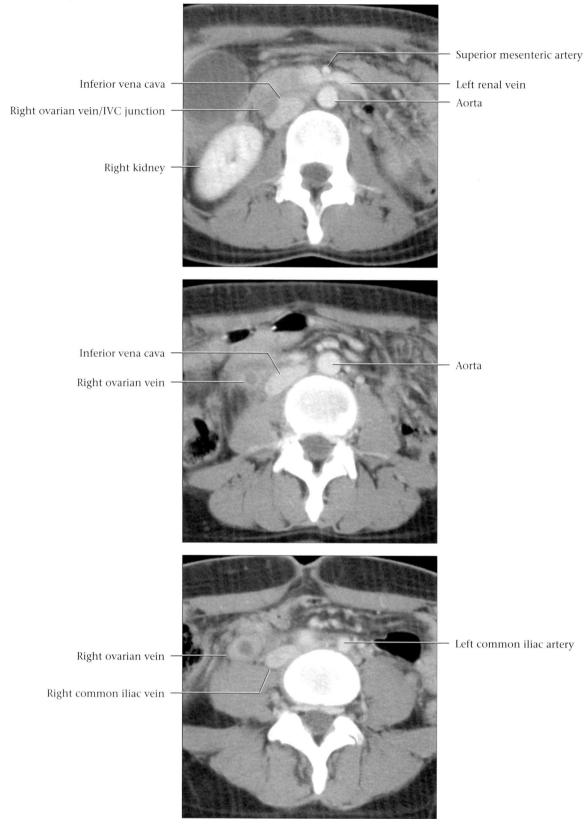

(Top) First of three axial CECT images in a postpartum woman with fever and right-sided ovarian vein thrombosis. On this most cephalad image, the thrombus is seen extending to the entrance of the right ovarian vein into the inferior vena cava. (Middle) The right ovarian vein is dilated and filled with thrombus. (Bottom) Thrombosis usually occurs secondary to pelvic infection. In addition to the thrombus itself, the vessel wall is thickened and there is a surrounding inflammatory reaction. Following the normal course of the vein up towards the IVC allows differentiation from other pelvic pathologies, such as appendicitis.

VESSELS, LYMPHATIC SYSTEM AND NERVES

AXIAL CECT, THROMBOSED LEFT OVARIAN VEIN

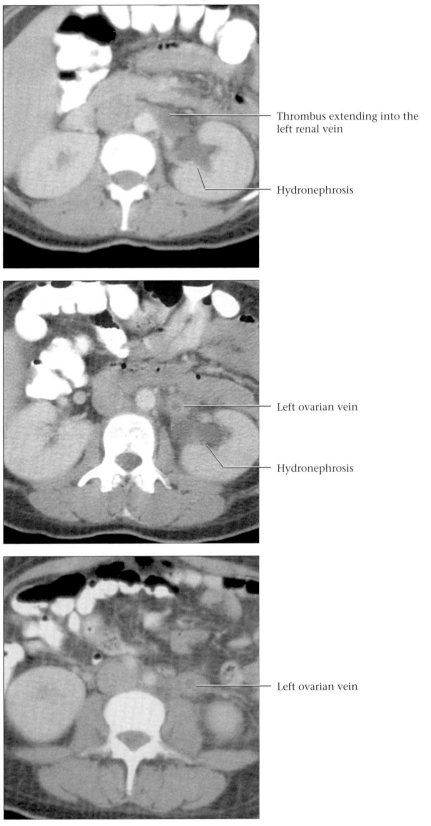

Thrombus extending into the left renal vein

Hydronephrosis

Left ovarian vein

Hydronephrosis

Left ovarian vein

(Top) First of three axial CECT images in a woman with postpartum thrombosis of the left ovarian vein. This image shows the thrombus extending into the non-opacified left renal vein. (Middle) Clot is present within the left ovarian vein and the wall is thickened, with surrounding inflammatory changes. (Bottom) The ovarian veins ascend along the psoas muscle and cross anterior to the ureters, near the confluence of the common iliac veins. Inflammation from ovarian vein thrombosis may also affect the ureter and result in hydronephrosis, as is seen in this case.

VESSELS, LYMPHATIC SYSTEM AND NERVES

PELVIC LYMPH NODES

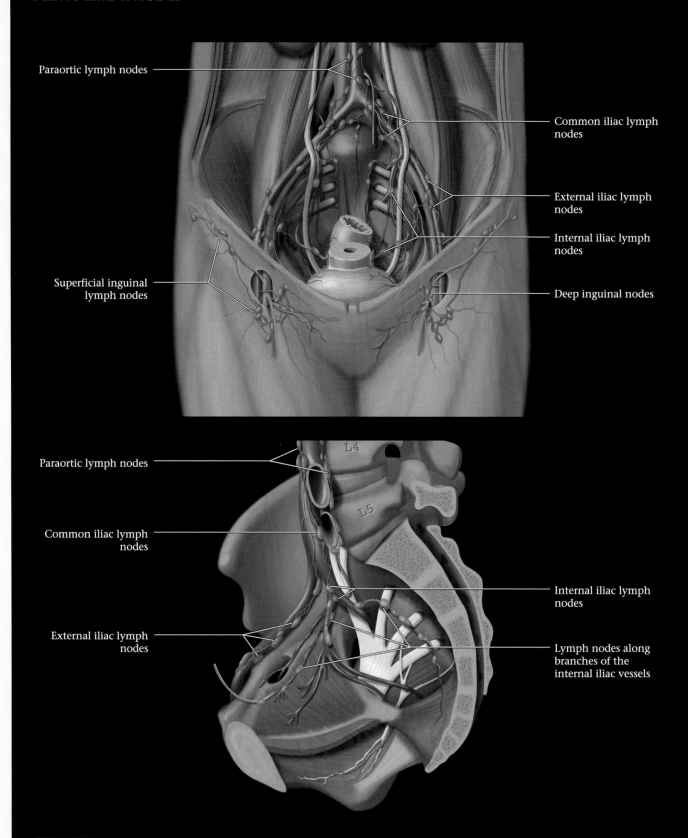

Paraortic lymph nodes

Common iliac lymph nodes

External iliac lymph nodes

Internal iliac lymph nodes

Deep inguinal nodes

Superficial inguinal lymph nodes

Paraortic lymph nodes

Common iliac lymph nodes

External iliac lymph nodes

Internal iliac lymph nodes

Lymph nodes along branches of the internal iliac vessels

(Top) Graphic of the lymph nodes of the pelvis. Generally the lymph nodes are located along, and named after, the iliac vessels. Two groups of inguinal lymph nodes are described: The superficial and deep group. The superficial inguinal nodes lie along the saphenous vein, superficial to the cribriform fascia which overlies the femoral vessels. There are approximately 10 superficial lymph nodes. The deep inguinal lymph nodes are located medial to the femoral vein and under the cribriform fascia. There are approximately 3-5 deep nodes. The most superior inguinal node is located under the inguinal ligament and is called the gland or node of Cloquet. **(Bottom)** Graphic of the side wall of the pelvis shows the lymph nodes along the corresponding iliac vessels.

VESSELS, LYMPHATIC SYSTEM AND NERVES

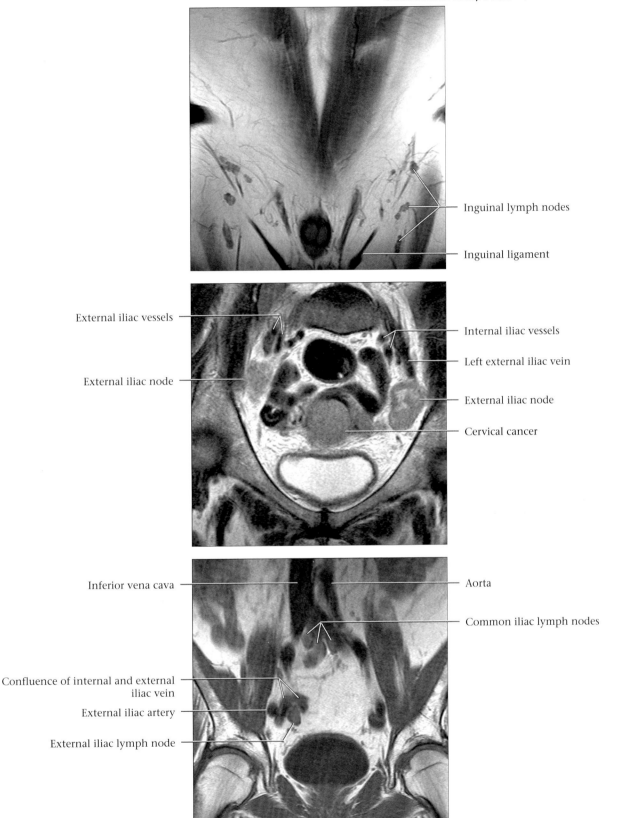

Inguinal lymph nodes

Inguinal ligament

External iliac vessels

Internal iliac vessels

Left external iliac vein

External iliac node

External iliac node

Cervical cancer

Inferior vena cava

Aorta

Common iliac lymph nodes

Confluence of internal and external iliac vein

External iliac artery

External iliac lymph node

(Top) Coronal T1 MR image shows the distribution of normal-sized inguinal lymph nodes along the inguinal ligament. **(Middle)** Coronal oblique T2 MR image of woman with cervical cancer shows enlarged external iliac lymph nodes from metastatic disease. **(Bottom)** Coronal T1 MR shows multiple enlarged pelvic lymph nodes in a patient with lymphoma.

PET CT, PELVIC LYMPH NODES

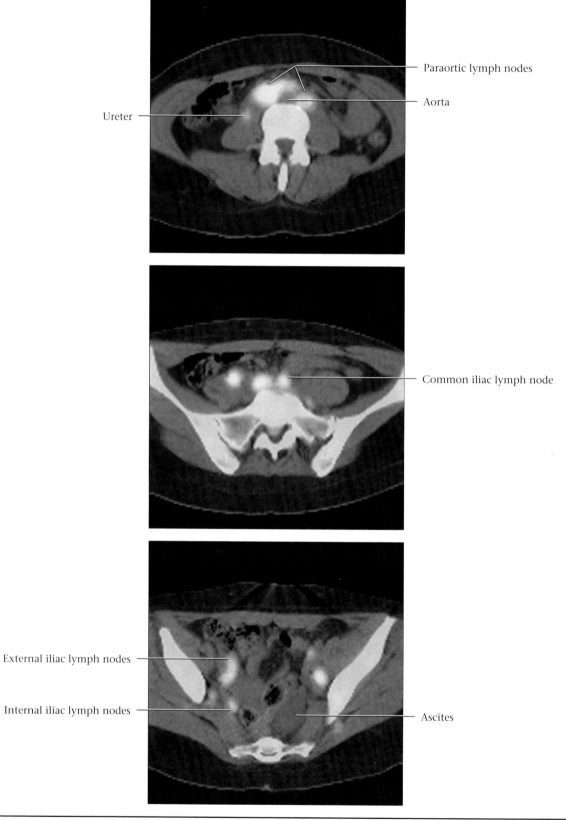

Paraortic lymph nodes

Aorta

Ureter

Common iliac lymph node

External iliac lymph nodes

Internal iliac lymph nodes

Ascites

(Top) First of six axial PET CT images, after injection of 18-F FDG, shows increased metabolic activity in multiple enlarged groups of lymph nodes in a young patient diagnosed with non-Hodgkin lymphoma. Image shows involvement of the para-aortic lymph nodes. Increased activity is seen in the right ureter due to excretion of 18-F FDG in urine. **(Middle)** Increased metabolic activity in the common iliac lymph nodes. **(Bottom)** Increased metabolic activity in the internal and external iliac lymph nodes on both sides.

VESSELS, LYMPHATIC SYSTEM AND NERVES

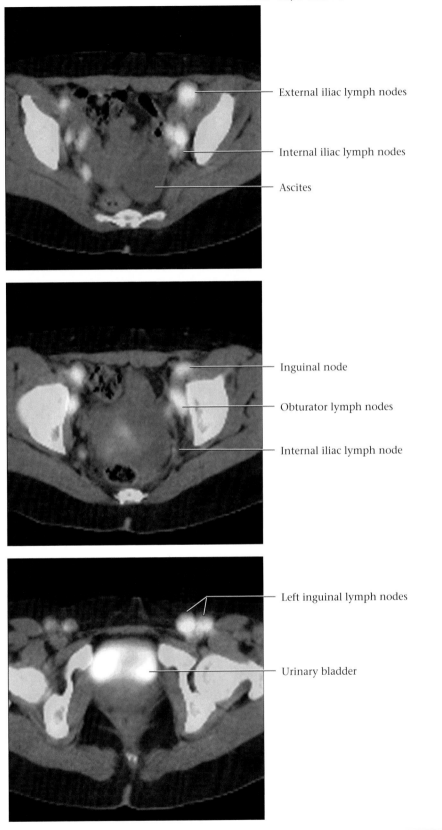

External iliac lymph nodes

Internal iliac lymph nodes

Ascites

Inguinal node

Obturator lymph nodes

Internal iliac lymph node

Left inguinal lymph nodes

Urinary bladder

(Top) The nodal chains are named for the vessels they accompany. **(Middle)** Obturator nodes lie adjacent to the obturator internus muscle and are a frequent site of metastases for pelvic malignancies. **(Bottom)** The superficial inguinal nodes drain the skin of the penis, lower abdomen, perineum, scrotum and part of the buttock area. The deep inguinal nodes located under the fascia lata are the main lymphatic drainage from the lower extremities, but they also receive small branches from the penis and efferent vessels from the superficial inguinal nodes.

VESSELS, LYMPHATIC SYSTEM AND NERVES

PET CT, PELVIC LYMPH NODES

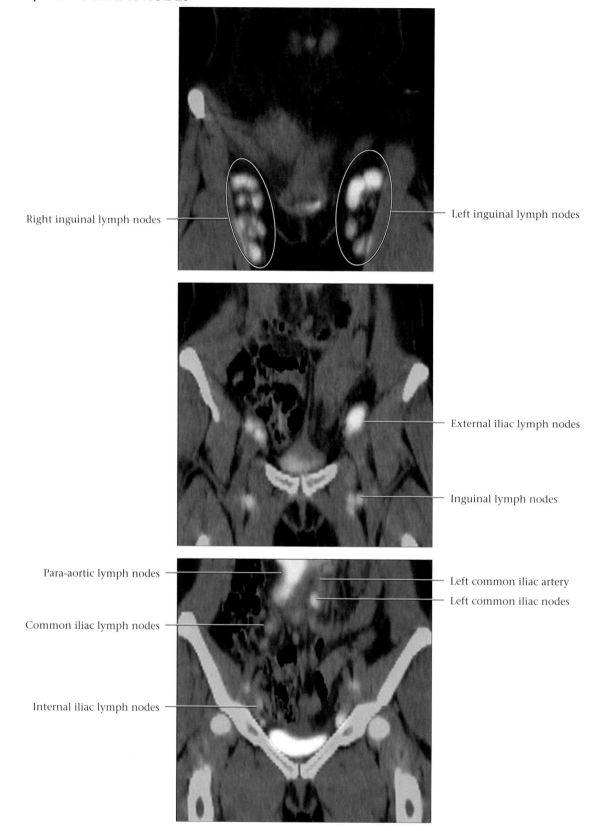

Right inguinal lymph nodes — Left inguinal lymph nodes

External iliac lymph nodes

Inguinal lymph nodes

Para-aortic lymph nodes — Left common iliac artery — Left common iliac nodes

Common iliac lymph nodes

Internal iliac lymph nodes

(Top) First of six coronal PET CT images in the same patient diagnosed with lymphoma shows enlarged metabolically active inguinal lymph nodes. **(Middle)** The external iliac nodes are above the inguinal ligament and are the primary drainage for the inguinal nodes. **(Bottom)** More posteriorly, metabolic activity is seen in internal iliac, common iliac and para-aortic lymph nodes.

VESSELS, LYMPHATIC SYSTEM AND NERVES

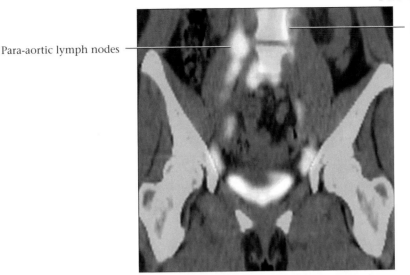

Para-aortic lymph nodes   Para-aortic lymph nodes

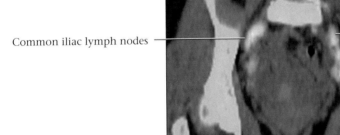

Common iliac lymph nodes   Common iliac lymph nodes

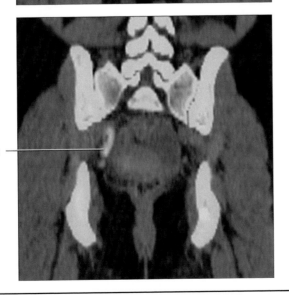

Internal iliac lymph nodes

(Top) This image shows the para-aortic lymph nodes. These nodes receive lymphatic drainage from the common iliac lymph nodes. In addition the para-aortic nodes receive drainage from the gonads. Typical patterns of spread in testicular cancer patients occur according to the side of the primary tumor. Right-sided testicular tumors spread initially to the aortocaval nodes, the right para-aortic nodes and the precaval nodes. Left-sided primaries metastasize to preaortic nodes and left para-aortic nodes just below the level of the renal vein. **(Middle)** The common iliac nodes receive lymphatic drainage from the internal and external groups of lymph nodes, and drain into the para-aortic lymph nodes. **(Bottom)** The internal iliac lymph nodes receive lymphatic drainage from the pelvic viscera and drain into the common iliac lymph nodes.

PELVIC NERVES

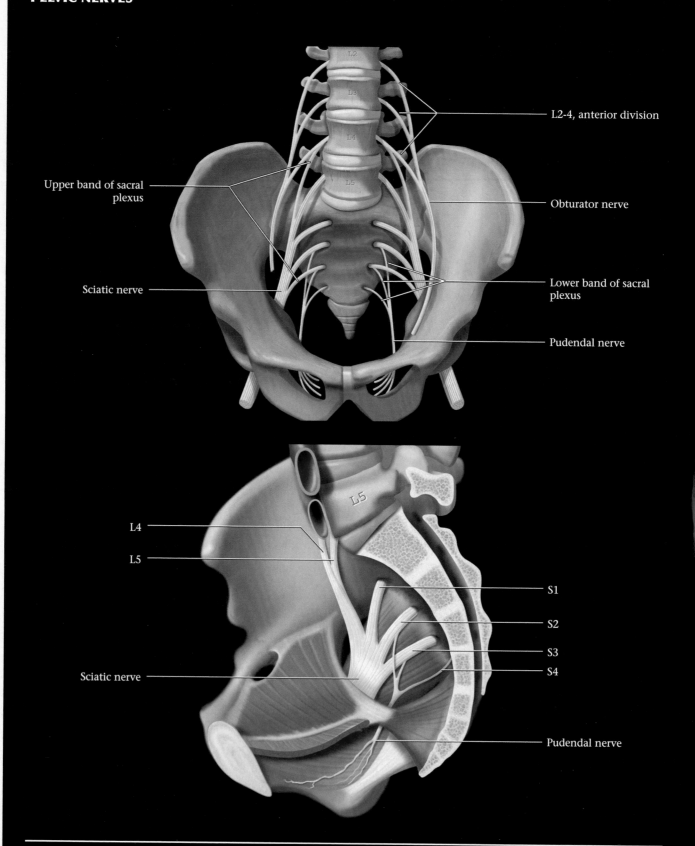

L2-4, anterior division

Obturator nerve

Upper band of sacral plexus

Lower band of sacral plexus

Sciatic nerve

Pudendal nerve

L4

L5

S1

S2

S3

S4

Sciatic nerve

Pudendal nerve

(Top) The ventral rami of L2-4 split into two divisions: A larger posterior division, which forms the femoral nerve (not shown) and a smaller anterior division, which forms the obturator nerve. The obturator nerve follows the obturator vessels, leaving the pelvis through the obturator foramen. The sacral plexus has a larger upper band (L4, L5, S1-3), which becomes the sciatic nerve and a lower band (S2-4), which becomes the pudendal nerve. **(Bottom)** The upper band of the sacral plexus coalesces into the sciatic nerve on the ventral surface of the piriformis muscle. The lower band forms the pudendal nerve, which exits the pelvis through the greater sciatic foramen. It then curves around the sacrospinous ligament to enter the perineum through the lesser sciatic foramen. The pudendal nerve is the primary innervation for the perineum and external anal sphincter.

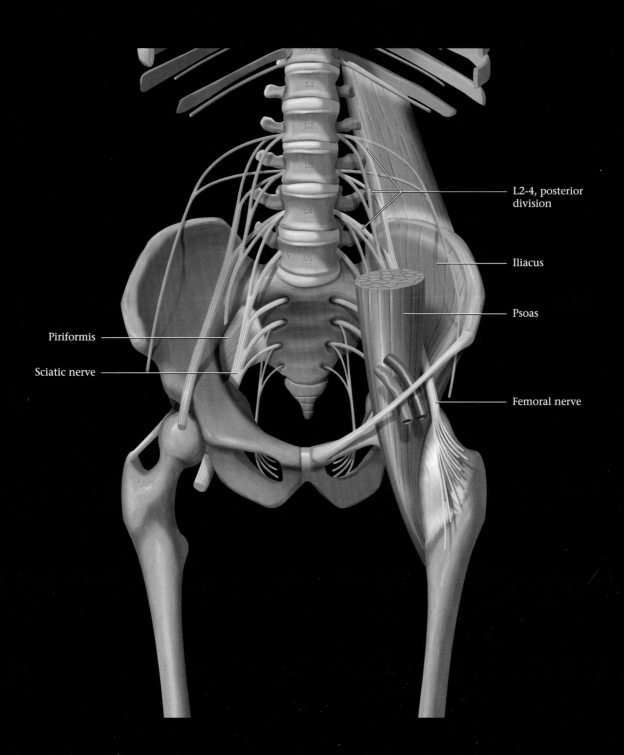

L2-4, posterior division

Iliacus

Psoas

Femoral nerve

Piriformis

Sciatic nerve

The femoral nerve is formed from the posterior division of the L2-4 ventral rami. It descends through the psoas major muscle and into the iliopsoas groove. It exits the pelvis beneath the inguinal ligament through the femoral canal. The well known acronym "NAVL" (nerve, artery, vein, lymphatic) describes the order of the femoral canal contents from lateral to medial. The femoral nerve innervates the anteromedial thigh. The sciatic nerve exits the pelvis through the greater sciatic foramen below the piriformis muscle to innervate the posterior thigh and leg.

SCIATIC NERVE

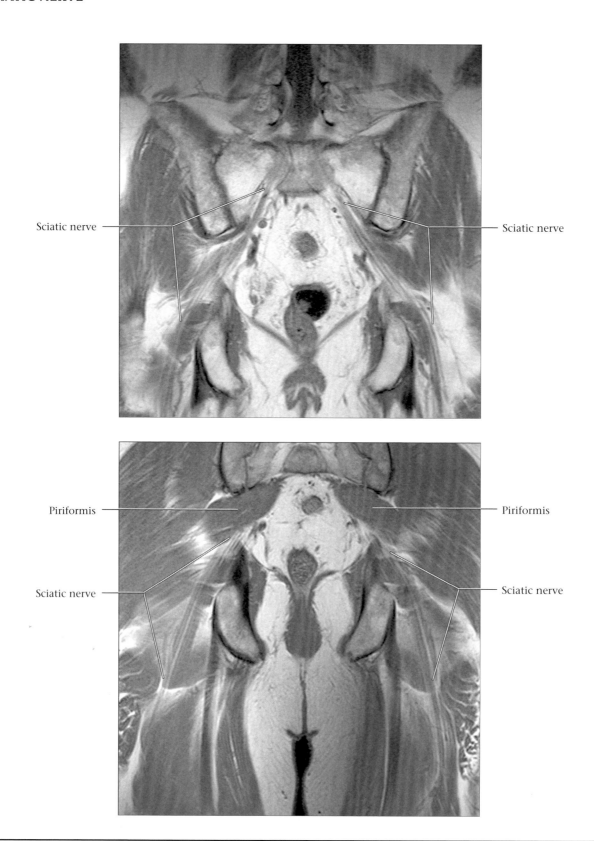

Sciatic nerve — ... — Sciatic nerve

Piriformis — ... — Piriformis

Sciatic nerve — ... — Sciatic nerve

(Top) Coronal T1 MR shows the nerves from the sacral plexus coalescing to form the sciatic nerve. The long fascicles composing this large nerve can be easily recognized. (Bottom) Coronal T1 MR shows the sciatic nerve passing beneath the piriformis muscle into the posterior thigh.

VESSELS, LYMPHATIC SYSTEM AND NERVES

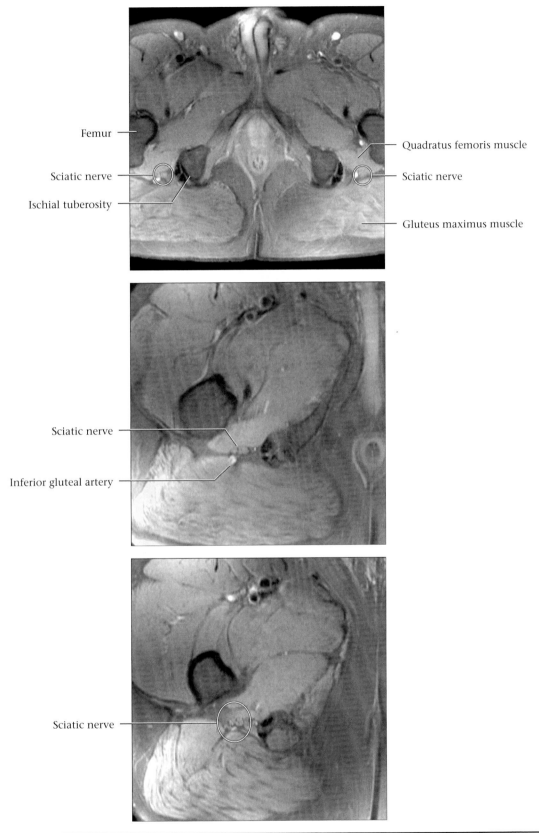

Femur — Quadratus femoris muscle

Sciatic nerve — Sciatic nerve

Ischial tuberosity

Gluteus maximus muscle

Sciatic nerve

Inferior gluteal artery

Sciatic nerve

(Top) First of three axial proton density, fat-saturated images shows the sciatic nerve. After it has left the pelvis, the sciatic nerve can be seen near the ischial tuberosities, between the gluteus maximus and quadratus femoris muscles. **(Middle)** As the sciatic nerve passes beneath the gluteus maximus muscle, it is accompanied by the inferior gluteal artery. **(Bottom)** The fascicular architecture of the nerve is very distinctive and permits differentiation from other soft tissues and vessels.

SCIATIC, FEMORAL NERVE

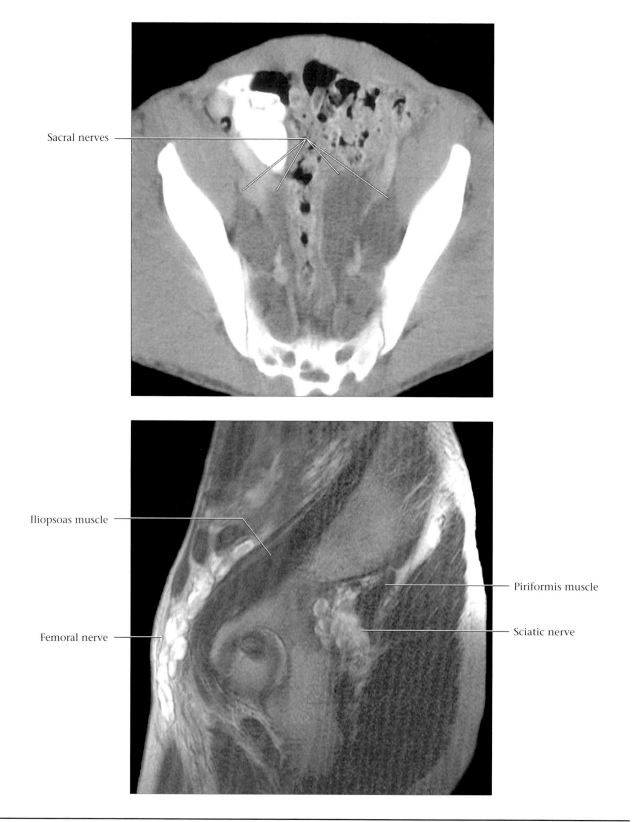

(Top) Axial CECT in a patient with neurofibromatosis type I. The sacral nerves, which form the sciatic nerve, are dramatically enlarged. (Bottom) Sagittal T2 image in a different patient, also with neurofibromatosis type 1. The sciatic nerve is dramatically enlarged, as it passes through the greater sciatic foramen, beneath the piriformis muscle. The femoral nerve is also grossly enlarged.

FEMORAL NERVE

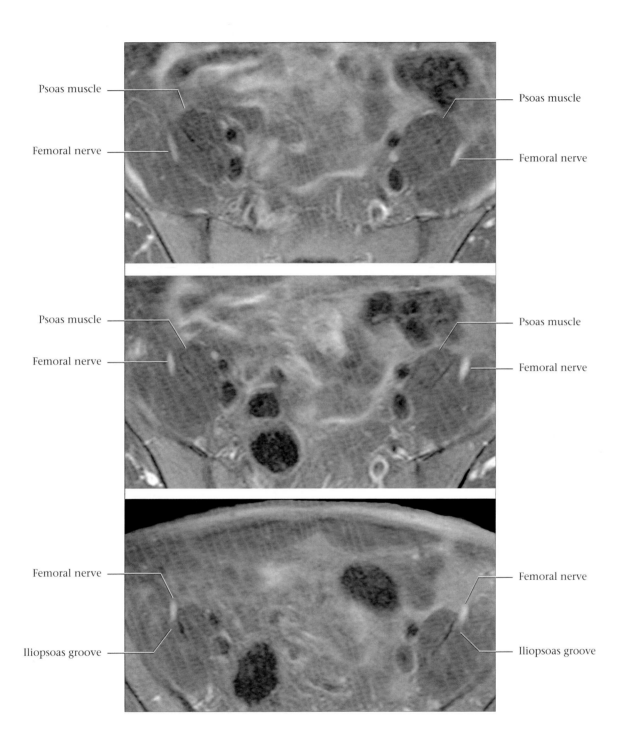

Psoas muscle

Femoral nerve

Psoas muscle

Femoral nerve

Psoas muscle

Femoral nerve

Psoas muscle

Femoral nerve

Femoral nerve

Iliopsoas groove

Femoral nerve

Iliopsoas groove

T2 fat-saturated MR in a patient with bilateral femoral nerve inflammation shows the course of the pelvic portion of this nerve. The femoral nerve is formed from the posterior division of the L2-4 ventral rami. It descends through the psoas muscle into the groove created between the psoas and iliacus muscles (iliopsoas groove). It maintains this position until it exits the pelvis beneath the inguinal ligament.

FEMORAL, OBTURATOR NERVES

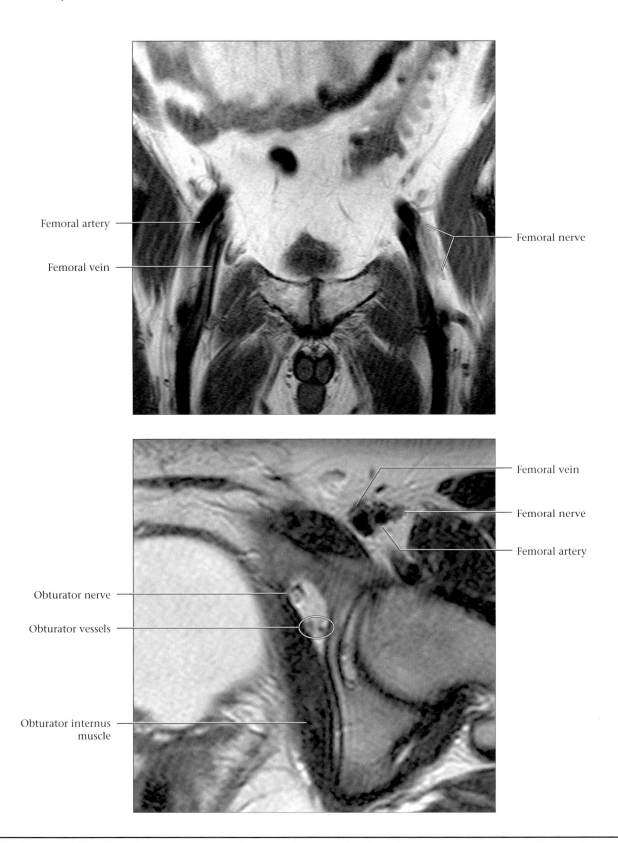

(Top) Coronal T1 MR of the femoral nerve. The femoral nerve exits the pelvis beneath the inguinal ligament where it is the most lateral component within the femoral canal. Branches of the femoral nerve innervate the anteromedial thigh. (Bottom) Axial T2 MR shows the obturator nerve, which runs anterosuperior to the obturator vessels to enter the upper part of the obturator foramen. Here it divides into an anterior and posterior division as it enters the thigh.

VESSELS, LYMPHATIC SYSTEM AND NERVES

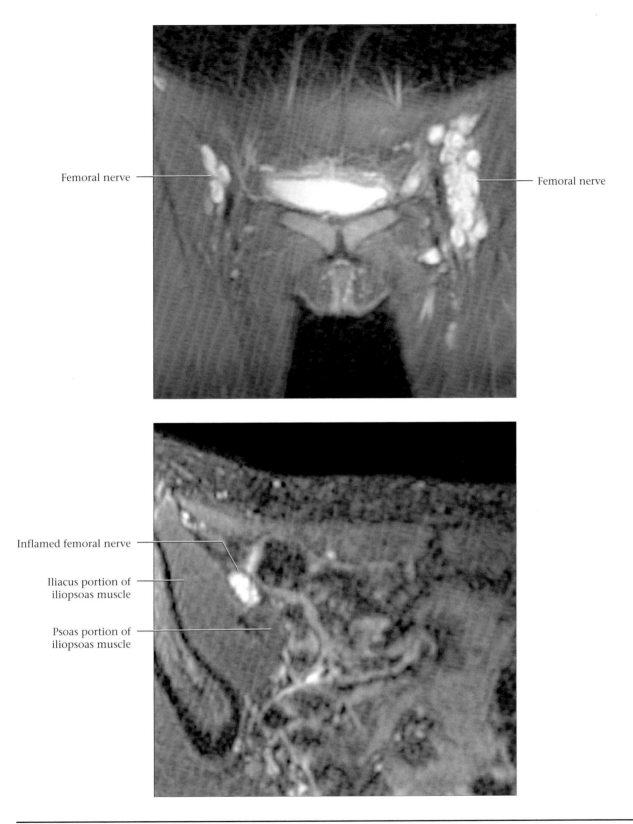

Femoral nerve

Femoral nerve

Inflamed femoral nerve

Iliacus portion of
iliopsoas muscle

Psoas portion of
iliopsoas muscle

(Top) Coronal STIR MR in a patient with neurofibromatosis type 1 shows involvement of both femoral nerves (left >
right). (Bottom) Axial STIR MR image shows an abnormal, inflamed, hyperintense right femoral nerve traveling in
the iliopsoas grove. The characteristic fascicular architecture of peripheral nerves is well shown. The femoral nerve
had been inadvertently sutured during herniorrhaphy.

FEMALE PELVIC LIGAMENTS AND SPACES

Imaging Anatomy

- All contents lie above levator ani except the vagina, which passes through it
- Reproductive organs
  - Uterus, cervix and fallopian tubes
  - Ovaries
  - Vagina
- Other pelvic organs (all extraperitoneal)
  - Distal ureters, bladder and urethra
  - Rectum
- **Supporting uterine ligaments**
  - These are **visceral ligaments** and contain vessels, nerves and lymphatics, as well as connective tissue
    - Similar function as bowel mesentery
    - Supportive role, connects viscera to pelvic wall
  - Peritoneum extends over bladder dome to anterior uterus
    - Reflects over uterus at lower uterine segment
    - Creates **anterior cul-de-sac** (vesico-uterine pouch)
  - Peritoneum sweeps over fundus, extends over posterior uterine surface to upper vagina, abutting posterior vaginal fornix
    - Creates **posterior cul-de-sac** (pouch of Douglas or rectouterine pouch)
    - Most dependent portion of female pelvis
- **Broad ligament** created from the two sheets of covering peritoneum
  - Extends laterally to pelvic sidewall
  - Very thin in superior portion and offers little support
  - Thickens at base to form major supporting ligaments
  - Nerves and vessels pass through broad ligament
- **Ovarian ligaments**
  - **Suspensory ligament of ovary** attaches ovary to pelvic wall and contains ovarian artery and vein
  - **Proper ovarian ligament** attaches ovary to uterine corpus
  - **Mesosalpinx** between fallopian tube and proper ovarian ligament
- **Round ligaments**
  - Arise from uterine cornu near fallopian tubes
  - Course anteriorly, through inguinal canal to insert on labia majora
  - Offer little support to uterus
  - Embryologic homologue to gubernaculum in male
  - **Canal of Nuck** is a peritoneal diverticulum (persistent processus vaginalis) created where round ligament enters inguinal canal
- **Cardinal ligaments**
  - Thickening of endopelvic fascia at **base of broad ligament**
  - Composed predominately of connective tissue and **transmits neurovascular structures**
  - Extend from cervix and vagina to lateral pelvic wall
  - Widen as they attach to pelvic wall
  - Important support function
- **Uterosacral ligaments**
  - Extend from cervix and vagina to sacrum
  - Extend around rectum and form lateral borders of pouch of Douglas
  - Composed predominately of smooth muscle and **transmits autonomic nerves**

- Important support function
- **Vesicouterine ligaments** course anteriorly
- **Vaginal support**
  - Multiple important attachments, which give support to all pelvic viscera
    - Cardinal ligaments, perineal body, levator ani, arcus tendineus, vesicovaginal and rectovaginal fascia
    - Failure of these supports results in cystocele, rectocele, enterocele and uterine prolapse
- **Spaces**
  - Many of these spaces are filled with loose connective tissue, and therefore serve as surgical dissection planes
  - **Space of Retzius**
    - Retropubic, prevesical space
    - Separated from anterior abdominal wall by transversalis fascia
  - **Vesicovaginal/vesicocervical space**
    - Between lower urinary tract and vagina/cervix
    - Distal portion of urethra fused with anterior vagina
  - **Rectovaginal space**
    - Rectovaginal fascia provides support for rectum and helps prevent rectoceles
  - **Paravesicle and pararectal spaces**
  - **Presacral (retrorectal) space**
    - Between rectum and sacrum/coccyx
    - Extends cephalad to aortic bifurcation
    - Contains autonomic (sympathetic and parasympathetic) nerves for pelvic viscera
  - **Parametrium**
    - Pelvic visceral fascia and contents adjacent to cervix (both uterosacral and cardinal ligaments)
- **Blood supply**
  - Extensive collateral supply
  - Ovarian arteries arise from aorta below renal arteries
  - Uterine, vaginal and pudendal arteries all arise from internal iliac artery
  - Right ovarian vein drains to inferior vein cava, while left drains to left renal vein
  - Remainder of veins drain into internal iliac veins
- **Lymphatic drainage**
  - Upper 2/3 of vagina and uterus drain into obturator, internal iliac and external iliac nodes
    - Uterine fundus may drain via lymphatic channels along round ligament to superficial inguinal nodes
  - Lower vagina drains to vulvar and inguinal nodes
  - Ovarian lymphatics follow ovarian veins and drain into aorto-caval and periaortic nodes

Clinical Implications

- Posterior cul-de-sac is most dependent portion of abdominal cavity
  - Common location for drop metastases from abdominal neoplasms
- Peritoneum over bladder is loose, and is used as an extraperitoneal surgical cleavage plane for cesarean section

FEMALE PELVIC LIGAMENTS AND SPACES

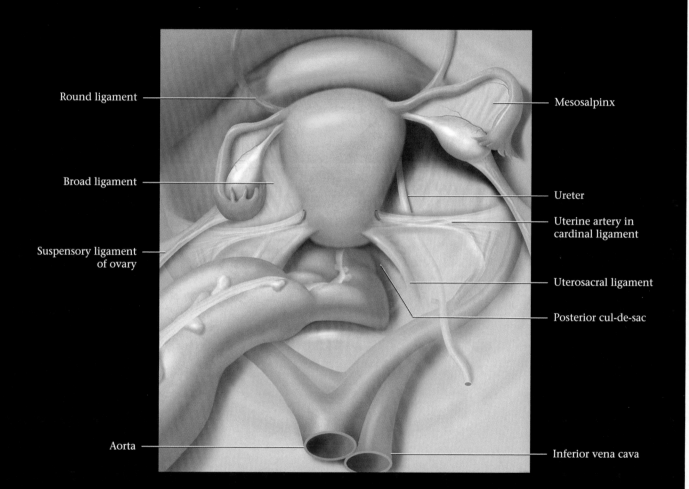

Round ligament

Broad ligament

Suspensory ligament
of ovary

Aorta

Mesosalpinx

Ureter

Uterine artery in
cardinal ligament

Uterosacral ligament

Posterior cul-de-sac

Inferior vena cava

Uterus viewed from above and behind shows its positioning and major ligaments. The uterus is covered by a sheet of peritoneum, creating a double layer (the broad ligament), which sweeps laterally to attach to the pelvic wall. Areas of thickening at its base are the cardinal ligament, which attaches to the lateral pelvic wall, and the uterosacral ligament, which attaches to the sacrum. The uterosacral ligaments form the lateral borders of the posterior cul-de-sac (rectouterine pouch or pouch of Douglas). The round ligaments arise from the cornu of the uterus and course anteriorly to pass through the inguinal canal and insert on the labia majora. They offer little support for the uterus. With a portion of the broad ligament removed (on the right), the uterine artery can be seen passing over the ureter to enter the uterus near the cervix.

FEMALE PELVIC LIGAMENTS AND SPACES

UTERINE LIGAMENTS

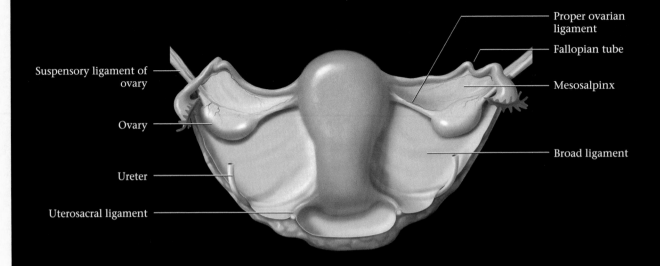

Proper ovarian ligament

Fallopian tube

Mesosalpinx

Suspensory ligament of ovary

Ovary

Ureter

Uterosacral ligament

Broad ligament

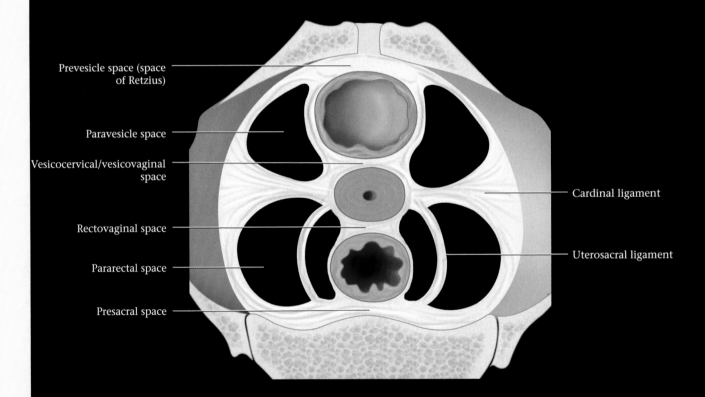

Prevesicle space (space of Retzius)

Paravesicle space

Vesicocervical/vesicovaginal space

Rectovaginal space

Pararectal space

Presacral space

Cardinal ligament

Uterosacral ligament

(Top) Illustration of the posterior aspect of the uterus and ovaries. The uterus and fallopian tubes are invested by peritoneum, which creates the broad ligament. The ovary is suspended from the pelvic side wall by the suspensory ligament of the ovary and from the uterus by the proper ovarian ligament. These ligaments separate the mesosalpinx above, from the broad ligament below. **(Bottom)** Schematic representation of the ligaments and spaces at the cervical/vaginal junction. The ligaments are visceral ligaments, which are composed of specialized endopelvic fascia and contain vessels, nerves and lymphatics. The main supporting ligaments for the uterus are the cardinal and uterosacral ligaments. The spaces are largely filled with loose connective tissue and are used as dissection planes during surgery.

FEMALE PELVIC LIGAMENTS AND SPACES

CUL-DE-SACS

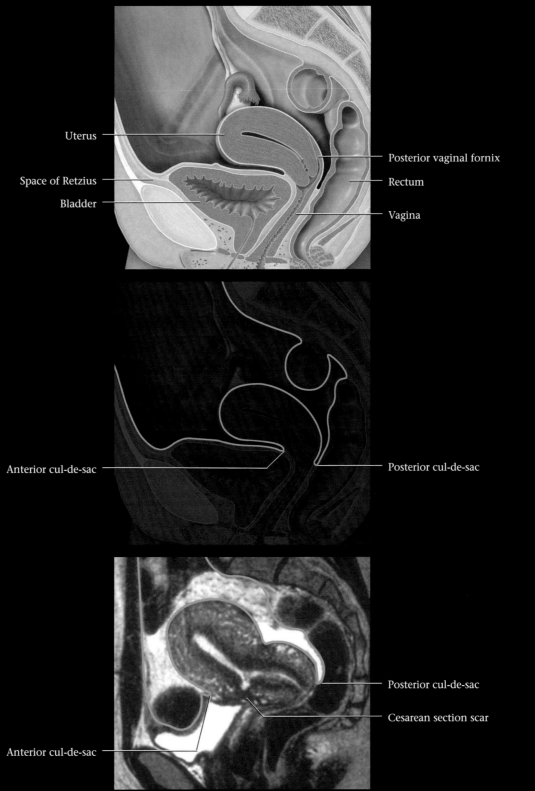

Uterus

Space of Retzius

Bladder

Posterior vaginal fornix

Rectum

Vagina

Anterior cul-de-sac

Posterior cul-de-sac

Posterior cul-de-sac

Cesarean section scar

Anterior cul-de-sac

(Top) Sagittal graphic of the female pelvis shows the bladder, uterus and rectum, all of which are extraperitoneal. **(Middle)** The peritoneum has been highlighted to show the cul-de-sacs. Posteriorly, the peritoneum extends along the posterior vaginal fornix, creating the posterior cul-de-sac (pouch of Douglas), the most dependent portion of the pelvis. Anteriorly, at the level of the lower uterine segment, the peritoneum is reflected over the dome of the bladder, creating the anterior cul-de-sac. **(Bottom)** Sagittal T2 MR image with the peritoneum outlined. Note that the scar from the prior cesarean section is actually extraperitoneal, lying below the anterior peritoneal reflection. The peritoneum over the bladder is loosely applied, allowing for filling of the bladder. This also allows it to be lifted, creating a surgical plane for a cesarean section.

FEMALE PELVIC LIGAMENTS AND SPACES

BROAD LIGAMENT

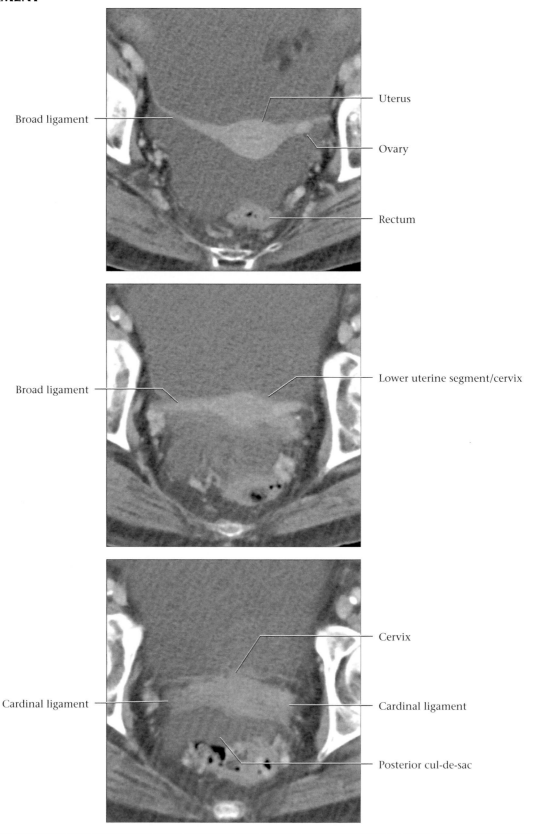

Broad ligament

Uterus

Ovary

Rectum

Broad ligament

Lower uterine segment/cervix

Cervix

Cardinal ligament

Cardinal ligament

Posterior cul-de-sac

(**Top**) First of three CT images in a woman with ascites showing the uterine ligaments. The broad ligaments represent peritoneal reflections that cover the uterus and adnexa, and extend laterally to the pelvic wall. They offer little structural support to the uterus. (**Middle**) Just caudal to the uterine arteries, the broad ligament begins to thicken, as it attaches to the cervix. (**Bottom**) The cardinal ligament attaches to the lateral margin of the cervix and vagina. It widens laterally to attach to the pelvic wall. Uterine ligaments are composed of specialized endopelvic fascia that provide support and transmit the neurovascular supply.

BROAD LIGAMENT

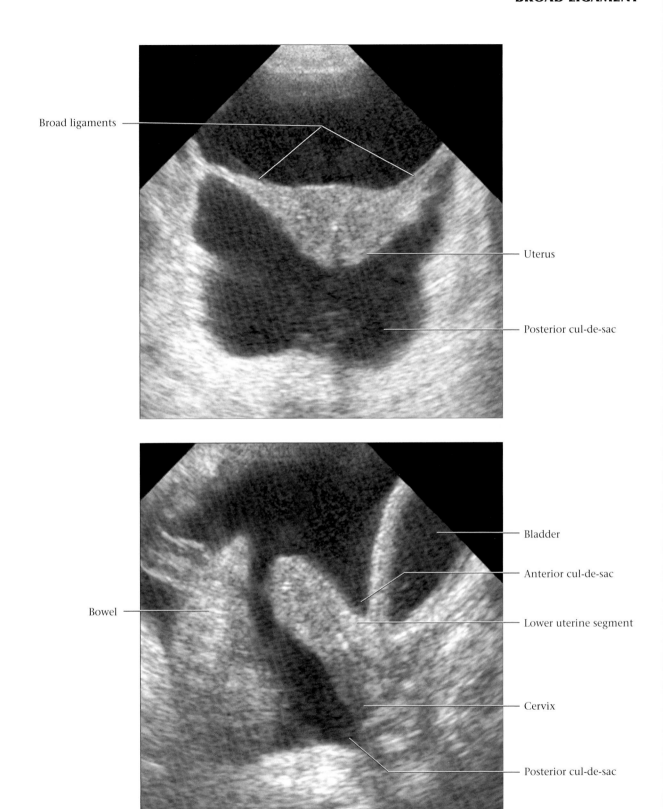

(Top) Axial transabdominal ultrasound in a patient with ascites shows the broad ligaments, attaching to the pelvic wall and suspending the uterus within the fluid. The uterine ligaments are analogous in function to the small bowel mesentery. (Bottom) In the longitudinal plane both the anterior and posterior cul-de-sacs are well demonstrated. The peritoneum reflects over the lower uterine segment to create the anterior cul-de-sac. Posteriorly, the peritoneum extends more inferiorly to the level of the posterior vaginal fornix, creating the posterior cul-de-sac. This is the most dependent spot in the pelvis.

FEMALE PELVIC LIGAMENTS AND SPACES

ROUND LIGAMENT

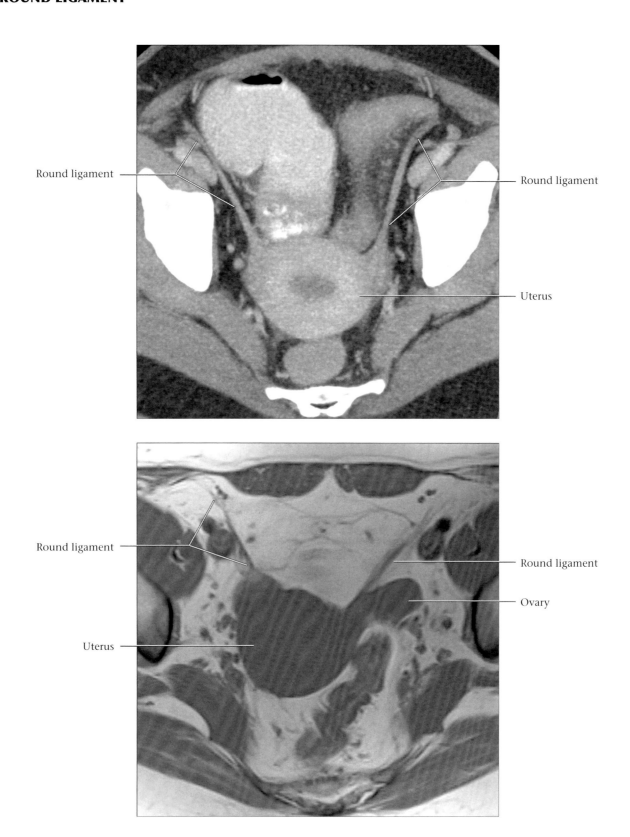

Round ligament

Round ligament

Uterus

Round ligament

Round ligament

Ovary

Uterus

(Top) CECT image of the round ligaments. The round ligaments arise anterior to the fallopian tubes and extend anteriorly. They pass through the inguinal canal and insert on the labia majora. They are the embryologic homologue to the gubernaculum in the male and offer little support to the uterus. **(Bottom)** Axial T1 MR image, also showing the round ligaments.

FEMALE PELVIC LIGAMENTS AND SPACES

IUD in cervix

Posterior cul-de-sac

Uterosacral ligament

Uterosacral ligament

Rectum

Ovary

Ovary

Uterus

Cervix

Uterosacral ligament

Uterosacral ligament

Cervical cancer

Thickened uterosacral ligament

Normal uterosacral ligament

(Top) Axial CT with rectal contrast in a patient with ascites. Free fluid is within the posterior cul-de-sac. The uterosacral ligaments can be seen forming the lateral borders of this space. (Middle) Normal axial T1 MR shows the uterosacral ligaments extending from the cervix posteriorly towards the sacrum. They are composed predominately of smooth muscle and convey the autonomic nerves to the pelvic organs. They, along with the cardinal ligaments and levator ani, are the main support for the uterus and cervix. (Bottom) An axial T2 MR image shows invasion of the right uterosacral ligament by cervical carcinoma. Cervical carcinoma commonly invades into the parametrium, which includes both the uterosacral and cardinal ligaments. These are very important areas to evaluate when staging cervical carcinoma.

FEMALE PELVIC LIGAMENTS AND SPACES

SPACES, PARAVESICLE/PERIRECTAL

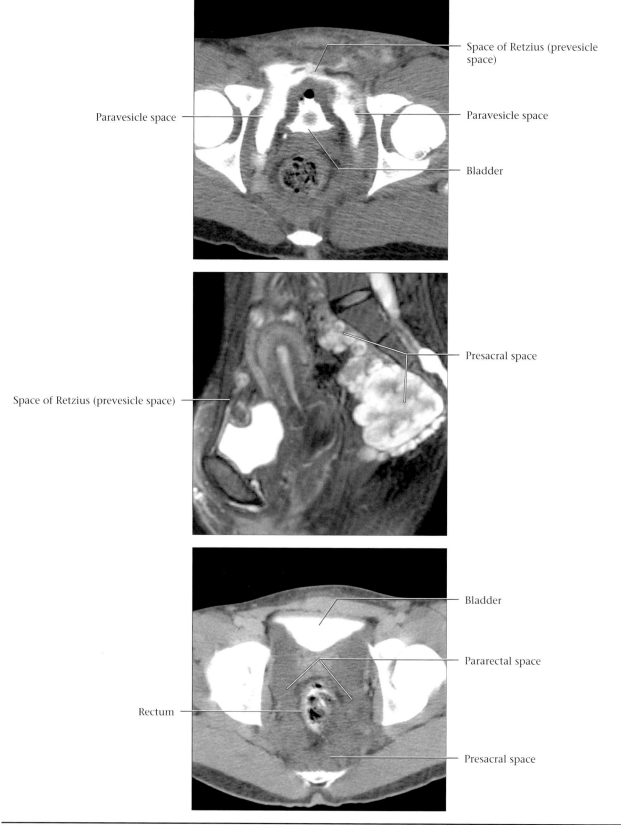

Space of Retzius (prevesicle space)

Paravesicle space

Paravesicle space

Bladder

Presacral space

Space of Retzius (prevesicle space)

Bladder

Pararectal space

Rectum

Presacral space

(Top) CT scan, after the instillation of contrast into the bladder, shows an extraperitoneal bladder rupture with contrast leaking into the prevesicle and paravesicle spaces. (Middle) Sagittal T2 FS MR in a patient with neurofibromatosis type I shows large neurofibromas in the prevesicle and presacral spaces. Note how the presacral space extends superiorly up to the level of the aortic bifurcation. (Bottom) Axial CECT in another patient with neurofibromatosis type I showing the pararectal, as well as the presacral spaces. Normally these pelvic spaces are filled with fat and connective tissue.

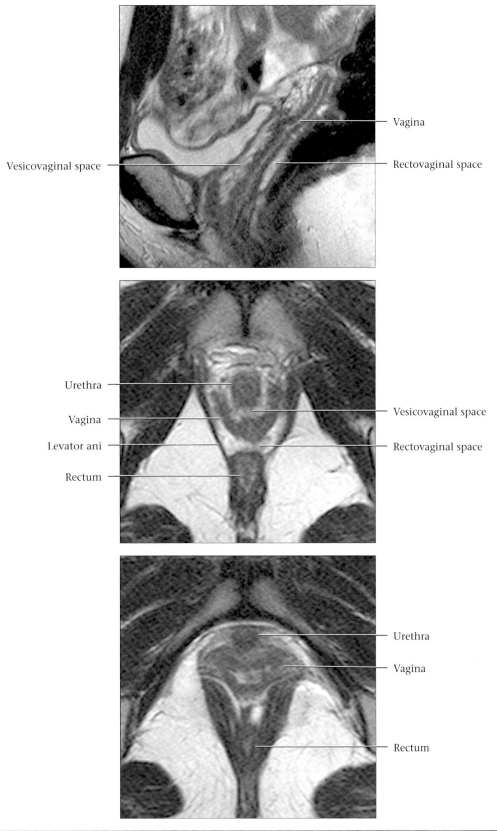

Vagina

Vesicovaginal space

Rectovaginal space

Urethra

Vagina

Levator ani

Rectum

Vesicovaginal space

Rectovaginal space

Urethra

Vagina

Rectum

(Top) First of three T2 MR images of the vagina in a woman who has had a hysterectomy. This sagittal image shows high-signal fluid/mucus separating the low-signal muscular walls of the vagina. The vagina is separated from the bladder by the vesicovaginal space and from the rectum by the rectovaginal space. The perivaginal venous plexus lies within these spaces and surrounds the vagina, and partially encircles the urethra and rectum. **(Middle)** Axial T2 MR shows the urethra, vagina and rectum as three separate structures. The high signal within the vesicovaginal and rectovaginal spaces represents the perivaginal venous plexus. **(Bottom)** The distal portion of the urethra is fused with the anterior wall of the vagina, and therefore, no distinct plane is seen between them.

SPACES, ANTERIOR CUL-DE-SAC

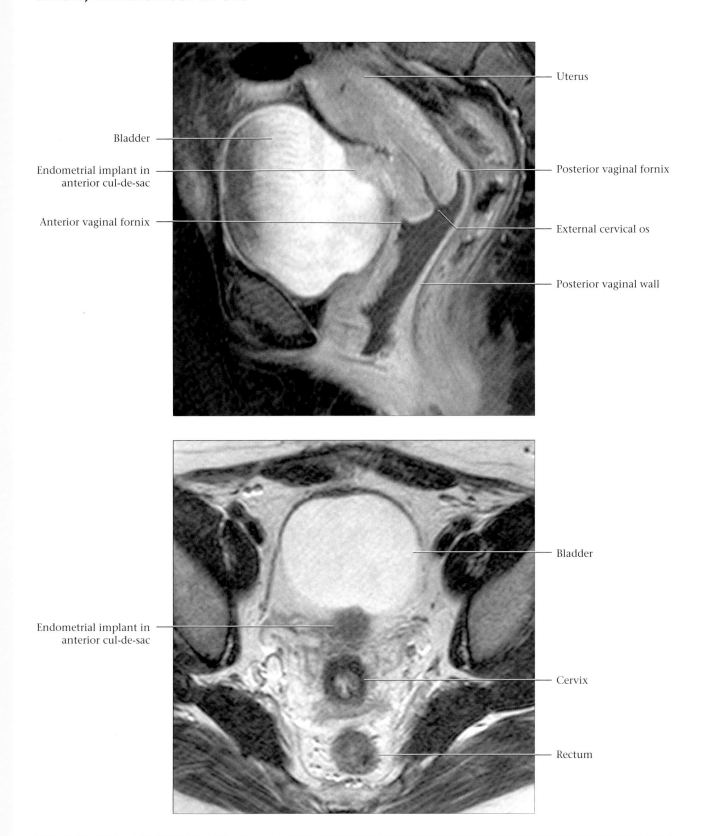

(Top) First of two images of an endometrial implant in the anterior cul-de-sac (vesico-uterine pouch). Sagittal T1 C+ FS MR image shows an enhancing endometrial implant in the anterior cul-de-sac. Gel has been instilled into the vagina, separating the walls. Note that the posterior ligainal fornix is higher than the anterior vaginal fornix. (Bottom) Axial T2 image showing the same endometrial implant. In the axial plane, it is often difficult to differentiate whether a mass is intraperitoneal (lying in the anterior cul-de-sac) or extraperitoneal (lying in the vesicocervical space). The sagittal plane is much better for making this determination.

Uterus — Bladder

Endometrial implants in posterior cul-de-sac

Uterus

Peritoneal implants

Peritoneal implants

Rectum

Uterus

Ectopic pregnancy

Blood in posterior cul-de-sac

(Top) Midline longitudinal ultrasound on a woman with endometriosis shows multiple, large implants within the posterior cul-de-sac. The posterior cul-de-sac is the most dependent spot in the female pelvis. Fluid, blood and peritoneal implants from both abdominal and pelvic pathologies can accumulate in this region making it a critical area to evaluate. **(Middle)** CECT image in a woman with gastric carcinoma and ascites shows both fluid and multiple peritoneal implants (drop metastases) within the posterior cul-de-sac. **(Bottom)** Longitudinal transvaginal ultrasound of the uterus in a woman with an ectopic pregnancy shows a large amount of echogenic blood within the posterior cul-de-sac (pouch of Douglas).

UTERUS

Gross Anatomy

Overview

- Thick-walled, fibromuscular organ composed of myometrium and endometrium
- Two major divisions
  - Body (corpus) and cervix
    - Fundus above ostia of fallopian tubes
- **Myometrium**
  - Interwoven layers of smooth muscle
- **Endometrium**
  - Simple, columnar epithelium forming numerous tubular glands supported by a thick vascular stroma
  - Composed of two distinct layers
    - **Stratum functionalis:** Superficial layer that grows under hormonal stimulation and sloughs with menstruation
    - **Stratum basalis:** Deep supporting layer, densely adherent to myometrium
- Cervix
  - Begins at inferior narrowing of uterus (**isthmus**)
    - Has a supravaginal and vaginal portion (ectocervix or portio vaginalis)
  - **Internal os:** Opening into uterine cavity
  - **External os:** Opening into vagina
  - Stroma is largely fibrous, with a high proportion of elastic fibers interwoven with smooth muscle
  - Endocervical canal lined by mucous secreting, columnar epithelium
    - Epithelium is in a series of small V-shaped folds (**plicae palmatae**)
  - Ectocervix lined by stratified squamous epithelium
  - **Squamocolumnar junction** near external os but exact position is variable, with continuous remodeling
- Appearance, size, shape and weight vary with estrogen stimulation and parturition
  - **Premenarche**
    - Cervix is larger than corpus (approximately 2/3 of uterine mass)
  - **Menarche**
    - Preferential growth of corpus in response to hormonal stimulation
    - Nulliparous women corpus and cervix roughly equal
    - Parous, non-pregnant women corpus is approximately 2/3 of uterine mass
  - **Postmenopausal**
    - Corpus decreases back to premenopausal size
- **Menstrual cycle**
  - **Proliferative phase**
    - End of menstruation to ovulation (~ day 14)
    - Estrogen induces proliferation of functionalis layer
    - Corresponds to follicular phase of ovary
  - **Secretory phase**
    - Ovulation to beginning of menstruation
    - Progesterone induces endometrium to secrete glycogen, mucous and other substances
    - Endometrial glands become enlarged and tortuous
    - Corresponds to luteal phase of ovary
  - **Menstrual phase**
    - Sloughing of functionalis layer of endometrium

Anatomic Relationships

- **Uterus is extraperitoneal**
  - Peritoneum extends over bladder dome to anterior uterus
    - Creates anterior cul-de-sac (vesico-uterine pouch)
  - Posteriorly, peritoneum extends more inferiorly to upper portion of vagina
    - Creates posterior cul-de-sac (pouch of Douglas, recto-uterine pouch)
    - Most dependent portion of female pelvis
- Supporting ligaments
  - Broad ligament
    - Formed by the two sheets of covering peritoneum
    - Extends laterally to pelvic wall and forms supporting mesentery for uterus
  - Round ligaments
    - Arise from uterine cornu near fallopian tubes
    - Course anteriorly, through inguinal canal to insert on labia majora
  - Ligaments formed from connective tissue thickening at base of broad ligament
    - Uterosacral ligaments posteriorly
    - Cardinal ligaments laterally
    - Vesicouterine ligaments anteriorly
- **Uterine position**
  - **Flexion** is axis of uterine body relative to cervix
  - **Version** is axis of cervix relative to vagina
  - Most uteri are anteverted and anteflexed
- **Fallopian tubes** connect uterus to peritoneal cavity
  - Attached to posterior broad ligament by mesosalpinx
  - 8-10 cm in length
  - Composed of four segments: **Interstitial, isthmus, ampulla and infundibulum**
  - **Interstitial or intramural portion**
    - Portion of tube which traverses uterine wall
    - ~ 1 cm in length
  - **Isthmus**
    - Narrow portion of tube, immediately adjacent to uterus
  - **Ampulla**
    - Tortuous, ectatic portion contiguous with isthmus
    - Fertilization usually occurs in this portion of tube
  - **Infundibulum**
    - Funnel-shaped opening, ringed by finger-like fimbriae
    - Adjacent to posterior surface of ovary, allowing it to "capture" ovulated ova
- Uterus has **dual blood supply**
  - **Uterine artery passes over ureter** at level of cervix ("**water under the bridge**")
    - Courses superiorly, along lateral margin of uterus and **anastomoses with ovarian artery**
  - Uterine arteries give rise to **arcuate arteries**, which run in outer third of myometrium
  - **Radial arteries** extend through myometrium terminating as **spiral arteries** in endometrium
- Venous drainage
  - Myometrial veins follow same course as arteries
  - Forms **complex venous network** in parametrium
  - Eventually drains to either uterine or ovarian vein

UTERUS

Imaging Anatomy

Ultrasound
- **Myometrium**: 3 layers usually discernible
  - Compacted, thin, hypoechoic inner layer forms **subendometrial halo**
  - Thicker, homogeneously echogenic middle layer
  - Thinner, hypoechoic outer layer
    - Portion of myometrium peripheral to arcuate vessels
- **Endometrial appearance varies** with phase of menstrual cycle
  - Thin, echogenic line early in proliferative phase
  - Progressive, hypoechoic thickening (4-8 mm) as proliferative phase progresses
    - Triple layer ("sandwich") appearance: Echogenic central line created where the 2 hypoechoic endometrial walls coapt
  - After ovulation (secretory phase), endometrium becomes thicker (7-14 mm) and more echogenic
- Sonohysterography
  - Study of choice for evaluating endometrial pathology
  - Balloon catheter inserted into cervix
  - Sterile saline infused while scanning
    - Separates endometrial walls, allowing for complete evaluation of endometrium
- 3D ultrasound
  - Allows multiple views to be reconstructed from single sweep through uterus

MR
- Uterus and cervix uniform intermediate signal on T1WI
- **Uterus has 3 distinct zones** on T2WI
  - High signal **endometrium**
  - Low signal **junctional zone**
    - Inner layer of myometrium with low water content, resulting in decreased signal
    - Normal thickness 2-8 mm
    - ≥ 12 mm abnormal (adenomyosis)
    - 9-11 mm equivocal
  - Intermediate signal myometrium
- Uterine appearance varies according to hormonal stimulation
  - **Premenopausal**
    - Endometrium thickens in secretory phase
    - Myometrial signal increases in secretory phase from increased water content and vascular flow
    - Low signal uterine contractions, which bulge the uterine contour may be seen
    - **Contractions** are transient and should not be confused with fibroids or adenomyosis
  - **Oral contraceptives**
    - Both endometrium and junctional zone become thin
  - **Postmenopausal**
    - Endometrium atrophies, junctional zone is absent
- **Cervical zonal anatomy** on T2WI
  - High signal endocervical canal
    - **Plicae palmatae** may be seen as a separate intermediate signal zone, on high resolution scans
  - Predominately low signal cervical stroma, secondary to large proportion of elastic fibrous tissue
    - Contiguous with junctional zone
  - An outer layer of intermediate signal smooth muscle may be variably present
  - **Nabothian cysts** are commonly seen
    - Represent obstructed, mucous-secreting glands
    - Low signal on T1WI, high signal on T2WI
- **Parametrium**
  - Low to intermediate signal intensity T1WI
  - Variable signal intensity T2WI
    - Round ligament and uterosacral ligament low signal intensity
    - Cardinal ligament and associated venous plexuses high signal intensity

Embryology
- Uterus is formed from paired paramesonephric (Müllerian ducts)
- These paired ducts meet in midline and fuse
  - Fusion forms uterovaginal canal (uterus and upper vagina)
  - Unfused portions remain as fallopian tubes
- Lower vagina formed from urogenital sinus

Clinical Implications

Müllerian Duct Anomalies
- Failure of Müllerian duct development and/or fusion leads to spectrum of congenital uterine anomalies
  - Class I: Agenesis or hypoplasia (10% of cases)
  - Class II: Unicornuate uterus (20% of cases)
    - Single uterine horn, may have accessory rudimentary horn
  - Class III: Uterus didelphys (5% of cases)
    - Two, separate, non-communicating horns
  - Class IV: Bicornuate uterus (10% of cases)
    - Concave or heart-shaped external uterine contour
  - Class V: Septate uterus (55% of cases)
    - Normal external contour
    - Dividing septum of variable lengths
- High association with **renal anomalies**
  - Check kidneys in every patient

Ectopic Pregnancy
- 95% of ectopic pregnancies are tubal
  - Ampullary portion of tube most common location
- 2-5% are interstitial
  - Located in intramural portion of fallopian tube
  - Can grow to larger size before rupture
  - **Interstitial line sign**: Echogenic line from endometrium to ectopic sac
    - Overlying myometrium is thinned
- Rare ectopics: Cervical, ovary, abdominal, cesarean-section scar

Hydrosalpinx
- Dilated, fluid-filled fallopian tube
- "Cogwheel" shape in cross section
  - Incomplete septae from mucosal folds

UTERUS

UTERUS

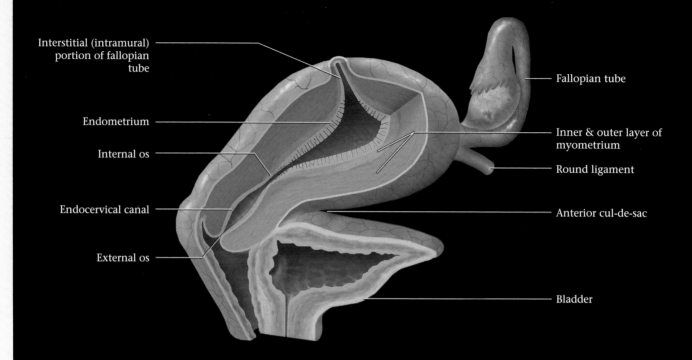

Interstitial (intramural) portion of fallopian tube

Endometrium

Internal os

Endocervical canal

External os

Fallopian tube

Inner & outer layer of myometrium

Round ligament

Anterior cul-de-sac

Bladder

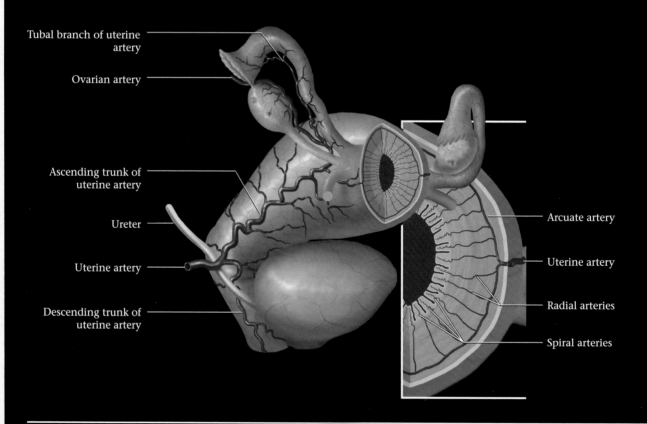

Tubal branch of uterine artery

Ovarian artery

Ascending trunk of uterine artery

Ureter

Uterine artery

Descending trunk of uterine artery

Arcuate artery

Uterine artery

Radial arteries

Spiral arteries

(Top) The uterus is composed of a glandular endometrium and muscular myometrium. The smooth muscle within the inner portion of the myometrium is more compacted and relatively hypovascular. **(Bottom)** The uterine artery arises from the anterior trunk of the internal iliac artery. It crosses the ureter as it courses medially to the lateral wall of the uterus. At the level of the cervix it bifurcates into an ascending and descending trunk. The ascending trunk forms the major blood supply to the uterus. It courses superiorly along the lateral wall of the uterus where it anastomoses with the ovarian artery, a branch of the aorta. Arcuate arteries course circumferentially in the outer third of the myometrium and give rise to the radial arteries and finally the spiral arteries, which supply the endometrium.

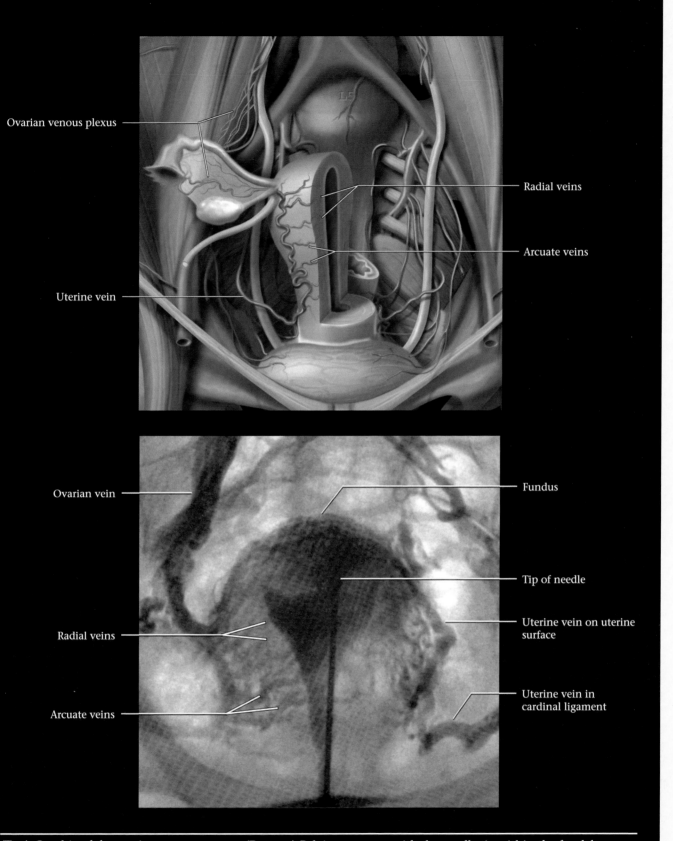

Ovarian venous plexus

Radial veins

Arcuate veins

Uterine vein

Ovarian vein

Fundus

Tip of needle

Uterine vein on uterine surface

Radial veins

Arcuate veins

Uterine vein in cardinal ligament

(Top) Graphic of the uterine venous system. **(Bottom)** Pelvic venogram with the needle tip within the fundal myometrium shows very fine radial veins extending from the endometrium and larger arcuate veins, which course around in a circular fashion in the outer third of the myometrium. Venous drainage may be via the uterine or ovarian veins. Note the presence of numerous small surrounding veins. These are part of the extensive venous plexus network within the pelvis. They form a rich collateral venous drainage system. Varices can develop within these vessels, causing pelvic congestion and chronic pelvic pain.

UTERUS

ARCUATE VESSELS

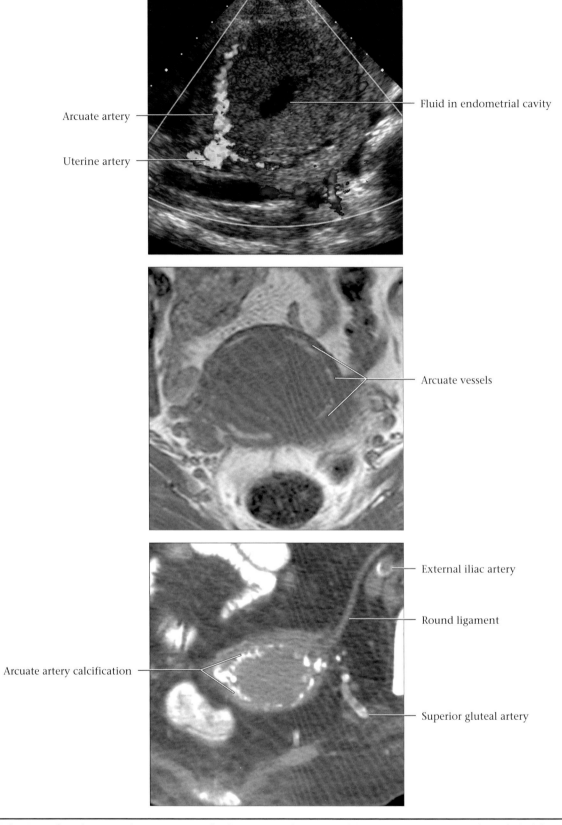

Arcuate artery

Uterine artery

Fluid in endometrial cavity

Arcuate vessels

External iliac artery

Round ligament

Arcuate artery calcification

Superior gluteal artery

(Top) Color Doppler ultrasound in a patient who has just undergone a dilatation and curettage for a failed first trimester pregnancy. There is very prominent flow in the arcuate arteries, which run in the outer third of the myometrium (Courtesy J. Wong, MD). **(Middle)** T1 MR of the uterus shows high signal within the arcuate vessels. This could represent either the arcuate veins or slow flow within the arcuate arteries. **(Bottom)** Unenhanced CT scan in a woman with renal failure shows prominent arcuate artery calcifications. The pattern and location of calcifications is characteristic and should not be confused with a pathologic entity, such as a calcified fibroid. Note calcifications within other pelvic vessels.

UTERUS

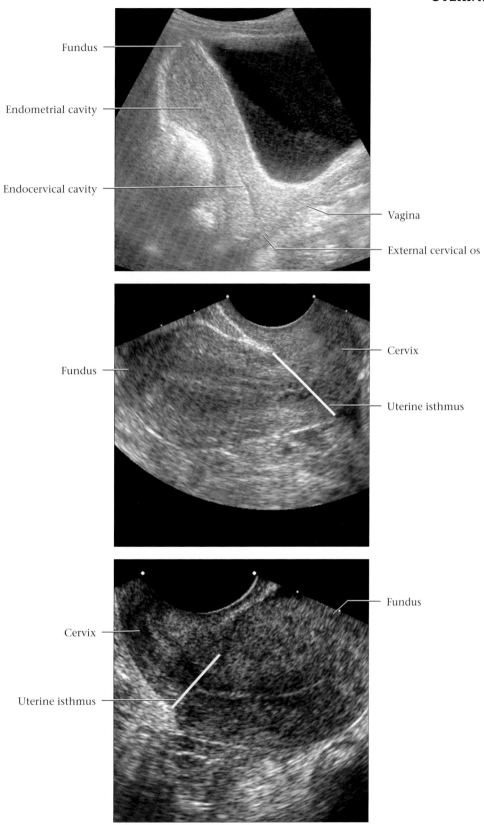

(Top) Transabdominal ultrasound of an anteverted uterus. Version refers to the angle the cervix makes with the vagina. In this case, the cervix is angled anteriorly and the uterus continues in a straight line with the cervix, making this anteversion. Uterine position can change with the degree of bladder filling. (Middle) Transvaginal ultrasound of an anteflexed uterus. Flexion refers to the angle the uterine corpus makes with the cervix (a line has been drawn across the uterine isthmus as a reference point). The uterine corpus is angled forward with respect to the cervix at this junction. (Bottom) Transvaginal ultrasound shows the cervix angling posteriorly with respect the probe, which is in the vagina (retroversion). In addition, the uterus is even more posteriorly angled with respect to the cervix (retroflexion). Retropositioned can be used generically for either of these positions.

UTERUS

ENDOMETRIUM, CYCLICAL VARIATIONS

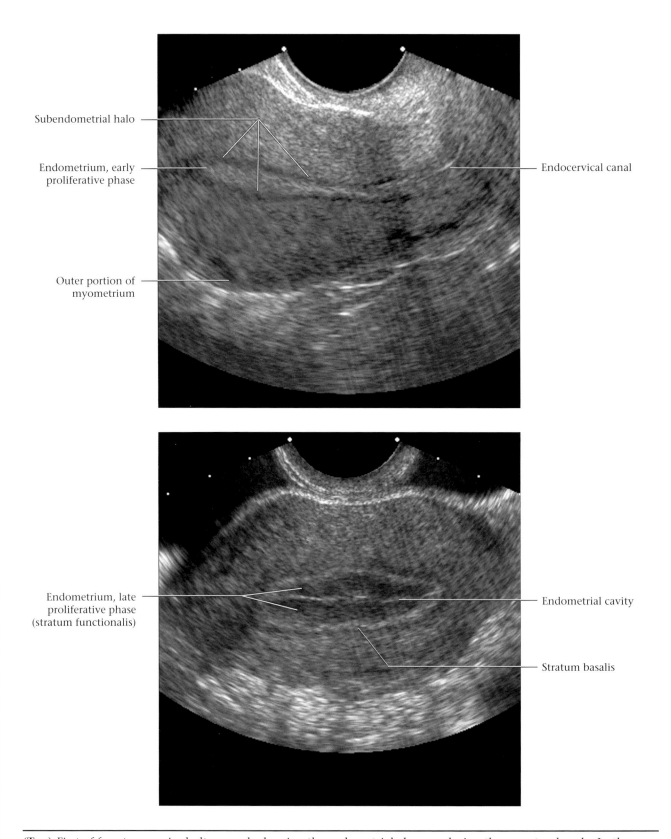

Subendometrial halo

Endometrium, early proliferative phase

Outer portion of myometrium

Endocervical canal

Endometrium, late proliferative phase (stratum functionalis)

Endometrial cavity

Stratum basalis

(Top) First of four transvaginal ultrasounds showing the endometrial changes during the menstrual cycle. In the early proliferative phase, the endometrium is thin and echogenic. This image also nicely demonstrates features of the myometrium. The smooth muscle within the inner band of myometrium is more compacted and relatively hypovascular, giving it a more hypoechoic appearance (subendometrial halo). The majority of the myometrium has a homogeneous echogenicity, with the outer portion (peripheral to arcuate vessels) sometimes being slightly less echogenic. **(Bottom)** In the late proliferative phase, the functionalis layer of the endometrium thickens and becomes hypoechoic (the basalis layer remains echogenic). A hyperechoic central line is created where the two endometrial walls coapt. This gives the endometrium a layered, "sandwich" appearance.

UTERUS

ENDOMETRIUM, CYCLICAL VARIATIONS

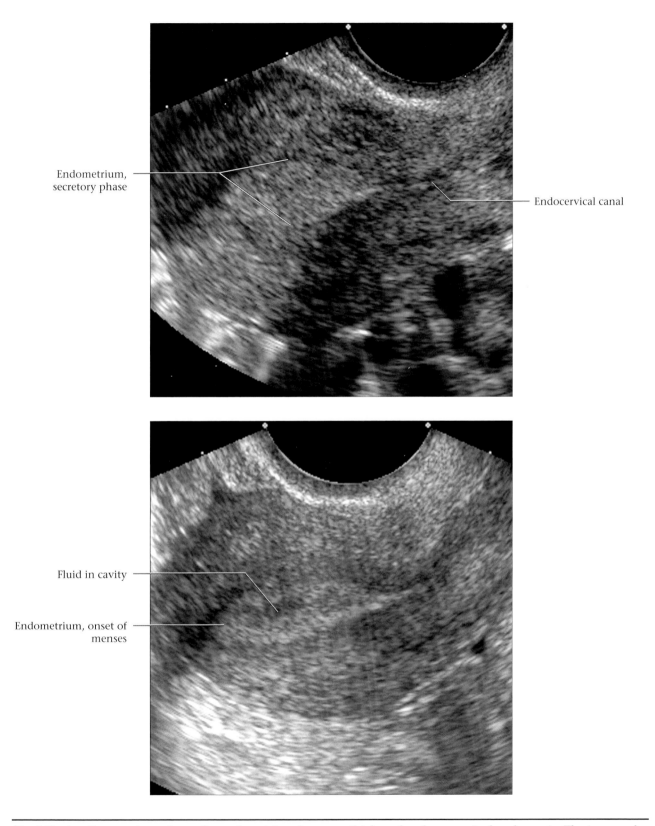

Endometrium, secretory phase

Endocervical canal

Fluid in cavity

Endometrium, onset of menses

(Top) During the secretory phase, the endometrium becomes thickened and progressively echogenic. The increased echogenicity is the result of the endometrial glands becoming enlarged and tortuous, and filled with glycogen, mucous and other substances necessary to sustain a pregnancy. **(Bottom)** If no pregnancy occurs, the functionalis layer of the endometrium begins to involute and slough off (menses). The endometrium becomes progressively thinner, and a small amount of fluid may be seen within the endometrial cavity.

SONOHYSTEROGRAPHY, ENDOMETRIUM

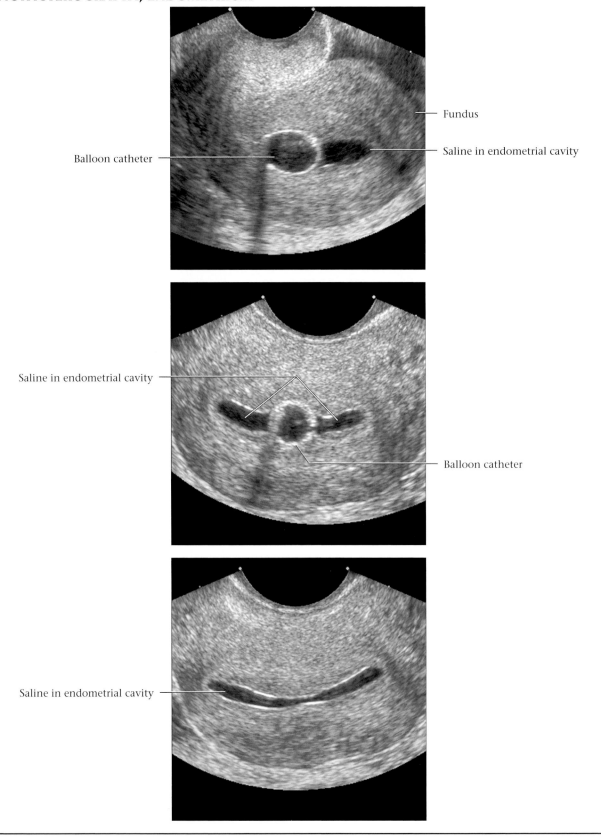

Fundus

Saline in endometrial cavity

Balloon catheter

Saline in endometrial cavity

Balloon catheter

Saline in endometrial cavity

(Top) First of three images from a sonohysterogram in a retroflexed uterus performed just after the cessation of menses. A balloon catheter is inflated in the lower uterine segment and sterile saline is infused while scanning. As the cavity distends, the uterine walls begin to separate and the endometrium can be evaluated. This longitudinal image at the beginning of the infusion shows the inflated balloon in place, and saline beginning to expand the endometrial cavity. (Middle) Transverse image through the lower uterine segment shows continued distention of the endometrial cavity. (Bottom) Near the fundus, the entire endometrium is well seen and has a normal, uniformly thin appearance. Sonohysterography is the imaging study of choice for evaluating endometrial abnormalities.

UTERUS

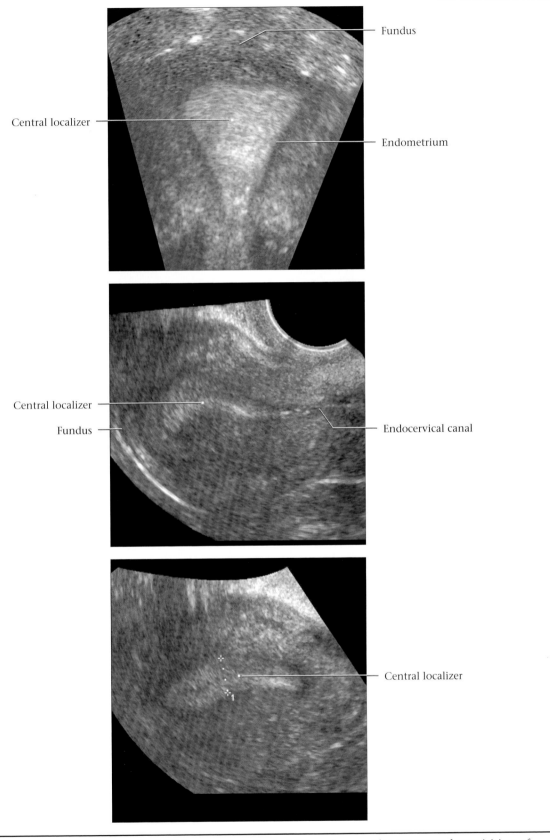

Fundus

Central localizer

Endometrium

Central localizer

Fundus

Endocervical canal

Central localizer

(**Top**) First of three simultaneously acquired 3D images. A dedicated 3D probe provides automated acquisition of ultrasound volume data. This data is displayed in 3 simultaneous orthogonal planes. Multiplanar and rendered images can be rotated and "sliced through" like CT and MR. A central localizer point on each image allows the operator to know the precise location in all three planes. In this coronal image the entire endometrial and fundal contour are displayed. This has particular utility in evaluating Müllerian duct anomalies. (**Middle**) Same 3D data set projected in the longitudinal plane. (**Bottom**) Same 3D data set projected in the transverse plane. The cursors are measuring the endometrial thickness.

UTERUS

MR, UTERUS

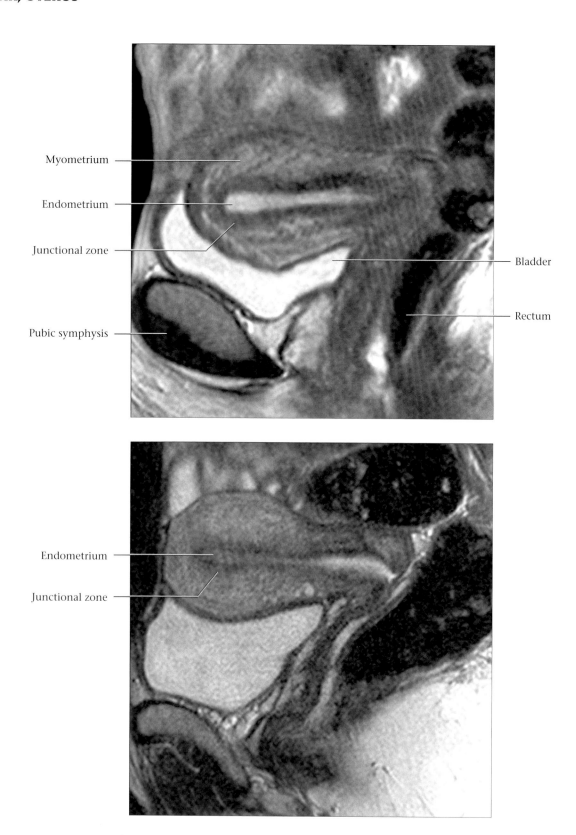

Myometrium

Endometrium

Junctional zone

Bladder

Rectum

Pubic symphysis

Endometrium

Junctional zone

(Top) Sagittal T2 MR of the uterus in a woman not on oral contraceptives shows the typical zonal anatomy, with a high signal endometrium, low signal junctional zone and intermediate signal myometrium. The junctional zone represents the inner most portion of the myometrium, which has a lower water content resulting in the lower signal. Maximum normal junctional zone thickness is 8 mm, with ≥ 12 mm diagnostic of adenomyosis. Measurements of 9-11 mm are in the equivocal range. **(Bottom)** Sagittal T2 MR of the uterus in a woman who is taking oral contraceptives shows a much less distinct zonal architecture. Both the endometrium and junctional zone have thinned, and are far less obvious. The endometrium no longer cycles so remains 1-2 mm in thickness, even before menses.

UTERUS

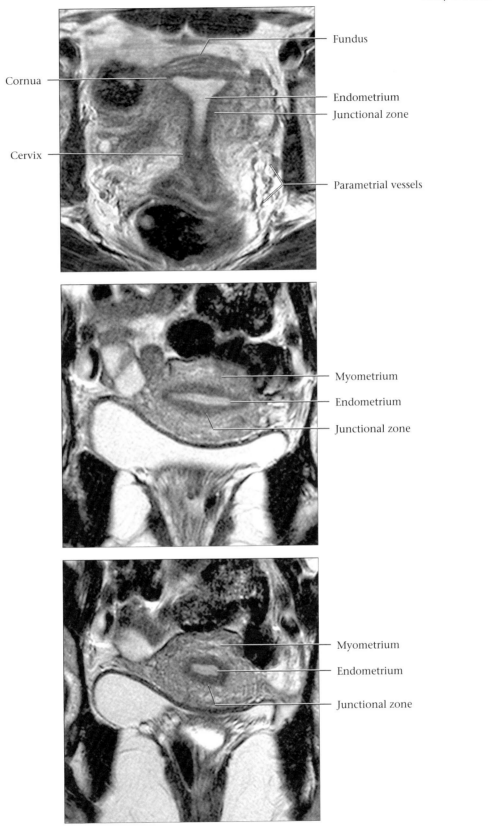

Fundus

Cornua

Endometrium

Junctional zone

Cervix

Parametrial vessels

Myometrium

Endometrium

Junctional zone

Myometrium

Endometrium

Junctional zone

(Top) Coronal T2 MR view of the uterus allows simultaneous viewing of the endometrial cavity and uterine fundus. This view is obtained by angling the scan plane along the long axis of the uterus. **(Middle)** First of two T2 MR images taken in an axial plane, with respect to the uterus (oblique coronal to the body). This first image is taken near the fundus. The uterus and endometrium have an elliptical contour at this level. **(Bottom)** In the lower uterine segment, the uterus and endometrium become more rounded in appearance.

UTERUS

CERVIX

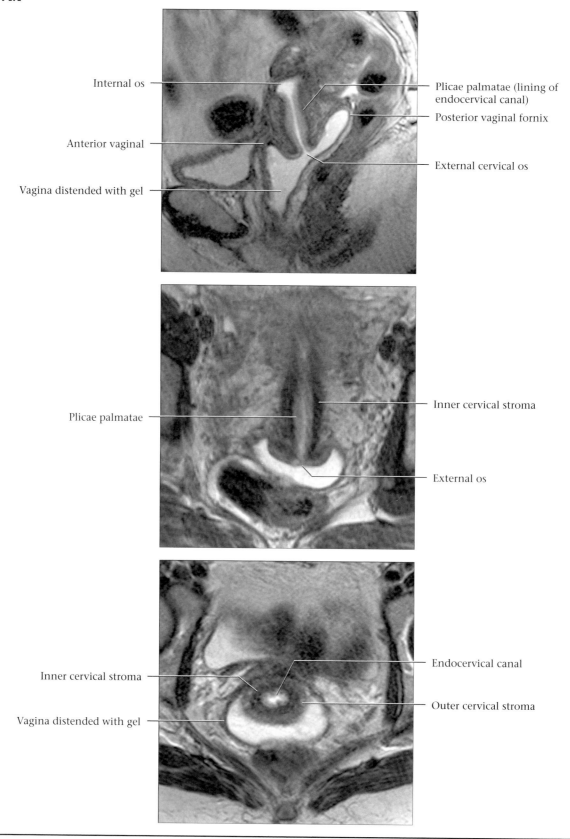

Internal os

Plicae palmatae (lining of endocervical canal)

Posterior vaginal fornix

Anterior vaginal

External cervical os

Vagina distended with gel

Plicae palmatae

Inner cervical stroma

External os

Inner cervical stroma

Endocervical canal

Outer cervical stroma

Vagina distended with gel

(Top) First of three T2 MR views of the cervix. This sagittal image shows the feathery appearance of the endocervical canal. The endocervical canal is lined by mucous-secreting, columnar epithelium. This epithelium is arranged in small V-shaped folds giving a "frond-like" appearance, and hence the name, plicae palmatae. **(Middle)** Image plane taken along the long axis of the cervix. **(Bottom)** Axial ("donut") view shows the high signal intensity endocervical canal surrounded by low signal intensity cervical stroma. The cervical stroma is largely fibrous, with a high proportion of elastic fibers interwoven with smooth muscle. A third intermediate signal outer layer of smooth muscle is also seen. This layer is of variable thickness and is not seen in all patients.

Ovarian cyst

Internal os

Posterior vaginal fornix

Line separating supravaginal cervix from ectocervix

Anterior vaginal fornix

External os

Endocervical canal

Cervical stroma

Coapted walls of cervix

Free fluid in posterior cul-de-sac

Bowel

Nabothian cysts

(**Top**) Sagittal T2 MR image of the cervix, with a line connecting the vaginal fornices. The supravaginal portion of the cervix is above this line and the ectocervix, or portio vaginalis, is below it. (**Middle**) Transvaginal ultrasound of the cervix shows a hypoechoic band within the central portion of the cervix, which is formed by glands and mucous secretions of the endocervical canal. An echogenic central line is created where the two cervical walls coapt. (**Bottom**) Transvaginal ultrasound of the cervix shows multiple small Nabothian cysts lining the endocervical canal. Nabothian cysts result from obstructed, mucous-secreting glands of the cervix. They are generally anechoic but can be hypoechoic or contain obvious debris. Most are small, measuring < 1.5 cm. They appear as well-defined, high signal cysts on T2-weighted MR images.

UTERUS

FALLOPIAN TUBE

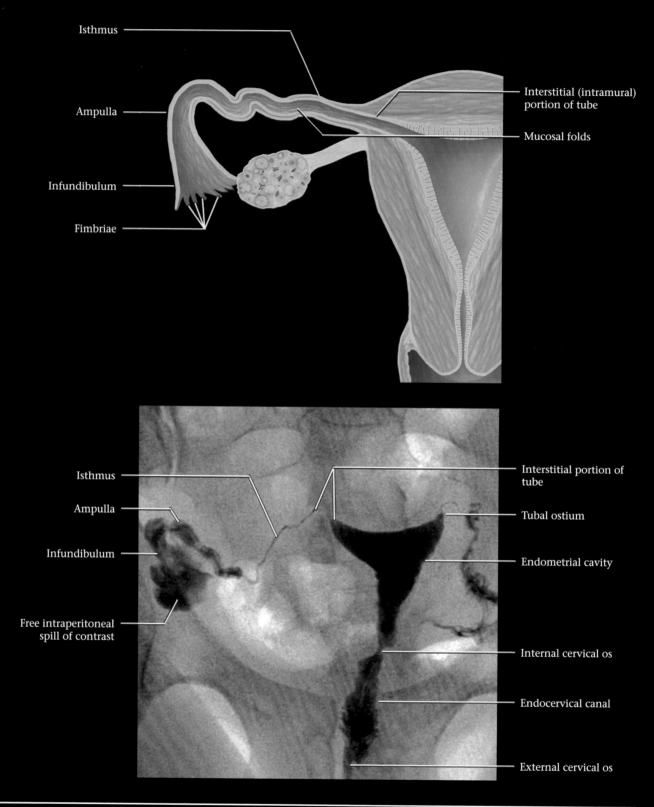

(Top) A graphic of the fallopian tube shows the four segments including the interstitial (intramural) portion, isthmus, ampulla and infundibulum, which is ringed by the fimbriae. (Bottom) A hysterosalpingogram shows the endocervical canal with a feathered appearance created by the endocervical glands (plicae palmatae). The uterine cavity has a triangular configuration. The interstitial portion of the tube traverses the myometrial wall at the cornua (approximately 1 cm in length). An acute angulation can often be seen between it and the isthmus. The fallopian tube widens at the ampulla and infundibulum, before opening into the peritoneal cavity adjacent to the posterior surface of the ovary.

UTERUS

ECTOPIC PREGNANCY

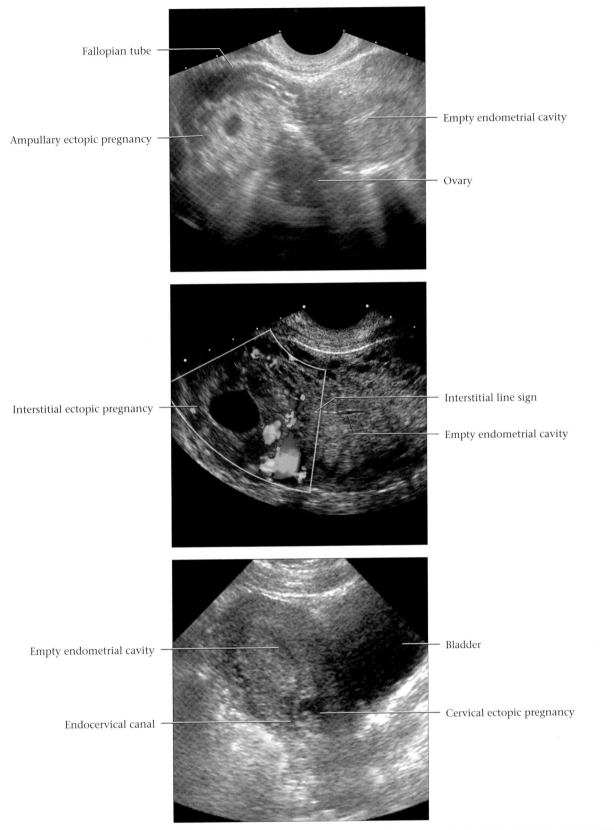

(Top) First of three different examples of ectopic pregnancy showing the relative position of the gestational sac to the fallopian tube and endometrial cavity. In this case, an ectopic gestation (thick echogenic ring) is seen in the ampullary portion of the fallopian tube. This is the most common ectopic location, although precise tubal localization is usually not possible. **(Middle)** Color Doppler image of an interstitial ectopic pregnancy. The endometrial cavity is empty. At the cornua, the proximal interstitial portion of the tube can be followed to the ectopic sac. This has been called the interstitial line sign. The ectopic pregnancy has dramatically enlarged the portion of the tube traveling through the uterine wall (interstitial portion) and there is essentially no surrounding myometrium. **(Bottom)** Transabdominal ultrasound of a cervical ectopic pregnancy.

UTERUS

HYDROSALPINX

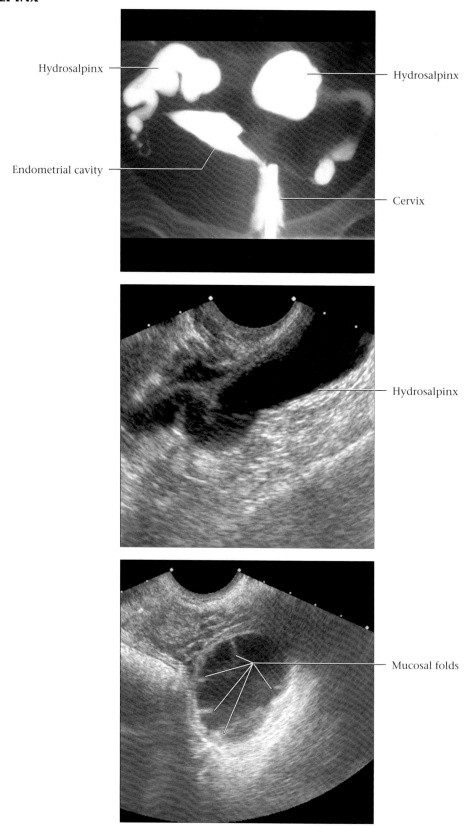

Hydrosalpinx — Hydrosalpinx

Endometrial cavity — Cervix

Hydrosalpinx

Mucosal folds

(**Top**) Hysterosalpingogram shows bilateral hydrosalpinges. The ampullary portion expands dramatically and there is no free intraperitoneal spill of contrast. (**Middle**) First of two transvaginal ultrasound images of a left-sided hydrosalpinx. During real-time scanning it is important to try to elongate the tube as in this image. This allows differentiation from a cystic ovarian mass. (**Bottom**) In the cross-sectional plane, a hydrosalpinx will often display a "cogwheel" appearance. The mucosal folds of the fallopian tube project into the lumen. As the hydrosalpinx becomes more chronic, these folds will become thick and nodular.

UTERUS

UTERINE EMBRYOLOGY

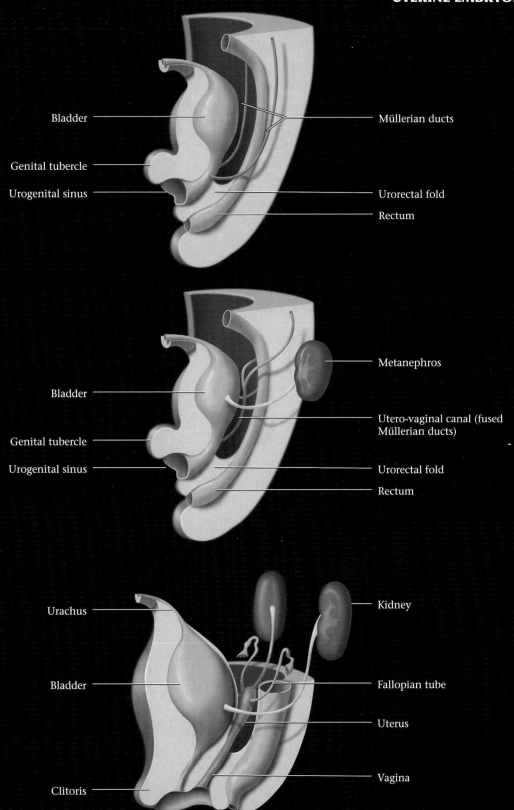

Bladder — Müllerian ducts

Genital tubercle

Urogenital sinus — Urorectal fold

— Rectum

— Metanephros

Bladder — Utero-vaginal canal (fused Müllerian ducts)

Genital tubercle

Urogenital sinus — Urorectal fold

— Rectum

Urachus — Kidney

Bladder — Fallopian tube

— Uterus

— Vagina

Clitoris

(Top) The fallopian tubes, uterus and upper vagina form from the paired Müllerian (paramesonephric) ducts, which develop on either side of the midline. **(Middle)** These ducts must meet in the midline and fuse to form the uterus and upper portion of the vagina (uterovaginal canal). The unfused portions will form the fallopian tubes. The development of the kidney (metanephros) is closely related to uterine development, and coexistent renal and Müllerian duct anomalies are common. **(Bottom)** The distal portion of the vagina is formed from the urogenital sinus, which splits to form the bladder and urethra anteriorly, and the vagina posteriorly.

UTERUS

UNICORNUATE UTERUS

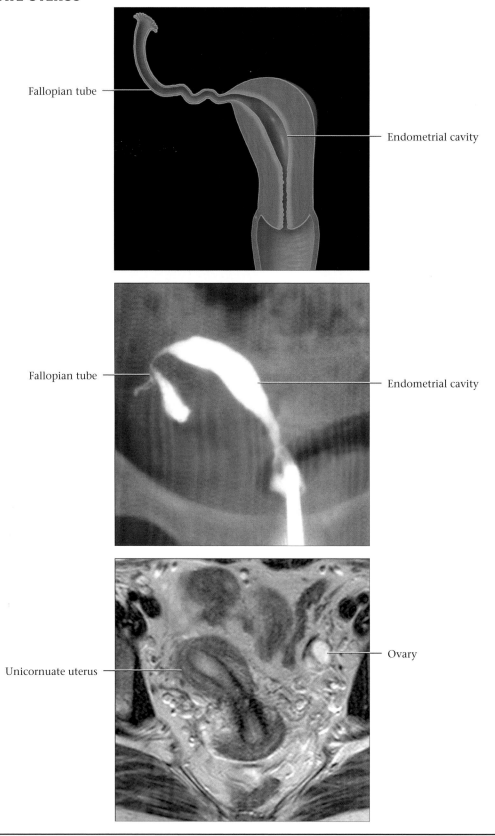

Fallopian tube

Endometrial cavity

Fallopian tube

Endometrial cavity

Unicornuate uterus

Ovary

(Top) Graphic of a unicornate uterus, which occurs if only one paramesonephric duct forms. **(Middle)** A hysterosalpingogram shows the characteristic "banana" or "cigar-shaped" endometrial cavity, with a single fallopian tube at the apex. **(Bottom)** T2 MR of a unicornuate uterus. Note the presence of a normal left ovary. The ovaries form independently from the uterus, and Müllerian duct anomalies are not associated with ovarian anomalies. They are, however, associated with congenital renal anomalies, particularly renal agenesis. Every patient with a Müllerian duct anomaly should have their kidneys evaluated.

UTERUS

UTERUS DIDELPHYS

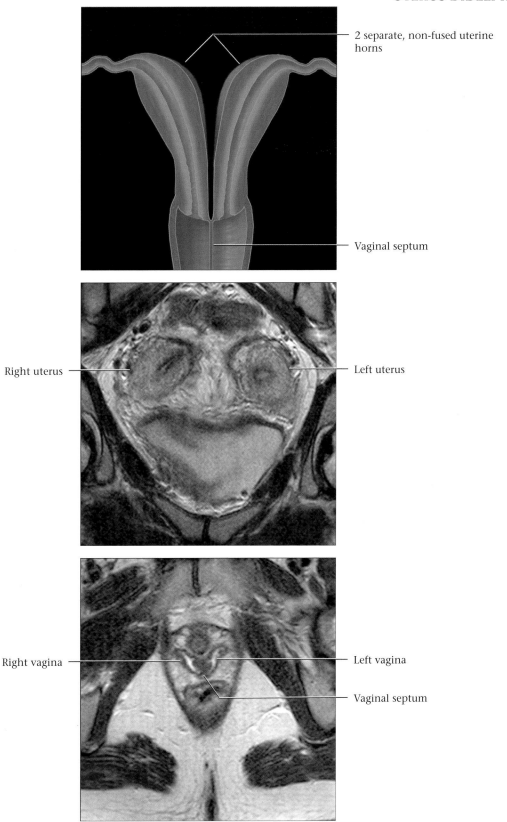

2 separate, non-fused uterine horns

Vaginal septum

Right uterus — Left uterus

Right vagina — Left vagina

Vaginal septum

(Top) Graphic illustration of a uterus didelphys. If both paramesonephric ducts form but fail to fuse, the result is a uterus didelphys. This malformation has the appearance of two unicornuate uteri side-by-side. A vaginal septum is seen in approximately 75% of cases. If the septum is transverse, it can cause an obstruction with blood products accumulating within the obstructed uterine cavity. **(Middle)** First of two T2 MR images of a uterus didelphys. Oblique image of the pelvis shows two separate uterine horns, each of which has a similar configuration to a unicornuate uterus. **(Bottom)** Axial image lower in the pelvis shows a thick vaginal septum, which is creating two separate vaginas.

UTERUS

BICORNUATE UTERUS

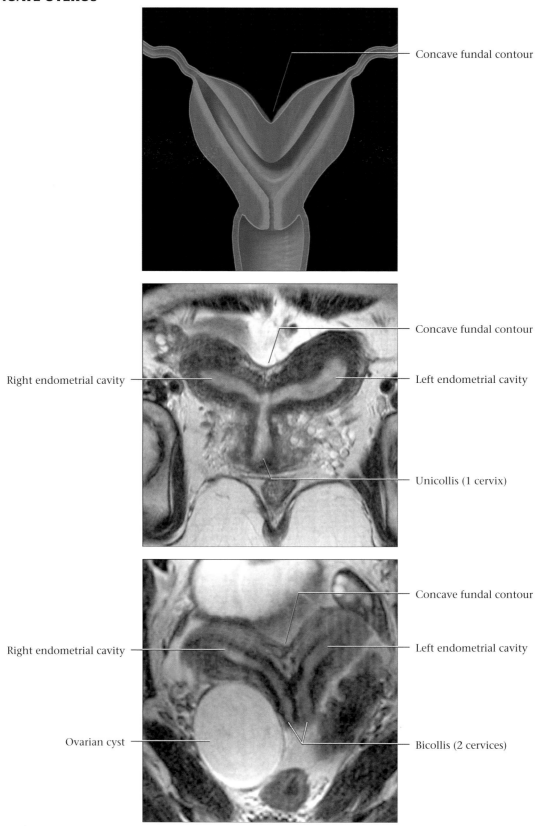

(Top) Graphic illustration of a bicornuate uterus. If the paramesonephric ducts only partially fuse, the external contour of the uterus will be concave or "heart-shaped", which is diagnostic of a bicornuate uterus. There may either be a single cervix (unicollis) or two cervices (bicollis). **(Middle)** Coronal T2 MR of the uterus shows the classic concave appearance of a bicornuate uterus. The two endometrial cavities communicate inferiorly and there is a single cervix (unicollis). **(Bottom)** Coronal T2 MR of the uterus also shows the classic concave appearance of a bicornuate uterus. In this particular case, the two endometrial cavities do not communicate and there are two separate cervices (bicollis).

UTERUS

SEPTATE UTERUS

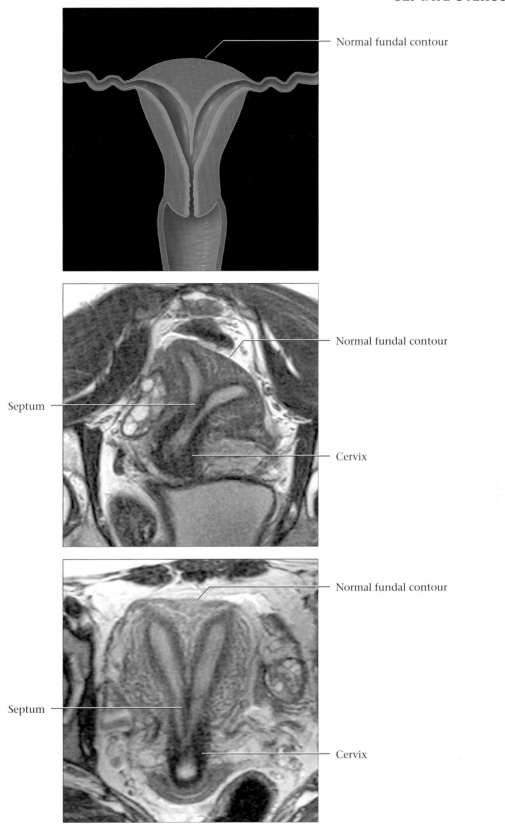

Normal fundal contour

Normal fundal contour

Septum

Cervix

Normal fundal contour

Septum

Cervix

(Top) Graphic illustration of a septate uterus. If the paramesonephric ducts fuse appropriately but the wall between them is incompletely resorbed, the result is a septate uterus, the hallmark of which is a normal fundal contour. The septum itself can be quite variable, and extend only partially into the endometrial cavity or all the way to the cervix, and even into the vagina. (Middle) Coronal T2 MR of the uterus shows a normal fundal contour, with the septum ending before reaching the cervix. (Bottom) Coronal T2 MR of the uterus shows a normal fundal contour. In this case, there is a complete septum which extend all the way down to the cervix. It is imperative when evaluating Müllerian duct anomalies to angle the scanning plane along the long axis of the uterus to simultaneously evaluate fundal contour and the endometrial cavities.

III

OVARIES

Gross Anatomy

Overview

- Ovaries located in true pelvis, although exact **position variable**
  ○ Laxity in ligaments allows some mobility
  ○ Location affected by parity, ovarian size and uterine size/position
  ○ Located within **ovarian fossa** in nulliparous women
    ▪ Lateral pelvic wall below bifurcation of common iliac vessels
    ▪ Anterior to ureter
    ▪ Posterior to broad ligament
  ○ Position more variable in parous women
    ▪ Ovaries pushed out of pelvis with pregnancy
    ▪ Seldom return to same spot
- Fallopian tube drapes over much of surface
  ○ Partially covered by fimbriated end
- Composed of a **medulla and cortex**
  ○ Vessels enter and exit ovary through medulla
  ○ Cortex contains follicles in varying stages of development
  ○ Surface covered by specialized peritoneum called **germinal epithelium**
- Ligamentous supports
  ○ **Suspensory ligament** of ovary (infundibulopelvic ligament)
    ▪ Attaches ovary to pelvic wall
    ▪ **Contains ovarian artery and vein**
    ▪ Positions ovary in craniocaudal orientation
  ○ **Mesovarium**
    ▪ Attaches ovary to posterior surface of broad ligament
    ▪ Transmits nerves and vessels to ovary
  ○ **Proper ovarian ligament** (utero-ovarian ligament)
    ▪ Fibromuscular band extending from ovary to uterine cornu
  ○ **Mesosalpinx**
    ▪ Extends between fallopian tube and proper ovarian ligament
  ○ **Broad ligament**
    ▪ Below proper ovarian ligament
- Dual blood supply
  ○ **Ovarian artery** is branch of aorta
    ▪ Descends to pelvis and enters suspensory ligament of ovary
    ▪ Continues through mesovarium to enter ovary
    ▪ Anastomoses with uterine artery
  ○ **Drainage via venous plexus** into ovarian veins
    ▪ Right ovarian drains to inferior vena cava
    ▪ Left ovarian vein drains to left renal vein
  ○ Both arteries and veins markedly enlarge in pregnancy
- Lymphatic drainage follows venous drainage

Physiology

- ~ 400,000 follicles present at birth but only 0.1% (400) mature to ovulation
- **Menstrual cycle**
  ○ **Follicular phase** (days 0-14)
    ▪ Several follicles (range 1-11, mean 5) begin to develop
    ▪ By days 8-12 a dominant follicle develops, while remainder start to regress
  ○ **Ovulation** (day 14)
    ▪ Egg extruded from ovary
    ▪ Dominate follicle typically 2.0-2.5 cm at ovulation
  ○ **Luteal phase** (days 14-28)
    ▪ Luteinizing hormone induces formation of corpus luteum

Imaging Anatomy

Ultrasound

- Scan between uterus and pelvic sidewall
  ○ Often seen by internal iliac vessels
- **Medulla mildly hyperechoic** in comparison to hypoechoic cortex
- Developing follicles anechoic
- Corpus luteum may have thick, echogenic ring
  ○ Hemorrhage common
    ▪ Variable appearance, with classic appearances of lace-like septations, fluid-fluid level and retracting clot
    ▪ No flow on Doppler ultrasound
- **Echogenic foci** common
  ○ Non-shadowing, 1-3 mm
  ○ Represent specular reflectors from walls of tiny unresolved cysts
  ○ More common in periphery
- **Focal calcification** may also be seen
- Doppler shows a low-velocity, low-resistance arterial wave form
- Volume (0.523 x length x width x height) more accurate than individual measurements
  ○ Premenopausal: Mean ~ 10 +/- 6 cc, max 22 cc
  ○ Postmenopausal: Mean ~ 2-6 cc, max 8 cc

MR

- T1WI: Uniform intermediate signal with low-signal follicles (unless hemorrhage)
- T2WI: Multiple high-signal follicles of varying sizes
  ○ Low-signal intensity capsule
  ○ Medulla higher signal intensity than cortex
- Postmenopausal ovaries usually homogeneous low signal on T1WI and T2WI

Clinical Implications

Clinical Importance

- Hemorrhagic cysts common & may be confused with an endometrioma, dermoid or epithelial neoplasm
  ○ Short term follow-up (~ 6 wks) if diagnosis not clear
- **Polycystic ovarian syndrome**
  ○ Failure of ovarian follicles to mature
  ○ Large ovaries with **multiple, small, peripheral follicles**
- **Theca lutein cysts**
  ○ Response to excessive human chorionic gonadotropic
  ○ **Multiple, large cysts** replace parenchyma and markedly enlarge ovaries
  ○ May be seen with gestational trophoblastic disease, triploidy, infertility treatment, multiple gestations

OVARIES

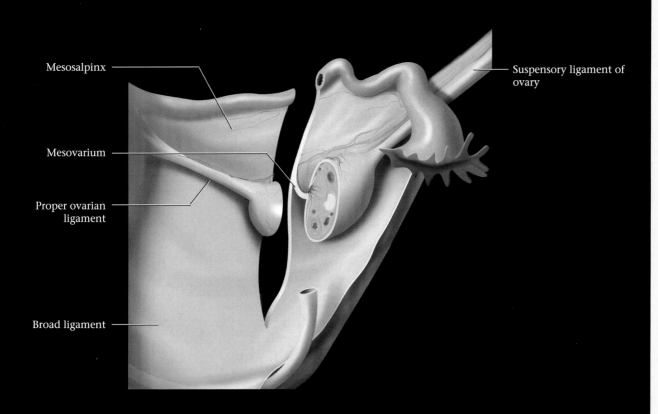

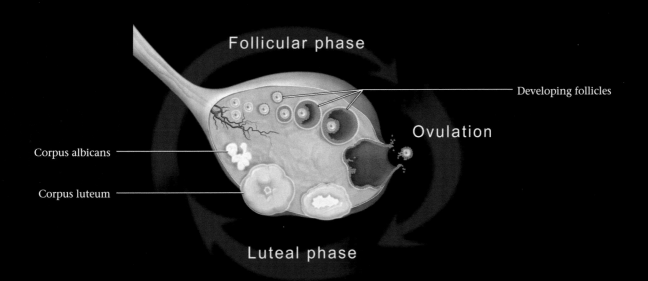

(Top) Posterior view of the ligamentous attachment of the ovary. The ovary is attached to the pelvic sidewall by the suspensory ligament (infundibulopelvic ligament) of the ovary, which transmits the ovarian artery and vein. These vessels enter the ovary through the mesovarium, a specialized ligamentous attachment between the ovary and broad ligament. The ovary is attached to the uterus by the proper ovarian ligament, which divides the mesosalpinx above from the broad ligament below. **(Bottom)** During the follicular phase of the menstrual cycle, several follicles begin to develop but by days 8-12 a dominant follicle has formed, and the remainder begin to regress. On day 14 the follicle ruptures and the egg is extruded. After ovulation, a corpus luteum forms, and if fertilization does not occur, the corpus luteum degenerates into a corpus albicans.

OVARY AND LIGAMENTS

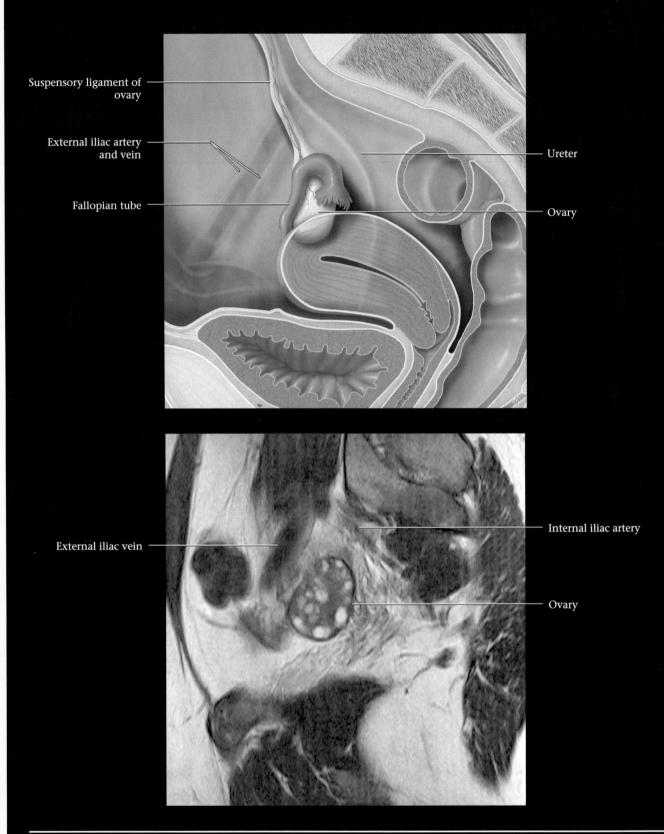

(Top) Graphic shows the location of the ovary in nulliparous women. It lies against the lateral pelvic wall within the ovarian fossa, which is the area below the iliac bifurcation, posterior to the external iliac vessels, and anterior to the ureter. With pregnancy, the ovaries are pushed out of the pelvis and seldom return to the same spot. **(Bottom)** Sagittal T2 MR of the lateral pelvic wall shows the ovary within the ovarian fossa, inferior to the iliac bifurcation.

OVARIES

OVARY AND LIGAMENTS

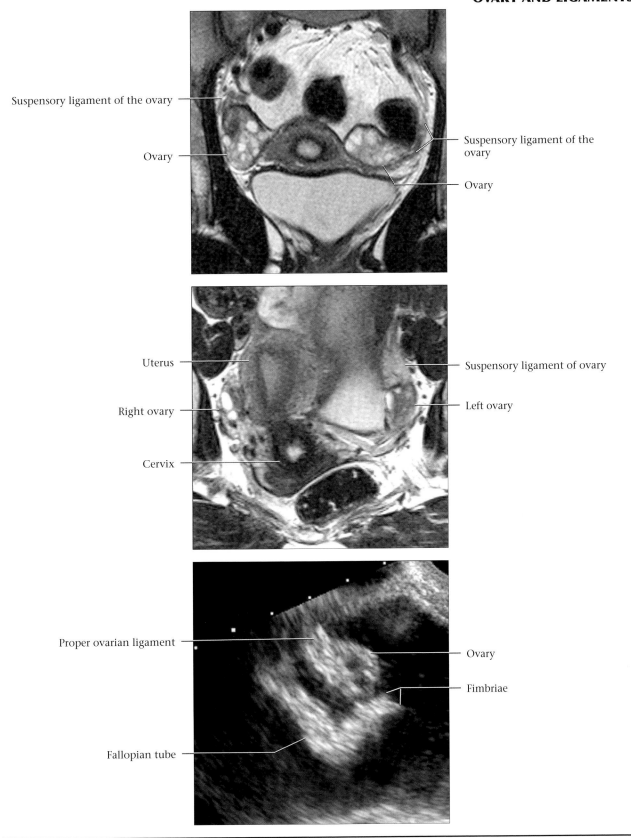

Suspensory ligament of the ovary

Ovary

Suspensory ligament of the ovary

Ovary

Uterus

Right ovary

Cervix

Suspensory ligament of ovary

Left ovary

Proper ovarian ligament

Fallopian tube

Ovary

Fimbriae

(Top) Coronal T2 MR of the ovaries. The suspensory ligament of the ovary attaches the ovary to the pelvic wall and transmits the ovarian artery, vein and lymphatics. It is an elongated, narrow band of tissue (best show on the left), which widens as it attaches to the ovary (best shown on the right). **(Middle)** Axial T2 MR showing the triangular configuration of the suspensory ligament as it attaches to the left ovary. **(Bottom)** Transvaginal ultrasound in a patient with ascites shows the fallopian tube arching around the superior aspect of the ovary. The fallopian tube "cradles" the ovary and the fimbriated end is in intimate contact with it, allowing the fallopian tube to "capture" the ova. The proper, or utero-ovarian ligament attaches the ovary to the uterine cornu. The proper ovarian ligament is inferior to the fallopian tube.

OVARIES

ULTRASOUND, NORMAL OVARY

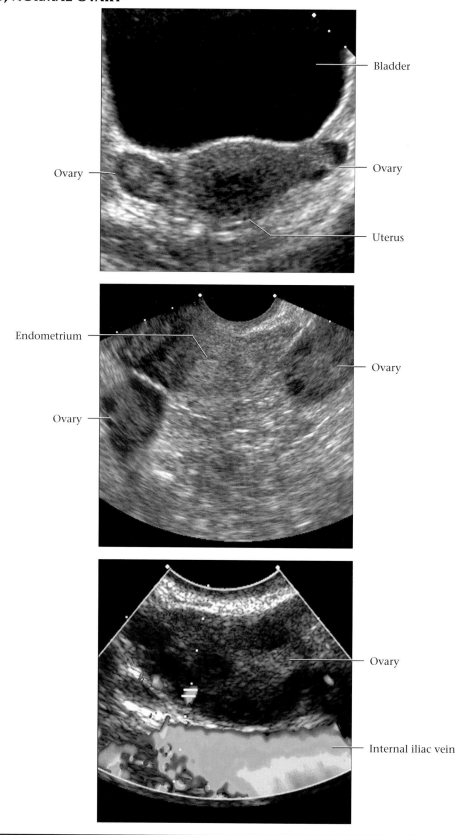

(Top) Transabdominal ultrasound shows the mildly hyperechoic ovarian medulla, compared to the hypoechoic cortex. The vessels and lymphatics enter and exit the ovary through the medulla. This complex series of acoustic interfaces results in increased echogenicity. **(Middle)** Transvaginal ultrasound showing both ovaries adjacent to the uterus. Ovarian ligaments can be lax, especially after childbirth, making ovarian position quite variable. Ovaries can be located from above the fundus to the posterior cul-de-sac. When looking for the ovaries it is best to start near the uterine fundus and follow the ligaments laterally to the pelvic sidewall. They can often be located by the iliac vessels. **(Bottom)** Transvaginal color Doppler ultrasound shows the ovary adjacent to the internal iliac vein. Color Doppler ultrasound is also helpful in differentiating pelvic vessels from ovarian follicles.

OVARIES

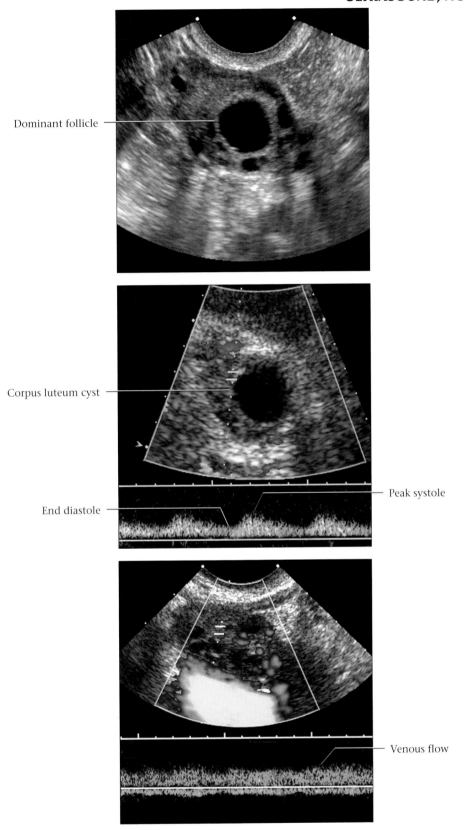

(Top) Transvaginal ultrasound of a woman on day 13 of the menstrual cycle. At this point, a dominant follicle has formed with multiple, smaller surrounding follicles. (Middle) Transvaginal color Doppler ultrasound of a different woman on day 20 of the menstrual cycle shows normal ovarian arterial blood flow. The ovary normally has a low-resistance, low-velocity wave form. Increased flow can be seen around a corpus luteum cyst, which can appear as a "ring of fire" on color Doppler. This should not be confused with a similarly-appearing "ring of fire", as seen in an ectopic pregnancy. (Bottom) Transvaginal power Doppler ultrasound shows normal venous flow. Venous flow is the first to be compromised in ovarian torsion, and therefore should be documented in all cases where torsion is suspected.

OVARIES

ECHOGENIC FOCI

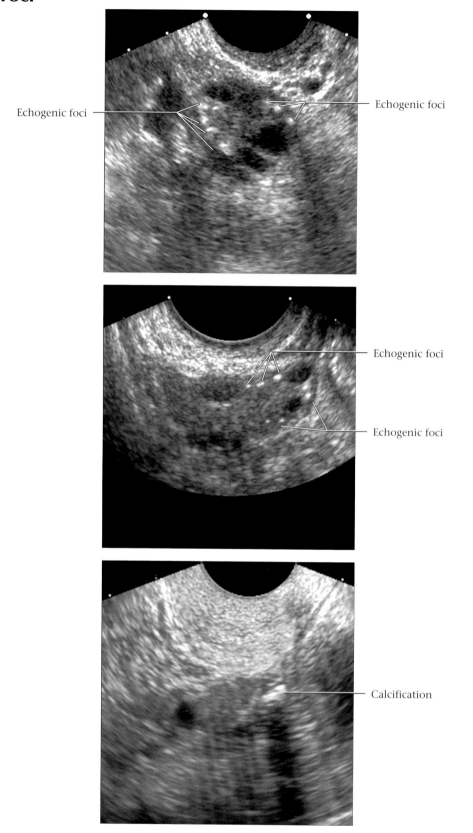

(Top) Transvaginal ultrasound showing multiple, peripheral echogenic foci. These are typically 1-3 mm and are non-shadowing, specular reflectors from unresolved cysts. They are of no malignant potential and should be considered a normal variant. **(Middle)** Transvaginal ultrasound in another example of echogenic ovarian foci. **(Bottom)** Ovarian calcification in a perimenopausal woman. Note the larger size and posterior shadowing when compared to the small echogenic foci. These too, may be seen in an otherwise normal ovary and are likely due to previous hemorrhage or infection. Care should be taken, however, as neoplasms may have calcifications. Follow-up scans should be done if there is any suspicion of a mass.

OVARIES

Left ovary

Uterus

Follicle in right ovary

Ovary

Uterus

Ovary

Bladder

Ovary

Dominant follicle

Medullary portion of ovary

(Top) Axial T1 MR of normal ovaries and uterus. Both the ovaries and uterus are of intermediate-signal intensity, similar to skeletal muscles. Fluid-containing ovarian follicles will be low-signal intensity. Lack of soft tissue contrast makes it difficult to differentiate the borders between the uterus and ovaries. On the right, it is difficult to differentiate the right ovary from surrounding bowel. (Middle) Coronal T2 MR shows the superior delineation of pelvic viscera using this sequence. The ovary is surrounded by a low-signal intensity capsule, aiding in differentiation from surrounding structures. The fluid-containing follicles are high-signal intensity and of variable size. (Bottom) Axial MR shows higher signal in the medullary portion of the right ovary. This is a common finding and represents the vessels, which enter and exit through this area.

OVARIES

HEMORRHAGIC CYST

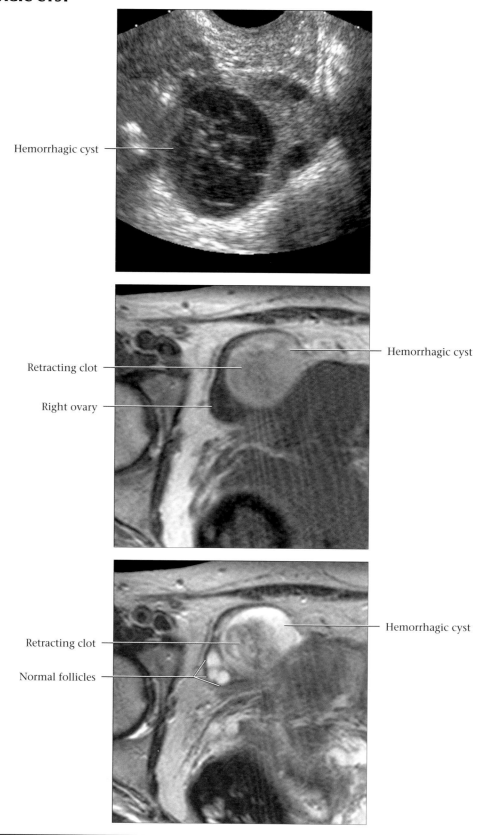

(Top) Transvaginal ultrasound shows the typical appearance of a hemorrhagic ovarian cyst. The cyst is filled with thin, fibrinous septations, which have no flow on Doppler imaging. **(Middle)** First of two axial MR images of a hemorrhagic cyst. T1 MR shows a moderately-high signal intensity cyst in the right ovary. A lower-signal area within it represents a retracting clot. There was no enhancement with gadolinium. **(Bottom)** On T2 MR, the organized clot is seen to better advantage. There are overlapping features with endometriomas, but the low signal seen in endometriomas (T2 shading), generally does not appear as organized as a retracting clot. Additionally, endometriomas are typically brighter on T1 than a hemorrhagic cyst. A follow-up ultrasound will show resolution of a hemorrhagic cyst.

OVARIES

RESOLVING HEMORRHAGIC CYST

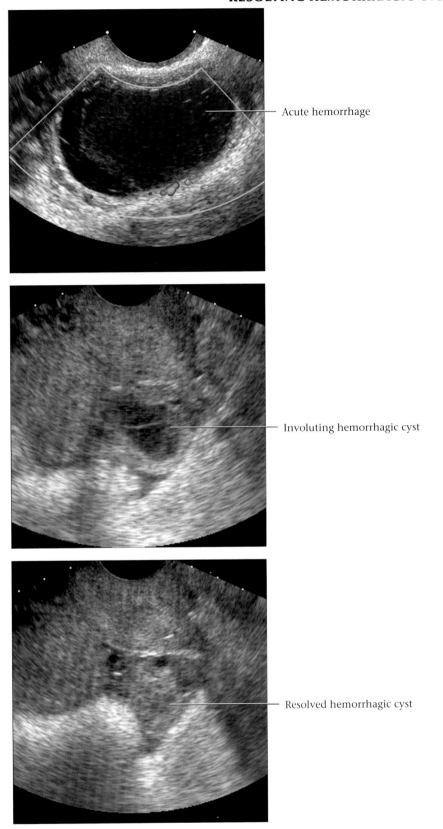

Acute hemorrhage

Involuting hemorrhagic cyst

Resolved hemorrhagic cyst

(Top) First of three transvaginal ultrasound images in a woman with acute left lower quadrant pain. The initial color Doppler image shows a large cyst, filled with low-level echoes. There is flow around the cyst but not within it. When cysts are large or atypical, a follow-up scan should be done to ensure resolution. (Middle) At 6 weeks, there has been marked involution of the cyst. (Bottom) At 10 weeks, it has essentially resolved with only a vague hypoechoic area where the cyst had been.

OVARIES

POLYCYSTIC OVARIAN SYNDROME

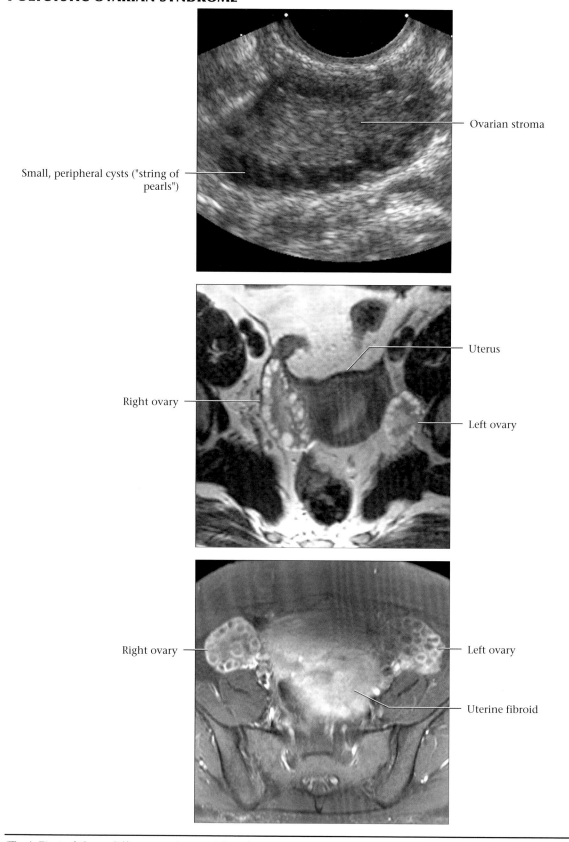

Ovarian stroma

Small, peripheral cysts ("string of pearls")

Right ovary

Uterus

Left ovary

Right ovary

Left ovary

Uterine fibroid

(Top) First of three different patients with polycystic ovarian syndrome (PCOS). Transvaginal ultrasound shows the classic appearance of small, peripherally-placed cysts, creating a "string of pearls" appearance. The ovarian size is increased and there is prominent ovarian stroma. **(Middle)** Axial T2 MR shows the high signal, peripheral cysts. These are primordial follicles, with failure of a dominant follicle to develop. Failure of follicular delvelopment results in anovulatory cycles. **(Bottom)** Axial T1 C+ FS MR image shows scattered small cysts within the ovarian stoma. Once again, no dominant follicle is present. This is another potential appearance of PCOS. Symptoms of PCOS vary, with the classic Stein-Leventhal syndrome (amenorrhea, hirsutism, sterility and obesity) being a severe form.

OVARIES

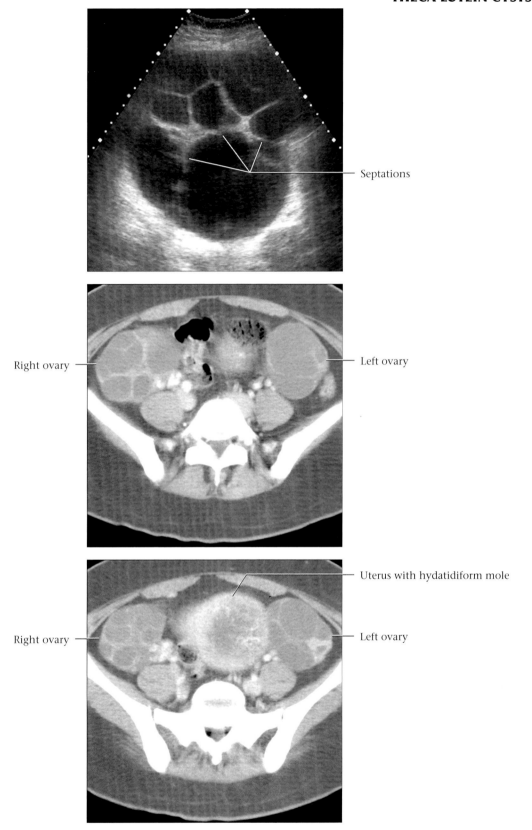

Septations

Right ovary — — Left ovary

Uterus with hydatidiform mole

Right ovary — — Left ovary

(Top) First of three images in a woman with theca lutein cysts and a hydatidiform mole. The ultrasound shows multiple, simple-appearing cysts, essentially replacing the ovarian parenchyma. Multiple prominent septae are seen separating these cysts. These have sometimes been described as having a "spoke-wheel" appearance. (Middle) Contrast-enhanced CT shows enhancement of the septae. Both ovaries are enlarged, which is typical. Occasionally there may be only unilateral enlargement. (Bottom) Inferiorly, the fundus of the enlarged uterus is seen. Theca lutein cysts are the result of increased stimulation from excessive human chorionic gonadotropin. This can be seen with gestational trophoblastic disease (hydatiform mole, invasive mole, choriocarcinoma), triploidy, infertility treatments and multiple gestations.

III
129

TESTES AND SCROTUM

Embryology and Histology

- **Testes form from genital ridges**, which extend from T6-S2 in embryo
- Composed of **3 cell lines**
  ○ Germ cells
  ○ Sertoli cells
  ○ Leydig cells
- **Germ cells**
  ○ Form in wall of yolk sac and migrate along hindgut to genital ridges
  ○ Form spermatogenic cells in mature testes
    ▪ Mature from basement membrane to lumen of seminiferous tubule (spermatogonia ⇒ spermatocytes ⇒ spermatids ⇒ spermatozoa)
- **Sertoli cells**
  ○ Supporting network for developing spermatozoa
  ○ Form tight junctions (**blood-testis barrier**)
  ○ Secrete Müllerian inhibiting factor
    ▪ Causes **paramesonephric (Müllerian) ducts** to regress
    ▪ Embryologic remnant may remain as **appendix testis**
- **Leydig cells**
  ○ Principal source of testosterone production
  ○ Lie within interstitium
  ○ Causes differentiation of **mesonephric (Wolffian) ducts**
    ▪ Each duct forms epididymis, vas deferens, seminal vesicle, and ejaculatory duct
    ▪ An embryologic remnant may remain as **appendix epididymis**
- **Scrotum** derived from labioscrotal folds
  ○ Folds swell under influence of testosterone to form **twin scrotal sacs**
    ▪ Point of fusion is median raphe, which extends from anus, along perineum to ventral surface of penis
  ○ **Processus vaginalis**, a sock-like evagination of peritoneum, elongates through abdominal wall into twin sacs
    ▪ Forms anterior to developing testes
    ▪ Aids in descent of testes, along with **gubernaculum** (ligamentous cord extending from testis to labioscrotal fold)
    ▪ Results in component layers of adult scrotum
- **Testicular descent**
  ○ Between 7-12th week of gestation, testes descend into pelvis
    ▪ Remain near internal inguinal ring until 7th month, when they begin descent through inguinal canal into twin scrotal sacs
    ▪ Testes **remain retroperitoneal throughout descent**
    ▪ Testes intimately associated with posterior wall of processus vaginalis
  ○ Component layers of spermatic cord and scrotum formed during descent through abdominal wall
  ○ Transversalis fascia ⇒ **internal spermatic fascia**
    ▪ Transversus abdominis muscle is discontinuous inferiorly and does not contribute to formation of scrotum
  ○ Internal oblique muscle ⇒ **cremasteric muscle and fascia**
  ○ External oblique muscle ⇒ **external spermatic fascia**
  ○ **Dartos muscle and fascia** embedded in loose areolar tissue below skin
  ○ Processus vaginalis closes and forms **tunica vaginalis**
    ▪ Mesothelial-lined sac around anterior and lateral sides of testis
    ▪ Visceral layer of tunica vaginalis blends imperceptibly with tunica albuginea

Gross Anatomy

Testis

- **Tunica albuginea** forms thick fibrous capsule around testis
- Densely packed seminiferous tubules separated by thin fibrous septae
  ○ **200-300 lobules** in adult testis
    ▪ Each has 400-600 seminiferous tubules
    ▪ Each tubule 30-80 cm long
    ▪ **Total length of seminiferous tubules 300-980 meters**
- Seminiferous tubules converge posteriorly to form larger ducts (**tubuli recti**)
  ○ Drain into **rete testis** at testicular hilum
- Rete testis converges posteriorly to form 15-20 **efferent ductules**
  ○ Penetrate posterior tunica albuginea at mediastinum to form head of epididymis
- **Mediastinum testis** thickened area of tunica albuginea where ducts, nerves, and vessels enter and exit testis

Epididymis

- Crescent-shaped structure running along posterior border of testis
- Efferent ductules form head (**globus major**)
  ○ Unite to form single, long, highly convoluted tubule in body of epididymis
- Tubule continues inferiorly to form epididymal tail (**globus minor**)
  ○ Attached to lower pole of testis by loose areolar tissue
- Tubule emerges at acute angle from tail as **vas deferens** (also know as ductus deferens)
  ○ Continues cephalad within spermatic cord
  ○ Eventually merges with duct of seminal vesicle to form ejaculatory duct

Spermatic Cord

- Contains vas deferens, nerves, lymphatics, and connective tissue
- Begins at internal (deep) inguinal ring and exits through external (superficial) inguinal ring into scrotum
- Arteries
  ○ **Testicular artery**
    ▪ Branch of aorta
    ▪ Primary blood supply to testis
  ○ **Deferential artery**

TESTES AND SCROTUM

- - Branch of inferior or superior vesicle artery
  - Arterial supply to vas deferens
  - ○ **Cremasteric artery**
    - Branch of inferior epigastric artery
    - Supplies muscular components of cord and skin
- • Venous drainage
  - ○ **Pampiniform plexus**
    - Interconnected network of small veins
    - Merges to form testicular vein
    - **Left testicular vein** drains to left renal vein
    - **Right testicular vein** drains to inferior vena cava
- • Lymphatic drainage
  - ○ Testis follows venous drainage
    - Right side drains to interaortocaval chain
    - Left side drains to left para-aortic nodes near renal hilum
  - ○ Epididymis may also drain to external iliac nodes
  - ○ Scrotal skin drains to inguinal nodes

Imaging Anatomy

Ultrasound
- • **Testes**
  - ○ Ovoid, homogeneous, medium-level, granular echotexture
  - ○ **Mediastinum testis** may appear as prominent echogenic line emanating from posterior testis
  - ○ **Blood flow**
    - Testicular artery pierces tunica albuginea and arborizes over periphery of testis
    - Multiple, radially-arranged vessels travel along septae
    - May have prominent transmediastinal artery
    - Low-velocity, low-resistance wave form on Doppler imaging, with continuous forward flow in diastole
- • Epididymis
  - ○ Isoechoic to slightly hyperechoic compared with testis
  - ○ Best seen in longitudinal plane
  - ○ Head has rounded or triangular configuration
  - ○ Head 10-12 mm, body and tail often difficult to visualize
- • Spermatic cord
  - ○ May be difficult to differentiate from surrounding soft tissues
  - ○ Evaluate for varicocele with color Doppler

MR
- • T1WI
  - ○ Testes uniform intermediate signal
  - ○ Epididymis isointense or slightly hypointense compared to testis
- • T2WI
  - ○ Testes moderately high signal
    - Tunica albuginea, low-signal capsule around testis
    - Mediastinum testis appears as linear band of low signal along posterior aspect of testis
    - Thin, low-signal septae can be seen radiating back toward mediastinum
  - ○ Epididymis hypointense relative to testis

Clinical Implications

Hydrocele
- • Fluid between visceral and parietal layers of tunica vaginalis
- • Small amount of fluid is normal
- • Larger hydroceles may be either congenital (patent processus vaginalis) or acquired

Cryptorchidism
- • Failure of testes to descend completely into scrotum
- • Most lie near external inguinal ring
- • Associated with **decreased fertility and testicular carcinoma**
  - ○ **Risk of carcinoma is increased for both testes**, even if other side is normally descended

Varicocele
- • Idiopathic or secondary to abdominal mass
  - ○ Idiopathic more common on left
- • Vessel diameter > **3 mm abnormal**
- • Always evaluate with provocative maneuvers, such as Valsalva

Scrotal Calculi
- • Free floating calcifications within tunica vaginalis
- • May result from torsion of appendix testis or epididymis

Torsion
- • Occurs most commonly when tunica vaginalis completely surrounds testis and epididymis
  - ○ Testis is suspended from spermatic cord like **"bell-clapper"**, rather than being anchored posteriorly
- • Normal grayscale appearance with early torsion
  - ○ Becomes heterogeneous and enlarged with infarction
- • Doppler required for diagnosis
  - ○ **Some flow may be seen even if torsed** but will be decreased compared to normal side
  - ○ Venous flow compromised first, then diastolic flow, finally systolic flow

Testicular Carcinoma
- • Most common malignancy in young men
  - ○ 95% are germ cell tumors
    - Seminoma (most common pure tumor), embryonal, yolk sac tumor, choriocarcinoma, teratoma
    - Mixed germ cell tumor (components of 2 or more cell lines) most common overall
  - ○ Remainder of primary tumors are sex cord (Sertoli cells) or stromal (Leydig cells)
  - ○ Lymphoma, leukemia and metastases more common in older men
- • Most metastasize via lymphatics in predictable fashion
  - ○ Right-sided first echelon nodes: Interaortocaval chain at second vertebral body
  - ○ Left-sided first echelon nodes: Left para-aortic nodes in area bounded by renal vein, aorta, ureter and inferior mesenteric artery

TESTES AND SCROTUM

TESTIS

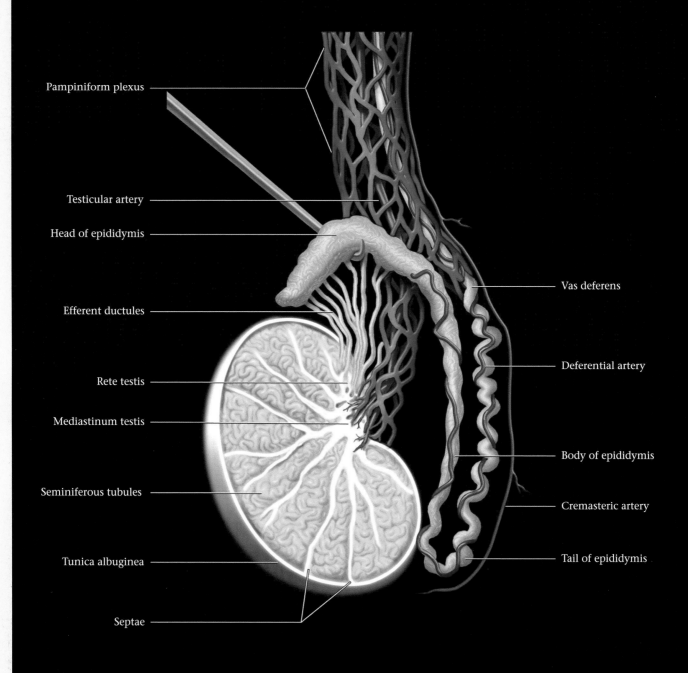

Pampiniform plexus

Testicular artery

Head of epididymis

Efferent ductules

Rete testis

Mediastinum testis

Seminiferous tubules

Tunica albuginea

Septae

Vas deferens

Deferential artery

Body of epididymis

Cremasteric artery

Tail of epididymis

The testis is composed of densely packed seminiferous tubules, which are separated by thin fibrous septae. These tubules converge posteriorly, eventually draining into the rete testis. The rete testis continues to converge to form the efferent ductules, which pierce through the tunica albuginea at the mediastinum testis and form the head of the epididymis. Within the epididymis these tubules unite to form a single, highly-convoluted tubule in the body, which finally emerges from the tail as the vas deferens. In addition to the vas deferens, other components of the spermatic cord include the testicular artery, deferential artery, cremasteric artery, pampiniform plexus, lymphatics and nerves.

TESTES AND SCROTUM

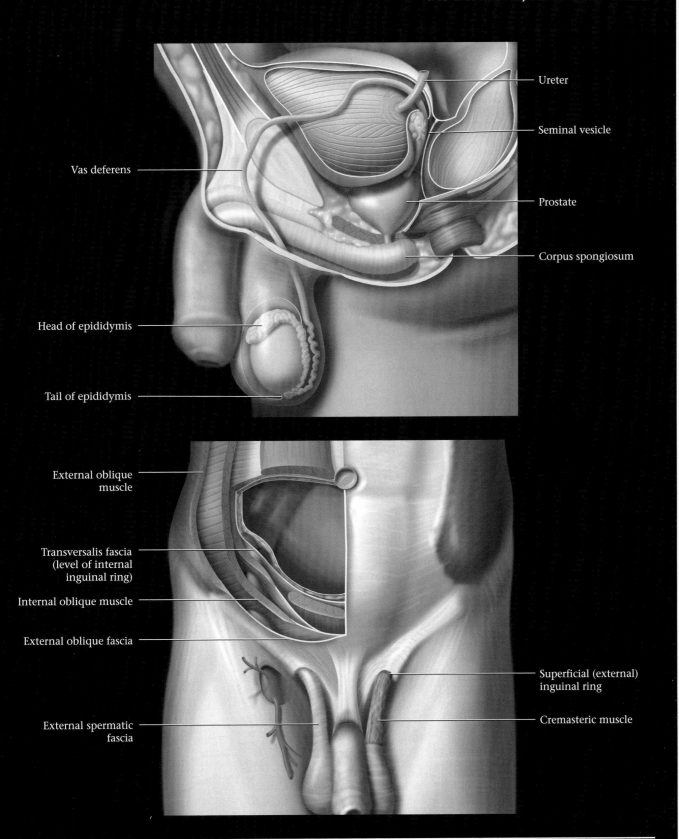

Ureter

Seminal vesicle

Vas deferens

Prostate

Corpus spongiosum

Head of epididymis

Tail of epididymis

External oblique muscle

Transversalis fascia (level of internal inguinal ring)

Internal oblique muscle

External oblique fascia

Superficial (external) inguinal ring

Cremasteric muscle

External spermatic fascia

(Top) The tail of the epididymis is loosely attached to the lower pole of the testis by areolar tissue. The vas deferens (also referred to as ductus deferens) emerges from the tail at an acute angle and continues cephalad as part of the spermatic cord. After passing through the inguinal canal, the vas deferens courses posteriorly to unite with the duct of the seminal vesicle to form the ejaculatory duct. These narrow ducts have thick, muscular walls composed of smooth muscle, which reflexly contract during ejaculation and propel sperm forward. **(Bottom)** The muscle layers of the pelvic wall have been separated to show the spermatic cord as it passes through the inguinal canal. The cremasteric muscle is derived from the internal oblique muscle, while the external spermatic fascia is formed by the fascia of the external oblique muscle.

TESTES AND SCROTUM

SCROTAL DEVELOPMENT

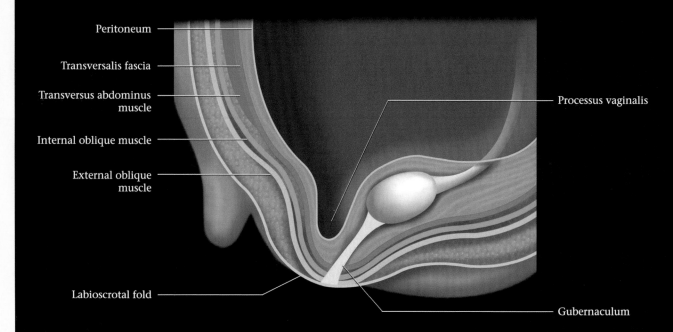

Peritoneum
Transversalis fascia
Transversus abdominus muscle
Internal oblique muscle
External oblique muscle
Labioscrotal fold
Processus vaginalis
Gubernaculum

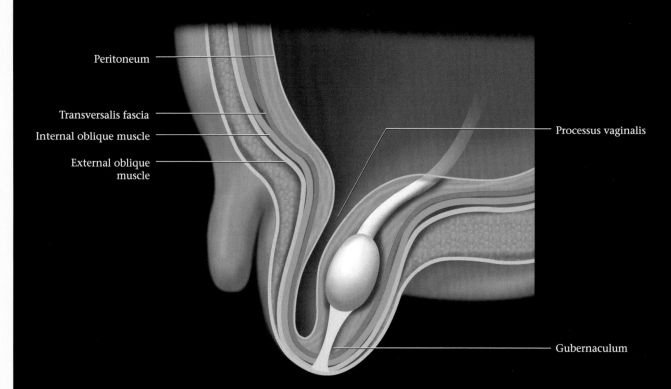

Peritoneum
Transversalis fascia
Internal oblique muscle
External oblique muscle
Processus vaginalis
Gubernaculum

(Top) The processus vaginalis is a sock-like evagination of the peritoneum, which elongates caudally through the abdominal wall. It forms on each side of the lower abdomen just anterior to the developing testes and, along with the gubernaculum (a ligamentous cord extending from the testis to the labioscrotal fold), aids in their descent. **(Bottom)** As the processus vaginalis evaginates, it becomes ensheathed by fascial extensions of the abdominal wall, which ultimately form the layers of the scrotum and spermatic cord. The transversus abdominis muscle is discontinuous inferiorly and does not contribute to the formation of the scrotum.

TESTES AND SCROTUM

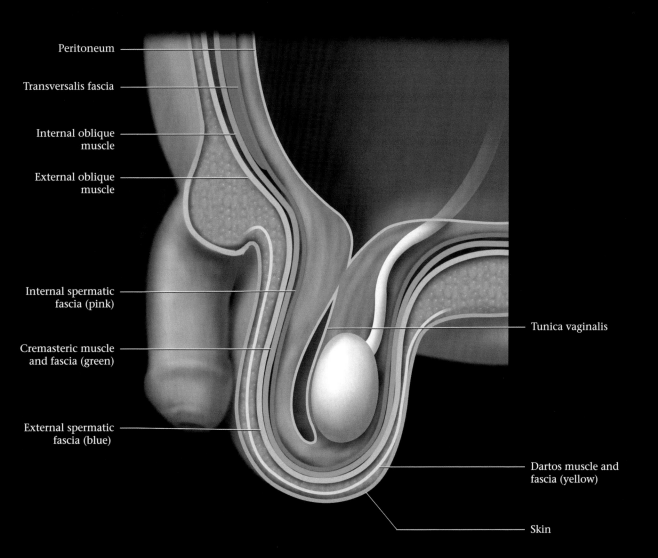

Peritoneum

Transversalis fascia

Internal oblique muscle

External oblique muscle

Internal spermatic fascia (pink)

Cremasteric muscle and fascia (green)

External spermatic fascia (blue)

Tunica vaginalis

Dartos muscle and fascia (yellow)

Skin

The abdominal wall derivative layers of the scrotum are as follows: Transversalis fascia ⇒ internal spermatic fascia, internal oblique muscle ⇒ cremasteric muscle and fascia, external oblique muscle ⇒ external spermatic fascia. The dartos muscle is embedded in the loose areolar tissue and is closely associated with the skin. Its primary function is to contract the skin and elevate the testes in response to cold. The various layers of the scrotum cannot usually be discerned with imaging. The superior portion of the processus vaginalis closes and forms an isolated mesothelial-lined sac, the tunica vaginalis. Failure of closure may result in a congenital hydrocele and is a risk factor for an inguinal hernia.

TESTES AND SCROTUM

ULTRASOUND, TESTIS

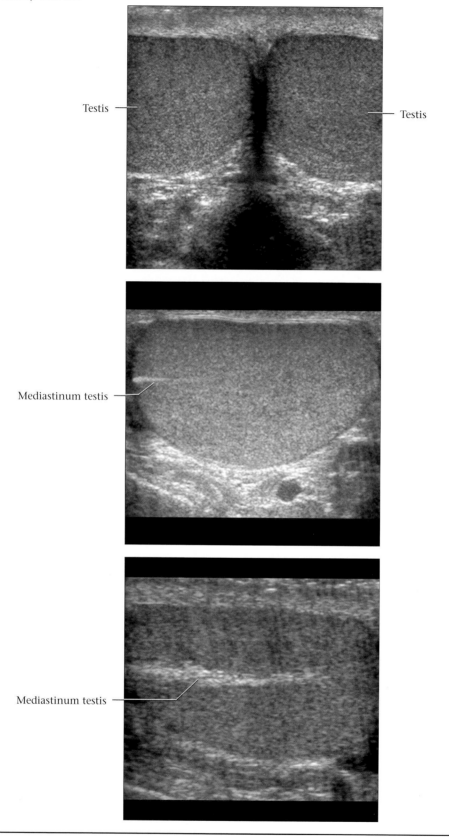

Testis — Testis

Mediastinum testis

Mediastinum testis

(Top) Transverse ultrasound showing both testes. The testes have a homogeneous, medium-level, granular echotexture. (Middle) Longitudinal ultrasound shows the ovoid shape. The tunica albuginea may form an echogenic linear band where it invaginates at the mediastinum testis. The mediastinum testis has a craniocaudal linear course and is where the efferent ductules, vessels and lymphatics pierce through the capsule. (Bottom) Longitudinal ultrasound of a prominent mediastinum testis. A transmediastinal artery may also sometimes be seen.

TESTES AND SCROTUM

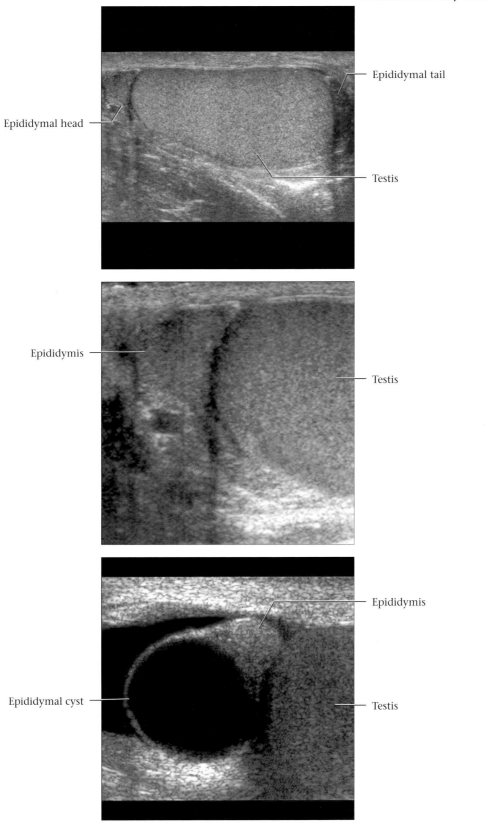

Epididymal tail

Epididymal head

Testis

Epididymis

Testis

Epididymis

Epididymal cyst

Testis

(Top) Longitudinal ultrasound shows both the epididymal head (globus major) and tail (globus minor). The epididymal head measures approximately 10-12 mm and is iso- to slightly hyperechoic compared to the testis. The body and tail are more difficult to visualize, and may be slightly less echogenic than the head. **(Middle)** Longitudinal ultrasound shows the epididymal head, which typically has a triangular or slightly rounded configuration. **(Bottom)** Longitudinal ultrasound of the epididymal head shows a well-defined, anechoic cyst. Epididymal cysts are common incidental findings and either represent true epithelial-lined cysts or spermatoceles. Differentiation is not clinically necessary as both are benign.

APPENDIX TESTIS, APPENDIX EPIDIDYMIS

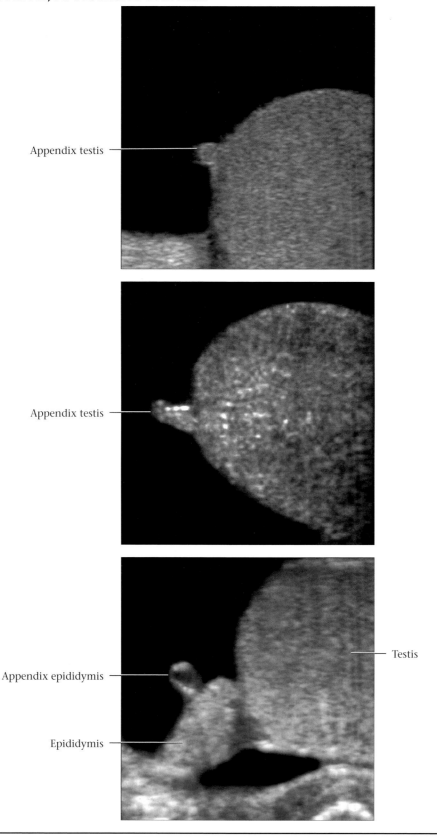

(Top) Ultrasound of the testis in a patient with a hydrocele shows a small, nodular protuberance from the surface of the testis. It is isoechoic to normal testicular parenchyma. This is the appendix testis, which is a remnant of the Müllerian system. **(Middle)** Ultrasound of a slightly larger appendix testis in a different patient. **(Bottom)** Longitudinal ultrasound of the upper testis and epididymis shows a small, cystic "tag" of tissue projecting from the epididymis. This is an appendix epididymis, which is a remnant of the Wolffian system. Both the appendix testis and appendix epididymis are usually not visible sonographically, unless there is a hydrocele. They are usually of no clinical significance; however, they can rarely torse and be a cause of scrotal pain.

SCROTAL CALCULI

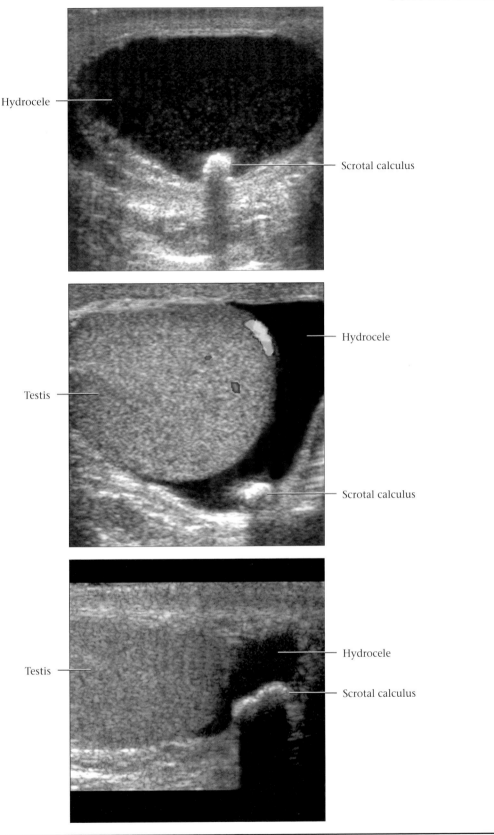

Hydrocele

Scrotal calculus

Hydrocele

Testis

Scrotal calculus

Testis

Hydrocele

Scrotal calculus

(Top) Ultrasound of a complex hydrocele (note low-level echoes throughout the fluid) and a small scrotal calculus. Scrotal calculi, also called scrotoliths or scrotal pearls, are free-floating calcifications within the tunica vaginalis. They may result from torsion of the appendix epididymis or appendix testis, or from inflammatory deposits on the tunica vaginalis that have separated from the lining. On ultrasound they appear as mobile, echogenic calculi with posterior shadowing. **(Middle)** Color Doppler ultrasound shows a small scrotal calculus with posterior shadowing. **(Bottom)** Longitudinal ultrasound shows a larger scrotal calculus by the inferior pole of the testis.

TESTES AND SCROTUM

NORMAL FLOW

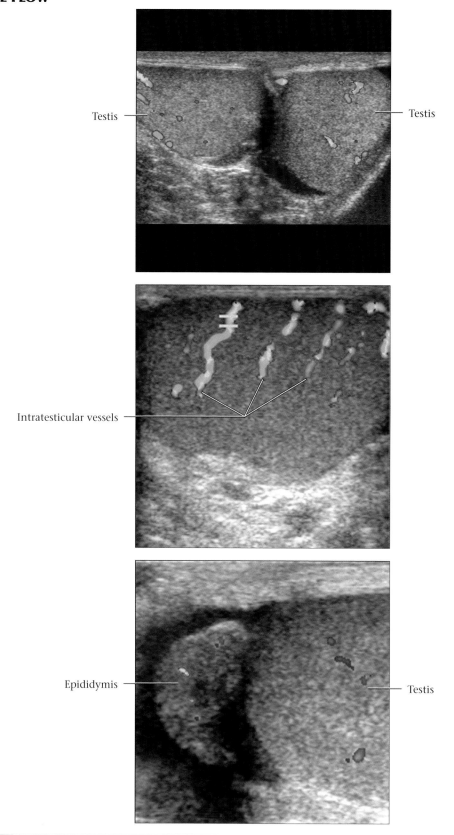

(**Top**) Transverse color Doppler ultrasound of the testes. It is important to compare flow between testes to determine if the symptomatic side has increased or decreased flow, when compared to the asymptomatic side. (**Middle**) Longitudinal color Doppler ultrasound shows prominent, radially-arranged vessels within the testis. (**Bottom**) Color Doppler ultrasound of the epididymal head and testis.

TESTES AND SCROTUM

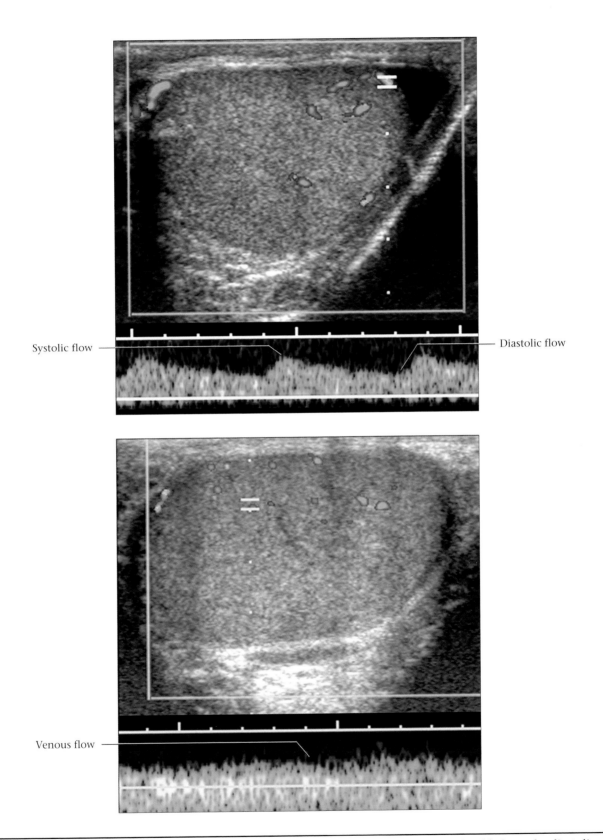

Systolic flow

Diastolic flow

Venous flow

(**Top**) Pulsed-wave arterial Doppler shows the normal, low-resistance wave form. There should always be diastolic flow present. (**Bottom**) Pulsed-wave venous Doppler shows normal venous flow. In evaluating an acutely painful testis, both arterial and venous flow should be documented, as incomplete torsion may compromise venous flow but not arterial flow.

TESTES AND SCROTUM

INCREASED FLOW, INFECTION

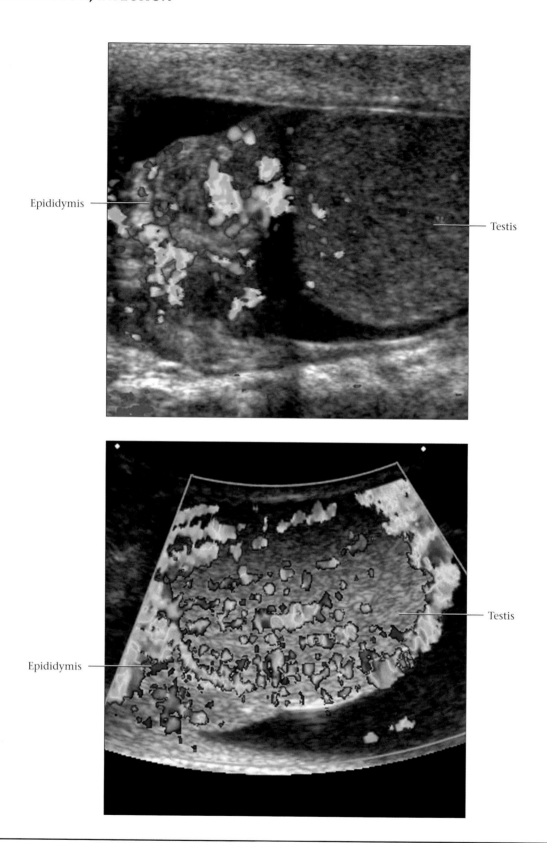

Epididymis — Testis

Epididymis — Testis

(Top) Color Doppler ultrasound of a patient with acute epididymitis. The epididymal head is enlarged and hyperemic, with a marked increase in color flow. The testis is normal and flow was symmetric with the other testis. Most infections occur from direct extension of pathogens retrograde, via the vas deferens, from a lower urinary tract source. Thus, the epididymis becomes infected before the testis. (Bottom) Color Doppler ultrasound of a different patient with acute epididymo-orchitis. There is dramatic increased flow in both the epididymis and testis. Approximately 20% of epididymitis cases are complicated by a coexistent orchitis. This is a potentially more serious condition, which can lead to vascular compromise with testicular ischemia, infarction and/or abscess.

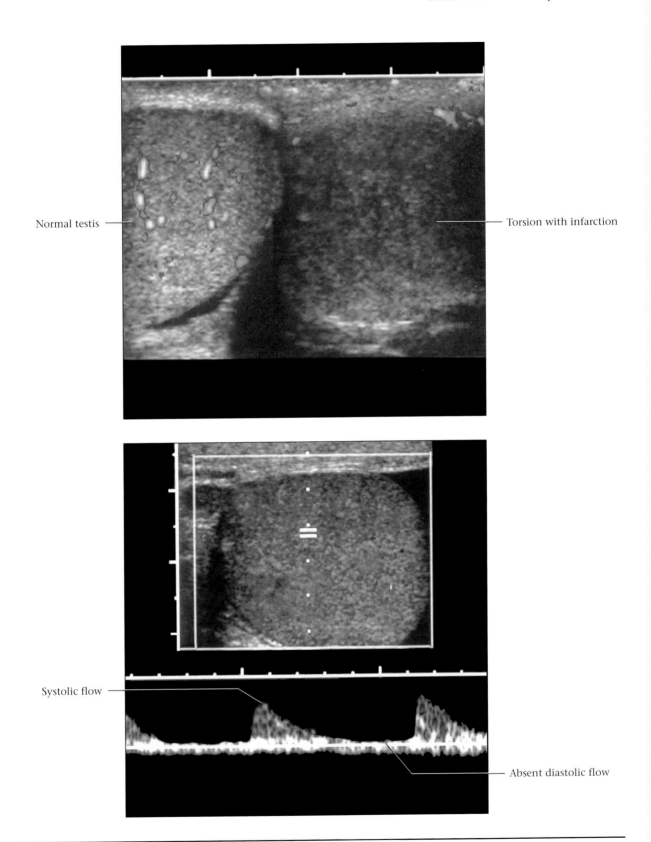

Normal testis — Torsion with infarction

Systolic flow — Absent diastolic flow

(Top) Transverse power Doppler ultrasound in a patient with left testicular torsion and infarction. The left testis is enlarged and hypoechoic compared to the normal side. Flow is seen in the surrounding scrotal skin but none is present within the testis itself. **(Bottom)** Color and pulsed-wave Doppler ultrasound in a different patient with testicular torsion. The grayscale appearance of the testis is normal. Flow was seen on color Doppler but was decreased when compared to the asymptomatic side. Pulsed-wave Doppler shows systolic flow but there is absent diastolic flow. Venous flow was absent as well. Because veins are more compressible, their flow is compromised first. This is followed by loss of diastolic flow and finally systolic flow. Complete loss of blood flow may not be seen unless the cord has twisted at least 540 degrees.

MR, NORMAL SCROTUM

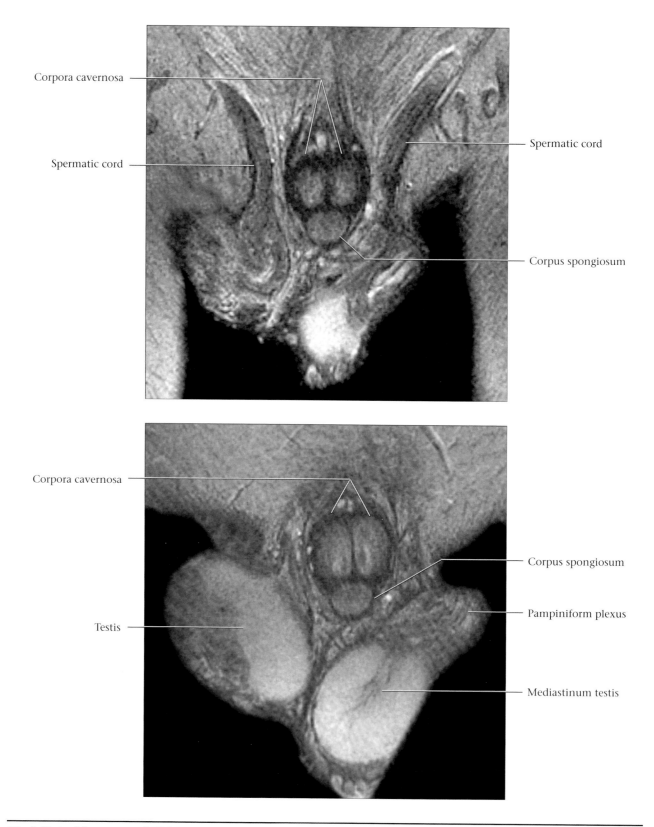

(Top) First of four coronal T2 MR images, presented from back to front, showing normal scrotal anatomy. (Bottom) The testes have a moderately-high signal intensity. The mediastinum testis is an invagination of the tunica albuginea along the posterior aspect of the testis. It is low signal intensity, with thin low signal septae radiating away from it.

TESTES AND SCROTUM

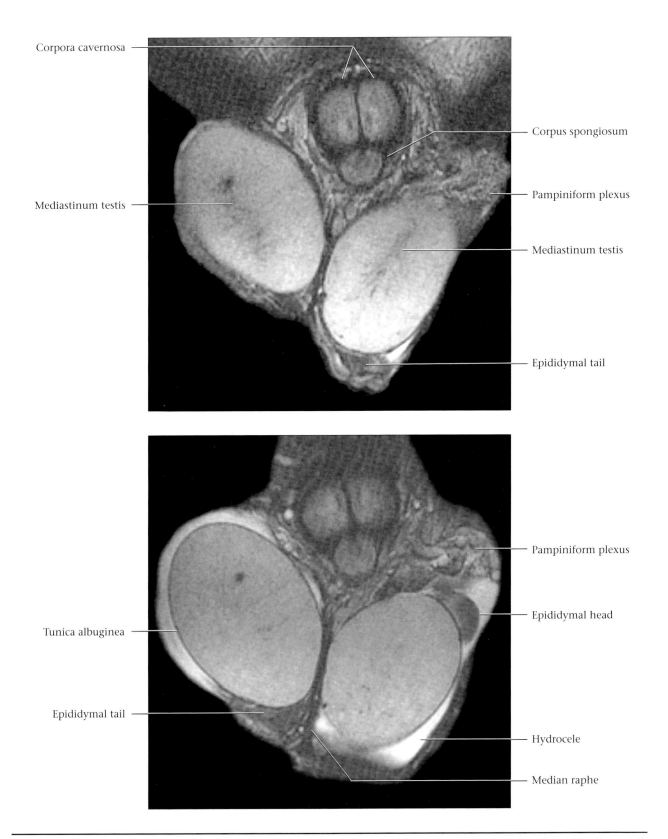

Corpora cavernosa

Corpus spongiosum

Mediastinum testis

Pampiniform plexus

Mediastinum testis

Epididymal tail

Tunica albuginea

Pampiniform plexus

Epididymal head

Epididymal tail

Hydrocele

Median raphe

(Top) The pampiniform plexus is a meshwork of interconnected veins. These generally have slow flow so will appear as an area of serpiginous high signal above the testis. (Bottom) The epididymis is relatively hypointense when compared to the testis. The tunica albuginea forms a distinct low signal capsule around the testis. The median raphe separates the twin scrotal sacs and extends in a linear fashion from the anus to the ventral surface of the penis.

TESTES AND SCROTUM

MR, HYDROCELE

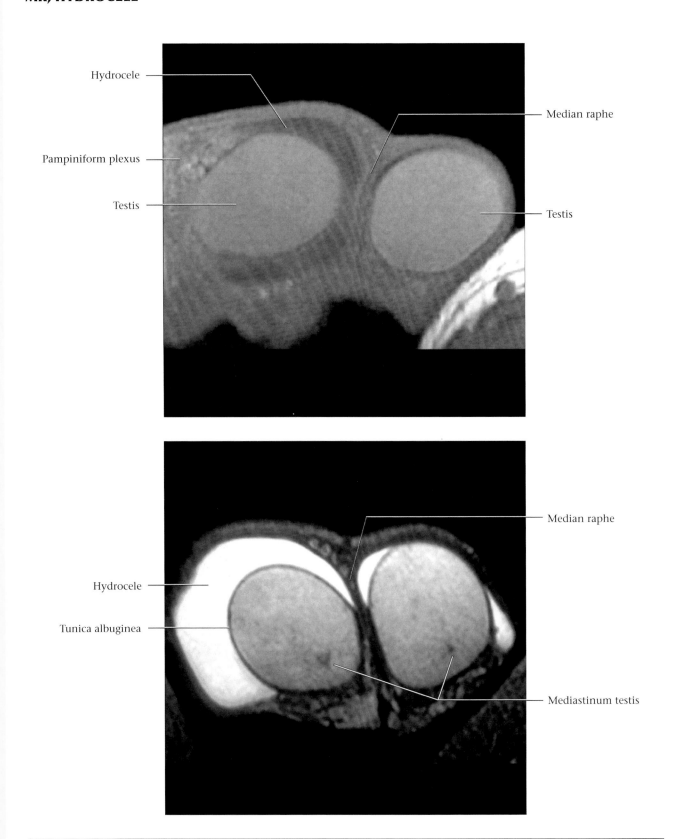

(Top) Axial T1 MR of the scrotum shows the intermediate signal testes and low-signal hydrocele. **(Bottom)** Axial T2 FS MR shows bilateral hydroceles (right > left). A hydrocele is an accumulation of fluid between the parietal and visceral layers of the tunica vaginalis. The tunica vaginalis surrounds all but the posterior aspect of the testis, which is attached to scrotal skin. If the tunica vaginalis completely surrounds the testis, it will be freely mobile ("bell-clapper" anomaly) and is predisposed to torsion.

TESTES AND SCROTUM

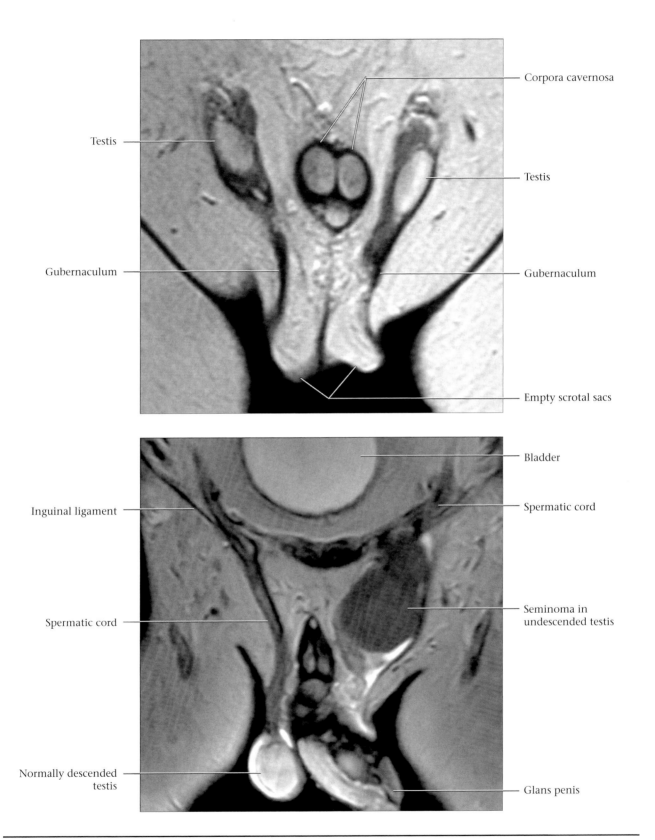

(Top) Coronal T2 MR of bilateral cryptorchidism. Most undescended testes lie within the inguinal canal, near the external ring, but can be anywhere along the path of testicular descent. Cryptorchidism is associated with testicular carcinoma, decreased fertility and other congenital genitourinary abnormalities. (Bottom) Coronal T2 MR shows a tumor (seminoma) in an undescended left testis, lying within the inguinal canal. It is important to be aware that the increased risk of carcinoma does not just apply to the undescended side but also to the normally descended testis. The increased risk may be from a generalized embryogenesis defect that results in bilateral dysgenetic gonads and a predisposition to tumor formation.

TESTES AND SCROTUM

RETE TESTIS

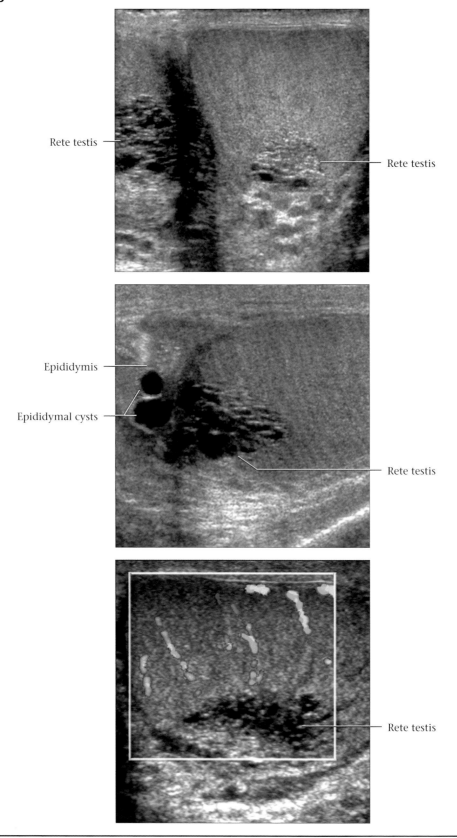

Rete testis — | — Rete testis

Epididymis —
Epididymal cysts —
| — Rete testis

| — Rete testis

(Top) First of three ultrasound images in a patient with tubular ectasia of the rete testis. Dilatation of the rete testis is thought to occur secondary to obstruction in the epididymis or efferent ductules. Tubular ectasia is located posteriorly by the mediastinum and is frequently bilateral. It may give an impression of a mass, but careful scanning shows the "mass" is actually a series of dilated tubules. (Middle) Longitudinal ultrasound of the right side shows two epididymal cysts. These are frequently associated with dilatation of the rete testis. (Bottom) Longitudinal color Doppler ultrasound of the left testis shows no flow within these cystic spaces.

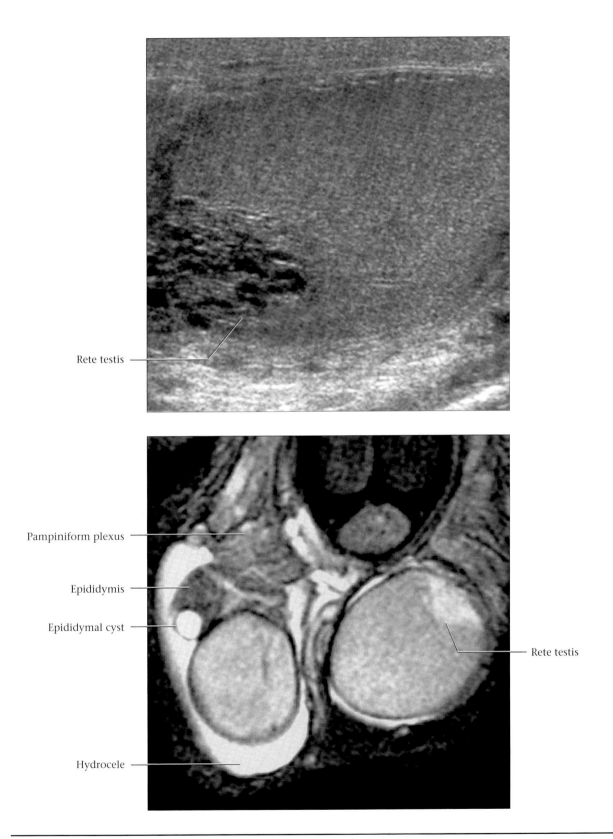

Rete testis

Pampiniform plexus

Epididymis

Epididymal cyst

Rete testis

Hydrocele

(Top) First of two images in a patient with a dilated rete testis. Longitudinal ultrasound of the left testis shows the typical appearance with multiple dilated tubules. **(Bottom)** Coronal T2 FS MR shows a triangular area of increased signal within the superior aspect of the left testis. This appearance helps to further differentiate tubular ectasia from a tumor, which is typically a round, low signal intensity mass on T2 MR.

TESTES AND SCROTUM

VARICOCELE

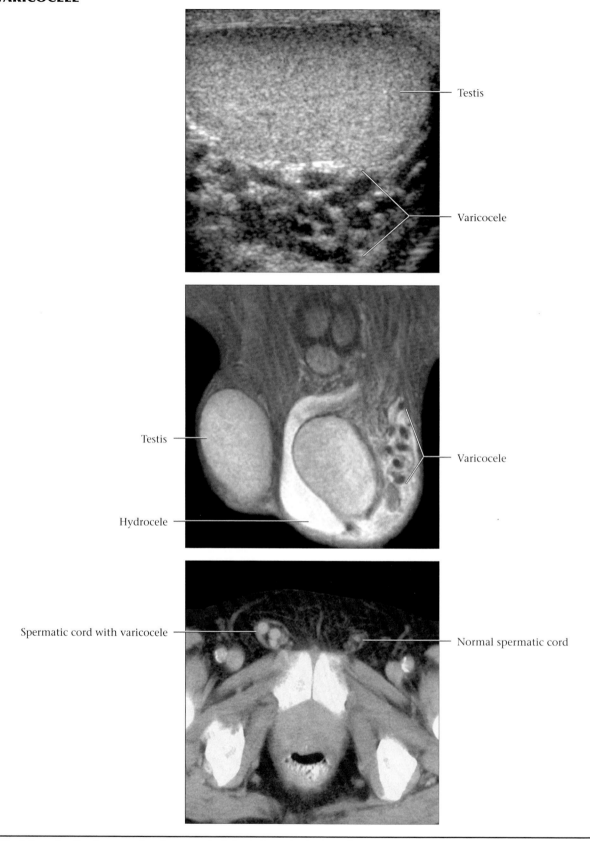

Testis

Varicocele

Testis

Varicocele

Hydrocele

Spermatic cord with varicocele

Normal spermatic cord

(Top) Longitudinal grayscale ultrasound of the left testis shows a large varicocele. Varicoceles are often idiopathic, particularly on the left side. Several anatomic factors predispose the left side: A) The left testicular vein has a longer course than the right. B) It has a perpendicular insertion into the left renal vein, while the right flows obliquely into the inferior vena cava. C) The left renal vein passes beneath the superior mesenteric artery creating a "nutcracker" effect. **(Middle)** Coronal T2 MR of a left-sided varicocele. The signal intensity may vary according to blood flow velocity. Fast-flowing varicoceles have a signal void, while slow-flowing ones will be intermediate to high signal. **(Bottom)** CECT of a right-sided varicocele in a patient with a right renal tumor. Varicoceles may be caused by compression or invasion of the renal vein or inferior vena cava.

TESTES AND SCROTUM

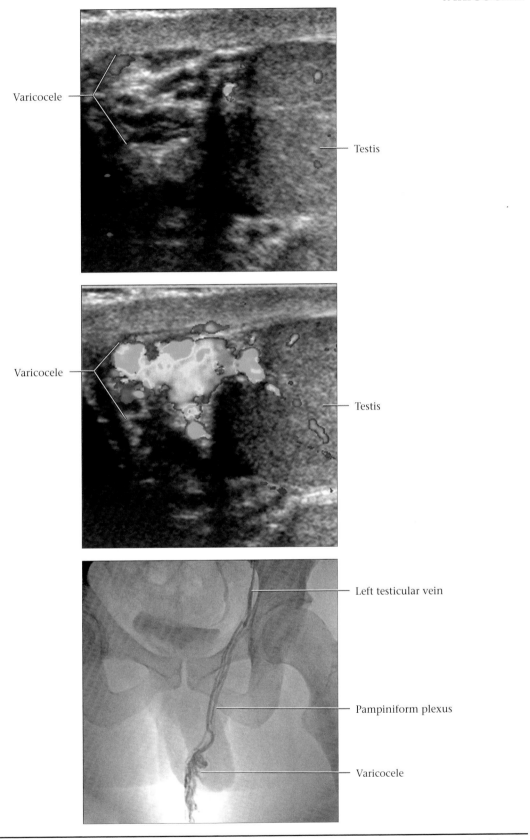

Varicocele —

— Testis

Varicocele —

— Testis

— Left testicular vein

— Pampiniform plexus

— Varicocele

(Top) First of three images in a patient with infertility and a left-sided varicocele. Normal vessel diameter should not exceed 3 mm. Color Doppler ultrasound at rest shows parallel channels with little to no flow. Often flow is so slow it is not discernible by Doppler. **(Middle)** Color Doppler shows filling of the varicocele with the Valsalva maneuver. Other provocative maneuvers, such as scanning in the upright position, can also be used to help make the diagnosis. **(Bottom)** Angiogram confirms the varicocele, which was subsequently embolized.

TESTES AND SCROTUM

RIGHT-SIDED LYMPHATIC DRAINAGE

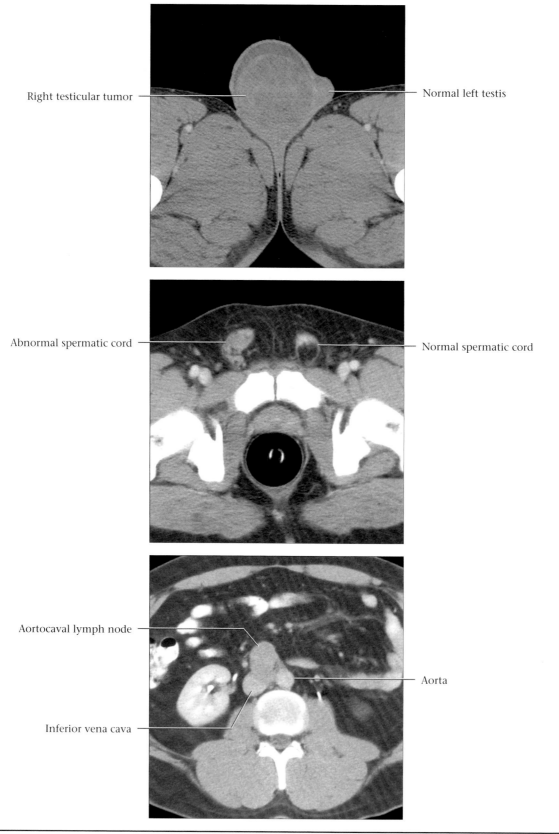

Right testicular tumor — Normal left testis

Abnormal spermatic cord — Normal spermatic cord

Aortocaval lymph node — Aorta

Inferior vena cava

(Top) First of three CECT images in a patient with a right-sided mixed germ cell tumor shows a large right testicular mass. **(Middle)** The right spermatic cord is enlarged and was invaded by tumor. **(Bottom)** A single enlarged aortocaval node is present. Most testicular tumors metastasize in a predictable fashion. Lymphatic drainage follows the testicular veins with the right side first metastasizing to the interaortocaval chain, at the level of the second lumbar vertebral body.

TESTES AND SCROTUM

LEFT-SIDED LYMPHATIC DRAINAGE

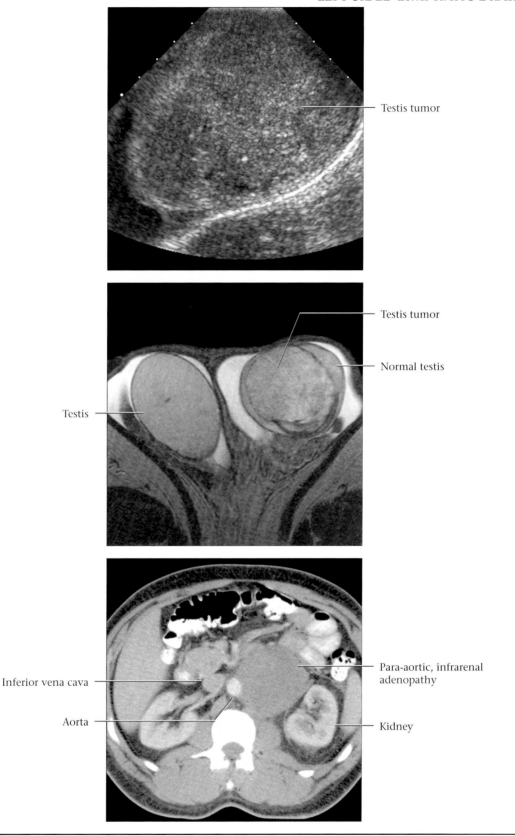

Testis tumor

Testis tumor

Normal testis

Testis

Inferior vena cava

Aorta

Para-aortic, infrarenal adenopathy

Kidney

(Top) First of three images of a patient with a left-sided seminoma. Longitudinal ultrasound shows a large, hypoechoic mass. (Middle) Axial T2 MR shows a large, lobular mass essentially replacing the left testis. A small amount of normal parenchyma remains in the periphery. (Bottom) CECT shows significant left-sided adenopathy. The first-echelon nodes for a left-sided testicular tumor are in an area bounded by the left renal vein, aorta, ureter, and inferior mesenteric artery.

PENIS AND URETHRA

Imaging Anatomy

Penis

- **Composed of three cylindrical shafts**
  - **Two corpora cavernosa**: Main erectile bodies
    - On dorsal surface of penis
    - Diverge at root of penis (**crura**) and are invested by **ischiocavernosus muscles**
    - Chambers traversed by numerous trabeculae, creating sinusoidal spaces
    - Multiple fenestrations between corpora, creating multiple anastomotic channels
  - **One corpus spongiosum**: Contains urethra
    - On ventral surface, in groove created by corpora cavernosa
    - Becomes **penile bulb** (urethral bulb) at root and is invested by **bulbospongiosus muscle**
    - Forms **glans penis** distally
    - Also erectile tissue but of far less importance
- **Tunica albuginea** forms capsule around each corpora
  - Thinner around spongiosum than cavernosa
- All three corpora surrounded by a deep fascia (**Buck fascia**) and a superficial fascia (**Colles fascia**)
- **Suspensory ligament** of penis (part of fundiform ligament) is an inferior extension of abdominal rectus sheath
- Main arterial supply from internal pudendal artery
  - **Cavernosal artery** runs within center of each corpus cavernosum
    - Gives off **helicine arteries**, which fill trabecular spaces
    - Primary source of blood for erectile tissue
  - **Paired dorsal penile arteries** run between tunica albuginea of corpora cavernosa and Buck fascia
    - Supplies glans penis and skin
  - Multiple anastomoses between cavernosal and dorsal penile arteries
- **Venous drainage** of corpora cavernosa
  - Emissary veins in corpora pierce through tunica albuginea ⇒ circumflex veins ⇒ deep dorsal vein of penis ⇒ retropubic venous plexus
  - Superficial dorsal vein drains skin and glans penis
- Primary innervation from terminal branches of internal pudendal nerve

Normal Erectile Function

- Neurologically mediated response eliciting smooth muscle relaxation of cavernosal arteries, helicine arteries and cavernosal sinusoids
- Blood flows from helicine arteries into sinusoidal spaces
- Sinusoids distend, eventually compressing emissary veins against rigid tunica albuginea
  - Venous compression prevents egress of blood from corpora, which maintains erection
- **Ultrasound** can be used to evaluate erectile function
  - Doppler evaluation of cavernosal arteries performed after injection of vasodilating agent
  - In flaccid state there is little diastolic flow
  - At onset of erection, there is dilatation of cavernosal arteries
    - Increase in both systolic and diastolic flow
  - At maximum erection, venous drainage is blocked
    - Waveform changes to high resistance with reversal of diastolic flow
  - **Normal measurements**
    - Peak systolic velocity > 30 cm/sec
    - Cavernosal artery diameter increase > 75%

Urethra

- Divided into four sections: Prostatic, membranous, bulbous and penile
  - **Posterior urethra**: Prostatic and membranous
  - **Anterior urethra**: Bulbous and penile
- **Prostatic urethra**
  - **Verumontanum** is 1 cm ovoid mound along ureteral crest (smooth muscle ridge on posterior wall)
  - Prostatic utricle, prostatic ducts and ejaculatory ducts enter in this segment
  - Lined by transitional cells
    - Remainder of urethra lined by columnar cells, except glans which has squamous epithelium
- **Membranous urethra**
  - Short course through urogenital diaphragm
    - Level of external urethral sphincter
  - Contains bulbourethral glands (Cowper glands)
    - Ducts travel distally ~ 2 cm to enter bulbous urethra
- **Bulbous urethra**
  - Below urogenital diaphragm to suspensory ligament of penis at penoscrotal junction
- **Penile urethra**
  - Pendulous portion, distal to suspensory ligament
  - **Fossa navicularis**: Widening at glans penis
  - Both penile and bulbous urethra lined by mucosal urethral glands (**glands of Littré**)
- **Two points of fixations**: Urogenital diaphragm (membranous urethra) and penoscrotal junction

Clinical Implications

- **Erectile dysfunction**
  - Complex and often multifactorial
  - Major causes include vascular, neurogenic and psychologic
  - Vascular etiology most common
  - Arteriogenic impotence effects inflow
    - Usually small vessels (internal pudendal, penile)
    - Blockage may be as high as distal aorta (**Leriche syndrome**)
  - Venogenic impotence effects outflow
    - Ineffective veno-occlusion with continuous outflow of blood from sinusoids
- **Peyronie disease**
  - Plaques formation on tunica albuginea
  - Causes painful erections, with shortening and curvature of penis
- **Trauma**
  - Most commonly involves **membranous urethra**
    - High association with pelvic fractures
  - **Straddle injuries** most commonly involve bulbous urethra
    - Urethral injury from compression against inferior pubic symphysis

PENIS AND URETHRA

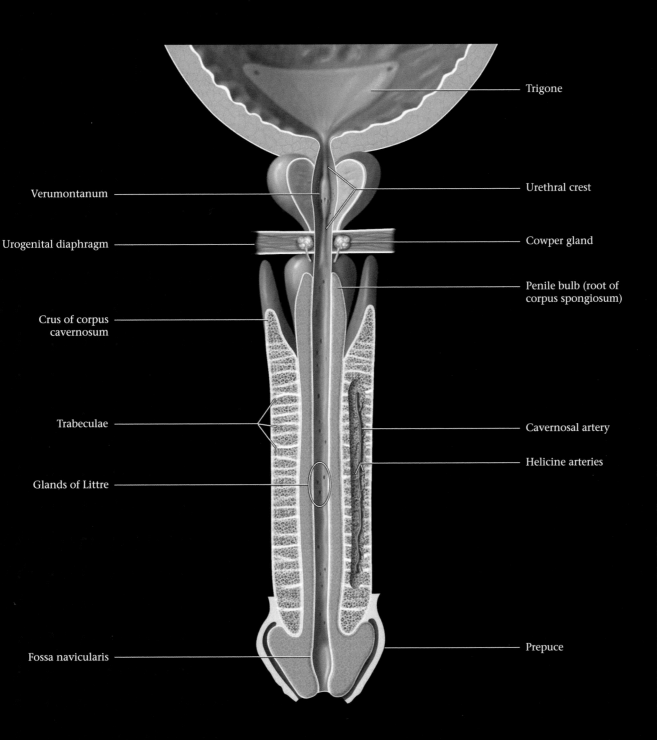

Verumontanum

Urogenital diaphragm

Crus of corpus cavernosum

Trabeculae

Glands of Littre

Fossa navicularis

Trigone

Urethral crest

Cowper gland

Penile bulb (root of corpus spongiosum)

Cavernosal artery

Helicine arteries

Prepuce

Graphic showing the posterior wall of the urethra from the bladder base to the fossa navicularis. The verumontanum is the most prominent portion of the urethral crest. The prostatic utricle (an embryologic remnant of the Müllerian system) enters in the center of the verumontanum, along with the ejaculatory ducts, which are just distal on either side. Cowper glands are within the urogenital diaphragm but their ducts course distally approximately 2 cm to enter the bulbous urethra. Multiple, small, mucosal glands (glands of Littré) line the mucosa of the anterior urethra. The corpora cavernosa are the primary erectile bodies. They are traversed by numerous trabeculae, creating sinusoidal spaces. The cavernosal artery runs within the center of each corpus cavernosum and gives rise to the helicine arteries, which flow into the sinusoids.

PENIS AND URETHRA

PENIS AND PERINEUM

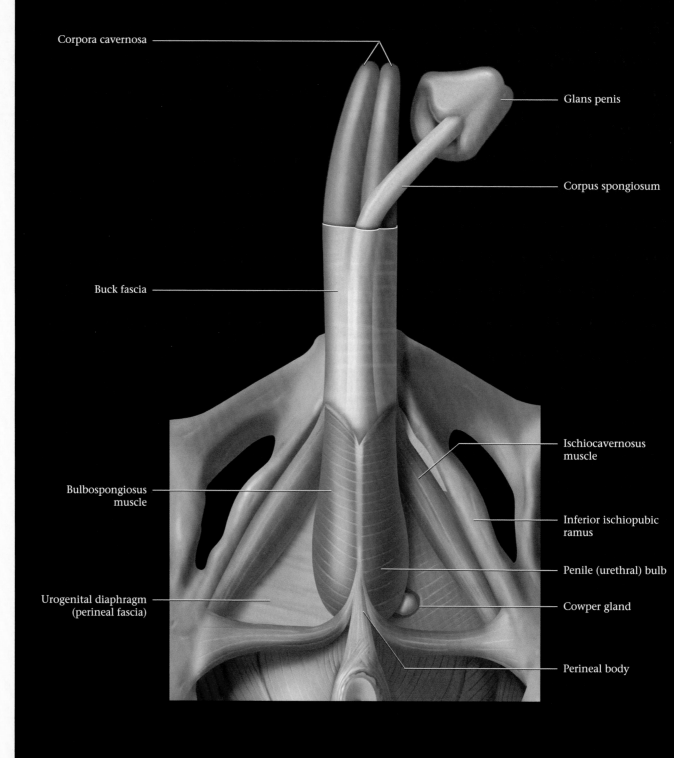

Corpora cavernosa

Glans penis

Corpus spongiosum

Buck fascia

Ischiocavernosus muscle

Bulbospongiosus muscle

Inferior ischiopubic ramus

Penile (urethral) bulb

Urogenital diaphragm (perineal fascia)

Cowper gland

Perineal body

At the root of the penis, the corpora split into a triradiate form. The crura of the corpora cavernosa diverge and each crus is invested by an ischiocavernosus muscle. The corpus spongiosum remains midline and is invested by the bulbospongiosus muscle. It widens at its attachment to the urogenital diaphragm and is called the penile or urethral bulb. The root of the penis is firmly anchored between the urogenital diaphragm above and Colles fascia below (cut away to show perineal muscles). Additional supports include fascial attachments to the medial surface of the pubic rami and and pubic symphysis.

PENIS AND URETHRA

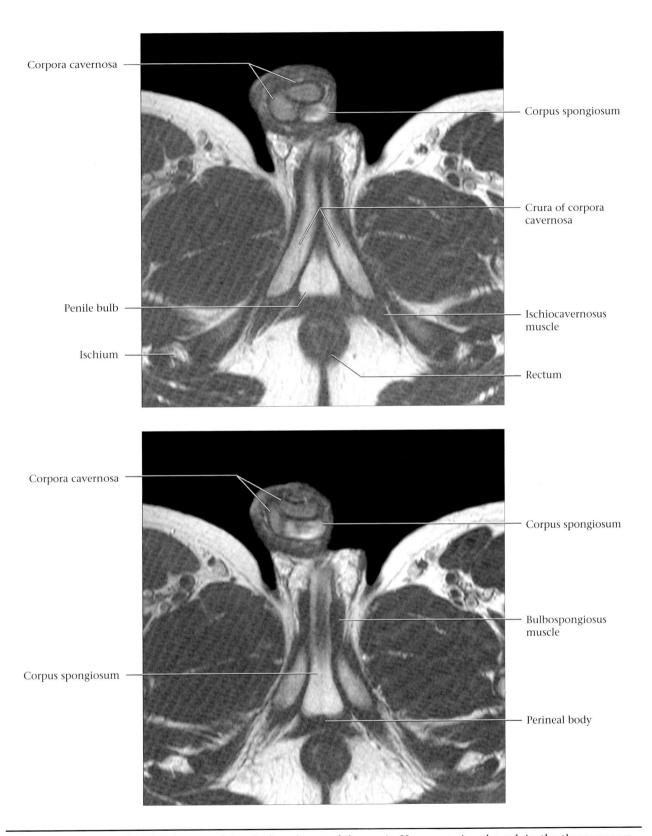

Corpora cavernosa

Corpus spongiosum

Crura of corpora cavernosa

Penile bulb

Ischiocavernosus muscle

Ischium

Rectum

Corpora cavernosa

Corpus spongiosum

Bulbospongiosus muscle

Corpus spongiosum

Perineal body

(Top) First of two axial T2 MR images of the shaft and root of the penis. Upon entering the pelvis, the three corpora are each invested within a muscle layer. The ischiocavernosus muscles surround the crura of the corpora cavernosa, and the bulbospongiosus muscle surrounds the root of the corpus spongiosum. These muscles are innervated by the perineal nerves and assist in erection, ejaculation and the sensation of orgasm. **(Bottom)** More distally in the pendulous portion of the penis, the corpora cavernosa begin to diminish in size, while the corpus spongiosum becomes larger and forms the glans of the penis.

PENIS AND URETHRA

ROOT OF PENIS

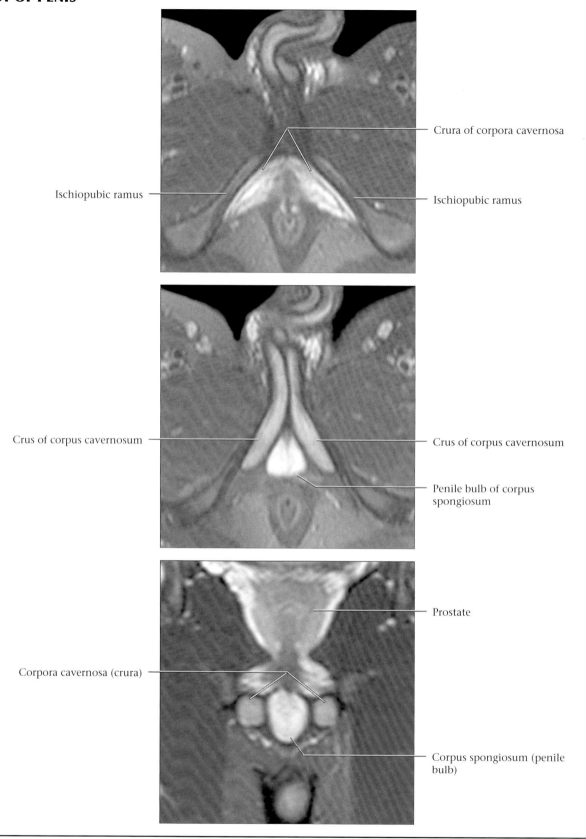

Crura of corpora cavernosa

Ischiopubic ramus

Ischiopubic ramus

Crus of corpus cavernosum

Crus of corpus cavernosum

Penile bulb of corpus spongiosum

Prostate

Corpora cavernosa (crura)

Corpus spongiosum (penile bulb)

(Top) First of two axial T2 FS images of the root of the penis presented from superior to inferior. The crura of the corpora cavernosa are firmly attached to the pelvic floor by the ischiocavernous muscles and by strong fascial attachments to the ischiopubic rami. **(Middle)** The root of the penis has a triradiate appearance, with the crura of the corpora cavernosa splaying and attaching to the inferior pubic rami, while the corpus spongiosum remains midline. **(Bottom)** Coronal STIR image, at the level of the prostate, shows all three corpora at the same level. The corpora cavernosa crura diminish in size as they continue to diverge and attach to the inferior ischiopubic rami. The corpus spongiosum remains midline and enlarges to form the penile bulb (also known as the urethral bulb).

PENIS AND URETHRA

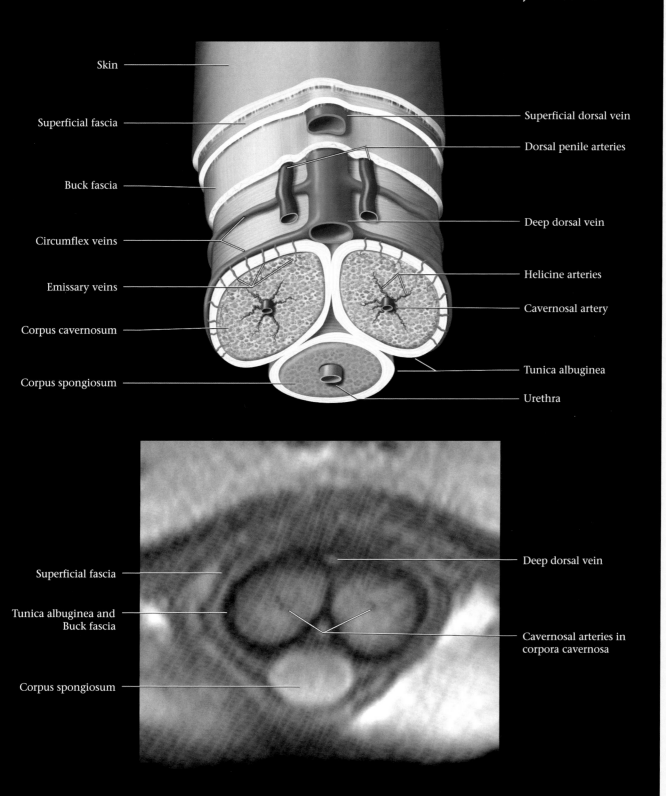

Skin

Superficial fascia

Buck fascia

Circumflex veins

Emissary veins

Corpus cavernosum

Corpus spongiosum

Superficial dorsal vein

Dorsal penile arteries

Deep dorsal vein

Helicine arteries

Cavernosal artery

Tunica albuginea

Urethra

Superficial fascia

Tunica albuginea and Buck fascia

Corpus spongiosum

Deep dorsal vein

Cavernosal arteries in corpora cavernosa

(Top) Cross-section of the penis viewed from above shows the three corpora, each of which is invested by a tunica albuginea. The three corpora are surrounded by Buck fascia. The cavernosal arteries run within the corpora cavernosa and give rise to the helicine arteries, which fill the sinusoids. Normal drainage is via the emissary veins ⇒ circumflex veins ⇒ deep dorsal vein of penis. With an erection, the emissary veins are compressed against the strong tunica albuginea, occluding venous drainage. The dorsal penile arteries and deep dorsal vein run beneath the Buck fascia. The penile arteries supply the glans and skin, but there are significant anastomoses between both the arterial and venous systems. **(Bottom)** T2 MR cross-section of the penis shows the low signal tunica albuginea surrounding each of the corpora (more prominent around the cavernosa). Buck fascia can not be separated from the tunica albuginea.

NORMAL ERECTILE FUNCTION

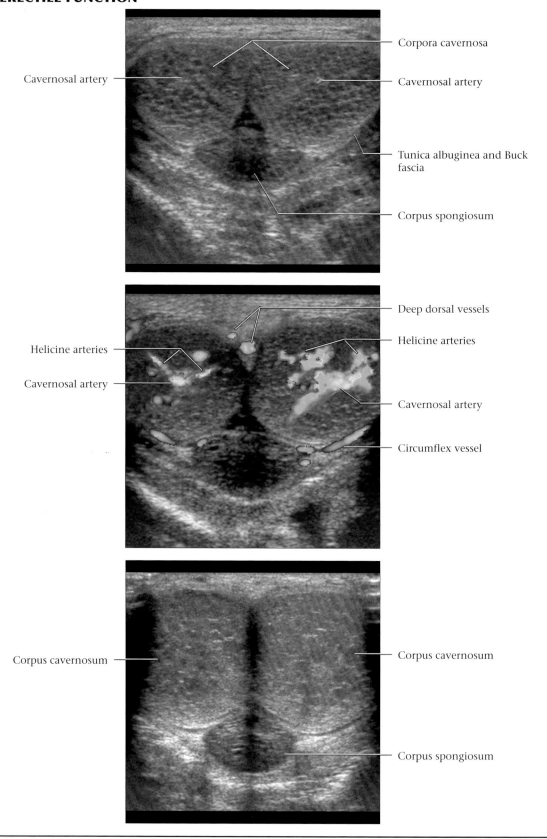

Corpora cavernosa

Cavernosal artery

Cavernosal artery

Tunica albuginea and Buck fascia

Corpus spongiosum

Deep dorsal vessels

Helicine arteries

Helicine arteries

Cavernosal artery

Cavernosal artery

Circumflex vessel

Corpus cavernosum

Corpus cavernosum

Corpus spongiosum

(Top) First of three cross-sectional ultrasound images of the penis showing the changing appearance during a normal erection. The paired corpora cavernosa are the primary erectile bodies. They are composed of a complex network of trabeculae, which create the sinusoids and give a "sponge-like" appearance on ultrasound. Each corpus is surrounded by a tough tunica albuginea, which appears as a thin echogenic line. Buck fascia, which surrounds all three corpora, is intimately associated with the tunica and cannot be distinguished as a separate structure. (Middle) Color Doppler at the onset of an erection shows arterial inflow. There is dilation of the cavernosal and helicine arteries, as they begin to fill the sinusoidal spaces. (Bottom) With continued arterial inflow and compressed venous outflow, the corpora become maximally distended and rigid.

PENIS AND URETHRA

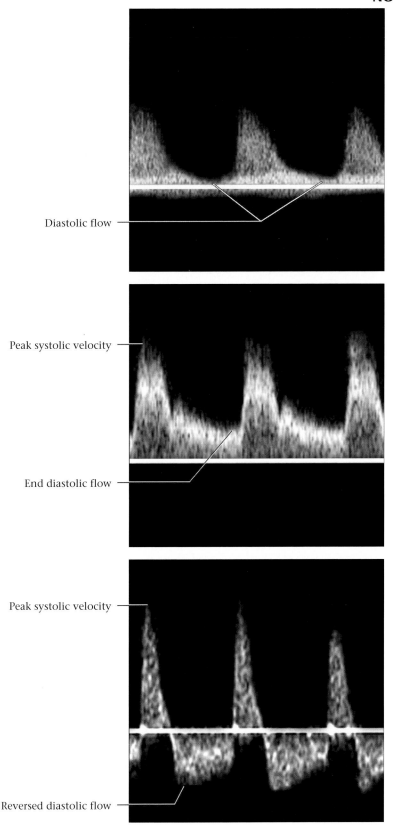

Diastolic flow

Peak systolic velocity

End diastolic flow

Peak systolic velocity

Reversed diastolic flow

(Top) First of 3 Doppler tracings showing the changing flow patterns during a normal erection. In the flaccid state, there is little to no diastolic flow. **(Middle)** At onset of erection, there is vasodilation of the cavernosal and helicine arteries (increased inflow), and smooth muscle relaxation within the sinusoids (decreased resistance). This causes a marked increase in both the peak systolic velocity (PSV) & end diastolic flow. **(Bottom)** In the fully erect state, the emissary veins are compressed against the rigid tunica albuginea, preventing outflow of blood. This dramatically increases the arterial resistance resulting in absent or reversed diastolic flow. A PSV > 30 cm/sec is considered normal, while < 25 cm/sec is strong evidence of arteriogenic impotence (25-30 borderline). Venogenic impotence is due to failure of draining vein occlusion. The Doppler tracing would show continuous forward flow in diastole.

PENIS AND URETHRA

NORMAL ERECTILE FUNCTION

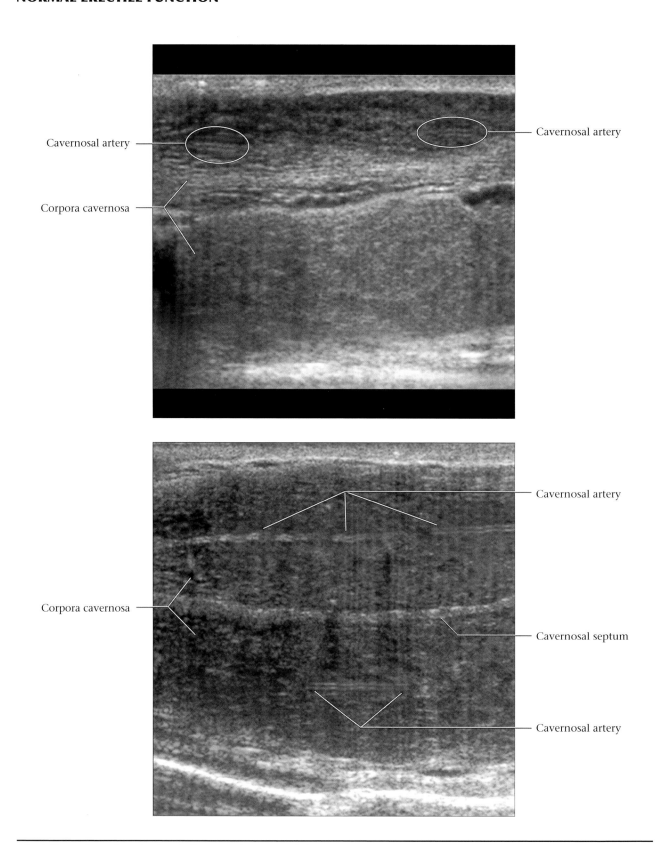

Cavernosal artery

Cavernosal artery

Corpora cavernosa

Cavernosal artery

Corpora cavernosa

Cavernosal septum

Cavernosal artery

(Top) First of two longitudinal ultrasound images of the corpora cavernosa. In the flaccid state the cavernosal arteries are tortuous, and therefore, can only be intermittently visualized in the longitudinal plane. **(Bottom)** In the erect state, the cavernosal arteries assume a straighter course and can be easily imaged. Magnified views of the cavernosal artery should be obtained to measure vessel diameter. Most measure < 1 mm in the flaccid state. The diameter should increase by 75% with an erection. Failure to increase in size, coupled with an abnormal Doppler waveform is strong evidence of arteriogenic impotence. Despite the fact that each corpora is sheathed within its own tunica albuginea, there is significant communication across the septum between the two corpora cavernosa. Therefore when performing a study, only one corpus cavernosum needs to be injected with the vasodilating agent.

PENIS AND URETHRA

PEYRONIE DISEASE

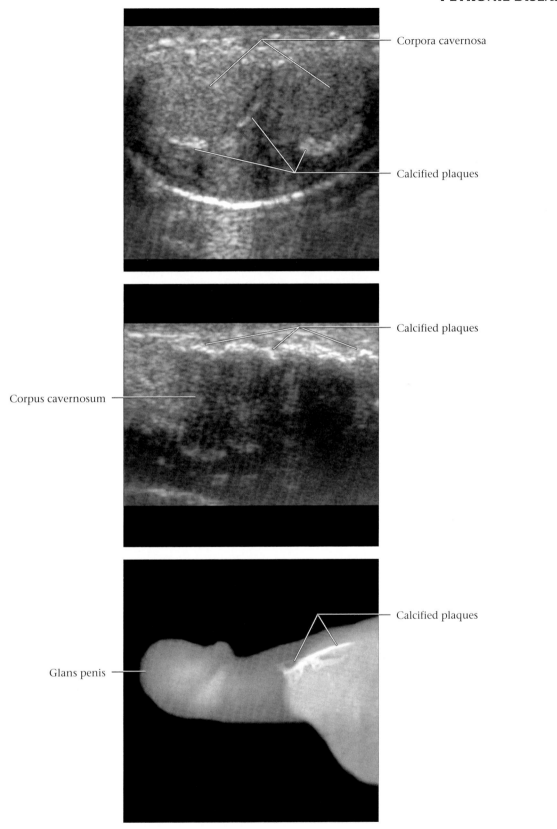

Corpora cavernosa

Calcified plaques

Calcified plaques

Corpus cavernosum

Calcified plaques

Glans penis

(Top) First of three images in a patient with Peyronie disease. Cross-sectional ultrasound shows calcified plaques within the tunica albuginea of the corpora cavernosa. (Middle) A longitudinal ultrasound of one corpus cavernosum shows densely calcified plaques, with significant posterior shadowing. (Bottom) Lateral radiograph of the penis shows not only the calcified plaques, but also shortening and upward curvature of the penis. Peyronie disease is an incompletely understood inflammatory process, with fibroblastic proliferation and calcification involving the tunica albuginea. It manifests as pain and deformity with erection. The penis may shrink in size with disease progression.

PENIS AND URETHRA

PENIS AND URETHRA

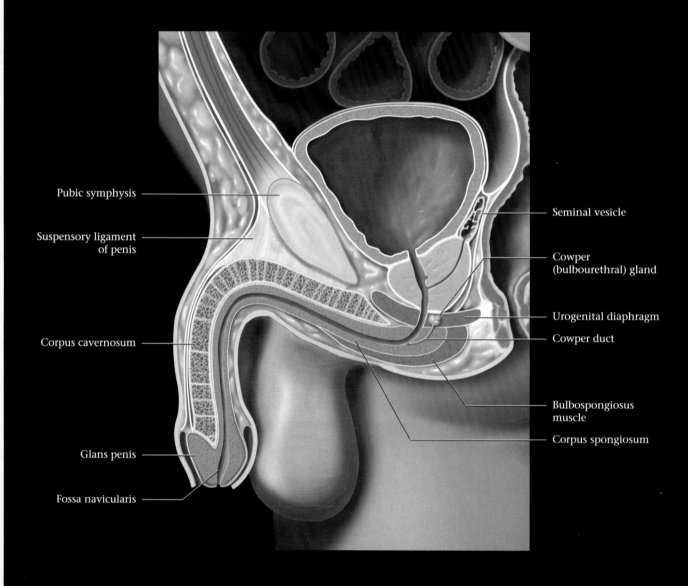

Pubic symphysis

Suspensory ligament
of penis

Corpus cavernosum

Glans penis

Fossa navicularis

Seminal vesicle

Cowper
(bulbourethral) gland

Urogenital diaphragm

Cowper duct

Bulbospongiosus
muscle

Corpus spongiosum

Sagittal midline graphic shows the course of the urethra. The anterior urethra runs within the corpus spongiosum.
The external (pendulous) portion of the penis begins below the pubic symphysis, at the penoscrotal junction. It is
fixed at this position by the suspensory ligament of the penis, which is part of the fundiform ligament, an inferior
extension of the rectus sheath. The proximal (internal) urethral sphincter extends from the bladder neck to above the
verumontanum. The distal, or external sphincter, has both intrinsic and extrinsic components. The intrinsic
component is composed of concentric smooth muscle extending from the distal prostatic urethra through the
membranous urethra. The surrounding extrinsic component is composed of striated muscle and is under voluntary
control.

PENIS AND URETHRA

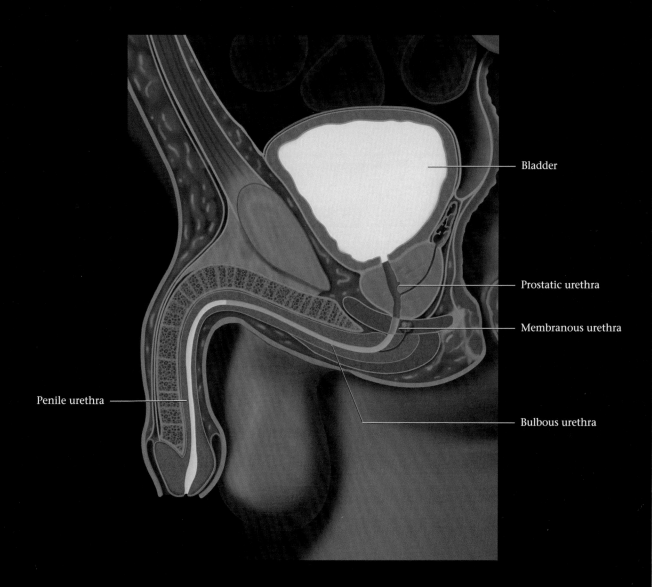

Bladder

Prostatic urethra

Membranous urethra

Penile urethra

Bulbous urethra

The urethra has two major divisions: The anterior and posterior urethra, each of which has two parts. The posterior urethra is composed of the prostatic and membranous portions, and the anterior urethra is composed of the bulbous and penile portions. The prostatic urethra begins at the bladder base and extends to the apex of the prostatic gland. The membranous urethra traverses the urogenital diaphragm. It is the shortest portion of the urethra but the area most vulnerable to injury. The bulbous urethra extends from the bottom of the urogenital diaphragm to the suspensory ligament of the penis. The penile urethra is distal to the suspensory ligament and travels through the pendulous portion of the penis. It widens into the fossa navicularis at the distal glans.

PENIS AND URETHRA

URETHRAL ANATOMY

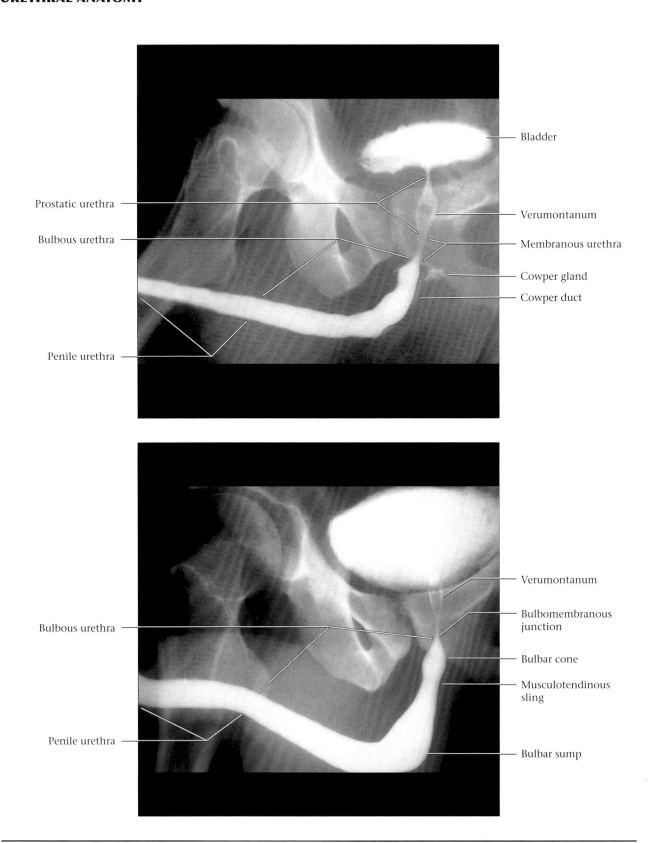

Bladder

Prostatic urethra

Verumontanum

Bulbous urethra

Membranous urethra

Cowper gland

Cowper duct

Penile urethra

Bulbous urethra

Verumontanum

Bulbomembranous junction

Bulbar cone

Musculotendinous sling

Penile urethra

Bulbar sump

(Top) The verumontanum is a smooth filling defect along the posterior wall of the prostatic urethra. The membranous urethra is the shortest segment (~ 1-1.5 cm) and passes through the urogenital diaphragm. The paired Cowper glands lie within the urogenital diaphragm but their ducts extend ~ 2 cm to enter the bulbous urethra. **(Bottom)** The bulbous urethra begins just below urogenital diaphragm at the bulbomembranous junction (BMJ). Just distal to the BMJ, there is a conical widening of the bulbous urethra called the "cone". A musculotendinous sling of the bulbospongiosus muscle may cause an indentation just distal to the cone. This should not be confused with a stricture. The proximal-to-mid bulbous urethra widens and is termed the "sump". There is a mild angulation of the urethra at the penoscrotal junction. The penile or pendulous urethra is distal to this point.

PENIS AND URETHRA

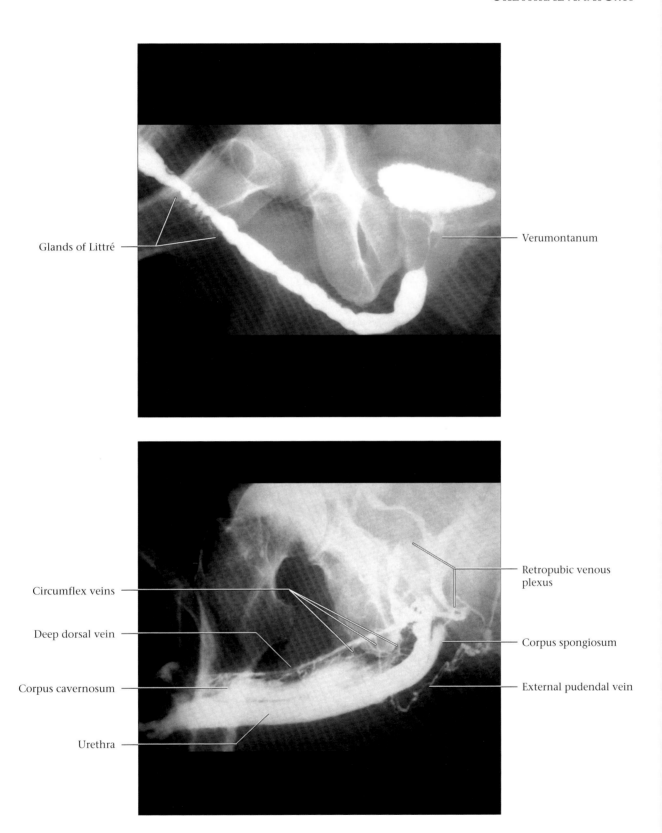

Glands of Littré

Verumontanum

Circumflex veins

Deep dorsal vein

Corpus cavernosum

Urethra

Retropubic venous plexus

Corpus spongiosum

External pudendal vein

(Top) Retrograde urethrogram in a patient with gonococcal urethritis shows irregularity of the penile and bulbous urethra, with filling of the glands of Littré. The glands of Littré are small, mucosal, mucus-secreting glands found predominately in the penile and bulbous portions of the urethra. Unlike Cowper glands, which may be seen in normal individuals (especially the elderly), filling of the glands of Littré is highly associated with an inflammatory/infectious process. **(Bottom)** Retrograde urethrogram of a complete anterior urethral disruption shows the venous drainage pattern of the penis. There is extravasation of contrast into the corpora spongiosum and cavernosa. The circumflex veins lie beneath Buck fascia and drain to the deep dorsal vein of the penis and finally into the retropubic venous plexus.

PENIS AND URETHRA

POSTERIOR URETHRAL TRAUMA AND STRICTURE

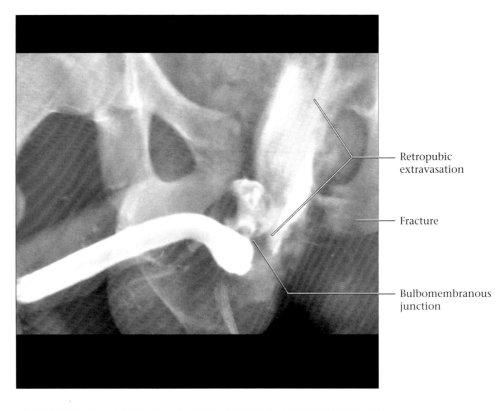

Retropubic
extravasation

Fracture

Bulbomembranous
junction

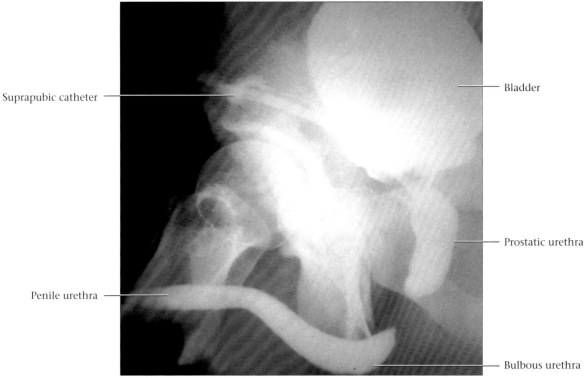

Suprapubic catheter

Penile urethra

Bladder

Prostatic urethra

Bulbous urethra

(Top) Retrograde urethrogram shows a posterior urethral injury, with complete disruption of urethra at the level of the urogenital diaphragm and extravasation of contrast into the retropubic space. Posterior urethral injuries have a high association with pelvic fractures. This was treated with a suprapubic catheter, and a subsequent urethral stricture developed. **(Bottom)** Combination retrograde urethrogram and bladder filling via suprapubic catheter shows the stricture, which extends from the bottom of the prostatic urethra to the bulbous urethra. This is the area of the urogenital diaphragm, which is the most common site of urethral injury in blunt abdominal trauma.

PENIS AND URETHRA

ANTERIOR URETHRA TRAUMA

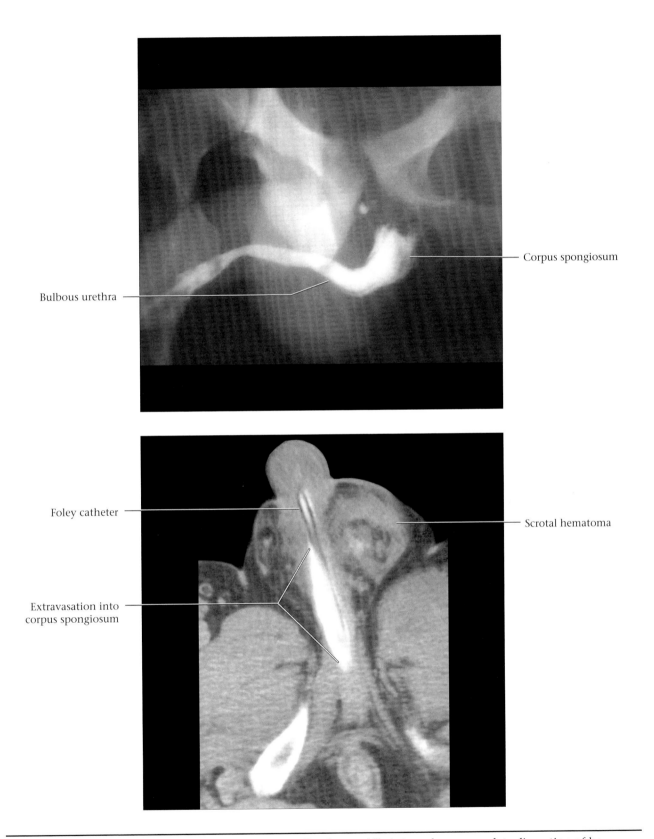

Corpus spongiosum

Bulbous urethra

Foley catheter

Scrotal hematoma

Extravasation into
corpus spongiosum

(Top) Retrograde urethrogram in a patient who has suffered a straddle injury shows complete disruption of he bulbous urethra with extravasation of contrast into the corpus spongiosum. Anterior urethral injuries occur when the urethra (usually bulbous) is forcefully compressed against the inferior pubic symphysis. Anterior urethral injuries are less likely to be associated with fractures than posterior urethral injuries. **(Bottom)** CT scan performed after a retrograde urethrogram in a patient with an incomplete tear of the anterior urethra shows extravasation of contrast into the corpus spongiosum. There is an associated scrotal hematoma, which is common in anterior urethral injury.

PROSTATE AND SEMINAL VESICLES

Terminology

Abbreviations

- Anterior fibromuscular stroma (AFMS)
- Central zone (CZ)
- Peripheral zone (PZ)
- Transitional zone (TZ)
- Neurovascular bundle (NVB)
- Benign prostatic hyperplasia (BPH)

Gross Anatomy

Prostate

- Walnut-sized gland located beneath bladder and in front of rectum
  - Above superior fascia of urogenital diaphragm
  - Surrounds uppermost part of urethra
  - Normal prostate ~ 3 cm craniocaudal x 4 cm wide x 2 cm anteroposteriorly
  - Surrounded by fibrous prostatic capsule
- Conical in shape with base, apex and anterior, posterior and two inferolateral surfaces
  - **Base** directed upward
    - Closely related to inferior surface of bladder
  - **Apex** directed downward
    - In contact with superior fascia of urogenital diaphragm
  - **Posterior surface** separated from rectum by rectovesical septum (**Denonvilliers fascia**)
    - Two **ejaculatory ducts** enter prostate through posterior surface
    - Posterosuperiorly, seminal vesicles lie between bladder base and rectum
  - **Anterior surface** separated from symphysis pubis by extraperitoneal fat and plexus of veins
    - Connected to pubic bone on either side by puboprostatic ligaments
  - **Inferolateral surfaces** separated from levator ani by periprostatic plexus of veins
- **Prostatic urethra**
  - Prostatic utricle, prostatic ducts and ejaculatory ducts enter prostatic urethra
  - **Urethral crest**
    - Narrow longitudinal ridge on posterior wall
    - Formed by elevation of mucosal membrane and its subjacent tissue
    - 15-17 mm in length, about 3 mm in height
  - **Verumontanum** (colliculus seminalis)
    - Median elevation of urethral crest below its summit
    - Openings of prostatic utricle and ejaculatory ducts
  - **Prostatic sinus**
    - Slightly depressed fossae on each side of verumontanum
    - Multiple openings of prostatic ducts
  - **Prostatic utricle**
    - Small vestigial blind pouch of prostate gland, about 6 mm long
    - Developed from united lower ends of atrophied Müllerian ducts
    - Homologous with uterus and vagina in female

- Prostatic urethra is divided into proximal and distal parts by verumontanum
  - Midway between prostatic apex and bladder neck
  - Sharp anterior angulation of urethra of approximately 35° at verumontanum
- **Neurovascular bundles (NVB)**
  - Lie posterolaterally to prostate
  - Separated from prostate by Denonvilliers fascia
  - Carries nerve and vascular supply to corpora cavernosa
    - Critical for normal erectile function
- **Arterial supply** derived from internal pudendal, inferior vesicle, and middle rectal arteries
  - All branches of internal iliac arteries
- **Prostatic venous plexus**
  - Receives blood from dorsal vein of penis
  - Drains into internal iliac veins
  - Prostatic venous plexus communicates with internal vertebral venous plexus (**Batson plexus**)
- **Nerve supply**
  - Parasympathetic fibers from pelvic splanchnic nerves (S2-4)
  - Sympathetic fibers from inferior hypogastric plexuses
- **Lymphatic drainage** chiefly to internal iliac and sacral lymph nodes
  - Some drainage from posterior surface joins with bladder lymphatics, and drains to external iliac lymph nodes

Zonal Anatomy (McNeal)

- Prostate is histologically composed of glandular (acinar) and nonglandular elements
- Two nonglandular elements: Prostatic urethra and AFMS
  - AFMS is contiguous with bladder muscle and external sphincter
    - ~ 30% of prostate volume
  - Proximal half of prostatic urethra is surrounded by cuff of smooth muscle ("**preprostatic sphincter**")
- **Glandular prostate** consists of outer and inner components
- **Inner prostate** has two parts: Periurethral glandular tissue and transitional zone
  - **Periurethral glands**
    - < 1% of normal glandular prostate
    - Small glands confined to submucosal layer of proximal prostatic urethra above verumontanum and deep to preprostatic sphincter
    - Ducts drain into proximal posterolateral wall of prostatic urethra in two rows
  - **Transitional zone**
    - ~ 5% of normal glandular prostate
    - Surrounds anterior and lateral aspects of proximal urethra
    - Involvement in BPH causes bladder outlet obstruction because of urethral compression
- **Outer prostate** has two parts: Central and peripheral zones
  - **Central zone**
    - ~ 25% of normal glandular prostate
    - Surrounds ejaculatory ducts

PROSTATE AND SEMINAL VESICLES

- Funnel-shaped with its widest portion making majority of prostatic base
- Tapered tip extends inferiorly to level of verumontanum
- Encloses both periurethral glands and TZ
- Ducts of CZ drain to region of verumontanum, clustered around entry of ejaculatory ducts
  ○ **Peripheral zone**
    - ~ 70% of the normal glandular prostate
    - Surrounds both CZ and distal prostatic urethra
    - Ducts of PZ drain exclusively to distal prostatic urethra
    - Ducts are arranged in two vertical lines along posterolateral urethral wall
  ○ **Prostate pseudocapsule** ("surgical capsule")
    - Visible boundary between CZ & PZ

Seminal Vesicles and Ejaculatory Ducts
- **Seminal vesicles**
  ○ Saclike structures located superolaterally to prostate
    - Between fundus of urinary bladder and rectum
  ○ **Secrete fructose-rich, alkaline fluid**, which is major component of semen
    - Secretions are energy source for sperm
    - **Do not store sperm**
  ○ **Arterial supply**
    - Inferior vesicle and middle hemorrhoidal arteries
  ○ **Venous drainage** accompanies arteries
  ○ **Lymphatic drainage**
    - Superior portion → external iliac nodes
    - Inferior portion → internal iliac nodes
- **Ejaculatory ducts**
  ○ Located on either side of midline
  ○ Formed by union of seminal vesicle duct and ductus deferens
  ○ ~ 2.5 cm long
  ○ Start at base of prostate and run forward and downward through gland
    - Terminate as separate slit-like openings close to utricle

Imaging Anatomy

Prostate
- MR
  ○ T1WI: Homogeneous intermediate signal intensity
    - Does not delineate zonal anatomy
  ○ **T2WI depicts zonal anatomy**
    - AFMS is low signal intensity
    - PZ is high signal intensity ≥ periprostatic fat
    - PZ is surrounded by thin, low signal true capsule
    - CZ and TZ are of similar T2 signal intensity, < PZ
  ○ MR spectroscopic imaging allows analysis of prostate gland metabolism
    - Helpful in mapping prostatic carcinoma
- Transrectal ultrasound (TRUS)
  ○ Zones of normal prostate are not sonographically evident
  ○ TZ becomes distinguishable in BPH as well-demarcated area of heterogeneity
    - May contain visible nodules, cysts, and calcifications
  ○ TRUS guided biopsy for suspected prostate cancer
- CT
  ○ Prostate has homogeneous density similar to muscles
  ○ Not used for evaluation of prostate because of poor tissue characterization
- Prostate volume measurement
  ○ Prolate ellipse volume for 3 unequal axes
    - Width x height x length x 0.523
  ○ 1 cc of prostate tissue ~ 1 g
  ○ Prostate weighs ~ 20 g in young men
  ○ Prostatic enlargement when gland is > 40 g

Seminal Vesicles and Vasa Deferentia
- MR is an excellent modality to evaluate seminal vesicles
  ○ Fluid-containing structures therefore low-signal intensity on T1WI, high-signal intensity T2WI
  ○ Evaluation of seminal vesicles is important during staging of prostate cancer
- Cystic appearance on TRUS
- **Vasography**
  ○ Injection of contrast into vas deferens to evaluate its patency
  ○ Performed intra-operatively or retrogradely during cystoscopy
- Seminal vesiculography
  ○ Injection of contrast material into seminal vesicle
  ○ Performed under TRUS-guidance
  ○ Largely replaced vasography for diagnosis of ejaculatory duct obstruction

Clinical Implications

Zonal Distribution of Prostatic Disease
- Prostatic diseases have zonal distribution
  ○ **Prostate carcinoma**
    - 70% of adenocarcinomas arise in PZ
    - 20% in TZ
    - 10% in CZ
  ○ **Benign prostatic hypertrophy (BPH)**
    - Originates in TZ
    - Compresses CZ & PZ

Spread of Prostate Carcinoma
- Predictors of extracapsular extension of prostatic carcinoma
  ○ Asymmetry of NVB
  ○ Obliteration of rectoprostatic angle
  ○ Irregular bulge in prostatic contour
- Rarely spreads posterior to seminal vesicles across Denonvilliers fascia to involve rectum
- 90% of prostatic metastases involve spine
  ○ Lumbar spine affected three times > cervical spine

Surgical Treatment for Prostatic Carcinoma
- Radical prostatectomy
  ○ Impotence in almost all patients due to division of NVB
- Nerve sparing radical prostatectomy spares NVB
  ○ Reserved for early localized disease not involving prostate base

PROSTATE AND SEMINAL VESICLES

PROSTATE GLAND

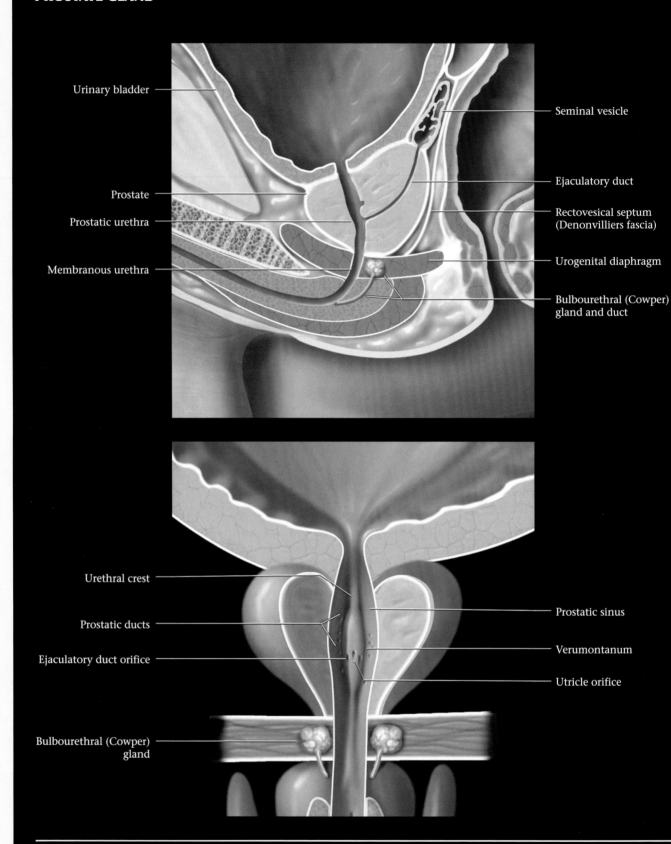

Urinary bladder

Seminal vesicle

Prostate

Ejaculatory duct

Prostatic urethra

Rectovesical septum (Denonvilliers fascia)

Membranous urethra

Urogenital diaphragm

Bulbourethral (Cowper) gland and duct

Urethral crest

Prostatic ducts

Prostatic sinus

Ejaculatory duct orifice

Verumontanum

Utricle orifice

Bulbourethral (Cowper) gland

(Top) Graphic illustrates the relationship between the prostate and the male pelvic organs. The prostate surrounds the upper part of the urethra (prostatic urethra). The base of the prostate is in direct contact with the neck of the urinary bladder and its apex is in contact with the superior fascia of urogenital veiaphragm. The posterior surface is separated from rectum by rectovesical septum (Denonvilliers fascia). **(Bottom)** Graphic illustrates the topography of the posterior wall of the prostatic urethra. The urethral crest is a mucosal elevation along the posterior wall, with the verumontanum being a mound-like elevation in the mid-portion of the crest. The utricle opens midline onto the verumontanum, with the ejaculatory ducts opening on either side. The prostatic ducts are clustered around the verumontanum and open into the prostatic sinuses, which are depressions along the sides of the urethral crest.

PROSTATE AND SEMINAL VESICLES

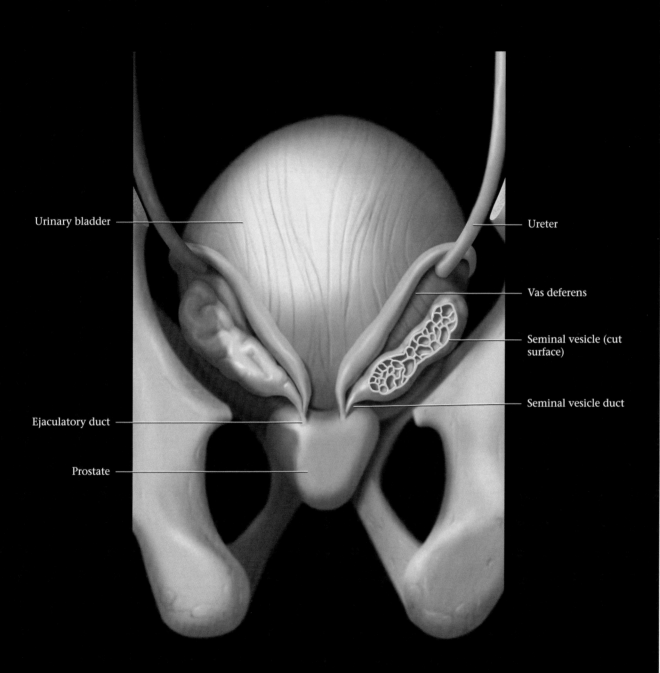

Urinary bladder

Ureter

Vas deferens

Seminal vesicle (cut surface)

Ejaculatory duct

Seminal vesicle duct

Prostate

Posterior view of the prostate gland and seminal vesicles. The cut surface of the seminal vesicle shows its highly convoluted fold pattern. The vas deferens crosses superior to the ureterovesical junction, continues along the posterior surface of the urinary bladder, medial to the seminal vesicle. In the base of the prostate, it is directed forward and is joined at an acute angle by the duct of the seminal vesicle to form the ejaculatory duct. The ejaculatory ducts course anteriorly and downward through the prostate to slit-like openings on either side of the orifice of the prostatic utricle.

PROSTATE AND SEMINAL VESICLES

PROSTATE ZONAL ANATOMY

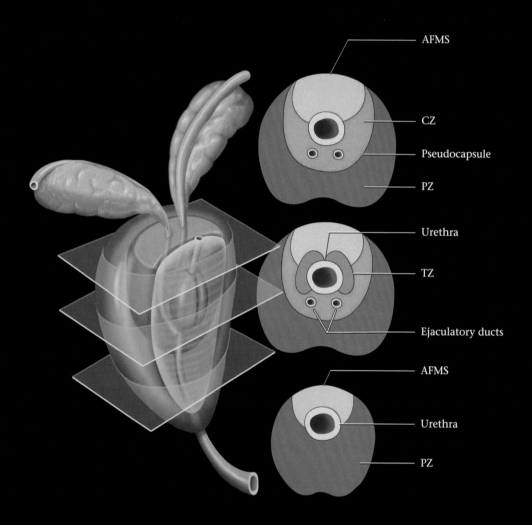

AFMS

CZ

Pseudocapsule

PZ

Urethra

TZ

Ejaculatory ducts

AFMS

Urethra

PZ

3D graphic depiction of the prostate with axial drawings of the zonal anatomy at three different levels. The TZ (in blue) is anterolateral to the verumontanum. The CZ (in orange) surrounds the ejaculatory ducts, and encloses the periurethral glands and the TZ. It is conical in shape and extends downward to about the level of the verumontanum. The PZ (in green) surrounds the posterior aspect of the CZ in the upper half of the gland and the urethra in the lower half, below the verumontanum. The prostatic pseudocapsule is a visible boundary between the CZ & PZ. The anterior fibromuscular stroma (in yellow) covers the anterior part of the gland and is thicker superiorly and thins inferiorly in the prostatic apex.

PROSTATE AND SEMINAL VESICLES

PROSTATE ZONAL ANATOMY

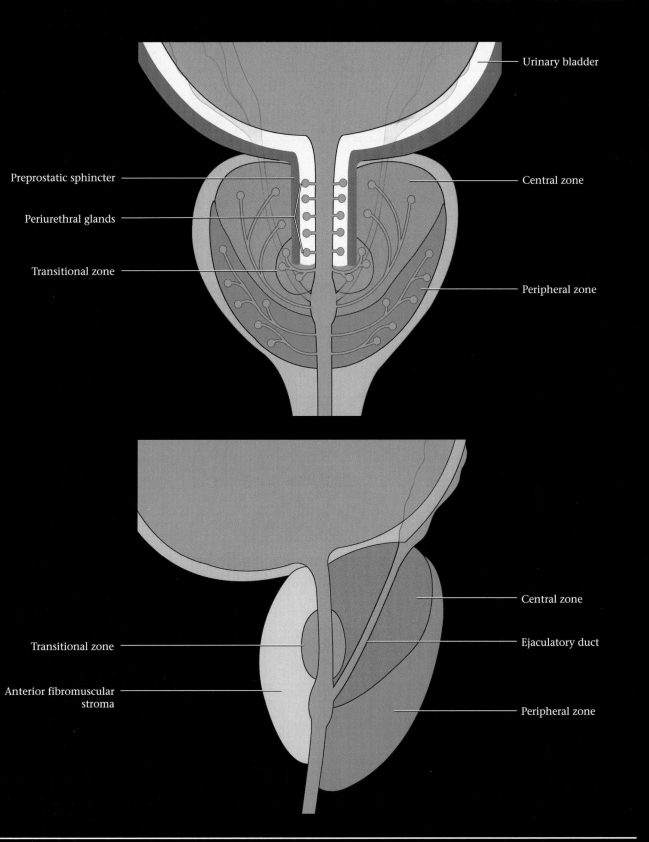

Urinary bladder

Preprostatic sphincter

Periurethral glands

Transitional zone

Central zone

Peripheral zone

Transitional zone

Anterior fibromuscular stroma

Central zone

Ejaculatory duct

Peripheral zone

(Top) Graphic illustrates the zonal anatomy of the prostate in the coronal plane. The proximal half of the prostatic urethra is surrounded by a cuff of smooth muscle, the preprostatic sphincter. This cuff extends inferiorly to the level of the verumontanum. The periurethral glands are confined to the urethral submucosa deep to the preprostatic sphincter. The TZ is a downward extension of the periurethral glands around the verumontanum. It surrounds the anterior and lateral portions of the proximal urethra in a horseshoe-like fashion. **(Bottom)** Graphic illustrates the zonal anatomy of the prostate in the sagittal plane. The outer prostate is composed of CZ and PZ. The CZ surrounds the proximal urethra posterosuperiorly, enclosing both the periurethral glands and the TZ. It forms most of the prostatic base. The PZ surrounds both the CZ and the distal prostatic urethra.

PROSTATE AND SEMINAL VESICLES

T1 MR, PROSTATE

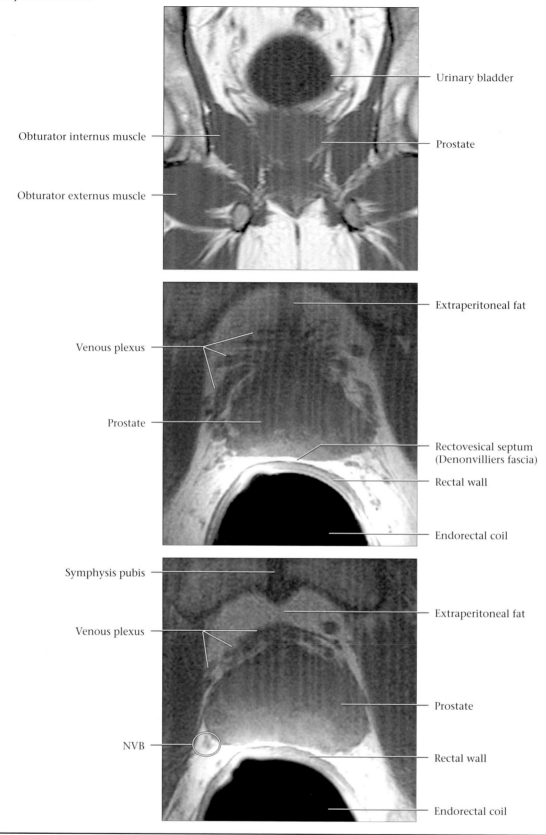

Urinary bladder

Obturator internus muscle

Prostate

Obturator externus muscle

Extraperitoneal fat

Venous plexus

Prostate

Rectovesical septum (Denonvilliers fascia)

Rectal wall

Endorectal coil

Symphysis pubis

Extraperitoneal fat

Venous plexus

Prostate

NVB

Rectal wall

Endorectal coil

(Top) Coronal T1 MR image of the prostate in a normal young adult shows the conical-shaped prostate, with the wide base in contact with the urinary bladder neck and the apex in contact with the urogenital diaphragm. (Middle) First of two axial T1 endorectal images of the prostate gland. This image is immediately below the bladder neck, just entering the base of the prostate gland. The anterior surface of the prostate is separated from the symphysis pubis by extraperitoneal fat and a venous plexus. Posteriorly it is separated from the rectum by the rectovesical septum (Denonvilliers fascia). (Bottom) Slightly inferiorly, the complete contour of the prostate is well seen. It is homogeneous intermediate-to-low signal intensity, similar to the pelvic floor muscles. T1 images are not helpful in depicting prostate zonal anatomy.

PROSTATE AND SEMINAL VESICLES

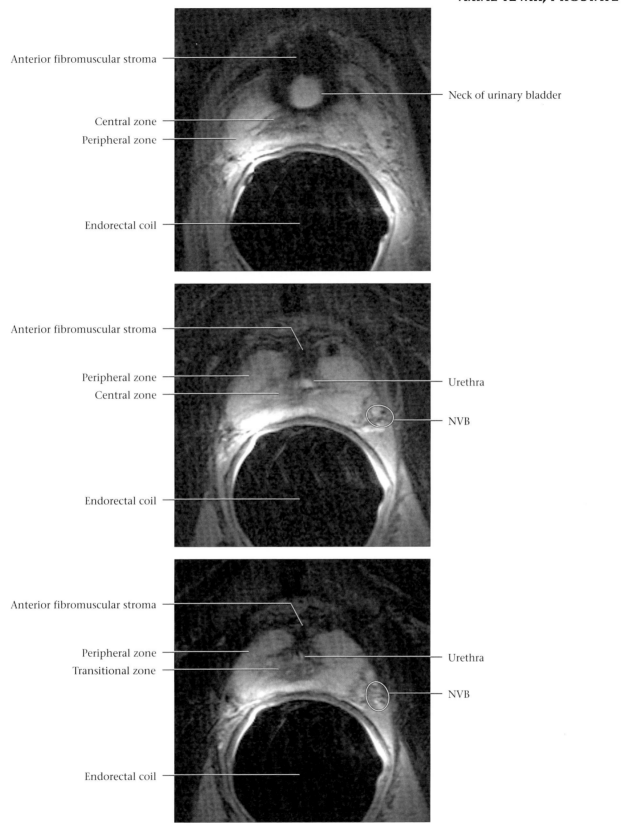

Anterior fibromuscular stroma

Neck of urinary bladder

Central zone
Peripheral zone

Endorectal coil

Anterior fibromuscular stroma

Peripheral zone
Central zone

Urethra

NVB

Endorectal coil

Anterior fibromuscular stroma

Peripheral zone
Transitional zone

Urethra

NVB

Endorectal coil

(Top) First of three axial T2 MR images of the prostate of a 45 year old man with mild prostatic obstructive symptoms. This image, at the level of the prostatic base, shows the AFMS continuous with the bladder muscle and external sphincter. The peripheral zone encloses the central zone which forms a large part of the prostatic base. **(Middle)** The tapered end of the funnel-shaped central zone extends to the level of verumontanum. The NVB lie posterolaterally to the prostate, at roughly the 5 and 7 o'clock positions. They supply to corpora cavernosa and are critical for normal erectile function. The periurethral glands are not discernible on imaging. **(Bottom)** At the level of the verumontanum, the slightly prominent transitional zone can be identified as an area of heterogeneous low signal intensity with scattered, small areas of high signal.

PROSTATE AND SEMINAL VESICLES

CT & ULTRASOUND, PROSTATE

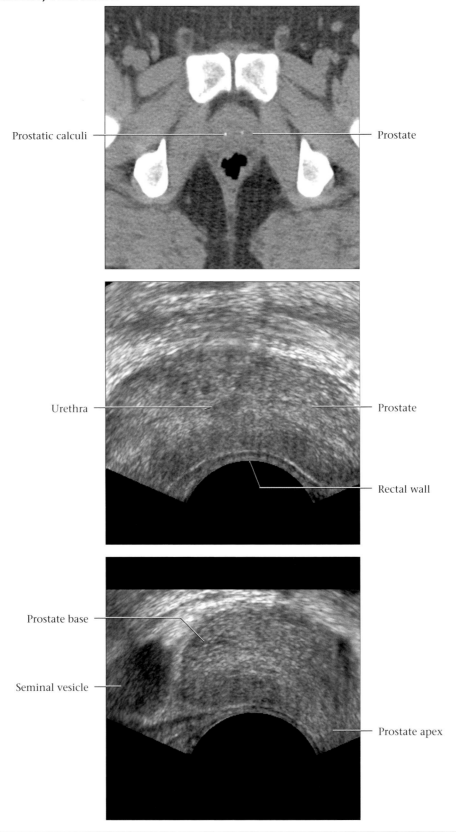

Prostatic calculi — Prostate

Urethra — Prostate

Rectal wall

Prostate base

Seminal vesicle — Prostate apex

(Top) Axial CT image of a normal-sized prostate shows prostatic calculi. Prostatic calculi are most often asymptomatic, but may be associated with some other disease process (BPH, prostatic carcinoma, metabolic abnormalities). They may be solitary but usually occur in clusters. CT images cannot show the zonal anatomy of the prostate but can show prostatic enlargement. **(Middle)** Transverse TRUS of the base of a normal prostate gland. The zonal anatomy of a normal prostate is not sonographically evident. **(Bottom)** Oblique sagittal TRUS shows the seminal vesicle adjacent to the base of the prostate.

PROSTATE AND SEMINAL VESICLES

MR, SEMINAL VESICLES

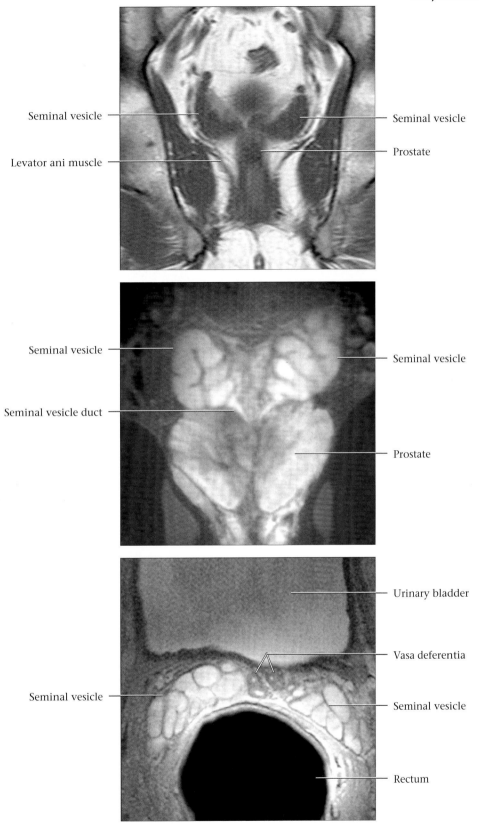

Seminal vesicle

Levator ani muscle

Seminal vesicle

Prostate

Seminal vesicle

Seminal vesicle duct

Seminal vesicle

Prostate

Urinary bladder

Vasa deferentia

Seminal vesicle

Seminal vesicle

Rectum

(Top) Coronal T1 MR shows the two seminal vesicles superior to the posterior margin of the prostate. The seminal vesicles are of intermediate signal intensity, similar to pelvic muscles. **(Middle)** Coronal T2 MR shows the "vesicular" appearance of the seminal vesicles with high signal intensity similar to fluid. The seminal vesicles secrete and store a fructose-rich, alkaline fluid, which is the major constituent of semen. They do not store sperm, which are transported from the testes via the vasa deferentia during ejaculation. The duct of the seminal vesicle and the vas deferens join to form the ejaculatory duct. **(Bottom)** Axial T2WI shows the seminal vesicles between the urinary bladder and the rectum. The distal vas deferens has a thickened, low signal wall and should not be confused with tumor extension from prostate carcinoma.

PROSTATE AND SEMINAL VESICLES

NORMAL PROSTATE & BPH

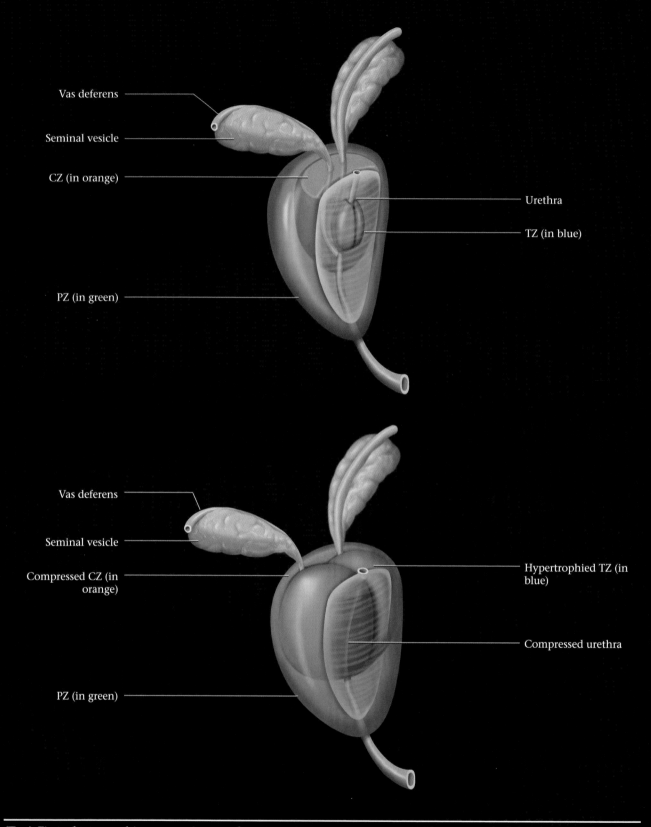

Vas deferens

Seminal vesicle

CZ (in orange)

Urethra

TZ (in blue)

PZ (in green)

Vas deferens

Seminal vesicle

Compressed CZ (in orange)

Hypertrophied TZ (in blue)

Compressed urethra

PZ (in green)

(Top) First of two graphics comparing zonal anatomy in a young man to an older man with BPH. The transitional zone in young men is small in size, comprising about 5% of the volume of the glandular tissue of the prostate. It surrounds the anterolateral aspect of the urethra at the level of verumontanum in a horseshoe fashion. **(Bottom)** With the development of BPH, there is enlargement of the transitional zone. This causes enlargement of the prostate and compression of the central and peripheral zones. BPH mainly involves the transitional zone, though other zones may also be involved. The enlarged transitional zone causes compression of the prostatic urethra, the primary reason for development of urinary obstructive symptoms in patients with BPH.

PROSTATE AND SEMINAL VESICLES

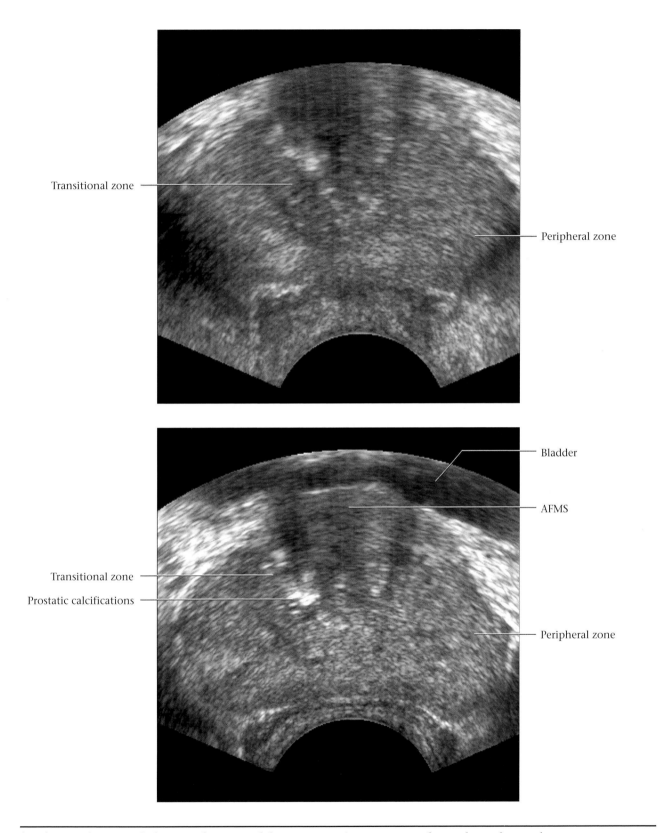

Transitional zone

Peripheral zone

Bladder

AFMS

Transitional zone

Prostatic calcifications

Peripheral zone

(Top) First of two axial ultrasound images of the prostate using a transrectal transducer shows a heterogeneous, slightly enlarged, transitional zone. As BPH begins to develop, the transitional zone becomes distinguishable by ultrasound. It has a heterogeneous echogenicity with visible cysts, nodules and calcifications. **(Bottom)** Focal areas of calcifications with shadowing are seen in this patient.

DIFFERENT GRADES OF BPH

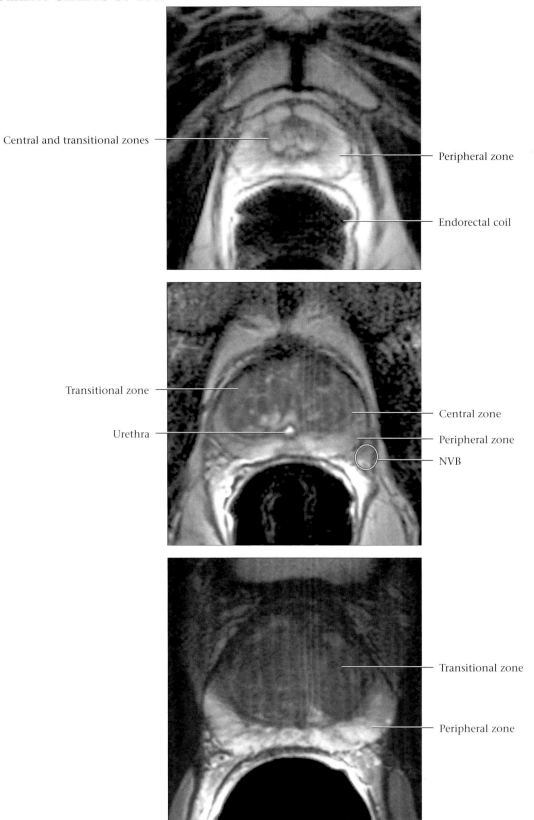

Central and transitional zones

Peripheral zone

Endorectal coil

Transitional zone

Urethra

Central zone

Peripheral zone

NVB

Transitional zone

Peripheral zone

(Top) First of six T2 MR images of the prostate showing varying degrees of BPH. This axial endorectal scan is of a young patient with a normal-sized prostate and mild degree of BPH. Note that it is not possible to differentiate the transitional zone from the central zone. **(Middle)** Axial endorectal image from a patient with moderate BPH. The hypertrophied transitional zone is heterogeneous, with areas of high and low signal. It is expanding the central zone and compressing it against the high signal intensity peripheral zone (Courtesy K. Hosseinzadeh, MD). **(Bottom)** More severe BPH with enlargement of the gland and further expansion of the transitional zone.

PROSTATE AND SEMINAL VESICLES

DIFFERENT GRADES OF BPH

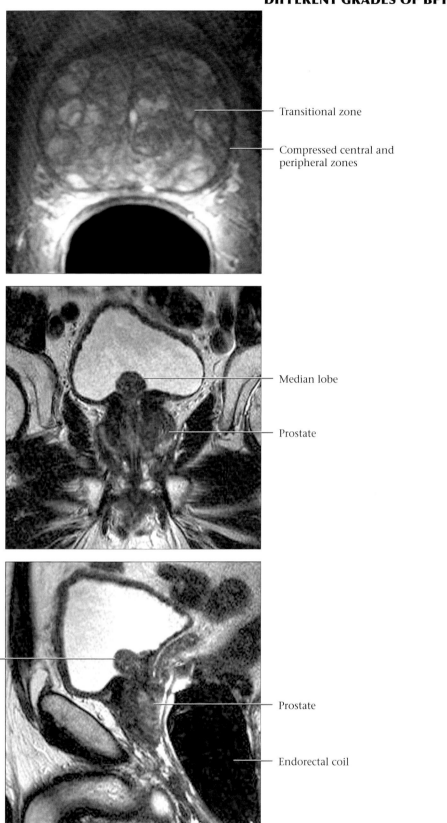

Transitional zone

Compressed central and peripheral zones

Median lobe

Prostate

Median lobe

Prostate

Endorectal coil

(Top) Severe BPH in a patient with severe obstructive symptoms shows diffuse enlargement of the prostate. There is a very large, nodular-appearing transitional zone, which is compressing and essentially obliterating the central and peripheral zones. (Middle) Coronal T2 MR image of the prostate shows a tear-drop shaped midline structure at the posterior bladder neck. This represents hyperplastic periurethral glands. The periurethral glands are less commonly involved with BPH but, when enlarged, can form what is termed a median lobe. This can cause severe obstructive voiding symptoms by creating a ball-valve into the urethra. (Bottom) Sagittal T2 MR image of median lobe hypertrophy.

PROSTATE AND SEMINAL VESICLES

POST TRANSURETHRAL RESECTION OF THE PROSTATE (TURP)

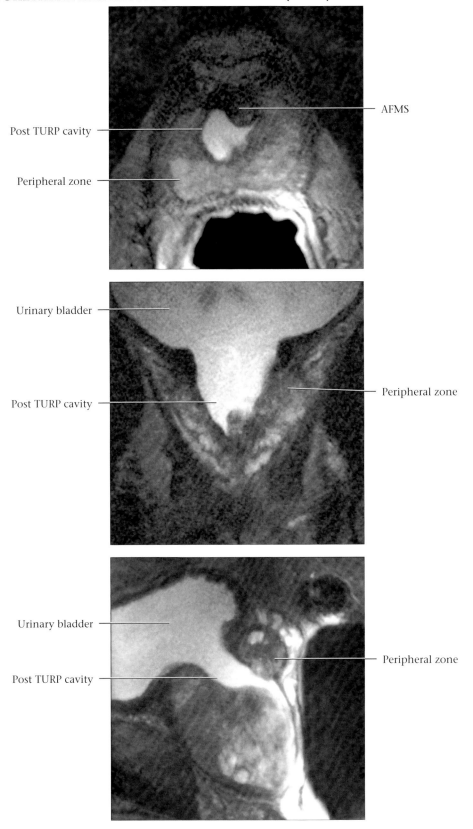

AFMS

Post TURP cavity

Peripheral zone

Urinary bladder

Post TURP cavity

Peripheral zone

Urinary bladder

Post TURP cavity

Peripheral zone

(Top) First of three endorectal T2 MR images of a patient who had a transurethral resection of the prostate (TURP). This axial image shows an irregular cavity within the prostate gland that is continuous with the bladder neck. During the procedure, much of the hyperplastic tissue around the proximal urethra is resected leaving this cavity. Part of the peripheral zone may also be resected. The cavity can be of variable size and shape, neither of which has a bearing on symptomatic outcome. **(Middle)** Coronal image shows the funnel-shaped cavity continuous with the bladder neck and surrounded by the peripheral zone. **(Bottom)** Sagittal T2 MR image also shows the funnel-shaped TURP defect.

PROSTATE CARCINOMA

Central/transitional zone

Peripheral zone

Tumor

Hypertrophied transitional zone

Peripheral zone

Tumor

Tumor

NVB

NVB

Extracapsular extension

Endorectal coil

(Top) Coronal endorectal T2 image shows a small, low signal intensity, nodular tumor in the lower part of the peripheral zone. It is confined to the gland and there is no evidence of extracapsular extension (Courtesy J. Wong, MD). (Middle) Axial, endorectal T2 MR image of a patient with a peripheral zone apical tumor. It is bulging the prostatic capsule, which is highly suspicious for extracapsular extension of tumor. (Bottom) Axial T2 MR image from another patient with a large peripheral zone tumor, which has extended into the inner gland. Also note the soft tissue irregularity where the tumor has breached the capsule and the close proximity to the right NVB (Courtesy K. Hosseinzadeh, MD). It is imperative to carefully examine the capsule and neurovascular bundles in all cases of prostatic carcinoma.

PROSTATE CARCINOMA

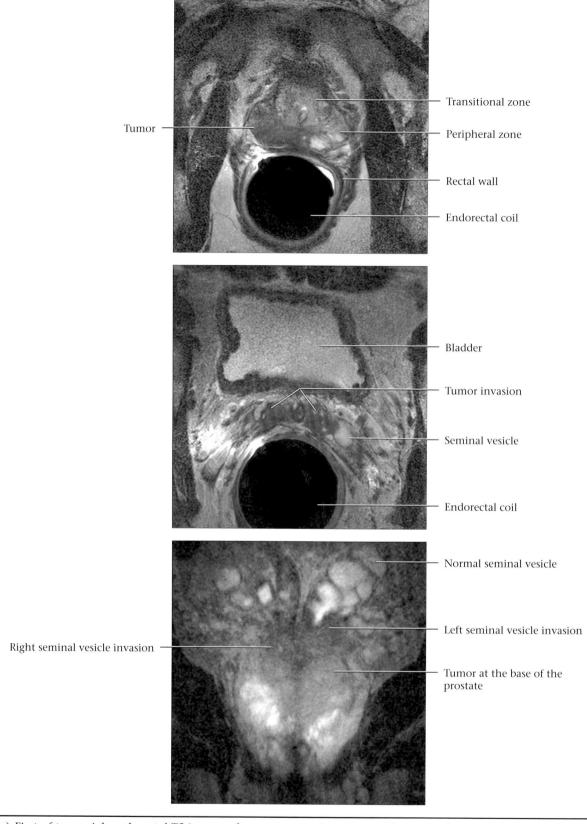

(**Top**) First of two axial, endorectal T2 images of a prostate carcinoma extending into the seminal vesicles. A large tumor is seen on the right side of the peripheral zone. (**Middle**) An image above the prostate shows the low signal tumor involving both seminal vesicles (Courtesy P. Choyke, MD). Seminal vesicle invasion is a common mode of spread for prostate carcinoma, therefore, the seminal vesicles should be thoroughly evaluated in every case. (**Bottom**) Coronal endorectal T2 MR image in a different patient shows a low signal tumor at the base of the prostate, with tumor invading both seminal vesicles.

PROSTATE AND SEMINAL VESICLES

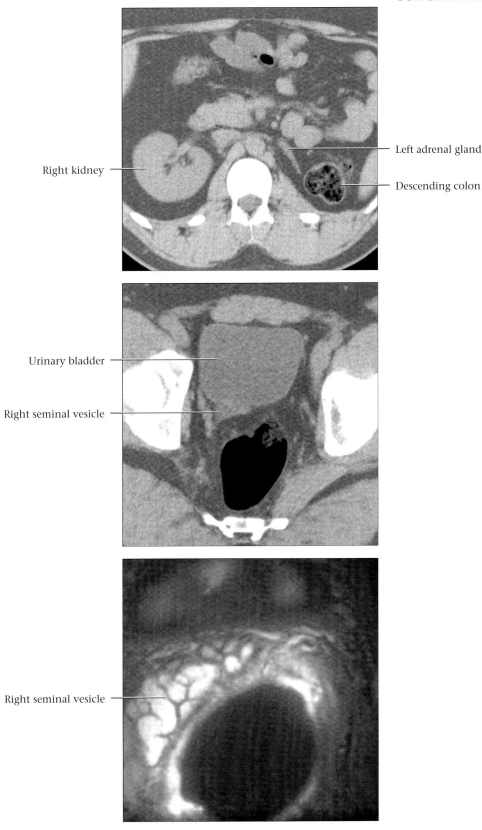

(Top) First of two images of a patient with congenital absence of the left kidney and left seminal vesicle. Axial CT at the level of the right kidney shows absence of the left kidney. The descending colon occupies the left renal fossa. Note the presence of the left adrenal gland, which has a separate embryological origin. (Middle) Axial CT image of the pelvis shows absence of the left seminal vesicle. The combination of absence of a seminal vesicle or seminal vesicle cysts and ipsilateral renoureteral agenesis is explained by the close embryologic development of these structures. (Bottom) Transrectal T2 MR image shows absence of the left seminal vesicle in an another patient with ipsilateral renal agenesis.

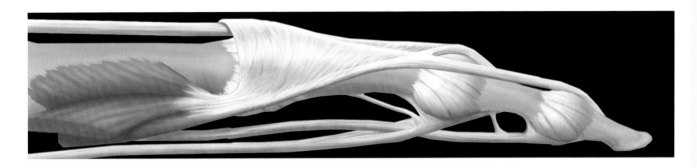

INDEX

INDEX

INDEX

INDEX

INDEX

INDEX

INDEX

INDEX

INDEX

INDEX

INDEX

INDEX

INDEX

INDEX

INDEX

INDEX

INDEX

INDEX

INDEX

INDEX

INDEX

INDEX

P

INDEX

INDEX

INDEX

INDEX

INDEX

INDEX

INDEX

INDEX

INDEX

INDEX

T

INDEX

INDEX

INDEX